Staying Healthy with Nutrition

The Complete Guide to Diet and Nutritional Medicine

Elson M. Haas, M.D.

Celestial Arts
Berkeley, California

Cover art by Mohammad Rezaiian
Cover design by Nancy Austin and Sarah Levin
Art direction by Neil Murray
Composition by Canterbury Press
Project direction by Bethany S. ArgIsle

The following books were used as sources for some icon designs:
Handbook of Pictorial Symbols. New York: Dover Publications, 1976.
Japanese Design Motifs. New York: Dover Publications, 1972.

FIRST PRINTING 1992

Library of Congress Cataloging-in-Publication Data

Haas, Elson M., 1947—
    Staying healthy with nutrition : the complete guide to diet and nutritional
      medicine / Elson M. Haas.
      p. cm.
    Includes bibliographical references and index.
    ISBN 0-89087-481-6
    1. Nutrition.   2. Diet therapy.   I. Title.
   QP141.H183   1990
   613.2—dc20
                                     90-38517
                                     CIP

7 8 9 10 11 — 01 00 99 98 97

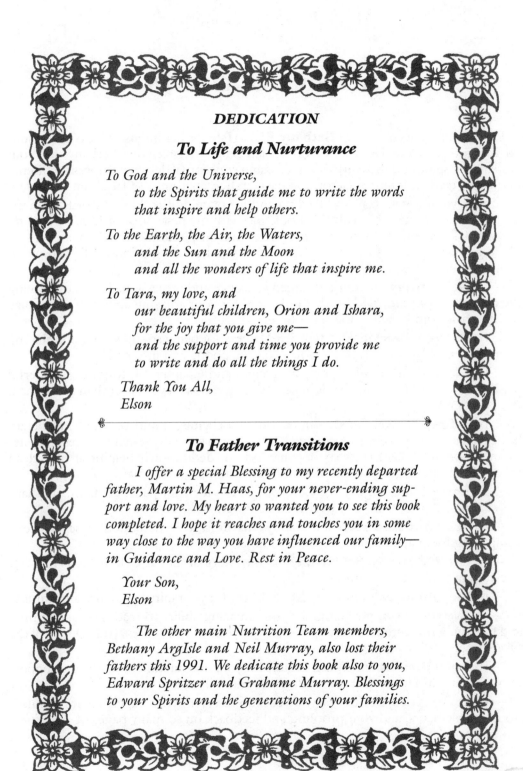

DEDICATION

To Life and Nurturance

To God and the Universe,
to the Spirits that guide me to write the words
that inspire and help others.

To the Earth, the Air, the Waters,
and the Sun and the Moon
and all the wonders of life that inspire me.

To Tara, my love, and
our beautiful children, Orion and Ishara,
for the joy that you give me—
and the support and time you provide me
to write and do all the things I do.

Thank You All,
Elson

To Father Transitions

I offer a special Blessing to my recently departed
father, Martin M. Haas, for your never-ending sup-
port and love. My heart so wanted you to see this book
completed. I hope it reaches and touches you in some
way close to the way you have influenced our family—
in Guidance and Love. Rest in Peace.

Your Son,
Elson

The other main Nutrition Team members,
Bethany ArgIsle and Neil Murray, also lost their
fathers this 1991. We dedicate this book also to you,
Edward Spritzer and Grahame Murray. Blessings
to your Spirits and the generations of your families.

ACKNOWLEDGEMENTS

First I want to acknowledge **Bethany S. ArgIsle** for her intense efforts and results on my behalf in the 15 years of our "blendship." Thank you, Bethany, for your guidance, inspiration, and work as a creator and conceptual designer, supporter, friend, interacter, reactor, fountain factor, question crafter, anatomist of laughter.

I thank you for your care and feeding and for opening the flow of words from my soul, for helping me both with this book and with my first, *Staying Healthy with the Seasons*. I know our readers will appreciate your inspired and humorous pearls of wisdom, anecdotes, and *emo-modulations* that you have so graciously allowed me to include in the pages of the text that follow.

—To **Neil Murray** for your continued brilliance and professionalism in overseeing the design of both *Staying Healthy* books, and for your amazing ability to harmonize with Bethany and myself at the same time!

—To **Cathren, Braelan,** and **Jennica Murray** for being so supportive and sharing your husband/dad with us so graciously on the phone and in your home.

—To **Eleonora Manzolini** for your recipes and Chapter 14, for your wonderful cuisine, devotion to your art, for doing everything you said even faster than I imagined. It's been a real joy!

—To **Jeffrey H. Reinhardt**—nutritional biochemist, mind of minds, planetary healer. Thank you for your support and knowledge in proofing so many pages and fine-tuning *Nutrition*. Thank you also for your work and dedication in helping all of us clean up our food, clean up our environment, and clean up our Karma!

—To **David Hinds**—guide of **Celestial Arts**—for your patience, faith, and hard work! King Allower, Gardener of the Edu-Flower.

—To **Mary Ann Anderson** and **Nancy Austin** for your dedicated perseverance in completing the many final details of this immense manuscript.

—To **Cynthia Harris, Sal Glynn,** and the editorial staff at Celestial Arts for your fine-tuning finale on *Nutrition*.

—To **Judy Johnstone** and **Patty Mote Lacey** for your initial guidance and editing.

—To **Evelyn Brown** for being, for your amazing ability to read my handwriting, and for typing this entire manuscript—that was years of work. Bless you! Queen of the Overcomers.

—To **Brian Breiling** and **Wing Hodas** for your encouragment, faith, and support in my life and in Health Harvest Unlimited, Inc.—Thanks!

—To **Dr. Stephen Levine** for your backup research, your expert advice in nutritional supplements, and your proofing and feedback on so many pages of *Nutrition*.

—To **Jonathan Rothschild** for your phone and reference support on many nutritional product questions.

—To **Richard Kunin, M.D.** for your knowledge and expertise in nutritional medicine and for taking the time to read some of my manuscript.

—To **Nancy Friedrich,** Nurse Midwife, for your review and input on *Pregnancy* and *Lactation* programs—it was a great labor!

—To **Sharon deBuren, N.P.**—nurse extraordinaire and creator of some fine nutritional supplements—thanks for your support and review of the women's health programs.

—To **Ifeoma Ikense, M.D.**—homeopathic pediatrician—thanks for your suggestions about nutrition for the young folks.

—To **Dr. Ed Bauman** for your review of the *Fasting* and *Detoxification* sections.

—To **Mohammad Rezaiian** for your incredible talent and the beautiful painting you did for the *Seasonal Food Guide* and this book. Was there one or two hairs on those brushes you used to paint all those fruits and vegetables?

—To **Richard Moffett** in celebration of ten years of production of *Staying Healthy with the Seasons* with your brilliant drawings, and for letting us use the seasonal borders in this *Nutrition* book.

—To **Cheryl Taylor**—partner in the *Seasonal Food Guide* poster and booklet—for working with me and seeing the painting done with Mohammad and for guiding some of the basic nutritional concepts in this book. Thanks!

—To **Rita Aero**—Tantric Tweaker aiming us toward this peak experience.

—To **Gene Shaparenko** of Aqua Technology in San Jose, California, for your input on the complex water story.

—To **Dr. Sondra G. Barrett**—for your support and input in reviewing immunological matters and for your persevering work on the questionnaires.

—To **Jeff Sherwin** for help in developing computer art and the iconographic grids.

—To **MMT Prepress, David** and **Debora**—for freeing the words and giving format to the entire manuscript.

—To **Faith, Felicity, Francine, Roberta,** and the whole staff at the Marin Clinic of Preventive Medicine and Health Education in San Rafael—for your support and love, and for pursuing excellence in health care!

—To **Martin** and **Shirley Haas**—my fabulous folks. Thank you for your support and for your love of food, and for feeding me so well all of our years.

I love and thank you all!

Elson

CONTENTS

PREFACE

I would like to say that I've never met a meal I didn't remember, although there have been a few I wouldn't mind forgetting. After digesting and assimilating many thousands of cuisine concoctions, I have metabolized them into the thousand-plus pages you now have before you.

When my writing muse tapped me for this immense nutritional treatise, my taste buds quivered. There I was, working on *Staying Healthy with Modern Medicine,* just finishing large sections on drugs and surgery, and planning to write a simple yet in-depth chapter on nutrition and its use in "new medicine" and a healthy hospital environment, and presto! four years later, we have *Staying Healthy with Nutrition.*

David Hinds, my very adaptable publisher at Celestial Arts, asked me, "Didn't you realize you were doing a whole new book?" "Who, me?" I retorted. Well, things do happen that way sometimes, even in the world of contracts.

Now, with all the writing, research, editing, writing, more editing, more writing, and hundreds of other steps—including calling on my Seasons team, Bethany S. ArgIsle and Neil Murray—here you have it! One of the largest and healthiest meals on the planet.

I hope you will enjoy this book as you would a fine meal. Please don't try to eat it all at once. Take your time, chew well, let it digest and assimilate—then you'll be able to use it for energy and health now and beyond.

ENJOY!
Elson M. Haas, M.D.

FOREWORD HO!

I love the keen sense of purpose contained etymologically within words, and the first syllable of nutrition speaks for itself. "Nut"—you've got to be one these days to find your own balance and direction in a sea of media maniacs and claims.

Dr. Elson's love of food has led him to write this traveler's guidebook for us to understand how we can use all the nutrients around us for our own best health. We are made of many mouths—these are the doors to the senses, and when harmonized the body's symphony is able to maintain its balance and participate fully in the joy of living, even sensing the right time to die. I have spent less time and money on problematic health since I became aware of the nutritional needs of all my mouths—the quality of food I eat, the sleep I enjoy, the body I wear and what it can do for me and others as I try to serve more often than I swerve.

When I was a child, my parents were upset that I wouldn't eat as much and as often as they desired, so they made a long-playing record at the Santa Monica Pier that repeated, over and over, on its thick red plastic skin—"Eat Bethany, Eat Bethany, Eat…" Of course, mother and father did their very best, and I'm healthfully here to write this scenario. Dad, a motion-picture theater manager fed me chocolates, sodas, and hot dogs. Mom tried a more earthy approach with meatloaf and stew, omelettes, my favorite spaghetti, some vegetables. She also fed my brain and taught me memory games, while father made sure I got my RDA of work and responsibility training at an early age. In the meantime, I noticed if people chewed their food right- or left-mouthed…if they ate fast or talked while they ate…if they gave thanks for their food as my family always does no matter where we eat or with whom.

Later I began my walk on the path to greater understanding and gave up everything "unnatural"—for eight years I became a vegetarian until that day I pulled a carrot out of the earth and it said to me, "All things are relative" (you see, this was an Einsteinian carrot), "life and death is not a moral issue in the natural sense…take what you need in deep respect and only use what you need." And so, I became a dedicated Nutrition Nut.

My lifestyle requires that I travel a great deal. In fact, as I am completing this foreword, I am packing for a three-week journey to Wales to record children's stories and songs I have co-authored. To "keep the healthy flow quite front row" in my life, I drink more water, carry my own supply—in fact, carry my own food whenever possible on planes, trains, and autos. Hunting and gathering the most naturally grown and prepared food possible is the challenge. If there is not much of a selection, I have a baked potato or a glass of lemon water until I meet a local gardener/farmer or I find a salad bar or restaurant with vital and well-prepared foods. I skip sauces and dressings or any food that I will taste long after the meal is over. I have paid dearly on the road for eating inappropriately, and as many of you who travel know, it is not convenient in any way to be ill or out-of-sync in a strange place.

The other obstacle is the all-too-accepted airport X-ray search. What really are the effects on my body and food supply? I always try to get my food through without the insta-radioactive special seasoning. With all of these porta-picnic methods I have devised, including filling my hotel rooms with the best water and fruits and vegetables available, the moment I arrive in a new location in the constellation, I have been quite able to maintain my health. When imbalance seemed to appear I have been able to bounce back more quickly than ever with several immune system boosters and hydrating tools. Resting up a bit before leaving is practical and inexpensive insurance toward optimum immunity and joyous traveling. Bon Voyage and Welcome Home!

As a consumer, interested in the economy of breathing, thinking, and being on this planet, our garden, I believe that the obvious common sense approach should be guiding us above all else to protect the Earth where our nutrition originates. At this time in history, many techno-advances have made the food industry mega-corporate. Although the United States has the potential to feed much of the world, a growing shadow has fallen on the way of life that founded this country—the farm and the family.

When we begin revering and honoring our teachers and our elders, as Asians and Hunzas do; when we begin to protect the careers of those who tend our food supply; when we begin insisting with our true vote, our dollar power that our food supply not be tampered with unnecessarily by abusing the elements and treatment of the soil, or through shipping and storing procedures; when we learn to keep our economy at one with our very lives—then and only then will we emerge beyond the control of a manipulative and destructive economic force that has devastated the spirit of the farm and family. Instead of protecting certain lands and waters, we have allowed corporate takeover of water sources and food supplies. There needs to be a health management team for each area which could make sure that our food sources are kept clean. Our energy is fueled by health to begin with, not by abuses, which will interupt our lives in the long run and escalate medical costs and the emotional devastation of a well-fed, yet starving nation. We must go beyond our own borders and accept our responsiblity to feed others rather than nurture differences and conflict. We all have one thing in common: this appetite for life. Thanks to all of the farmers and earth caretakers who against all odds—weather, economy, family conditions—have continued THE HARVEST OF HEALTH, WHICH IS UNLIMITED!

We must recreate a renewed world—where the future is not just republican, democrat, or bare "survivalcrat"; where the headlines are not "if it bleeds, it leads"; where headlines become heartvines and deadlines turn into lifelines; where it is not them or us, right or left brain. So what if we are black or white, young or old, rich or poor? We have the greatest opportunity to heal the Earth, to live the life here in the Garden of Eden. Now is the time to claim our right to breathe free...whether we live long or not, each moment is a treasure. A new world where honorable deeds are normal is a world where the forests and the waters are appreciated as our primary resource for life.

This time in history is an opportunity to grow, when doctors once more become students of the great and eternal teachings, the intuitive sciences and medicine coalesce, when those who teach us grow and know. We can become a culture that begins to stop grabbing for money and lying on our insurance forms...we will no longer set our elderly aside because we fear death...we will grow our food, such a bounteous opportunity to serve ourselves and others...we will begin to learn cooperation beyond compromise. As the Chinese have known for centuries—pay your doctor to keep you well but don't pay if you become ill...if, that is, you have done what you were supposed to do.

Please enjoy the concept of health...words do not make health, just as birds do not make sky....We, the NUT team, wish you well as you study your own life and balance your Conscientious Dietary Elements. We have turned ourselves inside out on these pages to provide you with the deepest level of information, organization, and guidance that we could access. NUTRITION is a key to seeing more clearly and being more available to assist in the coming changes, which are continuous and ever more challenging. Choose well; yours is the life God gave you to care for.

Bethany S. ArgIsle

"TREEDOM"*

TREES DON'T ASK WHY,
THEY JUST STRETCH OUT THEIR LIMBS AND HOLD UP THE SKY.

and now a moment from our sponsor — breathing...

Guns
and guitars
from dead trees,
skateboards and skis
from bygone trees
chairs and toilet seats
drums that keep the beat
wooden shoes, yesterday's news
boats that float
tables, labels, and fables
wooden soldiers, file folders
love letters, branches for birds
paper fans, lists, plans
soon, breathing may seem absurd
shopping bags, convention name tags
junk mail doth prevail, tax forms, paper storms
Self-help books (including this one)
lamp and amp stands, walking sticks
tent poles, chopsticks toothpicks, surfboards, coffins
try watering them and see if they'll grow
once our savings got loaned
and our high-yield oxygen bank
has nothing on account but stumps, holes,
cold coals
salad bowls
toilet paper rolls
from tree
to shiny tree
TREEDOM
TREEDOM
TREEDOM

© 1991 by Bethany S. ArgIsle

---

* Within two days recently, two dear friends both used the word "Treedom." This word says so much in so little space...Treedom for the human race.

Dear Breather,

During the years spent helping create this book, I became ever more aware that while healing planetary citizens (including myself), I had become one of the "users" of the "green" resource bank that needs so much to be replenished.

In this Spirit of Renewal, we have made a commitment (under the auspices of The "Green Pages" pledge) to replant trees in an amount equal to our use for this book, donating a portion of the profits from sales to the tree replanting program as outlined by Earth Island and Global Releaf. Please join us and replenish our global oxygen bank account for ourselves and the children of the future.

If you are a paper user, please donate as much time and re$ource$ as possible (especially on a local level) by contacting:

Green Pages
Earth Island Institute
300 Broadway, Ste. 28
San Francisco, CA 94133-3312
415-788-3666

Releaf
Trust for Public Land
116 New Montgomery, 3rd Floor
San Francisco, CA 94105
415-495-5660
HOTLINE: 800-TREE-GEO

For further family and classroom inspiration, I recommend the following delight-filled materials:

Video

Man of the Trees—The life of Richard St. Barbe Baker who dedicated 92 years to preserving the world's forests. Contact: Children for Old Growth, dedicated to "Saving Ancient Forests for the Future," P.O. Box 1090, Redway, CA 95560.

Film

Man Who Planted Trees—Academy Award (1987) "Best Animated Film," 30-minute color video or 16mm film available. For sales, rentals, and further information: Direct Cinema Limited Library, P.O. Box 69799, Los Angeles, CA 90069, U.S. Toll Free (800) FILMS 4-U, (213) 652-8000.

Books

Celtic Tree Oracle, Colin Murray (New York: St. Martin's Press, 1988).
Giving Tree, Shel Silverstein (New York: Harper & Row Junior Books, 1964).
Just a Dream, Chris Van Allsburg (Boston: Houghton Mifflin Co., 1990).
Little Green Book, Cherry Denman (New York: Stewart, Tabori & Chang, 1990).
Man Who Planted Trees, Jean Giono (Post Mills, VT: Chelsea Green Publishing Co., 1985). Winner (1986) New England Book Show.

HOW TO USE THIS BOOK

When Elson first brought me his skyscraper-sized stack of writing based on his nutrition research, I wondered how I, as a humanologist, might bring forth a vision that would be accessible in a commonsense, day-to-day lifestyle manner. Since many of the larger volumes I have purchased over the years have been used to hold open doors against the wind and adjust my slide projector's height, I realized I faced a challenge.

Fortunately, I acquired my first computer, a Macintosh Plus, at the same time Elson delivered his manuscript. At first resistant to techno-dependency, I became enamored of the overall organizational capabilities of the micro world and of the icon, a pictogram standing for a philosophy or an idea. We have all become used to this simplification tool, from NO SMOKING signs to road signs. Why, I asked, not develop iconographics that utilize the Macintosh's method of accessing information to organize this book? We constructed the hexagonal or beehive compartment to show the chapters included in each of the four parts. You will find these iconographs at the opening of each part as well as at the beginning of each chapter. When you begin a section, all chapter titles will have a white background. As you progress, the beehive is repeated, but the chapter you are entering will have a black background (reversed) and those you've already read or are saving for later will be shaded. We have also included running heads throughout so that you can easily find information.

Bethany S. ArgIsle

Staying Healthy with Nutrition is many books in one. It can be used in a variety of ways.

1. A Reference Guide that can be entered through
   a. The Table of Contents
   b. The Index
   c. Or, open it and see where you land.

For example, if you have a specific topic, concern, or condition you wish to look up, check the index and see if you can pinpoint the exact location of the information in the nutritional constellation. Having found your topic, you may find other areas of interest to which you then can progress.

2. A Textbook
   a. Designed as a course in basic nutrition that proceeds to nutritional medicine. For example, we begin with *Building Blocks,* then progress to *Foods and Diets,*

which is followed by a specific *Seasonal Diet Plan, The Ideal Diet,* and then to Part Four, with many examples of *Nutritional Application,* thus providing the individual experience.

3. A Special Interest Manual

a. If the environment is of special concern to you, and the various names of additives found in food or in your own cupboard are of interest, then you can look them up.

b. If your diet needs minor or major adjustments, you can seek inspiration and guidance in how to change your food choices. Furthermore, you may choose to follow the specific *Seasonal Diets* during a time cycle, such as a year.

4. A Questionnaire Extraordinaire

a. Lettuce say you like the look of this "masterpiece" and you're not sure if you need it at all.

b. The questions at the back are designed in three stages.

Make a copy if you wish to use them more than once or to give to family members or friends.

1. Biofeedback: To look at your own nutritional and health attitudes and experiences, to see that your health is a reflection of them.

2. Experiential Applications: For when one has made the decision to have a healing conversation with their refrigerator, their medicine chest, their cupboards, and their body, with concerns for the support of a balanced environment.

3. Beginning health professionals: How much do you know about the body— specific substances, minerals, dosages, and nutrient interaction?

The questionnaire has been designed so that you can take the "tests" many times during your nutritional journeying—once a year or every other year may indicate subtle transformations.

Bethany S. ArgIsle, Neil Murray, and Elson M. Haas, M.D.

General Book Disclaimers

There are many nutritional suggestions and special supplement programs contained in this book. It is written mostly to inform those interested in the various aspects of nutrition and lifestyle as they relate to both health and disease. Further, my intention is to assist you to act as a nutritional guide for yourself and for others seeking educational support.

This text is brought to you in the most up-to-date state based on my extensive research and experience; however, I am sure that there is a great deal more to learn and add. I could continue updating this book, especially Part Four, for all of my life. You may choose to keep abreast of the latest nutritional news from the various multimedia communication outlets. I hope you do, and apply it wisely to your daily life.

The suggestions in Part Four are not meant to replace your doctor (or your own intuitive guidance), and, specifically, are not meant as medical treatment. Also, please realize that the same nutritional plan, much like the same medicine, does not work the same for every individual. You are a unique person, not a disease. Thus, medicine is always experimental (sounds optimistic?), that is, even though we may have had previous experience treating a similar health concern, we do not know for sure how any specific remedy or program will work for a particular individual. For example, many people with asthma, a disease that is difficult to treat, will respond to my nutritional and supplemental program to varying degrees, yet I am confident that most shall see at least some benefit. I hope you can use my guidance as inspiration and support along the important path of improving your health.

Please use the suggestions in this book as educational tools to enhance your life. If you use this compendium to design your own individual treatment program, **you do so at your own risk** and with your conscience at peace with your nutritional adventures. Please see an appropriately trained (and healthy) professional if you have any questions about your health, have medical concerns, or need guidance for your life.

Good Luck and Wise Choices!

Tryptophan

I do not completely accept the "story" that tryptophan itself is the disease culprit for which it stands accused at the time of publication of this book (it was clearly a chemical contaminant that caused the "myalgia" problems); currently, it is not available. However, since I continue to believe that it is a potentially very useful nutritional medicine adjunct, I have not deleted the discussions and suggestions for its use from this text.

Footnoting

I have made a conscious decision to make this a book for the general reader rather than for researchers. Therefore, I have avoided extensive footnotes and article references. See the *Bibliography* for books and articles consulted, and the discussion of *Science and Nutrition* in the *Introduction*.

NUTRITION WHEEL

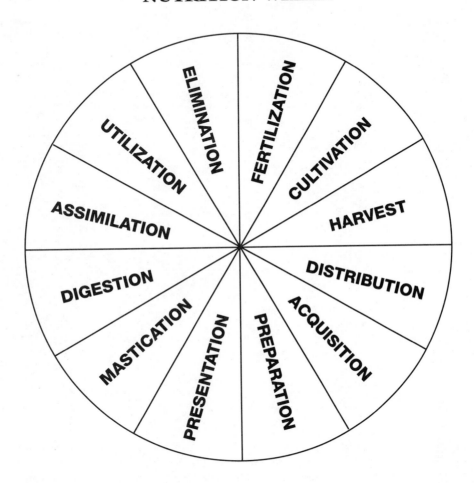

Dear Reader,

    If you have adjusted your nutritional program because of this book and have any observable results, please inform us.

    Write to Dr. Elson M. Haas

        c/o Celestial Arts
            P.O. Box 7123
            Berkeley, CA 94707

Staying Healthy with Nutrition

The Complete Guide to Diet and Nutritional Medicine

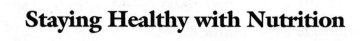

Staying Healthy with Nutrition

> *"The doctor of the future will give no medicines, but will interest his patients in the care of the human frame, in diet, and in the causes of disease."*
> —**Thomas Edison**

> *"Let food be your medicine."*
> —**Hippocrates**

These quotes might do well to be on the walls of medical schools, doctors' offices, and hospitals everywhere, since nutrition has been an important part of medicine from the time of Hippocrates and before; special foods, diets, fasting, and herbs were part of the ancient Greeks' medical care. Today as well, true health begins in our gardens, markets, and kitchens and follows our food choices and habits. Technology has created both new problems for us as well as many new and advanced medical, herbal, and nutritional products. A good diet and lifestyle are still our best medicine and safeguards for health!

Introduction

*S*taying Healthy with Nutrition comes out of the last decade of my experience in medical practice. Prior to the 1980s, I was more concerned with a philosopher-physician's understanding of disease and healing. I researched and applied the natural therapeutic approaches of traditional Chinese medicine, herbology, body therapies, guided imagery, and other inner healing processes in my practice. I still incorporate all of these modalities into my current work, but during most of the last decade I have focused my attention on the rapidly advancing field of nutritional medicine. Nutrition has also been an area of great interest to the general public, because, I believe, it is one we all have in common. Nutrition has been and continues to be a primary part of my life and practice, as well as my own personal challenge. Given the history of Western medicine to date, many people seek empowerment in the health care of themselves and their families; nutrition is really a basic component of preventive medicine and also an area that can be effective in corrective medicine for many common health problems.

My first book, *Staying Healthy with the Seasons* (Celestial Arts, 1981), dealt mainly with the overall concepts and guidelines for a healthy approach to nutrition and lifestyle. In recent years my knowledge and practice have evolved toward what I now term "Scientific Nutrition" and "Integrated Medicine." This is a balance of scientific and intuitive nutritional medicine. My medical clinic provides "patient-centered" medicine, offering an eclectic blend of services within the context of a general practice. We attempt to deal with as many levels and concerns as individuals bring with them. We directly involve "patients" in decision-making where that is relevant, inform and educate them where that is appropriate, and work together to achieve the clearest approach and best results for their state of disease, health, or evolution. Combining a wide range of laboratory evaluations and potential therapeutic approaches is, I believe, an advanced synthesis of medical practice, especially for disease prevention and support of health. Treatment options include both pharmaceutical and natural medicines (nutritional supplements, homeopathics, and herbal products), dietary changes, acupuncture, osteopathic care and massage therapy, stress management, and hypnotherapy. I believe that medical care should provide a full spectrum of services from crisis intervention and evaluation and treatment of illness to therapies and education that help people to grow in their daily lives and learn to stay healthy.

It is my intention in this book to investigate and substantiate the significance of food and nutrients as an integral and accepted part of the world of medicine and individual medical practice. Nutrition is a basic component of health, and certainly a factor in disease. A reasonable knowledge of nutritional biochemistry may help in the application of therapies that relieve many symptoms relating to or resulting from improper dietary habits. Furthermore, with the proper construction of a diet plan we can help rebuild a patient's health (or our own) after illness or surgery.

Medical schools and doctors are oriented to treating disease with drugs and surgery, and foods are not yet seen to be "powerful medicine." It is certainly true that nutrition plays a more important part in preventive medicine than it does in the treatment of disease, although we will see that an understanding of the body's functioning at the nutritional level can help in the treatment of a variety of problems.

Nutritional medicine is really a completely new field; it is also as ancient as medicine and healing itself. It is a specialty much like other medical specialties and should be considered as such. There is still a great deal to learn about nutrition and how it relates to illness and health, but this is true of all specialties.

It is important for each practitioner to be aware of the limits of his or her knowledge and its applications. If, when treating or screening patients, we do not have sufficient or appropriate knowledge to help them completely, then we should look for another doctor or practitioner to assist or advise us on further treatment. My own policy is to maintain an extensive referral list of helpful caregivers. It is the responsibility of patients to know something about nutrition and be concerned with the healthful feeding of themselves and their families, and, where appropriate, to be willing to keep discovering and readjusting their own balance.

Medical and Nutritional Training

To date, doctors have not been well trained in nutrition. I personally had fewer than ten hours of nutritional education in four years of study at a highly ranked medical school. I had about the same in grade school, and the information was no more advanced. The "four-food-group" idea of a balanced diet and concern over the significant and symptomatic vitamin/mineral deficiencies were the major focus. There was a separate study of biochemistry, but very little discussion of its practical application to nutritional physiology. Some information was given about the relevance of the metabolism of specific vitamins and minerals, although there was little understanding of how diet could affect health or disease. Twenty years ago when I was in medical school, there was a great deal less information available on the relationship of diet to major diseases such as cancer, cardiovascular disease, diabetes, and obesity. Yet even with the knowledge we have today, nutritional education is still belittled as secondary paramedical information in most medical centers.

Doctors in training are informed that there are nutritionists prepared to help them devise diets for sick people who need to change and/or limit their food intake to control their diseases. These nutritionists, formerly called "dieticians," are trained with the same limited knowledge—with emphasis on the American "four-food-group" diet (which is too high in fat, protein, and sugar) that has been and still is contributing to much of the chronic disease rampant in this country.

The basic components of the nutritionist's practice include diets to control diabetes by reducing simple sugars and refined carbohydrates, to encourage weight loss by restricting calories, to lower high blood pressure by reducing salt intake, to treat ulcers by recommending dairy products, and to manage heart disease by lowering cholesterol levels. Thus, basically these nutritionists assist doctors in the control of diseases after they have already occurred. For the most part, doctors and dieticians have neither taken the time to study and incorporate nor been willing to accept various special diets, such as vegetarianism and fasting therapy, or the power that specific nutrients have in the prevention and treatment of medical problems. If it hasn't been double-blind studied, or accepted in the medical community for a decade, then it "must be a fad."

Science and Nutrition

This book integrates experience, intuition, and research—all designed to simplify an enormous amount of nutritional information and inspire you to apply this guidance to your lives in positive ways. I have deliberately avoided the regular use of footnotes and related bibliography to keep the material simple, flowing, and easy to digest. Indigestion is one of the great symptoms of our society, and it is not only related to what we put into our mouths, but also to what enters our bodies through our eyes, ears, hearts, and minds. I hope this text will be a guide for you to create a healthier diet and lifestyle.

Research and our interpretation of many scientific studies still has a long way to go. Just because someone finds something to be "true" in a particular study doesn't make it so. It is just part of the learning process, which must involve both the seen and the unseen, the proven and yet-to-be proven. In many instances two research groups conducting similar studies come to opposite conclusions, depending upon factors such as the economic support for the study and the consciousness of the researchers. "As we think and feel is the way of truth revealed," notes Bethany ArgIsle.

Much of the nutritional scientific dilemma involves differences of interpretation between the "provers" and "experiencers." I believe that experience comes first, then proof.

Some of this book, and much of the current nutritional marketplace, is still "experience" waiting to be validated and accepted by the hard-core "scientists." Yet, we would not have the cutting edge in medicine if we waited for "provers" to accept everything before we could implement change.

Most pharmaceutical and natural remedies vary in effect from person to person. Thus, medicine is always partly experimental. The studies and information included in this book come from my own personal explorations, as well as twenty years of practice, combined with the knowledge and experience of my colleagues and patients. Research is important, but innovative medical care is on the cutting edge of experience. The practice of medicine is both a science and an art.

The first level of good medical care is to "do no harm," and then, to serve and support people in making positive changes toward better self-care in creating lifestyle balance and, subsequently, optimal health. Of course, I appreciate acceptance from the medical community. However, if doctors did only what was acceptable to the norm, medicine would still be in the Dark Ages and would not have continued to evolve toward its current credible and incredible levels of achievement. As technology and nutrition merge, as they do in this book, we shall continue to experience advances in medical care and the quality of life.

New Medicine

Happily, as the years pass, there are changes in attitudes and in the application of medical practice, however slow they may be. Out of the will to survive, the high and rising cost of medical care, and the potential help offered from food and supplement products, we have become more concerned and empowered in maintaining personal health—and nutrition clearly plays a big role here. As we maintain health through our own application of knowledge, we will not need to take drugs or have operations to correct problems that interfere with our lives. Clearly, economics come into play. If the majority of doctors and hospitals make money by treating sick people, and if proper nutrition and healthy living habits such as regular exercise, stress management, and positive attitude help prevent disease, then it would be ludicrous for physicans to promote these ideas for fear of financial ruin. Of course, this is an overstatement, although I believe it is one aspect of the overall attitude of the medical establishment.

As more people ask their doctors about nutrition, vitamin supplements, fasting, and so on, more doctors will attempt to learn about these areas or to add knowledgeable staff. These interested and motivated patients will find doctors or other practitioners to assist them in their journey toward more healthful living programs. There are always sick people, from those who abuse themselves to those who are aging, who wish to have and need medical care. Yet, as people become healthier, the medical profession will need to include more doctors who are educators and supporters of health. After all, the word doctor comes from the Latin *docere,* meaning "to teach."

A great deal of knowledge and experience has surfaced in the field of nutrition in the last decade. An incredible amount of research is being done on the effects of different diets and various supplements on health and disease. There are many new practitioners calling themselves "nutritionists" and more companies making very exacting and advanced products for dietary support and nutritional therapeutics (see *Appendix*). In recent years, many diseases have been described, such as premenstrual syndrome, candidiasis, and food allergy problems, which has instigated the development of new nutritional programs and a great many new products. Many of these trends, discoveries, and nutritional programs are discussed in this book.

Basic Western Nutrition

The public's basic knowledge of and focus on nutrition have also made a major shift in recent years. People's idea of the balanced diet has changed from the archaic "four-food-group" approach of meals containing a meat, a dairy food, a cereal grain, and fruits and vegetables to a more natural diet, lower in fat, protein, and refined carbohydrates. Whole foods, unprocessed and without chemical additives, as Nature herself presents them to us, are again becoming the mainstay of the "new American" diet. But, of course, as nature is continually polluted, so is our food.

Dietary habits, the ways people eat, have also changed. Choosing nourishing foods is becoming a top priority for many of us concerned with our optimum health. Meals are becoming simpler, containing fewer foods. Many people follow the basic principles of food combining—eating foods in certain combinations for best digestion and absorption. The time of the day when food is consumed, the setting, how we feel when eating, and how the food is prepared are all very important as well.

So, reader, let us each take the time to ask ourselves what the best diet is to help us improve and perpetuate our health. Poor nutrition is advertised and available to us everywhere, and restraint is not the strongest attribute of the American "I want it all now" public. When we are guided and conditioned early in life about good nutrition and schools require us to learn to nurture and harvest a garden, then Earth will nourish us in return with wholesome foods.

A healthy diet most obviously involves the application of common sense. Our body sends us messages to change our diet to attune to our real needs; the internal biofeedback system we have is superb if we cooperate with it rather than override it. Yet, many of us follow our desires and taste buds, eating the richer, sweeter, or saltier foods that industry promotes and packaged nutrition provides. It may not seem to matter a great deal in the short term that we follow our passions/addictions rather than our common sense. The sad part, though, is that this *does* affect how we feel and function now, and does make a difference over the long term.

The average American is overweight. To many people, the word "diet" means a special program developed to lose those extra pounds that we carry around, followed only until we lose them and can go back to eating the foods that produced the extra fat in the first place. The condition of our body, such as our weight, is an end result of how we live and, primarily, is a reflection of the food we eat and our activity levels. **Therefore, if we wish to change our weight permanently, we must change our lifestyle.** Usually this means eating less and exercising more—a dynamic duo that really cannot fail (unless one has a preexisting or particularly limiting condition). Specifically, this means eating less of the richer foods for which so many of us have developed a special taste; this often requires reprogramming ourselves to find "new," less fattening foods to replace our bad habits. Eating and weight also have a lot to do with one's emotions, psychological nature, and fear of creativity and change. In my own life, I have tended to "feed my face" and "stuff" myself to hold back feelings trying to flood from my subconscious. I now realize that permanent dietary and weight change do not come easily, but usually take some level of personal transformation, psychological and emotional expression, and new creative outlets, which for me includes writing these "health" books.

Many of us, very early in life, develop body shapes, dietary habits, and specific eating patterns that become deeply ingrained. Family tradition and individual upbringing influence each of us. The early connection between love, emotional bonding, or acceptance with eating food are common to most cultures, yet are particularly strong in American Jewish and Italian families, both of which possess a higher-than-average incidence of obesity. Chronic obesity contributes to many major illnesses and disease patterns, such as high blood pressure, heart disease, and diabetes.

Thus, it is possible that we inherit some disease through inheriting eating habits. When attempting to change diet and weight, these deeper patterns are the most difficult to recognize and transform but must be dealt with to bring about significant and lasting change. At times, uprooting unhealthy dietary habits and choices can bring a great deal of stress to traditional family relationships. When we cannot eat with our parents and other relatives because of dietary differences, the hardships become especially clear. I experienced this difficulty during my years of nutritional radicalism when I was eating a special vegetarian diet to overcome a weight problem that was rampant in my family because of excess consumption and many poor eating and emotional habits.

My association with the courageous Bethany ArgIsle was an inspiration and support for me to change. Her energy was (and is) more powerful than the force of my eating patterns and addictions, especially when she would place herself between me and the refrigerator and telephone when I would find myself ready to munch and chat when the frustration of the inner creative process would arise. When she said, "Go back to your desk and write, we'll eat later," I knew she was serving the higher good and that my task was to align with it. My weight loss and the other positive health changes that resulted from that hard work became an inspiration for family members, patients, and readers of *Staying Healthy with the Seasons*. Since then, the public's awareness of nutrition has grown and my parents' diet has even become healthier; at the same time my own dietary patterns have become balanced enough to allow me to eat the same meal as my family while at home or, on occasion, at a suitable wholesome restaurant.

The information available in recent years regarding the relationship of diet to disease has affected the nutritional trends of the American consumer, especially since it concerns the incidence of common chronic and deadly diseases, such as cancer and cardiovascular disease. *The Surgeon General's Report on Nutrition and Health—Summary and Recommendations* (U.S. Dept of Health and Human Services 1988) suggests the message is getting loud and clear—**diet influences disease and health in a major way.**

I have a theory that the body has three basic metabolic functions. These are *building* or tonification, *cleansing* or detoxification, and *maintenance* or balance. Maintenance is the main function, but occasionally the body clicks into a detoxification or purification cycle where it must eliminate previous buildup. The bowels become more active and the secreting cells and the mucous membranes work more; mucus may flow out of the body, from the sinuses and nose for example, often appearing as the result of a cold or flu. When we continue to eat a congesting or highly processed diet of meat, milk products, or breads, the condition may worsen. When we listen to our body and drink more liquids and eat lightly, emphasizing the cleansing fruits and vegetables, we may support the detoxification period and feel better. On the other hand, if the body is in a building or toning cycle and we are not feeding it the fuel and specific nutrients it needs, we may feel a lack of energy and not develop the strength required for future activity. This and other theories presented in this book have evolved into appropriate diets for each cycle. The yearly cycle of diet—introduced in my first book, *Staying Healthy with the Seasons*—is dealt with more thoroughly in Part Three of this text—*Building a Healthy Diet.*

Our dietary needs change not only with the seasons of the year, but also with the seasons of our lives. As children we need a wholesome, nutrient-rich, building diet to support growth. We use the extra nutrients, oils, and proteins to construct and expand tissues. In our 20s, 30s and later, after we have stopped growing physically, we can get into trouble if we continue with the childhood diet. We need to shift to a maintenance-oriented diet of lighter, more fiber-rich and nutrient-rich natural foods with occasional periods of fasting or detoxification. As we age even more, our metabolism and activity level often slow down and food requirements decrease further. Continuing the mid-life maintenance diet into later life will probably cause weight increase. Thus, responding to our dietary needs and using the nutrients we consume appropriately, both metabolically and through some type of aerobic/fitness activity, is an important day-to-day goal.

As I mentioned, psychological and emotional states also have a great deal to do with how well we utilize our nutrition. When we are under stress, we may not digest and absorb our nutrients as well and, at the same time, may need higher amounts of many vitamins and minerals. This is one situation where additional supplements may be necessary. Our appetite is often a result of inner contentment. Many people override their appetite mechanism through regular eating and do not really experience hunger. When we are emotionally upset, feeling insecure or depressed for example, we may lose our appetite, which is the appropriate response, since our body does not process food well at these times. Not eating allows us to go within more easily to explore our feelings or lets us express our emotions more freely. Being aware of the need for nourishment via hunger and then relaxing and preparing the body to receive wholesome food in a comfortable setting are important prerequisites for eating.

I hope that your journey through *Staying Healthy with Nutrition* will inspire you to use nutrition wisely to obtain and maintain your optimum health. I also hope that this book will inspire other doctors toward greater awareness and application of nutrition in their practices. Overall, my goal is to help each of us become our own nutritional doctor in order to best care for ourselves, our family and friends, and Planet Earth, the source of real nutrition.

Knowledge is the key. Open the door and explore the realms of your being. Yearn for and learn your soul's essence and manifest the life that you are meant to bring forth. Feeding yourself well, naturally, wholesomely, and in balance, will provide all the nutrients that you need to nourish your multi-dimensional self and the vital unfoldment of your path.

Good luck.

Rise and shine, embrace the Divine in You!

Elson M. Haas, M.D.

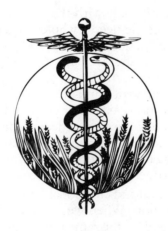

PART ONE
THE BUILDING BLOCKS

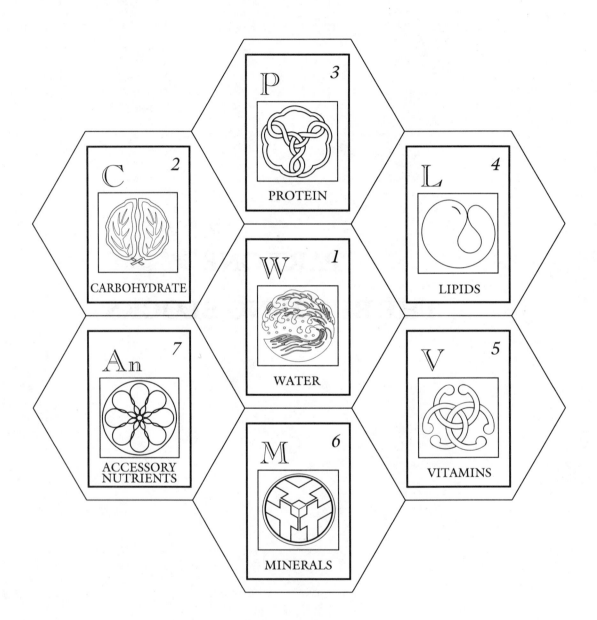

The human body needs food to function. Food is our body's fuel—our source of energy. We need food and its nutrients to maintain life and promote cell and tissue growth. The building blocks of our diet provide our sources for energy, biochemical support, and the medium in which our nutrients can function. These essentials for life include the macronutrients—*carbohydrates, proteins,* and *fats;* the micronutrients—*vitamins* and *minerals,* so important to our body chemistry; and *water*—the solvent for all soluble ingredients in the blood and cells. Water makes up by far the largest percentage of the body's volume. We get all these essential nutrients from fruits, vegetables, grains, legumes, nuts and seeds, dairy foods, and meats—the basic food groups that comprise our diet.

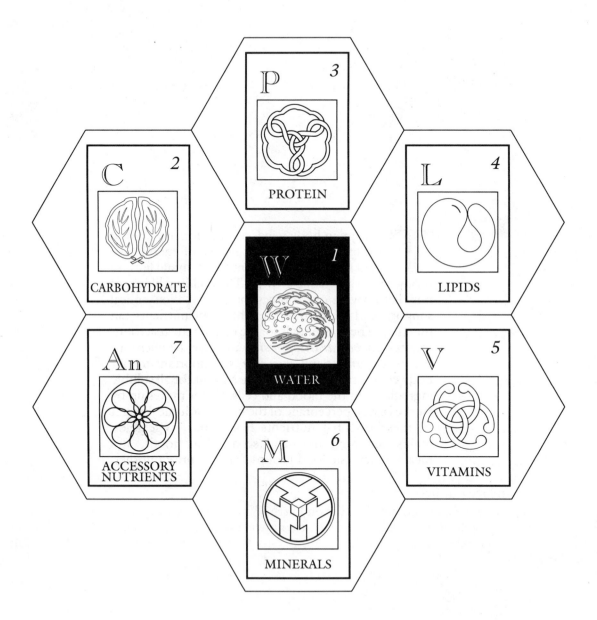

Chapter 1

Water

Water is the medium in which all other nutrients are found. Three simple molecules, two hydrogen and one oxygen, bind together to form each molecule of water, the most abundant and important substance on Earth and in the human body. Pure water does not exist naturally on our planet; water is the universal solvent, and most other substances present on Earth dissolve in it to different degrees. The earth's natural water varies in mineral content, as does the water found within our bodies.

Our bodies are at least 60 percent water. It is the primary component of all the bodily fluids—blood, lymph, digestive juices, urine, tears, and sweat. Water is involved in almost every bodily function: circulation, digestion, absorption, and elimination of wastes, to name a few. Water carries the electrolytes, mineral salts that help convey electrical currents in the body; the major minerals that make up these salts are sodium, potassium, calcium, magnesium, and chloride. Water requirements vary greatly from person to person. The climate in which we live, our activity level, and our diet all influence our need for water.

Water is fundamental to all life on Earth. Without clean water we cannot experience optimum health. Awareness of the urgent need to address the issue of water pollution is growing. Subsequently, healing our waters and providing safe and tasty drinking water are becoming a major industry—filtered water systems, international spring waters, designer water, flavored waters, juice waters, and more.

Recognizing the importance of clean water, I wrote this chapter to offer you a synergistic collation of the most current, usable information; however, I am aware that it is not the final word. Much water information is purported as "fact" by business interests, yet scientific study is lacking. Surely this will change, so look for upcoming data on this crucial subject.

Since water is an essential part of our basic life needs—life force if you will—we could spend more energy and dollars researching how to keep it safe for human consumption. My concern is that our governments will wait too long to correct our current water problems, much like modern Western medicine focuses on end-stage disease over preventive medicine. Keeping people well and learning more about the factors that affect this goal, such as the chemicals in our environment, deserve a great deal more attention. Healing and maintaining Earth's environment, keeping our basic elements—water, air, and food—clean and wholesome, is a good place to start!

Drinking water has become an issue of concern. In all too many cases it has been shown that tap water is not totally safe. We need to ask what role drinking tap water plays in our health. What is its subtle effect on biochemical processes in our body, and what is its relationship to symptoms of illness or chronic disease? Not enough research has come out to date showing how tap water and its contents influence our health. Many cities' water has a high sodium level, which has been correlated with an increased likelihood of high blood pressure and subsequent cardiovascular disease. Soft water, in which a high level of sodium has replaced biologically important minerals such as calcium and magnesium, has also been implicated in reducing our resistance to heart disease.

With the trend toward using pure and natural products in personal health care, city tap water has come to be considered a processed, unnatural substance, containing potentially hazardous chemical additives. No wonder bottled water has become a huge industry in the last decade! For the most part, city water is heavily chlorinated to kill germs, fluoridated to prevent tooth decay, and some cities add calcium hydroxide or other alkaline substances to change the pH (acidity) of the water so it does not corrode pipes. Chlorine and other additives used to treat water can react with other organic chemicals to produce chlorinated hydrocarbons that may act as carcinogens. For example, the chloramines including chloroform and other trihalomethanes, are formed in water from chlorine and organic matter such as ammonia or decaying leaves. Water pipes may contribute chemicals or metals such as copper or lead.

○ CHOOSING YOUR DRINKING WATER

I have urged people for many years to use special purified drinking water and to avoid the faucet. I have not drunk tap water in more than a decade; instead, I have used well water or spring water collected from mountain or underground sources (unfortunately these waters can be contaminated also) or, more recently, home-filtered tap water. But lately there have even been questions regarding the purity of bottled waters and the effectiveness of filters. What is the right thing to do? Clearly, scientific research and the marketing information of companies selling water and the various water cleaners may differ. After all, advertising has a big influence on our nutrition in general and certainly has and continues to be a hindrance that must be overcome to achieve a healthier diet and lifestyle. The government can only protect the consumer from gross misrepresentation and not subtle interpretation of "facts."

POSSIBLE CONTAMINANTS IN OUR DRINKING WATER
(MUNICIPAL AND WELL WATER)

Lead	Bacteria	Asbestos
Mercury	Viruses	Radon
Aluminum	Parasites	Nitrates
Cadmium	esp. Giardia	Chlorine
Organic Solvents	Industrial Chemicals	Fluoride
	Pesticides	Sodium

Let's look at our drinking water choices before we decide. We don't want to worry or be fanatic, but since water is second in importance only to air for sustaining life, we do want to do the best we can with the current knowledge and inner guidance we have. Taste and smell can help us assess if our water is good for us. However, the presence of negative health factors may not alter taste or smell. If there is a question about water safety, we can have our drinking supply, whatever it is, analyzed for bacteria, minerals, or chemical pollutants.

My goal in this section on water, since there is much technical information I cannot include here, is to give you the basics about drinking water so you can at least ask yourself what is best. Water is an important component of nutrition. The first step of good nutrition is to know the origin, processing, and contents of anything we take into our bodies. Now let's talk about the many sources of water available to us.

Tap Water

Most tap water comes from surface reservoirs formed from rivers, streams, and lakes, or from groundwater. Groundwater refers to the subterranean reservoirs that hold much of the earth's water and supply nearly all the rural drinking water and about half of city water supplies. The water from these sources goes through local treatment plants, many of which use a very old process of settling tanks, filtration through sand and gravel, and then chemicals to clean up the water so it is fit for human consumption.

Many minerals and chemicals are used for "purification," including chlorine, alum or sodium aluminum salts, soda, ash, phosphates, calcium hydroxide, and activated carbon. Yet this process may not clear all of the many environmental pollutants that can contaminate our water supplies, including animal wastes, local fertilizers, and insecticides; chemicals and wastes from industry; and air pollutants such as lead or radon. Toxic organic chemicals and petroleum spills can also pollute large amounts of water. Since much of this pollution affects groundwater as well as surface waters, most municipal or artesian well drinking waters are at risk and deserve our concern.

The January 1990 *Consumer Reports* analysis suggests that the three drinking water pollutants of most concern are lead, radon, and nitrates.

Lead may contaminate the water of more than 40 million Americans. It occurs mainly from corrosion of water pipes, from lead solder in plumbing, and from lead in brass faucets. The possibility of contamination is of greatest concern to people living in homes more than 30 years old whose pipes contain more lead, and for families with young children, who are more sensitive to lead toxicity (see Chapter 6, *Minerals*). Testing for lead is relatively easy and inexpensive. Reverse osmosis will remove lead; solid carbon filters may also remove it to some degree.

Radon is a radioactive gas by-product of uranium and is found in the earth's crust. High radon gas levels are associated with an increased risk of lung cancer. This carcinogenic element can be present in any home in levels high enough to cause concern but is more likely to be found in the northeast United States, North Carolina, and Arizona. Water that comes from wells and groundwater have a higher incidence of contamination. Municipal waters that come from lakes, rivers, and reservoirs are usually low in radon. When present in the water, radon can be released into the air with showering, laundering, and dishwashing. Radon in the air at home can be tested with several new devices available on the market. If present in the water in high amounts, radon can be removed with carbon filtration, but this system must be attached to the entire water system of the home.

Nitrates are suggested to be the third main risk in water. They are present mostly in groundwater sources that have agricultural contamination; these waters may also then have higher amounts of toxic pesticides and herbicides. High nitrate levels are of greatest risk to infants and seriously ill people. Nitrates are converted to nitrites by certain intestinal bacteria; these nitrites may alter the hemoglobin molecule, converting it to methemoglobin, which cannot carry oxygen. Rural families, especially those with infants and pregnant women, should test their water for nitrates. If it is present in high amounts, either reverse osmosis or distillation systems will help to clear the nitrate molecules.

Other major concerns in drinking water are the chemicals that are released into our waters by industry and the agricultural chemical pesticides, herbicides, and fertilizers that run off into local waters. These organic chemicals are more toxic and carcinogenic at lower levels than many other contaminants. The trihalomethanes (THMs) formed in chlorinated water are also a carcinogenic concern.

However, with all these possible health threats, the government would like us to believe that we should have no concerns about our drinking water. Clearly, tap water consumption usually does not cause immediate or significant health problems unless it is contaminated with infectious organisms. Millions of people drink water from this source every day, though many avoid drinking it straight because of the taste. However, more research studying the relationship of drinking water to chronic disease needs to be done. Until we know more about tap water (and even well water) and its long-range effects, it is better to be careful and not drink it. In some areas, chemical contamination from using tap water for cooking and bathing may even be a concern. It may be worthwhile to analyze questionable water for toxic chemicals and metals, as well as analyzing its mineral content, hardness, and pH. Several companies in the United States analyze water, including Water Test in New Hampshire, National Testing Labs in Ohio, and Suburban Water Testing Labs in Pennsylvania. They all have toll free 800-numbers.

In a television special, "The Poisoning of America," the danger that our water is now in, both in the earth and at the tap, was made very clear. Though some countries have concerns about infectious water, that problem is minimal for us in America. Our woes are problems of modern technology—toxic chemical wastes, farming wastes, and heavy metals. Yet, technology can also help us correct these difficulties. We have made some progress with filtration, purification, and distillation through more chemicals and water units, but we still have a ways to go. I believe we can do better. I also believe it is going to take a half century or more to clean up our waters and counteract the destruction we've done to our planet. The generation born now through the end of this century will need to be the "dismantlers," the "cleanup" generation. Let us hope this process is successful.

Well Water

Well water comes primarily from groundwater supplies and can vary greatly in its mineral content. Some is very low in most minerals while other well water is a rich source of beneficial nutritional minerals such as iron, zinc, selenium, magnesium, or calcium. Unfortunately, groundwater may also contain toxic heavy metals or agricultural and industrial chemical pollutants such as pesticides, herbicides, radon, asbestos, or hydrocarbons (gasoline by-products).

If your water source is a well, have the water analyzed for bacteria, mineral content, and organic chemical pollutants. With a clean bill of health, go ahead and use this potentially nutritious water freely.

Spring Water

This is the "natural" water found in surface or underground springs. Some companies retrieve and bottle this water. Other than being disinfected (chlorine may be used), this water is not processed. The water tastes very different from tap water and, to me, is a refreshing drink. The mineral content depends upon the region from which the water is taken and upon whether it is surface or underground water (surface spring water is relatively low in minerals). For example, the lakes, streams, and spring water from the southeastern and northwestern regions of our country are relatively low in minerals, and this "soft" water may increase the incidence of cardiovascular disease. The Midwest, in contrast, has high-mineral underground waters, and the farm people who drink this unchlorinated well water have a lower cardiovascular disease rate. Of course, there may be other lifestyle factors that contribute to this finding.

Just as groundwater can be polluted, spring water can also be contaminated. It is a good idea to have spring water checked out or to get full reports or summaries of tests from the company selling spring water. Ideally, these are independent lab reports performed yearly. Also, find out if the water is bottled at the source or transported and then treated and bottled. (Water bottled at the source is preferable.) Though spring water can be costly, it is high on the list of drinkable waters.

Martin Fox, in his book *Healthy Water for a Longer Life*, suggests that three ideal characteristics of drinking water are: (1) total dissolved solids of about 300 ppm. (parts per million), (2) hardness (containing at least 170 mg./l. of calcium carbonate), and (3) an alkaline pH (over 7.0), to reduce leeching of metals from pipes. Spring and well waters may fit into these categories.

Mineral Water

Really, most waters are mineral waters—that is, they contain minerals. In California, the standard for bottled mineral water is more than 500 ppm. of dissolved minerals. Underground bubbly water, called "natural sparkling water," usually contains lots of minerals, as well as carbon dioxide (CO_2). Many companies bottling this "mineral" water must inject CO_2 back into the water, since it is easily lost between the ground and bottle. Seltzer is any water that is carbonated with carbon dioxide; it is usually filtered tap water. Club soda is essentially the same, though it usually has more minerals added.

All of these types of waters can also be polluted, though any bottled carbonated water would be free of microorganisms, as they cannot live there. Generally though, they should be checked out for mineral levels and chemicals if you consume them in any quantity. I do not recommend, however, large amounts of these carbonated waters. The carbon dioxide can get into the blood and affect the acid-alkaline balance, although the body usually handles this easily through respiration or kidney filtration.

Filtered Water

Filtration, or purification, involves the removal of extraneous matter, be it chemicals, metals, or bacteria, from water. Legally, anything called a "purifier" must remove 99.75 percent of incoming bacteria. Americans are purchasing about two million home filtering systems yearly, and there are a great many models from which to choose. There are several types of filtration systems that can be used, including carbon filters, both granulated and solid, and reverse osmosis. (Distillation will be discussed separately, next.) It is a good idea to educate yourself about water filtration before purchasing a home unit. In the long run, home filters/purifiers are the least expensive and safest way to obtain good drinking water.

Activated Carbon (AC) is the most common type of filter. The carbon, used for centuries as a filtering substance, is "activated" by exposing it to chemicals at high temperatures and steam in the absence of oxygen. That gives the carbon a large surface on which to attach and absorb contaminants. Most carbon filtration units mechanically and biomagnetically (ionically) filter the water and remove the unpleasant appearance, odor, and taste by cleaning it of bacteria, parasites, most viruses, chlorine, and the heavier minerals and particulate matter. However, carbon is best at removing organic chemicals and chlorine, not perfect for all microorganisms and metals. Basically, they will filter out any particles or organisms over 0.04 microns, or whatever the size of the filter pores. The filters can, however, collect bacteria and sediment; as a result, there is some concern that they may breed bacteria and dump them back into the water. Hot water should not be run through carbon filters because it can cause contaminant release. Carbon is excellent at trapping the larger molecules, chemicals, and larger microorganisms; it is not good at removing inorganic minerals including fluoride bound strongly to sodium or calcium, the way it is added to municipal waters. However, solid carbon filtration is believed to be relatively effective (this is still controversial) at removing many of the toxic minerals with higher molecular weights, such as lead or mercury.

The two main types of carbon filters are granulated carbon and solid carbon block filters. The granulated carbon filter has air spaces between the carbon particles to trap bacteria and remove it from the water; however, the bacteria can multiply within the air spaces. Silver is used in most granulated filters to assist in killing the bacteria. These "silver-impregnated" filters do help reduce the bacterial growth within the filter, but there are concerns about ineffectiveness and silver toxicity. Though granulated carbon filters are economical, their use is short-lived, and their safety is definitely questionable; I do not recommend them.

The Solid Carbon Block with its surrounding filter alleviates the concern of microorganism contamination. Not only can the filtering surface area of this denser carbon bed clean much more water but, because there is very little oxygen or supply nutrients within the filter, the germs will not thrive; however, to be safe, if the filter is not used for a day or longer, let the water run through it for 10–20 seconds before drinking. Research has demonstrated that these units also trap more chemicals, organic pollutants, radon, and asbestos than the looser granulated carbon filters. Some companies that sell solid carbon block water filters are Multi-Pure, NeoLife, and Amway.

Carbon filters are rated by volume of water treated, since they can hold only a limited amount of sediment. They should be changed regularly to avoid dumping more bacteria and chemicals back into the drinking water and because the filtration slows down when they near the end of their effectiveness. The carbon filter may clean roughly 400–1,000 gallons, and each unit may vary depending on the amount of sediment in the incoming water. A unit should probably be changed at about 75 percent of its maximum capacity for best results. Figure your average daily usage and mark the time for change on your calendar. Activated carbon filters/purifiers, though more expensive than tap water, are usually less expensive than distillers or units that use reverse osmosis.

Reverse Osmosis (RO) is thought by some authorities to be the best way to purify water. Under pressure, usually from the tap, water flows through special membranes with microporous holes the size of the water molecule. These pores allow the water molecule to pass through while rejecting the larger inorganic and organic materials.

Reverse osmosis units usually have two or three filtering mechanisms. First is a sedimentation filter, which merely allows particulate matter to settle. Then comes the RO filter. It is followed by a carbon filter, which removes most any contaminants that may have passed through the RO membrane. With this system, virtually 100 percent of the organic material is removed, along with almost all the minerals.

Reverse osmosis units range from small home units to those of industrial size. Home units can make from three to ten gallons per day. They are energy efficient, as they require only tap water pressure, yet are not water efficient. Until recently, they were very expensive, but now there are good units available at competitive prices. Since the life of the RO filter is usually about five years, the price per gallon of water is approximately 20–30 cents. The carbon filter (and possibly the RO membrane) in this unit should be replaced every year or so, and this is relatively inexpensive. Disadvantages of RO units include their bulky size, the limitation of water production determined by the size of the holding tank (usually one to two gallons), and the time involved to prepare the water for drinking (often three to six hours per gallon). The units produce many gallons of "waste water" per gallon of drinking water because only 10–25 percent of the incoming water goes through the unit; waste can run between 2–30 gallons daily depending on the unit's efficiency. This is not ideal in droughts, though this waste water can be collected for other uses. RO units may not clear all bacteria and chemicals, though the addition of carbon filtration/purification makes them very efficient. Furthermore, RO units remove almost all minerals (high-calcium waters may clog their filters), which many authorities feel are an important component in our water. Concern over the same hazard of leaching body minerals from drinking distilled water exclusively is not yet well founded scientifically, though people drinking only these waters while fasting run the risk of depleting themselves more rapidly. Deionized water, though, different from RO or distilled, should not be used for drinking as it can deplete body minerals more readily.

Overall, reverse osmosis may be our key filtration system now and in the future, especially with more efficient and economical systems available. Reverse osmosis is best for removing dissolved solids, organic chemicals, and lead and other heavy metals.

Distilled Water

The distillation process involves vaporizing water (turning it into steam) in one chamber and then condensing it once again into liquid in a separate chamber. This removes all the minerals, organisms, and chemicals from the water. Distilled water should be pure H_2O. However, there is some concern that certain volatile organic chemicals will vaporize and recondense into the second chamber's water; therefore, distillation should be preceded by solid carbon filtration. There is also concern that heating water to 212 degrees Fahrenheit before drinking it changes the water so it has a different biochemical effect in the body. Home distillers are fairly expensive and require electrical energy to process a few gallons; furthermore, it takes significant time, usually five hours or more per gallon, for the water to be distilled, so this limits the amount available for use.

Distilled water contains no minerals (as mentioned, distillation takes out everything except volatile chemicals). Therefore, when consumed, it tends to attract minerals (and toxins) to balance with the other body fluids. The regular consumption of distilled water, especially by someone who may already be slightly deficient, can cause mineral deficiencies. Fasting for long periods exclusively on distilled water "to pull out toxins" is not recommended because of the potential mineral depletions it can create. However, when doing extractions, as in making herbal teas, distilled water may help bring out the most in the medicinal properties of the herbs. Also, during detoxification diets, distilled water may be suggested because it may be more effective for this process, having a stronger "magnetic" charge to pull out toxins.

Note on Demineralized Water. Many nutritional advocates, mostly the elders, recommend drinking demineralized water because they believe that the inorganic minerals contained naturally in some waters are not usable by the human body, that these naturally dissolved inorganic minerals may even cause problems. This is simply not true; many of the minerals we acquire are in the inorganic or salt state and are not part of organic tissues. They can still be assimilated and used by the body. The mineral levels in water, however, are not anywhere near sufficient to satisify body needs. Cooking foods in demineralized water pulls more minerals from them, whereas using water containing natural minerals will lessen this loss and possibly even improve food values. Furthermore, many of the dissolved solids, such as the trace minerals selenium, zinc, or silica, found in natural waters are associated with lower cancer rates in the people who consume them than in people who consume treated or demineralized water. Many of the cultures in which people live long healthy lives are located in regions with mineral-rich mountain waters. These waters have always tasted the best and felt the best to me when I have had the opportunity to drink them. Overall, I believe that the naturally occurring earth minerals contained in our water are beneficial to our health.

○ SO, WHAT DO WE DRINK?

Water is the substance we need most, and since good drinking water is so important to health we should know about the water we use and what it contains. Water contamination is inescapable, so we need help. If there is any question about the water we drink, we can have it checked for bacteria count, mineral content, and the presence of a wide number of chemical pollutants. Should there be concern over what it contains, we should then find a filtration and/or purification system that makes it safe and healthy or find another source of drinking water.

In the past I believed that the prime choice of drinking water was the uncontaminated (these may be extinct) natural springs or wells of the earth. Especially if this water comes from the area where we live, it puts us in harmony with our environment and often provides important minerals (though it should be checked for abnormally high mineral content). However, because of our current pollution problems, it may be essential for all of us to purify our drinking water adequately now or in the near future.

Most of us who live in cities provided with tap water from treatment plants must take appropriate steps to make our water the best it can be. Bottled water is expensive and may come in polyethylene containers, which raise their own health questions. Besides, the water is often chlorinated and may have been in the containers for months, if not longer.

I now believe that we need to create a cost-effective and water-efficient system to protect us from water pollution. Current technology is advancing, and it seems that the combination of solid carbon and reverse osmosis will be the wave of the future and are currently the best ways we have to obtain clean water. Solid carbon alone can help clear most bacteria, chlorine, and most of the chemical pollutants that infiltrate our water. I personally have a Multi-Pure stainless-steel unit hooked up to our kitchen faucet so that my family can have purified water to use for drinking, cooking, and washing food (including our sprouts). This type of system is the most economical for the quality of water it delivers. Of course, it is more expensive than drinking tap water, so we must decide that it is worth the five to ten dollars a month it costs over time to know that our water is free of bacteria, chlorine, toxic chemicals, and most heavy metals. Solid carbon may actually be the best system for removing chemicals, one of our biggest concerns in drinking water. An added advantage of solid carbon block filters over reverse osmosis and distillation, besides lower cost-per-gallon of water and easier accessibility, is that they leave the natural trace minerals that our bodies can use. However, if nitrate levels are high or if we want fluoride removed, reverse osmosis is necessary. We should remember that solid carbon filters are very different from carbon granule filters (often silver impregnated), which can harbor bacteria and then release them, and chemicals, back into the water in even greater concentrations.

To review, the three common, effective home treatment systems are solid carbon block filters, reverse osmosis, and distillation. Purchasing prebottled water is an

WATER SYSTEMS ANALYSIS

Contents	Source		Purification		
	Tap Water	Well or Spring	Solid Carbon	Reverse Osmosis	Distillation
Chlorine	yes	not unless treated	removed	not removed unless carbon used also	removed
Fluoride	if added	natural or if treated	not removed	removed	removed
Bacteria	unlikely	possibly removed	most likely	removed	removed
Parasites	possibly	possibly	removed	removed	removed
Chemicals	likely	likely	removed	removed	possibly*
Basic Minerals	some	likely	not removed	removed	removed
Heavy Metals	possibly	possibly	some removed	removed	removed
Energy Factors					
Electricity Used	no	probably	no	no	yes
Wastes Water	no	no	no	yes	some

* Potential volatilization of chlorinated hydrocarbons and other toxic chemicals.

unnecessary expense, and in many cases, the water is not as good and definitely not as fresh as water purified at home. All three systems will remove chlorine (not RO alone), bacteria, metals, and chemicals, though I have some concern about volatile chemicals left after distillation. (Distilled water should be prefiltered by solid carbon.) Because solid carbon filtration is more economical in time, water use, and dollars and very good at removing chemicals, this may be the best process for city folk unless you want the added fluoride taken out. Solid carbon will not remove the fluoride ions, which are strongly bonded to sodium or calcium. Natural spring or well water that is tested and clean may be the best choice for people living in the country. (See more on water quality and contamination in Chapter 11, *Environmental Aspects of Nutrition.*)

Traveler's Water

In the United States and much of the Westernized world, the greatest concern is contamination of water by pesticides and herbicides used in agriculture; by chemicals, such as hydrocarbons, from industry; and by the chlorine and other agents added to kill existing and potential germs in the water. When traveling to Third World countries and other areas that do not "treat" their water, or when hiking or camping in nature areas of this country, we may need to take measures to make the water safe from microorganisms.

There are always potential dangers from microbial contamination in water or food. Awareness and safety measures are important. Untreated water may harbor bacteria or parasites most commonly, or viruses on occasion. Our mountain rivers and streams or lake waters may contain giardia or parasitic amoeba, campylobacter or other bacteria, metals, chemicals, or radioactivity. Common organisms that may cause intestinal infection in Third World countries (or in contaminated food or water in this country) include salmonella, shigella, E. coli, giardia, amoebas, and cryptosporidium. Contracting hepatitis from water may also be a slight concern, but foods are a more common transmitter of infectious hepatitis.

We have a few options concerning drinking water when we travel. First, we may carry our own water, although this is limited to short trips or when camping with a vehicle. We may also avoid drinking water totally as some try, for example, when traveling to Mexico or South America. Drinking bottled carbonated beverages such as waters, sodas, or beer usually keeps us safe from germs, as they cannot exist in the high carbon dioxide levels. But food might be washed or ice cubes made with contaminated water.

Overall, when traveling (or anytime for that matter), there are three ways to clean water to make it safer. These treatments are heat, chemicals, and filtration. At sea level, boiling water for one minute will kill bacteria and parasites; boil ten minutes to destroy viruses. For every 1,000 feet of elevation, add one minute to the boiling time to clean the water of possible germs. So in the mountains, at 10,000 feet, water must be boiled for 10–20 minutes, dependent upon your concerns. Little heating coils or stoves may be used, but overall this process may be cumbersome, especially when larger amounts of water are needed.

Chemical treatment may be simplest and the least expensive, yet it has drawbacks— most people do not like the taste and for some there might be side effects or reactions. Both chlorine and iodine have been used effectively for this purpose. Halazone tablets release chlorine into the water. Five tablets per quart will effectively kill almost all microorganisms, but the taste is not very exciting. In my opinion iodine is preferable, used as 2 percent liquid—ten drops per quart and let it sit for 30 minutes to kill the germs. Globaline is a crystaline iodine. One tablet can be added to a quart of water and will work in ten minutes. Overall, I believe that chemical treatment is a last resort for water purification.

Our goal at home or when traveling is to have germ-free water without chemicals or chlorine. Filtration is the best way to do this. I have discussed home filters. There are also filters designed for travel and camping. These are small units that have pumps so lake or river waters can be used. Since the recent outbreaks of giardiasis contracted by drinking the crystal clear, good-tasting mountain stream waters in our country, even wilderness packers need to carry some type of water purification. With the difficulty of boiling at higher altitudes and the distaste of chemical purification, filtration is the best way to go for backpacking, especially if large amounts of water are needed.

Most hand filters are granulated carbon, often with silver added. Though these are not ideal for home use, they are simplest for travel. They will take out some chemicals, but our biggest concern is microorganisms. Here the pore size of the filter, which should be clearly stated in the product information, is the crucial factor in determining what germs will be removed. The following chart shows micron sizes of relevant organisms.

Organism	Size in microns
Giardia lamblia	10–20
Amoebas	10–50
Cryptosporidium	2–5
Campylobacter bacteria	.2–.3
CMV and Herpes virus	.15–.2
Retro virus (AIDS)	.1–.12
Hepatitis viruses	.025–.04

The pore size of available filters ranges from 0.2—2.0 microns. They all will remove parasites, some will remove bacteria, but most will not take out viruses. In drinking water our biggest concerns are from parasites and bacteria; viruses, more unlikely to survive in water, are really a lesser concern. The Katadyn unit, claiming a pore size of .2 microns, may remove some viruses as well. It is the most expensive of the travel-pump units. Most of the available travel filters can clean about one to two pints per minute. If the water is dirty or turbid, use a prefilter such as a coffee filter or clean cotton bandana, for example, and pour the water through one of these before pumping. Prefiltering extends the life of the carbon filter.

○ WATER REQUIREMENTS

Water is essential for all life, and drinking the right amount is important to health. All the beverages we drink—teas, coffee, sodas, beer—are basically water that contains other ingredients as well. Drinking good water is still the best way, I believe, to obtain our fluid requirements.

The amount of water we need is based upon a number of factors—our size; our activity level, which influences the amount of fluid we lose through sweat; the climate or temperature (higher environmental temperatures increase our fluid losses); and our diet. A diet high in fruits and vegetables provides more total fluids through food than a diet high in fat, meat, and dairy products, for example. Special circumstances in which increased amounts of water may be needed include fever, diarrhea, kidney disease, or any situation where excessive fluid losses occur through normal body elimination processes.

We lose water daily through our skin, urine, bowels, and lungs (as water vapor in the air). About half of our water losses can be replaced with the water content in our food. The remaining half requires specific fluid intake, primarily from drinking good water. Caffeinated beverages, such as coffee, tea, cocoa, or colas, and alcoholic beverages do not count as the same volume of water because they act as diuretics in the body, increasing fluid losses from the kidneys.

The average human requirement is about three quarts of water per day, including food and beverages. An inactive person in a cool climate may need less, while an athlete training in the desert will need much more. People who eat a lot of fruits and vegetables, which are high in water content, will require less drinking water than people who consume proportionally more meats and fats, which are more concentrated and require additional water to help utilize them. In addition to a healthy diet containing fresh fruits and vegetables, I recommend that the average person consume at least one and a half to two quarts of water daily, because I also suggest a physically active lifestyle with daily exercise.

Water is best consumed at several intervals throughout the day—one or two glasses upon awakening and also about an hour before each meal. Water should not be drunk with or just after meals, as it can dilute digestive juices and reduce food digestion and nutrient assimilation. Some people like to drink a glass or two in the evening to help flush out their systems overnight, even though this may result in getting up during the night to urinate. It is important to drink water to avoid problems such as constipation and dry skin. Drinking enough contaminant-free water is likely our most significant nutritional health factor. Water will keep us current, clean, and flowing through life.

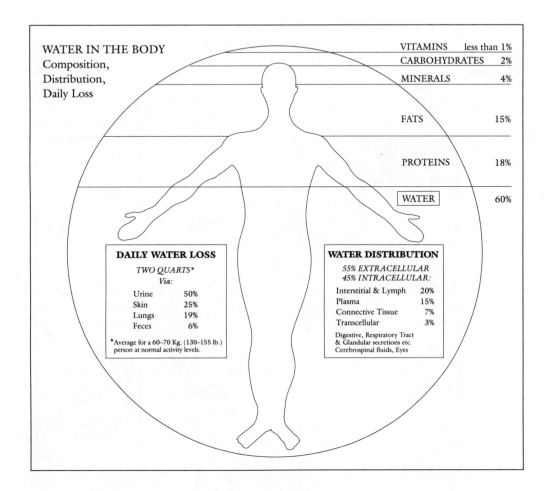

WATER IN THE BODY
Composition,
Distribution,
Daily Loss

VITAMINS	less than 1%
CARBOHYDRATES	2%
MINERALS	4%
FATS	15%
PROTEINS	18%
WATER	60%

DAILY WATER LOSS
TWO QUARTS*
Via:

Urine	50%
Skin	25%
Lungs	19%
Feces	6%

*Average for a 60–70 Kg. (130–155 lb.)
person at normal activity levels.

WATER DISTRIBUTION
55% EXTRACELLULAR
45% INTRACELLULAR:

Interstitial & Lymph	20%
Plasma	15%
Connective Tissue	7%
Transcellular	3%

Digestive, Respiratory Tract
& Glandular secretions etc.
Cerebrospinal fluids, Eyes

On the desk in my office, my purified drinking water is in
a special gold-amber bottle engraved with the slogan:

"Nectar of the Golden Life of Health and Vitality."

I believe water to be that substance.

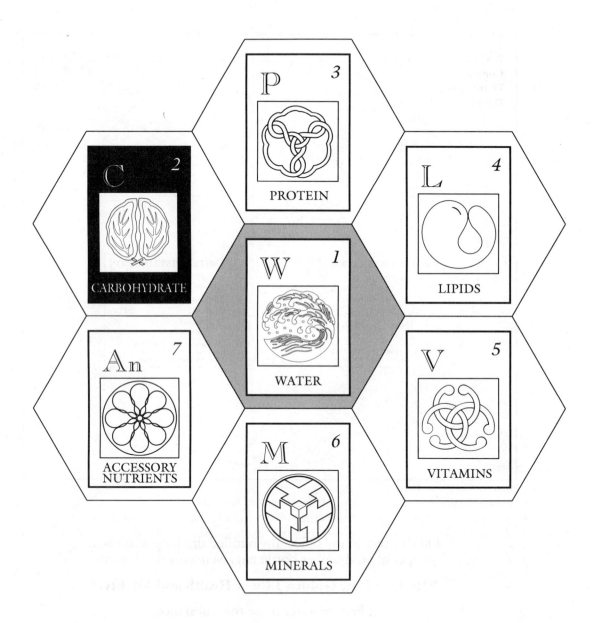

Chapter 2

Carbohydrates

Carbohydrates are probably the most important of the three main classes of foods since they are our main source of energy and should constitute at least 50–60 percent of the diet. There has been a shift in this century away from the healthful consumption of fresh fruits and vegetables and complex carbohydrates—the starches and fiber foods—toward a diet of more refined carbohydrates and simple sugars that are implicated in a variety of diseases, among them obesity, diabetes, cardiovascular problems, and tooth decay.

Carbohydrates are organic molecules; that is, they contain carbon and come from living sources. They are composed of carbon (C), hydrogen (H), and oxygen (O) (thus, the abbreviation CHO) in a 1:2:1 ratio. The basic relationship is that of carbon coupled with water molecules. Carbohydrates are a quick source of energy for the body, being easily converted to glucose, the fuel for the body's cells. Each gram of carbohydrate releases four calories, units of heat or energy, for the body.

Carbohydrates are produced by photosynthesis in plants. The carbohydrates are the primary source of energy in nature's plant foods—fruits, vegetables, grains, legumes, and tubers. These foods play a very important role in the functioning of the internal organs, the nervous system, and the muscles. They are the best source of energy for endurance athletics because they provide both an immediate and a time-released energy source as they are digested easily and then consistently metabolized in the bloodstream.

Carbohydrates are also needed to regulate protein and fat metabolism. With the proteins and fats, the carbohydrates help to fight infections, promote growth of body tissues such as bones and skin, and lubricate the joints. Many carbohydrate foods are also high in fiber, and the fiber content of foods is important in the bulking of the stool, which aids in regular elimination of waste materials through the colon. Indeed,

31

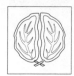
fiber is thought to be helpful in preventing colon diseases such as colon cancer and diverticulosis and is being prescribed by more doctors as a dietary necessity.

Three principal carbohydrates are present in foods. Carbohydrates are classified according to their structure. First are the sugars, both monosaccharides (simple sugars), such as those found in honey and fruits, and oligosaccharides (multiple sugars), such as table sugar and malt sugar, which both happen to be disaccharides (two-sugar molecules). Then there are the starches, or complex carbohydrates, found primarily in vegetables such as carrots and potatoes and in whole grains such as rice and corn. Finally, there is fiber, mainly cellulose and hemicellulose, the indigestible roughage found in most unprocessed, carbohydrate-containing foods.

○ SUGARS

The basic unit of the simple sugars (monosaccharides) is one hexose (containing six carbon atoms) or pentose (five carbon atoms) molecule. These simple sugars are easily and quickly digested and utilized by the body. They have the same chemical makeup but vary in structure. The disaccharides, such as table sugar or milk sugar, require some enzymatic breakdown but are easily converted into monosaccharides for digestion. The following represent the common basic sugars.

Monosaccharides

Glucose is the metabolized form of "sugar" in the body. It is found in some fruits, such as grapes. It can also be hydrolyzed from starch, cane sugar (sucrose), milk sugar (lactose), and malt syrup (maltose). Glucose is carried in the blood and is the principal sugar used by the tissues and cells for energy. Glucose can be measured by the "blood sugar" test, which reads the current concentration of glucose in the serum or plasma. A high glucose level can signal a diabetic condition; low blood sugar is called hypoglycemia. Both of these abnormalities can become chronic and even life-threatening. The adrenal and pancreatic hormones, adrenaline and insulin, are very important in sugar metabolism. High-sugar and refined-carbohydrate diets, stress, and lack of exercise can generate elevated glucose levels in both blood and tissue. Pregnancy is also a stress on carbohydrate metabolism because of its high metabolic demands.

Fructose is found in most fruits and fruit juices, as well as in honey and some vegetables. Fructose is sweeter than cane sugar and is absorbed directly into the blood. Cane sugar (sucrose) is metabolized into fructose and glucose. Fructose can be changed to glucose in the liver or in the small intestine for a quick source of energy.

Galactose comes from the metabolism of the milk sugar lactose, which breaks down into galactose and glucose. Galactose is converted to glucose in the liver and is synthesized in the mammary glands to make the lactose of mother's milk.

Disaccharides

These sugars can be hydrolyzed into two monosaccharides with the addition of a water molecule. They are all water soluble and will crystallize when dehydrated.

Lactose (milk sugar) is the only sugar of animal origin, the sugar of mother's milk. It is composed of one molecule each of glucose and galactose. Lactose is broken down by the enzyme *lactase*, which may be deficient or absent in some races of people, leading to problems with milk digestion.

Sucrose ("white sugar") is found in sugar cane and sugar beets, maple syrup, molasses, sorghum, and pineapple. Sucrose is composed of one molecule each of fructose and glucose. Sucrose is very sweet and can be metabolized in the body. Its crystalline form, table sugar, is used excessively in our society, not only as a sweetener on food and in beverages but also in cooking and "hidden" in preparation of many other common foods and condiments, such as catsup, mayonnaise, salad dressings, and baby foods. Addiction to sucrose begins early and is supported by millions of dollars of advertising. The average American consumes well more than 100 pounds of sucrose a year, and this particular disaccharide is responsible for a wide variety of problems. It has been implicated in obesity, tooth decay, diabetes, and many psychological and emotional problems, including premenstrual syndrome and stress/burnout syndromes. Using less sugar would be a boost to anyone's health.

Maltose (malt sugar) is a short chain of two glucose molecules. It is produced during the breakdown of starches in many cereal grains. Maltose is present in beers, malted snacks, and some breakfast cereals and is the sweetener of many crackers (read labels!). It is easily broken down into glucose molecules for quick utilization by the body.

O STARCHES

The second category of carbohydrates is the starches, or polysaccharides. These are also termed the complex carbohydrates, as they are composed of long chains of glucose molecules. Starches require amylase enzymes (other biochemical catalysts) to be broken down into simple sugars for digestion, absorption, and utilization.

Starch provides a more consistent blood sugar level than the simple sugars, which cause the glucose level in the blood to rise and fall rapidly. In the traditional diet, a high percentage of foods consumed included the complex carbohydrates of potatoes, vegetable roots, and whole grains such as wheat, rice, and corn. This was much healthier than the present-day preference for high-sugar and refined-flour diets, which are associated with degenerative tissue disease and aging.

There are several types of starches. If the polysaccharide chains are shorter and branched, the starch is called amylopectin—the most common one found in foods. Amylose has long chains of glucose molecules, which are easily separated by the enzyme *amylase*. Glycogen is the animal-source starch contained in muscle and liver. It is similar in structure to amylopectin and can be broken down to release glucose for energy needs or be formed from extra glucose and stored in the liver. Glycogen is really the form in which glucose is stored in our body. Dextrins are partially digested starches that are formed in the breakdown of starch.

○ FIBER

The third component of carbohydrates is fiber—mainly the indigestible cellulose commonly found in the skins of fruits and vegetables and in the coverings of cereal grains, such as wheat bran. This fiber in foods provides little energy or caloric value. As mentioned earlier, it fosters good intestinal function and elimination. Low-fiber diets are associated with constipation, gastrointestinal disorders, diverticulosis, and colon cancer, while a high-fiber diet may prevent these problems. Fiber in the diet may also reduce the risk of appendicitis.

Cellulose is the most common fiber contained in basic foods. Other fibers include the hemicelluloses, found in the cell walls of plants, which have a high ability to bind water. This helps in digestion and elimination. Psyllium seed husks are a good example of a hemicellulose. They are a popular fiber supplement used to provide bulk and to speed transit time through the bowels. Pectin is another hemicellulose, which, besides absorbing water, can lower the amount of fat absorption. This is the pectin found in the rind of citrus fruits and in the pulp of apples, which is also used in making jams.

Other fibers used in the diet include both agar and alginate (derived from seaweed) and carrageen, which comes from the Irish moss plant. All indigestible polysaccharides, they are used in food preparation and in cosmetics for their smooth gelatinous consistency. Carrageen is used commonly with dairy products such as yogurt to create a smooth consistency. Agar is used to bring a gelatinous quality to foods and desserts. Alginate can bind up minerals and metals, such as cadmium, mercury, lead, and arsenic, in the intestines and has been found useful in detoxification programs.

Several other high-fiber substances that have some use in the diet have been shown in preliminary research to help reduce cholesterol levels because of their ability to hinder fat absorption from the intestines. Guar gum may also be used to slow glucose uptake in the intestines and may be helpful in mild diabetes. Konjar root flour from Japan has also been shown in tests to have some influence in moderating diabetes, in lowering cholesterol levels, and in weight control. Chitosan, derived from oyster shells, has also been used to lower cholesterol levels. (For further discussion of the health aspects of fiber, see the beginning of Chapter 8, *Foods.*)

○ REQUIREMENTS

Although the carbohydrate-containing foods often constitute the majority of our diet, there are no specific requirements published for our carbohydrate needs. They are one of the best sources of energy and are simple for the body to use; however, since the body can make its own glucose from stored glycogen and the amino acid L-alanine, the government lists no minimum requirement. Yet, carbohydrate intake is important to health. Many of the carbohydrate foods contain essential vitamins and minerals as well as the dietary fiber necessary for colon health and proper elimination.

On the other hand, people can live without carbohydrate intake; in fact, in many weight loss programs carbohydrate consumption is severely limited. It is wise in these cases to consume supplemental fiber. Also, some people have a tendency to overeat carbohydrate foods, even to become "carb addicts." With this, weight may increase; obesity is associated most frequently with carbohydrate overindulgence. Allergies and emotional shifts, including "carbohydrate depression," have also been associated with sensitivity to overconsumption of this macronutrient.

Peoples of different cultures consume varying amounts of carbohydrates. Native or traditional diets may be very high in carbohydrates, while in cold climates, as with the Eskimo culture, people may consume very few carbohydrates. The average American diet includes about 40–50 percent carbohydrates; sadly enough, about half of that is from the refined and processed flours and sugars in breads, candies, cookies, and cakes. These foods deplete the body of many B vitamins and of minerals such as chromium. In addition to the already-mentioned diseases of obesity and tooth decay, it is possible that this type of diet (high in simple and refined sugars, high in fats, and low in complex carbohydrates) may be influencing the incidence of diabetes, high blood pressure, heart disease, anemia, skin problems, kidney disease, and cancer.

I feel that a diet of about 60–70 percent carbohydrate foods is ideal, especially when caloric consumption will support our best weight range. Intake of the refined carbohydrate foods should be minimal; primary intake should be the complex carbohydrates (many vegetables, whole grains, and legumes) and some simple "naturally occurring" sugars from the fruits and vegetables. For the adult, this higher carbohydrate/fiber diet, along with about 15–25 percent fat and 15–20 percent protein, is likely to be the best long-range healthy diet.

○ CARBOHYDRATE DIGESTION AND METABOLISM

Carbohydrates—sugars and starches—are broken down in the gastrointestinal tract by various enzymes for absorption into the blood. The disaccharides (lactose, sucrose, and maltose) are converted into their monosaccharides (glucose, fructose, and galactose). The polysaccharides (starches) are converted by salivary *amylase* in the mouth into dextrin, a shorter-chain starch; then the dextrins are reduced to maltose by pancreatic *amylase* released into the small intestine. The maltose is further broken down into glucose by *maltase* enzymes at the intestinal lining. Also in the small intestine, sucrose is changed into glucose and fructose by the enzyme *sucrase*, while *lactase* converts lactose, the milk sugar, into glucose and galactose. The monosaccharides, or simple sugars, such as glucose, galactose, and fructose, are the end products of carbohydrate digestion and are all absorbed into the bloodstream through the intestinal lining. The blood circulates to the liver, where fructose and galactose are easily converted into glucose, the fuel the body uses for energy.

The healthy liver regulates the use of glucose as it allows certain levels to circulate in the blood for use by the cells of the body. If the carbohydrate intake is higher than immediately needed, the liver will normally convert extra glucose into glycogen, a highly branched polysaccharide, and this glycogen can be stored in the liver or in the muscles. At a later time, if energy is needed when there are no dietary carbohydrates available, the liver will convert glycogen back to glucose and return it to the bloodstream, while the muscles may use the muscle glycogen directly for energy.

If we consume higher levels of carbohydrates than are immediately needed or can be converted to glycogen (that is, if there are already sufficient storage sources), then the liver will convert the excess glucose into fatty acids and then triglycerides that can be stored as body fat, a process termed lipogenesis. If carbohydrates are consumed in high quantities on a regular basis by a person with a sedentary lifestyle, weight gain occurs. Fat is a reserve source of energy. With decreased carbohydrate intake and increased activity levels, fat reserves are converted back to fatty acids for body fuel, a process called lipolysis. This generally produces weight loss.

Even when there is little or no intake of carbohydrates, the body attempts to maintain a steady blood sugar level through many mechanisms. Glucose is used by the liver as a source of energy to help synthesize a variety of essential substances. Insulin, a pancreatic hormone, regulates blood sugar levels by stimulating glucose uptake by the cells. Activity and exercise also can reduce blood sugar by increasing tissue glucose needs. A number of hormones influence the production of glucose when the body, and especially the brain, needs more energy. Epinephrine (adrenaline) stimulates glycogen breakdown and raises blood sugar. Steroids enhance conversion of fats and proteins into glucose, and adrenocorticotrophic hormone (ACTH) can interfere with insulin activity. Glucagon is produced in the pancreas and can raise blood sugar, while thyroid hormone may increase intestinal absorption of glucose as it attempts to stimulate metabolism.

CARBOHYDRATE DIGESTION AND METABOLISM CHART

CARBOHYDRATES

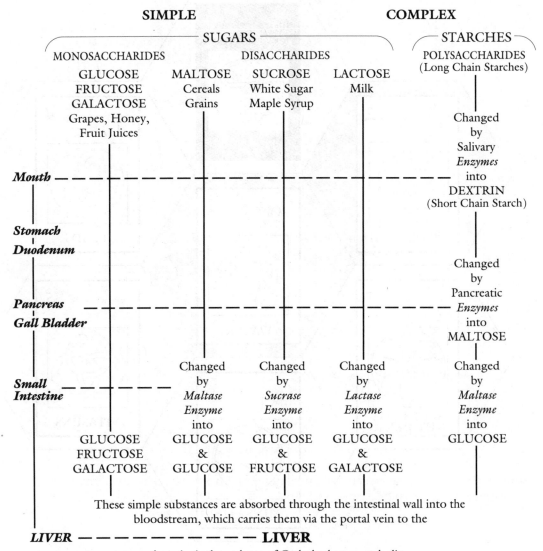

	SIMPLE			COMPLEX
	— SUGARS —			⌐ STARCHES ¬
	MONOSACCHARIDES	DISACCHARIDES		POLYSACCHARIDES (Long Chain Starches)
	GLUCOSE	MALTOSE	SUCROSE	LACTOSE
	FRUCTOSE	Cereals	White Sugar	Milk
	GALACTOSE	Grains	Maple Syrup	
	Grapes, Honey, Fruit Juices			Changed by Salivary *Enzymes* into
Mouth				DEXTRIN (Short Chain Starch)
Stomach *Duodenum*				
				Changed by Pancreatic *Enzymes* into MALTOSE
Pancreas *Gall Bladder*				
Small Intestine		Changed by *Maltase Enzyme* into	Changed by *Sucrase Enzyme* into	Changed by *Lactase Enzyme* into	Changed by *Maltase Enzyme* into
	GLUCOSE FRUCTOSE GALACTOSE	GLUCOSE & GLUCOSE	GLUCOSE & FRUCTOSE	GLUCOSE & GALACTOSE	GLUCOSE

These simple substances are absorbed through the intestinal wall into the bloodstream, which carries them via the portal vein to the

LIVER — — — — — — — — — **LIVER**

the principal regulator of Carbohydrate metabolism

37

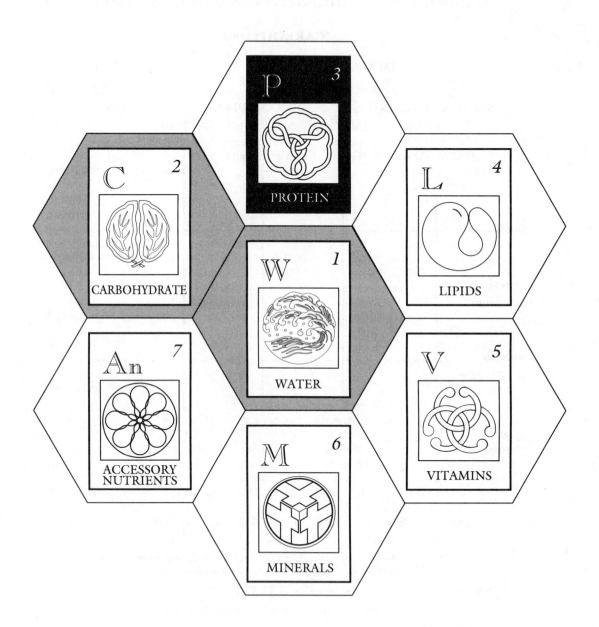

Chapter 3

Proteins

Protein is an essential part of nutrition, second only to water in the body's physical composition. Protein makes up about 20 percent of our body weight and is a primary component of our muscles, hair, nails, skin, eyes, and internal organs—especially the heart (muscle) and brain. Our immune defense system requires protein, especially for the formation of antibodies that help fight infections. Hemoglobin, our oxygen-carrying, red-blood-cell molecule, is a protein, as are many hormones that regulate our metabolism, such as thyroid hormone and insulin. Biochemical deficiency can occur when there is a lack of enzymes, the protein molecules that catalyze chemical reactions in the body. Protein is needed for growth and the maintenance of body tissues; it is vitally important during childhood or pregnancy and lactation. However, we can eat too much protein!

Protein molecules are composed of carbon, oxygen, hydrogen, and nitrogen, while fats and carbohydrates are made up of carbon, oxygen, and hydrogen only. All three macronutrients—proteins, fats, and carbohydrates—are organic (containing carbon) components that are part of the living tissues of plants and animals of Earth.

○ THE AMINO ACIDS

Proteins are complex molecules comprised of a combination of 22 naturally occurring amino acids. Proteins, each having its unique amino acid sequence and three-dimensional structure, exist as long chains, branched molecules, spheres, or helixes (as with DNA). The L- (levorotatory) forms of each amino acid are those found naturally in proteins, while the D- (dextrotatory) forms—which may be synthesized yet are not part of body proteins—are the mirror images of the amino acid molecules as they

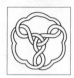

occur naturally. Twenty main L- amino acids and some other minor ones as well, are required to build bodily proteins.

Essential amino acids are those our body cannot synthesize on its own and which we must acquire through our diet. These eight are isoleucine, leucine, lysine, methionine, phenylalanine, threonine, tryptophan, and valine. Arginine and histidine are considered semiessential in that they are essential for children and may be needed in increased growth-demand states such as pregnancy. There are 12 (the number may vary in different texts) nonessential amino acids, which the body produces to build the proteins for muscles and hair and important molecules (hemoglobin, enzymes, and antibodies) and hormones (thyroid and insulin).

We may be deficient in some of these so-called nonessential amino acids when our diet is lacking in protein or in certain vitamins, minerals, or enzymes that are needed to produce enough of each amino acid. Then we may become deficient in the particular proteins made by those amino acids as well. The liver is the site for production and conversion of many nonessential amino acids. It needs pyridoxal-5-phosphate, the active form of vitamin B_6, to make the cofactor required by the transaminase enzymes, which can then generate the formation of certain nonessential amino acids. The concept of nonessential amino acid deficiency is not yet in the forefront of medicine, and it may not be applicable in light of the average protein-centered American diet, but it might be wise to analyze the amino acid levels of vegetarians, people on special diets, or those malnourished because of illness or digestive problems (see *Appendix* for a sample amino acid profile). Or, it is possible to supplement our diet with an L- amino acid mixture, taken after meals.

Amino acid therapy is relatively new to nutritional medicine, having begun with the ability to extract individual amino acids for supplementation in clinical situations. Also, as mentioned, some laboratories can run an amino acid profile to decipher the exact amino acid balance, or rather imbalance, that correlates with many disease states. A recent book entitled *The Healing Nutrients Within: Facts, Findings and New Research on Amino Acids*, by Eric Braverman, M.D., with Carl Pfeiffer, M.D. (Keats Publishing, 1987), adds some of the research performed at the Brain Bio Center in Princeton, New Jersey, to the existing information on amino acids. It is clear from my own experience and that of many other doctors and nutritionists that amino acid analysis and therapy has great possibilities in medicine and, as research continues, can be an important addition to medical care in the future.

The following pages offer individual discussions of each amino acid, along with their roles in body function and clinical uses where applicable. Amino acids are obviously most abundant in protein foods, yet all foods contain some. Animal foods such as beef, pork, lamb, chicken, turkey, eggs, milk, and cheese are known as complete proteins and usually contain all eight essential amino acids. Many vegetable proteins contain adequate levels of many of the essential amino acids, but may be low in one or two; grains and their germ coverings, legumes, nuts and seeds, and some vegetables fit into this category. The important topic of protein complementarity, that is, combining different vegetable proteins to acquire all the essential amino acids, will be discussed as will specific protein functions and requirements, following the individual amino acids.

AMINO ACIDS

Essential	*Nonessential*	*Others**
Isoleucine	Alanine	Carnitine
Leucine	Aspartic acid	Citrulline
Lysine	(Asparagine)	Gamma-aminobutyric acid
Methionine	Cysteine	(GABA)
Phenylalanine	Glutamic acid	Glutathione
Threonine	(glutamine)	(a tripeptide)
Tryptophan	Glycine	Ornithine
Valine	Homocysteine	Taurine
	Hydroxylysine	
Semiessential	Hydroxyproline	
Arginine	Proline	
Histidine	Serine	
	Tyrosine	

AMINO ACIDS COMMONLY
USED IN CLINICAL PRACTICE

Amino Acid	*Uses*
L-tryptophan	Sleep, anxiety
L-lysine	*Herpes simplex* treatment and prevention
DL-phenylalanine	Pain
L-carnitine	Weight loss, cardiovascular disease
L-arginine/L-ornithine	Bodybuilding
L-cysteine	Antioxidant, detoxifier
L-taurine	Depression, convulsions
L-glutamine	Alcohol and sugar cravings/addictions
L-tyrosine	Depression

*These are not found in body tissue structure, but contribute to human metabolism.

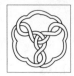

ESSENTIAL AMINO ACIDS

In the following discussion of the amino acids, these particular ones warrant a more in-depth review of their common uses, dosages, and success level in therapy. When taking any individual amino acid in the amount suggested, limit its use to six–eight weeks and then take a two- to three-week break before starting again, unless stated otherwise. This will avoid, as with B vitamin therapy, an imbalance of any amino acid, whose absorption may be inhibited by a higher intake of others. Another way to avoid a possible amino acid imbalance is to take a basic amino acid mixture that contains all the amino acids, essential and nonessential, along with the specific, appropriate ones, as demonstrated in many of the programs in Part Four of this book.

Isoleucine, available in most food sources, is particularly high in many fish and meats, in cheeses, and relatively high in wheat germ and most seeds and nuts. L-isoleucine is a branched amino acid found in high concentrations in our muscle tissues. It is used in the body to produce certain biochemical compounds that help in energy production and has been found experimentally to reduce twitching and tremors in animals. The branched-chain amino acids (BCAA)—isoleucine, leucine, and valine—have been used as supplements for body (muscle) building.

Leucine is also readily available in good concentrations in animal protein foods (poultry and red meats) and dairy products; wheat germ and oats also contain leucine. It is essential for growth, as it stimulates protein synthesis in muscle. Leucine may help stabilize or lower blood sugar, it can be metabolized to produce energy, as can isoleucine and valine, the other branched-chain amino acids during periods of fasting or starvation. A deficiency of leucine can cause a biochemical malfunction producing hypoglycemia in infants. Leucine is also helpful in healing wounds of the skin and bones.

Lysine is found in most protein food sources but is not as readily available from the grain cereals or peanuts. Lysine is particularly high in fish, meats, and dairy products and higher than most other amino acids in wheat germ, legumes, and many fruits and vegetables. Lysine has many functions. It is concentrated in muscle tissue and helps in the absorption of calcium from the intestinal tract, the promotion of bone growth, and the formation of collagen. Collagen is an important body protein that is the basic matrix of the connective tissues, skin, cartilage, and bone. Vitamin C is needed to convert lysine into hydroxylysine, which is then incorporated into collagen. Lysine is also metabolized by transaminase enzymes in the liver; its metabolism depends on vitamins B6, B3, B2, and C and on iron and glutamic acid. Dietary needs for lysine are estimated to be 750–1000 mg. daily. A deficiency may contribute to reduced growth and immunity along with an increase in urinary calcium. This latter fact suggests that adequate lysine may help prevent osteoporosis through better absorption and utilization of calcium.

Lysine has recently become popular in the prevention and treatment of *Herpes simplex* infections. Though research has been somewhat contradictory, most studies claimed good success, particularly for cold sores (herpes type 1). Nearly 80 percent of patients studied believed that taking 1–2 grams of L-lysine each day helped them reduce outbreaks and symptoms. The percentage was lower for genital herpes (type 2), a finding that my clinical experience supports. For people who seem to respond to lysine treatment, recent research suggests that an effective dose is 1500 mg. a day (usually 500 mg. three times daily) during an infection and 500 mg. daily when no symptoms are present. Please remember, though, that recurrent herpes outbreaks can be a complex problem relating to stress, weakened immunity, a diet too high in acid-forming foods, and nutritional deficiencies and that lysine therapy is not a substitute for dealing with these factors.

Another aspect of herpes infections involves the ratio of lysine to arginine in the diet. A higher lysine to arginine ratio seems to help many patients reduce the incidence of herpes outbreaks. Animal proteins provide a ratio of about 3 or 4:1, while vegetables are closer to a 1:1 ratio.

LYSINE-RICH FOODS		ARGININE-RICH FOODS
Meats	Yeast	Nuts
Milk	Beans	Chocolate
Cheese	Eggs	Grains
		Fish

Thus, in herpes prevention and treatment, avoiding arginine-rich foods and eating more lysine-rich foods may be helpful.

Interestingly, recent research has suggested that therapy using L-lysine and L-arginine (see later discussion) together is useful and possibly even better than the arginine/ornithine combination in stimulating growth hormone, muscle building, weight loss, and immune support. A dosage of 500 mg. twice daily, or 1000–1500 mg. taken before bed, of each amino acid would help in these functions.

Lysine has little or no toxicity. Not uncommonly, when one stops therapy for herpes, he or she has an outbreak. Lysine is fairly safe, although I do not believe that any amino acid should be used over a long time without a break or without supporting the diet with the other amino acids as well.

Methionine is of concern mainly because it is the limiting, or the least abundant, amino acid (see the following section on *Food, Protein, and Complementarity*) in many foods, particularly low in most legumes, soybeans, and peanuts. Though it is higher in dairy foods, eggs, fish, and meats, it is still present in lower concentration in many of these foods than are the other essential amino acids. Those eating vegetarian diets can obtain a fairly good proportion of methionine in the protein content of many nuts and seeds, as well as corn, rice, and other grains, which are naturally lower in tryptophan and lysine.

Methionine is one of the sulfur-containing amino acids (cysteine and cystine are others) and is important for many bodily functions. Through its supply of sulfur, it helps prevent problems of the skin and nails. It acts as a lipotropic agent (others are inositol and choline) to prevent excess fat buildup in the liver and the body, is helpful in relieving or preventing fatigue, and may be useful in some cases of allergy because it reduces histamine release. It also may help lower an elevated serum copper level. Methionine works as an antioxidant (free radical deactivator) through conversion to L-cysteine to help neutralize toxins. However, L-cysteine is used more often than methionine as an antioxidant because it seems to be better tolerated and has a wider range of protection.

Phenylalanine is a ringed amino acid that is readily available in most food sources, particularly meats and milk products, with lower levels found in oats and wheat germ. It is essential for many bodily functions and is one of the few amino acids that can cross the blood-brain barrier and thus directly affect brain chemistry. Phenylalanine is the precursor of the amino acid tyrosine, which cannot be reconverted, so

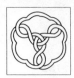

phenylalanine is essential in the diet. As a precursor of tyrosine, phenylalanine can form norepinephrine in the brain in addition to other catecholamines such as epinephrine, dopamine, and tyramine. Norepinephrine is an important neurotransmitter (that is, it conveys chemoelectric information at nerve synapses) and is apparently important for memory, alertness, and learning. Phenylalanine metabolism requires pyridoxine (B_6), niacin (B_3), vitamin C, copper, and iron. This amino acid is part of some psychoactive drugs as well as body chemicals such as acetylcholine, melanotropin, vasopressin, cholecystokinins, and the enkephalins and endorphins.

Phenylalanine has been used for treatment of depression in the D-, L-, or DL- forms, probably because it forms tyrosine, an excitatory neurotransmitter. Braverman and Pfeiffer, in *The Healing Nutrients Within*, suggest that L-phenylalanine works best in bipolar disorders (with manic and depressive states) in doses of 500 mg. twice daily up to 2–3 grams daily, along with 100 mg. of vitamin B_6 twice daily, whereas D- and DL-phenylalanine work better for affective (lack of positive attitude or emotional enthusiasm for life) depression. Phenylalanine is better absorbed than tyrosine and produces fewer headaches, so may be more useful in depression than L-tyrosine. Both DL- and D-phenylalanine are helpful pain relievers in certain musculoskeletal problems, and this is their primary use currently. Aspartame, the new nutrient sweetener, is synthesized from the combination of aspartic acid and phenylalanine. Aspartame is safe, except for pregnant women or people with phenylketonuria (PKU), a genetic problem of phenylalanine metabolism.

I have used phenylalanine in particular for patients with pain problems, most commonly back pain due to muscular or ligamentous irritation, though it may be helpful for any type of pain. It probably works for this purpose because of its function of increasing endorphins in the brain, but it is not really a treatment for the cause of the pain, such as inflammation or spasms. The endorphins are thought to give us a more positive outlook on life, to enhance alertness, and to improve vitality. (This may be a reason why phenylalanine works for depression.) Endorphins are the mysterious substances released when we exercise or when we experience positive emotions. They are also thought to make us less sensitive to or aware of pain. DL-phenylalanine blocks the enkephalinase enzymes that break down the endorphins and enkephalins, the natural pain relievers and mood elevators. However, this substance does not work all the time, nor is it a complete therapy; the underlying cause of the pain or depression should be discovered.

Some of the pain problems for which phenylalanine may be helpful are low back pain; neck pain; osteoarthritis; rheumatoid arthritis; menstrual cramps; and headaches, particularly migraines. However, patients suffering from migraines may have elevated phenylalanine levels, in which case supplementation would not help. L-tryptophan may work better in these patients.

On a trial basis, to see whether it will be helpful for pain, DL-phenylalanine can be taken in a dose of about 500–750 mg. two to three times daily. It really has no common side effects other than occasional headache or jitteriness. However, its catecholamine effect may raise blood pressure in some people, so this should be watched. Phenylalanine therapy is not recommended for long-term use; as with the other amino acids, it should not be taken for more than three weeks at a time without a break or without the support of the other amino acids.

 Threonine is somewhat low in corn and some grains, though it is not the limiting (that is, the lowest relative to making a complete protein) amino acid in these foods. There are good levels of threonine in most flesh foods, dairy foods, and eggs and moderate levels in wheat germ, many nuts, beans, and seeds, as well as some vegetables. Threonine is an important constituent in many body proteins and is necessary for the formation of tooth enamel protein, elastin, and collagen. It is found in high amounts in newborns, and requirements seem to decrease with age yet increase with stress. Threonine also has a minor role (a greater one when choline is deficient) as a lipotropic in controlling fat buildup in the liver.

Threonine has a mild glucose-sparing effect and is a precursor of amino acids glycine and serine. Threonine is one of the immune-stimulating nutrients (cysteine, lysine, alanine, and aspartic acid are others), as it promotes thymus growth and activity. A deficiency of threonine in rats has been associated with a weakened cellular response and antibody formation. One gram of threonine twice daily may also be helpful in some cases of depression.

I do not totally accept the "story" that tryptophan itself is the disease culprit for which it stands accused at the time of publication of this book; currently its use has been banned and it has been made unavailable. However, since I continue to believe that it is potentially a very useful nutritional medicine adjunct, I have elected not to delete the discussions and utilization suggestions from this text.

 Tryptophan is the lowest essential amino acid in corn, many cereal grains, and legumes. The dietary intake of tryptophan in general is lower than most other amino acids. It is not particularly high in any foods but is readily available in flesh foods, eggs, dairy products, and some nuts and seeds. It is present in the casein component of milk.

Functionally, tryptophan is very important, and it has been used effectively for a variety of medical problems. Vitamin B_6, vitamin C, folic acid, and magnesium are needed to metabolize tryptophan. It is the precursor for a vital neurotransmitter, serotonin, which influences moods and sleep, and serotonin levels are directly related to tryptophan intake. As other amino acids, such as tyrosine and phenylalanine, compete for absorption with tryptophan, tryptophan must often be taken as a supplement to increase its blood levels. It also acts differently than other amino acids, as it can exist free in the blood and can be carried by protein. In a sense tryptophan is really an essential vitamin since it is the precursor of vitamin B_3 (niacin); a deficiency of tryptophan, combined with inadequate dietary niacin, can cause the symptoms of pellagra: dermatitis, diarrhea, dementia, and death (the four D's; see the section on *Niacin* in Chapter 5, *Vitamins*). Low tryptophan levels are found in many patients with dementia and may have subclinical or subtle psychological effects.

Tryptophan has been used effectively to treat insomnia in many people. Serotonin is needed in the brain to induce and maintain sleep. Usually, 1–2 grams of L-tryptophan (the desired form) are needed to increase blood levels sufficiently to induce sleep. However, the lowest dose that works to aid sleep (often as little as 500 mg.) should be maintained. It can be repeated if the person wakes in the middle of the night. As an initial treatment, I suggest 1 gram of L-tryptophan taken 30–45 minutes before bed, which reduces the time it takes to fall asleep (sleep latency period). Some formulas contain vitamin B_6 and niacinamide, which improve tryptophan utilization. If 1 gram is insufficient, increase the dose 500 mg. each night, up to a total of 3000 mg., and add calcium, 300–600 mg., and magnesium, 200–400 mg., to your good-night supplements.

Tryptophan works better for acute insomnia than for chronic sleep problems. Patients with asthma or systemic lupus erythematosus should not take tryptophan. Generally, side effects are negligible, and tryptophan does

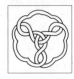

not distort sleep patterns until more than 10 grams are taken. Occasionally, some morning sluggishness may occur.

Tryptophan also has an antidepressant effect and is particularly effective in manic depression and depression associated with menopause. Many depressed patients have low levels of tryptophan. Tryptophan can be a useful and safe pain reliever. It has been shown most helpful for dental pain, headaches (migraines in particular), and cancer pain, often in conjunction with aspirin or acetaminophen. Tryptophan appears to increase the pain threshold. It may help treat anorexia by increasing the appetite. Since it is the precursor of niacin, tryptophan supplementation may help to lower cholesterol and blood fat levels. Other possible uses for L-tryptophan include parkinsonism, epilepsy, and schizophrenia, and with further research, we may find this important amino acid may provide help in other medical conditions.

 Valine is found in substantial quantities in most foods and is an essential part of many proteins. Other functions of valine are not really known, though it is thought to be somewhat helpful in treating addictions. A deficiency may affect the myelin covering of nerves. Valine can be metabolized to produce energy, which spares glucose. Like leucine and isoleucine, valine is a branched-chain amino acid with similar metabolic pathways. A potentially deadly hereditary disease, commonly called the "maple syrup urine disease," blocks the metabolism of these three amino acids. In children affected with this disease, keto acids are dumped into the urine, making it smell like maple syrup. The amino acid deficiencies that result cause problems with the nervous system, seizures, and a failure to thrive. Valine supplementation may be helpful in muscle building (along with isoleucine and leucine) and in liver and gallbladder disease.

SEMIESSENTIAL AMINO ACIDS

 Arginine is usually synthesized by adults in amounts sufficient to maintain the body proteins, but additional dietary arginine is needed during periods of growth, as in childhood or during pregnancy, and possibly during times of stress. Arginine is present in most proteins, including meats, nuts, milk, cheese, and eggs. In particular, nuts, grains, and chocolate have a high arginine to lysine ratio. These foods have been noted to increase the frequency of *Herpes simplex* attacks (both cold sores and genital lesions) in patients infected with this virus. (Eating foods high in lysine, L-lysine supplementation, or both, may help treat such outbreaks; see the section on *Lysine*.) Arginine deficiencies can exist in human beings and may occur during times of high protein demand; with trauma, low protein intake, or malnutrition; or from excess lysine intake, which may compete with arginine. Arginine deficiency can result in hair loss, constipation, a delay in the healing of wounds, and liver disease.

Arginine has several important functions. It is essential to the metabolism of ammonia that is generated from protein breakdown. It is also needed to transport the nitrogen used in muscle metabolism. Arginine is one of the body-building amino acids and also influences several hormone functions. L-arginine has been shown to stimulate the pituitary gland to produce and secrete human growth hormone in young males, at a dose of more than 3 grams daily. Human growth hormone helps in muscle building, leading to increased muscle strength and tone, and enhances fat metabolism (increases the burning of fats), which may help with weight loss. Growth hormone in general seems to increase metabolism and energy. L-arginine has a positive effect on the immune system, mainly by stimulating thymus activity, and also helps the body heal from wounds. Some research has shown that high doses of L-arginine may increase male fertility by increasing sperm production and motility.

L-arginine has several possible uses. The most common use, in part promoted by Pearson and Shaw's book *Life Extension*, is as a growth hormone stimulant. Body builders supplement L-arginine along with L-ornithine for its muscle-building effects. Recent research has suggested that L-arginine and L-lysine together have a similar effect, possibly at lower dosages. L-arginine supplementation, at a dosage of 4 grams daily, has been successful in improving fertility in men by increasing low sperm count and motility. Arginine has been shown to help speed wound healing in rats, possibly as an aid to collagen formation. Other possible uses for L-arginine as seen in animals are to improve decreased liver functions, to lower cholesterol levels, and to inhibit the growth of certain tumors (it may also stimulate the growth of certain tumors).

L-arginine, available in 500 mg. capsules, is usually well tolerated in doses as high as 3–6 grams, although side effects such as diarrhea, nausea, and, rarely, ataxia (unsteadiness) may occur in some people. Dosages of less than 2 grams daily are usually handled without problems. A dosage of 3–4 grams daily is needed for the growth hormone effect. L-arginine and L-ornithine, or L-arginine and L-lysine, can be supplemented at 500–1000 mg. of each twice daily, or 1000 to 1500 mg. of each before bed. To improve male fertility, a dosage of 2 grams twice daily is suggested. Children and teenagers should avoid supplementation of L-arginine for growth stimulation or body building. People with diabetes must be careful because of arginine's effect on insulin and carbohydrate metabolism. Supplementation should not be done continuously for a long period. I suggest that it be used for two to three weeks, followed by a break of one to two weeks. A balanced amino acid supplement can also be used.

 Histidine must also be obtained from diet during childhood and growth periods. It may be needed in malnourished or injured individuals, or whenever there is need for tissue formation or repair. Histidine is found in most animal and vegetable proteins, particularly pork, poultry, cheese, and wheat germ. Histidine is involved in a wide range of metabolic processes involving blood cell production (it is present in hemoglobin) and in the production of histamine, which is involved in many allergic and inflammatory reactions. Histidine has been used supplementally in the treatment of allergic disorders, peptic ulcers, anemia, and cardiovascular disease, as it has a hypotensive effect (that is, it lowers blood pressure) through the autonomic nervous system. Some cases of arthritis have improved with a supplemented dosage of 1000–1500 mg. taken three times daily. Histidine also acts as a metal chelating agent—that is, it can bind itself to metals— and can be given bound to minerals such as zinc or copper to improve their absorption.

NONESSENTIAL AMINO ACIDS

These are the amino acids that our bodies normally make and that are found in body proteins. (There are other important amino acids that are not found in proteins, which include carnitine, citrulline, taurine, and ornithine.) Nonessential amino acids are supposedly not needed in our diet; each one can be manufactured by the body. However, it is very possible that some people, because of metabolic deficiencies in their biochemical systems (which could also be based on dietary nutrient intake), may have low production levels of certain amino acids. In that case, the particular functions usually performed by them will not be fulfilled. Let us explore some of the functions and possible supplementary uses of these nonessential amino acids.

Alanine is an important part of human muscle tissue and is found readily in protein foods, including beef, pork, turkey, and cheese as well as wheat germ, oats, yogurt, and avocado. Glucose can be made from alanine in the liver or muscles when energy is needed, and thus it may help maintain the blood sugar level. Alanine deficiency has been seen in hypoglycemia, and alanine supplementation may be helpful in treating this condition. Alanine stimulates lymphocyte production and may help people who have immune suppression. It is also an inhibitory neurotransmitter in the brain and may decrease excitation, such as that found in epilepsy. Alanine is a big part of the cell walls of many bacteria, including *Streptococcus faecium*, a normal intestinal bacterium. Beta-alanine, a variant of natural L-alanine, is not a constituent of proteins but is part of pantothenic acid, vitamin B_5.

Aspartic acid, readily available in protein foods, is very active in many body processes, including the formation of ammonia and urea and their disposal from the body. It is found in high levels throughout the human body, especially in the brain, where it performs an excitatory function. Aspartic acid has been found in increased levels in people with epilepsy and in decreased amounts in some cases of depression. Aspartic acid also can help form the ribonucleotides that assist production of DNA and RNA and aids energy production from carbohydrate metabolism. Aspartic acid can help protect the liver from some drug toxicity and the body from radiation; it may also increase resistance to fatigue. Aspartic acid is employed to form mineral salts, such as potassium, calcium, or magnesium aspartate. Since aspartates are easily absorbed, they can actively transport these minerals across the intestinal lining into the blood and cells where they can be used for their particular functions, such as energy production or bone metabolism. Asparagine, formed from aspartic acid, aids the metabolic function of the cells of the brain and nervous system by releasing energy as it reverts back to aspartic acid.

Clinically, aspartic acid may be used to treat fatigue or depression. Its effect on the thymus gland lets it be used as a mild immunostimulant. A current popular use is in the sweetener, aspartame (see Chapter 11, *Environmental Aspects of Nutrition*), which is a combination of aspartic acid and phenylalanine. Aspartic acid is basically nontoxic.

Cysteine and Cystine are sulfur-containing amino acids that are synthesized in the liver and are involved in multiple metabolic pathways. Cysteine is formed from homocysteine, which comes from the essential amino acid methionine. Cysteine can be converted to cystine and taurine. Cystine itself is a disulfide, containing two cysteine molecules. Cysteine is contained in a variety of foods and is found mainly as cystine in poultry, yogurt, oats, and wheat germ, or in the sulfur foods that contain methionine and cysteine, such as egg yolks, red peppers, garlic, onions, broccoli, and brussels sprouts.

In recent years, findings about cysteine and its many functions in the body have been exciting. It can be used to help treat a variety of problems. Cysteine can form glutathione (along with glutamic acid and glycine), a powerful antioxidant and detoxifier that functions in many enzyme systems. Glutathione is a cofactor in many important enzymes that help protect us from the harm of heavy metals, chemicals, and smoke. Cysteine is becoming even more important as a useful antioxidant-detoxifier-protector with the increasing pollution and toxicity of this industrial age. A cell membrane stabilizer, it may reduce the hazards of smoking and alcohol consumption. It specifically helps neutralize the aldehydes produced by the liver as a by-product of the metabolism of alcohol, fats, air pollutants, and some drugs. It may also be helpful in this regard by minimizing free-radical effects, which also contribute to a variety of degenerative processes. Cysteine in sufficient levels will bind with metals—preferentially, the heavy metals lead, mercury, and cadmium bond most strongly—thus, cysteine aids the body's elimination of them. It helps promote tissue healing after surgery or burns, and it also may stimulate white blood cell activity to help in disease resistance and provide protection from mutagenesis of cells and the carcinogenic process, though further research is needed in these areas.

POSSIBLE USES OF L-CYSTEINE

Smokers*
Smoker's cough/bronchitis
Air pollution
Exposure to chemicals
Psoriasis (aids skin healing)
Surgery or injury (aids wound healing)
Hair loss
Infection (immune support, detoxifier)
Rheumatoid arthritis
Cataract (best in prevention)
Cancer prevention and treatment
　　(decreases toxicity of offending agents)
Mental illness
Asthma
Metal toxicity or exposure (lead,
　　mercury, cadmium)

---

* Protects alveoli from smoke damage, along with beta carotene, zinc, and selenium.

The overall idea, then, is that L-cysteine is one of the antiaging nutrients, as aging is thought to be due mainly to oxidation and free-radical damage. It may be helpful in actually increasing our life span and can be beneficial in those inflammatory problems caused by free radicals, such as arthritis and vascular irritation. L-cysteine also forms another amino acid, L-cystine, which is important in hair and nail tissues.

L-cysteine supplementation will be discussed in the specific programs in Part Four of this book. Basically it is used in amounts commonly ranging from 250–750 mg. daily, often taken in several portions throughout the day along with three times the vitamin C to prevent crystallization of excess cystine.

 Glutamic acid (glutamate) is simply converted to glutamine and is synthesized from arginine, ornithine, and proline. It is abundant in both animal and vegetable proteins and is found in high concentrations in the human brain. Glutamic acid, which is important to brain function, is the only amino acid metabolized in the brain. The conversion of glutamic acid to glutamine helps clear potentially toxic ammonia. Glutamic acid, with the help of vitamin B_6 and manganese, is also a precursor of GABA (gamma-aminobutyric acid), an important neurotransmitter in the central nervous system. Glutamic acid helps transport potassium into the spinal fluid and is itself an excitatory neurotransmitter. (GABA, however, is inhibitory.) Glutamic acid thus has been used in the treatment of fatigue, parkinsonism, schizophrenia, mental retardation, muscular dystrophy, and alcoholism. Supplemented as L-glutamine, it penetrates the blood-brain barrier and can be used as a brain fuel. Research has shown that L-glutamine, in a dose of 500 mg. four times daily, decreases the craving for alcohol. This amino acid is now commonly used in alcoholism clinics. L-glutamine also seems to reduce the craving for sugar and carbohydrates and so may be helpful for some people in dealing with obesity or sugar abuse. It may also help in the healing of ulcers.

Monosodium Glutamate (MSG) is a single sodium salt of glutamic acid. This seaweed

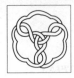

extract, now commonly produced chemically, may suggest the possible toxicity of glutamic acid as slightly neurologically irritating in high dosages. Some people seem to be particularly sensitive to glutamine and MSG. Otherwise, glutamine is relatively safe and is the best way to supplement this amino acid.

GABA itself has been used in the treatment of epilepsy, high blood pressure, and anxiety, as it helps in relaxation. GABA may also enhance the sex drive and reduce nighttime urination.

Glycine can be formed from choline in the liver or kidney and from the amino acids threonine and serine. It can be converted back to serine in the fasting state. Glycine is one of the few amino acids that helps spare glucose for energy by improving glycogen storage. It is important in brain metabolism, where it has a calming effect. Glycine is a simple amino acid needed for the synthesis of the hemoglobin molecule, collagen, and glutathione. It can also be converted to creatine, which is utilized to make DNA and RNA. Glycine is useful in healing wounds (orally or in a cream) and treating manic psychological states or problems of muscle spasticity. When the blood fats or uric acid levels are high, it helps to clear or utilize these substances. Glycine may also be helpful in reducing gastric acidity; in higher doses, 4–8 grams, it stimulates growth hormone release; and it is also used as a mild sweetener in foods or drugs.

Dimethylglycine (DMG) is a popular substance in today's nutritional products. It will also be discussed as a corollary for vitamin B_{15}, pangamic acid. DMG is an intermediary of cell metabolism, mainly from glycine and choline. As a precursor also to glycine, some of DMG's effects may be attributed to simple glycine, particularly in regard to its neuroinhibitory effect in problems such as epilepsy. DMG seems to be able to increase the immune antibody response and improve physical energy and has been used in the treatment of infections, immune suppression, fatigue, and poor endurance. Some people experience good results; others do not. More research is needed to properly understand dimethylglycine's role in clinical medicine.

Homocysteine is an intermediary metabolite of the amino acid methionine. Homocystine is a double molecule of homocysteine. These amino acids are known mostly for their use in genetic enzyme problems that cause a buildup of homocystine. The disease called homocystinuria can cause problems of the vascular system (advanced atherosclerosis), eyes, central nervous system, and also can create kidney stones. Excessive levels of these amino acids may also contribute to mental retardation or psychosis and have been implicated in speeding up the atherosclerotic process. Nutrients like B_6 (important in many amino acid conversions), B_{12}, folic acid, and cystine may reduce some of the problems of homocysteine genetic deficits.

Hydroxylysine is closely related to lysine and is important in the formation of collagen. It is also found in gelatin and in the digestive enzymes trypsin and chymotrypsin.

Hydroxyproline is an important component of collagen, which makes up the white, fibrous connective tissue and is part of the skin, bones, and cartilage. Hydroxyproline is converted from proline by hydroxylation only after proline gets into the amino acid chains that form body proteins.

Proline is one of the main amino acids of collagen and is also helpful to bone, skin, and cartilage formation. Proline can be formed from glutamine or the amino acid ornithine. In foods, it is found readily in dairy products and eggs, with some found in meats or wheat germ. Proline is helpful in maintaining joints and tendons, in tissue repair after injury, or for any type of wound healing.

Serine can be made in the tissue from glycine (or threonine) so it is nonessential, but its production requires adequate amounts of B_3, B_6, and folic acid. Serine is a constituent of brain proteins, including nerve coverings. It is also important in metabolism of purines and pyrimidines (part of the nucleic acids RNA and DNA), in the formation of cell membranes, and in creatine (part of muscle) synthesis. Serine has also been used as a natural moisturizer in skin creams. Serine is readily found in meats and dairy products, wheat gluten, peanuts, and soy products, many foods that can cause allergy. There is some concern that elevated serine levels (especially in sausage and lunch meats) can cause immune suppression and psychological symptoms, such as is seen in cerebral allergies.

Tyrosine is easily made in the body from phenylalanine and is very important to general metabolism, as it is a direct precursor of both adrenaline (as well as norepinephrine and dopamine) and thyroid hormones, all stimulants to metabolism and the nervous system. Folic acid, niacin, vitamin C, and copper are needed to support tyrosine metabolism into these and other important substances, which also include melanin, estrogen molecules, and the enkephalins (natural pain relievers). Tyrosine may stimulate growth hormone and can act as a mild appetite suppressant. It may also be useful in the control of anxiety or depression. Tyrosine is known as the "antidepressant" amino acid. It has a mild antioxidant effect, binding up free radicals (unstable molecules) that can cause damage to the cells and tissues, and is useful in smokers, people with stressful lives, or those exposed to chemicals and radiation. L-tyrosine has also been used, usually in a dose of 1–2 grams a day, for low sex drive, Parkinson's disease, and in programs for drug problems or weight loss. As an antidepressant,

500–1000 mg. of L-tyrosine can be taken two or three times during the day. Since tyrosine has a more stimulating antidepressant effect, taking 1000 to 1500 mg. of L-tryptophan (which is more tranquilizing) at night for sleep may be a good therapeutic combination to help in mild to moderate depression.

AMINO ACIDS
NOT FOUND IN BODY PROTEINS

Many other amino acids are found in nature and in food that, though not building blocks of human protein tissue, can be important and helpful in metabolic functions. Some of these amino acids are very similar to or are by-products of the previously discussed amino acids, such as asparagine (a variant of aspartic acid) or ornithine (available from arginine); others are separate in structure and functions. Some common ones are discussed here.

Carnitine has only recently been noted as an important amino acid (the L- form only) essential to our health. It is found in the diet and can also be made by the body, mainly in the liver and kidneys, from lysine with the help of vitamin C, pyridoxine, niacin, iron, and methionine. Among our foods, carnitine is found mainly in the red meats (thus, the name) with some found in fish, poultry, and milk products and less in tempeh (fermented soybeans), wheat, and avocados. Carnitine is stored primarily in the skeletal muscles and heart, where it is needed to transform fatty acids into energy for muscular activity. It is also concentrated in sperm and in the brain. Carnitine is utilized to transport fatty acids into the cell and across the mitochondrial membranes into our cellular energy factories, the mitochondria. It also increases the rate at which the liver oxidizes (uses) fats, an energy-generating process.

L-carnitine is the active form and can be taken as a safe supplement with positive benefits. With carnitine's effect on fatty acids and

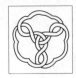
POSSIBLE USES OF L-CARNITINE

Ischemic heart disease
Angina pectoris
Cardiac arrhythmias
Elevated cholesterol and/or triglyceride
  levels
Low HDL cholesterol
Atherosclerosis
Muscle weakness
Muscle diseases
General fatigue
Overweight
Poor endurance
Immune suppression
Alcohol abuse
Pregnancy
Hypothroidism
Male infertility

energy production, especially in the heart and muscles, it is now known as a nutrient that protects us from cardiovascular disease. It has been shown to reduce blood triglycerides and cholesterol levels by increasing fat utilization; at the same time, carnitine can raise the HDL portion of the cholesterol, which reduces cardiovascular disease risk. L-carnitine also helps with weight loss, usually improves our exercise capacities (possibly through the oxidation of amino acids), and may possibly enhance our muscle building and endurance. These latter two aspects may be a result of the weight loss and better exercise. Many athletes have noted improved endurance with L-carnitine supplementation. In some studies, L-carnitine has been shown to improve the symptoms of angina, reducing pain and allowing more activity. It also may lessen the risk of fatty deposits in the liver associated with alcohol abuse.

Deficiencies of carnitine have been noted, more so recently with people avoiding red meats in the diet. These occur most often in vegetarians and during pregnancy or lactation. Vegetarians, though, often have low-fat diets and otherwise reduced cardiovascular disease risk. Deficiencies may increase symptoms of fatigue, angina, muscle weakness, or confusion. More research is needed to clarify and verify these deficiency states, as well as to establish whether the metabolic benefits of L-carnitine are clearly separate from correcting that deficiency.

The dosage of L-carnitine (not D- or DL-carnitine) suggested to improve fat metabolism and muscular performance is 1000–2000 mg. daily, usually divided into two doses. This is basically safe and can be taken over an extended period, although it probably should be stopped for one week each month, until its long-term safety as a supplement is more clearly established. The *Physician's Desk Reference* has recommended L-carnitine in the treatment of ischemic heart disease and hyperlipid states (specifically, Type IV hyperlipidemia) in a dosage of 600–1200 mg. three times daily. Carnitine is not recommended in people with active liver or kidney disease or with diabetes. However, it is definitely recommended for persons with heart problems such as ischemia or arrhythmia or with increased cardiovascular risk, such as high blood fats, and for problems with poor endurance, muscle weakness, or obesity. I am excited about the uses of L-carnitine and look forward to more positive research in the future.

Citrulline can be made in the body from ornithine by the addition of carbon dioxide and ammonia, and can also be converted in the body to arginine. Citrulline promotes the detoxification of ammonia (nitrogen) in the blood and is sometimes helpful in problems of fatigue. It is also thought to stimulate the immune defense system.

GABA is gamma-aminobutyric acid, an inhibitory neurotransmitter formed from glutamine. It is discussed under *Glutamic Acid*.

Glutathione (GTH) is actually a tripeptide composed of three amino acids—cysteine, glutamic acid, and glycine. Cysteine is the important amino acid here; it controls the amount of glutathione made in the liver and gives GTH its metabolic power as an antioxidant and detoxifier. Since GTH is not easily available or usable by its oral administration (it breaks down into the individual amino acids), L-cysteine is usually supplemented to enhance glutathione production by the liver. Since methionine can be converted to cysteine, it may also be helpful.

 Glutathione and the enzymes that it forms, such as GTH peroxidase, are essential to life and are present in all cells of both plants and animals. In humans, GTH is found in all tissues, with the highest levels found in the liver, lenses of the eyes, spleen, pancreas, and kidneys. It is a key protector from the potential damage by wastes and toxins and is effective in preventing aging. GTH functions as a:

Reducing agent—protects against oxidation.

Antioxidant (actually an antitoxin as part of an enzyme system that helps protect against environmental and metabolic toxins)—protects against peroxidation. Lipid peroxides alter unsaturated lipids in cell membranes. Peroxides are also potent free radicals. (Like hydrogen peroxide, H_2O_2, peroxides release oxygen, which can destroy bacteria and parasites, as well as our own cells if they are not protected by all of the nutritional antioxidants.) Some chemicals that increase peroxidation include pesticides, plastics, benzene, and carbon tetrachloride. Glutathione protects against these as well as heavy metals, cigarette smoke, smog, carbon monoxide from cars, drugs, solvents, dyes, phenols, and nitrates. GTH transferase helps to detoxify these chemicals into less toxic forms. It is possible that future uses will allow us to use some form of glutathione to clean up our environment.

An immune helper—GTH helps get nutrients and amino acids to the lymphocytes and phagocytes, thus helping cells combat immunity.

Aids integrity of red blood cells—and really the protection of all cells and membranes.

USES OF GLUTATHIONE (AS L-CYSTEINE)

Antioxidant
Cigarette smoke
Radiation exposure
Metal toxicity
Chemical exposure
Drug use
Alcoholism
Diabetes
Cataracts
Stroke and brain injury
Ulcers
Skin problems
Cancer

Glutathione's main uses are to combat all types of pollution and many irritated body states, often those generated by chemical use. As I said, due to cost and actual usability, GTH itself is not usually taken as a supplement (though available as such) but is obtained from L-cysteine or L-methionine (not the D- forms). Since L-cysteine is handled better and is a more direct precursor of GTH, it is supplemented in amounts of 500 mg. daily (250 mg. twice daily) up to 2–3 grams daily. Vitamin C is usually recommended by many authors in doses at least three times that of L-cysteine to facilitate the function of L-cysteine. In general, patients should not take more than 1 gram daily of L-cysteine without being monitored by a physician. Though not all the research is supportive of this method of generating glutathione, apparently it is currently the best way to increase glutathione

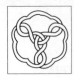
levels in the body. Up to 200–300 mcg. daily of extra selenium is also given for its antioxidant support, usually along with vitamin E, but not with vitamin C. Vitamin C may increase the conversion of selenite, a common form of supplemental selenium, to its more toxic form, elemental selenium.

 Ornithine can be made from arginine, and it in turn can proceed to form glutamic acid, citrulline, and arginine and further to proline and hydroxyproline. With arginine, ornithine is useful in nitrogen (ammonia) metabolism. It has been described as a stimulant for growth hormone release and is thought to help build the immune system, promote wound healing, and support liver regeneration. People who are poorly nourished or who lack protein in their diet may be deficient. Ornithine is usually supplemented along with arginine, as they have similar actions. The most common use is in body builders as a growth hormone stimulant. A dose of 1500–2500 mg. twice daily is required for this type of effect. Side effects might include insomnia.

 Taurine, a lesser known amino acid, is not part of our muscle protein yet is important in metabolism, especially in the brain. It is essential in newborns, as they cannot make it. Adults can produce sulfur-containing taurine from cysteine with the help of pyridoxine, B_6. It is possible that if not enough taurine is made in the body, especially if cysteine or B_6 is deficient, it might be further required in the diet. In foods, it is high in meats and fish proteins.

Taurine functions in electrically active tissues such as the brain and heart to help stabilize cell membranes. It also has functions in the gallbladder, eyes, and blood vessels and appears to have some antioxidant and detoxifying activity. Taurine aids the movement of potassium, sodium, calcium, and magnesium in and out of cells and thus helps generate nerve impulses. Zinc seems to support this effect of taurine. Taurine is found in the central nervous system, skeletal muscle, and heart; it is very concentrated in the brain and high in the heart tissues.

Taurine is an inhibitory neurotransmitter, and its main use has been to help treat epilepsy and other excitable brain states, where it functions as a mild sedative. Research shows low taurine levels at seizure sites and its anticonvulsant effect comes from its ability to stabilize nerve cell membranes, which prevents the erratic firing of nerve cells. Doses for this effect are 500 mg. three times daily.

The cardiovascular dosage of taurine is higher. In Japan, taurine therapy is used in the treatment of ischemic heart disease with supplements of 5–6 grams daily in three divided doses. Low taurine and magnesium levels were found in patients after heart attacks. Taurine has potential in the treatment of arrhythmias, especially arrhythmias secondary to ischemia. People with congestive heart failure have also responded to a dosage of 2 grams three times daily with improved cardiac and respiratory function. Other possible cardiovascular uses of taurine include hypertension, possibly related to effects in the renin-angiotensin system of the kidneys, and in patients with high cholesterol levels. Taurine helps gallbladder function by forming tauracholate from bile acids; tauracholate helps increase cholesterol elimination in the bile.

Other possible uses for taurine include immune suppression (by sparing L-cysteine), visual problems and eye disease, cirrhosis and liver failure, depression, male infertility due to low sperm motility, and as a supplement for newborns and new mothers. Overall, the dosage used may range from 500 mg. to 5–6 grams, with the higher amounts needed for the cardiovascular problems and possibly epilepsy. Possible symptoms of toxicity from taurine supplementation include diarrhea and peptic ulcers.

○ FOOD, PROTEIN, AND COMPLEMENTARITY

The importance of balancing the diet so as to get sufficient levels of all the essential amino acids cannot be overstated. It is essential to health. This is why a diet containing a variety of wholesome foods is important. Certain foods have one or two amino acids that are in lower proportions than the others, and if one of these foods, such as rice or corn, is a predominant part of the diet, it can mean that protein production and the significant functions that protein performs can be deficient.

Each food has a different mix of amino acids. Therefore, it is important to have an understanding of protein composition and to apply it to our diet. The meat foods (including fish and poultry), dairy foods, and eggs almost all have sufficient quantities of amino acids to sustain life; that is, they are complete proteins. When we eat these foods daily, we do not really need to worry about amino acid complementarity; in fact, there are concerns that overconsumption of protein foods (particularly meat and milk) in many societies contributes to some major illnesses, so we may not wish to consume these foods daily, or at all.

Vegetarians or other people on diets that limit certain foods may need to be more knowledgeable about combining food. Lacto-ovo-vegetarians, who eat eggs and dairy foods—both complete proteins—need have less concern than the pure vegetarian, or vegan. Of the essential amino acids, we have seen that lysine, methionine, and tryptophan are the deficient. They are present in all vegetable proteins, but at lower levels than other amino acids. Since they are not all low in the same foods, it is not as difficult as many think to obtain a good protein balance from vegetables, grains, nuts, and legumes. The simplest idea is to eat grains with some beans or seeds, for example, millet and aduki beans or brown rice and sunflower seeds. Other complete-protein combinations of vegetable sources include soybeans and rice or soybeans with sesame, corn, wheat, or rye; peanuts with grain or coconut; grain with legumes or leafy greens; beans and corn or rice (South American diet); and peas and wheat. *The Nutrition Almanac*, written by Nutrition Research, Inc. (McGraw-Hill, 1984) has a food-by-food breakdown of amino acid content that is very helpful in creating a diet to achieve proper protein intake.

The body will make protein only as long as it has sufficient levels of all necessary amino acids in the cellular "storage" pool. When one amino acid is deficient, we will not be able to produce most proteins, and then either muscle protein will be catabolized to obtain adequate amounts of the needed amino acid(s) or the metabolism will use protein for energy. The body breaks down an average of about 300 mg. (maybe much more under many stressful conditions) of protein per day, which it replaces if there are sufficient nutrients. If there are not, however, we experience net protein loss; thus the importance of consuming all the amino acids through a daily intake of 50–60 grams of "balanced" protein in forms that are easily digested and assimilated.

Protein foods have been classified according to their ability to be digested and used

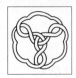

by the body; that is, their biological availability, or value. The measurement of this ability is termed net protein utilization (NPU); it is also called biological value (BV). Chicken eggs are considered to have the protein (ovalbumin) of highest known NPU. Following eggs, in descending order, are fish, cow's milk and cheese, brown rice, red meat, and poultry (Garrison and Somer, *Nutrition Desk Reference*, Keats Publishing, 1985). Again, this is not based on protein content but on biological value, how efficiently the body utilizes the protein in the food. Clearly, the amino acids in brown rice do not make it as complete a protein as the others, though the protein in it is readily usable. Here is where the vegetarian complementing with legumes may help as long as digestion and assimilation are functioning properly. (See more about protein complementarity in Chapter 9, *Diets*, in the discussion of *Lacto-ovo-vegetarian*.)

○ DIGESTION AND METABOLISM

Proteins are first broken down in the stomach by hydrochloric acid, *pepsin*, and *proteases* into peptides (amino acid chains) by splitting peptide bonds between the amino acid protein chains. In the first part of the small intestine, the duodenum, the pancreatic enzyme *trypsin* continues the conversion of the polypeptides into dipeptides (two amino acids) and tripeptides (three amino acids). Farther along the small intestine, amino *peptidases*, including *dipeptidases*, reduce the proteins to single amino acids. These individual amino acid molecules are then absorbed into the bloodstream through the intestinal wall and carried to the liver through the portal vein circulation.

The liver is the main site and regulator of amino acid metabolism, which may also take place throughout the body. Proteins are made and broken down daily. About 60–70 percent of amino acids available in the body are recycled from old tissue proteins. These recycled amino acids are called endogenous amino acids; new ones from the diet are termed exogenous. Each cell has the capability of building its needed proteins from either or both sources of amino acids.

Protein synthesis is a fairly complex though well-documented process that is described in detail in most biochemistry texts. DNA (deoxyribonucleic acid) controls and guides protein formation with the assistance of RNA (ribonucleic acid) through a duplication and replication process. Each protein has a specific sequence of amino acids used in the genetic code in our DNA.

Most of the amino acids, probably three-fourths, are used to form body proteins such as enzymes, hormones, antibodies, and the tissue proteins such as muscle. Some amino acids are metabolized into other tissue substances, such as melanin (pigmentation hormone), epinephrine, creatine, niacin, choline, and so on. Most often, protein is synthesized at the site in which it is to be used. Every day, protein is made (this process is called anabolism) and broken down (this is called catabolism). This daily process determines the nitrogen (found only in proteins, not fats or carbohydrates) balance of the body. With an increase in protein intake, the body will have a positive nitrogen balance and growth can occur. If we have deficient protein intake, the body will have a negative nitrogen balance. Most of our lives we want to have a neutral nitrogen balance. The average healthy adult synthesizes about 250–350 grams (this number may also be much higher) of protein daily. Depending on protein and amino acid intake, our activity, and protein utilization, we can move into positive or negative nitrogen balance and either build more protein or lose some, which influences body weight, shape, and tone. Excess protein can be turned into fat and stored in the body as potential fuel or as glycogen in the liver. A protein deficiency can cause weight loss and a wide variety of functional problems.

METABOLISM OF PROTEINS—FROM INGESTION TO THE LIVER

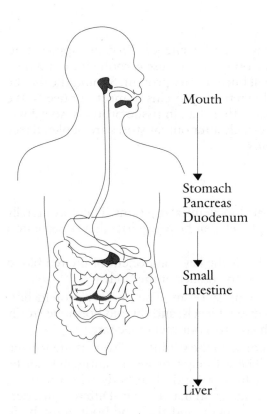

Mouth

Stomach
Pancreas
Duodenum

Small
Intestine

Liver

PROTEIN INTAKE
(long amino acid chains)

Hydrochloric Acid, Pepsin and *Proteases* (enzymes) split peptide bonds between amino acid chains —turning them into long chain polypeptides.

Pancreatic enzyme *Trypsin* turns long chain polypeptides into shorter chain polypeptides, tripeptides (3 amino acids) and dipeptides (2 amino acids).

Amino Peptidases and Dipeptidases turn polypeptides, tripeptides and dipeptides into single amino acids, which are actively transported through the wall of the intestines into the bloodstream and then via the portal vein to the LIVER, the principal site of PROTEIN metabolism.

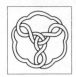

○ PROTEIN FUNCTIONS

Growth and Maintenance

We must have a constant supply of amino acids to build the proteins that create our body tissues. This is especially true in fetal formation during pregnancy and in growing children, but we are constantly rebuilding new tissue throughout our lives as well. Hair and nails are growing, and all cells in the body become worn out and need replacement, requiring amino acids. Red blood cells last about a month, as do skin cells, while cells that line our intestinal tract are replaced almost twice weekly. During times of healing, during illness, and after surgery, injuries, burns, or blood loss, we require more protein production to assist in bringing back the body's strength through regeneration of cells and tissues.

Energy

The body's main priority is satisfying the need for energy. Protein supplies four calories per gram, as does carbohydrate. The body will first use carbohydrate and then fats for energy; if these sources are low, it will burn dietary protein. Should the diet be deficient in energy sources, we will break down tissue proteins to meet our needs. We do not store extra amino acids (as we do fat) other than in tissue proteins, so we will destroy body protein when fuel is needed, usually after our fat stores are depleted (see the upcoming section, *Protein Requirements*).

Building Important Substances

Enzymes are protein catalysts that stimulate biochemical reactions. There are literally thousands of different enzymes within a single cell that help join together or separate a wide variety of substances.

Hemoglobin, an iron-bearing protein that is the key component of the red blood cell, is the molecule that carries the oxygen to the tissues of the body.

Hormones have a dynamic effect on our metabolism. The primary protein hormones are insulin, which regulates our blood sugar levels, and thyroid hormone (really an amino acid, tyrosine with iodine), which controls our metabolic rate.

Antibodies are proteins formed as a response to the stimulus of something foreign (usually a protein) that enters the body. These foreign proteins (antigens) can be bacteria, viruses, fungi, pollens, or protein from a food. The body will produce a specific antibody to bind with the foreign antigen and inactivate it. Different invaders require different proteins that are specific for them, and thus the body must be in constant surveillance and preparedness for production of new antibodies. Proteins are a big part of our immunity.

The immune response is the basis for using immunizations to create immunity to disease through recognition and response to an antigen. Giving a small dose of the disease-causing antigen allows the body to produce the antibody. Our immune system has near-perfect memory, so once we produce an antibody, it will always be available. Should we be contaminated with a polio or tetanus germ after being immunized, we would rapidly produce the antibody to deactivate the germs and not be infected. Thus, we must always have our protein-making capacities available.

This immune response, so important for maintaining health, can also cause problems, as when we react to tissue transplants or blood transfusions. Antibody responses to antigens can be the basis for some allergic reactions. We can also misguidedly make antibodies to our own tissues, a process called autoimmunity, which may lead to a number of serious and/or difficult-to-treat problems.

Fluid and Salt Balance

Proteins inside cells help keep the correct amount of water in the cells. Most proteins do not move in and out of cells, as can water, and large protein molecules attract water. The proteins in plasma help maintain the blood volume as well. When overall protein concentrations are low, we can get fluid imbalances. Proteins also help maintain the normal sodium and potassium balance, which is essential to life. Sodium is concentrated outside the cells, while potassium is mainly inside, a situation necessary for normal muscle and nerve cell function. Proteins push sodium out of the cell and potassium into it, thus aiding the heart, lungs, and nervous system to function optimally.

Acid-Alkaline Balance

Proteins can help normalize the acid-base balance by acting as buffers. The body constantly produces acids and bases from chemical reactions. Proteins help in the elimination of excess hydrogen ions, which are part of acids. In this way, the pH, the acid-base balance of the blood, is kept near constant at about 7.4.

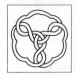

○ PROTEIN REQUIREMENTS

There are definitely specific requirements for proteins, though the exact amount is somewhat questionable. The Recommended Daily Allowance (RDA) of protein according to U.S. government standards is 0.8 gram per kilogram (1 kilogram equals 2.2 pounds) of ideal body weight for the adult. Ideal body weight is used in the calculation because amino acids are not needed by fat cells, only by the lean body mass. So an adult male who should weigh about 154 pounds, or 70 kilograms, requires 56 grams of protein daily. A female whose best weight is 110 pounds, or 50 kilograms, needs 40 grams a day. The RDA increases by 30 grams per day during pregnancy and 20 grams per day during lactation. During growth, different amounts are needed. For example, 2.2 grams of protein are needed per kilogram of body weight each day in the first six months of life, and 2.0 grams per kilogram for the next six months.

DAILY PROTEIN REQUIREMENTS

Age	RDA*
0–6 months	2.2
6 months–1 year	2.0
1–3 years	1.8
4–6 years	1.5
7–10 years	1.2
11–14 years	1.0
15–18 years	0.9
19 years and older	0.8

*(in grams per kilogram [2.2 pounds] of body weight)

These requirements are based on maintaining a positive nitrogen balance in children and an even to positive nitrogen balance in adults. Protein is the nitrogen-containing nutrient. As it is broken down for excretion, it must be replaced by dietary nitrogen so protein formation can continue. In the healthy adult, nitrogen equilibrium, or zero balance, is the ideal, while a positive nitrogen balance is needed during times of illness and healing. In children, when growth is occurring regularly, a positive nitrogen balance is necessary, as it is in pregnancy.

As discussed in the previous section, *Food Complementarity*, the protein requirements are also based on the protein quality, as measured by the biological value (BV). Protein is also measured by the way it supports growth; this measurement, called the protein efficiency ratio (PER), is determined by feeding an animal a particular protein food and measuring its growth.

The reference protein for determining the biological value of foods is that of eggs (ovalbumin), the food with the highest BV at 94 percent (although mother's milk is valued at 100 percent). Next are fish at 75–90 percent, rice at 86 percent, legumes at 70–80 percent, and meats and poultry at 75–85 percent. Corn, an incomplete protein, has approximately 40 percent biological value.

Protein Excess

There is definite concern that the developed countries are overconsuming protein, especially from meat and dairy foods. Since nearly 700 million people in the world are protein deficient, it seems ludicrous that Americans and people in other well-to-do countries consume so much. But we could be paying the price!

The RDA protein standards may be highly overestimated; and many people consume well over those guidelines, 100 or 200 grams of protein daily. The World Health Organization more conservatively puts our protein needs at about half of the U.S. government minimum levels, or 0.45 grams of protein per kilogram of ideal body weight.

The Western world definitely has less deficiency disease than parts of the Third World, such as Africa, the Near and Far East, and Central and South America. But we also have far more chronic and degenerative diseases, such as arthritis, diabetes, cardiovascular disease, and cancer. All of these problems have dietary correlations, some of which are shown in specific studies, but many that, in my opinion, will be discovered in future years with research into the nutritional components of disease. Eventually, through knowledge and behavior, we need to find the right balance in our diet.

Protein Deficiency

With all the worldly and space technology and the wealth of resources we possess, much of the world's population is yet impoverished and near starvation. Thousands of children and adults die daily from lack of nourishing food, and protein is of key importance. In areas where meats and milk products are not plentiful and where often only one or two food sources are available, such as rice, wheat, corn, or potatoes, people are not getting the complete balance of amino acids and protein needed to sustain the body. They go into negative nitrogen balance and begin to experience weight loss, fluid retention, weakness, hair loss, and the inability to heal wounds.

The name for protein deficiency disease is kwashiorkor, a Ghanian word for "the evil spirit that infects the child." Protein deficiency is a wasting disease that in its severe state leads to death. It is curable, of course, with consumption of complete protein foods or supplements. *Marasmus*, another protein deficiency disease associated with calorie or

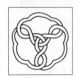

food deficiency, comes from a starvation diet and results in complete loss of energy and tissue wasting. Also called "protein-calorie malnutrition" (PCM), it is the world's most widespread and correctable malnutrition problem, killing millions yearly.

The Western world's example of protein deficiency is mirrored in the alcoholic, who obtains a large portion of his or her calorie intake from carbohydrates in the form of ethyl alcohol. Food and protein consumption may be minimal. Malnutrition and fat accumulation in the liver lead to rapidly advancing demise unless alcohol is reduced and nutrition is increased. Cirrhosis, scarring, and malnutrition of the liver is one of the top ten degenerative diseases leading to death in the United States.

Recently there has been worldwide concern over hunger, malnutrition, and starvation. It certainly seems that a primary part of our responsibility on this planet is to feed all the people adequately. After all, on an individual or family level, food, shelter, and clothing come before fancy cars, exclusive restaurants, and trips to the Caribbean. Donations to hunger projects, attending fundraising music concerts, and helping to raise money ourselves are short-term ways to feed some hungry people, but there are other approaches too. Currently, on a global level, higher precedence is given to using land for grazing meat-rendering animals than for growing grain for direct human consumption. Many acres of grain and plant proteins are used to feed a small number

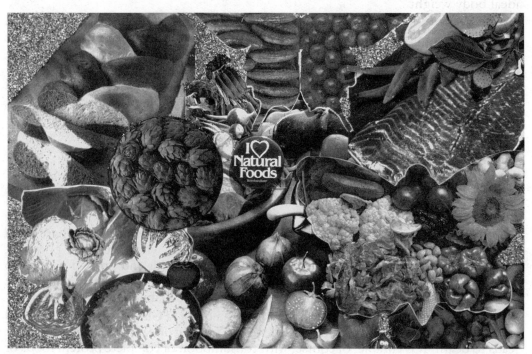

Bethany ArgIsle

of cattle and still more grain is used to feed poultry. This grain could feed many more people than can the meat of dead chickens! A reduction in animal meat production and an increased emphasis on vegetable and grain foods would help feed the impoverished everywhere. Yet perhaps the most important contibution we can make towards reducing hunger and starvation in the world is by helping and teaching people to plant and harvest their own food sources.

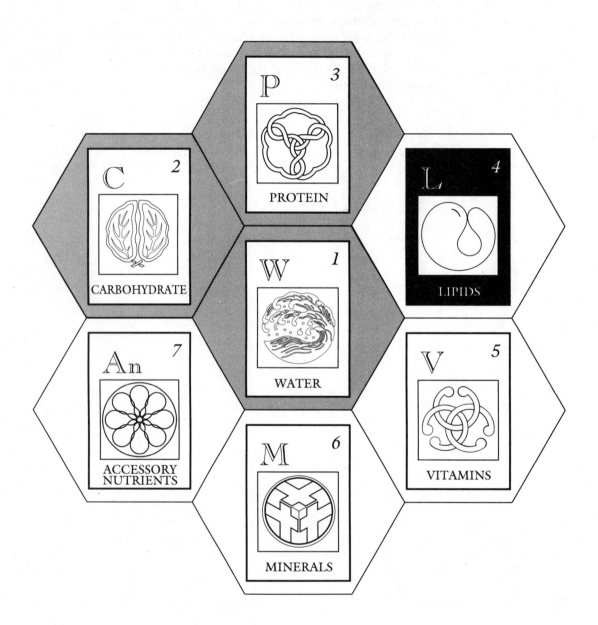

C 2
CARBOHYDRATE

P 3
PROTEIN

L 4
LIPIDS

W 1
WATER

V 5
VITAMINS

An 7
ACCESSORY NUTRIENTS

M 6
MINERALS

Chapter 4

Lipids: Fats and Oils

Fats, or lipids, are the third main class of the macronutrients needed in human nutrition. The lipids are found primarily in meats and dairy foods—at least, these are the most visible sources, but most foods contain some fat. Some of the richer vegetable sources of dietary fat are nuts and seeds, soybeans, olives, peanuts, and avocados, and these contain the needed or essential fatty acids (EFAs). Fats are an important component of our diet, and at least a minimum intake is essential. However, many problems are associated with excessive intake of dietary fat, including obesity, cardiovascular disease, and some forms of cancer.

Primarily a form of energy reserves and insulation in the body, fats can be burned to make energy when we need energy and are not getting enough from our diet. Fats are important in transporting other nutrients, such as vitamins A, D, E, and K—the "fat-soluble vitamins." Fats are also an essential component of the cell membrane, and internal fatty tissues protect the vital organs from trauma and temperature change by providing padding and insulation. Fatty tissue, in fact, even helps regulate body temperature.

An important component of lipids is the fatty acids. Three essential fatty acids are needed biochemically by our bodies and are available to us only from our diet: linoleic acid (LA), arachidonic acid, and linolenic acid (LNA). All are commonly contained in plant oils. Some sources describe linoleic acid as the only true essential fatty acid, as the others may be made from it. With more recent research it appears that this is true in plants but not in humans. We can make arachidonic acid from linoleic acid but not the important linolenic acid. Actually humans need higher amounts of alpha-linolenic acid than the other fatty acids, and luckily, these three fatty acids are commonly found together in food sources anyway. Most of our dietary intake of fat is in the form of triglycerides, which are composed of three fatty acids and a glycerol molecule. A less prevalent form of dietary fat is the phospholipids, such as lecithin, which is important to cell membranes and the brain and nerves. Cholesterol, a member of the sterol family, is both found in foods and manufactured by the body. It is essential to many body functions but has been implicated as a primary factor in heart and blood vessel disease.

Levels of fat intake are highly correlated with weight. High consumption of dietary fat is associated with both increased body fat and obesity. Fats are the most concentrated source of food energy, supplying nine calories per gram—more than double the calorie content of the proteins and carbohydrates. They provide about 42 percent of the calories in the average American diet. A diet that derives closer to 20–25 percent of total calories from fat is probably healthier. A range of 10–20 percent is also acceptable and may be helpful in reducing the incidence and progression of cardiovascular disease by lowering blood levels of triglycerides and cholesterol. Reducing fat intake to this level means cutting down greatly on consumption of red meats and dairy products such as milk, cheese, and butter. Restricting dietary fat (which usually reduces calorie intake as well) while maintaining adequate protein and complex carbohydrate intake is probably the best long-range approach to weight loss, maintenance of optimal body weight, and general good health.

○ CLASSIFICATION AND BIOCHEMISTRY

Fats, like carbohydrates, are composed of carbon, hydrogen, and oxygen; however, some phospholipids also contain nitrogen and phosphorus. The common property of all fats is that they are insoluble in water and dissolve only in the fat solvents. Tissue lipids (found in normal tissues such as liver or muscle and surrounding or covering the abdominal organs) make up about 10–15 percent of the average adult's weight; total body fat consists of all the tissue lipids plus the stored fat (this subcutaneous fat and brown fat can vary with weight and diet). Though we should keep our fat levels down, dietary fat is a high-energy food source and gives food a special flavor to which many people are attracted. The lipids include the triglycerides, the phospholipids, and the sterols.

Triglycerides and Fatty Acids

Triglycerides comprise about 95 percent of the lipids in food and in our bodies. They are the storage form of fat when we eat calories in excess of our energy needs. Burning up the stored fat allows us to live without food for periods of time, as I have done during my many fasts.

All triglycerides have a similar structure, being composed of three fatty acids attached to a glycerol molecule. Glycerol is a short-chained carbohydrate molecule that is soluble in water, and when triglycerides are metabolized, the glycerol can be converted to glucose. Fatty acids may differ in their length and their degree of saturation. They are commonly composed of a series of 16–18 carbon molecules attached to hydrogen molecules. The number of hydrogen molecules is what determines the saturation of the fat. When each carbon has its maximum number of hydrogens attached, the fat is said to be saturated—that is, filled to capacity with hydrogen.

Saturated fats, which are commonly found in animals, are hard at room temperature. Lard, suet, and butter are common saturated animal fats; coconut and palm oil are two saturated vegetable oils. Saturated fats are generally more stable than the unsaturated fats and go rancid (undergo an oxidative change in molecular structure) less easily.

Unsaturated fats are of two varieties—monounsaturated and polyunsaturated. If two adjoining carbon atoms are attached by a double bond, there is room for one more pair of hydrogen atoms, and the fatty acid is said to be monounsaturated. Oleic acid, present in olive oil, is a monounsaturated fat. When more than one area of the carbon chain can accept additional hydrogen atoms, the fat is said to be polyunsaturated. Linoleic acid, an essential fatty acid found in safflower oil, soybean oil, and other vegetable oils, is an example of a polyunsaturated fat. Other oils of this category include peanut, corn, and cottonseed oils.

Unsaturated fats are unstable at room temperature and sensitive to interaction with oxygen, light, and heat. This is why storage in dark glass or cans and/or under refrigeration is ideal. There are two other ways besides refrigeration to prevent rancidification (spoiling) of an oil. The first is to use antioxidants. (Points of unsaturation, the weak spots in the fatty acid, can be "attacked" by oxygen; antioxidants protect the molecules from oxidation.) Vitamin E is a common antioxidant; beta-carotene and the chemicals BHA and BHT are others.

Hydrogenation is another way of dealing with the spoilage problem of unsaturated oils. With chemically induced hydrogen saturation of the carbon bonds, the structure of the unsaturated oils is changed. This alters the way the body metabolizes these fats and often changes the physical form, as with margarines. Many manufacturers hydrogenate oils to make margarine and other spreads. These hydrogenated products are consumed in large amounts in the American culture and there is some question as to their carcinogenicity. Also, they no longer provide their once-available polyunsaturated fats and, since they are now saturated, tend to raise the level of blood cholesterol rather than lower it, increasing risk of cardiovascular disease.

The essential fatty acids (EFA) include linoleic, linolenic, and arachidonic acids, collectively termed vitamin F. They are all polyunsaturated fatty acids that cannot ordinarily be synthesized in the body; although, if sufficient quantities of linoleic acid (omega-6) are present, arachidonic acid can be made. Alpha-linolenic, an omega-3 fatty acid that is found in special oils such as linseed (flax), rapeseed (canola), and soybean, is also essential and is the precursor of other important omega-3 oils EPA and DHA commonly found in fish. Ideally we need more linolenic, about a 2:1 ratio, than linoleic. The essential fatty acids are important for normal growth, especially of the blood vessels and nerves, and to keep the skin and other tissues youthful and supple through their lubricating quality.

Linoleic acid is necessary for synthesis of prostaglandins in the E_1 and E_2 series; linolenic acid is the precursor of the E_3 series and other omega-3 fatty acids. Prostaglandins, hormonelike substances, have various effects on smooth muscle and inflammatory processes. The E_3 (PGE_3) series seems to reduce cholesterol levels as well as platelet aggregation and thrombosis and are generally anti-inflammatory. Prostaglandin E_2, related to arachidonic acid, tends to promote platelet aggregation, is more inflammatory, and may even be related to high blood pressure and cancer. PGE_1 is mildly inflammatory as it prevents release of arachidonic acid from the cells. Safflower oil is particularly high in linoleic acid, as are sunflower and corn oils; other vegetable oils, nuts, and seeds are also good sources. As stated, soybean, flaxseed, canola, as well as pumpkin and walnut are the best sources of alpha-linolenic acid. (See *Vitamin F*, Chapter 5, *Vitamins*.)

Another fatty acid recently shown to be beneficial is eicosapentaenoic acid (EPA). It is a polyunsaturated, omega-3 fatty acid found in high concentrations in cold-water fish. Where it is consumed in large amounts, as among Greenland Eskimos or in fishing villages in Japan, there is reduced cardiovascular disease. EPA seems to reduce serum triglycerides, raise HDL (good) cholesterol, and prolong bleeding time by reducing platelet aggregation, thus preventing thrombosis. Fish such as mackerel, sardines, and salmon are high in eicosapentaenoic acid. Consumption of cold-water fish once or twice a week seems to have a positive effect on cholesterol levels. When taken as a supplement such as MaxEPA (there are many products now available), which contains EPA and another omega-3 fatty acid, decosahexaenoic acid (DHA), may decrease the risk of vascular thrombosis and cardiovascular disease. (See more on *EPA* in Chapter 7, *Accessory Nutrients*.)

Phospholipids

Phospholipids, of which the most common is lecithin, are important in the structure of all membranes. Their structure is similar to that of triglycerides, but they contain only two fatty acids (both polyunsaturated). The third molecule attached to the glycerol is a phosphatidylcholine molecule (choline is one of the B vitamins). Certain phospholipids also contain inositol (another B vitamin) as phosphatidylinositol, as well as phosphatidylethanolamine, another phospholipid that has several functions, such as being a precursor to choline and acetylcholine. Lecithin is found in highest concentration in soybeans and egg yolks. Recently, egg lecithin has been used in the treatment of acquired immune deficiency syndrome (AIDS). There is some question as to whether supplemental lecithin helps to lower cholesterol levels. It seems to have a mild influence, perhaps due to its polyunsaturated nature. Because of their carbohydrate-fat construction, phospholipids move well in fats as well as in water and thus move easily

LIPID CHART*

Saturated Fats		*Monounsaturated Fats*	*Polyunsaturated Fats*	
Beef	Milk	Olive oil	Soybean	Corn
Pork	Butter	Canola oil	Safflower	Sesame
Lamb	Cheese	Almond oil	Sunflower	Peanut
Poultry	Yogurt		Cottonseed	Others
Coconut oil				

Linoleic Acid (Omega-6)	*Linolenic Acid (Omega-3)*
Soybean	Flaxseed
Safflower	Soybean
Sunflower	Rapeseed (canola)
Corn	Pumpkin
Wheat germ	Walnut
Sesame	

*These foods are listed under their primary lipid components.

ESSENTIAL FATTY ACID METABOLISM

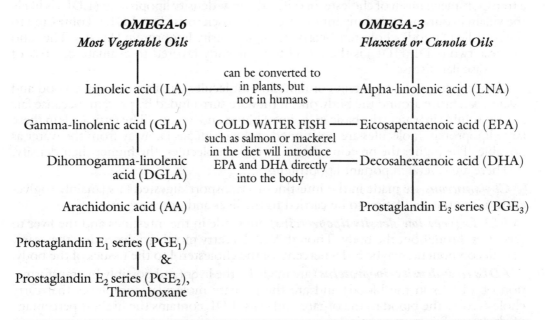

OMEGA-6		OMEGA-3
Most Vegetable Oils		*Flaxseed or Canola Oils*
Linoleic acid (LA) ——	can be converted to in plants, but not in humans	—— Alpha-linolenic acid (LNA)
Gamma-linolenic acid (GLA)	COLD WATER FISH ——	Eicosapentaenoic acid (EPA)
Dihomogamma-linolenic acid (DGLA)	such as salmon or mackerel in the diet will introduce EPA and DHA directly into the body ——	Decosahexaenoic acid (DHA)
Arachidonic acid (AA)		Prostaglandin E_3 series (PGE$_3$)
Prostaglandin E_1 series (PGE$_1$) & Prostaglandin E_2 series (PGE$_2$), Thromboxane		

in and out of cells. Another phospholipid, sphingomyelin, consists of glycerol, fatty acid, phosphate, choline, and an amino alcohol called sphingosine and is part of the tissues covering brain and nerve cells, as are the cerebrosides, phospholipids that contain galactose, fatty acid, and sphingosine.

Sterols/Cholesterol

Sterols, the third primary lipid, include cholesterol, phytosterols (plant sterols), and some of the steroid hormones. Cholesterol, the best known of the sterols, is the precursor of the bile acids and the sex hormones. Manufactured in the body, primarily in the liver, although all tissues of the body except the brain can make it, cholesterol is present in almost all cells and is particularly high in the liver, brain and nervous tissue, and the blood. Cholesterol, like lecithin, is also available in foods, such as egg yolk, meats, and other animal fats, including milk products. It is not readily available in most vegetable foods.

Cholesterol has been implicated in occlusive cardiovascular disease, causing plaque and obstruction of the arteries. The cholesterol in foods, however, is not really the villain. It is the oxidized cholesterol in the blood that causes the trouble, and the level of this is more a function of total dietary fat intake and genetically determined aspects of cholesterol metabolism, than of the amount of cholesterol in our food. In particular, a transport mechanism of cholesterol called the low-density lipoprotein (LDL) is likely the villain in our society's rampant disease—atherosclerosis. This LDL is contrasted to the so-called "good" cholesterol-carrying high-density lipoprotein (HDL). The ratio of these two (LDL:HDL) is the blood test currently favored to evaluate our risk of cardiovascular disease.

Lipoproteins, the fat-protein combination molecules circulating in our blood and tissues, can move around the body only if they are surrounded by protein, because fats are not soluble in water (the basic makeup of blood and lymph). The fatty acids in these large lipoprotein molecules are positioned at the inside, as far away from the water as possible. The higher the protein portion in these molecules, the higher their density.

There are several important lipoproteins.

Chylomicrons are made in the intestines to transport digested fats (mainly triglycerides) into the circulation to be carried to the liver and other organs.

VLDLs (very-low-density lipoproteins) are made in the intestines and the liver to carry fats throughout the body. Though VLDLs carry mostly triglycerides, they carry a small component, maybe 5–15 percent, of the cholesterol to the tissues of the body.

LDLs (low-density lipoproteins) are made by the liver (and possibly by transformation of VLDLs in the blood) and are the primary molecular complexes that carry cholesterol in the blood to the organs and cells. LDL contains the highest percentage of cholesterol in most people.

HDLs (high-density lipoproteins) are large, dense protein-fat molecules that circulate in the blood, picking up already used or unused cholesterol and cholesterol esters and taking them back to the liver as part of a recycling process. Where in the body HDL is made is not certain (probably in the liver), but it may be the most protective form of lipoprotein in preventing buildup of cholesterol. People with higher HDL levels have less risk of cardiovascular disease because their cholesterol is cleared more readily from the blood. It also appears that HDL may be able to collect cholesterol from artery plaque, thus reversing the atherosclerotic process that leads to heart attacks. HDL will deliver cholesterol to the VLDL, converting them to LDL, which have more density; the liver then removes the LDLs from the blood and converts their cholesterol into bile acids, which are then eliminated.

Estrogen helps raise HDL levels, and women have less cardiovascular risk than men, possibly because of this hormone. Smoking, obesity, and a sedentary lifestyle cause a low level of HDLs, whereas low dietary fat and cholesterol intake, aerobic exercise, and keeping weight near the ideal level are factors that help raise the HDL level and diminish cardiovascular risk.

○ DIGESTION AND METABOLISM

Because of their viscosity and insolubility in water, fats and oil require our bodies to take special care to digest and transport them to the cells and organs. The chewing process is the first act of digestion to help separate the fats. In the stomach, gastric lipase has a very minimal effect in beginning the breakdown of fats; other enzymes and hydrochloric acid do more to digest protein and carbohydrates and free the lipids from the food. Fats and oils are less dense than water; unless they are emulsified they rise and pool at the top of the gastric contents and so are acted upon last, thus taking the longest to digest and in some ways slowing the digestion. Fatty meals seem to satisfy us longer as they cause the stomach to empty more slowly.

When the fats move into the small intestine, their main place of digestion, bile is secreted from the gallbladder (bile is made by the liver and concentrated in the gallbladder). Bile first emulsifies the fats, that is, breaks down the fat globules into smaller groups of molecules so the other enzymes can actually work on the individual triglycerides to release the fatty acids. Pancreatic lipase is the main enzyme that splits the triglycerides into diglycerides and monoglycerides, which are ultimately hydrolyzed into their components, fatty acids and glycerol.

When the digestive system is working well, most (up to 95 percent) dietary fats are absorbed into the body. (Some are excreted through the colon.) Many of the fatty acids need now be altered in order to be absorbed and transported to the liver, the principal site of fat metabolism. The short-chained fatty acids, up to 12 carbons in length, are more hydrophilic, or attracted to water, and can be absorbed directly through the cell membranes of the small intestine villi (small protrusions into the intestinal lumen lined by epithelial cells and filled with capillaries; they increase the absorption surface of the small intestine). Within the villi, these short-chained fatty acids are picked up in the capillaries and transported through the bloodstream to the liver.

The longer-chained fatty acids with 14 carbons or more, and the mono- and diglycerides must be reconverted to triglycerides in the intestinal wall. These triglycerides are then surrounded with a protective protein coat (like rain gear) in order to be transported to the liver. These become large transporter molecules, the chylomicrons, which first go into the lymph circulation before entering the blood to go to the liver. VLDLs also carry some of the triglyceride molecules. Phospholipids and cholesterol are also incorporated into chylomicrons in order to get to the liver. After a fatty meal, the blood may be filled with chylomicrons, and the blood serum may have a milky appearance.

In the multifunctional liver, the chylomicrons are separated and the fats may be dismantled and reassembled into other needed fats. Lipids can also combine with proteins to make lipoproteins, with phosphate to make phospholipids, or with carbohydrates to form glycolipids. In the blood, free fatty acids, the active lipids for cell use, are bound to albumin, a protein. The other fats, such as cholesterol, are bound mainly to the high- and low-density lipoproteins. Each cell can take the triglycerides out of the lipoproteins and use the fatty acids for energy. Excess fat in the body is often stored in the fat cells. The adult human has a set number of fat cells, which enlarge to accommodate the increased triglyceride stores; an obese person's fat cells may be many times larger than a thin person's. These fat cells are formed at specific times of growth, such as infancy and adolescence. So later in life when we work to lose or gain weight, we are just shrinking or expanding our existing cells. And these fat cells are in a constant state of metabolism; they do not just sit there as many people think.

○ FUNCTIONS

Lipids perform many life-supporting functions in each cell of our body. They are part of every cell membrane and every organ and tissue. The fatty acids keep our cells strong to protect against invasion by microorganisms or damage by chemicals. Fats are very important to our nervous system and in the manufacture of the steroid and sex hormones and the important hormonelike prostaglandins. Cholesterol is responsible for some of these functions that support the health of the brain, nervous system, liver, blood, and skin.

Beside the fact that fats add a lot of the flavor to the foods that many of us are used to and savor, such as buttery treats, gravies, and juicy meats, fats serve three primary functions in the body. They are first and foremost a ready energy source, contributing nine calories for every gram of fat used, more than 4,000 calories per pound of fat.

METABOLISM OF LIPIDS, FATS AND OILS
From Ingestion to the Liver

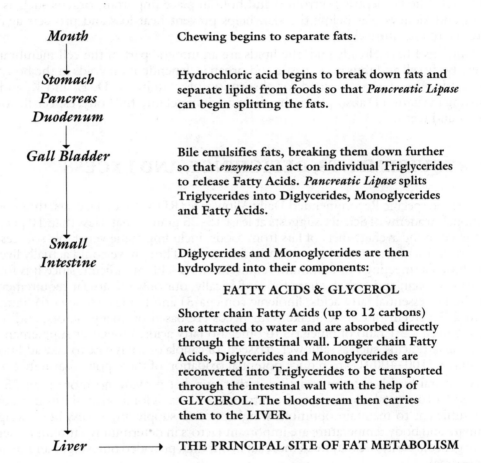

Mouth — Chewing begins to separate fats.

Stomach
Pancreas
Duodenum — Hydrochloric acid begins to break down fats and separate lipids from foods so that *Pancreatic Lipase* can begin splitting the fats.

Gall Bladder — Bile emulsifies fats, breaking them down further so that *enzymes* can act on individual Triglycerides to release Fatty Acids. *Pancreatic Lipase* splits Triglycerides into Diglycerides, Monoglycerides and Fatty Acids.

Small Intestine — Diglycerides and Monoglycerides are then hydrolyzed into their components:

FATTY ACIDS & GLYCEROL

Shorter chain Fatty Acids (up to 12 carbons) are attracted to water and are absorbed directly through the intestinal wall. Longer chain Fatty Acids, Diglycerides and Monoglycerides are reconverted into Triglycerides to be transported through the intestinal wall with the help of GLYCEROL. The bloodstream then carries them to the LIVER.

Liver ⟶ THE PRINCIPAL SITE OF FAT METABOLISM

That's a lot of potential energy we are carrying, both from dietary intake of those fatty foods and in the stored fat of our body. This stored fat helps give the body its curves and can be used for fuel during times of reduced food intake.

Fats in the body also act as a protective blanket shielding the organs from trauma and cold. The fat deposits surround and hold in place important organs such as the heart and kidneys. Fat below the skin helps prevent heat loss and protects against external temperature changes.

Third, as I have already said, the lipids are an integral part of the cell membranes. Every body cell and thus every tissue and organ is dependent on lipids in the body for its health. Also, fats are needed for absorption of vitamins A, D, E, and K, and by assisting in vitamin D absorption, they help calcium get into the body, especially to the bones and teeth.

◯ REQUIREMENTS, DEFICIENCY, AND EXCESS

There is no specific Recommended Daily Allowance (RDA) for dietary fats, though the National Academy of Science suggests at least 15–25 grams (that's less than 10 percent of the fat in the average diet) of fats from foods, including some vegetable sources, to obtain sufficient amounts of our essential fatty acids. Though we could actually live on very little fat, meeting our minimum requirements is seldom difficult, since it is found in many protein and carbohydrate foods. Basically, our only dietary fat requirement is for the key essential fatty acids, linolenic (omega-3) and linoleic (omega-6), ranging from 2–5 percent of calorie intake. Our needs are based on many factors, and most people need a 2:1 ratio of omega-3 to omega-6 fatty acids. Whenever supplementing essential fatty acids, such as safflower, flaxseed, or canola oils, it is wise to take additional vitamin E (100–400 IU) to reduce potential oxidation of these polyunsaturated oils.

A general health recommendation is that our diet provide no more than 25–30 percent* of our total calories from fat nutrients, and that is for food intake in an amount just sufficient to maintain optimum weight, not to supply any excess body weight. Climate and body temperature are important factors in determining fat requirements. If we get cold easily, we may need more fat in our diet, provided our weight and thyroid are normal.

Since linoleic and linolenic acids are polyunsaturated fats available mainly in vegetable sources, such as corn, safflower, and soybean oils, as well as many nuts and seeds, it is conceivable that we could eat solely animal fats and still not get our needed amounts of essential fatty acids. Deficiency of vitamin F (essential fatty acids) can lead to dryness, scaliness, or eczema of the skin, as well as to reductions in the oil-soluble

---

*This can be analyzed through a diet record (see *Appendix*). Since a gram of fat is 9 calories, a 2000-calorie daily diet could include 500–600 calories of fat, or 55–66 grams, daily.

vitamins A, D, E, and K. Also, if there is deficient fat intake during growth periods, a retardation in the growing process may occur. Fortunately, however, fat deficiencies are not very common, though obtaining the right balance of fats, particularly of alpha-linolenic acid, given the standard diet is not easy, but very important.

In most Western cultures, as in American society, the real concern is over an excess intake of fat. The average daily diet (higher than needed for ideal weight and health) includes about 150 grams of fat, providing 1,350 calories, well over 40–50 percent of needed daily dietary calories. This is an increase over fat consumption earlier in the century, which averaged about 120 grams per day. And much of this is from the so-called "unhealthy" fats—meat and its saturated fats, hydrogenated oils, such as vegetable shortening, and foods fried in cooking oils. In the last 10–15 years, however, there has been a great deal of public education about the high-fat diet and, as a result, a small reduction in average fat intake has occurred. In the early 1970s, fat intake was about 160 grams per day; now it has dropped to under 150 grams.

An analysis of fat consumption of the typical North American's diet was done by the Select Committee on Nutrition and Human Needs of the U.S. Senate. The reason for this study is the obvious role that dietary fat plays in disease. In 1977, they published their Dietary Goal for the United States, revealing that the average American con-sumed 42 percent of his or her calories from lipids, approximately 16 percent saturated fats, 19 percent monosaturated, and 7 percent polyunsaturated. To obtain a higher percentage of polyunsaturated fat and a lower percentage of fats in total, the Senate Select Committee has suggested the following:

- Reduce the consumption of red meats, organ meats, eggs, and dairy products in the diet.
- Choose low-fat protein sources, such as fish, turkey, chicken, and legumes (dried peas and beans).
- When consuming meats, use lean cuts and trim excess fats.
- Substitute skim and low-fat milk products for whole-fat dairy foods.
- Broil, bake, or boil foods instead of frying.
- Increase the consumption of fruits, vegetables, and whole grains in the diet.

More long-range and specific goals* for our fat consumption include:

- Reduce dietary fat consumption from about 40 percent to 30 percent of calorie intake.
- Reduce saturated fats to about 10 percent of intake, with approximately equal amounts of monounsaturated and polyunsaturated fats—that is, more vegetable-source lipids.
- Reduce cholesterol intake to about 300 mg. per day.

---

*There are more advanced and stringent guidelines for reducing problematic fat and oil intake discussed in other areas of this book.

○ DIETARY FAT AND DISEASE

A topic of great concern in modern nutritional medicine, which will be discussed throughout this book, is the correlation between increased dietary fat intake and disease. Research continues regarding the relationship between disease and cholesterol and the types of fats consumed. We now know that two aspects of diet must be considered: first, the total amount of fat intake—that is, the percentage of the total diet consisting of fats and oils, both saturated and unsaturated fats (mono- or polyunsaturated), and second, the types of fats consumed. Saturated and hydrogenated fats seem to be worse in regard to increasing cholesterol and causing vascular congestive problems than the vegetable-source unsaturated ones, which may actually improve cholesterol by reducing the LDL:HDL ratio and decreasing total cholesterol. Fried foods seem to be more difficult for the body to process, as well.

Of the diseases related to increased fat intake, number one is atherosclerosis. Clogging, or atherosclerosis, of the coronary arteries (the blood vessels that nourish the heart muscle itself with blood) is the disease process causing the most deaths in the Western "affluent diet" cultures. Clogging vital arteries with plaque (consisting of fat, mucopolysaccharides, calcium, platelets, and smooth muscle cells) decreases the delivery of life-supporting blood to the tissues and is related to a variety of other diseases. Narrowing and stiffness of the blood vessel resulting from arterial plaque leads to high blood pressure, or hypertension, which forces the heart to work harder to get the blood to the body. This constant extra effort can lead to enlargement of the heart, general heart disease, and congestive heart failure. Coronary artery disease leads to the physical limitations associated with angina pectoris and is the primary cause for the big business of coronary artery bypass surgery.

Two major types of cancer are associated with excessive dietary fat intake. The first one is the most common cancer in men and women combined, cancer of the colon and rectum. The other is the most common major female cancer, cancer of the breast. Both of these can be deadly, especially if they are not diagnosed early, and both are associated with a high-fat, low-fiber diet. There is also an association between prostate cancer in men and uterine and ovarian cancer in women and high dietary fat consumption, particularly saturated fats found in animal foods.

Obesity is much more likely in people who eat a high-fat diet, which is often a high-calorie diet, since each gram of fat contains nine calories instead of the four calories in each gram of protein or carbohydrate. With obesity comes an increased risk of all the previously mentioned diseases, such as atherosclerosis, hypertension, and certain cancers, besides a variety of other problems, including adult-onset diabetes.

I want to further delineate the role of fats in cardiovascular diseases. Saturated fats and hydrogenated vegetable oils, which contain high amounts of saturated fats in place of their once polyunsaturated oils, both raise serum cholesterol. The liver makes cholesterol from saturated fats. A number of factors can increase the risk of cardiovascular disease. The top three are **elevated serum cholesterol, smoking, and high blood pressure.** (For cholesterol, the most important factor is elevated LDL.) Anyone who smokes, has high blood pressure, and has a serum cholesterol level of more than 250, especially with a high LDL:HDL ratio, is almost certain to close off his or her arteries relatively rapidly. Other risk factors for the cardiovascular diseases include stress, obesity, gender (the female hormone estrogen is protective for women), heredity (for heart disease or for higher cholesterol levels), lack of exercise, and elevated blood triglyceride levels. We are in a position to reduce most of these risk factors by changing our lifestyles and dietary habits, and doing so will significantly reduce our chances of developing blood vessel and heart disease. **Overall, the best way to lower risks of cardiovascular disease is to reduce total and saturated fat intake, keep the blood pressure normal, not smoke, and exercise regularly.**

The current theory about the body's process of forming plaque in the arteries is rather complex. A simple version is as follows: The liver produces cholesterol mainly from the saturated fats. The LDLs are the primary carriers of cholesterol through the blood and to the plaques, so the higher the intake of saturated fats (increasing cholesterol and LDLs), the greater the potential for plaque formation. The smooth muscle cells in the middle layer of the arterial wall invade the inner wall to help form the plaques, which start from some irritation of the inner lining that may come from irritants such as smoking, viruses, chemicals in the diet, and increased stress. High blood pressure also causes increased stress on the artery walls. These irritations attract platelets and LDL cholesterols and thicken the wall with plaque. HDLs carry cholesterol away from plaque and out of the bloodstream back to the liver for reprocessing, so higher HDL levels reduce the likelihood of plaque formation.

An important key to preventing cardiovascular disease is lowering serum cholesterol and LDL levels and raising the HDL cholesterol in ratio to the total cholesterol and to LDL. This can be done by following my repeated suggestion, which is also that of the government and the American Heart Association: lower intake of saturated fats found in meats and animal foods, in milk products, and in hydrogenated oils and increase the proportion of mono- and polyunsaturated vegetable-source fats and oils in the diet. In general, a fat-modified diet can lower serum cholesterol from 20–40 percent, especially if exercise is included. Polyunsaturated fats specifically can lower cholesterol by reducing lipoprotein (LDL) synthesis and increasing lipoprotein breakdown, as well as by the effect of the essential fatty acid linolenic acid. Linolenic acid reduces plaque formation and thrombosis by decreasing platelet aggregation, promoting prostaglandin (E_3 series) synthesis (which also influences platelets), and decreasing LDLs. The essential fatty acids also influence the intravascular coagulation as well as energy metabolism within the myocardial muscle of the heart.

One of the main ways to raise HDL levels is exercise—that is, regular, prolonged, aerobic-type exercise. Females normally have higher levels of HDL and thus a reduced cardiovascular disease risk. Smoking lowers HDL, so stopping smoking will help raise it, besides reducing the increased risk caused by the vascular irritation of smoking. Also, the polyunsaturated fat level influences the HDL level, and the omega-3 fatty acids, particularly eicosapentaenoic acid (EPA) found in fish, help to raise HDL levels and reduce the risk of cardiovascular disease.

Factors that help lower LDL levels, besides reducing saturated fat and dietary cholesterol, include eating a relatively higher amount of mono- and polyunsaturated fats compared to the saturated or hydrogenated varieties; adding specific nutrients, such as sufficient dietary vitamin C (a deficiency of vitamin C can raise LDL); avoiding excess copper, sodium, and iron intakes, which can raise LDL; and getting sufficient chromium and natural dietary fluoride, as deficiencies can raise LDL. A diet high in animal protein can raise LDL, whereas eating a higher percentage of vegetable protein helps to lower it. Sufficient fiber in the diet, particularly from the legumes, vegetables, and fruits (such as apples that contain pectin), helps in lowering LDL as well.

With regard to nutrition and cancer (our second most prevalent deadly adult disease), it is likely that more than 50 percent (probably more) of cancer occurrences are related at least in part to diet. The Hunza tribes of Pakistan who are known for their longevity and have the lowest known cancer rates eat an exclusively natural, chemical-free diet of foods they grow themselves. High animal protein intake and low dietary fiber consumption are two important factors increasing cancer incidence, but the one that is being shown to be the most significant is increasingly high intake of fats, particularly the saturated animal fats, in the diet. Many chemicals in foods, used as preservatives or from herbicides and pesticides, may be carcinogenic in the body, especially in the gastrointestinal tract, and many of these chemicals are stored in animal fats. Artificial red dyes, cyclamate, nitrites and nitrates in processed meats, and saccharin have all been implicated in cancer.

The theory of how fat can cause cancer in the colon and rectum is based on the fact that fats in the diet cause release of bile acids from the gallbladder and liver into the intestine to help emulsify the fats. High-fat diets stimulate increased bile acid levels in the colon. Fat in the diet also weakens the metabolism of the normal colon bacteria which, when functioning optimally, may help protect the colon lining from carcinogens. These altered microflora interact with the bile acids to potentially create compounds that may cause cancer. An increased fiber content, even in a higher-fat diet, seems to be protective by increasing bowel motility, by diluting these carcinogenic substances through its bulking action, and by improving bacterial detoxification functions.

More than 100,000 new cases of cancer of the colon are diagnosed each year. The high-fat diet increases the incidence of this cancer, which, if diagnosed early, can usually be cured through major surgery—a drastic measure that could be prevented. The high-fat diet is also commonly associated with a higher fried-food component and lower fiber content, two other important dietary factors in carcinogenesis in the colon.

Numerous studies have shown the relationship of dietary fat to colon cancer. Research with the Seventh-Day Adventists who eat a vegetarian diet reveals that their incidence of colon cancer is much lower than average. They usually consume a diet higher in fiber and lower in fat than the average American. A study of the Mormon high-fiber diet has more clearly isolated dietary fats as the main connection to colon cancer incidence. Other nutritional qualities of the fruit and vegetable fiber foods seem to help inhibit cancer formation as well. Vitamins C and E, beta-carotene, and selenium, plus the plant sterols and antioxidant phenolic compounds like bioflavonoids from foods such as berries and citrus fruits, all seem to be beneficial factors. The cruciferous vegetables, such as broccoli and cabbage, seem to have other factors such as sulfhydryl-containing molecules besides the fiber that may protect against the development of cancer.

Cancer of the breast and a high-fat diet have been shown to be related for some time. It is thought that saturated fats generate more cholesterol and higher estrogen levels in women. This theory supports the dietary fat and breast cancer relationship as estrogen is particularly related to increased incidence of female breast cancer. Although the dietary fat and breast cancer question is not conclusively answered, it is generally agreed that, in regards to this disease, a low-fat, high-complex-carbohydrate diet minimizing alcohol, cigarettes, and preserved and chemical foods is still the best way to live to help prevent breast cancer. Countries, such as Japan, whose people traditionally eat a low-fat diet have a much lower incidence of breast cancer than countries eating higher quantities of animal fat, such as the United States, Australia, New Zealand, and the countries of Western Europe. Japanese who eat more Westernized diets in their own country or who move to a country eating a Western diet have a higher incidence of breast cancer. In the United States, Seventh-Day Adventist women on a vegetarian diet exhibit a lower incidence of this disease.

Not all recent studies correlate higher cancer incidence solely with total fat intake. There is some question as to whether certain fats are more significant than others. Milk fat and dairy foods have been implicated in several studies. The strongest correlation for breast cancer has been with the intake of the trans-fatty acids that are created when vegetable oils are hydrogenated to make margarine and solid vegetable shortening. There is even some concern with the polyunsaturated fats. Since they are less stable, they can go through peroxidation, which can lead to the formation of epoxides that may be cancer causing. This is especially true when these fats are heated. (Vitamin E and beta-carotene are two antioxidants which protect against the peroxidation process.) Because of this, I suggest using polyunsaturates moderately, along with some monosaturates, such as olive oil, which are more stable, while cutting down on the saturated fats.

CANCER PREVENTION

The specific cancer preventive diet put out in 1984 by the American Cancer Society's Medical and Scientific Committee includes the following suggestions:

1 **Avoid Obesity.** Obese people have higher incidences of many cancers, particularly of the breast, colon, stomach, gallbladder, and uterus.

2 **Reduce total fat intake.** As we have just discussed, dietary fat is mainly associated with increased risk of colon, breast, and prostate cancer. It also adds to obesity, another risk.

3 **Eat more high-fiber foods, particularly fresh fruit and vegetables and whole grains.** This is not conclusive, but it does seem that these nutrient rich, low-calorie and low-fat foods reduce the likelihood of cancer through a variety of means.

4 **Include in the diet those foods that are rich in vitamin A and vitamin C.** Beta-carotene, the precursor of vitamin A, is found in many fruits and vegetables, such as carrots, spinach, tomatoes, apricots, peaches, and melons. This nutrient is thought to help reduce carcinogenesis. Vitamin C, found in high amounts in citrus fruits and many vegetables, may also prevent cancer. It interferes with production of nitrosamine, a carcinogen formed from dietary nitrites in preserved foods.

5 **Include the cruciferous vegetables, such as broccoli, Brussels sprouts, cabbage, and cauliflower, in the diet.** Their actions are not known exactly, but these foods are thought to help prevent cancer.

6 **Minimize the consumption of alcoholic beverages.** Alcohol increases the risks for certain cancers, which are even more liable to occur in those who smoke.

7 **Avoid the consumption of salt-cured, smoked, and nitrate-treated foods.** Nitrates and nitrites can form nitrosamine, a carcinogen, in the digestive tract. Also, the smoking of foods can cause fats to be converted to polycyclic aromatic hydrocarbons, which are also carcinogenic.

CARDIOVASCULAR DISEASE
PREVENTION

The suggestions for reducing cardiovascular diseases include the following:

1. **Reduce the amount of total fats** in the diet from more than 40 percent (the current average) of total calories to approximately 30 percent or below.

2. **Specifically reduce the saturated-fat** intake by reducing consumption of red meats and whole milk products, such as cheeses and butter.

3. **Reduce intake of hydrogenated fat** (also saturated) found in cooking oils and margarine.

4. **Raise the ratio of poly-unsaturated fats to saturated fats in the diet** by maintaining or slightly increasing the dietary intake of polyunsaturated fats found in vegetable oils such as safflower, corn, and soybean oils and in most seeds and nuts. These also contain high amounts of the essential fatty acids, which are important to healthy body function.

5. **Eat more cold-water fish** (at least twice weekly), rather than red meats, for the omega-3 fatty acid content.

6. **Keep the blood pressure under control, do not smoke, and exercise regularly.**

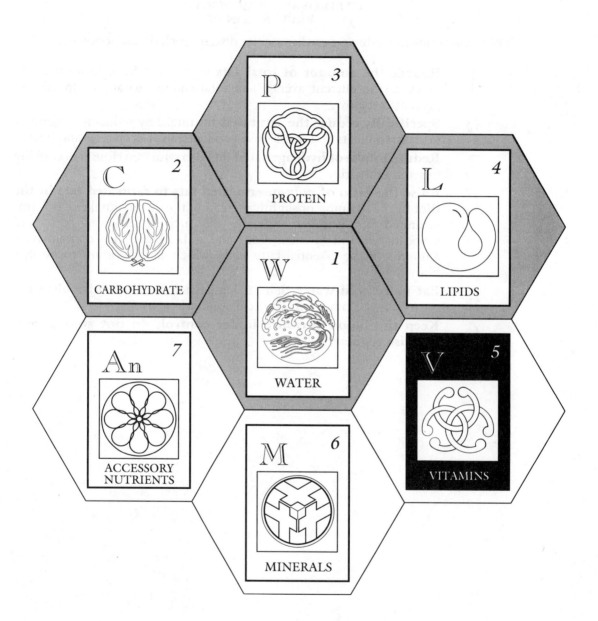

Chapter 5

Vitamins

Vitamins are one of two groups of substances classified as micronutrients (the other is minerals) that are essential in human nutrition. Vitamins are organic, meaning they contain the element carbon and are found in plant and animal substances in small amounts. We obtain them by eating the plants and animals that make them. Most vitamins cannot be manufactured in our body; exceptions are some of the B vitamins, which can be made by our intestinal bacteria, and occasional biochemical conversions from a precursor to the active form of the required vitamin, as when beta-carotene is converted to vitamin A. Vitamins, however, are not sources of energy (calories). We obtain our energy from the macronutrients—carbohydrates, proteins, and fats. In fact, vitamins help to convert these macronutrients to more bioavailable or metabolically useful forms. Vitamins function principally as coenzymes (in collaboration with enzymes) for a variety of metabolic reactions and biochemical mechanisms within our many bodily systems. Each enzyme is specific to one biochemical reaction. Enzymes are catalysts—that is, they speed up specific chemical reactions that would proceed very slowly, if at all, without them.

Vitamins themselves are not part of our body tissues; they are not building blocks but helpers in metabolism. We cannot live on vitamins but need food that provides energy and helps form the actual tissues of our body. In fact, we need food and certain minerals to best absorb any vitamin supplements we take. Vitamins are essential for growth, vitality, and health and are helpful in digestion, elimination, and resistance to disease. Depletions or deficiencies can lead to a variety of both specific nutritional disorders and general health problems, according to what vitamin is lacking in the diet.

Historically, vitamins were discovered primarily through the deficiency diseases caused by their absence in the diet. Many vitamins were discovered in naturally occurring human experiments and in laboratory studies using rats, mice, or birds fed specific diets lacking certain essential foods. It was not until the early 1900s that Sir Frederick Galen Hopkins published a paper suggesting that there were some "accessory nutrients" needed in our diet in small quantities to maintain good health. In 1911 the first vitamin was isolated from rice polishings (this vitamin was thiamine). It was found to be an amine (containing nitrogen), and thus was termed "vitamine"—that is "amine essential for life." In later years other vitamins were discovered that were not amines, and the term was converted to our current one, vitamin.

Back in the 1500s records were first made of nature's vitamin experiments and vitamin deficiency disease. The British Royal Navy at the time of Queen Elizabeth was fed a diet of dried or salted meat or fish, biscuits, butter, cheese, and beer. Many men developed a serious and painful disease, and more than 10,000 died during a period of 20 years. The disease, named "scurvy," was associated with rotten gums and tooth loss, painful jaws, swollen legs, aches and pains, and easy bruising. When the men were fed raw potatoes, watercress, raisins, or scurvy grass, sources of vitamin C, their pains and disease reversed rapidly. Likewise, beriberi, now known to be a thiamine deficiency, was a debilitating and deadly disease among Japanese sailors who ate a diet deficient in whole grain foods; contributing particularly to this disease was the processing that removed the outer covering of rice. Dietary adjustment was helpful in curing this disease. When rats were experimentally fed only proteins, starches, sugars, and fats without milk products or vegetables, the animals' eyes were affected and they failed to grow. Vitamin A was then isolated from milk, butter, liver, and egg yolks, and this substance was shown to reverse the eye problem and promote growth in the rats.

There are many more stories regarding experiments and discoveries of specific vitamins. I mention this because in the U.S. government's development of the commonly quoted Recommended Daily Allowances (RDAs), which will be discussed shortly, various experiments determine these suggested values.

Vitamins are usually classified into those that are water-soluble and those that are fat-soluble. They are further categorized by letters, groups, and individual chemical names.

Water-soluble vitamins include mainly the many B vitamins and vitamin C. They are stable in raw foods but may be lost easily during the cooking and processing. Commonly found in the vegetable foods, these vitamins are contained less so in most animal sources. The water-soluble vitamins are not stored in the body to a very large degree, so they are needed regularly in our diets; this makes them much less potentially toxic than the fat-soluble vitamins, which are stored when taken in higher dosages. Most of the water-soluble vitamins act in the body as coenzymes in combination with an inactive protein to make an active enzyme.

Fat-soluble vitamins are vitamins A, D, E, and K, which are found in the lipid component of both vegetable- and animal-source foods (the source varies for each vitamin). Grains, seeds, and nuts contain vitamin E, and many vegetables contain vitamin A, or, more commonly, its precursor beta-carotene. These fat-soluble vitamins can be stored in the body tissues, so we can function for longer periods of time without obtaining them from the diet than we can without the water-soluble ones. For this reason, toxic levels can occur more easily from regular increased intake of these vitamins, especially vitamin A; vitamins D and K can also cause problems when taken in high dosages. Toxicity is less likely with vitamin E, since it is used readily by the body as an antioxidant to help protect against the harmful by-products of metabolism and against outside pollutants. Vitamin A adds cellular protection as well as resistance to infection, while vitamin D aids in absorption of calcium from the gut and thus is important to skeletal health. Vitamin K helps make factors crucial to blood clotting to prevent bleeding.

○ RECOMMENDED DAILY ALLOWANCES (RDAS)

Set by a group of conservative doctors and nutritionists of the government's Committee on Dietary Allowances of the Food and Nutrition Board, the RDAs of vitamins are broad guidelines that establish the amounts of nearly 40 essential nutrients that are believed on the basis of currently available scientific knowledge "to be adequate to meet the known nutritional needs of practically all healthy persons." But what is a "healthy person?" How is that decided on a standard American scale? Many of us want to surpass the level that we see as "average health." And "practically all" is not quite everyone, is it? It is estimated that about 3 percent of people, even healthy ones, need more than the minimum RDA of each nutrient. With this information, it appears possible, or even likely, that each of us may not obtain our individual adequate levels of every nutrient from consuming only the RDAs. Remember, the RDAs apply only to "practically all healthy people" and guarantee only minimal, not optimal levels of nutrition.

These values may have nothing to do with maintaining vitality for a given individual. Nor is it likely that they are the amounts needed during recovery from serious disease or even minor sicknesses. And what about possible increased needs during times of extra stress or if we smoke cigarettes, drink a lot of alcohol or coffee, or eat sugar, all of which could deplete some vitamins or create extra needs? And what are our requirements if we are on a special diet or are planning surgery? No one knows for certain the answers to these questions, but many doctors and other people do not go by the RDAs in these situations. We recognize them as the minimum, not the optimum. And even these minimum levels may not be provided by diet alone, so many people take additional supplements for insurance against deficiency problems. On the other hand, vitamin advertisers and nutritional magazines promote all kinds of supplements. Consumers must be very aware of this and gain knowledge to make healthy choices. In my discussion here, I want to look more at the optimum levels of each nutrient, understand what each can do at these levels, explore potential deficiency problems, and list the food sources from which each can be obtained. Providing knowledgeable use of diet and nutritional supplements for each individual is my goal.

In the discussions of individual vitamins, I will give the specific RDAs, including those for children, adults, and the elderly when they are different, and special requirements during times when health is below normal. I will also provide optimum intake levels of the various vitamins. Vitamin levels for the fat-soluble nutrients A, D, E, and K are measured in international units (IUs) and for the water-soluble vitamins measurement is in either milligrams (mg., thousandths of a gram) or micrograms (mcg., thousandths of a milligram).

Other Nutritional Supplement Terms

Natural: Vitamins are considered natural when they are extracted exclusively from food sources and contain the specific mix of nutrients found in nature. Often, this mix includes other enzymes, catalysts, or minerals to aid the body's use of the vitamins. Yeast, liver, corn, soy, rosehips, and alfalfa are common sources from which vitamins and minerals are extracted. People who are allergic or sensitive to any of these foods may be reacting to the other ingredients but not to the vitamins themselves. The amounts of individual nutrients in purely natural vitamins are usually not very high, and thus many higher-dose "vitamins" contain a combination of natural and synthetic vitamins.

Synthetic: When vitamins are made chemically in the laboratory, rather than extracted from foods, they are termed "synthetic." The amounts of these vitamins can range from low to very high. Though synthetic vitamins able to perform the same functions and chemical reactions in the body as natural vitamins (since they have the same chemical structure), many people, especially those who are sensitive to chemicals, do not tolerate them as well. Synthetic vitamin products are more likely than those from natural sources to contain binders and fillers that might cause allergic reactions or gastrointestinal distress.

Organic: Scientifically speaking, all vitamins are organic, in that they contain carbon, but as with the term "natural," the health industry uses this term differently. Here, "organic" means that foods or supplements come from pesticide- and herbicide-free plant sources or naturally raised animals. In the body, nutrients can also be "organically" bound into tissues, for example, iron in the hemoglobin of the red blood cell. The agricultural term "organic" means that foods are grown without the addition of chemicals to the soil or the food. When vitamins are naturally derived from organically grown food, they can truly be called "organic" vitamins. As you can see, the term "organic" has become quite confusing.

Inorganic: Vitamins are organic, and minerals are inorganic—that is, they do not contain carbon. Within the meaning of our agricultural term, though, almost all nutritional supplements are "inorganic" (really nonorganic) in the sense that they are chemically manufactured or extracted from foods grown with chemicals.

Chelated: When minerals are bound to another molecule to enhance absorption from the digestive tract, they are said to be "chelated." This organic molecule must have a dicarboxylic acid with two negatively charged sites to hold the mineral. Many minerals, such as iron, calcium, zinc, and chromium, are more readily absorbed when they are chelated, because they have less competition for active absorption sites. Examples of chelated minerals are iron fumarate, calcium aspartate, and zinc citrate.

Time-release: In order to sustain blood and body levels of the water-soluble vitamins over a longer period of time, they may be manufactured in micropellets within the vitamin pill. These micropellets are digested and absorbed into the body more slowly—that is, time-released—usually over an 8–12 hour period.

Orthomolecular Medicine: Treating each individual's medical problems with the appropriate level or "right amount" of each nutrient, usually higher levels of the various vitamins and minerals than the RDAs, is termed "orthomolecular medicine." This term was coined by Linus Pauling. The objective of orthomolecular medicine is to achieve a balanced metabolism by having the appropriate nutrient or biochemical molecule in the appropriate location at the appropriate time.

Orthomolecular Psychiatry: This is a type of orthomolecular medicine where the large doses of vitamins and minerals are used in conjunction with therapy for psychiatric conditions, such as depression and schizophrenia.

Megavitamin Therapy: This is a simplistic extension of the orthomolecular approach, using dosages many times the RDAs to prevent problems, treat certain biological symptoms and potential genetic and nutritional deficiencies, and obtain optimum health. Megavitamin therapy has been advocated by many people, such as Adelle Davis, Richard Passwater in his book *Supernutrition: The Megavitamin Revolution*, Linus Pauling in regard to vitamin C, and Pearson and Shaw in their book *Life Extension*.

Vitamin Availability

Vitamins are available in a variety of forms: tablets, capsules, powders, and liquids.

Tablets are most common because of their convenience and longer shelf life. However, they usually have fillers, binders, or coatings to keep them more stable. Here, "natural" vitamins without these unnecessary additives may be more beneficial.

Capsules, which are also easy to take and probably more easily digested and absorbed than are tablets, are used for powdered formulas and the fat-soluble vitamins. Capsules may be opened easily and the contents can be sprinkled on foods, as powders, or applied to the skin, as with vitamin A or E oil. Most capsules are made from beef or pork gelatin. Though there is a very expensive vegetable gelatin, it is really not used yet in vitamin manufacturing. True vegetarian vitamins must be put into tablets or powdered; the powders and liquids are potentially the purest.

Powdered vitamins, usually mixed with water or juice, are suggested because of their rapid absorbability, but they are not always as convenient or palatable as tablets and capsules. They are especially helpful for people who have trouble swallowing pills, who have weak digestion, or who need higher levels of particular nutrients, most commonly vitamin C.

Liquid vitamins are most often used for infants and children and have the same advantages as powders for the adult. However, many are colored and sweetened, often artificially, as are the common children's chewables. With vitamin supplements, as with foods, reading labels may help us determine their origins and the manufacturing policies.

Many liquid injectable vitamins are available for use in treating certain illnesses. These can be used in the hospital, doctor's office, or, occasionally, at home for intramuscular injection. B-complex and vitamin B_{12} injections are commonly given. Intravenous vitamins are used by some doctors in the clinical setting.

O WHO NEEDS VITAMINS?

Vitamin supplements to our diet can be used as a preventive approach to maintain or improve health, characterized as a basic state of vitality and involvement—a many-leveled relationship—with life. Vitamins may also be used in the primary treatment or in the support of other treatments for a variety of symptoms, short-term illnesses, and chronic diseases. Nutritional supplements are being used increasingly by nutritionists, physicians, and individuals as treatment for a multitude of problems. And many times they are helpful. An extra positive benefit is that vitamins rarely ever make matters worse, although they may have many effects, even including diarrhea or other detoxification symptoms.

The use of supplements as medical treatment for specific problems will be described in this chapter, discussing each individual nutrient, while programs for specific illnesses and lifestyles will be detailed in Part Four of this book, entitled *Nutritional Application*. Often, when we refer to "vitamins," we do not mean the specific essential vitamins, such as A, B, and C, but the more general idea of "taking vitamins," which alludes to the minerals and other nutritional "pills" as well. In the following discussion, "vitamins" refers to the general concept of taking nutritional supplements.

Does everyone need "vitamin" supplements? While I do not believe that the average, basically healthy individual who has a sensible, balanced diet and low-stress lifestyle needs to take regular supplements, there are times in this healthy person's life when certain supplements or a general high-level nutritional program will be helpful on a daily, monthly, or yearly basis. Certain people taking "vitamins" will notice a big change in health or energy, particularly if they have been deficient in the elements they are supplementing. With an adequate level of the basic micronutrients—that is, a multiple vitamin/mineral—most active people will notice a difference. So when this healthy person is under more stress, or during times of change or early illness, or if symptoms or illnesses are coming more frequently, a specific supplement program may be helpful. These individual nutritional programs can be designed either to build up, balance, or to detoxify the body, as the situation requires.

Those of us who lead a busy, active life, drive a car in traffic regularly, live in the city, work at a busy or stressful job, or do not necessarily eat as well as we could may benefit from a daily basic regimen of nutritional supplements. This is really the "insurance" concept of "vitamin" usage; we take supplements to make sure we do not become deficient in any nutrient and to balance out the effects of a stressful lifestyle so we will not break down and become ill. And this works for a lot of people! So stress is one reason to take supplements. Illness, especially recovering and rebuilding from illness, is another reason to make sure we are getting our basic nutrient needs. Supplements, of course, do not replace a good diet. But often when we are ill, we do not feel much like eating or our digestion and absorption functions are not working well. After injury or before and after surgery, extra nutritional supplements may be very helpful in supporting rapid healing. Minimally, vitamin A, vitamin C, and zinc can help tissue repair and very likely lessen the chance of infection following injuries or surgery. A full supplement program may be even more helpful. I think that with proper application of supplements and observation, many surgeons would be impressed with general recovery and wound healing in their patients taking additional "vitamins" before and after surgery.

Those people who are dieting or go on special or limited diets because of allergies, a desire to lose weight, or from personal preference would do well to "cover" themselves with a basic general supplement program to ensure that all their essential micronutrient requirements are met. With unexplained weight loss, there may be a need for additional nutrient intake, as well as finding out the cause of the weight loss. Fatigue also has a variety of causes, but often a combination of nutrient supplements with a well-balanced diet and stress reduction may be very helpful in restoring and enhancing energy.

During all life transitions, I believe, it is wise to take additional supplements. During childhood, especially for children who do not eat a balanced diet or who consume sugar foods, which deplete body nutrients, an extra daily multivitamin/mineral is a good idea. For elderly people, whose digestive systems are not always working optimally and some of whose nutrient needs may be increased, especially for minerals such as calcium, magnesium, and potassium, extra supplementation may help with continued vitality and health. For many children or elders, more easily digested and absorbed supplements, such as a liquid or powdered vitamin/mineral combination, may be advantageous.

I mentioned sugar as a nutrient-depleting substance, devoid of its own nutrients. Those who have consumed lots of sugary foods or crave and eat refined sugar products need additional supplements for two reasons. First, they may replace any depleted nutrients from the generally poor diet; in terms of sugar craving, chromium is probably the most significant. Second, supplements such as the B vitamins, vitamin C, the amino acid glutamine, chromium, and other minerals may help to balance out the fluctuating blood sugar and reduce food cravings, especially for sweets. For example, one of my patients claims that when she takes calcium and magnesium, her intense craving for chocolate is reduced.

Those who smoke may also get some protection by taking nutritional supplements. Regular smoking of tobacco causes a lot of potential problems in the body, many of which result from inhalation of tars and other chemicals which lead to increased free-radical (unstable, irritating molecules) formation. General supplementation plus specific antioxidant therapy, which helps bind these potentially damaging free radicals, may reduce some harmful effects of smoking. Vitamin A or beta-carotene, vitamin C, vitamin E and selenium, and L-cysteine all have this antioxidant effect, and all may be required in higher amounts in smokers.

Regular alcohol use and abuse may also generate depletion of bodily nutrients. In the extreme case, an alcoholic can become malnourished when not consuming a proper diet and can suffer a number of vitamin and mineral deficiencies, as well as have problems with carbohydrate metabolism and maintaining blood sugar levels and with fat accumulation in the liver. A balanced diet and a supplement program including the B vitamins, beta-carotene, and minerals can give a little insurance against the effects of alcohol abuse. Extra minerals and fluids can help counteract the dehydrating effects of alcohol, and may reduce the morning-after doldrums.

Of course, if we all created our own healthy, balanced lifestyle and were not the victims of a busy, high-tech society, we would likely be able to obtain our needed nutrients completely from our fresh, homegrown vital foods. Breathing clean air and drinking fresh, noncontaminated water would be additional bonuses to our health. But for most of us, our high-demand, fast-paced, stressful lifestyle places extra requirements upon our body, and we need the additional support and protection that supplementation can give us. Even our natural fruits, vegetables, and whole grains may not be nourishing us in the way they used to because of the depletion of soil minerals and the additional stress on our body caused by chemical and pesticide exposure. Let's face it, with all the changes and stresses that our society is experiencing, we need all the help we can get—and nutritional support is an important ally.

○ SPECIAL SUGGESTIONS

Since vitamins and minerals are essential constituents of vegetable and animal foods, the first and most important suggestion is that they need to be viewed as "food supplements"—they are digested and assimilated best when taken with or following food. The B vitamins, vitamin C, and the minerals, all of which are water-soluble, especially need to be dissolved and digested with food before they can be assimilated and thereby used by the body. The fat-soluble vitamins can be utilized, as is often suggested, when taken alone either in the morning before breakfast or at bedtime.

They also can be taken after meals of fat-containing foods. Emulsified, water-dispersed forms of vitamins E and A, for example, that can be taken along with the other vitamins are also available.

Some authorities suggest taking all "vitamins" on an empty stomach because that way the body has a better chance to absorb them, though we would best separate the oil-soluble and water-soluble vitamins. No studies I know of demonstrate comparative blood levels of vitamins taken with or without food consumption. On the basis of my experience and sense, I suggest consuming "vitamins" as I have previously suggested, with food, usually after meals. Most healthy people with good digestive tracts handle this well. Sensitive people may need to isolate individual nutrients. People whose stomachs become upset when taking supplements or those with weak digestive systems notice that they do better taking supplements either with food or with digestive supplements, such as enzymes or hydrochloric acid.

Also, in general, I do not suggest big, time-release "horse pills." Our digestion, especially hydrochloric acid output, needs to be very efficient to utilize them. Young, healthy people seem to do fairly well with them, but during illness or other weakened states or in elderly people, I do not think this type of "multiple" is useful. Too many times I have received reports from radiologists who have seen whole "vitamin" pills in the intestines.

I also usually suggest simple, easy-to-absorb supplements and powdered formulas whenever possible, either in capsules or as straight powder to mix in water or juice. Their percentage of bioavailability is higher, I believe, than that of tablets. To obtain increased blood levels of vitamin C, for example, I suggest either a concentrated ascorbic acid powder or a mineralized (with calcium, magnesium, and potassium, for example) vitamin C powder to be taken every couple of hours throughout the day, because vitamin C gets used very rapidly in the body.

For people who have energy problems, such as fatigue, hyperactivity, or insomnia, I will often separate the supplement plan so they take their B vitamins early in the day with breakfast and lunch and their minerals, such as calcium and magnesium, later in the day and before bed. The B vitamins tend to be stimulating, while the minerals tend to be relaxing and balancing to muscles and nervous system.

I like to plan nutrient programs with patients after doing an analysis of the diet and of the blood levels of minerals or vitamins (see *Appendix*) so my suggestions can be tailored to the individual's needs. Then, at a later time, we can repeat certain tests to see whether the supplements have helped in achieving the appropriate balance. When I have people on nutritional supplements, I prefer to meet with them every few months, accompanied with all their bottles of whatever, to review their program. The patient might have read an article or talked to a friend and then added a new supplement. I feel that it is important to change programs occasionally and not get too rigid in the plan. Even if everything is working well, I think reassessment and change, at least every six months to a year, is a good idea. Often, certain nutrients are not really

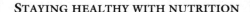

needed in the same amounts or a new supplement might be appropriate. Too often, people find supplements that work and may take them for years without checking to see if their biochemistry is balanced. Overall, I encourage individuals to learn and understand what they are doing nutritionally and to adapt some type of process for self-evaluation and "listening to their body" to make healthy choices at appropriate times.

Establishing a proper individual nutritional supplement program is a fine art. If we focus on a particular nutrient and take higher amounts of it, we may become deficient in other nutrients that have a similar process of absorption into the blood. The B vitamins are absorbed fairly well, so this is less a concern for them, although I still do not suggest supplementing just one. The main concern is for the different minerals that tend to compete for absorption sites—taking a high amount of one may limit utilization of the others. If we take a lot of zinc, we may absorb more zinc into our body, but then we may not absorb as much copper, manganese, or magnesium out of our food if we are not supplementing them also. Giving all our nutrients a "fair chance" will let the body's natural wisdom work more easily.

My main medical goal is to guide people in developing the skills to become their own best doctor, and thus be able to make more informed, conscious choices.

○ **THE INDIVIDUAL VITAMINS**

Following is a detailed discussion of each of the currently known vitamins. I have listed them in two groups alphabetically, and then the more numerous water-soluble ones. For each vitamin, the discussion is organized into the following categories:

• *General description*—what the vitamin is, how our body handles it, and its special features;

• *Sources*—the best food sources for the vitamin;

• *Functions*—what the vitamin does in our body;

• *Uses*—how we can use the vitamin in treatment or prevention of disease;

• *Deficiency and toxicity*—what problems are caused by too much of the vitamin, and what can happen if we do not receive sufficient amounts of it; and

• *Requirements or dosages**—ranging from the minimum requirements, or RDA, for each vitamin to the therapeutic and safe maximum dosages, and, wherever appropiate, what forms are available and which is best utilized by the body.

FAT-SOLUBLE VITAMINS
Vitamin A—Retinol and Beta-Carotene
Vitamin D
Vitamin E
Vitamin F—Essential Fatty Acids
Vitamin K

Note: Potential problems of toxicity may occur with overuse of these fat-soluble vitamins, more so than with higher intakes of the water-soluble vitamins, since oil-based nutrients are more readily stored in our body tissues. The range between efficacy and toxicity, especially for vitamins A and D, is much closer than for most other essential nutrients. Thus, caution is advised in supplementing higher amounts than suggested in the following discussions of these fat-soluble vitamins.

---

*I use the term "dosage" loosely to describe the suggested amount, not to infer a likeness to pharmaceutical prescriptions. Intake levels or requirements are more accurate terms.

Vitamin A, also known as beta-carotene or retinol, is a very important vitamin. Preformed vitamin A, as is found in fish liver oil, was the first vitamin officially named and was thereby given the letter A to identify it. Retinol, another name for preformed vitamin A, was so named because of its importance in vision. The rods of the eye, which are located within the retina, contain rhodopsin, or visual purple, and need vitamin A for proper vision. Several carotene pigments found in foods, mainly yellow and orange vegetables and fruits, can be converted to vitamin A in our body and thus are termed provitamin A. Beta-carotene is the most available and also the one that yields the highest amount of A.

Vitamin A is absorbed primarily from the small intestine. Absorption of this fat-soluble vitamin is reduced with alcohol use, with vitamin E deficiency, with cortisone medication, and with excessive iron intake or the use of mineral oil, as well as with exercise. As a fat-soluble vitamin, vitamin A can be stored in the body and used when there is decreased intake. About 90 percent of the storable vitamin A is in the liver; it is also stored in the kidneys, lungs, eyes, and the fat tissue. In addition to reducing absorption, alcohol use also depletes liver stores. The storage of vitamin A is decreased during times of stress or illness unless intake is increased. The body needs the mineral zinc to help release stores of vitamin A for use.

Vitamin A is needed at a level of at least 5,000 IUs (international units) per day, though this may vary due to many factors. Deficiencies of vitamin A are still fairly common worldwide and cause many difficulties. Actually, analysis of the average American diet reveals that it provides only about 4,000 units of vitamin A daily, so the many problems of vitamin A deficiency, such as visual changes, skin dryness, and increased infections, are more common than most people realize.

BETA-CAROTENE SOURCES

Leafy and Green Vegetables

Seaweed (nori)	Kale
Mustard greens	Asparagus
Brussels sprouts	Parsley
Spinach	Lettuce
Broccoli	

Other Vegetables	Fruits
Carrots	Apricots
Sweet potatoes	Peaches
Winter squash	Mango
Yams	Cantaloupe
Pumpkin	Papaya
Red cabbage	Cherries
	Watermelon

Sources: The two forms of vitamin A come from different food sources. Preformed A (retinol) is the main animal-source vitamin A. It is found in highest concentrations in all kinds of liver and fish liver oil, which is a common source for supplements. Egg yolks and milk products, such as whole milk, cream, and butter, are also good sources of vitamin A.

Provitamin A, mainly in the form of beta-carotene, is found in a wide variety of yellow- and orange-colored fruits and vegetables, as well as leafy green vegetables. Beta-carotene is actually a double molecule of vitamin A. It may be converted to vitamin A in the upper intestine before absorption; beta-carotene can also be converted to vitamin A in the liver. People with diabetes, low thyroid activity, and those who use a lot of polyunsaturated fatty acids (PUFA) without antioxidants such as vitamin E have lowered ability to convert beta-carotene to A. Assimilation of vitamin A and the carotenes is helped by the presence of bile salts and fatty acids in the intestine.

Functions: Vitamin A performs many important functions in the human body. The following are the most common.

Eyesight. Vitamin A is needed for the formation of rhodopsin, or visual purple, which allows us to see at night. When vitamin A is lacking, there is a lag period in regenerating visual purple and a resulting inability to see well at night, termed "night blindness." Vitamin A also helps maintain the health of the cornea, the eye covering. Vitamin A deficiency may allow irritation or inflammation of the eye tissue to occur more easily.

Growth and tissue healing. This vitamin is involved in laying down new bone during growth and promoting healthy teeth. After tissue injury or surgery, vitamin A is needed for repair of the tissues and to help protect the tissues from infection.

Healthy skin. Vitamin A stimulates growth of the base layer of the skin cells. It helps the cells differentiate normally (progress from less to more mature cell forms) and gives them their structural integrity. It does this for both the external skin cells and the body's inner skin, the mucous membrane linings of the nose, eyes, intestinal tract, respiratory lining, and bladder. By this function, it also helps protect these areas from cancer cell development.

By moisturizing the mucous lining cells, which helps proper secretion, and by maintaining their structural integrity, vitamin A helps the body fight off infectious agents and environmental pollutants. The epithelial tissues protected include the linings of the lungs, nose, throat, stomach, intestines, vagina, bladder, and urinary tract, as well as the eyes and skin.

Antioxidation. Vitamin A helps protect the body (particularly cell membranes and tissue linings) from the irritating effects of free radicals (unstable molecules) by neutralizing them. Beta-carotene also protects the tissues from the toxic singlet oxygen radical. This function usually requires an amount higher than the RDA dose, perhaps 10,000–20,000 IUs per day or more. Through its antioxidant effects, vitamin A and beta-carotene help protect the body from the irritating effects of smoke and other pollutants and may also be helpful in preventing problems like ulcers, atherosclerosis and its attendant complications, such as high blood pressure and stroke.

Lowering cancer risk. As discussed previously, vitamin A helps maintain the structural integrity of cells and the healthy functioning of the mucous linings. It also helps with proper cell differentiation of the surface cells. Recently, beta-carotene was shown to improve immune response by stimulating T-helper cell activity. In these ways, it seems to prevent the development of cancer, and a number of studies have shown reduced lung and colon cancer rates in people with higher intakes of beta-carotene.

Uses: With the many functions performed by vitamin A, it has a variety of uses in basic tissue and health maintenance, in clinical treatment for a number of problems (some of which may be vitamin A deficiency symptoms), and in the prevention of many illnesses and diseases. Vitamin A works better when there are sufficient body levels of zinc and an adequate intake of protein.

Infections. Vitamin A helps in many cases to protect tissues during infections and promote rapid recovery, primarily through its support of the health of the skin and mucous lining barriers and its stimulation of mucus production. It also appears to improve antibody response and white blood cell functions. In these ways, vitamin A may be even more helpful in the prevention of infections. By keeping the mucous membranes healthy, it also helps protect against the irritating effects of smoke and pollution.

Eye problems. Vitamin A is often suggested for a variety of eye problems. Night blindness may be an early sign of vitamin A deficiency, but vitamin A functions in many ways to support the health of the eye tissue. It has been used in the treatment of conjunctivitis, blurred vision, nearsightedness, cataracts, and glaucoma, but there is no hard scientific evidence, other than anecdotal, that vitamin A works for these conditions.

Because of its beneficial effects on the skin, vitamin A is used to treat a variety of skin problems, both by local application to rashes, boils, skin ulcers, and so on, and by increased intake to help the skin's internal healing process. It may have some effect in psoriasis and in periodontal disease. Vitamin A can be supplemented for all kinds of wound healing, including before and after surgery. Its use in healing acne has been controversial, with some studies showing very good results and other studies showing no demonstrable effects. The amount used is usually about 100,000 IUs per day, as 50,000 IUs twice daily, with doses up to 300,000 IUs per day having better success. Used with 800 IUs of vitamin E daily (doesn't need to be taken at the same time as an A supplement) the vitamin E promotes the activity of vitamin A. One hundred thousand IUs of vitamin A may help alleviate severe acne in many cases. Of course, with these higher doses of vitamin A, some signs of toxicity, such as frontal headaches, can develop and should be watched. If these occur, decreasing the amount of vitamin A will usually alleviate them. Retin A, a new pharmaceutical derivative of vitamin A, appears to help reduce wrinkles (and acne) by restoring skin tissue when applied topically.

Cancer prevention. By its influence in maintaining the cell integrity of the skin and the mucous membrane linings, as in the lungs, digestive system, and urinary and genital tracts, and by its support of proper cell differentiation, vitamin A as beta-carotene has been shown to be helpful in lowering lung cancer risks. It is likely, because of its effects on epithelial cell membranes, adequate beta-carotene intake will reduce risk of many other cancers. Likewise, a deficiency of vitamin A, beta-carotene, or both, increase the risk of cancers.

Pollution protection. The antioxidant function of vitamin A helps to protect the body tissues from the irritating effects of stress, smoke, air pollution, and chemical exposure.

Other uses. Vitamin A has also been tried with some success in treating a variety of other problems, including asthma, fibrocystic breast disease, plantar warts, sebaceous cysts, ulcers, and premenstrual syndrome. In fibrocystic problems, one small study showed a reduction in breast pain and lumps with 150,000 IUs daily, used under medical supervision.

Deficiency and toxicity: A number of difficulties can arise from a deficiency of vitamin A, many of which are based on impairments in the biochemical functions that this important nutrient performs. It is estimated that the diets of approximately 25 percent of the people in the United States are supplying less than the RDA for vitamin A. This commonly occurs in those who avoid the carotene-containing fruits and vegetables or when the diet is filled with processed foods that are depleted of vitamins. The fruits and vegetables are really the most important food groups for intake of the many vitamins and minerals, as well as for fiber and water content. The elderly, teenagers, and alcoholics are the three groups most commonly deficient in vitamin A. Worldwide, vitamin A deficiency is even more common than it is in the United States.

Night blindness, the inability to adapt the eyes to see clearly in the dark, is probably one of the first signs of vitamin A deficiency. Lack of general eye tissue health and vitality may occur, as can decreased vision, irritated, reddened, or dry eyes, and eyes that tire easily; in severe deficiency states, corneal ulcers may develop. Usually, supplemental vitamin A or beta-carotene will correct these problems; the RDA of vitamin A will prevent night blindness and these other eye problems.

Perhaps of greater significance, vitamin A and beta-carotene deficiencies may decrease our protection against infectious agents and the internal process of carcinogenesis. A depletion or deficiency of vitamin A reduces both T lymphocyte (cellular immunity) and B lymphocyte (antibody production) responses; severe vitamin A deficiency has been shown to cause atrophy of the thymus and spleen, both immunologically important organs, and to reduce the number of circulating lymphocytes. Low dietary levels of vitamin A have been associated with an increased risk of many cancers, including breast, cervical, lung, prostate, laryngeal, and stomach cancers, while beta-carotene deficiency has been clearly seen in patients with cancers of the cervix or lungs.

Vitamin A deficiency also affects the skin. Dry, bumpy skin may occur, especially on the backs of the arms. Since vitamin A promotes skin growth, moisture retention, and proper cell differentiation, a deficiency causes decreased skin tone and rapid aging of the skin and a variety of blemishes, acne, or boils. Vitamin A supports the mucous-secreting cells of the internal mucous membranes. Mucus protects these membranes from infection and irritants. When vitamin A is deficient, these internal epithelial cells secrete a protein (keratin) commonly found externally in hair and nails. This keratinization process makes the epithelial cells harder and dryer and thus less protecting.

Vitamin A along with adequate protein intake generates healthy hair. With a lack of A, the hair may lack luster and dandruff is more likely because of the loss of scalp skin moisture. Bone softness or abnormal menstruation may also develop from vitamin A deficiency. Fatigue and insomnia are also possible, as are a decrease in the appetite and some loss of smell and taste. When vitamin A is deficient, vitamin C seems to be lost more rapidly from the body. In addition to the lowered immune function and increased infection rate associated with vitamin A deficiency, periodontal disease, kidney stone formation, ear problems, and acne may occur more frequently.

A number of toxicity symptoms and difficulties may occur when we take too much vitamin A. Since it is stored in the body and is not readily excreted, toxicity may occur from mildly increased doses (say 50,000–100,000 IUs per day) over an extended time, such as a month or two, or from very high doses over a shorter period. Animal liver meats have the highest concentrations of vitamin A; beef liver has about 15,000 IUs per ounce, while polar bear liver has much higher concentrations than this and has been known to cause vitamin A toxicity from one serving. It is highly unlikely that one would get vitamin A toxicity from the diet alone (without lots of liver), since we receive much of it which must then be converted to active vitamin A. The synthetic vitamin A supplements, such as the palmitate or acetate forms, have a greater potential to produce toxic symptoms; high amounts of fish liver oil may produce side effects as well. The levels that cause symptoms vary from person to person, just as the proper optimum dosage does. Under high levels of stress, with illness or trauma, if we smoke or live in a polluted environment, or if we are pregnant or nursing, our vitamin A requirements are higher. When there is depletion or deficiency of vitamin A, higher amounts can be taken for up to a month without the usual risks of toxicity.

The only problem that may arise from high amounts of beta-carotene, as can occur with a high intake of yellow and orange fruits and vegetables and the leafy greens, is an orange-yellow discoloring of the skin. This occurs occasionally when people drink large amounts of carrot juice daily over time. It is of no real consequence and will clear when there is a reduction in carotene intake. Carotenosis can be differentiated from jaundice somewhat by the color and also by the fact that the white parts of the eyes do not turn color as they do with jaundice.

Too much vitamin A intake, however, can lead to slight swelling of the brain and resulting pressure headaches, which may be described as the feeling of a tight band around the forehead. Nausea and vomiting may also occur, as can irritability, dizziness, abdominal pain, and hair loss. Itchy, flaky, or dry skin can also result from too much vitamin A. Anorexia (loss of appetite) and resulting weight loss, liver enlargement, menstrual problems, bone abnormalities or stunted growth, and dry or bleeding lips may also occur. There may be an

RDAS FOR VITAMIN A (in IUS)

Infants	Under 1 year	1,500–2,000
Children	1–3 years	2,000–2,500
	4–6 years	2,500–3,000
	7–10 years	3,000–3,500
Males	11 years & up	5,000–6,000
Females	11 years & up	4,000–5,000
	Pregnant	5,000–6,000
	Lactating	6,000–7,000

increased risk of birth defects in pregnant women taking high amounts of vitamin A, say over 400 IUs per pound of body weight. (To be safe, I suggest that pregnant women limit their preformed vitamin A to 15,000 IUs, with additional amounts taken only as beta-carotene.) Children have lower requirements, and toxicity has been seen in babies given adult doses of vitamin A, 20,000–30,000 IUs per day.

Requirements: The Recommended Daily Allowance (RDA)—that is, the minimum dietary or supplemental amount to prevent vitamin A deficiency—is approximately 5,000 IUs per day for the adult. About 10,000–15,000 IUs of beta-carotene will probably convert to about 5,000 IUs of vitamin A in the body. Approximately two medium-sized carrots will give us that daily amount. Since this vitamin is fat soluble and stored in the body, daily sources are not absolutely necessary. Requirements, however, depend on body weight, so larger people need more A. Vitamin A needs are also increased with illness, infection, trauma, anxiety or stress, pregnancy, lactation, and alcohol use or smoking.

Approximately 10,000 IUs should be the average adult intake and is a safe amount to consume. The RDA amount will prevent most deficiency symptoms, such as night blindness, but for vitamin A's antioxidant properties, higher amounts are needed. About 20,000–30,000 IUs daily, preferably as beta-carotene, may be the best range, especially for those of us with some levels of anxiety and stress. If

vitamins C and E are used, slightly lower amounts of A are needed, since C and E help prevent the loss of stored vitamin A.

The upper intake, including diet and supplemental vitamin A, ranges from 50,000–100,000 IUs per day for short periods of a week or two. However, these amounts often produce some side effects over time. If no body deficiency or increased body needs of vitamin A are present, 50,000 IUs can cause problems. Infants and children can run into difficulty with doses as low as 10,000–25,000 IUs given over time, depending on their size. This is why it is important to know our food sources and supplement levels of preformed vitamin A (not beta-carotene, which is safe at higher levels), so that we can find the right amounts for each of us and our families.

 Vitamin D (Calciferol) refers to several related fat-soluble vitamin variants, all of which are sterol (cholesterol-like) substances. D_2, or activated ergocalciferol, is the major synthetic form of provitamin D; D_3, or cholecalciferol, is found in animals, mainly in fish liver oils. These are converted in the liver and kidneys to 25-hydroxycholecalciferol, and 1, 25-dihydroxylcholecalciferol, the major circulating active forms of vitamin D.

Vitamin D is also known as the "sunshine" vitamin because it is actually manufactured in the human skin when in contact with the ultraviolet light in the sun's rays. The sunlight interacts with 7-dehydrocholesterol to form cholecalciferol, which is then transferred to the liver or kidneys and converted to active vitamin D. Wintertime, clouds, smog, and darkly pigmented skin reduce the body's production of the "sunshine" vitamin.

This fat-soluble vitamin, when ingested, is absorbed through the intestinal walls with other fats with the aid of bile. Mineral oil binds vitamin D in the gut and reduces its absorption. From the blood, calciferol is taken mainly to the liver, where it is utilized or stored. Vitamin D is also stored in the skin, brain, spleen, and bones. Vitamin D intake must be more finely tuned in regard to the right therapeutic level than most other vitamins, and it is considered by many authorities to be the most potentially toxic vitamin. Symptoms of vitamin D toxicity can easily occur when vitamin D is taken in large amounts or with excessive sun exposure. (It is possible that part of sun poisoning symptoms are due to vitamin D toxicity.)

Sources: Provitamin D is found mainly in animal foods. D_3, or "natural" vitamin D, is found in fish liver oil, which is the traditional source of both A and D. Cod liver oil is a commonly used source. Egg yolks, butter, and liver have some D, as do the oily fish, such as mackerel, salmon, sardines, and herring. Most homogenized milk and some breakfast cereals are "fortified" with synthetic vitamin D to give children, particularly, sufficient amounts. The plant foods are fairly low in D, with mushrooms and dark leafy greens containing some. Strict vegetarians who do not get adequate exposure to sunlight need to be concerned about getting their 400 IUs of vitamin D daily.

Functions: Vitamin D helps to regulate calcium metabolism and normal calcification of the bones in the body as well as influencing our utilization of the mineral phosphorus. Calcium and phosphorus together with other minerals make up our bones. Vitamin D_3 helps increase the absorption of calcium from the gut, decreases excretion from the kidneys, stimulates resorption of calcium and phosphorus from bone, helps put them into teeth, and helps to maintain normal blood levels of calcium and phosphorus. With these functions, vitamin D is closely tied to the work of the parathyroid glands. Vitamin D is most important in regulating calcium metabolism in the body. Even with adequate calcium and phosphorus intake, if our vitamin D intake is low, we will have poor calcification of our bones; whereas, with good vitamin D intake,

we will have better calcification even with low calcium and phosphorus intake. This function is especially important in menopausal women, for whom many doctors prescribe straight calcium without vitamin D, which is not likely to do much good unless they are sunbathing, an activity that doctors no longer recommend. Actually, taking calcium, magnesium, and vitamin D all together is probably ideal for best bone health. Phosphorus is usually readily available in adequate amounts in most diets.

Because of its regulation of calcium and phosphorus metabolism, vitamin D is very important to growth in children, especially to healthy bones and teeth. It is also helpful in maintaining the nervous system, heart function, and for normal blood clotting—all of which are affected by calcium levels.

Vitamin D works together with parathyroid hormone for calcium metabolism. Functionally, vitamin D is actually more like a hormone than a vitamin; it is produced in one part of the body (the skin) and released into the blood to affect other tissues (the bones). There is a feedback system with the parathyroid to produce active vitamin D_3 when the body needs it, and this "vitamin" is closely related structurally to the body hormones estrogen and cortisone.

Again, vitamin D regulates bone formation. If D is low, blood levels of calcium and phosphorus decrease, and the body pulls these minerals from the bones. This creates demineralized, weak bones, a condition called osteomalacia (loss of bone mineral), or adult rickets. Osteoporosis involves loss of bone mass (minerals and proteins together). The decreased level of calcium in the blood also affects the heart and nervous system.

Uses: Vitamin D works best with adequate calcium and phosphorus intake. It is supplied primarily to prevent or to cure rickets, the vitamin D deficiency disease. It also is used to maintain healthy bones and dentition, as D is helpful in preventing tooth decay and gum problems. Calciferol supplementation may be used to aid the healing of fractures, osteoporosis, and other bone problems.

Taking vitamin D with vitamin A has been shown in some studies to reduce the incidence of colds. It has also been used in the treatment of diabetes, cataracts, visual problems, allergies, sciatica pain, and skin problems. Some success in treating myopia (nearsightedness) and conjunctivitis has been had with high doses of vitamin D. Vitamins A and D together have helped muscle spasms, especially when related to anxiety states. A and D have been used in the treatment of asthma and arthritis as well. Menopausal symptoms such as hot flashes and depression have been helped by the use of calcium and vitamin D together. However, other than the use in menopause, these other applications of vitamin D are not very common in recent years. Medically, high vitamin D supplementation is used to treat hypocalcemia (low blood calcium) secondary to such problems as hypoparathyroidism, which may occur after thyroid surgery.

Deficiency and toxicity: There are some toxicity problems related to hypervitaminosis D. These usually occur with high doses of more than 1,000–1,500 IUs daily for a month or longer in adults, more than 400 IUs in infants, or more than 600 IUs daily in children. These are not exact numbers, of course, and may vary between individuals, time of year, and specific needs; however, it is wise to be careful with supplemental vitamin D. I personally think the combination 1,000 IU D/ 25,000 IU A formulas are potential trouble if taken at all regularly. However, if some people have poor fat digestion and assimilation, they may handle higher amounts of oral vitamin D.

Excessive thirst, diarrhea, nausea, weakness, and headaches are the milder symptoms of vitamin D toxicity. There are also increased levels of calcium and phosphorus in the blood and urine, and abnormal calcification of soft tissues may occur. There is some suggestion that excess vitamin D speeds the atherosclerosis process. Most symptoms decrease and clear up after excessive doses of vitamin D are discontinued. Toxic doses of vitamin D can be made by the skin through prolonged sun exposure, especially before the body has adapted through pigmentation (tanning), which protects the deeper layers where the vitamin D is synthesized. I have personally wondered if the weakness, nausea, dizziness, or headaches from sun exposure may be related to vitamin D toxicity.

Most people do not take very large amounts of supplemental vitamin D but make sufficient amounts through the skin from exposure to the sun. There is more concern with toxicity from the fortified vitamin D, especially in milk. This synthetic, irradiated ergocalciferol (D_2) has decreased the incidence of rickets, but it may be contributing to calcification of the arteries, or atherosclerosis, from infancy through old age. The added 400 IUs per quart of milk is about 15 times the amount normally found in milk and may increase the amount of calcium in the circulation, which could be a problem.

Deficiency of vitamin D has not been a major problem of late. Older people are more prone to vitamin D deficiency (a blood level can be measured) since their skin production is lower, their digestion and absorption may be diminished, and their liver function may be reduced. Vitamin D may be deficient in people with gastrointestinal disease, such as ulcerative colitis. The sun's action on the skin to produce vitamin D is inhibited by pollution, clouds, clothing, window glass, skin pigmentation, and sunscreens. The occurrence of several of these factors together may make the development of the symptoms of rickets more likely.

The decreased absorption of calcium, along with the retention of phosphorus that usually accompanies it, leads to poor mineralization of bone and the inability of the bones to handle stress. This problem, called osteomalacia, is manifested by poor calcification and soft bones. Vitamin D deficiency in the elderly increases general bone loss and osteoporosis. Supplementing this vitamin improves calcium absorption and reduces bone loss. In children, the bone disorder from vitamin D deficiency is rickets. It is characterized by soft skull bones and fragility of other bones, with bowing of the legs, spinal curvature, and an increase in the size of the joints, such as the wrists, ankles, and knees. Muscular development may be diminished as well. Because of low calcium availability, the teeth may have poor structure, and there may be muscle spasms from a problem called tetany, which also causes tingling and weakness of the areas affected. Nearsightedness and loss of hearing may also develop from vitamin D deficiency because of the vitamin's influence on the eye muscles and from loss of calcium in the ear bones. Furthermore, one of the current theories of multiple sclerosis is that it may be influenced by low vitamin D levels in puberty.

Requirements: Vitamin D is best utilized with vitamin A. Most of our calciferol needs are met with some vitamin D in foods and regular sunlight exposure. If we live in smoggy cities or where tall buildings block the sunlight, we may need more vitamin D. Those who have darkly pigmented skin, work nights, or cover their bodies with lots of clothes, as do members of some religious orders, probably need more vitamin D than the avid sunbather. In winter, we usually require more D from supplements or from our foods.

The RDA for vitamin D is 400 IUs, or roughly 10 mcg., per day. Infants and growing children probably need more vitamin D relative to body size than do adults. During pregnancy and lactation, more D is needed than the 400 IUs. Therapeutic doses for problems treated with vitamin D are about 1,000–1,500 IUs maximum per day, though some doctors may prescribe even more, mainly of the natural vitamin D_3. In general, however, it is wise for adults to limit any supplemented vitamin D to the 400 IUs per day commonly found in multivitamins and to limit use of vitamin-D-fortified milk for a variety of reasons.

 Vitamin E (Tocopherol) is a light yellow oil, a fat-soluble vitamin, that is actually a family of compounds, the tocopherols, found in nature. Alphatoxopherol is the most common and the most active of the seven currently described forms—alpha, beta, gamma, delta, epsilon, and zeta. Specifically, d-alpha tocopherol is the most potent form, more active than the synthetic dl-alpha tocopherol.

Vitamin E was discovered in 1922 with experiments on rats. When fed a purified diet devoid of vitamin E, the rats became infertile. Wheat germ oil added to their diet restored their fertility. Later, the oil-based substance was isolated and called the "antisterility" vitamin. (*Tokos* and *phero* are the Greek words for "offspring" and "to bear," so tocopherol literally means "to bear children.") Though there is no clear deficiency disease in humans, vitamin E is well accepted as an essential vitamin. There is some question, however, as to whether vitamin E is needed for fertility. From general public experience, though, it seems to be clear that vitamin E makes a difference to many. The average diet today contains much less natural vitamin E than it did 50 years ago; we will see soon why, and what vitamin E actually does in the body.

Alpha-tocopherol is basically stable in heat and in acids; other forms are lost in heat, with storage or freezing, or when oxidized by exposure to the air. All vitamin Es are slightly unstable in alkali and are readily used up when in contact with polyunsaturated oils or rancid fats and oils, which are protected from oxidative destruction by vitamin E. Frying oils, the processing and milling of foods, the bleaching of flours, and cooking remove much of the vitamin E content of whole foods. During the refinement and purification of vegetable oils, vitamin E is lost; the vitamin E-rich by-products of this process are used to make some of the E used in supplements.

Vitamin E is absorbed from the intestines,

along with fat and bile salts, first into the lymph and then into the blood, which carries it to the liver to be used or stored. Vitamin E is not stored in the body as effectively as the other fat-soluble vitamins, A, D, and K. Over half of any excesses may be lost in the feces, but some vitamin E is stored in the fatty tissues and the liver and to a lesser degree in the heart, muscles, testes, uterus, adrenal and pituitary glands, and in the blood. Vitamin E is partially absorbed through the skin when used as an ointment or oil application. Intestinal absorption, however, is reduced somewhat with chlorine, inorganic iron, and mineral oil. Unsaturated oils and estrogen also deplete vitamin E, increasing the body's demand for it.

Sources: Vitamin E, as its various tocopherol forms, is found in both plant and animal foods. In general, the animal sources of E are fairly poor, with some being found in butter, egg yolk, milk fat, and liver. The best sources of vitamin E are the vegetable and seed or nut oils. It was first isolated from wheat germ oil, which is still a commonly used, rich source of vitamin E.

The oil component of all grains, seeds, and nuts contain tocopherol. The protective covering or germ part of the grains is what contains the E, and this is lost easily in the milling of flour or in the refinement of grains. For the vitamin E to be preserved, extraction of the oils from nuts and seeds must be done naturally, as by cold pressing, rather than by heat or chemical extraction, used commonly in food processing. Because of these forms of processing, the average American diet has lost many of its natural sources of tocopherols, and intake is commonly very low. The cold-pressed vegetable oils are really the best source of vitamin E, and these are most healthfully used in their raw form in salad dressings and sauces rather than in cooking, since most are polyunsaturated oils, which are adversely affected by heating. With refined or cooked polyunsaturates, more vitamin E is needed to prevent oxidation, which could lead to free radical for-

mation, the invisible, underlying cause of many diseases. Free-radical-induced changes occur at the cellular level, the primary processes leading to many chronic degenerative diseases. The vitamin E content of most foods is related to the content of linoleic and linolenic acids, our most essential fatty acids (see Chapter 4, as well as *Vitamin F*). Also, the content of active alpha-tocopherol varies among the different foods and oils. Safflower oil is one of the best sources, with about 90 percent of the E being the alpha variety. Corn oil has only about 10 percent alpha-tocopherol. Some other foods that contain significant amounts of vitamin E are soybeans, some margarines and shortenings made from vegetable oils, and a few vegetables, such as uncooked green peas, spinach, asparagus, kale, and cucumber; tomato and celery also have a little.

Functions: The primary function of vitamin E is as an antioxidant, which is very important, I believe, in our present-day society with widespread pollution, processed food diets, and chemical exposure. Vitamin E is protective because it helps reduce oxidation of lipid membranes and the unsaturated fatty acids and prevents the breakdown of other nutrients by oxygen. This protective, nutritional antioxidant function is also performed and enhanced by other antioxidants, such as vitamin C, beta-carotene, glutathione (L-cysteine), and the mineral selenium. Oxidation in our body of such substances as the fat molecules, particularly from polyunsaturated fats, and from eating other oxidized fats such as hydrogenated oils and rancid oils, causes the genesis of free radicals, unstable molecules that can lead to cellular and tissue irritation and damage, which leads to chronic inflammation, especially in the vascular lining. Excess free radical formation comes from a variety of chemical reactions in the body and is the biochemical basis of many diseases, such as atherosclerosis, heart disease, hypertension, arthritis, senility, and probably even cancer. A number of experiments have shown that the antioxidant nutrients such as vitamin E can protect the tissues from oxidation and free radicals.

Without vitamin E, cell membranes, active enzyme sites, and DNA are less protected from free radical damage. Oxidation by circulating peroxides and superoxides (two types of free radicals) is also reduced by enzymes such as *glutathione peroxidase and superoxide dismutase*. As does vitamin E, these antioxidant enzymes also protect, by indirect mechanisms, the polyunsaturated fatty acids and vitamin A from oxidative destruction. Fried foods have more oxidized fat by-products, which increase the requirement for vitamin E, but they do not contain any E. This is partly why they are so dangerous when consumed on a regular basis.

More specifically, vitamin E as an antioxidant helps to stabilize cell membranes and protect the tissues of the skin, eyes, liver, breast, and testes, which are more sensitive to oxidation. It protects the lungs from oxidative damage from environmental substances. And vitamin E helps maintain the biological activity of vitamin A, another very important oil-soluble vitamin. Vitamin E protects the unsaturated fatty acids in the body and prevents the oxidation of some hormones, such as those released from the pituitary and adrenal glands. Free radical formation and oxidation are tied to cancer development, so the family of nutritional antioxidants, including vitamin E, may help in preventing tumor growth. More definitive research is needed in regard to this important function.

In simple terms, vitamin E's key function is to modify and stabilize blood fats so that the blood vessels, heart, and entire body are more protected from free-radical-induced injury. Vitamin E also has some anticlotting (antithrombotic) properties and protects the red blood cells' membranes from oxidative damage. Because it helps heart and muscle cell respiration by improving their functioning with less oxygen, vitamin E may help improve stamina and endurance and reduce cardiovas-

cular disease (CVD) risk, especially in those with already existing CVD. Vitamin E has recently been shown to reduce platelet aggregation and platelet adhesiveness to collagen, even more so than aspirin. These platelet functions are linked to an increased risk of atherosclerosis and cardiovascular disease, especially in high-risk groups. Vitamin E has also been shown to neutralize free radicals generated during surgery, particularly cardiopulmonary bypass surgery. It would also protect against the toxicity of some of the gases used in anesthesia.

Although vitamin E was first discovered as the fertility, or at least the antisterility, nutrient, there is no clear evidence that it enhances fertility if there is not a specific deficiency prior to its use. Many people, especially men, take vitamin E with some claimed success in regard to sexuality and vitality. Much of this effect, however, may be due to the antioxidant function and improved circulation and oxygenation.

Uses: There is quite an extensive list of uses for this popular nutrient, most commonly in the middle-aged and older populations. And there are many positive effects. Some of these claims are backed by good research, and more investigation is being done on vitamin E by medical and nutritional scientists. There is hope that the results of this research will enable us to better understand its mechanisms and apply them most effectively to prevent and treat our industrial-age medical conditions.

The antioxidant function that we have discussed gives vitamin E a variety of uses. The protection of cells and tissues against oxidation and injury from unstable molecules, pollution, and fats may also be the basis for the prevention of aging and many chronic diseases. Claims about vitamin E's role in preventing premature aging and promoting longevity are big areas of investigation for vitamin E researchers. These claims are often made and with some good reason. Aging, tissue degeneration, and skin changes may be

103

brought about by the damage that free radicals cause to cells unprotected by antioxidant nutrients in the body. Cancer and heart and vascular disease may also be created in this way, and vitamin E therapy may help reduce the risks of these major illnesses. Decreased blood clotting and increased tissue oxygenation may also help reduce symptoms of heart and vascular limitations, such as angina pectoris, intermittent claudication (leg pain with walking due to insufficiency of blood and oxygen, for which vitamin E has clearly been helpful), and problems of arterial spasm. In both congenital and rheumatic heart diseases, vitamin E may help reduce symptoms caused by impaired tissue oxygenation.

Vitamin E may be of help in the prevention of atherosclerosis. Its antioxidant effect reduces thrombin formation and thus helps decrease blood clotting, and it also appears to minimize platelet (blood-clotting component) aggregation and stickiness, aspects that either generate or perpetuate the atherosclerotic process. Vitamin E was thought to raise HDL ("good") cholesterol levels, especially when they were low; however, recent research suggests it has a very mild, if any, effect in this regard. Vitamin A and E together can help to decrease cholesterol and general fat accumulation. To assist in healing and to minimize clotting, tocopherol is a useful nutrient before and after surgery, but is limited to dosages of 200–300 IUs per day (higher amounts may actually suppress the healing process). Also, pre- and postsurgery, vitamin E neutralizes free radical formation and thus reduces possible problems from that. Recently, this antioxidant effect of vitamin E was shown in cardiopulmonary bypass surgery. In regard to its healing powers, vitamin E is used most commonly both internally and externally to assist in the repair of skin lesions, ulcers, burns, abrasions, and dry skin and to heal and/or diminish the scars caused from injury or surgery. (Vitamin A also appears to work in this regard, possibly even better than E in some

POSSIBLE USES OF ORAL VITAMIN E

Muscle cramps
Osteoarthritis
Diabetes
Dermatitis
Menstrual pain
Peptic ulcers
Menopause
Shingles
Cataract prevention
Vascular fragility
Miscarriage prevention
Wound healing
Impotence
Autoimmune diseases
Premenstrual syndrome
Viral disease
Anemia
Herpes infection
Periodontal disease
Cancer
Intermittent claudication
Fibrocystic breast disease
Cerebral thrombosis prevention
Surgery, especially cardiovascular
Protects against toxic effects
    of smoke, alcohol, ozone,
    estrogen, and adriamycin

POSSIBLE USES OF TOPICAL VITAMIN E

Wound healing
Herpes infections
Lupus rash
Skin ulcers
Dermatitis

instances where skin and tissue healing are needed.) Decreasing scars internally may be important in resolving damage from inflammation of blood vessels and may reduce the potential for clotting and thrombophlebitis. Vitamin E, with the help of vitamins C and P (bioflavonoids), may be useful in preventing progression of varicose veins, more so than treating them once they have occurred.

Vitamin E may be very helpful to women. Research shows relief from menstrual pains, as well as general relief from various menstrual disorders. Many problems of menopause, such as headaches, hot flashes, or vaginal itching due to dryness, may be reduced with the use of supplemental vitamin E. When birth control pills are used, the tocopherols may help protect the body from their possible side effects. Estrogen may decrease the effect of vitamin E, so more is needed when estrogen therapy is used. Vitamin E has been used both topically and orally with some success in the treatment of fibrocystic breast disease, or cystic mastitis, likely due to its protective mechanisms against estrogen, which seems to potentiate this disease.

Vitamin E's antioxidant functions help to protect our cell membranes and lung tissue from pollution, particularly from ozone (O_3) and nitrogen dioxide (NO_2) in the air. Research in rats clearly showed their ability to tolerate increased ozone levels and to survive much longer with vitamin E. There is also some cardiac protection from smoke and alcohol with vitamin E, and it protects against the cardio-toxic effects of adriamycin, an anticancer drug.

Vitamin E has also been used to enhance immunity in the treatment of viral illness and to reduce the neurologic pain from shingles, a viral infection of the nerves and skin. It is also helpful in preventing eye problems, such as poor vision or cataracts, that may be due to oxidation of fatty tissues and free radical formation leading to areas of inflammatory damage. Headaches may sometimes be helped with tocopherol treatment, depending on the cause. Various kidney and liver diseases and muscular dystrophy have all been treated with vitamin E, though more immediate inflammatory problems, as in bursitis, gout, and arthritis seem to benefit more. Leg cramps and

circulatory problems associated with diabetes may be helped with vitamin E treatment. For various skin rashes, including those of lupus erythematosus, vitamin E, usually along with vitamin A, may be of some help.

Deficiency and toxicity: Vitamin E is not stored as readily as are the other fat-soluble vitamins. Excess intake is usually eliminated in the urine and feces, and most doses clear the body within a few days. For these reasons, toxicity from vitamin E use is unlikely. In animal studies, very high amounts of E have been shown to retard growth and decrease muscle tissue, decrease the red blood count, and cause poor bone calcification, though in humans these seem more likely to be signs of E deficiency. High intakes of the vitamin E oil can cause nausea, diarrhea, or flatulence in some people.

Large doses of vitamin E are generally avoided for people with high blood pressure as it has been thought to raise blood pressure, though this has not been easily reproduced experimentally. Usually, though, 400–600 IUs daily (the nonoily, water-dispersible vitamin E succinate may be preferable for patients with hypertension) can provide some antioxidant and circulatory benefits without increasing blood pressure. It is possible that large doses of vitamin E (over 1,200 IUs), may have a mild immune-suppressing effect; smaller doses seem to be immune supportive. There is also some concern about using higher doses of vitamin E in people with rheumatic heart disease and administering it to people undergoing digitalis or anticoagulant therapy, as vitamin E may increase the anticoagulant effects of these medicines. Its effects on blood clotting must be watched carefully in such cases. Vitamin E does not contribute to blood clots or abnormal lipid patterns as is sometimes thought.

Vitamin E deficiency is fairly rare with vague symptoms that are difficult to diagnose, causing some question as to its importance since there is no clear deficiency disease in humans as there is with deficiency of vitamin C or many of the B vitamins. Infertility as an effect of vitamin E deficiency has not been revealed as clearly in humans as it was in the rat study. It is likely that vitamin E deficiency is simply more difficult to diagnose symptomatically because of its wide range of effects on the nervous, reproductive, muscular, and circulatory systems and because other nutrients may mask vitamin E deficiencies. However, biochemically, low levels of vitamin E can be measured in the blood and have been seen in such conditions as acne, anemia, infections, some cancers, periodontal disease, cholesterol gallstones, neuromuscular diseases, and dementias such as Alzheimer's disease.

Deficiencies are more of a concern in premature babies, since there is no maternal-fetal vitamin E transfer; vitamin E depletion may also appear in newborns fed on cow's milk, which contains no vitamin E, instead of breast milk, which does contain some if the mother's diet is healthy. Deficiency is also more likely in adults with gastrointestinal disease, with poor fat digestion and metabolism, or with pancreatic insufficiency.

Iron, especially the inorganic form, depletes vitamin E absorption in the small intestine. The two should not be taken together, as this causes the absorption of both to be diminished. Chlorine, ferric chloride, and rancid oils also deplete or destroy vitamin E.

The first sign of vitamin E deficiency may be loss of red blood cells due to fragility caused by the loss of cell membrane protection. Oxidized polyunsaturated fatty acids may also weaken the red blood cell membranes and cause rupture. The generalized decrease in cell and tissue protection from free radical molecules may lead to abnormal fat deposits in muscles, muscle wasting, and problems in the kidneys and liver because of the circulating dead cells and toxins released. Men may have changes in the testicular tissue with vitamin E deficiency.

With increased oxidation, there is an increased requirement for vitamin E. Vitamin E deficiency may lead to free radical effects on the unsaturated fatty acids, inhibiting their functions in the health of cell membranes and tissues. Pituitary and adrenal function may be lowered, as these glands may suffer from the cumulative effects of oxidation. Degenerative changes produced by deficiency of vitamin E may not be corrected by vitamin E therapy.

There is some question as to whether tocopherol ("to bear children") deficiency reduces the ability to carry pregnancy to term and increases the likelihood of premature birth or causes problems in infants. Is it related to increased heart disease or atherosclerosis or even cancer? Surely, there is a lot more to learn about vitamin E.

Requirements: The amount of vitamin E required depends upon body size and the amount of polyunsaturated fats in the diet, since vitamin E is needed to protect these fats from oxidation. More is needed when any refined oils, fried foods, or rancid oils are consumed. Supplemental estrogen or estrogen imbalance in women increases the need for vitamin E, as does air pollution. And, as I have mentioned, vitamin E should not be taken with iron, especially inorganic iron, such as ferrous sulfate or the iron added to food products. Selenium, another important antioxidant, however, may increase the potency of vitamin E.

Even though the RDA for vitamin E is really quite low, many people do not consume this in their diet alone.

For the d-alpha tocopheral form of this vitamin, 1 mg. equals 1.49 IUs. The different forms of vitamin E have various potencies, with d-alpha the most active and most prevalent in nature. Vitamin E extraction, purity, and activity also vary. The best forms, in my opinion, are those that contain the natural, unesterified d-alpha tocopherol along with the other (beta, gamma, and delta) naturally occurring tocopherols. This type of E is not

RDAS FOR VITAMIN E (IN IUS)

	Conservative	*Liberal*
Infants	5–7	30
Children	8–12	30
Adolescents	12–15	30–50
Adult males	15	100
Adult females	12	50–100
Pregnant	15	100
Lactating	18	100

easy to find because it is more difficult and costly to produce. The vitamin E palmitates and acetates are synthetic water-dispersible forms of vitamin E that have a good level of activity and are often easier to take, as they can be taken with other vitamins. Vitamin E oil is taken ideally in the morning before breakfast or at night before bed. It can also be taken after meals containing some fat. Approximately 400–600 IUs is used preventively, whereas for therapeutic effects, an amount between 800–1600 IUs daily is suggested. With therapeutic uses of vitamin E, it is best to start with a low level and gradually increase it. Levels over 1,600 IUs per day are not recommended unless there is close medical supervision.

 Vitamin F (Essential Fatty Acids) The unsaturated or essential fatty acids in our diet come primarily from liquid vegetable oils. Some of these contain vitamin E as well, which protects them from oxidation. There are two essential fatty acids which the body does not make and thus must be obtained from the diet (many sources state three, but arachidonic can be made from linoleic acid in humans). These are linoleic (LA) and linolenic (LNA) acids, found mainly in seeds, wheat germ, cod liver oil, and the golden vegetable oils, such as soy, safflower, and corn. Flaxseed (linseed) oil is probably our best oil, being particularly high in both omega-3 as alpha-linolenic acid and

omega-6 fatty acids in the right balance for us. Evening primrose oil is high specifically in gamma-linolenic acid, an omega-6 fatty acid, and the fish oils are high in omega-3 fatty acids, particularly eicosapentaenoic acid (EPA).

The essential fatty acids (EFAs) are very important to the body for cell and organ respiration and to add resiliency and lubrication to the tissues. It is thought that the EFAs can increase the solubility of cholesterol deposited in the arterial walls and can support adrenal and thyroid gland activity. A relative increase in intake of the EFA oils (the polyunsaturates) in proportion to the saturated animal fats will help reduce blood cholesterol, an important factor in reducing the risk of cardiovascular disease. Linolenic acid is the most important EFA in humans. This omega-3 fatty acid is the precursor of the protective oils now known to be found in fish and flaxseed. Linolenic and the other omega-3 fatty acids are thought to be needed in a 2:1 ratio over the omega-6 fatty acids, including those derived from linoleic acid. Linolenic is also essential and is found in most vegetable oils, however, higher amounts of this fatty acid, which is the precursor of arachidonic acid, may be more inflammatory than linolenic acid. This is especially true when vitamins A and E are depleted.

Deficiency of the EFAs can reduce growth and skin, tissue, and joint lubrication. Low levels in the body have been seen in such conditions as prostate enlargement, psoriasis, anorexia nervosa, hyperactivity, and multiple sclerosis. Deficiency problems of EFAs may include acne, diarrhea, dry skin, eczema, alopecia (hair loss), gallstones, and slow growth and wound healing.

Vitamin F has been used in the treatment of eczema, psoriasis, skin allergies, prostatitis, and asthma. It is required in amounts equaling in at least 2 percent of caloric intake, 1–2 teaspoons a day depending on weight. (The essential fatty acids are discussed in more detail in Chapter 4, *Lipids.*)

Vitamin K, a group of three related substances, is the last of the fat-soluble vitamins, completing the family that also includes vitamins A, D, E, and F. This nutrient, both found in nature and made in the body, helps bloodclotting, or coagulation, in humans. Phylloquinone, the natural vitamin K found in alfalfa and other foods, was discovered in Denmark and labeled vitamin K for the Danish word Koagulation. Food-source phylloquinone is termed K_1, while the menaquinone produced by our intestinal bacteria is labeled vitamin K_2. A synthetic compound with the basic structure of the quinones is menadione, or vitamin K_3. It has twice the activity of the natural Ks and is used therapeutically in people who may not use natural vitamin K well, such as those with decreased bile acid secretion.

All vitamin K variants are fat soluble and stable to heat. Alkalis, strong acids, radiation, and oxidizing agents can destroy vitamin K. It is absorbed from the upper small intestine with the help of bile or bile salts and pancreatic juices and then carried to the liver for the synthesis of prothrombin, a key blood-clotting factor. High intake (as with supplementation) of vitamin E or calcium may reduce vitamin K absorption. Vitamin K is stored in small amounts; most is excreted after therapeutic doses.

Yogurt, kefir, and acidophilus milk may help to increase the functioning of the intestinal bacterial flora and therefore contribute to vitamin K production. Antibiotics that reduce these bacteria will diminish vitamin K synthesis in the colon. Rancid oils and fats, X-rays, radiation, aspirin, air pollution, and freezing of foods all destroy vitamin K, and mineral oil binds with K and rapidly eliminates it from the intestines.

Sources: Vitamin K is found in both plant and animal sources in nature. Good supplies are found in the dark leafy greens, most green plants, alfalfa, and kelp. Blackstrap molasses and the polyunsaturated oils, such as safflower, also contain some vitamin K. In animal-source foods, K is found in liver, milk, yogurt, egg yolks, and fish liver oils. The best source for humans is that made by the intestinal bacteria. It is important for the production of many nutrients that we keep our "friendly" colon bacteria active and doing their job; to aid this process we should minimize our use of oral antibiotics, avoid excess sugars and processed foods, and occasionally evaluate and treat any abnormal organisms interfering in our colon, such as yeasts or parasites.

Functions: Vitamin K is necessary for normal blood clotting. It is required for the synthesis of prothrombin and other proteins (Factors IX, VII, and X) involved in blood coagulation. Vitamin K also helps prothrombin convert to thrombin with the aid of potassium and calcium; thrombin is the important factor needed for the conversion of fibrinogen to the active fibrin clot.

Coumarin, which comes from sweet clover, acts as an anticoagulant (decreases blood clotting) by competing with vitamin K at its active sites. Coumarin or synthetic dicumarol is used medically primarily as an oral anticoagulant to decrease prothrombin. The salicylates, such as aspirin, increase the need for vitamin K.

Uses: Vitamin K is used commonly by physicians in the treatment of clinical problems. It should not be taken routinely without the ability to monitor its effects on blood clotting. Currently, its most regular application in Western medicine is to inject newborns with vitamin K to prevent hemorrhage and other minor bleeding problems. Vitamin K is not transferred from the mother, nor are there colon bacteria to make it in newborns since the gastrointestinal tract is usually sterile for a few days after birth. The production of vitamin K and, therefore, prothrombin usually begins by the fourth day of life, giving babies their ability to clot blood when necessary.

Vitamin K is also sometimes given by injection to women prior to labor (a deficiency can occur during pregnancy) or to patients before or after surgery to prevent hemorrhage. Higher doses of vitamin K than are needed by the body do not cause excessive blood clotting, so this is not a concern. Additional K is given at times to women with heavy menstrual flow, to help relieve menstrual pain, or to reduce the nausea and vomiting of pregnancy. It is also used to promote blood clotting in people with liver disease, jaundice, or malabsorption problems. Those people who bruise easily or whose blood clots slowly after injury sometimes benefit from supplemental vitamin K, as do some sufferers of rheumatoid arthritis, where K may reduce irritation in the synovial linings of the joints.

An occasional use of vitamin K that can be lifesaving is the treatment of people who have taken too much of the anticoagulant Coumadin. People with strokes, heart attacks, thrombophlebitis, or pulmonary embolism or who are at risk of having problems related to abnormal blood clotting may receive this type of anticoagulant therapy. As I described previously, the coumarol medications reduce blood clotting by competing with vitamin K sites and reducing prothrombin formation. If bleeding problems occur in patients on Coumadin therapy, an injection of vitamin K may help correct it rapidly. Vitamin K is also used at times as a preservative in foods; it helps control fermentation. If vitamin K deficiency is suspected, it is usually wise to consume more foods high in this vitamin before using supplements.

Deficiency and toxicity: Toxicity rarely occurs from vitamin K from its natural sources—that is, from foods or from production by the intestinal bacteria—but toxic side effects are more likely from the synthetic vitamin K used in medical treatment. Natural vitamins K_1 and K_2 are easily stored or eliminated, whereas menadione, or K_3, can build up in the blood and cause some toxicity. Hemolytic anemia, a reduction in red blood cells due to destruction, is a possible problem. This usually increases the bilirubin, one of the breakdown products of hemoglobin in the blood, more of

a problem in infants, who have a harder time handling high levels of bilirubin. Symptoms of adult toxicity may include flushing, sweating, or a feeling of chest constriction; however, problems arising from vitamin K use are rare.

Deficiency of vitamin K is also uncommon. It is more likely with poor intestinal absorption, with low dietary intake or decreased production in the intestines, or when the liver is not able to use vitamin K (which may be caused by either a genetic condition or liver disease). Deficiency of vitamin K is also more common in sprue or celiac disease (intestinal malabsorption problems), in colitis, in ileitis, or after bowel surgery. I mentioned that for a few days the newborn baby is at risk of bleeding because of lack of vitamin K; vitamin K deficiency may also be a problem in the elderly, when the diet is poor or when antibiotic use or other factors decrease intestinal bacterial production.

The problems that may occur from vitamin K deficiency involve abnormal bleeding, as in nosebleeds and internal hemorrhage, which can be severe if it occurs in the brain or internal organs. Miscarriage may occur secondary to bleeding problems from vitamin K deficiency in pregnancy. Fortunately, this is uncommon.

Requirements: There is no official RDA for vitamin K (there may be one soon), as there is usually sufficient supply from foods and intestinal bacteria. An average diet will usually provide at least 75–150 mcg., which is the suggested minimum, though 300 mcg. daily may be optimal. Absorption may vary from person to person, estimated from 20–60 percent of intake. Overall, suggested needs are about 2 mcg. per kilogram (2.2 pounds) of body weight.

Newborns need about 1–5 mg. daily to prevent bleeding. Usually a 10 mg. injection is given at birth. Vitamin K is not available over the counter and must be given by prescription; for those who wish to consume more vitamin K, alfalfa tablets are a good source.

109

WATER SOLUBLE VITAMINS

Thiamine   Riboflavin   Niacin   Pantothenic   Pyridoxine   Cobalamin
                                        Acid

Biotin   Choline   Folic Acid   Inositol   PABA

Orotic Acid   Pangamic Acid   Laetrile

Ascorbic   Bioflavonoids   The Love   Vitamin T   Vitamin U
Acid   Vitamin

B Complex Vitamins

I wish to give a brief overview of the whole B vitamin group before dealing with each specifically. They are all water soluble and are not stored very well in the body. Thus, they are needed daily to support their many functions. Deficiencies of one or more of the B vitamins may occur fairly easily, especially during times of fasting or weight-loss diets or with diets that include substantial amounts of refined and processed food, sugar, or alcohol.

As a group they are named the B complex vitamins because they are commonly found together in foods and have similar coenzyme functions, often needing each other to perform best. Certain of the B vitamins can also be made in the body by inhabitant microorganisms, primarily in our large intestine. Bacteria, yeasts, fungi, and molds are all capable of producing B vitamins.

These vitamins are fairly easily digested from food or supplements and then absorbed into the blood, mainly from the small intestine. When the amount of Bs taken exceeds the body's needs, the excess is easily excreted in the urine, giving it a dark yellow color. Excesses of certain B vitamins, such as thiamine (B_1), are also eliminated in our perspiration. Since there are many deficiencies and no known toxicities of the B vitamins, taking modest excesses is really of no concern and may be helpful to many people. However, taking huge quantities is probably not needed under most conditions.

Sources: The B vitamins are found in many foods, and they often occur together. Actually, in nature, there is no B vitamin found in isolation. Heating, cooking, acid, and alkali affect each vitamin differently, so check the sections on individual Bs for this information.

The richest natural source containing the largest number of B vitamins is brewer's yeast, or nutritional yeast. Yeast is a common source used to make B vitamin supplements as well.

However, this is not necessarily an ideal food for many people, since sensitivities to yeast may cause digestive tract problems or allergy. Different yeasts may also vary in their concentrations of specific B vitamins.

The germ and bran of cereal grains are good sources of these vitamins, as are some beans, peas, and nuts. Milk and many leafy green vegetables may also supply small amounts of B vitamins. Liver is an excellent source of the B complex vitamins. Other meats, such as beef, are fairly low, except for B_{12}, which is found mainly in animal foods. Check the discussion of each individual B vitamin for its best sources. And remember, the B vitamins are produced by human intestinal bacteria, which seem to work best with the milk sugar and fats in our diet, though most foods can provide a source for this biodynamic B vitamin production in the colon. Antibiotics such as sulfa drugs and tetracyclines, which kill the intestinal bacterial flora, also lower our potential to produce B vitamins. Replacing the lactobacillus intestinal bacteria after taking antibiotics is important in maintaining the health and microbial ecosystem in the colon.

Functions: The B vitamins are the catalytic spark plugs of our body; they function as coenzymes to catalyze many biochemical reactions. B vitamins help provide energy by acting with enzymes to convert carbohydrates to glucose and also are important in fat and protein/amino acid metabolism.

The B complex vitamins are very important for the normal functioning of the nervous system and are often helpful in bringing relaxation or energy to individuals who are stressed or fatigued. The health of the skin, hair, eyes, and liver is influenced by the B vitamins, as is that of the mucosal linings, especially in and around the mouth. The general muscle tone of the gastrointestinal tract is also enhanced with proper levels of B vitamins, allowing the bowels to function most efficiently.

Uses: The functions of the B vitamins are so interrelated that it is suggested they be taken

111

combined in B complex food supplements. They are usually part of any multiple vitamin and are often taken in increased amounts for problems of stress, fatigue, anxiety and nervousness, insomnia, and hyperactivity. B vitamins are also used for many kinds of skin problems, especially dry or itchy dermatitis rashes, or cracks at the corners of the mouth. Some cases of vitiligo may be helped by B complex supplements, including higher amounts of PABA. Premenstrual and menopausal problems may be helped with additional B complex vitamins. Treatment of alcoholism and withdrawal from alcohol may be aided by taking large amounts of the B vitamins.

A wide range of various B vitamin deficiency symptoms can be treated with supplemental Bs. The natural food extract supplements are often preferred over the synthetic B complex because they seem to work more harmoniously and are more easily tolerated; in addition, it is likely that there are other enzymes, cofactors, and possibly even undiscovered B vitamins within the natural supplements.

Deficiency and toxicity: There are basically no real toxicity problems with any of the B vitamins, even in large amounts, since the body readily eliminates the excesses. There may be, of course, some subtle problems from taking high-dose individual B vitamins for too long. One such problem with taking large amounts of a single B vitamin is that this may cause a depletion of other Bs. Therefore, it is best to take a complete B complex supplement whenever taking any individual B vitamin regularly in higher amounts.

At least thirteen B vitamins are found in our food. Some may be lacking in many Americans' diets because of the consumption of refined flour products, sugar, coffee, and alcohol, which can deplete B vitamins. Deficiency symptoms include fatigue, irritability, nervousness, depression, insomnia, loss of appetite, sore (burning) mouth or tongue, and cracks at the corners of the mouth. Some deficiencies may also reduce immune functions or estro-

gen metabolism; other potential problems are anemia, especially from vitamin B_{12} or folic acid deficiency, constipation, neuritis, skin problems, acne, hair loss, early graying of the hair, increased serum cholesterol, and weakness of the legs, to name a few.

Requirements: The daily amount required for each of the B vitamins varies, and the RDA is not very high for any of them. (For specific values, see the separate discussions of the various Bs.) The overall recommended minimums may be too low, and most people who take B vitamins take much higher amounts than the RDA. Since the body does not store much of the B complex vitamins and many commonly used, diet-related substances such as sugar, coffee, and alcohol deplete B vitamins in the body, these B vitamins should be taken daily. B vitamins are needed for growth, so increased amounts are also suggested for children and for pregnant or breast-feeding women. Stress, infections, and high-carbohydrate diets also may cause greater requirements of B vitamin supplements.

Vitamin B_1 (Thiamine or thiamin), the first B vitamin by Earl Mindell in *Vitamin Bible* (Warner Books, 1979) because of the support it gives to the nervous system and mental attitude. Its odor and flavor are similar to those of yeast. Thiamine can be destroyed by the cooking process, especially by boiling or moist heat, but less by dry heat, such as baking.

Like most other B vitamins, thiamine is needed in regular supply, though after its absorption from the upper and lower small intestine, some B_1 is stored in the liver, heart, and kidneys. Most excess thiamine is eliminated in the urine; some seems to be excreted in the sweat as well.

Sources: Since thiamine is lost in cooking and is depleted by use of sugar, coffee, tannin from black teas, nicotine, and alcohol, it is necessary to insure that intake of thiamine is optimal. There are a number of food sources for thiamine; however, they may not be the everyday fare for many people. Good sources of vitamin B$_1$ include the germ and bran of wheat, rice husks (outer covering), and the outer portion of other grains. With the milling of grains and use of refined flours and white or "polished" rice, many of us are no longer getting the nourishment of thiamine that is available when we eat wholesome, unprocessed foods.

Other good sources of thiamine besides wheat germ and bran, whole wheat or enriched wheat flour, and brown rice are brewer's yeast and blackstrap molasses. Oats and millet have modest amounts, as do many vegetables, such as spinach and cauliflower, most nuts, sunflower seeds, and legumes, such as peanuts, peas, and beans. Of the fruits, avocado is the highest in vitamin B$_1$. Pork has a high amount of this B vitamin. Many dried fruits contain some thiamine, though the sulfur dioxide often added as a preservative seems to destroy this vitamin.

Functions: Thiamine helps a great many bodily functions, acting as the coenzyme thiamine pyrophosphate (TPP). It has a key metabolic role in the cellular production of energy, mainly in glucose metabolism. Thiamine is also needed to metabolize ethanol, converting it to carbon dioxide and water. B$_1$ helps in the initial steps of fatty acid and sterol production. In this way, thiamine also helps convert carbohydrate to fat for storage of potential energy.

Thiamine is important to the health of the nerves and nervous system, possibly because of its role in the synthesis of acetylcholine (via the production of acetyl CoA), an important neurotransmitter. With a lack of vitamin B$_1$, the nerves are more sensitive to inflammation. Thiamine is linked to individual learning capacity and to growth in children. It is also important to the muscle tone of the stomach, intestines, and heart because of the function of acetylcholine at nerve synaptic junction. It is conceivable that adequate thiamine levels

may help prevent the accumulation of fatty deposits in the arteries and thereby reduce the progression of atherosclerosis.

Uses: Vitamin B$_1$ is, of course, used to treat any of the symptoms of its deficiency or its deficiency disease beriberi (discussed below). It is used in the treatment of fatigue, irritability, low morale, and depression and to prevent air- or seasickness. It seems to help the nerves, heart, and muscular system function well. By aiding hydrochloric acid production, thiamine may help digestion or reduce nausea, and it can remedy constipation by increasing intestinal muscle tone. Thiamine is used commonly to improve healing after dental (or, often, any) surgery.

Increased thiamine intake may be suggested for numerous mental illnesses and problems that affect the nerves. These include alcoholism and its nerve problems, multiple sclerosis, Bell's palsy (a facial nerve paralysis), and neuritis. Treatment with thiamine, for example, has been helpful in decreasing the sensory neuropathy that accompanies diabetes and in lessening the pain of trigeminal neuralgia. Thiamine also has a mild diuretic effect and is supportive of heart function, so it is suggested in the treatment program for many cardiovascular problems.

Since thiamine is eliminated through the skin somewhat, doses of over 50–100 mg. per day may help repel insects such as flies and mosquitos from those with "sweet blood." Other uses for increased thiamine include treatment of stress and muscle tensions, diarrhea, fever and infections, cramps, and headaches.

Deficiency and toxicity: There is no known toxicity in humans from thiamine taken orally. People have taken hundreds of milligrams daily without any harmful effect, although some may become more stimulated than others. Thiamine injections, however, have occasionally been associated with trauma or edema.

Prolonged restriction of thiamine intake may produce a wide variety of symptoms,

113

particularly affecting the general disposition, nervous system, gastrointestinal tract, and heart. With thiamine deficiency, as with deficiency of most any essential nutrient, symptoms range from mild to moderate depletion disorders to the serious disease state that RDA amounts usually prevent.

Beriberi is the name given to the disease caused by thiamine deficiency. There are three basic expressions of beriberi, namely childhood, wet, and dry beriberi. Childhood beriberi stunts the growth process, and in infants high-pitched scream and rapid heartbeat are associated with the disease. Wet beriberi is the classic form with edema (swelling) in the feet and legs, spreading to the body, and associated decreased function of the heart. Dry beriberi is not accompanied by swelling but seems to be manifested by weight loss, muscle wasting, and nerve degeneration. Another thiamine deficiency disease involves degeneration of the brain and affects the general orientation, attitude, and ability to walk. This has been termed the Wernicke-Korsakoff syndrome and is usually seen in people who have been addicted to alcohol for many years.

These severe problems can and do lead to death when they are not corrected with dietary change or supplemental thiamine. Before vitamin B_1 was discovered, this affected many people who ate a diet consisting mainly of polished rice. Today, deficiency of this vitamin is still quite common. Although it does not usually lead to beriberi, a number of symptoms can result from a depletion of thiamine body levels. A low-B_1 diet consisting of polished rice or unenriched white flour is not often the culprit in our culture. The diet that contributes to deficiency today, especially among teenagers, is high in colas, sweets, fast foods, and many other empty-calorie foods. This diet can also lead to skin problems and symptoms of neurosis, almost like a Jekyll-and-Hyde disposition.

With a deficiency of thiamine, carbohydrate digestion and the metabolism of glucose are diminished. There is a build-up of pyruvic acid in the blood, which can lead to decreased oxygen utilization and therefore mental deficiency and even difficulty in breathing. While B_1 is needed for alcohol metabolism, alcohol abuse is often associated with a poor diet and poor B_1 absorption. The poor perceptions, mental states, and nerve problems that come with alcoholism may be associated with thiamine deficiency.

The first symptoms of thiamine deficiency may be fatigue, instability. These may be followed by confusion, loss of memory, depression, clumsiness, insomnia, gastrointestinal disturbances, abdominal pain, constipation, slow heart rate, and burning chest pains. As the condition progresses, there may be problems of irregular heart rhythm, prickling sensation in the legs, loss of vibratory sensation, and the muscles may become tender and atrophy. The optic nerve may become inflamed and the vision will be affected.

Generally, with low B_1 the central nervous system—the brain and nerves—does not function optimally. The gastrointestinal and cardiovascular systems are also influenced greatly. Vitamin B_1 levels have been shown to be low in many elderly people, especially those that experience senility, neuroses, and schizophrenia. We might question how much of the degeneration and disease of old age may be a result of withering digestion and assimilation, leading to deficiencies of various vitamins and other necessary nutrients.

Requirements: The RDA for vitamin B_1 is about 1.2 mg. per day, or 1.4 mg. during pregnancy or lactation. Infants need more per body weight though less in total, about 0.5 mg. per day. Thiamine needs are based on many factors; given good health, we need about 0.5 mg. per 1,000 calories consumed, since B_1 is required for energy metabolism. So our needs are based on body weight, calorie consumption, and the amount of vitamin B1 synthesized by intestinal bacteria, which can vary greatly from person to person.

Thiamine needs are also increased with higher stress levels, with fever or diarrhea, and during and after surgery. Those who smoke, drink alcohol, consume caffeine or tannin from coffee or tea, or who are pregnant, lactating, or taking birth control pills all need more thiamine, possibly much more than the RDA, for optimum health.

Thiamine is needed in the diet or in supplements daily. There are some stores in the heart, liver, and kidneys; however, these do not last very long. The minimum B_1 intake for those who are very healthy is at least 2 mg. per day. A good insurance level of thiamine is probably 10 mg. a day, though even higher levels may be useful in some situations. When we do not eat optimally, have any abusive substance habits (especially alcohol abuse), or are under stress, increased levels of thiamine are recommended. An example is the B complex 50 products—that is, 50 mg. of B_1 along with that amount of most of the other B vitamins—suggested as a daily regimen. The upper intake levels of thiamine should not be much more than 200–300 mg. daily. Often B_1, B_2 (riboflavin), and B_6 (pyridoxine) are formulated together in equal amounts within a B-complex supplement. When people take higher amounts of the B vitamins, many feel a difference in energy and vitality. (Note: Riboflavin taken for any length of time is best limited to 50 mg. daily.)

 Vitamin B_2 (Riboflavin) is an orange-yellow crystal that is more stable than thiamine. B_2 is stable to heat, acid, and oxidation. It is, however, sensitive to light, especially ultraviolet light, as in sunlight. So foods containing even moderate amounts of riboflavin—for example, milk—need to be protected from sunlight. Only a little of the B_2 in foods is lost in the cooking water.

Vitamin B_2 is easily absorbed from the small intestine into the blood which transports it to the tissues. Excess intake is eliminated in the urine, which can give it a yellow-green fluorescent glow, commonly seen after taking B complex 50 mg. or 100 mg. supplements. Riboflavin is not stored in the body, except for a small quantity in the liver and kidneys, so it is needed regularly in the diet.

Intestinal bacteria produce varying amounts of riboflavin; this poses some questions regarding different people's needs for B_2 and may minimize the degree of riboflavin deficiency, even with diets low in riboflavin intake. Though there are many deficiency symptoms possible with low levels of B_2 in the body, no specific serious deficiency disease is noted for riboflavin, as there is for vitamins B_1 and B_3 (niacin). Riboflavin-5-phosphate, a form of riboflavin, may be more readily assimilated by some people.

Sources: Riboflavin is found in many of the foods that contain other B vitamins, but it is not found in high amounts in very many foods. For this reason, dietary deficiency is fairly common, and supplementation may help prevent problems. Brewer's yeast is the richest natural source of vitamin B_2. Liver, tongue, and other organ meats are also excellent sources. Oily fish, such as mackerel, trout, eel, herring, and shad, have substantial levels of riboflavin, too. Nori seaweed is also a fine source. Milk products have some riboflavin, as do eggs, shellfish, millet and wild rice, dried peas, beans, and some seeds such as sunflower. Other foods with moderate amounts of riboflavin are dark leafy green vegetables, such as asparagus, collards, broccoli, and spinach, whole or enriched grain products, mushrooms, and avocados. Lower levels of vitamin B_2 are found in cabbage, carrots, cucumbers, apples, figs, berries, grapes, and tropical fruits.

Functions: Riboflavin functions as the precursor or building block for two coenzymes that are important in energy production. Flavin mononucleotide (FMN) and flavin adenine dinucleotide (FAD) are the two coenzymes that act as hydrogen carriers to help make energy as adenosine triphosphate (ATP) through the metabolism of carbohydrates and fats. Riboflavin is also instrumental in cell respiration, helping each cell utilize oxygen most efficiently; is helpful in maintaining good vision and healthy hair, skin, and nails; and is necessary for normal cell growth.

Uses: Supplemental riboflavin is commonly used to treat and help prevent visual problems, eye fatigue, and cataracts. It seems to help with burning eyes, excess tearing, and decreased vision resulting from eye strain. Riboflavin is also used for many kinds of stress conditions, fatigue, and vitality or growth problems. For people with allergies and chemical sensitivities, riboflavin-5-phosphate may be more readily assimilated than riboflavin. Riboflavin is given for skin difficulties such as acne, dermatitis, eczema, and skin ulcers. B_2 is also used in the treatment of alcohol problems, ulcers, digestive difficulties, and leg cramps, and supplementing it may be advantageous for prevention or during treatment of cancer. There is, however, not much published research to support these common uses.

Deficiency and toxicity: There are no known toxic reactions to riboflavin, though high doses may cause losses, mainly from the urine, of other B vitamins. Like most of the B vitamins, deficiency is a much greater concern. Some authorities claim that riboflavin, or vitamin B_2, deficiency is the most common nutrient deficiency in America. But because of its production by intestinal bacteria, it may not cause symptoms as severe as other vitamin deficiencies. Insufficient levels of riboflavin are provided by diets that do not include riboflavin-rich foods such as liver, yeast, and vegetables; special diets for weight loss, ulcers, or treatment of diabetes; or the diets of people who have bad eating habits and consume mostly refined foods and fast foods. Riboflavin deficiency is more commonly seen in persons with alcohol problems, in the elderly and the poor, and in depressed patients.

Symptoms of vitamin B_2 deficiency include sensitivity or inflammation of the mucous membranes of the mouth; cracks or sores at the corners of the mouth, called cheilosis; a red, sore tongue; eye redness or sensitivity to light, burning eyes, eye fatigue, or a dry, sandy feeling of the eyes; fatigue and/or dizziness; dermatitis with a dry yet greasy or oily scaling; nervous tissue damage; and retarded growth in infants and children. Cataracts may occur more frequently with B_2 deficiency. Hair loss, weight loss, general lack of vitality, and digestive problems are also possible with depletion or deficiency states of vitamin B_2; these problems may begin when daily intake is 0.6 mg. or less.

RDAS FOR VITAMIN B_2

Infants	0.4–0.6 mg.
Children ages 1–3	0.8 mg.
Children ages 4–6	1.0 mg.
Children ages 7–10	1.4 mg
Men	1.6 mg.
Women	1.2 mg.
Pregnant	1.5 mg.
Lactating	1.7 mg.

Requirements: The RDA of vitamin B_2 is based on weight, state of metabolism and growth, and protein and calorie intake. Riboflavin is related closely to energy metabolism. There are only small tissue reserves, and these may be lost when the calculated daily intake is lower than 1.2 mg.

Women who take estrogen or birth control pills, people on antibiotics such as sulfa, and those under stress need additional amounts of riboflavin. Specific amounts must be determined for each individual. Riboflavin may be taken in amounts between 25 and 50 mg. Many B vitamin supplements offer 100 mg. per day, of riboflavin which may be excessive; 10 mg. daily is considered a good insurance level.

Vitamin B$_3$ (Niacin) is used commonly to refer to two different compounds, nicotinic acid and niacinamide. B$_3$ was first isolated during oxidation of nicotine from tobacco and was thus given the name nicotinic acid vitamin, shortened to niacin. It is not, however, the same as or even closely related to the molecule nicotine. Niacin, as nicotinic acid or niacinamide, is converted in the body to the active forms, nicotinamide adenine dinucleotide (NAD) and a phosphorylated form (NADP).

Niacin is one of the most stable of the B vitamins. It is resistant to the effects of heat, light, air, acid, and alkali. A white crystalline substance that is soluble in both water and alcohol, niacin and niacinamide are both readily absorbed from the small intestine. Small amounts may be stored in the liver, but most of the excess is excreted in the urine.

Another important fact about vitamin B$_3$ is that it can be manufactured from the amino acid tryptophan, which is essential (needed in the diet). So niacin is not truly essential in the diet when enough protein, containing adequate tryptophan, and other nutrients are consumed. When niacin is not present in sufficient amounts, extra protein is needed. Also, when we are deficient in such nutrients as vitamins B$_1$, B$_2$, and B$_6$, vitamin C, and iron, we cannot easily convert tryptophan to niacin. Many foods that are low in tryptophan are also low in niacin or, as in corn, the niacin is not readily available. Corn is low in tryptophan and its niacin is bound, so it must receive special treatment. Native Americans knew this and would soak corn in ash water before or after grinding to release the niacin. Even when they subsisted almost solely on corn, they did not experience the serious niacin deficiency disease called pellagra. In the time around the American Civil War, in the South poor white farm workers subsisted on "quick cornmeal," the poorly prepared white people's version, and pellagra was epidemic until the discovery that it was a dietary deficiency disease. Pellagra, the disease of the "three Ds"—diarrhea, dermatitis, and dementia—historically has been a problem of corn-eaters, whereas beriberi has been a disease most correlated with rice-eating cultures.

Sources: Only small to moderate amounts of vitamin B$_3$ occur in foods as pure niacin; other niacin is converted from the amino acid tryptophan, as just discussed. The best sources of vitamin B$_3$ are liver and other organ meats, poultry, fish, and peanuts, all of which have both niacin and tryptophan. Yeast, dried beans and peas, wheat germ, whole grains, avocados, dates, figs, and prunes are pretty good sources of niacin. Milk and eggs are good because of their levels of tryptophan. Though B$_3$ is stable, the milling and processing of whole grains can remove up to 90 percent of the niacin. Thus, manufacturers will often "enrich" their products by adding niacin.

Functions: Niacin acts as part of two coenzymes, nicotinamide adenine dinucleotide (NAD) and nicotinamide adenine dinucleotide phosphate (NADP), that are involved in more than 50 different metabolic reactions in the human species. They play a key role in glycolysis (that is, extracting energy from carbohydrate and glucose), are important in fatty acid synthesis and in the deamination (nitrogen removal) of amino acids, are needed in the formation of red blood cells and steroids, and are helpful in the metabolism of some drugs and toxicants. Thus, niacin is a vital precursor for the coenzymes that supply energy to body cells.

Basically, the coenzymes of niacin help break down and utilize proteins, fats, and carbohydrates. Vitamin B$_3$ also stimulates circulation, reduces cholesterol levels in the blood of some people, and is important to healthy activity of the nervous system and normal brain function. Niacin supports the health of skin, tongue, and digestive tract tissues. Also, this important vitamin is needed for the synthesis of the sex hormones, such as estrogen,

117

progesterone, and testosterone, as well as other corticosteroids.

Niacin, taken orally as nicotinic acid, can produce redness, warmth, and itching over areas of the skin; this "niacin flush" usually occurs when doses of 50 mg. or more are taken and is a result of the release of histamine by the cells, which causes vasodilation. This reaction is harmless; it may even be helpful by enhancing blood flow to the "flushed" areas, and it lasts only 10–20 minutes. When these larger doses of niacin are taken regularly, this reaction no longer occurs because stores of histamine are reduced. Many people feel benefit from this "flush," but if it is not enjoyable, supplements that contain vitamin B_3 in the form of niacinamide or nicotinamide can be used, as they will not produce this reaction. (Note: When vitamin B_3 is used to lower cholesterol levels, the nicotinic acid form must be used; the niacinamide form does not work for this purpose.)

Uses: Niacin is used to support a variety of metabolic functions and to treat a number of conditions. Many niacin deficiency symptoms can be treated by adjusting the diet and by supplementing B_3 tablets along with other B complex vitamins. Many uses of niacin are based primarily on positive clinical experience and are not as well supported by medical research, although more studies are being done.

Niacin helps increase energy through improving food utilization and has been used beneficially for treating fatigue, irritability, and digestive disorders, such as diarrhea, constipation, and indigestion. It may also stimulate extra hydrochloric acid production. Niacin, mainly as nicotinic acid, helps in the regulation of blood sugar (as part of glucose tolerance factor) in people with hypoglycemia problems and gives all of us a greater ability to handle stress. It is helpful in treating anxiety and possibly depression. B_3 has been used for various skin reactions and acne, as well as for problems of the teeth and gums. Niacin has many other common uses. It is sometimes

helpful in the treatment of migraine-type headaches or arthritis, probably in both cases through stimulation of blood flow in the capillaries. This vitamin has also been used to stimulate the sex drive and enhance sexual experience, to help detoxify the body, and to protect it from certain toxins and pollutants. For most of these problems and the cardiovascular-related ones mentioned below, the preference is to take the "flushing" form of niacin, or nicotinic acid, not niacinamide.

Nicotinic acid works rapidly, particularly in its beneficial effects on the cardiovascular system. It stimulates circulation and for this reason may be helpful in treating leg cramps caused by circulatory deficiency; headaches, especially the migraine type; and Meniere's syndrome, associated with hearing loss and vertigo. Nicotinic acid also helps reduce blood pressure and, very importantly, acts as an agent to lower serum cholesterol. Treatment with about 2 grams a day of nicotinic acid has produced significant reductions in both blood cholesterol and triglyceride levels. To lower the LDL component and raise the good HDL cholesterol, people usually take 50–100 mg. twice daily and then increase the amount slowly over two or three weeks to 1500–2500 mg. Generally, for those with high cholesterol levels it has been used to help reduce the risk for atherosclerosis. Because of its vascular stimulation and effects of lowering cholesterol and blood pressure, vitamin B_3 has been used preventively for such serious secondary problems of cardiovascular disease as myocardial infarctions (heart attacks) and strokes. Also, some neurologic problems, such as Bell's palsy and trigeminal neuralgia, have been helped by niacin supplementation. In osteoarthritis, to help reduce joint pain and improve mobility, niacinamide has been used in amounts beginning at 500 mg. twice daily up to 1,000 mg. three times a day along with 100 mg. daily of B complex.

Niacin has been an important boon to the field of orthomolecular psychiatry for its use in a variety of mental disorders. It was initially well demonstrated to be helpful for the neuroses and psychoses described as the "dementia of pellagra," the niacin deficiency disease. Since then, it has been used in high amounts, well over 100 mg. per day and often over 1,000 mg. per day (up to 6,000 mg.), to treat a wide variety of psychological symptoms, including senility, alcoholism, drug problems, depression, and schizophrenia. Niacin has been helpful in reversing the hallucinatory experience, delusional thinking or wide mood and energy shifts of some psychological disturbances. Though this therapy has its skeptics, as does all application of nutritional medicine, some studies show promising results in treatment of schizophrenia with niacin and other supplements. Other studies show little or no effect. More research is definitely needed on niacin's effect in mental disorders.

People on high blood pressure medicines and those who have ulcers, gout, or diabetes should be very careful taking higher-dose supplements of niacin because of its effect of lowering blood pressure, its acidity, its liver toxicity, its potential to raise uric acid levels, and its effect in raising blood sugar—though recently niacin has been shown to have a positive effect on glucose tolerance (it is part of glucose tolerance factor) and, thereby, on diabetes as well. Exercise and niacin are helpful for people with adult diabetes through their positive effects on blood sugar and cholesterol.

Deficiency and toxicity: As with the other B vitamins, there are really no toxic effects from even the high doses of niacin, though the "niacin flush" previously described may be uncomfortable for some. However, with the use of high-dose niacin in recent years, the occasional person experiences some minor problems, such as irritation of the gastrointestinal tract and/or the liver, both of which subside with decreased intake of niacin. In addition, some people taking niacin experience sedation rather than stimulation.

Deficiency problems have been much more common than toxicity, and for a long period of history, the niacin deficiency disease, pellagra, was a very serious and fatal problem. Characterized as the disease of the "three Ds," pellagra causes its victims to experience dermatitis, diarrhea, and dementia. The fourth D was death.

As described previously, the classic B₃ deficiency occurs mainly in cultures whose diets rely heavily on corn and where the corn is not prepared in a way that releases its niacin. One of the first signs of pellagra, or niacin deficiency, is the skin's sensitivity to light, and the skin becomes rough, thick, and dry (pellagra means "skin that is rough" in Italian). The skin then becomes darkly pigmented, especially in areas of the body prone to be hot and sweaty or those exposed to sun. The first stage of this condition is extreme redness and sensitivity of those exposed areas, and it was from this symptom that the term "redneck," describing the bright red necks of eighteenth- and nineteenth-century niacin-deficient fieldworkers, came into being.

In general, niacin deficiency affects every cell, especially in those systems with rapid turnover, such as the skin, gastrointestinal tract, and nervous system. Other than photosensitivity, the first signs of niacin deficiency are noted as decreased energy production and problems with maintaining healthy functioning of the skin and intestines. These symptoms include weakness and general fatigue, anorexia, indigestion, and skin eruptions. These can progress to other problems, such as a sore, red tongue, canker sores, nausea, vomiting, tender gums, bad breath, and diarrhea. The neurological symptoms may begin with irritability, insomnia, and headaches and then progress to tremors, extreme anxiety, depression—all the way to full-blown psychosis. The skin will worsen, as will the diarrhea and inflammation of the mouth and intestinal tract. There will be a lack of stomach acid production (achlorhydria) and a decrease in fat digestion and, thus, lower availability from food absorption of the fat-soluble vitamins, such as A, D, and E.

Death could occur, usually from convulsions, if the niacin deficiency is not corrected.

Niacin deficiency symptoms can be seen in diets with niacin intake below 7.5 mg. per day, but often this is not the only deficiency; vitamin B_1, vitamin B_2, and other B vitamins, as well as protein and iron may be low. To treat pellagra and niacin deficiency disorders, vitamin B_3 supplements should be taken along with good protein intake to obtain adequate levels of the amino acid tryptophan. As described earlier, about 50 percent of daily niacin comes from the conversion in our livers of tryptophan to niacin with the help of pyridoxine (vitamin B_6).

Requirements: Many food charts list only sources that actually contain niacin and do not take into account tryptophan conversion into niacin. Approximately 60 mg. of tryptophan can generate 1 mg. of niacin. But tryptophan is available for conversion only when there are more than sufficient quantities in the diet to synthesize the necessary proteins as tryptophan is used in our body with the other essential amino acids to produce protein.

Niacin needs are based on caloric intake. We need about 6.6 mg. per 1,000 calories, and no less than 13 mg. per day. Women need at least 13 mg. and men at least 18 mg. per day. The RDA for children ranges from 9–16 mg.

Niacin needs are increased during pregnancy, lactation, and growth periods, as well as after physical exercise. Athletes require more B_3 than less active people. Stress, illness, and tissue injury also increase the body's need for niacin. People who eat much sugar or refined, processed foods require more niacin as well.

Realistically, 25–50 mg. per day is adequate intake of niacin if minimum protein requirements are met. On the average, many supplements provide at least 50–100 mg. per day of niacin or niacinamide, which is a good insurance level. For treatment of the variety of conditions described previously, higher amounts of niacin may be needed to really be helpful, and levels up to 2–3 grams per day are not uncommon as a therapeutic dose. The other B vitamins should also be supplied so as to not create an imbalanced metabolic condition.

Vitamin B_5 (Pantothenic Acid), another of the B complex vitamins, is a yellow viscous oil found usually as the calcium or sodium salt—that is, calcium pantothenate. It is present in all living cells and is very important to metabolism where it functions as part of the molecule called coenzyme A or CoA. Pantothenic acid is found in yeasts, molds, bacteria, and plant and animal cells, as well as in human blood plasma and lymph fluid.

B_5 is stable to moist heat and oxidation or reduction (adding or subtracting an electron), though it is easily destroyed by acids (such as vinegar) or alkalis (such as baking soda) and by dry heat. Over half of the pantothenic acid in wheat is lost during milling, and about one-third is degraded in meat during cooking. In many whole foods, vitamin B_5 is readily available.

Sources: The name pantothenic acid comes from the Greek word *pantos,* meaning "everywhere," referring to its wide availability in foods. Therefore, it is easily accessible in the diet, and deficiency is uncommon, except in those with a highly processed diet, since much of the available vitamin B_5 activity is lost during refinement of foods. Good sources of pantothenic acid include the organ meats, brewer's yeast, egg yolks, fish, chicken, whole grain cereals, cheese, peanuts, dried beans, and a variety of vegetables, such as sweet potatoes, green peas, cauliflower, and avocados. Vitamin B_5 is also made by the bacterial flora of human intestines, another source for this important metabolic assistant or coenzyme.

Functions: Pantothenic acid as coenzyme A is closely involved in adrenal cortex function and has come to be known as the "antistress" vitamin. It supports the adrenal glands to increase production of cortisone and other adrenal hormones to help counteract stress and enhance metabolism. Through this mechanism, pantothenic acid is also thought to help prevent aging and wrinkles. It is generally important to healthy skin and nerves. Through its adrenal support, vitamin B_5 may reduce potentially toxic effects of antibiotics and radiation.

As the coenzyme, pantothenic acid is important in cellular metabolism of carbohydrates and fats to release energy. As coenzyme A, it supports the synthesis of acetylcholine, a very important neurotransmitter agent that works throughout the body in a variety of neuromuscular reactions. Coenzyme A is vital in the synthesis of fatty acids, cholesterol, steroids, sphingosines, and phospholipids. It also helps synthesize porphyrin, which is connected to hemoglobin.

Uses: Pantothenic acid, found in a wide range of sources, is used in a wide variety of conditions. Again, it is known as the "anti-stress" vitamin and is used to relieve fatigue and stress and the many problems induced by stress, through its support of the adrenal glands. Allergies, headaches, arthritis, psoriasis, insomnia, asthma, and infections have all been treated with some effectiveness using vitamin B_5, possibly through its adrenal support and adequate production of adrenocorticosteroids.

Vitamin B_5 has also been used after surgery when there is paralysis of the gastrointestinal (GI) tract to stimulate GI peristalsis. It has been helpful in many cases for people who grind their teeth at night, a problem called bruxism. Other conditions treated by this vitamin are nerve disorders such as neuritis, epilepsy, and multiple sclerosis and various levels of mental illness and alcoholism. Of course, the effectiveness may vary in all these situations according to amount supplemented, length of time used, and individual responsiveness. Sound research to support the use of pantothenic acid in many of these treatments or for its energy-enhancing or antiaging effects is lacking, although some research has

shown positive results from the use of calcium pantothenate in reducing arthritis symptoms of joint pain and stiffness.

Deficiency and toxicity: As with other B vitamins, there are no specific toxic effects from high doses of pantothenic acid. Over 1,000 mg. daily has been taken for over six months with no side effects; when 1,500 mg. or more is taken daily for several weeks, some people experience a superficial sensitivity in their teeth. However, it is possible that if B_5 is taken without other B vitamins, it may create metabolic imbalance.

Fatigue is probably the earliest and most common symptom of pantothenic acid deficiency, though it is an unlikely vitamin deficiency because of the availability of B_5 in many foods, plus the fact that it is also produced by our intestinal bacteria. A diet high in refined and processed foods or a reduction or destruction of intestinal flora, most commonly by antibiotic use, can lead to a vitamin B_5 deficiency. Teenagers are more likely to experience a deficiency, because their diets often include high amounts of "fast foods" sugars, and refined flours (all low in B vitamins). And the problem may be compounded because the acne often associated with this type of diet is commonly treated with tetracycline antibiotics, which reduce the intestinal bacteria and thereby the production of pantothenic acid in the colon.

Studies of pantothenic acid deficiency in rats showed increased graying of the fur, decreased growth, and, in the extreme, hemorrhage and destruction of the adrenal glands. In humans, the decreased adrenal function caused by B_5 deficiency can lead to a variety of metabolic problems. Fatigue is most likely; there may also be physical and mental depression, a decrease in hydrochloric acid production and other digestive symptoms, some loss of nerve function, and problems in blood sugar metabolism, with symptoms of hypoglycemia (low blood sugar) being the most common. Pantothenic acid affects the function of cells in all systems, and a deficiency may reduce immunity, both cellular and antibody responses. Other symptoms of B_5 deficiency include vomiting, abdominal cramps, skin problems, tachycardia, insomnia, tingling of the hands and feet, muscle cramps, recurrent upper respiratory infections, and worsening of allergy symptoms.

Requirements: The RDA for pantothenic acid is about 5 mg. for children and 10 mg. for adults. Many other sources feel the minimum needs are more likely to be about 25–50 mg., and 50–100 mg. is probably a good "insurance" range. Therapeutic ranges are more like 250–500 mg. daily and even higher, taken, of course, along with the other B complex vitamins. Individual needs vary according to food intake, degree of stress, and whether one is pregnant or lactating. Those people who eat a diet of processed foods, have a stressful lifestyle, or have allergies require higher amounts of pantothenic acid. For all of the problems discussed here, 250–500 mg. taken twice daily is a safe and beneficial amount.

Vitamin B_6 (Pyridoxine*) is a very important B vitamin, especially for women. It seems to be connected somehow to hormone balance and water shifts in women. Vitamin B_6 is actually three related compounds, all of which are found in food— pyridoxine, pyridoxal, and pyridoxamine. Pyridoxal is the predominant biologically active form; however, in vitamin supplements, pyridoxine is the form used because it is the least expensive to produce commercially. Vitamin B_6 is stable in acid, somewhat less stable in alkali, and is fairly easily destroyed with ultraviolet light, such as sunlight, and during the processing of food. It is also lost in cooking or with improper food storage.

*And pyridoxal-5-phosphate (P5P), the active coenzyme form of vitamin B_6.

Pyridoxine is absorbed readily from the small intestine and used throughout the body in a multitude of functions. Fasting and reducing diets usually deplete the vitamin B_6 supply unless it is supplemented. Usually within eight hours, much of the excess is excreted through the urine; some B_6 is stored in muscle. It is also produced by the intestinal bacteria.

Sources: Vitamin B_6 in its several forms is widely available in nature, though not many foods have very high amounts. Since it is lost in cooking and in the refining or processing of foods, it is not the easiest B vitamin to obtain in sufficient amounts from the diet, especially if we eat much processed food, as it is not one of the vitamins replaced in "enriched" flour products such as cereals and pastries.

The best sources of vitamin B_6 are meats, particularly organ meats, such as liver, and the whole grains, especially wheat. Wheat germ is one of the richest sources. Besides meat, good protein sources of B_6 include fish, poultry, egg yolk, soybeans and other dried beans, peanuts, and walnuts. Vegetable and fruit sources include bananas, prunes, potatoes, cauliflower, cabbage, and avocados. As examples of how easily vitamin B_6 is lost in the processing of food, raw sugar cane has a good amount, while refined sugar has none; whole wheat flour contains nearly 0.5 mg. of pyridoxine (wheat germ and wheat flakes have much more), while refined wheat flour has almost none, and even whole wheat bread has lost nearly all of its vitamin B_6.

Functions: Pyridoxine and its coenzyme form, pyridoxal-5-phosphate, have a wide variety of metabolic functions in the body, especially in amino acid metabolism and in the central nervous system, where it supports production of gamma-aminobutyric acid (GABA). Many reactions, including the conversion of tryptophan to niacin and arachidonic acid to prostaglandin E_2 require vitamin B_6. The pyridoxal group is important in the utilization of all food sources for energy and in facilitating the release of glycogen (stored energy) from the liver and muscles. It helps as well in antibody and red blood cell production (hemoglobin synthesis) and in the synthesis and functioning of both DNA and RNA. By helping maintain the balance of sodium and potassium in the body, vitamin B$_6$ aids fluid balance regulation and the electrical functioning of the nerves, heart, and musculoskeletal system; B$_6$ is needed to help maintain a normal intracellular magnesium level, which is also important for these functions. The neurotransmitters norepinephrine and acetylcholine and the allergy regulator histamine are all very important body chemicals that depend on pyridoxal-5-phosphate in their metabolism. Also, the brain needs it to convert tryptophan to serotonin, another important antidepressant neurotransmitter.

Pyridoxine is especially important in regard to protein metabolism. Many amino acid reactions depend on vitamin B$_6$ to help in the transport of amino acids across the intestinal mucosa into the blood and from the blood into cells. By itself and with other enzymes, pyridoxal-5-phosphate helps build amino acids, break them down, and change one to another and is especially related to the production and metabolism of choline, methionine, serine, cysteine, tryptophan, and niacin.

The body has a high requirement for vitamin B$_6$ during pregnancy. It is important for maintaining hormonal and fluid balance of the mother and for the developing nervous system of the baby. Pyridoxine may somehow be related to the development and health of the myelin covering of the nerves, which allows them to conduct impulses properly.

Uses: With its many functions, there is also a wide range of clinical uses of vitamin B$_6$, clearly being most helpful when symptoms and diseases are related to a pyridoxine/pyridoxal-5-phosphate depletion or deficiency. Recently there has been widespread use of higher doses of B$_6$, usually from 50–200 mg. per day (though some studies use 500 mg. per day of pyridoxine in time-release form) for premenstrual symptoms, especially water retention, which can lead to breast soreness and emotional tension. Pyridoxine has been very helpful in this role, probably because of its diuretic effect through its influence on sodium-potassium balance and its mysterious influence on the hormonal system. Vitamin B$_6$ also helps with the acne that often develops premenstrually, as well as with dysmenorrhea, or menstrual pain; magnesium is usually used as well in all of these menstrual-related problems. In pregnancy, B$_6$ has been helpful in many women for controlling the nausea and vomiting of morning sickness, which some authorities feel is highly related to vitamin B$_6$ deficiency.

Linda B., a 33-year-old wife and mother of two, came to see me complaining of premenstrual irritability along with severe breast swelling and pain, all of which interfered with her life. She began a simple supplement regimen that included vitamin B$_6$ 50 mg. three times daily. She felt remarkably better during her next two menstrual cycles. Follow-up care included some diet shifts, weight loss, and a continued supplement program. She began feeling better throughout the month, and her well-being has continued for years. My office still receives thank-you notes from her.

It seems that whenever there are increased levels of estrogen in the body, more B$_6$ is required. This occurs not only in pregnancy but also for women who take birth control pills and those postmenopausal women on estrogen treatment as well. It is likely that some of the emotional symptoms experienced by many women on the pill, such as fatigue, mood swings, depression, and loss of sex drive, may be related to a deficiency of B$_6$ and thereby helped by supplementation.

Vitamin B$_6$ is used for people with stress conditions, fatigue, headaches, nervous disorders, anemia, and low blood sugar or diabetes, and in men for prostatitis, low sex drive, or hair loss. Pyridoxal-5-phosphate (P5P) is occasionally used in formulas or as an individual supplement for certain conditions. As the active coenzyme of pyridoxine, P5P can go more directly into the metabolic cycles and does not have to be converted; thus, it may be more helpful than pyridoxine alone in such problems as fatigue, allergies, viral disease, chemical sensitivities, mental illness, and cancer. Pyridoxine supplementation is also used for a variety of skin problems—dandruff, eczema, dermatitis, and psoriasis. In regard to the nervous system, vitamin B$_6$ has been supportive in cases of epilepsy, Parkinson's disease, multiple sclerosis, and neuritis. Vitamin B$_6$ therapy, from 100–300 mg. daily for 8–12 weeks, appears to reduce carpal tunnel syndrome and increase the ability to use the hands in most patients.

Pyridoxine is a natural diuretic and is often helpful not only for the previously mentioned premenstrual problems but also in overweight and fluid-retaining people and as an adjunct to blood pressure control. Vitamin B$_6$ (along with magnesium) has received some note in regard to preventing the formation of kidney stones or the recurrence of stones in those who have had them. In his book *Nutrition and Vitamin Therapy* (Grove Press, 1980), Michael Lesser, M.D., states that in a study reported in 1974 by the *Journal of Urology*, 10 mg. of vitamin B$_6$ and 300 mg. of magnesium oxide prevented recurrence in about 80 percent of patients with a long history of kidney and urinary tract stone formation. Dr. Lesser also noted that the B$_6$-magnesium combination helps in some hyperactive kids and those with fits or problems of autism. He states that pyridoxine in fairly large doses will stimulate dream activity as well as reduce the potential toxicity of barbiturate drugs, carbon monoxide and some other chemical expo-

POSSIBLE CLINICAL USES OF VITAMIN B$_6$

*Important uses

Fatigue*
Anxiety
Allergies
MSG reactions
Premenstrual syndrome*
Nausea associated with pregnancy*
Acne, especially premenstrual
Toxemia of pregnancy
Water retention*
Estrogen therapy*
Birth control pills*
Female infertility
Dysmenorrhea
Joint pain
Muscle pain*
Muscle fatigue
Atherosclerosis
Stress ulcers
Drug use
Asthma
Neuritis
Carpal tunnel syndrome*
Sickle-cell anemia
Other anemias
Depression
Learning disabilities
Hyperkinesis
Epilepsy
Parkinsonism
Autism
Schizophrenia
Immune suppression
Chemical and radiation protection
Kidney stones (mainly calcium oxalate)*
Any effect from improper amino acid
   metabolism*

LOW B₆ STATES

Elderly	Alcoholism
Pregnancy	Asthma
Birth control pills	Peptic ulcer
Depression	Malabsorption
Immune suppression	Crohn's disease
Multiple sclerosis	Cervical cancer

sures, and irradiation. Vitamin B₆ works best when taken with magnesium, zinc, riboflavin, and brewer's yeast or the other B vitamins.

Pyridoxine, probably more than the other B vitamins except folic acid, is supportive of healthy immune function. B₆ deficiency can produce immune weakness, and B₆ treatment may be helpful against infections and cancer. Recent studies have shown that pyridoxine can inhibit the growth of some cancer cells, specifically mice and human melanoma cells. Further research with B₆ will likely find an even wider range of uses.

Deficiency and toxicity: There is basically no toxicity with pyridoxine at reasonable daily dosages, though there has been some recent concern about this. Regular oral intake of 200 mg. and intravenous doses of 200 mg. have shown no side effects. Usually, the toxic doses are much higher, between 2–5 grams. Some recent reports in the medical literature show that regular usage of over 2,000 mg. per day, which some women especially have been taking, are correlated with episodes of peripheral neuritis. Although the experience of weakness or tingling of arms or legs has been transient and mostly correctable by decreasing the B₆ dosage, this does warrant some concern about excessive use of B₆, especially long-term use. Since part of the neuropathy problem comes from the liver's inability to convert all of the pyridoxine to active P5P, this concern can be lessened by supplementing some of the B₆ as pyridoxal-5-phosphate (as I have done in many of my programs), especially when the dose of vitamin B₆ exceeds 200 mg. per day. In addi-

tion, using increased amounts of magnesium with the higher levels of vitamin B₆ will reduce the occurrence of the peripheral neuritis.

Deficiency, as usual, is a bigger concern with vitamin B₆, as it is with all the B vitamins. So many functions are performed by pyridoxine that its deficiency affects the whole body. Most of these deficiency symptoms are fairly vague. Muscle weakness, nervousness, irritability, and depression are not uncommon. Many of the symptoms are similar to those of both niacin and riboflavin deficiencies; depression is common in all of them.

Metabolically, pyridoxine deficiency has a dramatic effect on amino acid metabolism, with a decreased synthesis of niacin from tryptophan, a decrease in neurotransmitter chemicals, and a decrease in hemoglobin production. Fatigue, nervous system symptoms, and anemia are all influenced by deficiency. Further nerve-related problems include paraesthesia, incoordination, confusion, insomnia, hyperactivity, and, more severely, neuritis, electroencephalogram (EEG) changes, and convulsions. Other problems include dermatitis or cracks and sores at the corners of the mouth and eyes and visual disturbances.

There is special concern about deficiency during pregnancy, when vitamin B₆ needs are higher, as it may cause water retention and the nausea and vomiting of morning sickness and has been correlated with a higher incidence of common problems of later pregnancy, such as toxemia (preeclampsia, high blood pressure, edema, and hyper-reflexes) and eclampsia (those same symptoms plus seizures). B₆ deficiency in later pregnancy can be associated with birthing difficulties. There is also an increased likelihood of diabetic and blood sugar problems in pregnancy when vitamin B₆ is deficient.

Overall, vitamin B₆ deficiency can cause a variety of nervous symptoms, skin problems, and amino acid/protein metabolic abnormalities. These can lead to the more common expressions—headache, dizziness, inability to

125

concentrate, irritability and epileptic-type activity, labile depression, and weakness. Water retention is common. Nausea, vomiting, and dry skin, especially extensive dandruff and a cracked sore mouth and tongue are also more likely with vitamin B_6 deficiency.

Requirements: Vitamin B_6 intake, though based on many factors, is determined primarily by protein intake, because it is so important to protein metabolism. The RDA for adults is a minimum of 2 mg. of B_6 per 100 grams of protein consumed. In children, it ranges from 0.6–1.2 mg. per 100 grams of protein.

However, the need for vitamin B_6 increases in a variety of situations. During pregnancy and lactation and with birth control pill or estrogen use, higher levels are required. For those who eat a high-sugar or processed-food diet or a high-protein diet, requirements for B_6 are greater and deficiencies or depletion are more common. When there is impairment of the digestive system, cardiac failure, or radiation use, or even just the aging process, needs for vitamin B_6 are increased.

Drugs that influence needs for B_6 are oral contraceptives, isoniazid (for tuberculosis), hydralazine (for high blood pressure), amphetamines, reserpine (for high blood pressure), and some antibiotics. More B_6 is utilized with an increased intake of the amino acid methionine. Adequate magnesium in the body is important to the functions of vitamin B_6.

A safe, basic intake for vitamin B_6 is probably 10–15 mg. per day, though much higher daily amounts are easily tolerated. B_6 should also be taken along with other B vitamins to prevent metabolic imbalance. For therapeutic purposes, amounts between 50–100 mg. (this is the quantity pyridoxal-5-phosphate usually comes in) are most common, and up to 200–500 mg. per day in time-release forms is used for some conditions, such as premenstrual problems and depression. With the current questions about neurologic side effects associated with megadoses of vitamin B6, particularly as pyridoxine hydrochloride, I suggest

limiting regular daily intake to 500 mg. daily or 1,000 mg. for a short course of treatment, such as one to two weeks; also, take some additional magnesium, 200–300 mg., which may help reduce any neurologic concerns.

Vitamin B_{12} (Cobalamin) is named the "red vitamin," as it is a red crystalline compound. B_{12} is unique in that it is the only vitamin that contains an essential mineral—namely, cobalt. Cobalt is thereby needed to make B_{12} and so is essential for health. B_{12} is unique also in that it is required in much tinier amounts than the other B vitamins. Only 3–4 mcg. (micrograms, or thousandths of a milligram) are needed at minimum; however, higher levels, up to 1 mg., are often used therapeutically.

Vitamin B_{12} is a very complex molecule. Besides cobalt, it also contains carbon, oxygen, phosphorus, and nitrogen. Cobalamin is stable to heat, though sensitive in heated acid or alkali solution, slightly sensitive to light, and destroyed by oxidizing and reducing agents and by some heavy metals.

Vitamin B_{12} was isolated in 1926 as the factor that treated a feared disease, pernicious anemia—termed "pernicious" because it could be fatal, most often from neurologic degeneration. But the substance cobalamin, when given orally (actually liver was used as the cure; it contains high amounts of B_{12}), did not cure all of the people with the disease, and some people still developed pernicious anemia. It was later found that a mucoprotein enzyme produced by the stomach (by the parietal cells that also make hydrochloric acid) was also needed for vitamin B_{12} to be absorbed into the body from the intestines. This enzyme has been termed the "intrinsic factor," while vitamin B_{12} is the "extrinsic factor." Aging, stress, and problems with the stomach or stomach surgery weaken the body's ability to produce the "intrinsic factor"; also, some people appear to have a genetic predisposition that makes them more prone to pernicious anemia. Hydrochloric acid helps the absorption of B_{12}; if acid production is weak, the absorption is lessened. Calcium and thyroid hormone assist as well. Pregnancy, absorb this important vitamin. Aging more likely lessens some of the many factors needed for ideal absorption of B_{12}, so deficiency symptoms are more common in older people.

Cobalamin is absorbed primarily from the last part of the small intestine, the ileum. In the blood, it is bound to a protein globulin to be carried to the various tissues. The body actually stores vitamin B_{12}, so any deficiencies may take several years to develop. The highest concentrations of B_{12} are found in the liver, heart, kidney, pancreas, brain, testes, blood, and bone marrow—all active metabolic tissues. The "red vitamin" is very important to the blood.

Cobalamin is made in nature by microbial synthesis—produced by bacteria in the intestinal tracts of animals and stored in their tissues. Some B_{12} is made during fermentation of foods as well. Cobalamin is the naturally occurring vitamin B_{12}. Cyanocobalamin, as B_{12} is often known, is actually the commercial variety of B_{12} and contains a cyanide molecule attached to the cobalt. B_{12} is not synthesized but, like penicillin, must be grown in bacteria or molds and then processed. Other forms of B_{12} include hydroxycobalamin (technically, vitamin $B_{12}a$), aquacobalamin (vitamin $B_{12}b$), and nitrocobalamin (vitamin $B_{12}c$).

Sources: Vitamin B_{12} is found in significant amounts only in the animal protein foods. B_{12} is also manufactured by bacteria in the human intestines, but it is not known how much we can naturally absorb and utilize from that source. In general, digestion and absorption must be good for adequate B_{12} to be obtained. Many laxatives and overuse of antacids can reduce absorption and deplete stores of B_{12}.

Our primary food sources of vitamin B_{12} include meat, most fish, especially the oily ones (trout, herring, and mackerel), crabs and oysters, eggs (the yolk), and milk products,

especially yogurt. Organ meats such as liver, heart, and kidney are particularly high. The vegan—that is, the strict vegetarian who consumes no animal-source foods—is not getting the necessary vitamin B_{12} from diet (although tempeh, a fermented soybean product, and some sprouts may contain some vitamin B_{12}); thus, vegans will often need an additional supplement (which absorbs well) or periodic injections.

Functions: Although vitamin B_{12}, cobalamin, apparently does not have as many functions as some of the other B vitamins, it has some very important ones. It is essential for the metabolism of the nerve tissue and necessary for the health of the entire nervous system. It stimulates growth and increases appetite in children. Cobalamin, along with iron, folic acid, copper, protein, and vitamins C and B_6, is needed for the formation of normal red blood cells.

Vitamin B_{12} is the "energy" vitamin, as it often increases the energy level, whether obtained from eating the B_{12} foods or from supplemental use. There may be several reasons for this. Cobalamin stimulates the utilization of proteins, fats, and carbohydrates. It also helps iron function better in humans and is important for the synthesis of DNA and RNA, as well as for production of choline, another B vitamin, and methionine, an amino acid.

Uses: Vitamin B_{12} is generally known as the longevity vitamin, possibly because it helps the energy level and activity of the nervous system of the elderly. B_{12} injections (the main therapeutic use of this vitamin) have been a common practice of many doctors for the treatment of fatigue, and, in my experience, it works very often. However, it would only be a "cure" when the tiredness is a result of B_{12} deficiency. There are many reasons for fatigue. As we age, our digestion and absorption are not usually as finely tuned as when we were young, particularly when we eat and live the way most of us late twentieth-century

127

beings do. And vitamin B_{12}, even though it is needed in such small doses, is one of the most difficult vitamins to acquire through diet and to metabolize. The "red vitamin" is the main "antifatigue" vitamin; often given along with folic acid, it helps energy and prevents most anemia, provided there is good iron absorption and hydrochloric acid production. Medically speaking, it is wise to check patients with fatigue for anemia and to measure vitamin B_{12} and folic acid levels before embarking on a treatment regimen.

B_{12}, given intramuscularly, usually in doses of 500–1,000 mcg. (0.5–1.0 mg.), is used once, twice, or three times weekly for a period of time to both give energy and, in adults, help with appetite suppression in weight loss programs. These amounts also replenish the vitamin B_{12} stores. It has a mild diuretic effect as well and may be used premenstrually to diminish water retention symptoms.

In the treatment of pernicious anemia and the earlier symptoms of vitamin B_{12} deficiency, injections of cobalamin or its variants are usually necessary because most everyone with deficiency has poor absorption. It is difficult to become B_{12} deficient from diet alone, unless we are on a strict vegan diet for years. In any anemia, really, it is wise to supplement B_{12}, because it helps the red blood cells develop to a point where protein, folic acid, iron, and vitamin C can then complete their maturation so that we can better carry oxygen and energy to all of our cells.

Vitamin B_{12} will stimulate growth in many malnourished children. In older people, it has helped with energy levels as well as psychological symptoms, including senile psychosis. B_{12} has also been used to help treat osteoarthritis and osteoporosis and for neuralgias, such as Bell's palsy, trigeminal neuralgia, or diabetic neuropathy. It has likewise been used in the treatment of hepatitis, shingles, asthma, other allergies, allergic dermatitis, urticaria, eczema, and bursitis. Cobalamin has been used for many other symptoms be-

sides fatigue, including nervousness and irritability, insomnia, memory problems, depression, and poor balance. Vitamin B_{12} is something to keep in mind when we are not "feeling our oats."

Deficiency and toxicity: There have been no known toxic effects from megadoses of vitamin B_{12}. Thousands of times more than the RDA have been injected both intravenously and intramuscularly without any ill consequences. On the contrary, there is often some benefit.

Vitamin B_{12} deficiency usually results from a combination of factors. Restricted diets, as seen in vegetarians or poor nations, can be very limited in B_{12}. Since the absorption into the body is so finely tuned, depletion and deficiency occur even more commonly from poor digestion and assimilation, or from deficient production of intrinsic factor. That is why it is so important to be aware of B_{12} and use some sort of supplementation once a deficiency has been diagnosed. Vitamin B_{12} blood levels, along with folic acid levels, are the most common vitamin tests performed by doctors. As we age, it is more likely that we may become B_{12} deficient. Also, alcoholics and people with malabsorption or dementia may have low B_{12} levels. Since the body stores vitamin B_{12}, it may take several years to become deficient with dietary restriction or a decrease in intrinsic factor.

The strict vegetarian has more concern than the average meat- and dairy-eating person. B_{12} is not found in the vegetable kingdom other than in foods fermented by certain bacteria; thus most fermented foods have some vitamin B_{12}. However, in vegetarians, there is usually a high folic acid intake, and since folic acid and B_{12} work similarly in the body, a B_{12} deficiency may be masked for a period of time, and then more pronounced symptoms may occur. If B_{12} is deficient in an animal eater, then we pretty much know there is a problem in absorption of the vitamin.

Most problems of B_{12} deficiency affect the blood, energy level, state of mind, and nervous system. Often, subtle symptoms may start with the nervous system. Vitamin B_{12} nourishes the myelin sheaths over the nerves, which help maintain the normal electrical conductivity through the nerves. Soreness or weakness of the arms or legs, decreased sensory perceptions, difficulty in walking or speaking, neuritis, a diminished reflex response, or limb jerking may result from B_{12} deficiency. Psychological symptoms may include mood changes with mental slowness may be one of the first symptoms.

With B_{12} deficiency, the body forms large, immature red blood cells, resulting in a "megaloblastic" anemia. Pernicious anemia refers to the deficiency in blood cells as well as the myriad of psychological and nerve symptoms. The anemia usually generates more fatigue and weakness. Menstrual problems, even amenorrhea (lack of menstrual flow), may also occur in B_{12}-deficient women.

The problems related to the nervous system caused by vitamin B_{12} deficiency can lead to permanent damage, not correctable by B_{12} supplementation. This irreversible nerve damage may occur when the B_{12} deficiency effect on the red blood cells is masked by adequate levels of folic acid, as I mentioned. More severe pernicious anemia can cause a red, sensitive tongue, referred to as "strawberry tongue," which may even ulcerate, and nerve or brain and spinal cord degeneration, which can cause weakness, numbness, tingling, shooting pains, and sensory hallucinations. Paranoid symptoms may even occur. In the early part of this century, pernicious anemia was often a fatal disease.

Requirements: Vitamin B_{12} is essential but required only in minute amounts; 3–4 mcg. is needed in most adults to prevent deficiency, and at least that amount is required by pregnant or lactating women, as well as infants and growing children. From 10–20 mcg. daily is a good insurance level, although certain people may need increased amounts with higher protein intake. Vitamin B_{12} is often taken in higher doses, 500–1000 mcgs. per day, to relieve fatigue. Injections of B_{12} in these amounts are used to treat a variety of low-energy and mental symptoms previously described as well as during some weight loss programs. When there is fatigue or anemia, it is a good idea to get the blood level of B_{12} checked by a doctor. It may lead to a very simple and successful treatment.

Other B Vitamins

I include here other very important B vitamins that are known only by their chemical names. These are **biotin, choline, folic acid, inositol,** and **para-aminobenzoic acid (PABA)**. Biotin, choline, and inositol are often thought of together because of their similar functions. Folic acid is closely related to amino acid metabolism and maturation of blood cells and vitamin B_{12}, and folic acid deficiency is possibly one of the more common deficiencies of the B vitamin family. PABA is popularly used to promote healthy hair and as a sunscreen to protect the skin from burning.

In general, these vitamins are commonly found in those foods that contain other B vitamins, such as brewer's yeast, liver, wheat germ, and whole grains. Folic acid is also abundant in the dark, leafy green vegetables. Deficiencies of these important nutrients like those of other B vitamins, can affect the skin, nervous system, and mental and physical energy levels and attitudes.

After discussion of these essential five, I will mention three other substances, orotic acid, pangamic acid, and amygdalin or laetrile. These are not B vitamins in the strict sense nor are they essential, but they have become known as vitamins B_{13}, B_{15}, and B_{17}, respectively. Let's look into these vitamins further.

129

Biotin, a fairly recently named B vitamin, was discovered by the deficiency symptoms created through consuming large amounts (about 30 percent of the diet) of raw eggs. Avidin, a protein and carbohydrate molecule in the egg white, binds with biotin in the stomach and decreases its absorption. Cooking destroys the avidin, so the only concern about this interaction is with raw egg consumption. Otherwise, biotin is one of the most stable of the B vitamins.

Sources: Many foods contain biotin, but most have only trace amounts. It is hard to obtain enough biotin from the diet. Luckily, our friendly intestinal bacteria (lactobacillin) produce biotin. This vitamin is found in egg yolks, liver, brewer's yeast, unpolished rice, nuts, and milk.

Functions: The biotin coenzymes participate in the metabolism of fat. Biotin is needed for fat production and in the synthesis of fatty acids. It also helps incorporate amino acids into protein and facilitates the synthesis of the pyrimidines, part of nucleic acids, and therefore helps the formation of DNA and RNA.

Uses: A common use of biotin is to help normalize fat metabolism and utilization in weight-reduction programs, and to help reduce blood sugar in diabetic patients, with a dosage of between 200–400 mcg. per day. Biotin has also been in wide use to prevent or slow the progression of graying hair or baldness. This may work, however, only when these symptoms are related to biotin deficiency; although, because of the nutrient and protein support of biotin, it may indeed have some hair-stimulating effect.

Biotin is often used for problems such as dermatitis or eczema, especially in infants, most often with appropriate intake of other B vitamins, such as riboflavin, niacin, and pyridoxine and vitamin A. It has also been used to treat muscle pains, though skin and hair are the main focus of supplementation. More recently, biotin has been used for diabetics and those with an overgrowth of intestinal yeast.

Deficiency and toxicity: There is no known toxicity with biotin, even in high amounts. Excesses are easily eliminated in the urine. Deficiency symptoms are also uncommon. Unless we are on a raw-egg diet or have taken a lot of antibiotics, especially sulfa, which diminish our biotin-producing intestinal bacteria, we are usually secure against biotin deficiency.

The raw-egg study generated symptoms such as fatigue, nausea, loss of appetite, muscle pains, and depression. Other symptoms that have since been seen with biotin deficiency include dry and flaky skin, loss of energy, insomnia, increases in cholesterol, sensitivity to touch, inflamed eyes, hair loss, muscle weakness, and impaired fat metabolism. Several enzymes depend on biotin to function properly. Without them, we cannot utilize our foods as well.

Biotin deficiency is sometimes seen in babies when a biotin-deficient formula is used or there is some problem with intestinal biotin synthesis. If this occurs, hair loss, muscle weakness, irritated eyes, and a scaly rash may result. In some studies in juveniles, biotin deficiency was seen to result in hair loss and occasional balding. With more advanced biotin deficiency in people of all ages, elevation in cholesterol, anemia, or changes in the electrocardiogram may occur.

Requirements: The recommended level of biotin needed in the diet ranges from 150–300 mcg., depending on how well it is produced by the intestinal bacterial flora. Probably 300–400 mcg. is a safer range. We need extra biotin if we consume raw eggs or have used antibiotics, especially the sulfa drugs. Biotin requirements are also higher during pregnancy and lactation. Infants require at least 50 mcg. per day. The need rises to an RDA of 120 mcg. at ages 7–10; after age 11, it is over 200 mcg. A common amount of biotin in vitamin B supplements is 400 mcg.

Choline is one of the "lipo-tropic" B vitamins—that is, it helps the utilization of fats in the body and thereby supports weight loss. This vitamin is widely available in food but is sensitive to water and may be destroyed by cooking, food processing, improper food storage, and the intake of various drugs, including alcohol, estrogen, and sulfa antibiotics.

Choline is easily absorbed from the intestines and is one of the only vitamins that crosses the blood-brain barrier into the spinal fluid to be involved directly in brain chemical metabolism. Choline is referred to as the "memory" vitamin, as it is an important part of the neurotransmitter acetylcholine.

Sources: Choline is present in all living cells and is widely distributed in plants and animals. Humans can synthesize choline from the amino acid glycine. The highest amount of choline is present in lecithin, usually obtained from soybeans. Other good sources include egg yolk, brewer's yeast, wheat germ, fish, peanuts, some leafy greens, and liver and other organ meats. Choline is probably also manufactured by intestinal bacteria.

Functions: Choline as phosphatidylcholine, is a basic component of soy lecithin and thereby helps in the emulsification of fats and cholesterol in the body, by helping form smaller fat globules in the blood and aiding the transport of fats through the smaller vasculature and in and out of the cells. Choline is combined with fatty acids glycerol and phosphate to make lecithin (see more on lecithin in Chapter 4, *Lipids*), an important part of cell membranes.

Choline is also an integral part of the neurotransmitter acetylcholine. Its availability preserves the integrity of the electrical transmission across the gaps between nerves, and this helps the flow of electrical energy within the nervous system. It is also important to the health of the myelin sheaths covering the nerve fibers. Choline helps the liver and gallbladder function and is vital to brain chemistry, as it seems to aid thinking capacity and memory.

Uses: There are a great many uses for this important B vitamin. Choline may be helpful in the treatment of nerve conduction problems, memory deficiencies, muscle twitching, heart palpitations, and Alzheimer's disease, where it seems to help brain function and slow the progression of the disease. Evidence has been mixed, however, as to effectiveness of phosphatidylcholine/lecithin treatment for Alzheimer's disease; it has certainly not been shown to be a great panacea.

Choline has also been used for many kinds of liver and kidney problems, especially hepatitis and cirrhosis, by improving fat emulsification, transport, and utilization. It may actually help with general body detoxification by "decongesting" the liver of excess fats. Choline has been helpful in reducing some side effects of the phenothiazine drugs, which may cause abnormal facial muscle twitching and spasms, a syndrome called "tardive dyskinesia." It probably works by increasing acetylcholine function, thus promoting the transmission functions at nerve synapses. Recently, purified egg lecithin, which contains choline, has been used in the treatment of AIDS.

Other possible uses for choline are for headaches, dizziness, insomnia, constipation, glaucoma and other eye problems, abnormal ear noises such as tinnitis (ringing), hypoglycemia, and alcohol problems. Choline may be helpful for fatigue, and athletes have benefited from choline supplementation. With high cholesterol and high blood pressure, two important factors in cardiovascular disease, phosphatidylcholine (lecithin) may be helpful in reducing the progression of atherosclerosis. It seems to be effective as a fat and cholesterol emulsifier, and supplementation has been shown to reduce some gallstones. Choline has also been used with some benefit in stroke patients.

Deficiency and toxicity: There are no known toxic effects from choline, though high doses

131

could aggravate epileptic conditions because of its nerve stimulation potential. Neither is there a common deficiency problem, though the therapeutic amounts utilized are usually much higher than those acquired through food or made in the body. There are not any specific symptoms attributed to choline deficiency. When choline is depleted, fat metabolism and utilization may be decreased, conceivably leading to fat accumulations. However, the main concern could involve loss of cell membrane integrity and the effects on the myelin covering of the nerves.

Requirements: No specific minimums for dietary choline are listed. The average needs seem to be about 500 mg. per day, which is about the least amount consumed in an average diet. It is often supplemented at 500 mg. along with the same amount of inositol because both are necessary for membrane integrity. Soy lecithin is the most common source for choline supplementation. One capsule of lecithin contains about 40–50 mg. of choline, while a tablespoon (5 grams) of lecithin has about 500 mg. of choline.

Therapeutic amounts of choline are usually in the 500–1,000 mg. area. More than this may produce some side effects and is likely not needed, although some experiments have utilized higher amounts. It is best taken with other B vitamins. If large amounts of lecithin are taken, more calcium is usually needed to balance the phosphorus contained in the lecithin. Additional choline may be needed when higher amounts of niacin, such as 1–3 grams daily, are taken to lower cholesterol levels Recently, high-quality, concentrated phosphatidylcholine capsules have become available for specific use of this nutrient in place of the more variable lecithin.

Folic Acid (Folacin or Folate) is another of the key water-soluble B vitamins. It received its name from the Latin word *folium,* meaning "foliage," because folic acid is found in nature's leafy green vegetables, such as spinach, kale, and beet greens. Folacin, a derivative of folic acid, is a dull yellow crystalline substance made up chemically of a pteridine molecule, para-aminobenzoic acid (PABA), and glutamic acid. It is actually a "vitamin within a vitamin," with PABA as part of its structure.

Folic acid is very sensitive and is easily destroyed in a variety of ways, such as by light, heat, any type of cooking, or an acid pH below 4; it can even be lost from foods when they are stored at room temperature for long periods. The potency of this B vitamin is diminished in most food processing and food preparation.

When folic acid is consumed, it is actively transported into the blood from the gastrointestinal tract, where it acts as a coenzyme for a multitude of functions and often is converted to its active form, tetrahydrofolic acid (THFA), in the presence of the niacin coenzyme (NADPH) and vitamin C. In the body, folic acid is found mainly as methyl folate, and vitamin B_{12} is needed to convert it back to the active THFA. Extra folic acid is stored in the liver, enough for six to nine months of vitamin for body use before deficiency symptoms might develop.

Folic acid deficiency, however, may still be one of the most common vitamin deficiencies. It is more likely to be a problem in the elderly, in alcoholics, in psychiatric patients, in epileptics, in women on birth control pills, and with drug therapy such as the sulfa antibiotics and tetracyclines that deplete folic acid-producing bacteria in the colon. Pregnancy is a time for concern about sufficient folic acid intake (the RDA doubles during pregnancy). Also, those eating the standard American diet that is high in fats, meats, white flour, white sugar, and desserts may develop folic acid deficiency. Eating some fresh or lightly cooked vegetables daily will allow us to maintain normal folate levels.

Folic acid was discovered in 1931 as a "cure" for the anemia of pregnancy. Eating extra yeast also seemed to relieve the symptoms of pernicious anemia, but the neurological symptoms of this disease either were not resolved or appeared later on, confirming some doctors' feelings that there were two different problems involved. In 1945, folic acid was isolated from spinach; we now know that B_{12} and folic acid produce two very similar deficiency problems. B_{12} deficiency may lead to progressive and irreversible neurological damage, whereas a lack of folic acid will not, but taking a lot of folic acid may cover up the B_{12} anemia and other symptoms until it is too late for effective treatment with vitamin B_{12}. Therefore, vitamin tablets of folic acid with over 400 mcg. have been taken off the market and are available by prescription only. If megaloblastic (enlarged red blood cells) anemia occurs, both folic acid and vitamin B_{12} levels should be checked to assure proper treatment and follow-up.

Sources: The best source of folic acid is foliage, the green leafy vegetables. These include spinach, kale, beet greens and even beets, chard, asparagus, broccoli, sources are liver and kidney and brewer's yeast. Starchy vegetables containing some folacin are corn, lima beans, green peas, sweet potatoes, artichokes, okra, and parsnips. Bean sprouts, such as lentil, mung, and soy, are particularly good, as are wheat germ or flakes and soy flour. Whole wheat bread, other natural, whole grain baked goods, and milk also have some folic acid. And many fruits have folic acid, such as oranges, cantaloupe, pineapple, banana, and many berries, including loganberries, boysenberries, and strawberries.

Remember, folic acid is available from fresh, unprocessed food, which is why it is so commonly deficient in our culture's processed-food diet. Luckily, though, it is easily absorbed, used, and stored by our body. It is also manufactured by our intestinal bacteria, so if colon flora is healthy, we have another good source of folic acid.

Functions: Folic acid, or more specifically, its coenzyme tetrahydrofolic acid (THFA), has functions very similar to those of cobalamin, vitamin B_{12}. Folic acid aids in red blood cell production by carrying the carbon molecule to the larger heme molecule, which is the iron-containing part of hemoglobin (the oxygen-carrying molecule of the red blood cells).

With B_{12} and vitamin C, THFA helps in the breakdown and utilization of protein. With B_{12}, it assists in many amino acid conversions, such as the methylation of methionine, serine, histidine, and even the B vitamin choline. Folic acid is also used in the formation of the nucleic acids for RNA and DNA. Actually, the anemia that results from folic acid deficiency comes from the lack of THFA and decreased synthesis of the purines and pyrimidines that make up the DNA. So folic acid has a fundamental role in the growth and reproduction of all cells.

Since folic acid is important to the division of cells in the body, it is even more essential during times of growth, such as pregnancy. Pregnancy is a time of rapid cell multiplication. If there is a deficiency of folic acid, there is decreased nucleic acid synthesis, and cell division is hampered. This deficiency can lead to low birth weight or growth problems in infants.

Uses: Folic acid is, of course, used to restore its deficiencies and treat the problems resulting from them. People who are very stressed or fatigued or who have any loss of adrenal gland function may benefit from additional folic acid. Those who drink alcohol or take high amounts of vitamin C also require more of this vitamin. Also, epileptics on drug therapy require more folic acid, which may help them by improving mood and mental capacities. In patients with psoriasis, folate is used rapidly by the skin, thus is needed in increased amounts. Teenagers on poor diets with no vegetables and the elderly often are helped by folic acid supplementation.

POSSIBLE CLINICAL USES OF FOLIC ACID

Seborrheic dermatitis	Elderly
Pregnancy	Skin ulcers
Restless leg syndrome	Lactation
Depression	Diarrhea
Alcoholism	Poor appetite
Cervical dysplasia	Fatigue
Cervical cancer	Anemia
Neuropathy	Canker sores
Birth control pills	Gout
Atherosclerosis	Viral hepatitis
Immune weakness	Acne
Dementia	Infection
Organic brain syndrome	Gingivitis
Periodontal problems	Osteoporosis
Estrogen supplementation	

With increased estrogen, as in pregnancy or when taking birth control pills, folic acid supplementation helps prevent deficiency symptoms. More is also required during lactation, which it also aids. Folic acid is often used when there are any menstrual problems. The "restless leg syndrome," which is characterized by creeping, irritating sensations in the legs and occurs most commonly in later pregnancy, is often helped by increasing folic acid, as it may specifically be a deficiency problem.

With both folic acid deficiency anemia and pernicious anemia, folic acid is usually supplemented along with vitamin B_{12}. The fatigue, easy bruising, and inflammation of the tongue that may go along with anemia are often helped as well. Treatment of various blood diseases, osteoporosis, and atherosclerosis has been supported with folic acid. There is some suggestion that it helps in ischemia, with reports of improved blood flow to the eyes and improved vision in those with circulatory deficits.

Folic acid has been used for chronic diarrhea or malabsorption problems and to stimulate a depressed appetite. It may also be helpful in some cases of depression, dementia and brain disorders, epilepsy, or neuropathies, especially when deficient. Folic acid supports healthy skin and may help in healing skin ulcers, particularly of the leg, or sebborheic dermatitis. Usually 1 mg. tablet daily or an oral folate solution may be helpful in treating gingivitis or other periodontal diseases. It has been suggested and used with varying results, usually along with PABA and pantothenic acid, to prevent the graying of hair. Higher doses may have some use in healing dysplasia (precancerous cell changes) of the cervix, which is often associated with lowered folate levels. Further research is needed to substantiate some of these uses.

Deficiency and toxicity: There are no specific toxic symptoms from folic acid intake, at least up to 5 mg. daily. However, excess folic acid in the face of a B_{12} deficiency, when B_{12} is not supplemented and absorbed, may lead to serious consequences. Folic acid will mask the B_{12}-related anemia and early symptoms of vitamin B_{12} deficiency by helping the synthesis of DNA and red blood cell production, but folic acid has no effect on the myelin sheath covering the nerves, so nerve damage may occur where folic acid covers up a B_{12} deficiency. Higher doses of folate may also depress B_{12} levels. In recent research where higher levels (15 mg. daily) of folate have been used, some side effects developed after a month of treatment. These included gastrointestinal symptoms, insomnia, irritability, and malaise.

Folic acid deficiency is fairly common. It generates a picture similar to that of a B_{12} deficiency—anemia, fatigue, irritability, anorexia, weight loss, headache, sore and inflamed tongue, diarrhea, heart palpitations, forgetfulness, hostility, and a feeling of paranoia. Often, the mental symptoms occur before the anemia, with poor memory (possibly from decreased RNA synthesis), general apathy, withdrawal, irritability, and a decrease in basic mental powers.

Folic acid-deficiency anemia is not correctable with iron, and as it progresses, it will appear very different from iron-deficiency anemia. The blood will show large, irregular red blood cells, while low iron causes small red blood cells. In pregnancy, this megaloblastic anemia is of great concern. Folic acid deficiency is very common during pregnancy, when the requirements are at least double those for the nonpregnant state. Since folic acid stores in the liver can last several months, deficiency symptoms are more likely in later pregnancy. The fetus can readily draw on the folic acid of the mother, and deficiencies can cause problems in both. The mother's folacin-deficiency mental symptoms of indifference, lack of motivation, withdrawal, or depression may be passed over as hormonal. The anemia may likewise not be considerd a matter for concern. Serious problems can result from a major deficiency. Toxemia of pregnancy, premature birth, and hemorrhage are all possible in addition to the anemia of the mother. The fetus could develop birth deformities, brain damage, or show poor growth as a child. **It is very important to supplement folic acid during pregnancy.**

In general, folic acid deficiencies can result from:

- Inadequate nutrition, particularly lack of fresh fruits and vegetables;
- Poor absorption, as in malabsorption, with intestinal problems, with pellagra, or after stomach or intestinal surgery;
- Metabolic problems, such as those created by alcohol or drug use; and
- Excessive demands by tissues, as with stress, illness, or pregnancy.

We should be concerned about folate deficiency primarily in pregnancy, during breast-feeding, and in the elderly. Folic acid absorption seems to diminish with age, and deficiency is common in the elderly, especially those in rest or nursing homes, who are unlikely to get fresh vegetables or supplements.

Often, the first manifestation of a low folate level is feeling depressed. Folic acid deficiency is more common in people with depression or other psychological symptoms in mental institutions. Alcoholics have had serious problems maintaining proper folic acid levels. Teenagers with poor diets, who do not eat green vegetables or many vegetables at all other than fried potatoes, may more easily become folic acid deficient. If we suspect deficiencies, it is wise to get a blood folate level as well as a B_{12} level before treatment with supplements. A red-blood-cell folate level may more accurately reflect body stores of folic acid.

Besides causing mental symptoms, folate deficiency can also affect the skin. As in vitamin B_2 (riboflavin) deficiency, cracks or scaling at the lips and corners of the mouth (cheilosis) may occur. Also possible with deficiency are decreased growth, fatigue, and more rapid graying of the hair. More recently, folid acid deficiency (along with vitamin A deficiency) has been associated with cervical dysplasia and cancer.

Requirements: The RDA for folic acid is 400 mcg. in adults, 800 mcg. during pregnancy, and 600 mcg. during lactation. And many factors increase the minimum requirement for folic acid. But the average American diet contains only about half of this, about 220 mcg. This reveals why disorders involving folic acid deficiency are so common.

Between 180 and 200 mcg. of folic acid are needed daily to maintain the tissue stores of folate. During pregnancy, times of stress or illness, or with alcohol use, the demands are increased, and a 200 mcg. daily intake is not sufficient for supporting folic acid functions and maintaining tissue stores. Deficiency symptoms may then occur.

Other things besides stress, illness, and alcohol use create greater need for folic acid. Birth control pills may reduce absorption of this vitamin by 50 percent. Other drugs besides estrogen may interfere with absorption or metabolism. These include the sulfa antibiot-

RDAS FOR FOLIC ACID

Infants	30–50 mcg.
1–3 years	100 mcg.
4–6 years	200 mcg.
7–10 years	300 mcg.
14 years older	400 mcg.
Pregnant women	800 mcg.
Lactating women	600 mcg.

ics, phenobarbital, and antiepileptic drugs such as Dilantin and Mysoline. Consumption of more than 2,000 mg. of vitamin C per day also increases the need for folic acid. Anyone in these situations needs supplements of folic acid.

Most vitamin formulas contain 400 mcg. of folic acid. Higher amounts, such as 1 mg. (1,000 mcg.), 1.5 mg., or even 10 mg., are available only by prescription because of the concern of masking vitamin B_{12} deficiency. Injectable folate, in doses from 1–10 mg., may also have a place in nutritional medicine. Some doctors describe impressive results in many patients, especially the elderly, with injections of 1,000 mcg. of B_{12} and 10 mg. of folic acid. The suggested therapeutic dosages for most uses of folic acid or treating deficiency problems is about 1 mg. twice daily; it may take several months for this vitamin therapy to correct the deficiency and replenish stores of folic acid. Some studies are researching folic acid doses of 5–15 mg., and even up to 60 mg. daily.

The elderly, the pregnant, and women on birth control pills should definitely take additional folic acid. And the alcoholic also needs extra folic acid supplementation.

Inositol, also part of the B vitamin complex, is closely associated with choline. Like choline, inositol (as phosphatidylinositol) is also found in lecithin, though in lesser amounts than choline, and acts as a lipotropic agent (milder than choline) in the body, helping to emulsify fats. The body can produce its own inositol from glucose, so it is not really essential. We have high stores of inositol; its concentration in the body is second highest of the B vitamins, surpassed only by niacin.

Sources: Inositol is present in both plants and animals. It is part of phospholipids in animals; in plants, it is contained in phytic acid, which can bind calcium and iron. It is not totally clear how inositol is produced by the body; it may be made by intestinal bacteria. It is stored in the body, but drinking lots of coffee can deplete these stores. Inositol is found in the whole, unprocessed grains, citrus fruits (except lemons), cantaloupe, brewer's yeast, unrefined molasses, and liver. It is also available in wheat germ, lima beans, raisins, peanuts, cabbage, and some nuts. And, of course, lecithin is a good source.

Functions: Inositol, as phosphatidylinositol, has its primary function in cell membrane structure and integrity. Other functions of phosphatidylinositol are somewhat obscure. With choline, it may help in brain cell nutrition. Inositol is especially important for the cells of the bone marrow, eye tissue, and intestines. And it may also have something to do with hair growth.

Uses: Although inositol has been used to treat and prevent progression of athero-sclerosis throughout the body and to help reduce cholesterol, there is no good evidence from human studies that inositol lowers cholesterol and protects against cardiovascular disease. As a mild lipotropic agent, though, it is commonly used by overweight people to help with weight loss, and it may help in redistributing body fat. Exercise helps, too, of course.

Inositol helps promote healthy hair and skin. It has been used to treat eczema, and it may help the hair, especially if there is an inositol deficiency. For sleep, 500 mg. of inositol before bed has a mild antianxiety effect (placebo?) as well as possibly helping to utilize fat and cholesterol during sleep.

Inositol has also had some success therapeutically in improving the nerve function in diabetic patients with pain and numbness due to nerve degeneration. Generally, diabetic people should take extra inositol. People with multiple sclerosis may also receive some benefit with inositol supplementation, as there seems to be a higher percentage of inositol deficiency in nerve cell membranes in those patients.

Deficiency and toxicity: There is no known toxicity with inositol even in amounts of 50 grams, which are much higher than normal uses. Deficiencies are also uncommon, since inositol is so available in foods and the body also makes it. Caffeine, however, can produce an inositol deficiency. Some problems that have been associated with low levels of inositol in the body are eczema, constipation, eye problems, hair loss, and elevations of cholesterol. There may also be a greater propensity for fatty plaques to form in the heart and arteries and more likelihood for cardiovascular disease.

Requirements: There is no specific RDA for inositol, since it can be made in our bodies. We usually obtain it readily from food in an amount of about 1 gram daily. A therapeutic dosage is usually about 500 mg.; however, it should be taken with choline and other B vitamins and mainly as lecithin, which contains the natural balance of phospholipids. I do not recommend taking separate inositol capsules. Needs are increased with regular coffee consumption of more than two cups daily. Soy lecithin contains about 40 mg. of phosphatidylinositol per capsule.

Para-aminobenzoic Acid (PABA) is also a member of the B vitamins, and is part of the folic acid molecule. PABA itself is readily available in food and is made by our intestinal bacteria. It is known specifically for its nourishment to hair and its usefulness as a sunscreen.

Sources: PABA is found in liver, brewer's yeast, wheat germ, whole grains such as rice, eggs, and molasses. It is stored in body tissues and is also synthesized by the natural bacteria flora in our intestines.

Functions: Para-aminobenzoic acid, as part of the coenzyme tetrahydrofolic acid, aids in the metabolism and utilization of amino acids and is also supportive of blood cells, particularly the red blood cells. PABA supports folic acid production by the intestinal bacteria. PABA is important to skin, hair pigment, and intestinal health. Used as a sunscreen, it also can protect against the development of sunburn and skin cancer from excess ultraviolet light exposure.

Uses: Although PABA has been much used in attempts to stimulate hair growth and to turn gray hair back to its natural color, it has not had wide success in such uses. It may work in some cases that are related to a PABA deficiency. If graying of hair is caused by vitamin deficiency, it is likely a deficiency of a combination of vitamins, mostly the various Bs. PABA is usually used along with biotin, pantothenic acid, and folic acid in the restoration of hair, often with vitamin E as well. PABA is also used to reduce aging of the skin and lessen wrinkles. Vitiligo, a skin depigmenting condition, which could result from deficient hydrochloric acid, vitamin C, or pantothenic acid, may be helped somewhat by PABA, both orally and as a cream. PABA ointment is used commonly to prevent and treat sunburns and, with vitamin E, is often applied to other burns.

Deficiency and toxicity: It is possible that high doses of PABA can be somewhat irritating to the liver; in addition, nausea and vomiting have occurred, as have anorexia, fever, skin rash, and even vitiligo. Deficiency problems are not very common; they occur more frequently with the use of sulfa or other antibiotics that alter the functioning of intestinal bacteria and, therefore, the production of PABA. General fatigue, irritability, depression, nervousness, graying hair, headache, and constipation or other digestive symptoms may occur. Several patients have told me that they are "sensitive" to PABA in vitamin formulae and, thus, cannot take them (most vitamin combinations contain PABA). I do not know what this reaction is unless it is some allergy to the para-amino-benzoic acid molecule.

Requirements: No RDA is listed for PABA. It is available in supplements of 50–1,000 mg. Up to 1,000 mg. are used therapeutically in a time-released capsule, although the common treatment amount is usually about 50–100 mg. three times daily. If we take antibiotics, we might increase our intake of PABA for a while, although PABA taken with sulfa antibiotics may reduce their effectiveness. A therapeutic approach used by some authorities to attempt to restore normal hair color is 1,000 mg., time-released, daily for six days a week, taken with 400 mcg. of folic acid.

Vitamin B₁₃ (Orotic Acid)

I mention this substance here only for the sake of completeness. It is not really recognized as a vitamin, but it may be an accessory nutrient.

Actually, there is not much information about orotic acid. It has been used recently as orotate salts combined with such minerals as calcium, magnesium, and potassium. This is based on the work by German doctor Hans Nieper. Dr. Nieper's work has included treatment of multiple sclerosis and other chronic diseases with these mineral orotates. His experience concluded that orotate salts were active transporters of these minerals into the blood from the gastrointestinal tract. The salts then separate from the mineral in the blood, allowing the mineral to be used and leaving orotic acid available.

Orotic acid is found in a few natural food sources—for example, milk products and some root vegetables, such as carrots, beets, and Jerusalem artichokes. Orotic acid is a nucleic acid precursor and is needed for DNA and RNA synthesis. The body can make orotic acid for this purpose from its amino acid pool. As long as protein nutrition is adequate, the body can carry on nucleic acid synthesis. Neither toxicity or deficiency of orotic acid are likely a concern.

Recently, many medical claims for orotates have been made by foreign markets and the U.S. health industry. Due to this reason and possibly other political-economic ones, the U.S. Food and Drug Administration (FDA) has recently asked for the removal of orotates from the U.S. marketplace.

Vitamin B₁₅ (Pangamic Acid)

This is still a fairly controversial "vitamin." The quotation marks suggest that we are not sure whether it is a vitamin. It has not yet been shown to be essential in the diet (vitamins must be supplied from external sources), and no symptoms or deficiency diseases are clearly revealed when consumption is restricted. The FDA has been concerned about the wide range of medical conditions treated with it, primarily in other countries, and therefore pangamic acid is not readily available to the U.S. consumer. Because most of the information about pangamic acid is dated and is mainly from European and Soviet research, I discuss this substance here mainly for completeness.

The Soviet Union has been the most enthusiastic about pangamic acid, feeling that it is a very important nutrient with physiological actions that can treat a multitude of symptoms and diseases. Soviet scientists have shown that pangamic acid supplementation can reduce the buildup of lactic acid in athletes and thereby lessen muscle fatigue and increase endurance. It is used regularly and commonly in the Soviet Union for many problems, including alcoholism and drug addiction; mental problems such as those of aging and senility, minimal brain damage in children, autism, and schizophrenia; heart disease and high blood pressure; diabetes; skin diseases; liver disease; and chemical poisonings.

As I said, the FDA has taken pangamic acid products off the market. Dimethyl glycine (DMG) has been used by some people as a substitute as it is thought to increase pangamic acid production in the body. Dimethyl glycine combines with gluconic acid to form pangamic acid. It is thought that the DMG is the active component of pangamic acid.

Sources: Pangamic acid was first isolated in 1951 by Drs. Ernest Krebs, Sr. and Jr., from apricot kernels, along with laetrile, termed vitamin B$_{17}$. At that time, as today, they were not sure whether it was essential to life.

Pangamic acid is also found in whole grains such as brown rice, brewer's yeast, pumpkin and sunflower seeds, and beef blood. Water and direct sunlight may reduce the potency and availability of B$_{15}$ in these foods.

Functions: Pangamic acid is mainly a methyl donor, which helps in the formation of certain amino acids such as methionine. It may play a role in the oxidation of glucose and in cell respiration. By this function, it may reduce hypoxia (deficient oxygen) in cardiac and other muscles. Like vitamin E, it acts as an antioxidant, helping to lengthen cell life through its protection from oxidation. Pangamic acid is also thought to offer mild stimulation to the endocrine and nervous systems, and by enhancing liver function, it may help in the detoxification process.

Uses: Although many of these uses are not proven, there have been reports of pangamic acid or DMG providing some benefits for a wide range of symptoms, diseases, and metabolic problems. It may be useful for such symptoms as headaches, angina and musculoskeletal chest pain, shortness of breath, insomnia, and general stress—to be used, of course, only after specific medical conditions are ruled out.

B$_{15}$ has been shown to lower blood cholesterol, so it could provide some nutritional support for those with high serum cholesterol or cardiovascular problems or to reduce heart and blood vessel disease risks. It may also help improve circulation and general oxygenation of cells and tissues, so it may be used with any decreased cardiac or brain functions. Pangamic acid may be helpful in general for atherosclerosis and hypertension, America's most common diseases.

In Europe vitamin B$_{15}$ has been used to treat premature aging, because of both its circulatory stimulus and its antioxidant effect. It is felt to be a helpful protectant from pollutants, especially carbon monoxide. Pangamic acid (and possibly DMG) support for anyone living in a large polluted city or with a high-stress lifestyle could be a wave of the future.

In Russia, a big use of pangamic acid has been for treating those with alcohol problems, possibly reducing the craving. It has been reported to diminish hangover symptoms when alcohol has been abused. B$_{15}$ has also been used to treat fatigue, as well as asthma and rheumatism, and it may even have some antiallergic properties. Some child psychiatrists have reported good results using pangamic acid in disturbed children; it may help by stimulating speaking ability and other mental functions. B$_{15}$ may also be useful in problems of autism.

More studies regarding all claims of the benefits of pangamic acid must be done, of course, to see which ones may be valid. But as of now, it certainly is a "vitamin" or supplemental nutrient with potential health benefits and research interest.

Deficiency and toxicity: There are no known toxic effects from even high amounts of pangamic acid; 50–100 mg. (and even more) taken three times daily have revealed no side effects. There are reports of initial mild nausea with use of pangamates at high levels, but this only lasts a few days.

There is limited information about deficiencies of pangamic acid. There are no clear problems when it is absent in the diet, though some diminished circulatory and oxygenation functions are possible. Decreased cell respiration—that is, decreased oxygen use by cells—may influence many other cellular functions which may lead to effects on the heart.

Requirements: There is no RDA for pangamic acid. At the time of this writing, it is not legal to distribute B_{15} in the United States, though it was used as a supplement for some time in the 1970s. The most common form of pangamic acid was calcium pangamate, but currently it is dimethyl glycine (DMG), which may even be the active component that has been hailed in the Soviet Union. Pangamic acid or DMG, when used, is often taken with vitamin E and vitamin A. A common amount of DMG is 50–100 mg. taken twice daily, usually with breakfast and dinner. This level of intake may improve general energy levels, support the immune system, and is also thought to reduce cravings for alcohol and thus may be very helpful in moderating chronic alcohol problems.

Vitamin B_{17} (Laetrile)

Vitamin B_{17}, also known as laetrile and amygdalin, is another controversial "vitamin," as its source, the apricot kernel, becomes a focus of increasing interest. As with pangamic acid, B_{17} was also discovered by Dr. Ernest T. Krebs Sr., who thought it a vitamin essential to health, and who first tried amygdalin therapeutically. Laetrile is a nitriloside compound composed of four molecules: two sugar, one benzaldehyde, and one cyanide. It is likely the cyanide that accounts for the controversy over this substance, particularly in regard to cancer

therapy. Using laetrile—amygdalin, vitamin B_{17}, nitriloside, whatever we call it—as a treatment for cancer is now illegal in the United States. Some people seeking such treatment go to Mexico or other laetrile-supportive countries.

Arguments against laetrile as a therapy cite concerns about possible cyanide toxicity as well as studies that show it is not effective as a cancer treatment. Studies, however, cannot be completely objective, especially on a subject as complex as cancer, which is influenced by so many factors. The proponents of laetrile claim that cyanide is a natural molecule found in food and is not toxic in normal doses; laetrile treatment itself is not known to have any side effects in usual dosages. But, obviously, considering Western medicine's use of chemotherapy, radiation, and surgery, side effects are not the main concern when treating a life-threatening disease. The proof in any treatment is, ultimately, whether it works.

Amygdalin is not digested in the stomach by hydrochloric acid, but passes into the small intestine where it is acted on by enzymes that split it into various compounds, which are then absorbed.

Sources: Laetrile is found primarily in apricot kernels and comprises about 2–3 percent of the kernel. It is also available in the kernels of other fruits, such as plums, cherries, peaches, nectarines, and apples. The fruit kernels or seeds generally have other nutrients as well—some protein, unsaturated fatty acids, and various minerals. B_{17} is not found with other B vitamins in yeasts. Many plants do, however, contain some B_{17}, with the sprouting seeds, especially mung bean sprouts, containing the highest amount.

Functions: The specific theoretical function of laetrile is its effect on cancer cells. Normal cells have an enzyme, rhodanase, that inactivates the cyanide molecule of the laetrile compound. Cancer cells do not possess this enzyme. In fact, they have an enzyme, beta-glucosidase, that releases the cyanide, which then poisons the cancer cells.

Uses: The main use for laetrile is in the treatment of cancer, particularly to reduce tumor size and further spread, and to alleviate the sometimes severe pains of the cancerous process. As I stated, more well-designed research needs to be done to determine whether this compound in its natural form is effective. Other uses reported for laetrile have been in the treatment of high blood pressure and rheumatism.

Deficiency and toxicity: There are no known problems caused by not consuming this "vitamin," other than, theoretically, a deficiency could increase the likelihood of developing cancer. There are, however, concerns over toxicity, due to the cyanide within the vitamin or possibly from other metabolic effects. Usually, treatment amounts are limited to 1 gram to reduce potential side effects, which initially are most likely gastrointestinal in nature. Toxicity of this molecule must be researched further.

Requirements: This nutrient is not required as far as we know; in fact, it is against the law in the United States. When used, laetrile is administered at 250–1,000 mg. (1 gram) daily. Higher amounts—up to 3 grams per day— have been used, but divided into several smaller dosages, each usually limited to 1 gram. If the source is whole apricot kernels, the quantity is usually about 10–20 kernels per day; 1–2 cups of fresh mung bean sprouts may provide an equivalent amount. If apricot kernels are blended or pulverized, it is suggested that they be consumed immediately.

 Vitamin C (Ascorbic Acid) is a very important essential nutrient—that is, we must obtain it from diet. It is found only in the fruit and vegetable foods and is highest in fresh, uncooked foods. Vitamin C is one of the least stable vitamins, and cooking can destroy much of this water-soluble vitamin from foods.

In recent years, the C of this much-publicized vitamin has also stood for controversy. With Linus Pauling and others claiming that vitamin C has the potential to prevent and treat the common cold, flus, and cancer, all of which plague our society, concern has arisen in the medical establishment about these claims and the megadose requirements needed to achieve the hoped-for results. Some studies suggest that these claims have some validity; however, there is more personal testimony from avid users of ascorbic acid than there is irrefutable evidence. There has also been some recent research that disproves the claims about treatment and prevention of colds and cancer with vitamin C. However, in most cases, studies showing vitamin C to be ineffective used lower dosages than Dr. Pauling recommended. Overall, vitamin C research is heavily weighted to the positive side for its use in the treatment of many conditions, including the common cold.

C also stands for citrus, where this vitamin is found. It could also stand for collagen, the protein "cement" that is formed with ascorbic acid as a required cofactor. Many foods contain vitamin C, and many important functions are mediated by it as well.

Vitamin C is a weak acid and is stable in weak acids. Alkalis, such as baking soda, however, destroy ascorbic acid. It is also easily oxidized in air and sensitive to heat and light. Since it is contained in the watery part of fruits and vegetables, it is easily lost during cooking in water. Loss is minimized when vegetables such as broccoli or Brussels sprouts are cooked over water in a double boiler instead of directly in water. The mineral copper, in the water or in the cookware, diminishes vitamin C content of foods.

Ascorbic acid was not isolated from lemons until 1932, though the scourge of scurvy, the vitamin C deficiency disease, has been present for thousands of years. It was first written about circa 1500 B.C. and then described by Aristotle in 450 B.C. as a syndrome character-

141

ized by lack of energy, gum inflammation, tooth decay, and bleeding problems. In the 1700s, high percentages of sailors with the British navy and other fleets died from scurvy, until James Lind discovered that the juice of lemons could cure and also prevent this devastating and deadly disease. The ships then carried British West Indies limes for the sailors to consume daily to maintain health, and thus these sailors became known as "limeys." Other cultures of the world discovered their own sources of vitamin C. Powdered rose hips, acerola cherries, or spruce needles were consumed regularly, usually as teas, to prevent the scurvy disease.

In earlier times, humans consumed large amounts of vitamin C in their fresh and wholesome native diet, as apes (another species that does not make vitamin C) still do. Most other animals, except guinea pigs, produce ascorbic acid in the liver from glucose, and in relative amounts much higher than we get from our diets today. For this reason, Dr. Pauling and others feel that our bodies need somewhere between 2,000 and 9,000 mg. of vitamin C daily. These amounts seem a little high to me, given the basic food values of vitamin C. Some authorities feel we need 600–1,200 mg. daily based on extrapolations from the historical herbivore, early-human diet. These levels can be obtained today by eating sufficient fresh food; a diet that includes foods with high levels of vitamin C can provide several grams or more per day.

Ascorbic acid is readily absorbed from the intestines, ideally about 80–90 percent of that ingested. It is used by the body in about two hours and then usually out of the blood within three to four hours. For this reason, it is suggested that vitamin C supplements be taken at four-hour intervals rather than once a day; or it may be taken as time-released ascorbic acid. Vitamin C is used up even more rapidly under stressful conditions, with alcohol use, and with smoking. Vitamin C blood levels of smokers are much lower than those of non-

smokers given the same intakes. Other situations and substances that reduce absorption or increase utilization include fever, viral illness, antibiotics, cortisone, aspirin and other pain medicines, environmental toxins such as DDT, petroleum products, or carbon monoxide, and exposure to heavy metals such as lead, mercury, or cadmium. Sulfa antibiotics increase elimination of vitamin C from the body by two to three times.

Some ascorbic acid is stored in the body, where it seems to concentrate in the organs of higher metabolic activity. These include the adrenal glands (about 30 mg.), pituitary, brain, eyes, ovaries, and testes. A total of about 5 grams is available from our body tissues, or about 30 mg. per pound of body weight. We likely need at least 200 mg. a day in our diet to maintain body stores—much more if we smoke, drink alcohol, are under stress, have allergies, are elderly, or have diabetes.

Vitamin C is a very complex and important vitamin. The recommended amounts vary more widely than those for any other nutrient, ranging from 100–80 or 100 grams daily, depending on the condition. C is also the most commonly supplemented vitamin among the general public, because of either the popular press or its good effect, or because of the other common C—the "cold."

Sources: The best-known sources of vitamin C are the citrus fruits—oranges, lemons, limes, tangerines, and grapefruits. The fruits with the highest natural concentrations are citrus fruits, rose hips, and acerola cherries, followed by papayas, cantaloupes, and strawberries. Good vegetable sources include red and green peppers (the best), broccoli, Brussels sprouts, tomatoes, asparagus, parsley, dark leafy greens, cabbage, and sauerkraut. There is not much available in the whole grains, seeds, and beans; however, when these are sprouted, their vitamin C content shoots up. Sprouts, then, are good foods for winter and early spring, when other fresh fruits and vegetables are not as available. Animal foods contain almost no vitamin C; though fish, if eaten raw, has enough to prevent deficiency symptoms.

Natural vitamin C supplements are usually made from rose hips, acerola cherries, peppers, or citrus fruits. Vitamin C can be synthesized from corn syrup, which is high in dextrose, much as it is made from glucose in most other animals' bodies. Synthetic ascorbic acid, though it can be concentrated for higher doses than natural extracts, is still usually made from food sources. Sago palm is another fairly new source of vitamin C supplements. It is used primarily as a lower allergenic source than the corn-extracted ascorbic acid.

Functions: One important function of vitamin C is in the formation and maintenance of collagen, the basis of connective tissue, which is found in skin, ligaments, cartilage, vertebral discs, joint linings, capillary walls, and the bones and teeth. Collagen, and thus vitamin C, is needed to give support and shape to the body, to help wounds heal, and to maintain healthy blood vessels. Specifically, ascorbic acid works as a coenzyme to convert proline and lysine to hydroxyproline and hydroxylysine, both important to the collagen structure.

Vitamin C also aids the metabolism of tyrosine, folic acid, and tryptophan. Tryptophan is converted in the presence of ascorbic acid to 5-hydroxytryptophan, which forms serotonin, an important brain chemical. Vitamin C also helps folic acid convert to its active form, tetrahydrofolic acid, and tyrosine needs ascorbic acid to form the neurotransmitter substances dopamine and epinephrine. Vitamin C stimulates adrenal function and the release of norepinephrine and epinephrine (adrenaline), our stress hormones; however, prolonged stress depletes vitamin C in the adrenals and decreases the blood levels. Ascorbic acid also helps thyroid hormone production, and it aids in cholesterol metabolism, increasing its elimination and thereby assisting in lowering blood cholesterol.

Vitamin C is an antioxidant vitamin. By this function, it helps prevent oxidation of water-soluble molecules that could otherwise create free radicals, which may generate cellular injury and disease. Vitamin C also indirectly protects the fat-soluble vitamins A and E as well as some of the B vitamins, such as riboflavin, thiamine, folic acid, and pantothenic acid, from oxidation. Ascorbic acid acts as a detoxifier and may reduce the side effects of drugs such as cortisone, aspirin, and insulin; it may also reduce the toxicity of the heavy metals lead, mercury, and arsenic.

Vitamin C is being shown through continued research to stimulate the immune system; through this function, along with its antioxidant function, it may help in the prevention and treatment of infections and other diseases. Ascorbic acid may activate neutrophils, the most prevalent white blood cells that work on the frontline defense in more hand-to-hand combat than other white blood cells. It also seems to increase production of lymphocytes, the white cells important in antibody production and in coordinating the cellular immune functions. In this way also, C may be helpful against bacterial, viral, and fungal diseases. In higher amounts, ascorbic acid may actually increase interferon production and thus activate the immune response to viruses; it may also decrease the production of histamine, thereby reducing immediate allergy potential. Further research must be done for more definitive knowledge about vitamin C's actions in the prevention and treatment of disease.

Uses: There are a great many clinical and nutritional uses for ascorbic acid in its variety of available supplements. C for the common cold is indeed used very widely; its use in the treatment of cancer is more controversial, probably because of the seriousness of the disease and the political environment within the medical system—anything nutritional or alternative in regard to cancer therapy is looked upon with skepticism by orthodox physicians. For the prevention of cancer, there is reason for more optimism about the usefulness of vitamin C (as well as the other antioxidant nutrients—vitamin E, selenium, beta-carotene, and zinc) because of its effect in preventing the formation of free radicals (caused mainly by the oxidation of fats), which play a role in the genesis of disease.

Given the functions of vitamin C alone, it has a wide range of clinical uses. For the prevention and treatment of the common cold and flu syndrome, vitamin C produces a positive immunological response to help fight bacteria and viruses. Its support of the adrenal function and role in the production of adrenal hormones epinephrine and norepinephrine can help the body handle infections and stress of all kinds. Because of this adrenal-augmenting response, as well as thyroid support provided by stimulating production of thyroxine (T_4) hormone, vitamin C may help with problems of fatigue and slow metabolism. It also helps counteract the side effects of cortisone drug therapy and may counteract the decreased cellular immunity experienced during the course of treatment with these commonly used immune-suppressive drugs.

Because of ascorbic acid's role in immunity, its antioxidant effect, the adrenal support it provides, and probably its ability to make tissues healthy through its formation and maintenance of collagen, vitamin C is used to treat a wide range of viral, bacterial, and fungal infections and inflammatory problems of all kinds. I have used vitamin C successfully in many viral conditions, including colds, flus, hepatitis, *Herpes simplex* infections, mononucleosis, measles, and shingles. Recently, vitamin C has been shown in some studies to enhance the production and activity of interferon, an antiviral substance produced by our bodies. To affect these conditions, the vitamin C dosage is usually fairly high, at least 5–10 grams per day, but it is possible that much smaller doses are as effective. Vitamin C is also used to treat problems due to general inflammation from microorganisms, irritants, and/or decreased resistance; these problems may include cystitis, bronchitis, prostatitis, bursitis, arthritis (both osteo- and rheumatoid), and some chronic skin problems (dermatitis). With arthritis, there is some suggestion that increased ascorbic acid may improve the integrity of membranes in joints. In gouty arthritis, vitamin C improves the elimination of uric acid (the irritant) through the kidneys. Ascorbic acid has also been helpful for relief of back pain and pain from inflamed vertebral discs, as well as the inflammatory pain that is sometimes associated with rigorous exercise. In asthma, vitamin C may relieve the bronchospasm caused by noxious stimuli or when this tight-chest feeling is experienced during exercise.

Vitamin C's vital function in helping produce and maintain healthy collagen allows it to support the body cells and tissues and bring more rapid healing to injured or aging tissues. Therefore, it is used by many physicians for problems of rapid aging, burns, fracture healing, bedsores and other skin ulcers and to speed wound healing after injury or surgery. Peptic ulcers also appear to heal more rapidly with vitamin C therapy. The pre- and postsurgical use of vitamin C supplementation can have great benefits. With its collagen function, adrenal support, and immune response support, it helps the body defend against infection, supports tissue health and healing, and improves the ability to handle the stress of surgery. Vitamin A and zinc are the other important pre- and postsurgical nutrients shown by research to reduce hospitalization time and increase healing rates, thereby preventing a number of potential complications.

Vitamin C is also used to aid those withdrawing from drug addictions, addictions to such substances as narcotics and alcohol, as well as nicotine, caffeine, and even sugar—three very common addictions and abuses. High-level ascorbic acid may decrease withdrawal symptoms from these substances and increase the appetite and feeling of well-

VITAMIN C USES

Colds	Anemia
Flus	Atherosclerosis
Hepatitis	Herpes infections
Arthritis	Hypertension
Bursitis	Depression
Allergies	Infertility
Asthma	Surgery recovery
Glaucoma	Fatigue
Bruising	Peptic ulcer
Varicose veins	Skin ulcers
Cancer prevention	Gout
Cataract prevention	Diabetes
High cholesterol levels	Cervical dysplasia
High triglyceride levels	Chemical exposure
Periodontal disease	Gallbladder disease
Immune suppression	

being. For this reason, it may be helpful in some depression and other mental problems associated with detoxification during withdrawal. Vitamin C also may reduce the effects of pollution, likely through its antioxidant effect, its detoxifying help, and its adrenal and immune support; specifically, it may participate in protecting us from smog, carbon monoxide, lead, mercury, and cadmium.

Vitamin C is a natural laxative and may help with constipation problems. In fact, the main side effect of too much vitamin C intake is diarrhea. For iron-deficiency anemia, vitamin C helps the absorption of iron (especially the nonheme or vegetable-source iron) from the gastrointestinal tract. In diabetes, it is commonly used to improve the utilization of blood sugar and thereby reduce it, but there is no clear evidence that regular vitamin C usage alone can prevent diabetes. There are some preliminary reports that ascorbic acid may help prevent cataract formation (probably through its antioxidant effect) and may be helpful in the prevention and treatment of glaucoma, as well as certain cases of male infertility caused from the clumping

together of sperm, which decreases sperm function.

Vitamin C has a probable role in the prevention and treatment of atherosclerosis and, thereby, in reducing the risks of heart disease and its devastating results. It has been shown to reduce platelet aggregation, a factor important in reducing the formation of plaque and clots. Ascorbic acid has a triglyceride- and cholesterol-reducing effect and, more important, may help to raise the "good" HDL. This action needs further investigation, though the research is supportive so far. I haven't even mentioned the prevention of scurvy, which really takes very little vitamin C, about 10 mg. per day. This disease used to be a big concern and was often fatal unless the victim ate some citrus or other fresh fruit and vegetables containing a small amount of vitamin C.

I do not really want to approach the cancer and vitamin C issue; it deserves a book by itself. However, if we closely analyze the functions (antioxidant, immune support, interferon, tissue health and healing) that vitamin C performs in the body, along with the still mysterious influences of higher-dose ascorbic acid intake, we can see how vitamin C may have a positive influence in fighting and preventing cancer, our greatest twentieth-century medical dilemma.

Deficiency and toxicity: For most purposes, vitamin C, or ascorbic acid, in its many forms of use is nontoxic. It is not stored appreciably in our body, and most excess amounts are eliminated rapidly through the urine. However, amounts over 10 grams per day that some people use and some doctors prescribe are associated with some side effects, though none that are serious. Diarrhea is the most common and usually is the first sign that the body's tissue fluids have been saturated with ascorbic acid. Most people will not experience this with under 5–10 grams per day, the amount that is felt to correlate with the body's need and use. Other side effects include nausea, dysuria (burning with urination), and skin

145

sensitivities (sometimes sensitivity to touch or just a mild irritation). Hemolysis (breakage) of red blood cells may also occur with very high amounts of vitamin C. With any of these symptoms, it is wise to decrease intake.

There is some concern that higher levels of vitamin C intake may cause kidney stones, specifically calcium oxalate stones, because of increased oxalic acid clearance through the kidneys due to vitamin C metabolism. This is a rare case, if it does exist, and I personally have not seen, nor do I know any doctors who have seen, kidney stone occurrence with people taking vitamin C. Only people who are prone to form kidney stones or gout should give this any thought. If there is concern, supplementing magnesium in amounts between half and equaling that of calcium intake (which should be done anyway with calcium supplementation) would reduce that risk, at least for calcium-based stones. I usually suggest using a buffered vitamin C preparation with calcium and magnesium, which alleviates this concern.

As far as deficiency problems go, the once fairly common disease called scurvy is very rare these days. However, early symptoms of scurvy or vitamin C deficiency are more likely in formula-fed infants with little or no C intake or in teenagers or the elderly who do not eat any fresh fruits and vegetables. Smokers with poor diets and people with inflammatory bowel disease more often have lower vitamin C blood levels. Other people commonly found to be low in ascorbic acid include alcoholics, psychiatric patients, and patients with fatigue.

The symptoms of scurvy are produced primarily by the effects of the lack of ascorbic acid on collagen formation, causing reduced health of the tissues. The first signs of depletion may be related to vitamin C's other functions as well, where deficiency could lead to poor resistance to infection and very slow wound healing. Easy bruising and tiny hemorrhages, called petechiae, in the skin, general weakness, loss of appetite, and poor digestion may also occur. With worse deficiency, nosebleeds, sore and bleeding gums, anemia, joint tenderness and swelling, mouth ulcers, loose teeth, and shortness of breath could be experienced. During growth periods, there could be reduced growth, especially of the bones. The decrease in collagen may lead to bone brittleness, making the bones more fragile. The progression and health of the teeth and gums are also affected. In breastfeeding women, lactation may be reduced. With the elderly, vitamin C deficiency could enhance symptoms of senility. The bleeding that comes from capillary wall fragility may lead to clotting and increased risk of strokes and heart attacks.

An important note is that many medical problems have been found to be associated with low blood levels of vitamin C. These problems include various infections, colds, depression, high blood pressure, arthritis, vascular fragility, allergies, ulcers, and cholesterol gallstones.

Most of these symptoms and problems can be easily avoided with minimal supplementation of vitamin C or a diet well supplied with fresh fruits and vegetables. Since the average diet has much less vitamin C than that of our ancestors, it is important for us to be aware of our ascorbic acid intake.

Requirements: The RDA for adults is considered to be 60 mg. We need only about 10–20 mg. to prevent scurvy, and there is more than that in one portion of most fruits or vegetables. Infants need 35 mg.; about 50 mg. between ages one and fourteen and 60 mg. afterward are the suggested minimums. During pregnancy, 80 mg. are required; 100 mg. are needed during lactation. Realistically, between 100–150 mg. daily is a minimum dosage for most people.

Vitamin C needs, however, are increased with all kinds of stress, both internal (emotional) and external (environmental). Smoking decreases vitamin C levels and increases minimum needs. Birth control pills, estrogen for menopause, cortisone use, and aspirin also increase ascorbic acid requirements. Both nicotine and estrogen seem to increase copper blood levels, and copper inactivates vitamin C. In general, though, absorption of vitamin C from the intestines is good. Vitamin C (as ascorbic acid) taken with iron helps the absorption of iron (and many minerals) and is important in treating anemia, but the iron decreases absorption of the ascorbic acid. Overall, it is probably best to take vitamin C as it is found in nature, along with the vitamin P constituents (discovered later)—the bioflavonoids, rutin, and hesperidin. These may have a synergistic influence on the functions of vitamin C, although there is no conclusive research on humans to support this theory.

Vitamin C is the most commonly consumed nutrient supplement and is available in tablets, both fast-acting and time-released, in chewable tablets, in powders and effervescents, and in liquid form. It is available as ascorbic acid, L-ascorbic acid, and various mineral ascorbate salts, such as sodium or calcium ascorbate. One of my favorite formulas, which was developed by Stephen Levine at Nutricology in San Leandro, California, is a buffered powder made from sago palm that contains 2,350 mg. of vitamin C per teaspoon, along with 450 mg. of calcium, 250 mg. of magnesium, and 99 mg. of potassium. It gets into the body quickly and is very easy on and often soothing to the stomach and intestinal lining. The potassium-magnesium combination can often be helpful for fatigue, and this formula is a good vehicle for fulfilling calcium needs.

Vitamin C works rapidly, so the total amount we take over the day should be divided into multiple doses (four to six) or taken as a time-released tablet a couple of times a day. When increasing or decreasing vitamin C intake, it is best to do so slowly because our body systems become accustomed to certain levels. Some nutritionists describe a problem of rebound scurvy in infants, especially when a high amount is taken by the mother during preg-nancy but then the infant gets very little after birth and so suffers some deficiency symptoms. I have seen nothing confirming this in the literature. Overall, though, it is probably wise to reduce vitamin C intake slowly after taking high amounts, rather than to drop abruptly.

My basic suggestion for vitamin C use is about 2–4 grams per day with a typical active and healthy city lifestyle. Based on previous levels in our native diets, Linus Pauling feels that the optimum daily levels of vitamin C are between 2,500 and 10,000 mg. Clearly, requirements for vitamin C vary and may be higher according to state of health, age (needs increase with years), weight, activity and energy levels, and general metabolism. Stress, illness, and injuries further increase the requirements for ascorbic acid. Many authorities suggest that we take at least 500 mg. of vitamin C daily to meet basic body needs.

During times of specific illnesses, especially viral infections, doctors who use megadose vitamin C treatment suggest at least 20–40 grams daily, some of it intravenously. Vitamin C has been used safely and effectively in dosages of 10 grams or more dripped slowly (over 30–60 minutes) into the blood to reach optimum tissue levels before excretion, so as to bathe the cells in vitamin C. Some doctors prescribe what is called "bowel tolerance" daily intake of vitamin C—that is, increasing the oral dose until diarrhea results and then cutting back. This level can vary greatly from a few grams to 100 grams or more. The claim is that our body knows what we need and will respond by changing the water balance in the colon when we have had enough. Physician Robert Cathcart has used vitamin C this way in his practice for years to treat many problems, with claimed good success; yet, I do not have the experience to make an adequate conclusion. This practice does, however, add further mystery to the vitamin C controversy. More research is definitely needed regarding ascorbic acid, and new discoveries will likely be made.

147

Vitamin P (Bioflavonoids) are the water-soluble companions of ascorbic acid, usually found in the same foods. Vitamin P includes a number of components that work together—citrin, hesperidin, rutin, flavones, flavonals, and catechin and quercetin, which will also be discussed in Chapter 7, *Accessory Nutrients.* Their association with vitamin C is the reason that natural forms of vitamin C are more effective than are synthetic ascorbic acids without the bioflavonoids in the equivalent amounts.

Vitamin P was first discovered in 1936 by Soviet scientist Dr. Albert Szent-Gyorgyi, who found it within the white of the rind in citrus fruits. It is contained mainly in the edible pulp of the fruits rather than in the strained juices. The letter P, for permeability factor, was given to this group of nutrients because they improve the capillary lining's permeability and integrity—that is, the passage of oxygen, carbon dioxide, and nutrients through the capillary walls.

The bioflavonoids are easily absorbed from the intestinal tract, as is vitamin C. Some is stored in the body, though most of the excess is eliminated in the urine and perspiration.

Sources: The main source of bioflavonoids is the citrus fruits—lemons, grapefruits, oranges, and, to a lesser extent, limes. Rose hips, apricots, cherries, grapes, black currants, plums, blackberries, and papayas are other fruit sources of vitamin P. Green pepper, broccoli, and tomatoes are some good vegetable sources of bioflavonoids. The buckwheat plant, leaf and grain, is a particularly good source of bioflavonoids, especially the rutin component.

Functions: The bioflavonoids are helpful in the absorption of vitamin C and protect the multifunctional vitamin C molecule from oxidation, thereby improving and prolonging its functioning. Therefore, the bioflavonoids are indirectly, and possibly directly, involved in maintaining the health of the collagen that holds the cells together by forming the basement membranes of cells, tissues, and cartilage.

The main known function of the bioflavonoids is to increase the strength of the capillaries and to regulate their permeability. The capillaries link the arteries to the veins. They deliver oxygen and nutrients to the organs, tissues, and cells and then pick up carbon dioxide and waste and carry them through the veins and back to the heart. By its support of the capillaries, vitamin P helps to prevent hemorrhage and rupture of these tiny vessels, which could lead to easy bruising. Also, capillary strength may help protect us from infection, particularly viral problems. Bioflavonoids also can reduce the amount of histamine released from cells; quercetin is definitely strong in this function.

Uses: The main use of the bioflavonoids is to provide synergy in the utilization of vitamin C; therefore they contribute to many vitamin C applications—for example, the treatment of colds and flus. Bioflavonoids themselves are often supplemented for problems where improved capillary strength is needed, such as bleeding gums, easy bruising, and duodenal bleeding ulcers, which may be worsened by weak capillaries. The rutin component is particularly good for decreasing bleeding from weak blood vessels. In hemorrhoids, varicose veins, spontaneous abortions, excess menstrual bleeding (menorrhagia), postpartum hemorrhage, nosebleeds, the bleeding problems of diabetes, and generally during pregnancy, the bioflavonoids may be helpful in maintaining capillary health and reducing bleeding concerns. For women who have repeated spontaneous abortions or premature labor, supplementing citrus bioflavonoids—for example, 200 mg. three times daily—may be helpful in remedying these problems. Vitamin P has been used also in asthma, allergies, bursitis and arthritis, and eye problems secondary to diabetes and as protection from the harmful effects of radiation.

After all that, though, there is not much scientific evidence to support these clinical uses of bioflavonoids. Though they were touted very highly for a while, further research must be done to substantiate these claims.

Deficiency and toxicity: There is no known toxicity from any of the components of the bioflavonoids. Deficiency is fairly unlikely, although, as with vitamin C, an increased tendency to bruise or bleed is possible with vitamin P deficiency. Also, the protection that vitamin C gives against inflammatory problems, as in arthritis, may be lost when the bioflavonoids are not in the diet or supplemented. In my medical experience a question arises: if people respond to bioflavonoid (or any nutrient) supplementation, does that suggest a deficiency or depletion was present?

Requirements: There is no RDA for the bioflavonoids, perhaps because they naturally occur with vitamin C. When they are supplemented, 500 mg. bioflavonoids—containing 50 mg. rutin and 50 mg. hesperidin—is usually taken from one to three times daily. Supplements of 125 or 250 mg. of bioflavonoids are also commonly available and can be taken daily with the same frequency.

 Vitamin L (The Love Vitamin) is commonly known as the "universal" or the "love" vitamin, as coined by humanologist, Bethany ArgIsle. One of the most important nutrients for optimum health is a daily dose (or more) of Love. This vital human emotion/expression/experience is necessary for the optimal functioning of people and all of their cells, tissues, and organs. It is found in most of nature—in foods, domestic animals, friends, and family—and is used to heal a wide variety of diseases. There are no toxic effects, but deficiency can cause a wide range of ailments.

Sources: As stated, L is found in a great variety of sources but must be developed and nurtured to be available. Fear, anger, worry, self-concern, and many other human emotions can destroy vitamin L. It is found readily in most moms and dads and is very highly concentrated in grandmothers and grandpas. Sisters and brothers may be a good source of vitamin L, though often this is covered up in early years, develops in the teens, and is more available in adulthood. Massage therapy is a particularly good source of vitamin L.

Vitamin L is also found in cats, dogs, and horses; in flowers and birds; and in trees and plants. In food, it is especially found in home-cooked or other meals where vitamin L is used consciously as an ingredient. It is digested and absorbed easily and used by the body in its pure state, being eliminated almost unchanged; in this, it is unique among the vitamins. It is also made by friendly bacteria and all positive reactions and attitudes in the body.

Functions: This vitamin acts as the "universal" vitalizing energy. Vitamin L helps to catalyze all human functions and is particularly important to heart function and the circulation of warmth and joy. Digestion is very dependent on appropriate doses of vitamin L, as is the function of the nervous system. Adrenaline, the brain endorphins (natural tranquilizers and energizers), and other hormones are enhanced by vitamin L as well. A wide variety of other bodily and life functions are dependent on vitamin L, and it is extremely important to the healing process.

Uses: The list of uses is even longer than that of the functions. Vitamin L is an important nutrient in all human relations, domestic to international. We should definitely put it in the drinking supply! It is a vital ingredient in all health practitioners, doctors, clinics, and hospitals. Besides being referred to as the "universal" vitamin, Love is also known as the catalytic "vitamin of healing." It can pass through the energy vibrations of the healer to the recipient. It should be used in all heart problems and a wide variety of medical conditions. Vitamin L is also particularly helpful in all kinds of psychological disturbances. Depression, sadness, anger, fear, worry, pain, concern over world affairs, and many stresses of life can be helped by vitamin L therapy. It is particularly important in resolving relationship difficulties. Fear, one of the more difficult problems to treat, usually requires megadoses of vitamin L, as does greed.

Deficiency and toxicity: There are rarely any serious problems from excess intake of vitamin L. Side effects, however, may include swooning, a strange feeling in the center of the chest, goosebumps, and staring blankly into space. Usually, though, amounts many times the minimum requirements offer no difficulty and are often helpful.

Deficiency, as with many of the vitamins, cause a great many more problems than overdoses. Fatigue, muscle tension, increased likelihood of stress conditions, digestive upset, drug problems, and sexual aberrations are only a few of the possible effects of vitamin L deficiency. Diseases of the heart are of particular concern. Vitamin L can become deficient easily in people under great demand to perform, such as doctors, nurses, and other hospital workers or in people whose jobs are very cerebral, such as businesspersons, accountants, and stockbrokers.

Abrupt withdrawal from regular vitamin L use could be hazardous, as the love vitamin is somewhat addicting. People have varying sensitivities to decreases in vitamin L, and deficiency symptoms may occur easily. It is wise to replace any reductions with vitamin L from other sources (a key reason for having compassionate health practitioners). Increased amounts of vitamin L are more easily tolerated by most people, though huge increases should be taken slowly to prevent the side effects mentioned previously.

Requirements: The requirements may vary from person to person according to a wide range of factors. There are no specific RDAs for vitamin L, although infants and small children usually require fairly large doses. The suggested minimum from the Chinese culture is four hugs per day to maintain health. Recently, though, the International Hug Association (IHA) has changed its guidelines and suggests that a minimum of four hugs daily is needed to prevent vitamin L deficiency, six hugs a day for maintenance, and ten hugs per day for growth.

Vitamin T

 Known as the "sesame seed factor," vitamin T is found in sesame seeds and egg yolks. We do not yet know exactly what this substance is, but it is thought to be helpful in preventing anemia and the hemolysis of red blood cells. Halvah, a high-protein food made from sesame seeds, helped keep the armies marching in the time of Alexander the Great.

Vitamin U

 As with vitamin T, not much is known about vitamin U either. It is found in raw cabbage, has no known toxicity, and may be helpful in healing ulcers of the skin and intestinal tract. This nutrient is probably allantoin, which has tissue-healing power, and is found in herbs such as comfrey root, which is known to help heal and soothe the gastrointestinal mucosa. Cabbage, commonly consumed in longevity cultures such as the Hunzas, has been thought to be a very important enzyme food.

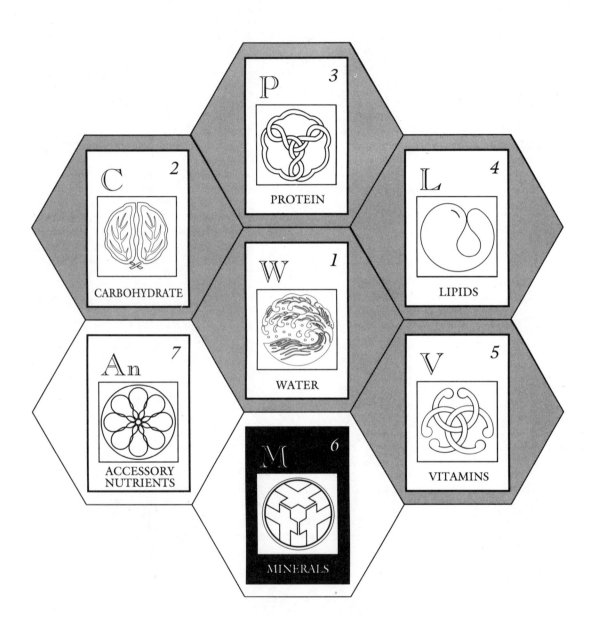

Chapter 6

Minerals

Minerals are what remain as ash when plant or animal tissues are burned or decompose completely after death. These "minerals" are actually the inorganic elements, of which there are approximately 103 currently known, listed on the chemistry periodic table. Minerals, or elements, come from the earth and eventually return to the earth and can most simply be defined as chemical molecules that cannot be reduced to simpler substances.

Minerals are basic constituents of all matter. They are part of living tissue as well as existing in their inorganic form in the earth. Approximately 4–5 percent of our body weight is mineral matter, and most of that is in our skeleton. Minerals are also present in tissue proteins, enzymes, blood, some vitamins, and so on. If the human body were left to decompose completely, most of the organic tissues—which are made up of proteins, carbohydrates, and fats (themselves composed of carbon, oxygen, hydrogen, and nitrogen)—would break down into water (H_2O), carbon dioxide (CO_2), and nitrogen (N_2) and either evaporate into the atmosphere or enter the soil. What was left would be about five pounds of elemental mineral ash. Of this, about 75 percent would be calcium and phosphorus, mostly from the bones; there would be about a teaspoon of iron, a couple of teaspoons of salt (sodium and chloride), and a little more of potassium; and the rest of the ash would contain numerous other elements.

In *Nutrition and Vitamin Therapy*, Michael Lesser, M.D., describes our body composition: The average human body is made up of 65 percent oxygen (O), 18 percent carbon (C), 10 percent hydrogen (H), and 3 percent nitrogen (N), which is contained in the proteins. Approximately 90 percent of the oxygen and 70 percent of the hydrogen combine to make the body's water, which constitutes two-thirds of our body weight. The remaining elements form the organic constituents—proteins, fats, and carbohydrates (by definition, organic molecules contain carbon). Much of the body's inorganic minerals is incorporated into organic matter as well.

The main elements, each of which makes up more than 0.01 percent of total body weight, are termed the bulk minerals, or macrominerals. These are calcium (1.5 of body weight), phosphorus (1), potassium (0.35), sulfur (0.25), sodium (0.15), chloride (0.15), magnesium (0.05), and silicon (0.05). (Silicon is not often listed as an essential element, though in recent years we have begun to realize its importance.) Most of the calcium and phosphorus is in the bones, but some is also present in the blood and in every cell. Calcium particularly is vital to heart and muscle function and nerve conductivity. The remaining phosphorus and most of the sulfur mix with the four primary elements to form the fats, proteins, and nucleic acids.

The next group of elements, though found only in minute amounts in the body, are also essential to health. By definition the trace minerals, or trace elements, constitute less than 0.01 percent of our total body weight. Many of these are measured in micrograms (mcg.) or in milligrams (mg.), as are the macrominerals (1 gram = 1,000 mg.; 1 mg. = 1,000 mcg.; thus, 1 million micrograms per gram). Historically, and again recently, our minerals were measured in parts per million (ppm) of body weight (1 ppm = 1 mcg. per gram).

Most of the trace elements discussed here are essential for life and health. Of these, iron is the most prevalent (60 ppm). Next is fluoride (37 ppm). There is some controversy about whether fluoride is actually essential and, though it does seem to prevent tooth decay when applied directly to the teeth or supplied in drinking water, there is clearly some danger of toxicity (fluorosis) from its regular use. Zinc follows fluoride at 33 ppm; the rest of the elements are present in considerably lower concentrations. Rubidium and strontium are both measured at 4.6 ppm; neither is regarded as essential. Bromine (2.9 ppm) is possibly essential, and copper (1.2 ppm) is definitely needed by our bodies. The remainder of the trace elements (some will be noted later as ultratrace elements) are boron (0.7 ppm), barium (0.3), cobalt (0.3), vanadium (0.3), iodine (0.2), tin (0.2), manganese (0.2), selenium (0.2), molybdenum (0.1), arsenic (0.1), and chromium (0.09). Of these, we know cobalt, iodine, manganese, selenium, molybdenum, and chromium are absolutely essential.

Other elements contained in the body include some of the toxic metals, which may cause harm in relatively high concentrations. These are primarily lead (1.7 ppm), aluminum (0.9), cadmium (0.7), and mercury (0.17). Through mining the earth, we have removed and used many of these toxic minerals, the heavy metals. They are now found more often in the atmosphere (for example, lead from car exhausts), in the rivers, in our food sources, and in many industrial products.

Metal poisoning primarily affects the metabolic enzymes, brain, and nervous system, but it can affect many other bodily functions as well. In addition to these toxic metals, some essential elements, such as copper, arsenic, iodine, selenium, chromium, and even iron and calcium, are more likely than other minerals to cause health problems when high levels are present in the body, resulting either from excessive intake or reduced ability to eliminate them.

ELEMENTAL COMPOSITION OF THE HUMAN BODY
(70Kg/155lbs)

Macrominerals	*Key Function*	*Grams*
OXYGEN	Cell and tissue respiration, water	43,000
CARBON	Protoplasm	12,000
HYDROGEN	Water, tissue	6,300
NITROGEN	Protein tissue	2,000
CALCIUM	Bone and teeth	1,100
PHOSPHORUS	Bone and teeth	750
POTASSIUM	Intracellular electrolyte	225
SULFUR	Amino acids, hair and skin	150
CHLORIDE	Electrolyte	100
SODIUM	Extracellular electrolyte	90
MAGNESIUM	Metabolic electrolyte	35
SILICON	Connective tissue	30
Microminerals		*Mg.*
IRON	Hemoglobin, oxygen carrier	4,200
FLUORIDE	Bones and teeth	2,600
ZINC	Metallo-enzymes	2,400
STRONTIUM	Bone integrity	320
COPPER	Enzyme cofactor	90
COBALT	Vitamin B_{12} core	20
VANADIUM	Lipid metabolism	20
IODINE	Thyroid hormones	15
TIN	Unknown	15
SELENIUM	Enzyme, antioxidant, detoxification	15
MANGANESE	Metallo-enzymes	13
NICKEL	Unknown	11
MOLYBDENUM	Enzyme cofactor	8
CHROMIUM	Glucose tolerance factor	6

This chart is adapted from a paper entitled "Essential Trace Elements, An Overview" by Dewitt Hunter M.D. and is based on percent body weights and parts per million (ppm) in this text. 1 ppm = 1 mcg. (microgram) per gram, 1000 mcg. = 1 mg. (milligram), 1000 mg. = 1 g. (gram).

What do minerals do for us? Like the vitamins, they contain no calories or energy in themselves but assist the body in energy production. Although our bodies can manufacture some vitamins, we make no minerals. Our natural minerals come from the earth. If a mineral nutrient is not contained in the soil, it will not be in the food grown there and thus will not be provided to us when we consume that food. Loss of topsoil,

155

continual replanting without enriching the soil, and the farmer's use of fertilizers that contain only nitrogen, phosphorus, and potassium (all of which stimulate plant growth) and not the other important macro- and micro- (trace) minerals, mean that our food may not contain all the minerals it once did. Fruits and vegetables grown in rich, well-nourished soils obviously will have more of the essential minerals we need for our health and vitality. Unfortunately, refinement and processing of foods decrease the mineral content even more.

Yes, obtaining the full spectrum of essential minerals is very important. In fact, in clinical, nutritional medicine, minerals may be even more important than vitamins. Deficiencies of many vital minerals are more common than deficiencies of vitamins since our body does not manufacture minerals and foods may be enriched with vitamins. Also, minerals are harder to liberate from food complexes during digestion—thus, lower amounts are absorbed; there is also more uptake competition between minerals, and compared to vitamins, a lower percentage of minerals move passively from the gastrointestinal tract to the blood. Like vitamins, minerals are essential to our physical and mental health and are a basic part of all cells, particularly blood, nerve, and muscle cells, as well as our bones, teeth, and all soft tissue. Minerals offer us both structural and functional support. The special electrolyte minerals—sodium, potassium, and chloride—help regulate the fluid and acid-base balance of our bodies. Other minerals are part of enzymes that catalyze biochemical reactions and aid the production of energy or participate in metabolism. Some minerals also help in nerve transmission, muscle contraction, cell permeability, and blood and tissue formation.

What does it mean for a mineral to be "essential"? Like other nutrients, when our bodies cannot produce them or produces them in quantities insufficient to support the functions in which they are used, they are said to be essential. Most commonly, a mineral is considered essential if deficiency symptoms are seen when it is lacking in the diet and the symptoms resolve when it is resupplied. This is easy to demonstrate with many of the body's bulk minerals, such as calcium, magnesium, sodium, and potassium; many problems arise when these are not supplied in the diet. But essentiality of the trace minerals is more difficult to determine; however, recent research has shed a great deal of light on many important subtleties of the trace minerals. Chromium and selenium, for years primarily the subject of toxicity concerns, now are known to be essential to carbohydrate metabolism and blood sugar regulation (GTF-chromium) and to proper immune function, heart function, and cancer prevention (selenium).

Other methods have been used to determine whether a mineral is essential to the body. If it is a necessary component of another essential nutrient, as is cobalt within vitamin B_{12}, it is considered essential. If it is a necessary part of tissues, fluids, or an enzyme used in a metabolic or bioenergetic process, it may be deemed essential.

There are approximately 17 essential minerals. (The primary elements carbon, hydrogen, oxygen, and nitrogen, part of all living tissue and food, are not included here.) The eight macrominerals are calcium (Ca), phosphorus (P), sodium (Na), potassium (K), chloride (Cl), sulfur (S), magnesium (Mg), and silicon (Si). Silicon is prevalent in the environment and seems to be important in some body functions and many body tissues, such as teeth, bones, and elastic tissue. Though silicon, or silica, deficiency does not seem to occur in humans, making its essentiality questionable, it is likely one of the "unsung" macrominerals.

The trace minerals that are known to be essential are iron (Fe), zinc (Z), copper (Cu), cobalt (Co), iodine (I), manganese (Mn), chromium (Cr), molybdenum (Mo), and selenium (Se). Vanadium (V), boron (B), and tin (Sn) are most likely essential. Research on lithium (Li) and rubidium (Rb) indicates that they are also probably essential. Strontium (Sr), nickel (Ni), fluoride (F), bromine (Br), barium (Ba), and arsenic (As) are all possibly essential in very small amounts. Probably nonessential are gold (Au), silver (Ag), aluminum (Al), mercury (Hg), cadmium (Cd), and lead (Pb); the latter four, possibly along with bismuth (Bi), beryllium (Be), and higher amounts of arsenic (As) are considered the toxic minerals.

Through several mechanisms, the body fine-tunes the levels of most of the minerals to maintain optimum functioning. Absorption from the gastrointestinal tract, the first step in getting the mineral into the circulation, can be a fairly complex process. Elimination through the kidneys through the urine or from the liver and bile or other digestive juices through the intestinal tract is the primary way to reduce mineral levels. The body can utilize a mineral in metabolic functions or store it in the tissues. Also, the body may control absorption of one mineral by preferentially absorbing a similar one, according to current needs. Many of the minerals compete with each other when naturally present in our diet or when we supplement them. For example, large amounts of calcium can reduce absorption of magnesium, phosphorus, zinc, and manganese. Zinc can reduce iron, copper, and phosphorus absorption, while phosphorus when taken in excess can interfere with absorption of a great many minerals.

Minerals are available to the body in a variety of forms. A common form is inorganic salts, such as sodium chloride or ferrous phosphate. They can also be part of organic salts or contained in plant or animal tissues, as mineral chelates, or bound to amino acids or protein molecules, as iron is in hemoglobin. *Chelation*, from the Greek word for "claw," refers to holding or "grabbing" a mineral by a special type of chemical bonding. Many minerals are chelated by organic molecules in nature; this is a natural process which enables a mineral to be better absorbed into the body.

Many minerals may be found in water in their free ionic states—that is, as positively or negatively charged particles. The salts that are the major components of seawater also provide the general matrix of cellular life. The main cations (positively charged ions)— sodium, potassium, calcium, and magnesium—combine with the negatively charged anions chloride, phosphate (phosphorus and four oxygen atoms), and carbonate (carbon and four oxygen atoms). The minerals may be in solution, such as calcium, magnesium, sodium, or potassium in water, or they may be present as free metals. The charge, or valence, of a mineral describes its balance between protons (positively

157

charged particles) and electrons (negatively charged particles), which determines the mineral's capacity to combine and whether it acts as an acid or a base in the body. The monovalent ions, those with one extra proton or electron (sodium(+), potassium(+) and chloride(-)), are absorbed more easily through the intestinal wall than the divalent ions, which have two extra protons, or a plus-two charge (calcium and magnesium). The lining of the gastrointestinal tract is also both electrically and ionically charged and, thus, may not allow other ions to pass through easily. That is why chelated minerals or mineral salts (positive and negative ions joined together) may be absorbed more easily.

Iron is a good example of the complexity of mineral absorption. Iron is found in two positive ionic forms, ferrous (2+) and ferric (3+). Ferric iron, as in iron pellets, is not very stable in nature or usable by the body, so iron supplements commonly contain ferrous forms, such as ferrous sulfate. The ferrous salts themselves vary in solubility. Vitamin C can help convert ferric ions to the more usable ferrous ones. Ferrous sulfate is potentially more irritating to the digestive tract than many other forms and may cause irritation, "gripping," and constipation. Other salts, such as ferrous gluconate or ferrous fumarate, are handled more easily by most people.

Minerals are available in water and, of course, in food, when they are in the soil in which it is grown. Minerals commonly found in water include calcium, magnesium, sodium, potassium, chloride, phosphates, and sulfates, and, depending on the source of the water, it could include iron, zinc, or copper as well. It is wise to investigate the mineral levels of our drinking water because imbalances or toxicities could develop from regular use of water from some sources. "Soft" water, which has had most of the minerals removed, is usually higher in sodium, which is not particularly healthy, especially for people with high blood pressure and cardiovascular problems. "Hard" water usually has more of the other minerals, such as calcium and magnesium, which may be helpful in those same diseases.

The mineral content of foods gives each food the potential for being acid or alkaline in the body. (Acid and alkaline diets are further discussed in chapters of Part Three, *Building a Healthy Diet.*) When food decomposes or is incinerated, either an acid or a base ash is left. Thus, a food can be either acid-forming or alkaline-forming. Our basic body acid-base balance (pH) is slightly alkaline, so more of our diet should consist of alkaline-forming foods, primarily the fruits and vegetables. Interestingly enough, these foods usually have a relatively high mineral content. Even though many people think of citrus foods as "acidic," they are actually alkaline in function—that is, they create an alkaline residue. Meats, dairy foods, and most nuts, seeds, and grains decompose with an acid residue, so too much of these may throw off the body's pH.

In general, most minerals are only moderately well absorbed even when the digestive system is functioning well. With digestive difficulties, trace minerals such as chromium and zinc may be absorbed poorly, and deficiency symptoms may develop quite rapidly. Most minerals are not destroyed by heat, but some are soluble in water and therefore are lost or leached out during the cooking process. I have already mentioned a number

MINERALS LOST THROUGH FOOD PROCESSING*

Wheat Milling			Refining Sugarcane	
Mineral	*Loss*		*Mineral*	*Loss*
Manganese	88%		Magnesium	99%
Chromium	87%		Zinc	98%
Magnesium	80%		Chromium	93%
Sodium	78%		Manganese	93%
Potassium	77%		Cobalt	88%
Iron	76%		Copper	83%
Zinc	72%			
Phosphorus	71%			
Copper	63%			
Calcium	60%			
Molybdenum	60%			
Cobalt	50%			

* Compiled from information found in *The Trace Elements and Man* (Devon-Adair Co., 1973), by Henry Schroeder, M.D.

of agricultural (modern farming), environmental (pollution and depletion), and food-processing (refined and nutritionally deficient) factors that cause the loss of even more of the once-prevalent elemental substances essential to human life.

Henry Schroeder, M.D., in *The Trace Elements and Man* (Devon-Adair Co., 1973), describes the losses of essential trace minerals through food processing. Milling of wheat has been the subject of the most research, and the findings are listed in the above table. But similar losses arise with polishing rice and refining cornmeal. Raw cane sugar has a wide range of trace elements, almost all of which are lost when white sugar is made; figures for these losses are also given below. The molasses left after refining sugar, which is rich in minerals, is usually fed to animals; the same is true of the "mill feed" pulled out of wheat and other grains. Similar losses occur for most of the vitamins.

Many minor and major problems can arise from mineral deficiencies. Well known is osteoporosis, a loss of bone minerals due mainly to long-term, low calcium intake (and vitamin D deficiency). Low calcium and, probably, low magnesium levels may contribute to hypertension, as does high sodium with lower potassium levels. Magnesium deficiency has also been associated with muscular spasms and nerve-related pain and, more recently, with acute heart attacks. Low zinc or selenium levels may hinder the immune system and make us prone to infection. The list goes on.

Even though many of these minerals are essential to life, there are RDA minimums for only a few—calcium, phosphorus, iron, iodine, zinc, copper, and magnesium. RDA minimums need to be established for many others, and the awareness of subtle, undiagnosed mineral deficiency states needs to increase. Even the minerals for which RDAs have been established need to be reevaluated; for instance, I believe that magnesium warrants much more attention and research. Further investigation to increase knowledge about the mineral content of foods and requirements in the diet should result in a new focus on this area not only by the government and the food industry but by the public as well.

All the macrominerals are needed in doses of over 100 mg. daily, with sodium requirements somewhere between 2–5 grams, potassium 3–4 grams, phosphorus about 1–2 grams, calcium 1–1.5 grams, and magnesium probably about 0.5–1 gram. The trace minerals are needed in much smaller amounts. To be on the safe side, daily intake of iron and zinc should probably be about 15–30 mg.; manganese about 5–10 mg.; and copper about 2 mg. Other trace minerals, such as chromium, selenium, molybdenum, cobalt, and iodine are needed in amounts of less than 1 mg. per day. (See discussions of the individual minerals for the specific requirements.)

The healthiest approach for assuring optimum mineral levels is to get the majority of them from wholesome foods. Eating a variety of foods, with a lot of organic, local produce and grains is a good start. Nourishing the soil is necessary to begin to get these basic elements into, and then back from, the earth. Picking and eating fresh vegetables from our own composted gardens would be ideal. Avoiding refined and processed foods that have poor mineral content, or high-sugar foods, caffeine, and alcohol, all of which can "flush" or deplete body minerals, is also a helpful habit. Eating a calcium-rich diet has been confused with drinking lots of milk, which poses potential health concerns related to fat intake. Raw nuts and seeds, whole grains, and leafy greens can provide adequate amounts of calcium. If we orient ourselves to the healthiest of diets—eating a variety of wholesome foods—we will assure ourselves the basics of good mineral nutrition.

THE MACROMINERALS

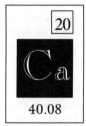

20
Ca
40.08

CALCIUM

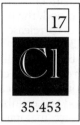

17
Cl
35.453

CHLORIDE

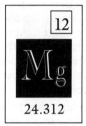

12
Mg
24.312

MAGNESIUM

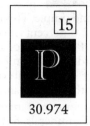

15
P
30.974

PHOSPHORUS

19
K
39.102

POTASSIUM

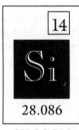

14
Si
28.086

SILICON

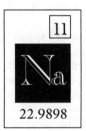

11
Na
22.9898

SODIUM

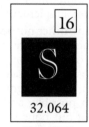

16
S
32.064

SULFUR

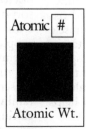

Atomic #

Atomic Wt.

Calcium is the most abundant mineral in the human body and one of the most important. The calcium topic is huge and complex; let me try to make it concise and simple. This mineral constitutes about 1.5–2.0 percent of our body weight. Almost all (98 percent) of our approximately three pounds of calcium is contained in our bones, about 1 percent in our teeth, and the rest in the other tissues and the circulation.

Calcium and magnesium are the "earth alkali" minerals found in the earth's crust, usually as salts that are fairly insoluble. (The word calcium comes from the Latin *calc*, meaning "lime," as in limestone, a calcium carbonate substance.) Dolomite, a calcium-magnesium earth mineral combination that is a little more soluble and usable by the body than some other forms, is a commonly used calcium supplement.

Many other nutrients, vitamin D, and certain hormones are important to calcium absorption, function, and metabolism. Phosphorus as well as calcium is needed for normal bones, as are magnesium, silicon, strontium, boron possibly, and the protein matrix—all part of our bone structure. The ratio of calcium to phosphorus in our bones is about 2.5:1; the best proportions of these minerals in our diet for proper metabolism are currently under question.

Calcium works with magnesium in its functions in the blood, nerves, muscles, and tissues, particularly in regulating heart and muscle contraction and nerve conduction. Vitamin D is needed for much calcium (and phosphorus) to be absorbed from the digestive tract. Along with parathyroid hormone and calcitonin secreted by the thyroid, vitamin D helps maintain normal blood calcium levels.

Maintaining a balanced blood calcium level is essential to life, especially for cardiac function. A normal blood calcium level is about 10 mg. percent—that is, about 10 mg. per 100 milliliters (ml.) of blood. Of that, approximately 5.5 mg. are in ionic form as Ca^{++}, about 4 mg. are bound to carrier proteins, and about 0.5 mg. is combined with phosphate or citrate. If there is not enough calcium in the diet to maintain sufficient amounts of calcium in the blood, the parathyroid glands will be activated to release more parathyroid hormone (PTH), which will then draw calcium out of the bones as well as increase intestinal absorption of available calcium. So even though most of our body's calcium is in the bones, the blood and cellular concentrations of this mineral are maintained first. This is why, with nearly 30 percent of people in this country eating calcium-deficient diets, osteoporosis (a loss of bone substance) is so prevalent.

Elderly people usually have less calcium in their diets than others do, and calcium deficiency particularly affects postmenopausal women. But low dietary calcium is only one factor in the huge and complex topic of calcium bioavailability from foods, calcium absorption, and osteoporosis. Many factors are involved in making calcium available for its many essential functions. Vitamin D is, of course, most essential to calcium absorption, though this may be less necessary when the calcium chelates, such as calcium aspartate or calcium citrate, are used. Some clinical studies need to be done to see which calcium supplements are readily transported into the body and how vitamin D may affect them. Many doctors do not consider this important absorption issue and prescribe an oyster shell or a dolomite or bonemeal source as a calcium supplement. Frequently, calcium lactate or calcium carbonate (such as Tums) pills—which are more alkaline and slowly absorbed—are prescribed without suggesting additional vitamin D and magnesium, so important for calcium balance and metabolism. A woman who needs more calcium could be taking an extra gram a day without really getting much of it into her blood or bones.

In general, calcium absorption becomes less efficient as we age. During infancy and childhood, 50–70 percent of the calcium ingested may be absorbed, whereas an adult might use only 30–50 percent of dietary calcium in his or her body. It is likely this is based on natural body needs. Various factors can improve our calcium absorption. Besides vitamin D, vitamins A and C can help support normal membrane transport of calcium. Protein intake helps absorption of calcium, but too much protein may reduce it. Some dietary fat may also help absorption, but high fat may reduce it. Lactose helps calcium absorption, and because of this as well as the protein-fat combination, the calcium content of milk is a reliable source of easily assimilated calcium. For other reasons, though, milk is not an ideal food for many people, especially the homogenized variety fortified with synthetic vitamin D, making milk a less-than-perfect (and definitely not the only) source of calcium. Nonfat milk does not improve calcium absorption and, in fact, may decrease it.

Gastric hydrochloric acid helps calcium absorption. The duodenum is the main location for absorption of calcium because farther down the small intestine the local environment becomes too alkaline. A fast-moving intestinal tract can also reduce calcium absorption. Exercise has been shown to improve absorption, and lack of exercise can lessen it. Stress also can diminish calcium absorption, possibly through its effect on stomach acid levels, digestion, and intestinal motility. Though calcium in the diet improves the absorption of the important vitamin B_{12}, too much of it may interfere with the absorption of the competing minerals magnesium, zinc, iron, and manganese.

Many dietary factors also reduce calcium absorption. Foods that are high in oxalic acid, such as spinach, rhubarb, chard, and chocolate, can interfere with calcium absorption by forming insoluble salts in the gut. Phytic acid, or phytates, found in whole grain foods or foods rich in fiber, may reduce the absorption of calcium and other minerals as well. Protein,

FACTORS AFFECTING CALCIUM ABSORPTION

Increased by:

- Body needs—growth, pregnancy, lactation
- Vitamin D
- Milk lactose
- Acid environment—hydrochloric acid, citric acid, ascorbic acid (vitamin C)
- Protein intake and amino acids such as lysine and glycine
- Fat intake
- Exercise
- Phosphorus balance

Decreased by:

- Vitamin D deficiency
- Gastrointestinal problems
- Hypochlorhydria (low stomach acid)
- Stress
- Lack of exercise
- High fat intake
- High protein intake
- Oxalic acid foods (beet greens, chard, spinach, rhubarb, cocoa)
- Phytic acid foods (whole grains)
- High phosphorus intake

fat, and acid foods may help calcium absorption, but high-protein diets may increase calcium elimination through the intestines. Calcium absorption is sensitive and requires energy to transport it into the body. Calcium is often chelated with proteins or amino acids (specifically, glutamic or aspartic acid) to make it more absorbable.

Because of the many complex factors affecting calcium absorption, anywhere from 30–80 percent may end up being excreted. Some may be eliminated in the feces. The kidneys also control calcium blood levels through their filtering and reabsorption functions.

Excess salt intake can lead to increased calcium losses in the urine. Sugar intake may reduce the reabsorption of calcium and magnesium and cause more to be eliminated. The table on the previous page summarizes the factors affecting calcium absorption.

Overall, we need good sources of calcium in our diets, good nutritional habits, and a diet that promotes healthy gastrointestinal function. Taking calcium and magnesium at bedtime or between meals, when the stomach may be more acidic, is often helpful for better absorption. Regular exercise, good nutrition, and lots of vegetables are important basics for providing the essential calcium we need and good health in general.

Sources: Calcium is found in many foods but is in high amounts in only a few. Even in light of my previous discussion, milk should be considered a good source of calcium as well as containing protein and fat and having a good balance of magnesium and phosphorus (a balanced calcium-phosphorus ratio is important). The lactose in milk also helps calcium absorption, but about 70 percent of blacks and 6 percent of Caucasians are lactose-intolerant—drinking milk makes them sick. An eight-ounce glass of whole milk contains about 300 mg. of calcium. Most other milk products also give good supplies of calcium—yogurt, most cheeses, and buttermilk, for example.

Many green, leafy vegetables are good sources of calcium, but some contain oxalic acid, so their calcium is not easily absorbed. Spinach, chard, and beet greens are not particularly good sources of calcium, whereas broccoli, cauliflower, and many peas and beans offer better supplies. (Pinto, aduki, and soybeans are good sources of calcium.) Many nuts, particularly almonds, brazil nuts, and hazelnuts, and seeds such as sunflower and sesame contain good amounts of calcium; though their phosphorus content is about double that of their calcium, this is much more of a concern with meats, which often

CALCIUM SOURCES

Food	Portion	Calcium (mgs.)
Swiss cheese	2 oz.	530
Jack cheese	2 oz.	420
Cheddar cheese	2 oz.	400
Other cheeses	2 oz.	300–400
Yogurt	6 oz.	300
Broccoli, cooked	2 stalks	250
Sardines (w/bones)	2 oz.	240
Goat milk	6 oz.	240
Cow's milk	6 oz.	225
Collard greens, cooked	6 oz.	225
Turnip greens, cooked	6 oz.	220
Almonds	3 oz.	210
Brazil nuts	3 oz.	160
Soybeans, cooked	6 oz.	150
Molasses, blackstrap	1 Tbl.	130
Corn tortillas (4, w/lime)	2 oz.	125
Carob flour	2 oz.	110
Tofu	3 oz.	110
Dried figs	3 oz.	100
Dried apricots	3 oz.	80
Parsley	1½ oz.	80
Kelp	¼ oz.	80
Sunflower seeds	2 oz.	80
Sesame seeds	2 oz.	75

contain 20–30 times as much phosphorus as calcium. Molasses is fairly high in calcium, while some fruits, such as citrus, figs, raisins, and dried apricots, have modest amounts.

When the diet is high in phosphorus, we can lose extra calcium through the urine, resulting in calcium being pulled out of the bones. Phosphorus is very plentiful in meat foods and is of particular concern in soda pops that have added phosphoric acid (phosphate). This phosphorus-calcium imbalance may lead to kidney stones and other calcification problems, as well as increased atherosclerotic plaque. This issue is fairly complex and is under investigation. It is currently felt that the best calcium-phosphorus ratio in the diet is about 1:1.

Sunlight increases the manufacture of vitamin D in the body, and is like having an extra calcium source because vitamin D improves absorption of any available dietary calcium. Calcium supplements could be taken in the first couple of hours after sunbathing to improve utilization.

Dolomite and bonemeal (ground cattle bones) are good sources of calcium and magnesium. In recent years, however, both of these natural sources have been found to be contaminated with lead and other heavy metal toxicants. It is probably wise not to take these supplements in large amounts or over prolonged periods of time unless they are tested for contamination. Calcium found in "hard" water may also be an important source for maintaining body levels.

Functions: Calcium has some very important life-supporting functions; the best known is the development and maintenance of bones and teeth. Our need for calcium is critical during the growth years of infancy and childhood, but it is also important lifelong to keep our bones healthy. Exercise, vitamin D, and many other nutrients, such as phosphorus and magnesium, are also needed to maintain our skeleton. Bones are primarily calcium phosphate and a protein matrix. Tooth enamel is the hardest substance in the body, made up of 99 percent minerals, primarily calcium.

Bones are not only our most basic physical support structure, they are the main reservoir for calcium. Most minerals are in a state of dynamic activity and function, and even the calcium in bones is being added to and removed depending on the calcium balance in the body. The bones provide calcium to the blood and other tissues when we are not getting sufficient amounts from our diet. Vitamin D, parathyroid hormone, and calcitonin are responsible for maintaining this balance.

Circulating calcium also performs many other vital functions. Ionized (Ca^{++}) calcium is needed for muscle contraction, as in muscular activity and in regulating the heartbeat. Heart function is mediated by several minerals: calcium stimulates contraction, magnesium supports the relaxation phase, and sodium and potassium are also important in generating the electrical impulse. Exercise can improve the circulation of calcium as well as that of all the other nutrients and thereby help the tone and function of the muscles, heart, and nervous system.

With regard to the nervous system, calcium is important in nerve transmission. Calcium ions influence nerve and cell membranes and the release of neurotransmitters. Calcium activates some enzyme systems, such as *choline acetylase*, which helps generate acetylcholine, an important neurotransmitter. Norepinephrine and serotonin are also affected by calcium. Calcium is said to be calming to the nerves, as higher concentrations tend to decrease nerve irritability.

Calcium plays an important role in the cells as well; it is necessary in cell division. Calcium is needed to activate prothrombin, which helps convert fibrinogen to fibrin and is essential to blood coagulation.

Uses: Calcium is one of the minerals most commonly prescribed by medical doctors (potassium is the other main one) because calcium deficiency is common and causes bone weakness through loss of bone calcium in the disease called osteoporosis. Osteoporosis is more common in the elderly population and occurs four times as often in women as in men. It can also occur at younger ages with chronic dietary insufficiency of calcium or with early menopause. Good evidence shows that there is a relationship between decreased calcium intake and osteoporosis; lack of exer-

165

cise also increases bone loss. Moderate daily exercise as well as supplementing calcium and vitamin D results in reduced to restore a positive calcium balance. The best way to combat osteoporosis is to prevent it with regular exercise, a calcium-rich diet not too high in phosphorus, calcium supplements, and for menopausal women considering estrogen therapy. Exercise can actually stimulate bone renewal by improving bone uptake of calcium and other minerals.

Osteoporosis (the term literally means "porous bones") is actually a loss of bone mass as the result of the loss of both minerals and protein; this differs slightly from osteomalacia, the bone problem seen in adults with vitamin D deficiency, which involves a softening of bones due to mineral loss alone. Rickets is the childhood equivalent of osteomalacia and is also caused by vitamin D deficiency. Extra calcium can help alleviate these problems somewhat, but the body needs supplemental vitamin D to get appreciable levels of calcium into the blood, tissues, and bones.

Calcium is the primary substance used in the prevention and treatment of osteoporosis, though estrogen used in menopausal hormone replacement therapy can reduce the likelihood of this disease in women. Since osteoporosis is found mainly in menopausal and postmenopausal woman, calcium is commonly seen as a treatment for problems of menopause. It does, in fact, reduce a number of the potential symptoms. Calcium not only helps the bones, especially when supplemented with magnesium and vitamin D, but may also reduce the headaches, irritability, insomnia, and depression sometimes associated with menopause. It is likely that a high percentage—as much as 70–90 percent—of bone fractures in people over 60 years of age are due to osteoporosis. These fractures are often more serious than an average fracture, because demineralized bones shatter when they break and take longer to heal. Actually, because osteoporotic fractures usually occur in the

elderly and are so disabling, about one in six people dies within three months after sustaining them. Therefore, by helping to retard osteoporosis, calcium can prevent some fractures.

Osteoporosis is most common in elderly white women with a history of borderline calcium intake. Calcium is often drained from the bones during pregnancy and nursing and becomes hard to replace in later years, especially with reduced consumption of milk products and a lower calcium intake in general. Calcium supplementation can be helpful in reducing the leg cramps of pregnancy and the fatigue and depression after delivery. Children's leg cramps are usually reduced by giving them calcium and magnesium. Calcium supplements tend to stimulate retention of calcium and decrease urinary excretion.

Calcium is often helpful for menstrual problems, particularly menstrual cramps, irritability or apprehension, and muscle cramps that occur around menstruation. The recently recognized premenstrual syndrome is often helped in part with additional calcium, though magnesium supplementation may be even more important. In some cases, however, reducing calcium intake can be helpful. Generally, muscle cramps or leg and foot cramps can be helped by calcium and vitamin D. Also, some cases of hyperkinesis in children, when associated with calcium deficiency, may be helped by supplementation.

Other problems related to bone health affect the mouth, jawbone, and teeth. In some cases, calcium may be helpful for problems of loose teeth, gingivitis (gum inflammation), and periodontal disease. Usually 1,000 mg. of calcium supplemented in the diet along with a dietary intake of phosphorus ranging from 1,000–2,000 mg. is suggested.

Calcium is often used to reduce heart irregularity; along with magnesium, it helps regulate heart contraction and relaxation. Through increasing contractility, calcium can help in congestive heart failure. Additional calcium may protect us from the toxicity of cadmium, rubidium, or mercury exposure by competing for absorption. Proper calcium intake may reduce the incidence of colon and rectal cancers through forming insoluble soaps with some mild carcinogens produced in the body, including bile acids and free, ionized fatty acids. A good calcium-phosphorus ratio in the diet also reduces the risk of cancer in the large intestine.

Deficiency and toxicity: In general, a high calcium intake for brief periods does not cause any problems, as excesses are usually eliminated in the urine and intestines. With magnesium deficiency, though, high amounts of calcium or vitamin D can lead to calcification of the soft tissues or to kidney stone formation. It is possible that prolonged high amounts of calcium (higher than a 2:1 calcium-phosphorus ratio) and supplemental vitamin D can lead to abnormal calcification of long bones in children or to hypercalcemia (high blood calcium levels) and soft tissue calcification in adults, as well as a decrease in bone strength. Also, if the parathyroid glands are not functioning well, calcium can accumulate and cause problems.

Calcium itself is thought to be one of the concerns in atherosclerosis, forming part of the plaque laid down in the arteries. Guy Abraham, M.D., who is known for his work in premenstrual syndrome, expressed a real concern over routine calcium supplementation in our society as he feels it exacerbates the degenerative process in the blood vessels, kidneys, and other organs and tissues. It is possible that these problems of calcium excess are not specifically related to dietary calcium but rather to calcium's metabolism in relationship to the endocrine system. More research is clearly needed in this area. This potential toxicity concern makes me realize that it is important to be very aware of calcium metabolism and individual needs and to not just blindly supplement it as is so common recently.

Still, though, calcium deficiency is a more common concern in our culture than is excess calcium. This is especially true for the elderly, for alcoholics, for pregnant women, and for people with gastrointestinal disease. The "standard" American diet does not meet the normal calcium requirements; part of this problem is due to high phosphorus levels in the diet. Phosphorus is found in most foods, but soda pops, diet pops, meats, eggs, and processed foods such as lunch meats and cheese spreads contain especially high amounts. The ideal dietary phosphorus-calcium ratio is about 1:1. The ratio in the average American diet is often greater than 2:1 and sometimes even 4:1 or 5:1. At those levels, excess calcium is removed from bone and eliminated, blood levels are reduced, and there is bone demineralization. A diet high in phosphorus and low in calcium has been shown to cause bone loss and increase tissue calcification.

The skeletal system suffers most from calcium deficiency. Teeth minerals are more stable, though there is a possibility of poor dentition with insufficient calcium. Tooth loss, periodontal disease, and gingivitis can be problems, especially with a high phosphorus intake, particularly from soft drinks. All kinds of bone problems can occur with prolonged calcium deficiency, which causes a decrease in bone mass. Rickets in children, osteomalacia (decreased bone calcium) in adults, and osteoporosis (porous and fragile bones) can occur when calcium is withdrawn from bones faster than it is deposited. Fractures are more common with osteoporosis—almost eight million yearly in the United States are related to this prevalent nutritional deficiency disease. Although there must be loss in bone mass of almost 40 percent before it is visible by X-ray, the problem may be detected earlier through diet history or blood and nutritional tests. A program of regular exercise and calcium intake through diet and supplements, while limiting phosphorus intake, is a good way to prevent bone loss in the first place.

Calcium deficiency in the blood can cause a wide range of other symptoms, such as tox-

RDAS FOR CALCIUM

Infants

Birth–6 months	360 mg.
6 months–1 year	540 mg.

Children

1–10 years	800 mg.
11–18 years	1,000 mg.

Adults

Men and women	800 mg.
Pregnant women	1,200 mg.
Lactating women	1,200 mg.
Postmenopausal women (not taking estrogen)	1,200 mg.

emia of pregnancy, anxiety, hyperkinesis, otosclerosis, and alcoholism. One theory about multiple sclerosis correlates it with calcium and vitamin D deficiency in puberty. Mild calcium deficiency can cause nerve sensitivity, paresthesias, muscle twitching, brittle nails, irritability, palpitations, insomnia, confusion, or a feeling of chronic depression. As it progresses, leg and foot or other muscle cramps, heart palpitations, numbness, tingling, and, finally, tetany, the sustained contraction of some muscles causing severe pain, may all occur. Evidence shows that drinking soft water, which is high in sodium and low in calcium can lead to increases in cardiovascular disease. Hard water supplies extra calcium and magnesium, which may protect the heart.

Requirements: Since absorption of calcium is so variable, it is difficult to determine the right amount of calcium for all people. Many factors regarding absorption come into play. And the body can adapt to lower levels of calcium, even as low as 200 mg. per day, and still maintain calcium balance, though this adjustment usually needs to be started in childhood. In most Western cultures, with average absorption rates ranging from 30–50 percent, even the 800 mg. RDA may not be enough to prevent osteoporosis and other calcium deficiency problems. Possibly half of the population is getting less than the RDA, and many people are consuming a diet that supplies less than two-thirds of the RDA for calcium. An additional concern is that absorption usually decreases with age and with excessive use of antacids. But, luckily, humans are adaptable. Lower intake may lead to greater absorption efficiency, and higher intake usually leads to more elimination in the urine and feces. And the body may naturally guide us to calcium foods that we can use.

The RDAs for calcium, shown in the table, are based on an absorption rate of approximately 40 percent and average daily losses of an estimated 320 mg.

A more liberal (or, really, conservative) suggestion is 1,000 mg. (1 gram) daily in adults. In pregnancy and during nursing, 1.5 grams per day of calcium are suggested, especially in the last two months of pregnancy when over half of the baby's calcium needs are supplied. The calcium intake suggested for postmenopausal women has recently been changed to 1.5 grams per day with some additional magnesium and vitamin D because of higher elimination and decreased absorption in these women.

People with high-protein, high-fat, or high-phosphorus diets need even more calcium. When we increase calcium, we should also increase our magnesium intake, keeping it at about one-half the calcium supply. Magnesium helps calcium stay more soluble, and thereby may reduce the risk of kidney stone formation and other calcifications. For phosphorus, an intake of about 800–1,000 mg. is recommended when the calcium intake is 1,000–1,200 mg.

Calcium is not absorbed well in an alkaline environment because it is less soluble. It is best taken between meals or in the absence of foods when the stomach is more acidic. Taking calcium with vitamin D and extra hydrochloric acid also increases absorption. Supplements of calcium or of calcium and magnesium are often taken at night before bed to help absorption and to prevent the extra loss of body calcium that can occur during the night. And calcium with magnesium is a good evening tranquilizer.

Other ideas for maximizing use of dietary calcium are spreading out calcium intake in balanced portions throughout the day; consuming protein, vitamin D, and vitamin C foods or supplements; adding more calcium-rich foods to the diet, especially in place of junk foods or phosphorus-rich soda pops; and taking supplemental calcium as part of a total mineral balance with magnesium, zinc, and manganese, for example. Recently, the trace mineral boron has been shown to help in calcium utilization and bone health.

The form in which calcium is supplied is also very important. Bonemeal and dolomite are good natural calcium and magnesium sources. They do not contain vitamin D but are still reasonably absorbable, though less so than other forms. There is some concern over lead and other toxic metals contaminating both dolomite and bonemeal. The form that I most highly recommend is aspartate or citrate salts of calcium, which are probably the most absorbable. Calcium aspartates are between 50–90 percent absorbable, which will likely place us in a positive calcium balance—exactly where we wish to be. Chelated calcium with amino acids are also easily absorbed. Calcium gluconate is the next choice, followed by calcium carbonate and lactate, which are also absorbable sources.

 Chlorine/Chloride The element chlorine itself is a poisonous gas that is soluble in water; in nature and in our body, it exists primarily as the chloride anion, the negatively charged ion that joins with cations such as sodium to make salt (sodium chloride) and with hydrogen to make

stomach acid (hydrochloric acid). Chloride makes up about 0.15 percent of our body weight and is found mainly in the extracellular fluid along with sodium. Less than 15 percent of the body chloride is found inside the cells, with the highest amounts within the red blood cells. As one of the mineral electrolytes, chloride works closely with sodium and water to help the distribution of body fluids.

Chloride is easily absorbed from the small intestine. It is eliminated through the kidneys, which can also retain chloride as part of their finely controlled regulation of acid-base balance. Chloride is also found along with sodium in perspiration. Heavy sweating can cause the loss of large amounts of sodium chloride, as well as some potassium.

Chlorine gas is used by many water-treatment plants as an agent to kill microorganisms in the water. It has been a great public health addition for eradicating disease in contaminated areas. But is it overused? Many are concerned with the levels of residual chlorine in drinking water because excess chlorine is thought to combine with certain organic water pollutants to form toxic chemicals and carcinogens (see Chapter 1, *Water*).

Sources: Chloride is obtained primarily from salt, such as standard table salt or sea salt. It is also contained in most foods, especially the vegetables. Seaweeds (such as dulse and kelp), olives, rye, lettuce, tomatoes, and celery are some examples of good chloride-containing foods. Potassium chloride (KCl) is also found in foods or as the "salt substitute."

Functions: Chloride travels primarily with sodium and water and helps generate the osmotic pressure of body fluids. It is an important constituent of stomach hydrochloric acid (HCl), the key digestive acid. Chloride is also needed to maintain the body's acid-base balance. The kidneys excrete or retain chloride mainly as sodium chloride, depending on whether they are trying to increase or decrease body acid levels. Chloride may also be helpful in allowing the liver to clear waste products.

Uses: Chloride is commonly used as sodium chloride, such as in salt tablets, to help replace the sodium and chloride lost in perspiration on hot days or with exercise. Chlorine is used in treating drinking water, swimming pools, hot tubs, and so on to kill bacteria and other microorganisms.

Deficiency and toxicity: Neither problem is very common nor worthy of much concern. Large amounts of chloride intake (more than 15 grams per day), usually in salt, may cause some problems with fluid retention and altered acid-base balance (although the main problem lies with the sodium). Chlorine itself, as gas or liquid, can be very irritating and toxic.

Chloride deficiency can arise from diarrhea, vomiting, or sweating. It can lead to metabolic alkalosis (body fluids becoming too alkaline), low fluid volume, and urinary potassium loss. This can cause further problems in acid-base balance. Infant formulas without chloride can cause some of these problems, which are alleviated when chloride is given.

Requirements: Chloride is so readily available in our normal high-salt food supply that there is no RDA. Infants probably need about 0.5–1 gram daily. The amount increases with age; adults needs are the range of 1.7–5 grams daily, but many people consume much more because of the salt content of their diet.

Magnesium is a very important essential macromineral, even though there are only several ounces in the body (0.05 percent of body weight). It is involved in several hundred enzymatic reactions, many of which contribute to production of energy and cardiovascular function. The great amount of research on magnesium done in the last decade has resulted in major changes in our knowledge. Decreases in magnesium intake have been more prevalent in our American diet with additions of supplemental vitamin D and calcium, dietary phosphorus, and refined or processed carbohydrate foods.

Drinking soft water decreases magnesium intake, while diuretic drugs cause magnesium loss, as do alcohol, caffeine, and sugar. Decreased blood and tissue levels of magnesium have been shown to be related to high blood pressure, kidney stones, heart disease and, particularly, heart attacks due to coronary artery spasm (magnesium helps relax and dilate coronary arteries). Studies have indicated that a decreased concentration of magnesium is found in the heart and blood of heart attack victims, though it is not clear whether this is a cause or a result of the problem. Magnesium's role in alleviating premenstrual syndrome (PMS) has made big news as well.

Magnesium, like calcium, is an earth alkali mineral. The word magnesium comes from the name of the Greek city, Magnesia, where large deposits of magnesium carbonate ($MgCO_3$) were found. This "salt" was first used as a laxative; magnesium carbonate and magnesium sulfate are still used in this way. Magnesium is the "iron" of the plant world— as iron is to hemoglobin, magnesium is to chlorophyll, the "blood" pigment of plants. The central atom of the chlorophyll structure is magnesium.

About 65 percent of our magnesium is contained in the bones and teeth. As with calcium, the bones act as a reservoir for magnesium in times of need. The remaining 35 percent of magnesium is contained in the blood, fluids, and other tissues; there is a high concentration, actually higher than in the blood, in the brain. Magnesium is present in significant amounts in the heart Most of it, like potassium, is inside the cells.

The process of digestion and absorption of magnesium is very similar to that of calcium. The suggested ratio of intake of these two vital nutrients is about 2:1, calcium to magnesium. Magnesium also requires an acidic stomach environment for best absorption, so taking it between meals or at bedtime is recommended. Meals high in protein or fat, a diet high in phosphorus or calcium (calcium and magnesium can compete), or alcohol use may decrease magnesium absorption. It is possible that some of the hangover symptoms related to alcohol are in part due to magnesium depletion. Taking this mineral with some thiamine (B_1) and drinking extra water can help prevent hangover symptoms.

Usually, about 40–50 percent of the magnesium we consume is absorbed, though this may vary from 25–75 percent depending on stomach acid levels, body needs, and dietary habits. Stress may increase magnesium excretion, and the resulting temporary magnesium depletion may make the heart more sensitive to electrical abnormalities and vascular spasm that could lead to cardiac ischemia. The kidneys can excrete or conserve magnesium according to body needs. The intestines can also eliminate excess magnesium in the feces. Otherwise, magnesium absorption is generally affected by the factors shown in the table (see *Calcium*) entitled *Factors Affecting Calcium Absorption*.

Sources: Almost all of our magnesium supplies come from the vegetable kingdom, though seafood has fairly high amounts. As a component of chlorophyll, this mineral is important to plant photosynthesis; therefore, the dark green vegetables are good sources of magnesium. Most nuts, seeds, and legumes have high amounts of magnesium; soy products, especially soy flour and tofu, and nuts such as almonds, pecans, cashews, and brazil nuts are good examples. The whole grains, particularly wheat (especially the bran and germ), millet, and brown rice, and fruits such as avocado and dried apricot are other sources. Hard water can also be a valuable source of magnesium. Dolomite and bonemeal are good sources of magnesium, as they are of calcium.

Many factors affect magnesium availability from foods. One is the amount of magnesium in the soil in which the food is grown. Much magnesium can be lost in the processing and refining of foods and in making oils from the magnesium-rich nuts and seeds. Nearly 85 percent of the magnesium in grains is lost during the milling of flours. Soaking and boiling foods can leach magnesium into the water, so the "pot liquor" from cooking vegetables may be high in magnesium and other minerals. Oxalic acid in vegetables such as spinach and chard and phytic acid in some grains may form insoluble salts with magnesium, causing it to be eliminated rather than absorbed. For these reasons and those previously discussed, many people get insufficient magnesium from their diets.

Functions: Magnesium is considered the "antistress" mineral. It is a natural tranquilizer, as it functions to relax skeletal muscles as well as the smooth muscles of blood vessels and the gastrointestinal tract. (While calcium stimulates muscle contraction, magnesium relaxes them.) Because of its influence on the heart, magnesium is considered important in preventing coronary artery spasm, a significant cause of heart attacks. Spasms of the blood vessels lead to insufficient oxygen supply through them and pain, injury, or death of the muscle tissue that they nourish. To function optimally, magnesium must be balanced in the body with calcium, phosphorus, potassium, and sodium chloride. For example, with low magnesium, more calcium flows into the vascular muscle cells, which contracts them—leading to tighter vessels and higher blood pressure. Adequate magnesium levels prevent this.

Magnesium, like potassium, is primarily an intracellular nutrient. It activates enzymes that are important for protein and carbohydrate metabolism, and it is needed in DNA production and function. Magnesium also modulates the electrical potential across cell membranes, which allows nutrients to pass back and forth. It helps in the release of energy by transferring the key phosphate molecule to adenosine triphosphate (ATP), an energy source generated by the cytochrome system.

In summary, even though it is not as prevalent as the other macrominerals, magnesium

171

has many essential metabolic functions in the body. It is important in the production and transfer of energy, in muscle contraction and relaxation, in nerve conduction, in protein synthesis, and in many biochemical reactions as a cofactor to enzymes. Magnesium is also thought to dilate the blood vessels.

Uses: As time goes on, magnesium is recommended and used in more and more treatments. Prevention or treatment of myocardial infarctions (MIs), prevention of kidney stones, and in treatment of premenstrual syndrome are some important recent uses. Magnesium has been used with some success in relieving certain kinds of angina and reducing the risks of coronary artery spasms, which can lead to angina or, more severely, heart attack. Deficient magnesium levels have been found in the blood and hearts of cardiac victims. Besides preventing heart attacks, magnesium has a mild effect on lowering blood pressure and so is used to treat and prevent hypertension and its effects. Magnesium supplementation can reduce many of the symptoms of mitral valve prolapse, such as palpitations or arrhythmias, and it may help in other cardiac arrythmias such as atrial tachycardia or fibrillation, or those caused by taking excess digitalis, a cardiac drug. It may also reduce the bronchoconstriction in asthma by relaxing the muscle around the bronchial tubes. Intravenous solutions containing magnesium and other nutrients have been used successfully to break acute asthma attacks.

Magnesium sulfate has been used specifically to lower blood pressure in pregnant women with preeclampsia, which is characterized by edema, hypertension, and hyperreflexia. These problems could become more severe and lead to seizures (then termed "eclampsia") as well. Magnesium sulfate also acts as a mild anticonvulsant in this case. Through its nerve- and muscle-relaxing effect, magnesium may be helpful in reducing epileptic seizures caused by nerve excitability.

By increasing calcium solubility, especially

PROBLEMS THAT MAY BE HELPED BY MAGNESIUM

Atherosclerosis	Kidney stones
Arrhythmias	Menstrual pain
Angina pectori	Alcoholism
Hypertension	Fatigue
Bronchial asthma	Fatigue
Epilepsy	Osteoporosis
Autism	Anxiety
Hyperactivity	Insomnia
Premenstrual syndrome	Muscle cramps

in the urine, magnesium can help prevent kidney stones, especially calcium oxalate stones. Research has shown this effect in a high percentage of people who form kidney stones regularly. Actually, it is thought that calcium oxalate stones are most likely to form in people who are magnesium deficient, so we may just be correcting that deficiency. Through this same effect, magnesium is helpful in preventing other tissue and blood vessel calcification (and thereby atherosclerosis), as well as some problems of the teeth, including cavities. For these purposes, a daily dose of 50 mg. of vitamin B_6 and 200–300 mg. of magnesium oxide is often given.

Supplementing magnesium has been shown to be very helpful in alleviating many symptoms related to the menstrual period. Menstrual cramps, irritibility, fatigue, depression, and water retention have been lessened with magnesium, usually given along with calcium and often with vitamin B_6. Magnesium is often at its lowest level during menstruation, and many symptoms of premenstrual syndrome (PMS) are relieved when this mineral is replenished. Supplementing magnesium in the same amount (or more) as calcium (about 500–1,000 mg. daily) is currently recommended for premenstrual problems.

Fatigue is often reduced with magnesium (and potassium) supplementation. The many enzyme systems that require magnesium help restore normal energy levels. Because of this function and its nerve and muscle support, magnesium may also be helpful for nervousness, anxiety, insomnia, depression, and muscle cramps. Magnesium is also given as part of a treatment for autism or hyperactivity in kids, usually along with vitamin B_6. Getting children and fatigued adults to eat more green vegetables and chlorophyll is often helpful for supplying additional naturally-occurring magnesium. People tend to sleep better after taking magnesium before bed. Alcoholics tend to have low magnesium levels, and this mineral can be helpful during withdrawal and to prevent or reduce hangover symptoms.

When given orally, magnesium sulfate (Epsom salts) is not absorbed but attracts water into the colon and thus acts as an effective laxative. Epsom salts in a bath are absorbed slightly and are known to be relaxing. For injuries, a concentrated solution is used as a compress to help drain toxins. Magnesium is also thought to reduce lead toxicity and its buildup, possibly through competing for absorption. Since magnesium is an alkaline mineral, it is used in several over-the-counter antacids.

Deficiency and toxicity: Toxicity due to magnesium overload is almost unknown in a nutritional context, as excesses are usually eliminated in the urine and feces. However, symptoms of magnesium toxicity can occur more likely if calcium intake is low. These symptoms may include depression of the central nervous system, causing muscle weakness, fatigue, sleepiness, or even hyperexcitability. In extreme states, magnesium overload can cause death.

Magnesium deficiency is actually fairly common; however, it is usually not looked for, and therefore, not found or corrected. Deficiency is more likely in those who eat a processed-food diet; in people who cook or boil all foods, especially vegetables; in those

who drink soft water; in alcoholics; and in people who eat food grown in magnesium-deficient soil, where synthetic fertilizers containing no magnesium are often used. Deficiency is also more common when magnesium absorption is decreased, such as after burns, serious injuries, or surgery and in patients with diabetes, liver disease, or malabsorption problems; and when magnesium elimination is increased, as in people who use alcohol, caffeine, or excess sugar, or who take diuretics or birth control pills.

Early symptoms of magnesium deficiency can include fatigue, anorexia, irritability, insomnia, and muscle tremors or twitching. Psychological changes, such as apathy, apprehension, decreased learning ability, confusion, and poor memory may occur. Tachycardia (rapid heartbeat) and other cardiovascular changes are likely with moderate deficiency, while severe magnesium deficiency may lead to numbness, tingling, and tetany (sustained contraction) of the muscles as well as delirium and hallucinations.

Arterial spasm, specifically of the coronary arteries, is a significant recent concern with magnesium deficiency. This could lead to angina symptoms or even a heart attack. Blood pressure can rise with magnesium deficiency, while an increased likelihood of kidney stones and other tissue calcification is possible.

Requirements: The current Recommended Daily Allowance (RDA) is about 300–350 mg. for adults—350 mg. for men and 300 mg. for women, increasing to about 450 mg. during pregnancy and lactation. The minimum is also expressed as about 6 mg. per kg. (2.2 pounds) of body weight. Many authorities feel that the RDA should be doubled, to about 600–700 mg. daily. An average diet usually supplies about 120 mg. of magnesium per 1,000 calories, for an estimated daily intake of about 250 mg. Unless absorption is great, that is not going to produce adequate tissue levels of magnesium for most people.

Magnesium chelated with amino acids is

173

probably the most absorbable form. Less absorbable forms include magnesium bicarbonate, magnesium oxide, and magnesium carbonate. Magnesium oxide is probably somewhat better than magnesium carbonate (dolomite). The newly available salts of magnesium aspartate or citrate, both known as mineral transporters, have a better percentage of absorption.

Calcium-magnesium balance is important. It is usually suggested that when we supplement calcium we take about half that amount in magnesium. If we increase calcium intake, we should likewise increase magnesium. We should also increase magnesium intake when we consume more phosphorus, vitamin D, or protein or when we have higher blood cholesterol. Those on birth control pills or diuretics, postmenopausal women, and those who drink alcohol need more magnesium.

The levels of magnesium used by physicians are commonly in the range of 600–1,000 mg.; however, the researchers in the kidney stone studies used only 200–300 mg. of supplemental magnesium oxide. Calcium and magnesium are both alkaline minerals, so they are not taken with or after meals, as they can reduce stomach acid as well as being absorbed poorly when taken with food. They are absorbed better when taken between meals or on an empty stomach, especially with a little vitamin C as ascorbic acid. Many calcium-magnesium combinations are formulated with hydrochloric acid and vitamin D to aid the mineral absorption. And taking them before bedtime may be very helpful in increasing utilization of both these important minerals and lead to a sleep-filled night.

 Phosphorus, the second most abundant element (after calcium) present in our bodies, makes up about 1 percent of our total body weight. It is present in every cell, but 85 percent of the phosphorus is found in the bones and teeth.

In the bones, phosphorus is present in the phosphate form as the bone salt calcium phosphate in an amount about half that of the total calcium. Both these important minerals are in constant turnover, even in the bone structure.

The body uses a variety of mechanisms to control the calcium-phosphorus ratio and metabolism. The ratio of these two elements in the diet has been the subject of much recent interest. The typical American diet provides too much phosphorus and not enough calcium, leading to reduced body storage of calcium; thus, many of the problems of calcium deficiency discussed earlier may develop. Phosphorus and calcium can compete for absorption in the intestines. High consumption of meats or soft drinks increases phosphorus intake and may contribute to this imbalance. The ideal ratio of calcium to phosphorus in the diet is 1:1.

Phosphorus is absorbed more efficiently than calcium. Nearly 70 percent of phosphorus is absorbed from the intestines, although the rate depends somewhat on the levels of calcium and vitamin D and the activity of parathyroid hormone (PTH), which regulates the metabolism of phosphorus and calcium. Most phosphorus is deposited in the bones, a little goes to the teeth, and the rest is contained in the cells and other tissues. Much is found in the red blood cells. The plasma phosphorus measures about 3.5 mg. (3.5 mg. of phosphorus per 100 ml. of plasma), while the total blood phosphorus is 30–40 mg.. The body level of this mineral is regulated by the kidneys, which are also influenced by PTH. Phosphorus absorption may be decreased by antacids, iron, aluminum, or magnesium, which may all form insoluble phosphates and be eliminated in the feces. Caffeine causes increased phosphorus excretion by the kidneys.

Sources: Since phosphorus is part of all cells, it is readily found in food, especially animal tissues. Most protein foods are high in phosphorus. Meats, fish, chicken, turkey, milk, cheese, and eggs all contain substantial amounts. Most red meats and poultry have much more phosphorus than calcium—between 10 and 20 times as much—whereas fish generally has about 2 or 3 times as much phosphorus as calcium. The dairy foods have a more balanced calcium-phosphorus ratio. Seeds and nuts also contain good levels of phosphorus (although they have less calcium) as do the whole grains, brewer's yeast, and wheat germ and bran. Most fruits and vegetables contain some phosphorus and help to balance the ratio of phosphorus to calcium in a wholesome diet.

In recent years, the increased consumption of soft drinks, which are buffered with phosphates, has been a concern. There may be up to 500 mg. of phosphorus per serving of a soft drink, with essentially no calcium. In 1970, the average per capita intake of soft drinks was 23 gallons, whereas in 1981, 39 gallons a year were consumed by the "average" person. Since some people do not drink any of these "beverages," quite a number of people are drinking even more than the average amount of soda pops, and thus consuming a lot of phosphorus.

Functions: Phosphorus is involved in many functions besides forming bones and teeth. Like calcium, it is found in all cells and is involved in some way in most biochemical reactions. Phosphorus is vital to energy production and exchange in a variety of ways. It provides the phosphate in adenosine triphosphate (ATP), which is the high-energy carrier molecule in the body's primary metabolic cycles. Phosphorus is important to the utilization of carbohydrates and fats for energy production and also in protein synthesis for the growth, maintenance, and repair of all tissues and cells. As inorganic phosphate in ATP, it is needed in protein synthesis and in the production of the nucleic acids in DNA and RNA, which carry the genetic code for all cells.

Phosphorus is also a component of the phospholipids, fat molecules essential to cell membranes; lecithin is the best-known phospholipid. It helps in fat emulsification and in other body functions. In the cell membranes, the phospholipids help maintain both fluidity and permeability, allowing the nutrients to pass in and out of the cells. The sphingolipids, involved in nerve conduction, also contain phosphorus. Phosphorus is combined with the B vitamins to assist their functions in the body; furthermore, phosphoproteins are contained in many enzyme systems.

In addition to its role in these processes and in skeletal growth and tooth development, phosphorus has a number of other functions. It helps in kidney function and acts as a buffer for acid-base balance in the body. Phosphorus aids muscle contraction, including the regularity of the heartbeat, and is also supportive of proper nerve conduction. This important mineral supports the conversion of niacin and riboflavin to their active coenzyme forms. As mentioned, parathyroid hormone regulates the phosphorus blood level and helps it carry out all these essential functions.

Uses: Phosphorus by itself is used in only a few medically significant conditions. It is not needed as frequently as calcium to balance the ratio between these two minerals. However, phosphorus has been used to treat many kinds of bone problems; it (along with calcium) helps in healing fractures by minimizing calcium loss from bones. It is used in the treatment of osteolmalacia, where there is decreased bone mineral content, and in osteoporosis, where total bone mass is decreased. Rickets has also been treated with phosphorus, as well as with calcium and vitamin D.

Rebalancing the calcium-phosphorus ratio in the diet can help reduce stress and many problems relating to calcium metabolism, arthritis being one example. Tooth and gum problems can be alleviated with dietary phosphorus, again in balance with calcium. Cancer research has revealed that cancer cells tend to lose phosphorus more readily than do normal cells, so phosphorus may be useful in the nutritional support of cancer patients; however, a high phosphorus-to-calcium intake is to be avoided.

Deficiency and toxicity: There is no known toxicity specific to phosphorus; however, high dietary phosphorus, as is found in a diet with meats, soft drinks, and other convenience foods, can readily affect calcium metabolism. Potential calcium deficiency symptoms may be more likely when the phosphorus intake is very high. A low calcium-to-phosphorus ratio in the diet increases the incidence of hypertension and the risk of colon-rectal cancer.

Problems of phosphorus deficiency are fairly uncommon, since it is so readily obtained in the diet; it is usually consumed in greater amounts than calcium and is readily absorbed. Relative deficiency of phosphorus can be caused by very high calcium intake or by taking a lot of antacids which can bind phosphorus. Aluminum, magnesium, and iron can interfere with phosphorus absorption. Low vitamin D intake can also lead to deficient body phosphorus.

Symptoms of phosphorus deficiency may include anorexia, weakness, weight loss, irritability, anxiety, stiff joints, paresthesias, bone pain, and bone fragility. Decreased growth, poor bone and tooth development, and symptoms of rickets may occur in phosphorus-deficient children. In adults, as mentioned, a low calcium-to-phosphorus ratio is most likely to generate problems. Osteoporosis (bone resorption) is often brought on by high phosphorus and low calcium intake. Other adult problems include skin disease, tooth decay, and even arthritis.

Requirements: The RDA for phosphorus is the same as that for calcium, 800 mg. for adults. However, the average dietary intake of calcium is low, at about 500 mg.; that for phosphorus is more like 1,500 mg. In pregnancy and lactation, as well as in children aged 11–18, the RDA is higher, at 1,200 mg. If the phosphorus intake is high or body levels are increased, we may need to take more

calcium to achieve the desired 1:1 ratio to maintain biochemical homeostasis.

Phosphorus in small amounts like 100–200 mg. is often contained in multimineral or multivitamin formulas. It is unlikely that anyone takes phosphorus as a separate supplement.

 Potassium is a very significant body mineral, important to both cellular and electrical function. It is one of the main blood minerals called "electrolytes" (the others are sodium and chloride), which means it carries a tiny electrical charge (potential). Potassium is the primary positive ion (cation) found within the cells, where 98 percent of the 120 grams of potassium in the body is found. The blood serum contains about 4–5 mg. (per 100 ml.) of the total potassium; the red blood cells contain 420 mg., which is why a red-blood-cell level is a better indication of an individual's potassium status than the commonly used serum level.

Magnesium helps maintain the potassium in the cells, but the sodium and potassium balance is as finely tuned as those of calcium and phosphorus or calcium and magnesium. Research has found that a high-sodium diet with low potassium intake influences vascular volume and tends to elevate the blood pressure. Then doctors may prescribe diuretics that can cause even more potassium loss, aggravating the underlying problems. The appropriate course is to shift to natural, potassium foods and away from high-salt foods, lose weight if needed, and follow an exercise program to improve cardiovascular tone and physical stamina. The natural diet high in fruits, vegetables, and whole grains is rich in potassium and low in sodium, helping to maintain normal blood pressure and sometimes lowering elevated blood pressure. The body contains more potassium than sodium, about nine ounces to four, but the American diet, with its reliance on fast foods, packaged convenience foods, chips, and salt has become high in sodium (salt). Because the body's biochemical functions are based on the components found in a natural diet, special mechanisms conserve sodium, while potassium is conserved somewhat less.

Potassium is well absorbed from the small intestine, with about 90 percent absorption, but is one of the most soluble minerals, so it is easily lost in cooking and processing foods. Most excess potassium is eliminated in the urine; some is eliminated in the sweat. When we perspire a great deal, we should replace our fluids with orange juice or vegetable juice containing potassium rather than just taking salt tablets.

The kidneys are the chief regulators of our body potassium, keeping the blood levels steady even with wide variation in intake. The adrenal hormone aldosterone stimulates elimination of potassium by the kidneys. Alcohol, coffee (and caffeine drinks), sugar, and diuretic drugs, however, cause potassium losses and can contribute to lowering the blood potassium. This mineral is also lost with vomiting and diarrhea.

Sources: Potassium is found in a wide range of foods. Many fruits and vegetables are high in potassium and low in sodium and, as discussed, help prevent hypertension. Most of the potassium is lost when processing or canning foods, while less is lost from frozen fruits or vegetables.

Leafy green vegetables such as spinach, parsley, and lettuce, as well as broccoli, peas, lima beans, tomatoes, and potatoes, especially the skins, all have significant levels of potassium. Fruits that contain this mineral include oranges and other citrus fruits, bananas, apples, avocados, raisins, and apricots, particularly dried. Whole grains, wheat germ, seeds, and nuts are high-potassium foods. Fish such as flounder, salmon, sardines, and cod are rich in potassium, and many meat foods contain even more potassium than sodium, although they often have additional sodium added as salt.

Functions: Potassium is very important in the human body. Along with sodium, it regulates the water balance and the acid-base balance in the blood and tissues. Potassium enters the cell more readily than does sodium and instigates the brief sodium-potassium exchange across the cell membranes. In the nerve cells, this sodium-potassium flux generates the electrical potential that aids the conduction of nerve impulses. When potassium leaves the cell, it changes the membrane potential and allows the nerve impulse to progress. This electrical potential gradient, created by the "sodium-potassium pump," helps generate muscle contractions and regulates the heartbeat.

Potassium is very important in cellular biochemical reactions and energy metabolism; it participates in the synthesis of protein from amino acids in the cell. Potassium also functions in carbohydrate metabolism; it is active in glycogen and glucose metabolism, converting glucose to glycogen that can be stored in the liver for future energy. Potassium is important for normal growth and for building muscle.

Uses: In medicine, potassium is one of the most commonly prescribed minerals. It is also commonly measured in biochemical testing and is supplemented if it is low. Because potassium is crucial to cardiovascular and nerve functions and is lost in diuretic therapy for edema or hypertension, a prevalent American disease, it must be added as a dietary supplement frequently. As stated before, the average American diet has reversed the natural high potassium—low sodium intake, and a shift back to this more healthful balance will help reduce some types of elevated blood pressure. Supplementing potassium can be helpful in treating hypertension specifically caused by a hyperresponse to excess sodium.

Pharmacological preparations of potassium are commonly prescribed for many of these conditions. A 10 percent potassium chloride solution is often given, but its taste is unpleasant. More easily used formulas are tablets that are swallowed or effervescent tablets. K-Lor,

177

Slow-K, K-Lyte, and Kaochlor are common preparations. Time-release formulas such as Micro-K are also available.

Potassium chloride has occasionally been helpful in treating infant colic, some cases of allergies, and headaches. During and after diarrhea, potassium replacement may be necessary, and many people feel better taking potassium during weight-loss programs. Fatigue or weakness, especially in the elderly, is often alleviated with supplemental potassium, along with magnesium. Additional potassium may also be required for dehydration states after fluid losses and may be used to prevent or reduce hangover symptoms after alcohol consumption.

Deficiency and Toxicity: Elevations or depletions of this important mineral can cause problems and, in the extreme, even death. Maintaining consistent levels of potassium in the blood and cells is vital to body function.

Even with high intakes of potassium, the kidneys will clear any excess, and blood levels will not be increased. For elevated potassium levels, called hyperkalemia, to occur, there must usually be other factors involved; decrease in renal function is the most likely cause. Major infection, gastrointestinal bleeding, and rapid protein breakdown also may cause elevated potassium levels. Cardiac function is affected by hyperkalemia; electrocardiogram changes can be seen in this condition.

Deficiency of potassium is much more common, especially with aging or chronic disease. Some common problems that have been associated with low potassium levels include hypertension, congestive heart failure, cardiac arrythmias, fatigue, and depression and other mood changes. Many factors reduce body levels of potassium. Diarrhea, vomiting, and other gastrointestinal problems may rapidly reduce potassium. Infants with diarrhea must be watched closely for low blood potassium, termed hypokalemia. Diabetes and renal disease may cause low as well as high potassium levels. Several drugs can cause hypokalemia—diuretic therapy is of most concern; long-term use of laxatives, aspirin, digitalis, and cortisone may also deplete potassium. Heat waves and profuse sweating can cause potassium loss and lead to dehydration, with potassium leaving the cells along with sodium and being lost in the urine. This can generate some of the symptoms associated with low potassium; most people are helped rapidly with potassium supplements or potassium-rich foods. People who consume excess sodium can lose extra urinary potassium, and people who eat lots of sugar also may become low in potassium.

Fatigue is the most common symptom of chronic potassium deficiency. Early symptoms include muscle weakness, slow reflexes, and dry skin or acne; these initial problems may progress to nervous disorders, insomnia, slow or irregular heartbeat, and loss of gastrointestinal tone. A sudden loss of potassium may lead to cardiac arrythmias. Low potassium may impair glucose metabolism and lead to elevated blood sugar. In more severe potassium deficiency, there can be serious muscle weakness, bone fragility, central nervous system changes, decreased heart rate, and even death. Potassium is the most commonly measured blood mineral in medicine, and deficiencies must be watched for carefully and treated without delay with supplemental potassium.

Requirements: There is no specific RDA for potassium, though it is thought that at least 2–2.5 grams per day are needed, or about 0.8–1.5 grams per 1,000 calories consumed. The average American diet includes from 2–6 grams per day.

In cooking or canning foods, potassium is depleted but sodium is increased, as it is in most American processed foods as well. It is suggested that we include more potassium than sodium in our diets; a ratio of about 2:1 would be ideal. When we increase sodium intake, we should also consume more potassium-rich foods or take a potassium supplement.

Over-the-counter potassium supplements usually contain 99 mg. per tablet. Prescription potassium is usually measured in milliequivalents (meq.); 1 meq. equals about 64 mg. About 10–20 meq. (640–1280 mg.) per day may be recommended as a supplement to the individual's diet.

The inorganic potassium salts are found as the sulfate, chloride, oxide, or carbonate. Organic salts are potassium gluconate, fumarate, or citrate. These organic molecules are normally part of our cells and body tissues. Potassium liquids and salt substitutes containing potassium chloride (KCl) are other ways to obtain additional sources of this mineral. Potassium is well absorbed, so it is available to the body in most forms.

 Sodium is the primary positive ion found in the blood and body fluids; it is also found in every cell although it is mainly extracellular, working closely with potassium, the primary intracellular mineral. About 60 percent of body sodium is in the fluids around cells (extracellular), 10 percent is inside the cells, and around 30 percent is found in the bones. Sodium is one of the electrolytes, along with potassium and chloride, and is closely tied in with the movement of water; "where sodium goes, water goes." Sodium represents about 0.15 percent of the body weight. Approximately 90–100 grams are present in the body, most of which occurs in combination with chloride as salt, or sodium chloride.

Sodium chloride is present in solution on a large part of the earth's surface in ocean water. In common usage, the word "salt" refers mainly to sodium chloride, but in chemistry, a salt is any combination of a positive and a negative ion in crystalline form or in solution. Sodium chloride is only 75 percent of the salt in seawater, which also contains potassium chloride (KCl), calcium chloride ($CaCl_2$), and calcium phosphate ($Ca(CPO_4)_2$), as well as other mineral salts.

Sodium, or salt, has been valued throughout history. The word "salt" is the source of the English word "salary," which originally referred to money paid to soldiers to buy salt. Yet this value placed on salt has possibly led to its overuse in industrial society. For millions of years, the human species lived on a natural diet containing less than 1 gram per day of sodium, and elevated blood pressure was very rare. Nowadays, 6–12 grams and even higher amounts of salt per day are consumed by people eating processed and snack foods or as salt added in cooking and preparing foods. Salt itself is 40 percent sodium and 60 percent chloride. Therefore, 5 grams of salt (about one teaspoon) contain approximately 2 grams of sodium.

High blood pressure is now epidemic in our society as well as in all other cultures eating high-salt diets. Where natural foods are the only source of sodium, there is almost no hypertension. These foods contain more potassium, which is found in high amounts in plant cells as well as in human cells. There is still some controversy about the relationship between salt and high blood pressure; the sodium-potassium ratio may be even more important in controlling blood pressure than the actual amount of sodium. Certain people seem to be more sensitive to sodium and its effects on blood pressure, although it is not clear whether this is due to genetic or other physiologic factors. Restricting sodium may significantly help the estimated 20–30 percent of the population that is salt sensitive. Reducing salt intake may have less effect on the blood pressure of other people. In any event, eating a low-sodium diet on a long-term basis may be one of the best ways to prevent hypertension; this will likely be even more effective if the diet is low in fat as well. Research indicates that other minerals, including calcium, magnesium, and chloride, may also be implicated in high blood pressure.

Sodium, like potassium, is very soluble and, therefore, is easily absorbed from the stomach and small intestine—nearly 100 percent of the sodium consumed gets into the body. It goes into the blood and is circulated through the kidneys, which can reabsorb or eliminate it in order to maintain stable blood sodium levels. About 90 percent of the sodium consumed in the average diet is in excess of body needs and must be eliminated in the urine. Therefore, urine levels reflect dietary intake. Aldosterone, a hormone made and secreted by the adrenal cortex, acts on the kidneys to regulate sodium metabolism.

Some sodium is stored in the bones and is available if needed. Sodium can be lost with excessive sweating and with vomiting or diarrhea. When this happens, we naturally crave water and salt. Should we then consume only water, we may experience "water intoxication," wherein water goes into the cells and causes swelling, which may lead to symptoms such as headaches, weakness, loss of appetite, or poor memory. More commonly, though, we first crave salt and then become thirsty for water to dilute or, rather, balance the osmotic effects of sodium, and help it to be eliminated. This is all carefully regulated by our masterful kidneys and adrenal glands.

Sources: Almost all foods contain some sodium, particularly as sodium chloride. It is found in high amounts in all seafood, in beef, and in poultry, and some sodium is in many vegetables, including celery, beets, carrots, and artichokes. Kelp and other sea vegetables are fairly high in sodium.

No wholesome natural food has a high salt content. It is only the Westernized diet of processed foods that has significant salt content, and many people consume these foods as their primary "diet." In many respects the standard American diet is sad! Breads, crackers, chips, cheeses, especially the processed types, some peanut butter, and salt-cured foods such as olives and pickles may constitute a good percentage of a typical unhealthy diet.

Lunch meats and processed or cured meats such as bacon, bologna, corned beef, and hot dogs are particularly high in salt and other preservatives such as nitrates and nitrites. Luckily, most people can clear excess sodium chloride from their bodies, but it creates additional work for the kidneys. After many years, the kidneys may weaken from this chronic stress and be unable to clear the salt as well, which may lead to more problems including high blood pressure.

Sodium can also come from nonsalt sources, such as baking soda (sodium bicarbonate), monosodium glutamate (MSG), sodium propionate, or any other ingredient listed on a package as soda or sodium "something." Soy sauce, or tamari, has high amounts of sodium as well, but the sodium is less concentrated than in crystal salt. "Softened" water also has extra sodium added to replace the naturally occurring magnesium and calcium that are removed. This is done because the more soluble sodium can wash clothes better and "bubble" and "soap" more for daily cleaning and bathing, but when this water is used as a drink, it adds to the already excessive sodium levels.

Functions: Along with potassium, sodium helps to regulate the fluid balance of the body, both within and outside the cells. Through the kidneys, by buffering the blood with a balance of all the positive or negative ions present, these two minerals help control the acid-base balance as well. The high blood levels of sodium contribute to the osmolarity (concentration of solutes in solution) and thereby regulate the fluid volume of the body and blood. The shifting of sodium and potassium across the cell membranes helps to create an electrical potential (charge) that enables muscles to contract and nerve impulses to be conducted. Sodium is also important to hydrochloric acid production in the stomach and is used during the transport of amino acids from the gut into the blood.

Since sodium is needed to maintain blood

fluid volume, excessive sodium can lead to increased blood volume and elevated blood pressure, especially when the kidneys do not clear it efficiently. It is easier to prevent hypertension with low salt intake than to treat it by lowering salt in the diet. Hypertension is more frequent in people who have a high salt intake, especially in people with low levels of potassium in their diets. Fresh fruits and vegetables are high in potassium and low in sodium, and research shows that increased potassium can balance out some of the effects high sodium intake has on blood pressure. Elderly people and the black population are more prone than others to elevated blood pressure. In cultures that consume low-sodium diets, there is very little, if any, hypertension.

Uses: There is not really a physiologic need for added salt or sodium in our diet. Our bodies tolerate and, in fact, probably do best on a much lower sodium intake than is provided by the average Westernized diet. So far more problems are caused by excess sodium—high blood pressure, premenstrual symptoms, and water retention, for example—than there are low-sodium difficulties that require treatment with sodium. Low sodium levels can, however, result from habitually avoiding sodium or from hot weather and severe perspiration; extra salt or sodium can help here. Potassium may also be needed. Preventing and treating heatstroke and leg cramps are occasional uses for sodium. It is possible that low sodium levels can cause blurred vision, edema, and even high blood pressure or, on the other hand, decreased fluid volume and low blood pressure. In these situations, additional sodium may be helpful. Salt is also employed to preserve foods, protecting them from oxidation and breakdown from microorganism activity.

Deficiency and toxicity: In the case of sodium, there is more of a concern with toxicity from excesses than with deficiencies. Some people, as many as 30 percent, are sensitive to high levels of dietary sodium and develop

HIGH-SALT FOODS TO AVOID

- Salt from the shaker, in cooking or at the table
- All smoked, salted meats, such as bacon, hot dogs, bologna, and sausage
- Food from Chinese restaurants with salt, soy sauce, and MSG
- Brine-soaked foods, such as pickles, olives, and sauerkraut
- Canned and instant soups unless salt-free (watch out for MSG, too)
- Salted and smoked fish and caviar
- Processed cheeses
- Commercially prepared condiments such as catsup, barbecue sauce, mayonnaise, salad dressings, mustard, and steak sauce.
- Most ready-made gravies and sauces
- Snack foods such as chips, salted peanuts and popcorn, pretzels, and the majority of crackers
- Any foods with added soda or sodium salts, such as sodium phosphate

hypertension from too much salt. However, hypertension is only one of the problems related to excess sodium; premenstrual problems may become more severe with too much salt, and toxemia of pregnancy is correlated with dietary sodium levels.

Consumption of more than 12 grams a day of salt is not uncommon; to limit salt intake to about 5 grams per day, which provides about 2 grams of sodium. To reduce sodium intake, eat more potassium-rich fruits and vegetables, and prepare foods without adding salt prior to eating.

Sodium deficiency is less common than excess sodium, as this mineral is readily available in the diet, but when it does occur, as with excessive sweating and sodium losses, deficiency can cause problems. The body can lose up to 8 grams per day of sodium through sweat; however, a loss of this amount usually requires about two to three quarts of sweat. Other causes of sodium deficiency include low intake, diarrhea or vomiting, and general malnourishment, particularly of carbohydrates. The deficiency is usually accompanied by water loss. When sodium and water are lost together, the extracellular fluid volume is depleted, which can cause decreased blood volume, increased hematocrit (blood count), decreased blood pressure, and muscle cramps. Other symptoms include nausea and vomiting, dizziness, poor memory and impaired concentration, somnolence, and muscle weakness. More seriously, circulatory collapse and shock may occur. Debilitating or wasting diseases such as cancer or tuberculosis may also produce low-sodium states.

When sodium is lost alone, water flows into the cells, causing cellular swelling and symptoms of water intoxication. These may include anorexia, fatigue, apathy, and muscle twitching. With low sodium, there is also usually poor carbohydrate metabolism.

When we lose sodium through sweat, the best treatment is not just replacement with salt tablets but by drinking salt solution prepared by adding about one-fifth teaspoon (1 gram) of salt to a quart of water; this will replenish us with a concentration similar to that in perspiration. Most salt tablets contain 1 gram of salt. One tablet can be taken with a quart of water, or two or three tablets with two or three quarts of water to replace greater fluid losses. It is ideal to add some potassium as well, about 500 mg. per quart.

Requirements: There is no specific RDA for sodium because almost everyone consumes more than needed. The Senate Select Committee on Nutrition and Human Needs suggests about 5 grams of salt, which provides about 2 grams of sodium, per day. We really need only about 0.5 gram to maintain the body's salt concentration and probably 1–2 grams to be safe, unless we perspire a great deal or are active exercisers.

Most people consume excess sodium. The average American diet contains about 3–6 grams of sodium, or about 7–15 grams of salt, per day. There are tribes that cook their food in seawater and consume huge amounts of salt, up to 40 grams per day. These people have a higher incidence of hypertension.

Another way to evaluate salt intake is to break down how it comes into the diet. The average diet derives about 3–4 grams of naturally occurring salt in food, 4–5 grams from eating processed foods, and another 3–4 grams from salt added in cooking or at the table. That adds up to about 10–13 grams of sodium chloride, or approximately 4–5 grams of sodium, per day, twice the suggested level. Higher sodium intake has evolved in the last century or two as a result of habit, taste, and social customs. It is probably most helpful to limit sodium to 1–3 grams per day and to obtain at least as much potassium as sodium, although the ideal potassium intake is double that of sodium. These precautions reduce the risk of sodium-sensitive hypertension and other effects of excess sodium. Potassium chloride as a salt substitute may be one helpful way to maintain this sodium-potassium balance. Eating more fresh fruits and vegetables is a good safeguard against problems with high blood pressure or diseases of the cardiovascular system.

 Sulfur is an interesting nonmetallic element that is found mainly as part of larger compounds. It is not discussed much in nutrition books, mainly because it has not been thought to be essential—that is, sulfur deficiency does not cause any visible problems.

Sulfur represents about 0.25 percent of our total body weight, similar to potassium. The body contains approximately 140 grams of sulfur—mainly in the proteins, although it is distributed in small amounts in all cells and tissues. Sulfur has a characteristic odor that can be smelled when hair or sheep's wool is burned. Keratin, present in the skin, hair, and nails, is particularly high in the amino acid cystine, in which sulfur is found. The sulfur-sulfur bond in keratin gives it greater strength.

Sulfur is present in four amino acids: methionine, an essential amino acid; the nonessential cystine and cysteine, which can be made from methionine; and taurine, which is not part of body tissues but does help produce bile acid for digestion. Sulfur is also present in two B vitamins, thiamine and biotin; interestingly, thiamine is important to skin and biotin to hair. Sulfur is also available as various sulfates or sulfides. But overall, sulfur is most important as part of protein.

Sulfur has been used commonly since the early 1800s. Grandma's "spring tonic" consisted mainly of sulfur and molasses. This also acted as a laxative. Sulfur has been known as the "beauty mineral" because it helps the complexion and skin stay clear and youthful. The hydrogen sulfide gas in onions is what causes tearing. This gas can also be made by intestinal bacteria and is absorbed by the body or released as gas with a characteristic odor.

Sulfur is absorbed from the small intestine primarily as the four sulfur-containing amino acids or from sulfates in water or fruits and vegetables. It is thought that elemental sulfur is not used by the human organism. Sulfur is stored in all body cells, especially the skin, hair, and nails. Excess amounts are eliminated through the urine or in the feces.

Sources: As part of four amino acids, sulfur is readily available in protein foods—meats, fish, poultry, eggs, milk, and legumes are all good sources. Egg yolks are one of the better sources of sulfur. Other foods that contain this somewhat smelly mineral are onions, garlic, cabbage, brussels sprouts, and turnips. Nuts have some, as do kale, lettuce, kelp and other seaweed, and raspberries. Complete vegetarians (those who eat no eggs or milk) and people on low-protein diets may not get sufficient amounts of sulfur; the resulting sulfur deficiency is difficult to differentiate clinically from protein deficiency, which is of much greater concern.

Functions: As part of four amino acids, sulfur performs a number of functions in enzyme reactions and protein synthesis. It is necessary for formation of collagen, the protein found in connective tissue in our bodies. Sulfur is also present in keratin, which is necessary for the maintenance of the skin, hair, and nails, helping to give strength, shape, and hardness to these protein tissues. Sulfur is also present in the fur and feathers of other animals. The cystine in hair gives off the sulfur smell when it is burned. Sulfur, as cystine and methionine, is part of other important body chemicals: insulin, which helps regulate carbohydrate metabolism, and heparin, an anticoagulant. Taurine is found in bile acids, used in digestion. The sulfur-containing amino acids help form other substances as well, such as biotin, coenzyme A, lipoic acid, and glutathione. The mucopoly-saccharides may contain chondroitin sulfate, which is important to joint tissues.

Sulfur is important to cellular respiration, as it is needed in the oxidation-reduction reactions that help the cells utilize oxygen, which aids brain function and all cell activity. These reactions are dependent on cysteine, which also helps the liver produce bile secretions and eliminate other toxins. L-cysteine is thought to generally help body detoxification mechanisms through the tripeptide compound, glutathione.

Uses: In its elemental form, sulfur was used for many disorders during the nineteenth century. In the twentieth century, the focus is more on the sulfur-containing amino acids, used internally; or as elemental sulfur-containing ointments used for skin disorders such as eczema, dermatitis, and psoriasis. Psoriasis has been treated with oral sulfur along with zinc. Other problems of the skin or hair have been treated with additional sulfur-containing compounds.

Joint problems may be helped by chondroitin sulfate, which is found in high amounts in the joint tissues. For centuries, arthritis sufferers have been helped by bathing in waters that contain high amounts of sulfur. Oral sulfur as sulfates in doses of 500–1,000 mg. may also reduce symptoms in some patients. Magnesium sulfate, which is not absorbed, has been used as a laxative. Taurine, another sulfur-containing amino acid, has been used in epilepsy treatment, usually along with zinc. A physiologic form of sulfur called methyl-sulfonyl methane (MSM) has recently become available and may be helpful in patients with allergies (see Chapter 7, *Accessory Nutrients*).

If we need additional sulfur, we can get it by eating an egg or two a day or eating extra garlic or onions, as well as other sulfur foods. There is no real cause for concern about the cholesterol in eggs if the diet is generally low in fat and blood cholesterol level is not elevated.

Deficiency and toxicity: There is minimal reason for concern about either toxicity or deficiency of sulfur in the body. No clearly defined symptoms exist with either state. Sulfur deficiency is more common when foods are grown in sulfur-depleted soil, with low-protein diets, or with a lack of intestinal bacteria, though none of these seems to cause any problems in regard to sulfur functions and metabolism.

Requirements: There is no specific RDA for sulfur other than the amino acids of which they are part are needed to meet protein requirements. Our needs are usually easily met through diet. About 850 mg. are thought to be needed for basic turnover of sulfur in the body. There is not much information available on sulfur content of foods, nor are there supplements specifically for sulfur. I have found that it is not really a nutritional concern.

 Silicon is another mineral that is not commonly written about as an essential nutrient. It is present in the soil and is actually the most abundant mineral in the earth's crust, as carbon is the most abundant in plant and animal tissues. Silicon is very hard and is found in rock crystals such as quartz or flint. Silicon dioxide (SiO_2) is an "active" form of silicon and is used to make glass. Silicon molecules in the tissues, such as the nails and connective tissue, give them strength and stability. Silicon is present in bone, blood vessels, cartilage, and tendons, helping to make them strong. Silicon is important to bone formation, as it is found in active areas of calcification. It is also found in plant fibers and is probably an important part of their structure. This mineral is able to form long molecules, much the same as is carbon, and gives these complex configurations some durability and strength. It represents about 0.05 percent of our body weight.

Silicon is currently considered a research macromineral, as it has been since the early 1970s. Studies have revealed retarded growth and poor bone development in young rats fed a silicon-deficient diet. Rabbits showed more atherosclerotic arterial plaques when fed diets low in silicon. I am sure that we will find further information regarding silicon and its functions in coming years.

Sources: Silicon is widely available in food. It is part of plant fibers (though not of cellulose) and is found in high amounts in the hulls of wheat, oats, and rice, in sugar beet and cane pulp, in alfalfa, and in the herbs horsetail, comfrey, and nettles. Horsetail, *Equisetum arvensa*, is a common source used to make supplemental silica. Silicon is also present in lettuce, cucumbers, avocados, strawberries, onions, and dandelions and other dark greens. The pectin in citrus fruits and alginic acid in kelp also contain small amounts of silicon. Hard drinking water may also be a good source.

This mineral is lost easily in food processing. Only about 2 percent of the original silicon is left in milled flour. Soil may also become deficient in silicon, and it is not being replaced; this loss could affect inherent plant structure.

Functions: Silicon promotes firmness and strength in the tissues. It is part of the arteries, tendons, skin, connective tissue, and eyes. Collagen contains silicon, helping hold the body tissues together. This mineral is also present with the chondroitin sulfates of cartilage, and it works with calcium to help restore bones.

Silicon is also thought to radiate or transmit energy in its crystalline structure, as in quartz crystal. It is thought by some to be able to deeply penetrate the tissues and help to clear stored toxins. The "silicea" tissue salt, a homeopathic remedy, is described poetically as acting like a "microscopic surgeon."

Uses: Silicon is often used in herbal remedies to promote strength in the hair, skin, and nails. It helps maintain the elasticity of the skin, so it may be one of our antiaging nutrients. Other possible uses of silica or silicon that are under investigation are to reduce the risk of atherosclerosis and heart disease, to treat arthritis and other joint or cartilage problems, gastric ulcers, and other conditions where tissue repair and healing are needed. Silicon is thought to help heal fractures and may have some role in the prevention or treatment of osteoporosis.

Deficiency and toxicity: There is little information on these areas, especially for toxicity. Deficiency problems are under investigation. Results of studies on animals suggest that silicon may be essential in humans. Decreased growth and deficient bone and tooth structure were found in rats with silicon-deficient diets. Silicon deficiency may increase atherosclerosis and heart disease; however, or it may not be a cause and effect relationship, but rather a result or association of these diseases. It would seem that the essential strength and stability this mineral provides to the tissues should give them protection from disease. Other research reveals that silicon levels affect physical endurance, with low tissue levels correlating with lowered stamina.

Requirements: There is no RDA for silicon since it is not considered essential. The average diet provides about 1–1.5 grams of this mineral, but eating a diet high in processed foods and avoiding the basic vegetable and grain foods may diminish our intake of silicon. To get extra silicon, eat more whole grains and fresh vegetables or use herbs, such as horsetail, or alfalfa or comfrey tablets.

185

THE ESSENTIAL TRACE MINERALS

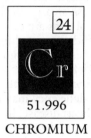

CHROMIUM

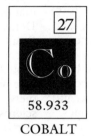

COBALT

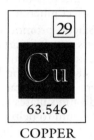

COPPER

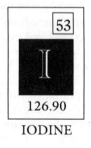

IODINE

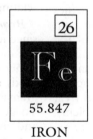

IRON

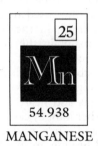

MANGANESE

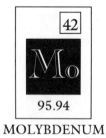

MOLYBDENUM

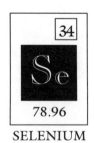

SELENIUM

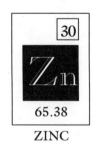

ZINC

Chromium has become a subject of much interest in recent years, and we continue to learn more about it. Chromium was long thought to be a toxic mineral until it was discovered in 1957 to be the essential part of glucose tolerance factor (GTF). GTF (and thus chromium) is a vital molecule in regulating carbohydrate metabolism by enhancing insulin function for proper use of glucose in the body. GTF is composed of one chromium molecule in the trivalent state (a +3 charge), two niacin molecules, and three amino acids—glycine, cysteine, and glutamic acid.

Trivalent chromium is the biologically active form. Hexavalent chromium (+6) is fairly unstable and is potentially toxic in the body. Chromium is not found in nature as a free metal, so it must be reduced to its elemental form to make the "chrome" used in the auto industry. This form, however, is not available to the body, so we cannot meet our daily chromium needs by sucking on car bumpers. The chromium in the blood is in the organic active form in the trivalent state, as part of GTF or carried with a beta-globulin protein.

Chromium is really considered an "ultratrace" mineral, since it is needed in such small quantities to perform its essential functions. The blood contains about 20 parts per billion (ppb), a fraction of a microgram. Even though it is in such small concentrations, this mineral is important to health. There are about 6 mg. of chromium stored in the bodies of people who live in the United States; tissue levels of people in other countries are usually higher, and those higher levels tend to be associated with a lower incidence of diabetes and atherosclerosis. There is less hardening of the arteries in people of Asian countries, who it is estimated have five times higher chromium tissue levels than Americans. People of Near Eastern countries who have about four times the average U.S. levels and African people who have twice our chromium levels seem to experience less diabetes than Americans. These higher tissue levels of chromium are due primarily to better soil supplies and a less refined diet. Chromium may be only one of the factors accounting for the differences in rates of diabetes and atherosclerosis between cultures, but it is probably a major one.

Chromium is a difficult mineral to absorb. Figures range from 0.5–3 percent absorption for the inorganic chromium salts often found in food. The organic complexes of chromium, such as GTF, are absorbed better, at about 10–20 percent. The kidneys clear any excess from the blood, while much of chromium intake is eliminated through the feces. This mineral is stored in many parts of the body, including the skin, fat, brain, muscles, spleen, kidneys, and testes.

Tissue levels of chromium tend to decrease with age, which may be a factor in the increase of adult-onset diabetes, a disease whose incidence has risen more than sixfold in the past 50 years. This increase may mirror the loss of chromium from our diets because of soil deficiency and the refinement of foods. Much of the chromium in whole grains and sugarcane is lost in making refined flour (40 percent loss) and white sugar (93 percent loss). In addition, there is some evidence that refined flour and sugar deplete even more chromium from the body. Reduced absorption related to aging, diets that are stressful to the digestive system, and the modern refined diet all contribute to chromium deficiency. Higher fat intake also may inhibit chromium absorption. If chromium is as important as we think it is to blood sugar metabolism, its deficiency may be in part responsible, along with the refined and processed diet, for the third leading cause of death (more than 300,000 yearly) in this country, diabetes mellitus, and this figure does not reflect other deaths that may be related to chromium deficiency, since high blood sugar levels seen in diabetes also increase the progression of atherosclerosis and cardiovascular disease, our number one killer.

187

Diagnosing and treating chromium deficiency is simple and should be done as early as possible, as it is much easier to prevent diabetes than to treat it.

Sources: Food refinement, and the loss of topsoil through poor agricultural practices reduce the level of chromium in foods. There are, however, still many good food sources. Since GTF is better absorbed than inorganic chromium, the level and activity of GTF in foods affect how well they supply us with this mineral. GTF activity may not always correspond to the actual amount of chromium in foods; however, many foods with good GTF activity also have good amounts of chromium. Hard water often contains some chromium; it may supply up to half of the daily needs of an adult.

Brewer's yeast is likely the best available source of chromium as well as having the highest GTF activity. About two tablespoons, or six tablets, per day supply most of our chromium needs; however, many people, maybe 30–40 percent, do not tolerate yeast very well and find that it causes digestive upset or bloating. If yeast is tolerated, it supplies a great many nutrients and is a low-calorie and low-fat source.

Following yeast in chromium concentration are beef, liver, whole wheat, rye, fresh chilies, oysters, potatoes, wheat germ, green peppers, eggs, chicken, apples, butter, bananas, and spinach. Yeast (44 ppm), black pepper (10 ppm), and molasses (2 ppm) are good sources of chromium, but since they are usually consumed in small quantities, it is best to have other chromium foods in the diet. In general, the whole grains, meats, shellfish, chicken, wheat germ and bran, and many vegetables, especially potato skins, are adequate sources. Beets and mushrooms may contain chromium.

Functions: Chromium is an essential mineral—that is, it is not made by the body and must be obtained from the diet. As the central part of GTF, it enhances the effect of insulin in the body. GTF is necessary for proper insulin function in the utilization of glucose and is needed in both human and animal nutrition for carbohydrate metabolism. Specifically, chromium/GTF improves the uptake of glucose into the cells so it can be metabolized to produce energy (ATP). GTF is thought to bind both to insulin and to the cell receptors to utilize glucose and thus help lower the blood sugar. This function of the glucose tolerance factor prevents continued elevations of blood sugar, which can lead to diabetes. If glucose does not enter the cells, the excess circulating sugar can cause damage to the cells, the retina of the eye, and the arteries, for example. Therefore, proper control of blood sugar may help to prevent atherosclerosis and its subsequent problems.

Chromium recently has been shown to lower blood cholesterol while mildly raising HDL (high-density lipoprotein), the good portion of cholesterol. This lowers the risk ratio for coronary artery disease. (Exercise is a key factor in raising HDL cholesterol and reducing coronary artery disease risk. Exercise also promotes the efficiency of insulin-mediated uptake of glucose into cells.)

Uses: Chromium and GTF are used in the treatment of both hypoglycemia and diabetes mellitus, two problems of blood sugar utilization and metabolism. Preventing chromium deficiency is the key here. The earlier treatment is begun, especially with potential diabetes, the more helpful it may be. Preformed GTF is not readily available, though formulas that contain all of its components seem to work better than chromium alone, and small amounts given daily have been shown to both increase glucose tolerance and decrease blood fats, both cholesterol and triglycerides, as well as to raise HDL. Chromium also does this and has been used along with niacin (also a part of GTF) in the treatment of high blood cholesterol.

Henry Schroeder, M.D., who has done numerous studies with chromium, has shown that 2 mg. of inorganic chromium given daily reduced cholesterol levels by about 15 percent. He has produced diabetes in lab animals by feeding them chromium-deficient diets. Such a diet raises not only blood sugar but blood cholesterol as well; both conditions return to normal with chromium supplementation. When Dr. Schroeder fed rats a chromium-rich diet, they showed improved longevity along with a reduction of atherosclerotic plaque found in the blood vessels at death. Chromium is used to help reduce atherosclerosis in people, especially in those who show low chromium levels. Cultures with higher tissue levels of chromium also appear to have lower incidences of atherosclerosis and heart disease.

Deficiency and toxicity: Because of the low absorption and high excretion rates of chromium, toxicity is not at all common in humans, especially with the usual forms of chromium used for supplementation. The amount of chromium that would cause toxicity is estimated to be much more than the amount commonly supplied in supplements.

Chromium deficiency is another story, however, with an estimated 25–50 percent of the U.S. population deficient in chromium. The United States has a greater incidence of deficiency than any other country, because of very low soil levels of chromium and the loss of this mineral from refined foods, especially sugar and flours. Deficiencies are more common in both the elderly and the young, especially teenagers on poor diets. Even though chromium is needed in such small amounts, it is difficult to obtain. Given these factors, and the fact that the already-low chromium absorption rate decreases even further with age, chromium deficiency is of great concern. It may even be the missing link in the development of adult-onset diabetes, a serious problem increasing rapidly in our culture. Nearly one in five adult Americans now develops diabetes.

A high-fat, high-sugar diet that contains refined flour products is probably the most important risk factor for diabetes. Such a diet tends to be low in chromium content and also causes more insulin to be produced, which requires even more chromium. Milk and other high-phosphorus foods tend to bind with chromium in the gut to make chromium phosphates that travel through the intestines and are not absorbed.

Even mild deficiencies of chromium can produce symptoms other than problems in blood sugar metabolism, such as anxiety or fatigue. Abnormal cholesterol metabolism and increased progress of atherosclerosis are associated with chromium deficiency, and deficiency may also cause decreased growth in young people and slower healing time after injuries or surgery. Most important, the low chromium levels seen in the United States are associated with a higher incidence of diabetes and arteriosclerosis. Further research is needed to confirm these associations and to determine whether correcting the chromium deficiency would actually reduce the incidence of these diseases.

Requirements: There is no specific RDA for chromium. Average daily intake may be about 80–100 mcg. We probably need a minimum of 1–2 mcg. going into the blood to maintain tissue levels; since only around 2 percent of our intake is absorbed, we need at least 100–200 mcg. in the daily diet. A safe dosage range for chromium supplementation is between 200–300 mcg. Children need somewhat less. Many vitamin or mineral supplements contain about 100–150 mcg. of chromium. Some people take up to 1 mg. (1,000 mcg.) per day for short periods without problems; this is not suggested as a long-term regimen but rather to help replenish chromium stores when deficiency is present. All of the precursors to the active form of GTF are used in some formulas, but usually with chromium in lower doses, such as 50 mcg., since it is thought to be better absorbed with niacin and the amino acids glycine, cysteine and glutamic acid.

189

TO AVOID DEFICIENCY AND MAINTAIN A GOOD INTAKE OF CHROMIUM:

- Avoid sugar and sugar products, soda pops, candy, and presweetened breakfast cereals.
- Avoid refined, white flour products, such as white breads and crackers.
- Use whole wheat products, wheat germ, and/or brewer's yeast.
- Eat whole foods.
- Take a general supplement that contains chromium, approximately 100–200 mcg. daily.

Cobalt is another essential mineral needed in very small amounts in the diet. It is an integral part of part of vitamin B_{12}, cobalamin, which supports red blood cell production and the formation of myelin nerve coverings. Some authorities do not consider cobalt to be essential as a separate nutrient, since it is needed primarily as part of B_{12}, which is itself essential.

Cobalt, as part of vitamin B_{12}, is not easily absorbed from the digestive tract. The body level of cobalt normally measures 80–300 mcg. It is stored in the red blood cells and the plasma, as well as in the liver, kidney, spleen, and pancreas.

Sources: Cobalt is available mainly as part of B_{12}. There is some question as to whether inorganic cobalt is actually usable in the human body. Meat, liver, kidney, clams, oysters, and milk all contain some cobalt. Ocean fish and sea vegetables have cobalt, but land vegetables have very little; some cobalt is available in legumes, spinach, cabbage, lettuce, beet greens, and figs.

Functions: As part of vitamin B_{12}, cobalt is essential to red blood cell formation and is also helpful to other cells.

Uses: Cobalt, as part of B_{12}, is used to prevent anemia, particularly pernicious anemia; vitamin B_{12} is also beneficial in some cases of fatigue, digestive disorders, and neuromuscular problems. There are no other known uses except for the radioactive cobalt-60 used to treat certain cancers.

Deficiency and toxicity: Toxicity can occur from excess inorganic cobalt found as a food contaminant. Beer drinker's cardiomyopathy (enlarged heart) and congestive heart failure have been traced to cobalt introduced into beer during manufacturing. Increased intake may affect the thyroid or cause overproduction of red blood cells, thickened blood, and increased activity in the bone marrow.

Deficiency of cobalt is not really a concern if we get enough vitamin B_{12}. Vegetarians need to be more concerned than others about getting enough cobalt and B_{12}. The soil is becoming deficient in cobalt, further reducing the already low levels found in plant foods. As cobalt deficiency leads to decreased availability of B_{12}, there is an increase of many symptoms and problems related to B_{12} deficiency, particularly pernicious anemia and nerve damage.

Requirements: No specific RDA is suggested for cobalt. Our needs are low, and vitamin B_{12} usually fulfills them. The average daily intake of cobalt is about 5–8 mcg. It is not usually given in supplements.

Copper has been known to be an essential trace mineral for some time. In recent years there has been more concern about copper toxicity than about getting the small amounts we need to make hemoglobin and perform other functions. Copper is present in all body tissues. The total amount in our bodies is about 75–100 mg., less than that contained in a copper penny.

Copper is found in many foods in small amounts (oysters and nuts are the richest sources). The standard amount available in our diet, whether or not it is excessive or deficient, is a controversial topic; the naturalist in me feels that if it is in wholesome foods, it must be the right amount. This mineral is present in water that flows through copper piping. Increases in estrogen hormone levels, from taking birth control pills or during pregnancy, for example, often increase serum copper levels to more than double normal values, while red blood cell levels, where copper is important, may actually be lower. This may contribute to some of the psychological or other symptoms seen during pregnancy or with birth control pill use. Increased copper levels have been associated with schizophrenia, learning disabilities, and senility, although none of these associations have been demonstrated with certainty. Depression and other mental problems, premenstrual syndrome, and hyperactivity have also been correlated with high copper levels, often in combination with low zinc levels.

Zinc and copper have a seesaw relationship in the body, competing with each other for absorption in the gut. Both zinc deficiency and copper toxicity have increased since the switch from zinc (galvanized) to copper water pipes. We can avoid this problem by not drinking tap water. Some studies of schizophrenics have revealed high blood copper with low urinary copper (showing that copper is being retained) and low blood zinc. In some of these cases, zinc was helpful as an antianxiety agent.

About 30 percent of copper intake is absorbed into the body from the stomach and upper intestine; it is fairly rapidly absorbed, usually within 15 minutes. Copper is transferred by albumin across the gut wall and carried to the liver, where it is formed into ceruloplasmin, a copper-protein complex. About 90 percent of the average 100 mcg. of copper in the blood is in the form of ceruloplasmin. As a balancing mechanism to minimize copper toxicities, absorption of copper is decreased when ceruloplasmin levels are adequate. Vitamin C, zinc, and manganese all interfere with copper absorption. Protein and fresh vegetable foods have been shown to improve copper absorption.

About 100 mg. of copper are stored in the body, with the highest concentrations in the liver and brain tissues, which account for about one-third of the total. Muscles contain approximately another third, with the remaining copper in the other tissues. At birth, a high amount is contained in the liver; by about age ten, the normal adult level of copper is reached, both in the liver and the rest of the body. Excess copper is eliminated mainly through the liver into the bile and is lost through the intestines. A minimal amount is excreted in the urine.

Sources: Copper is available in most natural foods. Some authorities believe that our average intake is higher than our actual needs, that low intakes are uncommon, and that toxicity is a potential problem. The other school of thought holds that low intake is common because soil depletion has decreased the copper level in many foods and because many people avoid natural, copper-containing foods.

Foods with good supplies of copper are the whole grains, particularly buckwheat and whole wheat; shellfish, such as shrimp and other seafoods; liver and other organ meats; most dried peas and beans; and nuts, such as Brazil nuts, almonds, hazelnuts, walnuts, and pecans. Oysters have high amounts, about five times as much as other foods. Soybeans supply copper, as do dark leafy greens and some dried fruits, such as prunes; cocoa, black pepper, and yeast are also sources. In addition to food sources, copper can come from water pipes and cookware.

Functions: Copper is important as a catalyst in the formation of hemoglobin, our oxygen-carrying molecule. Copper in the red blood cells is bound to erythrocuprein, a substance thought to have *superoxide dismutase* (SOD) activity, which is energy enhancing. Copper is also part of the cytochrome system for cell respiration, an energy-releasing process. It also helps oxidize vitamin

191

C and works with C to form collagen (part of cell membranes and the supportive matrix in muscles and other tissues), especially in the bone and connective tissue. It helps the cross-linking of collagen fibers and thus supports the healing process of tissues and aids in proper bone formation. An excess of copper may increase collagen and lead to stiffer and less flexible tissues.

Copper is found in many enzymes; most important is the cytoplasmic *superoxide dismutase*. Copper enzymes play a role in oxygen-free radical metabolism, and in this way have a mild anti-inflammatory effect. Copper also functions in certain amino acid conversions. Being essential in the synthesis of phospholipids, copper contributes to the integrity of the myelin sheaths covering nerves. It also aids the conversion of tyrosine to the pigment melanin, which gives hair and skin their coloring. Copper, as well as zinc, is important for converting T_3 (triiodothyronine) to T_4 (thyroxine), both thyroid hormones. Low copper levels may reduce thyroid functions.

Copper, like most metals, is a conductor of electricity; in the body, it helps the nervous system function. It also helps control levels of histamine, which may be related to allergic and inflammatory reactions. Copper in the blood is fixed to the protein cerulosplasmin, and copper is part of the enzyme *histaminase*, which is involved in the metabolism of histamine.

Uses: Some nutritional doctors feel that copper should not be supplemented because of the narrow line between the therapeutic and toxic doses. Copper has, however, been used in cases of anemia, vitiligo, fatigue, allergies, and stomach ulcers where low levels of copper have been found. Whenever copper is deficient, which it can be for many reasons, it should be supplemented. Copper can be measured in the blood, both plasma and red blood cell levels, to help determine the amount of copper to be supplemented.

The use of copper bracelets in the treatment of arthritis has a long history, and wearers continue to claim positive results. The copper in the bracelets reacts with the fatty acids in the skin to form copper salts that are absorbed into the body. The copper salts may cause a blue-green stain on the skin, but this can be removed with soap and water. Recent research suggests that copper salicylate used to treat arthritis reduces symptoms more effectively than either copper or aspirin alone.

In a Danish study, arthritis patients who were treated with injections of *superoxide dismutase*, an enzyme containing copper (or manganese and zinc) that is found within the cells, obtained relief from many of their symptoms, such as joint swelling, pain, and morning stiffness. SOD is available in tablets in the United States; however, it is not thought to be stable in the stomach and small intestine, so it may not be of any help for arthritis when taken orally. Additional research with enteric-coated tablets of active SOD may provide new insights into oral SOD treatment of arthritis and other inflammatory disorders.

Deficiency and toxicity: Copper toxicity has been the subject of great concern in recent years. High copper levels, especially when associated, as they often are, with low zinc levels, have been described in a wide variety of conditions. Whether this is incidental, a cause of these problems, or a result of them is not known for certain. Problems of copper toxicity may include stress and anxiety states, joint and muscle pains, psychological depression, mental fatigue, poor memory, lack of concentration, insomnia, manic depression, schizophrenia, senility, epilepsy, autism, hypertension, stuttering, hyperactivity in children, premenstrual syndrome, preeclampsia of pregnancy, and postpartum psychosis. Until further research clarifies the problems of copper toxicity, it is wise to check levels of copper (and zinc) in people with these conditions as well as those with alcoholism, cancer, and infectious diseases. The World Health Organization (WHO) still states that copper is nontoxic.

Hair levels of copper are not very helpful in

detecting increased body copper because external contamination from the fungicides and algicides used in swimming pools or hot tubs may leave copper on the hair, causing misleading test results. However, hair copper is suggestive of body state, such that if hair (or blood copper) levels are elevated, it is wise to check the 24-hour urine copper level or the blood ceruloplasmin level. Red blood cell copper levels may be a good test to measure increased copper levels as well; serum copper levels may be easier for detecting deficiency.

Symptoms of mild copper toxicity may be classified as hypochondriac or "neurotic" ones. Fatigue, irritability, nervousness, depression, and learning problems are some common symptoms. Higher levels of copper intoxication can lead to nausea, vomiting, diarrhea, liver damage, gingivitis, dermatitis, or a discoloration of the skin and hair. In their book *Trace Elements, Hair Analysis and Nutrition* (Keats Publishing, 1983), Drs. Richard Passwater and Elmer Cranton describe a case of three women who lived together in a house with copper pipes. All presented symptoms of fatigue, irritability, muscle and joint aches, and headaches, and all had elevated copper levels. They were treated successfully with increased levels of zinc and manganese, which compete with copper for absorption and also help eliminate copper through the bile and urine. Carl Pfeiffer, M.D., suggests using zinc (50 mg.), manganese (3 mg.), and vitamin B_6 (50 mg.) daily without supplemental copper to increase copper excretion. If copper levels are very high, treatment with penicillamine or chelation therapy with ethylenediaminetetraacetic acid (EDTA) may be needed. In Europe, a compound called Dimeval (di-mercapto-succinic acid) may be used to lower copper levels.

A genetic disorder called Wilson's disease affects copper metabolism and leads to low serum and hair copper with high liver and brain copper levels. This can be a serious and even fatal problem unless treated by chelating agents; penicillamine is most often used as it binds copper in the gut and carries it out. A low-copper diet and more zinc and manganese in the diet and as supplements will also help reduce copper levels. Menke's disease is a rare problem of copper malabsorption in infants. In this condition, which can often be fatal, decreased intestinal absorption causes copper to accumulate in the intestinal lining.

Copper deficiency has long been considered unlikely even with a suboptimal diet because it was thought to be readily available from foods. Newer surveys seem to suggest that, with soil deficiency and poor diet, the average dietary intake is now less than 1 mg. per day. Our bodies require more than this. A recent study revealed that 75 percent of those evaluated had less intake than the 2 mg. RDA. Many authorities feel that intake below 2 mg. is still sufficient, especially when drinking water from copper pipes.

Copper deficiency is commonly found together with iron deficiency, especially with iron deficiency anemia. Fatigue, paleness, skin sores, and edema may appear with this, as may slowed growth, hair loss, anorexia, diarrhea, and dermatitis. High zinc levels or intake can lead to lower copper levels and some symptoms of copper deficiency. The reduced red blood cell function and shortened red cell life span can influence energy levels and cause weakness and labored respiration from decreased oxygen delivery. Low copper levels may also affect collagen formation and thus tissue health and healing. Reduced thyroid function, weakened immunity, cardiovascular disease, increased cholesterol, skeletal defects related to bone demineralization, and poor nerve conductivity, including irregular heart rhythms, might all result from copper depletions. Copper deficiency results in several abnormalities of the immune system, such as reduced cellular immune response, reduced activity of white blood cells, and, possibly, reduced thymus hormone production, all of which may contribute to an increased infection rate. Infants fed an all-dairy (cow's milk) diet without copper supplements may develop copper deficiency. Some children with iron deficiency show reduced levels of copper as well. It is also likely that during pregnancy copper will be deficient unless supplemented with at least 2 mg. daily.

Requirements: The RDA for copper in adults is 2 mg. (liberally, 2–3 mg.) per day. For children it is 1–2 mg. and for infants about 0.5–1 mg. The average adult intake had been estimated at 2.5–5 mg. per day, although recent reports suggest lower levels.

Many nutritionists do not supplement copper at all or at least not more than 2 mg. per day in a general supplement because of the concern about toxicity and because excess copper can interfere with absorption of zinc. Zinc deficiency can cause a great number of problems, such as hair loss, menstrual problems, and weakened immunity. If the soil in which our food is grown is known to be high in copper or if we drink water from copper pipes, we should probably avoid copper supplements. If we eat a diet that includes whole grains, nuts, and leafy green vegetables or eat much liver, we are probably obtaining sufficient levels from our diet. Overall, if we do supplement zinc, we should also take copper in a ratio of 15–30 mg. zinc to 2 mg. copper, unless of course, we are trying to reduce copper or correct a zinc deficiency. Likewise, if we take copper we should add zinc, unless we are treating high zinc levels or copper deficiency.

Iodine is a good example of a trace mineral whose deficiency creates a disease that is easily corrected by resupplying it in the diet. Goiter, an enlargement of the thyroid gland, develops when this important metabolic gland does not have enough iodine to manufacture hormones. As it increases its cell size to try to trap more iodine, the whole gland increases in size, creating a swelling in the neck. Without supplemental iodine, a hypothyroid condition re-

sults, likely leading to fatigue and sluggishness, weight gain, and coldness of the body; at this stage, the condition may be harder to treat with iodine alone and thyroid hormone supplementation may be needed.

Goiter was first noted in the Great Lakes region; the "goiter belt" included that area and the midwestern and Plains states. In the 1930s, approximately 40 percent of the people in Michigan had goiter, due mainly to iodine-deficient soil; glacier melting had washed away the iodine. Areas by oceans or in the vicinity of ocean breezes usually contain enough iodine to prevent goiters. In 1924, iodine was added to table salt, a substance that was already in wide use (our salt problem has been going on for a long time). Iodized salt was first introduced in Michigan; by 1940, it was in general use. Even today, iodine deficiency is still a problem, and many people in the United States have goiter. Cretinism, another condition caused by iodine deficiency, is characterized by mental retardation and other problems. It may be present in iodine-deficient babies or children born to women who are lacking iodine. It is a serious and nonreversible problem that should be avoided by proper iodine intake.

Iodine itself is a poisonous gas, as are the related halogens chlorine, fluorine, and bromine. However, as with chlorine, the salts or negatively charged ions of iodine (iodides) are soluble in water, and iodine is essential to life in trace amounts. Plants do not need iodine, but humans require it for the production of thyroid hormones that regulate the metabolic energy of the body and set the basal metabolic rate (BMR).

The body contains about 25 mg. of iodine. A small percentage of this is in the muscles, 20 percent is in the thyroid, and the rest is in the skin and bones. Only 1 percent is present in the blood. The concentration of iodine in the thyroid gland is very high, more than 1,000 times that in the muscles. Approximately one-fourth of thyroid iodine is in the two main thyroid hormones, T_4 (thyroxine) and T_3 (triiodothyronine). Thyroxine itself is nearly two-thirds iodine. The remainder is in the precursor molecules of these two important hormones.

Iodine is well absorbed from the stomach into the blood. About 30 percent goes to the thyroid gland, depending on the need. Iodine is eliminated rapidly. Most of the remaining 70 percent is filtered by the kidneys into the urine. Our bodies do not conserve iodine as they do iron, and we must obtain it regularly from the diet. There is recent concern that perhaps iodine is being overconsumed, especially in iodized salt. The incidence of goiter has been rising again, however, so there may be factors other than iodine involved in this problem.

Sources: The life from ocean waters provides the best source of iodine. Fish, shellfish, and sea vegetables (seaweed) are dependably rich sources. Cod, sea bass, haddock, and perch are a few examples of iodine-rich sea animals consumed by humans; kelp is the most common, high-iodine sea vegetable. Kelp in particular is rich in other minerals and low in sodium and thus is a good seasoning substitute for salt.

The use of iodized salt has certainly reduced most iodine deficiency. It contains about 76 mcg. of iodine per gram of salt. The average person consumes at least 3 grams of salt daily, exceeding the RDA for iodine of 150 mcg. Many authorities feel (and I believe) that commercial iodized salt is overused and has other drawbacks. It contains aluminum and other unneeded chemicals and may contribute to other problems. Fast foods may be very high in iodine because of the added salt. Adding iodine to salt is part of the paternalistic thinking of the industrial age, not counting on people to learn or adapt, "just put it in their food or water and save them from their own ignorance." There are healthier ways to obtain iodine than in table salt; eating fish, especially fresh ocean fish, is probably the best, as it also may help reduce cholesterol and cardiovascular disease risk. Sea salt from the ocean water is

a natural source of iodine, although it is not nearly as high in this mineral as "iodized" salt.

Dietary iodine content may vary widely, depending on the iodine content in the soil in which food grows. Plants grown in or animals grazed on iodine-rich soil will contain substantial amounts of iodine. Milk and its products may be sources of iodine when the cows have an iodized salt lick in their pasture. Eggs may also be a good source when iodine is in the chicken feed. Bakers may add iodine to dough, so some may be present in bread. Other foods that may contain iodine, especially when the soil is good, are onions, mushrooms, lettuce, spinach, green peppers, pineapple, peanuts, cheddar cheese, and whole wheat bread. More and more, people are eating wholesome, natural foods, avoiding iodized salt, so they must eat more of the iodine-rich foods, such as the sea vegetables, or obtain iodine from a general vitamin-mineral supplement to make sure they are getting adequate amounts.

Functions: Iodine is an essential nutrient for production of the body's thyroid hormones and therefore is required for normal thyroid function. The thyroid hormones, particularly thyroxine, which is 65 percent iodine, are responsible for our basal metabolic rate (BMR)—that is, the body's use of energy. Thyroid is required for cell respiration and the production of energy as ATP and further increases oxygen consumption and general metabolism.

The thyroid hormones, thyroxine and triiodothyronine, are also needed for normal growth and development, protein synthesis, and energy metabolism. As thyroid stimulates the energy production of the cellular mitochondria and affects our BMR, it literally influences all body functions. Nerve and bone formation, reproduction, the condition of the skin, hair, nails, and teeth, and our speech and mental state are all influenced by thyroid as well. Thyroid and, thus, iodine also affect the conversion of carotene to vitamin A and of ribonucleic acids to protein; cholesterol synthesis; and carbohydrate absorption.

195

Iodine is picked up by the thyroid and combines with the thyroid hormones and amino acid tyrosine to make the thyroid hormone precursors diiodotyrosine, diiodothyronine, and monoiodotyrosine and, then, the hormones T_3 and T_4. These hormones are then carried through the body by a protein called thyroid binding globulin (TBG).

Uses: Supplemental iodine may be helpful in correcting hypothyroidism and goiter caused by deficient iodine intake, and it may reverse many of the symptoms of cretinism if given soon after birth. Thus, iodine's main use is really in the prevention or early treatment of its deficiency diseases.

Iodine has also been used to help increase energy level and utilization in cases of fatigue, mental sluggishness, and weight gain caused by hypothyroidism. Iodine itself will not help with weight loss if there is normal thyroid function. If weight gain results from iodine deficiency causing decreased thyroid activity, this hypothyroid condition may be improved with iodine followed by thyroid supplementation.

Iodine solutions, such as iodine tincture or Betadine, are commonly used as antiseptics and can actually kill bacteria and fungi.

Because of the thyroid's role in fat and cholesterol metabolism, sufficient iodine and thus normal thyroid levels are thought to help reduce atherosclerosis potential. Also, iodine and thyroid may help maintain healthy hair, skin, and nails. It is possible that iodine deficiency increases the risk of certain cancers, such as breast, ovary, and uterus. Iodine levels may be low in people with fibrocystic breast disease; in this case, supplementation may improve this condition.

Potassium iodide has been used medicinally for problems of the skin and as an expectorant for bronchial congestion. Silver iodide has been used to seed clouds to bring rain, but this practice is considered ecologically unsound. Iodine supplements may help prevent uptake of radioactive iodine if that is present in the environment or in medical diagnostic procedures. If the thyroid were saturated with normal iodine, it would eliminate the radioactive molecules more rapidly.

Deficiency and toxicity: There is no significant danger of toxicity of iodine from a natural diet, though some care must be taken when supplementing iodine or using it in drug therapy. High iodine intake, however, may actually reduce thyroxine production and thyroid function. Excessive quantities of iodized salt, taking too many kelp tablets, or overuse of potassium iodide expectorants such as SSKI can cause some problems, but regular elevated intake of iodine is needed to produce toxicity. Some people have allergic reactions, mainly as skin rashes, to iodine products. Iodine supplementation may also worsen acne in some cases.

Deficiencies of iodine have been very common, especially in areas where the soil is depleted, as discussed earlier. Several months of iodine deficiency can lead to goiter and/or hypothyroidism. With decreased iodine, the thyroid cells and gland enlarge, creating a goiter, which may be noticed mainly by the swelling it causes in the base of the neck.

Goiter is usually associated with hypothyroidism, which is decreased thyroid function that leads to slower metabolism, fatigue, weight gain, sluggishness, dry hair, thick skin, poor mental functioning, decreased resistance to infection, a feeling of coldness, and a decrease in sexual energy. More advanced hypothyroidism may worsen these symptoms as well as create a hyperactive, manic state and hypertension, which is paradoxical because this may occur with an overactive thyroid as well. Iodine by itself usually will not cure goiter and hypothyroidism but often will slow their progression.

Goitrogens are substances that can induce goiter, primarily by interfering with the formation and function of thyroglobulin. Some natural goitrogens are soybeans, cabbage, cauliflower, and peanuts, especially when they

RDAS FOR IODINE
(in mcg.)

Infants	40—50
Ages 1—3	70
Ages 4—6	90
Ages 7—10	120
Age 11 older	150
Pregnant women	175
Lactating women	200

come from iodine-deficient soils. Millet has recently been described as having goitrogenic tendencies. Certain drugs, such as thiouracil and sulfonamides, also act as goitrogens.

Some early studies correlate low iodine levels with an increased risk of breast cancer. These low levels usually correlate with low selenium levels as well, more classically associated with cancer. A higher incidence of breast cancer has been shown to occur in the goiter belt, whereas areas with high soil levels of iodine and selenium show a lower incidence.

Requirements: The RDA for iodine in adults is 150 mcg. The amount necessary to prevent goiter is about 1 mcg./kg.—that is, about 50–75 mcg. for most adults. Average intake from diet ranges from 65 mcg. to about 650 mcg. Much of that may come from iodized salt, which is not highly recommended; however, it is very difficult to avoid salt completely in our culture because it is added to so many prepared foods and by restaurants and mothers everywhere. A 6-ounce portion of ocean fish contains about 500 mcg. of iodine, more than is contained in one teaspoon of salt but without the extra 2 grams of sodium. Ideally, we can meet our iodine requirements by eating seafood, seaweed, and vegetables grown in iodine-rich soil. A typical mineral or complete vitamin supplement will contain the RDA, 150 mcg., of iodine per day. More iodine is needed during pregnancy and lactation. People on low-salt diets may need supplemental iodine.

 Iron is a well-known trace mineral with a long history. It may well have been the very first mineral to be incorporated into living tissue and is clearly a very important mineral. About 5 percent of the mineral content of the earth's crust is iron. Iron is found in every cell of the body, almost all of it combined with protein. There is a total of about 4 grams, or one-tenth teaspoon, of iron in an average 150-pound person. The hemoglobin molecule, essential for carrying oxygen throughout our system, contains 60–70 percent of the body's iron. If we lack iron, we will produce less hemoglobin and therefore supply less oxygen to our tissues. Besides being part of hemoglobin, iron is also stored in the liver, spleen, and bone marrow, which can be drawn on to supply extra iron for hemoglobin production.

Iron deficiency anemia is a well-known and all-too-common problem, even with our modern knowledge about the condition and the attention given to preventing it. The preanemia state is not easy to diagnose. Decreasing iron stores and a relative decrease in serum iron levels and protein-bound iron may cause symptoms before low tissue iron levels or anemia are measurable. More of this important mineral is needed during growth; iron deficiency is more common in infancy, childhood, adolescence, and pregnancy. Even the elderly may become deficient due to poorer absorption and diet. Women in their reproductive years have a greater problem with iron deficiency because of losses in menstrual blood and higher requirements. Minority and low-income people tend to have a higher incidence of low iron-related problems, primarily caused by dietary deficiency. Women in their childbearing years require at least 18 mg. of iron daily, but more than 25 percent of them probably obtain less than this amount. Usually, when the body needs more iron, absorption improves through an increase in iron-carrying proteins in the blood, called iron transferrin.

Iron absorption from the intestinal tract is a very subtle process; poor absorption is one of the main reasons, along with low-iron diets, that iron deficiency is so prevalent. Along with calcium, which is also difficult to absorb, iron and zinc are the minerals most commonly deficient in our diet.

Average iron absorption is about 8–10 percent of intake. All vegetable sources contain the "nonheme" form of iron, which is poorly absorbed and utilized. "Heme" iron, a special formulation of iron, is found only in flesh foods, beef and liver being the best sources. Between 10 and 30 percent of heme iron is absorbed. Combining heme foods with nonheme foods improves the absorption of iron from the nonheme foods. This is why complete vegetarians have trouble obtaining sufficient iron from the diet alone. Phytates present in whole grains and oxalates found in certain vegetables may bind up some of the iron and make it unabsorbable. Meat foods improve absorption, possibly by stimulating increased stomach acid production and by the fact that the iron contained is already bound into muscle and blood tissue, the iron proteins myoglobin and hemoglobin.

Iron absorption is a slow process, usually taking between two and four hours. The food-natural ferrous (+2) ion is absorbed much better than iron in the ferric (+3) form. Vitamin C in the gut along with iron converts any ferric iron to ferrous and thus improves absorption. Iron absorbed into the blood is usually bound to the protein transferrin and goes mainly to the bone marrow, where it can be used to make red blood cells. Some also goes to the liver and spleen. About 25 percent of body iron is stored bound to the protein ferritin and as the iron complex hemosiderin. Ferritin has good iron-binding capacity. A fully saturated ferritin molecule, which is actually ferric oxide surrounded by the protein apoferritin, can contain about 4,000 iron atoms. Ferritin stored in the liver, spleen, and bone marrow, for example, provides a good

reserve of iron to meet body needs. Measuring serum ferritin levels is a fairly new medical test that provides a good indication of iron storage levels. A normal value is 15–200 mcg. A level below 15 mcg. suggests very depleted iron reserves. Iron toxicity may show ferritin levels in the thousands.

About three-quarters of the iron in our bodies is active. Of that, about 70 percent is in hemoglobin, 5 percent is in myoglobin (muscle oxygenating protein), and the rest is part of iron cofactors and enzymes such as catalases, peroxidases, and the cytochromes. Some is also in transition, attached to transferrin, which transports iron to the bone marrow, liver, and other tissues for its functions in processing hemoglobin, myoglobin, and various enzymes. Fortunately, the body conserves iron very well, though this increases the possibility of toxicity. Toxicity has not been a great concern until recently, when the possibility of liver irritation and the increased risk of heart disease in men and postmenopausal women due to the oxidant effect of iron was suggested. About 1 percent of red blood cells are recycled each day (their average life span is 120 days), and we use the iron from them (about 30–50 mg. daily) to manufacture new cells. The recycled iron provides about 90 percent of the iron required to make new cells and to carry out other functions; therefore, we need only a little more for full functioning, unless, of course, there is blood loss.

Iron lost from the body must be replaced through dietary iron, but this often takes time and requires a regular source from food or supplements. A pint of blood contains about 200 mg. of iron. Even though iron absorption increases with increased need, it can still take several months to replenish the iron lost when we donate blood. About 30–40 mg. of iron will be lost during an average female menstrual cycle; this is why menstruating women need a consistently higher iron intake than men, a minimum of 18 mg. per day. During breast-feeding, the nursing mother will lose about 1–2 mg. per day. In pregnancy, the mother transfers 500–1000 mg. of iron to her growing baby, most of that (500–700 mg.) during the last few months. Since there are usually less than 500 mg. stored in the bone marrow and other tissues, the mother needs a regular, good dietary and supplemental intake of iron, or she will become very depleted and will be less able to obtain the extra oxygen she requires during pregnancy, labor, and delivery of her baby. After delivery, iron depletion could cause her to feel run-down and to have difficulty caring for her infant.

Many factors can increase iron absorption from the intestines and improve our chances of maintaining adequate body levels. Absorption improves when there is increased need for iron, as during growth periods, pregnancy, and lactation or after blood loss. Acids in the stomach, such as hydrochloric acid, and ascorbic acid (vitamin C) in the small intestine help change any ferric iron to the more easily absorbable ferrous form. Citrus fruits and many vegetables contain vitamin C and therefore help our iron absorption. The animal flesh foods have the more easily absorbed "heme," or blood, iron and also provide amino acids, which stimulate production of hydrochloric acid in the stomach. Cooking with an iron skillet will add iron to the food and make more of it available for absorption. Copper, cobalt, and manganese in the diet also improve iron absorption.

Likewise, many factors can reduce the body's iron absorption. Low stomach acid or taking antacids or other alkalis will diminish iron absorption. Rapid gastric motility reduces the chance to absorb iron, which is a slow process anyway. Phosphates, found in meats and soft drinks; oxalates, in spinach, chard, and other vegetables; and phytates, in the whole grains, all can form insoluble iron complexes or salts that will not be absorbed. Soy protein is being researched, as it may also reduce iron absorption. The caffeine and tannic acid in coffee and tea lower absorption of iron. Low copper in

FACTORS AFFECTING IRON ABSORPTION

Increased by:
- Body needs during growth, pregnancy, and lactation
- Hydrochloric acid
- Vitamin C
- Blood loss or iron deficiency
- Meats (heme iron)
- Protein foods
- Citrus fruits and vegetables
- Iron cookware
- Copper, cobalt, manganese

Decreased by:
- Low hydrochloride acid
- Antacids
- Low copper
- Phosphates in meats and soft drinks
- Calcium
- Phytates in whole grains
- Oxalates in leafy green vegetables
- Soy protein
- Coffee and black tea
- Fast gastrointestinal motility

the gut and in the body reduces iron absorption, and high calcium can compete with iron. Supplementing calcium with iron may create a more alkaline digestive medium, which further reduces iron absorption. Iron absorption usually decreases with age as well.

Any unabsorbed iron is eliminated in the feces. Otherwise, only minute amounts are lost in the urine, sweat, nail clippings, and hair. Other than through blood loss, most body iron is retained fairly well. Normal iron loss in the average person is about 1 mg. per day.

When we have plenty of iron, we can say we're "in the pink." Usually we will have good circulation, with rosy cheeks, pink earlobes, and pink tongue. (Yet we can also be "too pink" or red, with excess iron and blood cells.) If the tongue or the mucosal lining of the mouth is pale, we should look for anemia, so it is good for us to know what we can about iron, especially where we can find it in our foods.

Sources: Some of our soil is iron deficient, so the plants grown or the animals grazed there may contain relatively smaller amounts, though this is not yet a major concern. The milling of grain removes about 75 percent of the iron present in whole grains, as much of the iron is found in the outer bran and germ. The fortified or enriched grain foods, such as cereals and breads, contain some iron (plus vitamins B_1, B_2, and B_3), but this iron is in the poorly absorbed ferric state. Cooking in iron pots or skillets will add absorbable iron to food, but if this is done excessively over time, iron toxicity is a possibility.

Heme iron, as found in meats, is generally thought to be the iron that is best absorbed, several times more absorbable than the nonheme iron found in the vegetable kingdom. This does not mean that we need to eat meats in order to get sufficient iron, though that is often recommended in cases of iron deficiency. The 18 mg. of iron a day needed by a woman in the childbearing years is not always easy to obtain through diet. Though eating 22 slices of whole wheat bread or 13 cups of cooked kale would supply 18 mg., these are obviously not desirable ways to get it. In addition to beef, liver, and other organ meats that have relatively high amounts of absorbable iron, pork, lamb, chicken, and shellfish such as clams and oysters contain reasonable iron levels. Egg yolks are fairly good sources, and salmon is the best of the other seafood.

From the vegetable world, whole grains are the overall best source. Wheat, millet, oats, and brown rice are all iron-containing grains. The legumes—dried peas and beans—are good; lima beans, soybeans, kidney beans, and green peas are examples. Nuts, such as almonds and Brazil nuts, and most seeds contain iron. Green leafy vegetables such as spinach, kale, and dandelion are good sources, as are broccoli and asparagus. Dried fruits such as prunes, raisins, and apricots have a good amount of iron. Prune juice often gives us additional iron. Unsulfured molasses is concentrated in iron; one tablespoon contains about 3 mg. Tomatoes, strawberries, and many other fruits and vegetables contain some iron, so it is possible to obtain adequate amounts of iron from dietary sources without consuming a lot of meat by eating wholesome foods, especially whole grains, green vegetables, and the legumes, nuts, and seeds.

Functions: The primary function of iron in the body is the formation of hemoglobin. Iron is the central core of the hemoglobin molecule, which is the essential oxygen-carrying component of the red blood cell (RBC). In combination with protein, iron is carried in the blood to the bone marrow, where, with the help of copper, it forms hemoglobin. The ferritin and transferrin proteins actually hold and transport the iron. Hemoglobin carries the oxygen molecules throughout the body. Red blood cells pick up oxygen from the lungs and distribute it to the rest of the tissues, all of which need oxygen to survive. Iron's ability to change back and forth between its ferrous and ferric forms allows it to hold and release oxygen. Each hemoglobin molecule can carry four oxygen molecules. This large protein molecule makes up approximately 30 percent of the RBCs. Amazingly, there are some 20 trillion RBCs in the average human body (men have more than women), and about 115 million red blood cells are made every minute. As mentioned before, approximately 90 percent of the iron needed to make those cells comes from recycled RBCs that are normally destroyed by the spleen at the end of their 120-day life span.

Myoglobin is similar to hemoglobin in that it is an iron-protein compound that holds oxygen and carries it into the muscles, mainly

FOODS MOST CONCENTRATED IN IRON*

Mgs. Iron/100 g.**	Edible Food
100.0	kelp
17.3	brewer's yeast
16.1	blackstrap molasses
14.9	wheat bran
11.2	pumpkin seeds
10.5	sesame seeds, whole
9.4	wheat germ
8.8	beef liver
7.1	sunflower seeds
6.8	millet
6.2	parsley
6.1	clams
4.7	almonds
3.9	dried prunes
3.8	cashews
3.7	lean beef
3.5	raisins
3.4	Brazil nuts
3.4	Jerusalem artichokes
3.3	beet greens
3.2	Swiss chard
3.1	walnuts
3.0	dates
2.9	pork
2.7	cooked soybeans
2.4	pecans
2.3	eggs
2.1	lentils
2.1	peanuts
1.9	lamb
1.9	tofu
1.8	green peas
1.6	brown rice
1.6	ripe olives
1.5	chicken
1.3	artichokes
1.3	mung bean sprouts
1.2	salmon
1.1	broccoli
1.1	whole wheat bread
1.1	cauliflower

*From *The Nutrient Content of Foods* (Mineralab, Hayward, CA, 1979)

**About 4 oz.

the skeletal muscles and the heart. It provides our ability to work by increasing oxygen to our muscles with increased activity. Myoglobin also acts as an oxygen reservoir in the muscle cells. So muscle performance actually depends on this function of iron, besides the basic oxygenation by hemoglobin through normal blood circulation.

Hemoglobin—and therefore iron—really does give us our strength and the look of good health—our "rosy cheeks." One of the first symptoms of low iron is weakness, fatigue, or loss of stamina. Anemia results only after longer deficiency of iron or other nutrients; then, less hemoglobin and usually fewer red blood cells are made, and our ability to carry oxygen through the body is diminished. Iron and hemoglobin improve our respiratory activity. Many of the oxygen-dependent diseases (diseases that have symptoms based on circulation and the delivery of oxygen to tissues), such as coronary artery disease and vascular insufficiency, are worsened with iron deficiency. Many other symptoms, both psychological and physical, occur when we do not have enough iron. On the other hand, Jerome Sullivan, a researcher on iron metabolism, has recently shown that excess iron intake and storage may increase our risk of atherosclerosis and heart disease.

Iron is needed by some important enzymes for energy production and protein metabolism. The cytochrome system (a class of protein molecules that play a role in oxidative processes) depends on iron enzymes, which may work within the mitochondria (energy factories) of the cells to produce energy. The iron cytochromes, *iron catalase*, and *iron peroxidase* probably help protect our tissues and cells from oxidative damage, although most of the research in this area has been done on animals, and it is not clear yet whether the findings are analogous in humans, or if, in fact, iron can be an irritant to the vascular lining. Research is also being done on iron's role in the formation and health of tissue collagen and elastin and the involvement of iron in the immune system's health. When iron in the body is low, there seems to be an increased incidence of infections, possibly because of a decrease in lymphocyte proliferation and other white blood cells' ability to kill microorganisms. Iron also is helpful in the production of carnitine, a nonessential amino acid important for the oxidation and utilization of fatty acids.

Uses: Of course, the main use of iron is in the prevention and treatment of iron deficiency and iron deficiency anemia, whether caused by blood loss, pregnancy, or a low-iron diet. When total body iron or circulating iron is low, fatigue, learning difficulties, irritability, and other subtle symptoms may occur long before actual anemia is seen. Many emotional symptoms may occur in children as well.

Iron is used routinely during pregnancy and breastfeeding to prevent iron deficiency. Because of increased iron needs during these times, it is difficult to obtain all the required iron from the diet alone. The infant will usually get enough iron but will pull stores from the mother, who could become very depleted. Also, whenever there are menstrual periods with more than normal amounts of bleeding (medically called menorrhagia), iron is often suggested as a regular supplement. Iron has also been helpful in reducing pain in some women who have painful menstrual periods.

Sometimes fatigue, especially muscle fatigue and poor physical stamina, will respond to iron supplements. Subtle oxygen-deficit respiratory problems may be helped by attaining adequate iron levels, probably because the iron provides increased hemoglobin production and improved oxygenation of the tissue. There is some question as to whether iron acts as a mild antioxidant, protecting the cells and tissues from oxidative damage, or whether it actually stimulates oxidation and can cause problems.

Deficiency and toxicity: There is a controversy about iron toxicity—is everyone sensitive to iron overload from supplements, or does it affect only people who are genetically pre-disposed to iron accumulation and irritation? Iron overload is seen most commonly in older men because they tend to take supplements or iron tonics though losses may be small and through the years tend to accumulate iron stores, primarily in the liver. Usually, it takes moderately high amounts over a long period with minimal losses of this mineral to develop any iron toxicity problems. Further research by Jerome Sullivan suggests that iron overload is a factor in the development of atherosclerosis. A high-meat diet, separate iron supplements, or even the extra 18 mg. of iron that is contained in the average RDA-type multivitamin is more than many people, particularly men, require. Men lose very little iron, since the body recycles most of it; their needs are only about 10 mg. daily. Consuming much more than this may increase the risk of atherosclerosis and heart disease by an as-yet-undetermined mechanism, possibly through increased oxidation and free-radical formation. Women in the menstruating years seem to be protected from this increased risk, though they lose this protection after menopause, when their risk of heart disease rises to a level close to men's.

Children have been known to develop acute toxicity from eating extra vitamins or finding some of mother's ferrous sulfate or other iron supplement. Each year there are about ten deaths reported of young children who eat more than ten 300 mg. iron tablets—that is, more than 3 grams of iron—at one time.

It is unlikely that one would develop any iron toxicity from dietary sources alone, even with 50–75 mg. per day intake, unless all food is prepared in iron cookware, as is done in some African tribes, or unless the genetic iron storage disease called hemochromatosis is present. If this disease occurs, tissue damage may result from iron deposits in the liver, pancreas, spleen, skin, or heart. These iron deposits can cause cirrhosis of the liver, fibrosis of other tissues, a bronze color to the skin, and diabetes due to pancreatic disease, as well as joint problems or cardiac insufficiency. Hemochromatosis, a genetic metabolism problem that probably affects the regulation of iron absorption, can be discovered through blood tests and occurs in about 1 person in 20,000. Treatment includes a low-iron diet, avoidance of iron supplements, and giving regular donations of blood so that the iron stores will be used to make new red blood cells.

The term for excess iron storage in the body is hemosiderosis, or siderosis. Here an amorphous brown pigment called hemosiderin (about 35 percent iron as ferric hydroxide) is deposited in the liver and other tissues, which is not usually a problem unless there are excessive amounts. These increased iron stores usually come not from diet but from iron supplements or blood transfusions. Symptoms of iron toxicity include fatigue, anorexia, weight loss, headaches, dizziness, nausea, vomiting, shortness of breath, and a grayish hue to the skin. Iron has been found in increased levels in joints of patients with rheumatoid arthritis and may contribute to inflammation through increased hydroxyl free radicals. Supplementation should be avoided by patients with arthritis unless a proven iron deficiency is present.

Our digestion does not really screen excess iron, and our elimination is low after we absorb it. Therefore, it is fairly easy to get iron overloads in the body, although it is much easier to develop an iron deficiency.

Those most vulnerable to iron deficiency are infants, adolescents, pregnant or lactating women, vegetarians, people on diets, premenopausal women, and people with bleeding problems. People taking certain drugs, such as allopurinol for gout, tetracyclines, or high amounts of aspirin, may have impaired absorption of iron and thus may develop iron deficiency over time.

Both iron deficiency anemia and iron deficiency without anemia occur fairly commonly when a rapid growth period increases iron needs which are often not met with additional dietary intake. Several studies have shown that often more than half of children aged 1–5, teenagers, and women aged 18–44 had iron intakes below the RDA.

Females need more iron than men but often consume less. Iron deficiency is particularly common in pregnancy, especially later pregnancy, when the fetus needs about 7–8 mg. per day. Even though there is better absorption at this time than the average 10–20 percent of intake, the average diet supplies only 15–25 mg. per day, which is not enough to meet the needs of both mother and child.

Iron deficiency anemia is characterized as microcytic (the RBCs are small) and hypochromic (the RBCs are pale because of decreased hemoglobin). This type of anemia can be determined by doing a complete blood count and checking the hemoglobin, hematocrit, and red blood cell count, along with the RBC indices—the MCV (mean corpuscular volume), MCH (mean corpuscular hemoglobin), and MCHC (mean corpuscular hemoglobin concentration). The doctor or lab technician can also easily see small, pale red blood cells under the microscope. Iron deficiency can occur and generate vague symptoms before clinical anemia actually occurs. This state may be assessed by checking the serum iron concentration. If this is low, it may suggest iron deficiency, usually from low intake or increased losses. Even before serum iron is low, iron saturation, serum transferrin (iron-carrying protein), total iron binding capacity (TIBC), or, more recently, the ferritin level may be measured to detect low iron stores. The body will draw on these muscle and tissue stores to maintain normal serum levels.

Anemia is basically defined as a reduction in the number of red blood cells. Other factors besides iron, such as low copper, manganese, zinc, pyridoxine (vitamin B_6), folic acid, and vitamin B_{12} may also affect the RBCs. Vitamin B_6 and zinc deficiency may mimic iron deficiency, but giving iron may lead to iron toxicity problems in these cases. Measuring serum iron is the best way to ensure that the problem is actually iron deficiency, and measuring B_6 and zinc levels can help diagnose those hidden, though common, deficiency problems as well. So iron deficiency is but one cause of anemia. I have discussed the B_{12} and folic acid vitamin deficiency anemias in Chapter 5, *Vitamins*; copper, zinc, and manganese are some minerals whose deficiency can cause other forms of anemia. Thyroid problems or lead toxicity may cause anemia as well. We also need adequate protein, calcium, and vitamins E and C to keep our red blood cells healthy. Thus, many nutritionally related problems can lead to anemia; decreased production or increased destruction of RBCs and bleeding, however, are the most common causes. Overall, it is wise to diagnose and treat the definitive cause of anemia, not just give iron.

Many symptoms may arise from iron deficiency. Fatigue and lack of stamina usually arise first, caused by fewer red blood cells, low hemoglobin, and a reduced ability to hold and carry oxygen. Children who are iron deficient may experience psychological problems, learning disabilities based on hyperactivity or a decreased attention span, and even a lower IQ, besides other symptoms of anemia. Headaches, dizziness, weight loss from decreased appetite, constipation, and lowered immunity (a weakened resistance) may occur. With anemia, paleness of the skin, cheeks, lips, and tongue may occur, as can a sore tongue, canker sores in the mouth, hair loss, itching, and brittle nails. Not uncommon is a general state of apathy, irritability, and/or depression—a lack of enthusiasm for life—which can, however, improve rapidly with iron supplementation. Decreased memory may also occur. In children particularly, iron deficiency may cause a strange symptom called "pica"—eating and sucking on inedible objects, such as toys, clay, or ice. This usually disappears with iron treatment. In pregnancy, morning sickness may occur more frequently with low iron,

RDAS FOR IRON

Children

0–6 months	10 mg.
6 months–1 year	15 mg.
1–3 years	15 mg.
4–6 years	10 mg.
7–10 years	10 mg.

Men

11–18 years	18 mg.
19 years and older	10 mg.

Women

11–50 years (during years of menstruation)	18 mg.
51 years and older (or non-menstrual years)	10 mg.
Pregnant women	45–60 mg.
Lactating women	45–60 mg.

perhaps because of the relatively low oxygen distribution to cells. It can take several months for improved absorption and increased intake to catch up to needs.

In general, it is wise to discover the cause of iron deficiency. Is it from low intake? If so, the diet should be evaluated. Or is it due to poor absorption? Then check the absorption factors such as low stomach acid. Or is there some bleeding problem, especially a slow blood loss? Intestinal bleeding, as in colitis, ulcers, or even hemorrhoids, is not uncommon. Excess menstrual bleeding, often with the presence of uterine fibroids, is a common cause of iron loss in women. Parasites can cause iron deficiency anemia, as can cancer. Donating blood too frequently can lead to anemia and iron deficiency symptoms. Supplementing iron may help over time, but it is especially important to rule out any internal bleeding.

Requirements: The RDA for adult men and postmenopausal women is 10 mg. per day; for teenagers and women of childbearing age, it is 18 mg. per day. This is based on an average absorption of 10 percent to replace daily losses and to maintain iron storage levels of about 500 mg.

Iron needs increase with growth and development, when more red blood cells and body tissues are being made; during pregnancy, when extra iron is going to the growing fetus; and for at least several months postpartum during lactation, when losses through milk are high. But the average daily intake is only about 6 mg. per 1,000 calories consumed, so a 2,000-calorie diet supplies only 12 mg., which is less than is needed by most teenagers and women, especially during pregnancy and lactation. Luckily, when body needs increase, iron absorption improves, and we usually develop a craving or taste for iron-containing foods as part of our natural survival and health instincts.

Most people, especially women, should be aware of iron intake and absorption. Eating vitamin C-containing foods along with the high-iron foods or taking an ascorbic acid supplement, even 50–100 mg., improves the absorption of iron in supplements. Protein foods improve absorption and usually have a higher iron content, so eating more of these foods, such as meats and legumes, as well as leafy greens, helps get more iron into the body.

Iron supplements are strongly recommended when there are increased requirements, as with teenagers and most women, especially with heavy or long menstrual flow and definitely during pregnancy and lactation, when iron needs may triple. Most men, however, unless there is some bleeding problem, do not require additional iron. When there is sufficient iron intake, more will not necessarily help; in fact, it could lead to problems associated with excess iron storage over a period of time.

The ferrous (2+) forms of iron, not the ferric (3+) state, are the forms to have in supplements. Ferrous sulfate is the most commonly prescribed form of iron, although ferrous fumarate and gluconate are also prescribed by doctors. As an example, 325 mg. (5 grains) of ferrous sulfate contains about 120 mg. of elemental iron. With at least a 10 percent absorption rate, that allows more than 12 mg. of iron per tablet to get into the body; if these are taken several times daily in pregnancy or in anemia, as some doctors recommend, this may be excessive.

To improve iron absorption, take the iron with 250 mg. of vitamin C and between meals, if tolerated. During pregnancy, the increased need will also improve the percentage absorbed. Ferrous sulfate is often used because it is inexpensive and fairly assimilable for most women, though it can also be irritating to the gastrointestinal tract and cause constipation or blackening of the stools, which could cover up an intestinal bleeding problem (blood in the stool can also cause it to be black). Ferrous gluconate and fumarate are considered organic irons (as found in living tissues) and are also inexpensive and have good absorption, and they tend to cause fewer symptoms (constipation, intestinal upset) than the inorganic ferrous sulfate. The dosages are similar; 325 mg. of ferrous gluconate taken two or three times daily during pregnancy or to treat iron deficiency or blood losses. These amounts should not be taken regularly as a preventive or safeguard.

The form that probably is best assimilated and easiest on the intestinal tract is the hydrolyzed protein chelate of iron—that is, "chelated" iron. Usually about 50 mg. of chelated elemental iron taken once or twice daily will satisfy most iron needs during pregnancy or with iron deficiency. This can be used until the iron and red blood cell levels are normalized. The choice of form for iron supplements is based on absorption and gentleness. In order of preference, the suggested forms are chelated iron, such as iron aspartate, ferrous succinate, and ferrous fumarate, followed by ferrous gluconate and ferrous lactate. Ferrous sulfate is commonly used but produces more symptoms than the other forms.

There is some concern about vitamin E's interaction with iron. It can bind the iron to a nonutilizable form, which then can oxidize and thus inactivate the vitamin E when the two are taken together, though this occurs more so with the ferric forms of iron. Ferrous sulfate has some interaction with E. The organic forms of iron—gluconate, aspartate, and fumarate—as well as the chelated iron have little effect on reducing vitamin E. But, to be safe, it is best not to take vitamin E with iron but to take it by itself at night or in the morning.

Overall, iron is a very important mineral of which we must be constantly aware. Extra iron is not needed by everyone, but when it is required, we must increase iron foods or take supplemental iron to prevent loss of energy and enthusiasm for life and the many other problems caused by iron deficiency.

 Manganese, little known and underrated by both doctors and the general public, is an essential mineral important to many enzyme systems in carrying out such functions as energy production, protein metabolism, bone formation, and the synthesis of L-dopamine, cholesterol, and mucopolysaccharides.

The human body contains a total of about 15–20 mg. of manganese. About half of that is in the bones, and the remainder is found in the liver, pancreas, pituitary gland, adrenal glands, and kidneys—the active metabolic organs. Manganese is present in many enzymes in body cells, particularly in the mitochondria (or energy factories) as manganese-containing *superoxide dismutase*, an antioxidant enzyme.

In the food chain, most manganese is present in plant tissues, mainly in nuts, seeds, and whole grains, but in most vegetables as well, particularly the dark leafy greens. Like that of iron, our absorption of manganese is low; utilization of manganese from the diet has been estimated in the range of 15–30 percent

efficiency. Absorption may be influenced by body manganese levels. Alcohol and lecithin cause slight increases in manganese absorption.

Large amounts of calcium and/or phosphorus will interfere with manganese absorption. Heavy milk drinkers, meat eaters, or consumers of soda beverages may therefore need additional manganese. Magnesium, as is found in antacids, may interfere somewhat with manganese absorption. Iron definitely has a see-saw interaction with manganese; too much of either mineral will interfere with absorption of the other. In other words, taking extra manganese can interfere with iron absorption and lead to deficiency, which must then be corrected by taking extra iron. Zinc, cobalt, and soy protein may also interfere with manganese absorption into the blood from the intestines. Manganese can interfere with copper absorption and can decrease copper levels. Optimal absorption of manganese occurs when it is taken in the absence of other minerals or food and in its protein-chelated form.

After absorption, manganese is transported to the liver and then to other organs, such as the kidneys, for storage. A globulin protein called transmangamin carries the manganese molecules in the blood. Manganese is eliminated mainly through the feces after being excreted in the bile. The kidneys clear only a small amount. A manganese blood level (whole blood) can be measured; this level is often low in a person who eats the average American diet.

Sources: Nuts and whole grains are the best sources of manganese. Most animal foods have low levels, though egg yolks are a decent source. Seeds, legumes (peas and beans), and leafy greens, especially spinach, are all good sources of manganese if there is manganese in the soil in which these plants are grown. Alfalfa is high, and black teas and coffee beans have some manganese.

A number of factors, however, can affect dietary manganese levels. As I just implied, food manganese levels may vary greatly because of soil deficiencies; the leafy greens are particularly sensitive to this. Soil mineral losses related to runoff and high-tech farming have created manganese and other mineral depletion problems. Lime added to the soil binds manganese, and, though it may make nice greens, it will result in most foods having a lower manganese content.

Also, though the whole grains, such as barley, whole wheat, millet, and oats, all have good levels of manganese, most of it is in the bran and germ, and these outer parts are often stripped away through milling and refining. Nearly 90 percent of manganese is lost in the refinement of wheat to white flour. Ideally, we should eat whole and unprocessed foods from healthy, balanced soil to get sufficient amounts of manganese and many other minerals.

Functions: Manganese is involved in many enzyme systems—that is, it helps to catalyze many biochemical reactions. These and its other functions, shown to be essential in animals, are still under investigation for humans, but we are finding out that manganese also has some very important roles in the human body. There are some biochemical suggestions that manganese is closer to magnesium in more than just name. It is possible that magnesium can substitute for manganese in certain conditions when manganese is deficient.

Manganese activates the enzymes necessary for the body to use biotin, thiamine (B$_1$), vitamin C, and choline. It is important for the digestion and utilization of food, especially proteins, through *peptidase* activity, and it is needed for the synthesis of cholesterol and fatty acids and in glucose metabolism. As a cofactor in glycolysis, manganese aids glucose metabolism. By activating the *arginase* enzyme, manganese helps form urea, the end product of protein and ammonia breakdown cleared by the kidneys. Manganese may also be important in the growth and development of normal bone structure and in the formation of mucopolysaccharides, which are needed for healthy joint membranes.

Manganese may function as a protective antioxidant, especially in its +2 valence state. Divalent manganese, commonly found in the brain and other tissues as part of the enzyme *superoxide dismutase* (SOD), can bind oxygen free radicals, thus protecting the cell membranes and tissues from degeneration and disruption. Those areas in danger of oxidative damage are the cell membranes, nerve coverings (myelin), and tissue linings, and these are mainly protected by the antioxidant nutrients and enzymes. The manganese present in SOD is found in the "energy factories," the mitochondria, within the cells, and this enzyme protects the mitochondrial membrane from destruction, especially from superoxide free radicals. Trivalent (+3) manganese may be a prooxidant, meaning that it may generate oxidation and unstable molecules. This role as well as manganese's antioxidant functions are still being researched.

Also still under study is manganese's role in the production of thyroxine, essential for thyroid function; its role in normal lactation, in bone health, and in glucose metabolism; and its importance in reproduction. Since manganese seems to be needed in cholesterol synthesis, which is important to sex hormone formation, it may be essential in normal sexuality and reproduction. The idea that manganese is important to some enzymes that seem to stimulate maternal instincts is vague and difficult to research, and there is currently no proof to support this contention.

Uses: Manganese has been used as a therapeutic nutrient, but other than preventing problems of manganese deficiency, its influence on certain disease states seems only anecdotal to date; further research will provide us with more evidence. The *superoxide dismutase* enzymes, only one of which contains manganese (others utilize zinc or copper), have an anti-inflammatory effect in the body, and this function may be relevant to many of the possible uses suggested here.

Manganese has been helpful in some cases

of fatigue (possibly by enhancing certain enzymes), poor memory (by protecting brain tissue and helping oxygenation), and nervousness, irritability, or dizziness. In his book *Mental and Elemental Nutrients*, Carl Pfeiffer, M.D., suggests that manganese along with zinc will help decrease copper levels by both decreasing absorption and increasing urinary losses. He feels that copper in higher than normal amounts can cause psychological problems and even some forms of schizophrenia (see the earlier section on Copper). Also, by some unknown mechanism, manganese may help reduce some of the parkinsonian symptoms, such as muscle rigidity and twitching, secondary to phenothiazine drug use. Manganese supplementation may also help in some cases of epilepsy.

Whether manganese is useful in the treatment of diabetes by helping glucose metabolism or in people with osteoarthritis by stimulating mucopolysaccharide production to heal joints is still undemonstrated and questionable. It is more likely that a manganese deficiency reduces our ability to handle glucose and may thus worsen a diabetic condition. Manganese has also been tried in treatment for multiple sclerosis and myasthenia gravis. When given with B vitamins, manganese may alleviate fatigue or weakness by enhancing nerve impulses. Research has found most tumors and cancer cells to be very low in this mineral, which suggests a possibility that manganese may have a role in preventing cancer cell production and protecting against cancer growth.

Deficiency and toxicity: From a nutritional point of view, manganese may be one of the least toxic minerals. There is no known natural toxicity from manganese in food or from taking reasonable amounts in supplements. Lung problems can be caused, however, by breathing in the dust when mining the inorganic mineral.

In Chile, where much manganese is mined, workers sometimes develop a strange syndrome they call *locura manganica*, or "manganese madness." The first symptoms may be anorexia, weakness, and apathy. However, there may be an initial manic phase, characterized by inappropriate laughter, increased sexuality, insomnia, and even delusions or hallucinations. Violence and other mental change may occur. The earlier mania may shift to depression, impotence, and excessive sleeping. Parkinsonian symptoms such as tremors and muscle rigidity may also appear in the later stages. These symptoms may appear, as in Parkinson's disease, from a loss of dopamine in the brain cells. L-dopa, which converts to dopamine in the brain, is used in the treatment of manganese toxicity to reduce symptoms. Avoiding further manganese inhalation is obviously also suggested.

Manganese deficiency in animals has been studied extensively. In rats, manganese deficiency can lead to sterility or, if occurring during pregnancy, to poor growth in the offspring and decreased lactation in the mother. There is decreased bone growth, especially in length. Poor brain function may occur from decreases in several manganese activities. A decreased threshold for seizures has also been measured. Poor bone and cartilage health and spinal disc degeneration are possible with low manganese. The relevancy of these findings to humans is currently only theoretical and needs further documentation.

In children, severe manganese deficiency may lead to convulsions, paralysis, or blindness. In adults, dizziness, weakness, and problems with the hearing, such as strange ear noises, are associated with manganese deficiency. Decreased strength and ataxia (unstable gait) have also been related; in addition, weight loss, irregular heartbeat, and skin problems have been described by some authors.

Manganese deficiency may cause decreased glucose tolerance, or ability to remove excess sugar from the blood, as occurs also with chromium or zinc deficiency. Low manganese levels may even cause decreased function of the pancreatic cells, and this problem might be helped by manganese supplementation. Research on this relationship between manganese and glucose tolerance and other suggested effects of manganese deficiency is at a preliminary stage, and, to my knowledge, none of these effects has yet been proved. Whether the decreased manganese levels found in cancer are indicative of a causal relationship (which implicates a role of SOD in cancer) or a result of increased nutrient use is of great interest as well.

Requirements: There is no specific RDA for manganese; however, we probably need somewhere from 2.5–5 mg. per day. The average diet contains about 4 mg., depending on manganese soil levels, and intakes from food may range from 3–9 mg. per day. To be safe, I believe that we should get at least 4–5 mg. per day. When we take extra calcium and/or phosphorus, we probably also need extra manganese. However, taking supplemental manganese may decrease iron utilization and storage, so we need to make sure we get enough iron as well.

Since dietary manganese is relatively nontoxic, even 10–20 mg. per day is safe. Multivitamin/mineral supplements usually contain from 2–4 mg., but the amount may range from 1–9 mg. Separate manganese supplements are available in the chelated form or as manganese sulfate or gluconate. These are best absorbed when taken between meals and without other minerals, as these may interact with manganese and reduce its absorption. We should probably limit our intake of additional manganese to 10–15 mg. per day on a regular basis. Up to 50 mg. daily has been used in some research studies without negative effects.

 Molybdenum, though its name may be one of the more difficult to pronounce, is not generally well known. However, this mineral's importance has been discovered in recent years. Molybdenum is now considered one of our essential trace minerals. It has been found to be essential in most mammals, as well as in all plants. We obtain it primarily from foods, but since it is often scarce in the earth's crust and therefore deficient in many soils, molybdenum deficiency can be a problem. In fact, it was recently discovered that molybdenum deficiency in the soil in an area of China was responsible for the highest known incidence of esophageal carcinoma over many generations.

In nature, molybdenum is found as part of other metal complexes. In the soil, it serves as a catalyst to the nitrogen-fixing process; thus, decreased soil molybdenum can lead to deficient plant growth.

The body contains minute amounts, about 9 mg., of molybdenum. It is found mainly in the liver, kidneys, adrenal glands, bones, and skin, but it is present in all tissues. It is important to several enzyme systems, most significantly that of *xanthine oxidase*, which supports many functions, including uric acid metabolism and mobilization of iron from the liver for body use. Molybdenum is fairly easily absorbed from the gastrointestinal tract, though it competes with copper at absorption sites. It is eliminated through the urine and the bile.

As with chromium, depletions or deficiencies of molybdenum are common, and its availability in foods is decreased through soil depletion and food technology. This mineral has come to the nutritional forefront in the last decade with the recognition of its essential nature and the concern about deficiency.

Sources: The food levels of molybdenum depend largely on soil content. The amount in food may be increased a hundredfold with molybdenum-rich soil; in certain areas, hard water may contain some molybdenum. Soft water and refined foods contain hardly any. Whole grains, particularly the germ, usually have substantial amounts; oats, buckwheat, and wheat germ are some examples of grains containing molybdenum. Many vegetables and legumes are also good sources; these include lima beans, green beans, lentils, potatoes, spinach and other dark leafy greens, cauliflower, peas, and soybeans. Brewer's yeast also has some, and liver and organ meats are often fairly high in molybdenum.

Functions: Molybdenum is a vital part of three important enzyme systems—*xanthine oxidase, aldehyde oxidase*, and *sulfite oxidase*—and so has a vital role in uric acid formation and iron utilization, in carbohydrate metabolism, and sulfite detoxification as well. In the soil and possibly in the body, as the enzyme *nitrate reductase*, molybdenum can reduce the production or counteract the actions of nitrosamines, known cancer-causing chemicals, especially in the colon. Found more in molybdenum-deficient soils, nitrosamines have been associated with high rates of esophageal cancer.

Xanthine oxidase (XO) helps in the production of uric acid, an end product of protein (purine) metabolism. Though an excess of uric acid is known to cause gout, recent studies show that, in proper concentrations in the blood, it has antioxidant properties and helps protect the cells and tissues from irritation and damage caused by singlet oxygens and hydroxyl free radicals. This protection may prevent tissue wear and aging, in addition to other free-radical diseases discussed throughout this book. Thus, uric acid has a new image as being an important part of balanced human function and not just a waste product. With its different effects, uric acid is somewhat like cholesterol in its biochemistry. As with cholesterol, it is both made in the body and obtained through the diet; some people are genetically inclined to elevated levels; and, whereas the right amount is essential to important functions, excesses can lead to problems (cholesterol appears to be much more of a concern on this count than uric acid). *Xanthine oxidase* may also help in the mobilization of iron from liver reserves.

Aldehyde oxidase helps in the oxidation of carbohydrates and other aldehydes, including acetaldehyde produced from ethyl alcohol. *Sulfite oxidase* helps to detoxify sulfurs in the body, particularly sulfites, which are used to preserve food. These potentially toxic and harmful substances can cause nausea or diarrhea and precipitate asthma attacks in sensitive individuals. The "salad bar" syndrome is caused by sulfite sprays used on vegetables to keep them "fresh" longer. It is possible that adequate tissue levels of molybdenum keep the *sulfite oxidase* activity levels high enough to counteract this chemical and reduce potential symptoms; molybdenum deficiency may be a factor in those people who are more sensitive to sulfites. Luckily, though, the use of sulfites in food preservation is being made illegal.

Uses: Since molybdenum's activities in humans are so newly known, it does not have wide usage. Even the uses suggested in some nutritional texts are under question and require more research. Molybdenum may help prevent anemia by helping mobilize iron, provided there are sufficient iron stores. The suggestions that it protects the teeth from dental caries and that it prevents sexual impotence are not yet supported by definitive research. Molybdenum deficiency may reduce uric acid formation; this was not previously thought to be a problem, but it may be important to supplement molybdenum to maintain uric acid levels in midnormal range for the antioxidant function as well as possible others.

There are few research findings to suggest that molybdenum may play a role in preventing cancer and definitely none to support its use in cancer treatment. Adding molybdenum to the soil and diet has helped reduce the incidence of esophageal cancer in the Lin Xian area of China's Hunan Province, which had the highest incidence in the world of this deadly disease. It is unlikely, however, that lack of molybdenum in the soil and, thus, in the diet was a direct cause of the cancer; it was probably due to the production of nitrosamines in the soil that could not be metabolized because of a deficiency in the plants' roots activity of the molybdenum enzyme, *nitrate reductase*. Nitrates and nitrites, such as those in hot dogs, lunch meats, and other cured meats, also increase food levels of nitrates, which can lead to the formation of carcinogenic nitrosamines in the stomach. Both vitamin C, which helps detoxify nitrosamine, and *nitrate reductase*, which needs molybdenum to function, can help reduce the levels of this carcinogenic chemical as it has done for the Chinese esophageal cancer rates secondary to low soil molybdenum. It is also possible that molybdenum can help protect the body from nitrosamine formation after consumption of foods high in nitrates or nitrites, such as lunch meats.

Deficiency and toxicity: Molybdenum, like most trace minerals, is required in a specific narrow range of daily intake; amounts much greater than this may be toxic. Animals given large amounts experience weight loss, slow growth, anemia, or diarrhea, though these effects may be more the result of low levels of copper, a mineral with which molybdenum competes. In people who are sensitive to it, high doses of molybdenum may lead to high uric acid levels and gouty arthritis symptoms related to increased action of the enzyme *xanthine oxidase*.

Information about molybdenum deficiency is limited as well. Low soil levels of molybdenum lead to increased soil and plant levels of nitrates and nitrosamines, which increase risk of cancer, especially in the esophagus and stomach. Increased sensitivity to sulfites used in foods may be related to low molybdenum and deficient *sulfite oxidase* enzymes. In animals, molybdenum-deficient diets seem to produce anorexia, weight loss, and decreased life span. In humans, deficiency may lead to visual problems, rapid heart rate and breathing, and depression of consciousness.

Requirements: As with other newly recognized trace minerals, there is no specific RDA for molybdenum. The amount provided by the average diet ranges widely, from 50–500

mcg. a day. A safe and sensible amount of added molybdenum is from 150–500 mcg. for adults and 50–300 mcg. for children. A molybdenum-rich yeast may be available as an added nutrient, which usually contains a lot of other minerals and B vitamins. Sodium molybdate, which recently has come on the market, can be taken by people who want more molybdenum, though intake should be limited to 500 mcg. daily. It is probably best to take molybdenum in a general multivitamin and to take 2–3 mg. of copper daily as well, because of the potential copper loss with molybdenum supplementation. Further research is required, but it appears that molybdenum is very important for optimum health and longevity.

 Selenium has become one of the most exciting nutrients of the 1970s and 1980s. Once classified solely as a toxic mineral, it is now regarded as an essential one, needed in small daily amounts. Selenium functions as a component of the enzyme *glutathione peroxidase*, which accounts for its antioxidant function and thus its important contribution to the prevention of the twentieth-century plagues, cancer and cardiovascular disease.

Low soil levels of selenium are associated with higher cancer rates, and soil-rich areas have below-average cancer rates for a number of body systems, particularly the breasts, colon, and lungs. Keshan disease, a form of heart disease prevalent in children and is characterized by an enlarged heart and congestive heart failure, may be a direct result of selenium deficiency, as it has responded well to selenium treatment. People in Keshan, China, where the disease was discovered, treat it with a common herb called Astragalus, which accumulates selenium from the soil.

As in the Keshan area of China, the soil in many parts of the United States is very low in this important mineral. Here, the western states generally have higher selenium levels than the eastern; South Dakota has the highest and Ohio the lowest. Ohio has more than twice South Dakota's rate of a number of common cancers. Most states with high levels of soil selenium show a decreased rate of cancer deaths. There is some concern, though, that high amounts of selenium, particularly elemental selenium and inorganic sodium selenite, may be toxic in areas where it is found in high concentrations in the water and soil, such as South Dakota.

Selenium and vitamin E work together synergistically in that they carry out antioxidant and immunostimulating functions better together than individually; however, their mechanisms of action are probably not the same. Both of these nutrients are part of the "antiaging" or "longevity" group, which may be directly attributable to their antioxidant functions because tissue oxidation by free radicals may be the contributing factor to degenerative disease.

Despite its importance, there is less than 1 mg. of selenium in our body, most of it in the liver, kidneys, and pancreas and, in men, in the testes and seminal vesicles. Men have a greater need for selenium, which may function in sperm production and motility. Some selenium is lost through the sperm as well as through the urine and feces. It is absorbed fairly well from the intestines, with an absorption rate of nearly 60 percent.

Sources: Soil levels of selenium vary greatly from state to state and even within local regions across the United States, as well as from country to country throughout the world. So the amount of selenium in our food sources, whether consumed directly as plants or as meat from animals that have eaten the vegetation, varies according to the soil levels. Further, most selenium in foods is lost during processing, such as when making white rice or white flour.

Many natural foods contain selenium, mainly an organic form that is much less toxic than sodium selenite and definitely less so than elemental selenium. Selenium may be present in some drinking water, and it is sometimes even added to drinking water where it is deficient. We may see this more in the future as a general disease-prevention measure. Mother's milk usually has several times more selenium than cow's milk. Selenium is also used in some shampoos and skin lotions, and it is possible that we absorb small amounts of selenium from these products.

Brewer's yeast and wheat germ, both regarded as "health foods," usually contain high concentrations of selenium. Animal sources such as liver, butter, most fish, and lamb have adequate amounts. Many vegetables, whole grains, nuts, and molasses are fairly good selenium foods. Brazil nuts have high amounts; barley, oats, whole wheat, and brown rice are also good sources; and shellfish such as scallops, lobster, shrimp, clams, crab, and oysters are all rich in selenium. Garlic and onions, mushroom, broccoli, tomatoes, radishes, and Swiss chard may be good selenium sources if the soil in which they are grown contains it. Therefore, if we want to make sure we get adequate amounts of selenium and other minerals, it is best to eat a varied diet of wholesome foods.

Functions: Selenium has a variety of functions, and research is revealing new information. Its main role is as an antioxidant in the enzyme *selenium-glutathione peroxidase*. Selenium is part of a nutritional antioxidant system that protects cell membranes and intracellular structural membranes from lipid peroxidation. It is actually the selenocysteine complex that is incorporated into *glutathione peroxidase* (GP), an enzyme that helps prevent cellular degeneration from the common peroxidase free radicals, such as hydrogen peroxide. (Selenomethionine can be supplemented to generate the organically complexed and active selenocysteine.) GP also aids red blood cell metabolism and has been shown to prevent chromosome damage in tissue cultures.

Solidification of tissue membranes may occur through the oxidation of fatty acids. As an antioxidant, then, selenium in the form of selenocysteine prevents or slows the biochemical aging process of tissue degeneration and hardening—that is, loss of youthful elasticity. This protection of the tissues and cell membranes is enhanced by vitamin E. The antioxidant effect may also benefit the cardiovascular system and protect against cancer. We need adequate daily amounts of selenium for the maintenance of these antioxidant functions and for selenium's other cellular functions as well.

Selenium also appears to help stimulate antibody formation in response to vaccines. This immunostimulating effect is also enhanced by vitamin E; the presence of these two nutrients can increase antibody formation by 20–30 times, as shown by research.

Selenium is thought to offer protection against cardiovascular disease, possibly by its antioxidant function but possibly by another, as yet, unknown mechanism. Epidemiological studies show an increased incidence of strokes and other cardiovascular problems in many low-selenium areas.

Selenium is also being found to have an anticarcinogenic effect; its blood or tissue levels may correlate more closely with cancer risk than those of any other substance. Public health research shows this relationship in many cases; good selenium levels correlate with low cancer rates and low levels with increased cancer rates. I do not yet know exactly how this works other than possibly through the antioxidant function. Perhaps selenium decreases cell division or helps cell repair, or perhaps it protects against mutagenic changes in the first place.

Selenium also seems to protect us from the toxic effects of heavy metals and other substances. People with adequate selenium intake have fewer adverse effects from cigarette smoking, alcohol, oxidized fats, and mercury and cadmium toxicity. Aside from the likely antioxidant influence, the specific mechanism by which selenium affords this protection is not known, though the effect is confirmed by some research.

Selenium may also aid in protein synthesis, growth and development, and fertility, especially in the male. It has been shown to improve sperm production and motility. Thus, selenium may prevent male infertility; however, we do not know whether selenium deficiency will actually cause male infertility. These are only some of the conjectures about other selenium functions.

Uses: A growing number of clinically effective uses of selenium have been developed, and others are being tested for possible value. As part of nutritional antioxidant therapy with vitamin E, zinc, beta-carotene, and vitamin C, selenium, as selenomethionine (will form the active selenocysteine), may be beneficial in treating a variety of inflammatory problems and may be helpful in most acute or degenerative diseases to moderate the inflammatory process. Its use in treating arthritis and some autoimmune problems, such as lupus erythematosus or vasculitis, shows promise but needs further study. Selenium is known to help prevent cardiovascular disease and decrease the risk of complications such as strokes and heart attacks (possibly by reducing platelet aggregation) related to our number one disease process, atherosclerosis. This use, along with selenium's confirmed ability to reduce the incidence of certain cancers, makes this trace mineral quite important.

Where selenium is abundant in the soil or when it is added to the diet, it has an anticarcinogenic effect. These conditions are associated with both decreased cancer rates and decreased cancer mortality, especially regarding the number one female cancer, that of the breast, but also cancer of the colon/rectum, prostate, lung, ovary, bladder, pancreas, and skin. This is a wide range. In animal studies, 1–4 ppm of selenium added to the food or water is clearly associated with decreased cancer rates. High breast cancer rates are associated with areas of low soil selenium in the United States, and human epidemiological studies confirm these findings throughout the world.

Because of selenium's immunostimulating function, it's very useful in the treatment of many immunosuppression diseases. With its antioxidant properties, selenium, especially along with vitamin E, may become a routine and powerful nutritional of treatment in the medical world. Autoimmune diseases, recurrent illnesses or infections, and other inflammatory problems may be helped by restoring adequate selenium levels in the body. Selenium can help us prevent disease by increasing our resistance. In some cases, selenium promotes more rapid recovery from many basic disease processes. More controlled human studies related to specific illnesses will need to be done to generate greater acceptance by the medical establishment of selenium's important role.

Selenium's postulated antiaging effect offers another possible use of the mineral; this cell-membrane-protecting influence on improving tissue elasticity also needs further research. With vitamin E, selenium also appears to be helpful in treating acne. Selenium sulfide used topically seems to help in certain skin conditions, such as dandruff and dermatitis, and to improve skin health. It is also a helpful treatment for the mild skin fungus tinea versicolor.

There are even more exciting possibilities for selenium's use in heart diseases. One angina study showed reduced symptoms in nearly 100 percent of the patients when selenium was used in a dosage of 1 mg. per day with 200 IUs of vitamin E, whereas the placebo group reported little benefit. Selenium supplementation helps correct the serious symptoms of Keshan disease, a cardiomyopathy (heart muscle disease with heart enlargement) associated with congestive heart failure and the resulting symptoms

of body swelling, shortness of breath, and eventual circulatory collapse. This disease has been more prevalent in China, where it was first reported, but with our new knowledge, more cases are being found in other areas. It may simply be a disease of selenium deficiency. The antioxidant function of selenium likely decreases vascular clogging of inflamed artery linings by soothing irritation and binding free radicals; thus, selenium may play a role in reducing or preventing atherosclerosis at its initial biochemical level.

Some evidence suggests that selenium supplementation is also helpful in reducing menopausal symptoms. In addition, it has been suggested, with vitamin E, for male impotency. Although these uses need further study, it is certainly possible that selenium can increase sexual potency and fertility by improving sperm production and motility and by protecting against oxidative damage in the testes and related organs. (Fertility, potency, and sexuality are, however, more intricate than just these physiological processes.) I am sure that we will find more uses for selenium in the near future.

Deficiency and toxicity: Just 20 years ago, selenium was considered a nonessential toxic mineral. There is still justifiable concern over elemental selenium toxicity, but we are finding that the value of inorganic selenium salts, such as sodium selenite, and organically bound selenomethionine at appropriate levels far exceeds the potential to cause problems. Actually, selenium can be tolerated for short periods in higher amounts than was previously thought. Inorganic selenium, usually as sodium selenite, is the common form found in nature and can be more toxic in the short term than the organically bound selenium in the form of selenomethionine. While more than 1 mg. per day of sodium selenite is likely to produce symptoms, we may tolerate several milligrams daily of organic selenium without toxicity problems occurring. However, it is possible that the organic forms of selenium accumulate in the body and may be of long-term concern. Different authorities provide different figures for selenium intake and divergent viewpoints as to the question of toxicity; some sources state that toxicity is possible when 2,000 mcg. (2 mg.) are taken daily by people who already have total body stores of over 2.5 mg. (the normal level is 1 mg.), or when the water or food regularly contains over 5–10 ppm. Selenium is thought to interfere with sulfur compounds and even replace the sulfur in the body, as these two minerals are very similar biochemically, and thus may decrease a number of enzyme actions. The complexity of these issues in regard to selenium point out the importance of individual assessment and monitoring when taking certain supplemental products.

There is no clearly defined syndrome of selenium toxicity. Cattle that graze on selenium-rich soil have exhibited visual, muscular, and heart problems. Similar symptoms of toxicity have been found in humans living in high-selenium areas. Long-term ingestion of high amounts may cause problems with tooth enamel and strength, as higher selenium levels seem to increase tooth decay. One highly speculative theory is that selenium competes with fluoride in teeth, decreasing their strength. Other problems may include loss of hair, nails, and teeth, as well as skin inflammation, nausea, and fatigue. Some subtle symptoms that have been experienced include a garlic odor, metallic taste, or dizziness. Acute selenium poisoning can lead to fever, anorexia, gastrointestinal symptoms, liver and kidney impairment, and even death if the levels are high enough.

None of these symptoms should occur when selenium is taken in a therapeutic amount. There has been some fear of mutagenicity (that is, ability to cause developmental defects) of selenium in higher amounts. This might be true of the sodium selenite form, which may have both mutagenic and antimutagenic properties, depending on the amount. This theory needs further detailed study.

Selenium levels are frequently low in the soils of some regions and in certain Western diets. There appears to be problems associated with selenium deficiency; however, no clearly defined selenium deficiency syndrome has been accepted, although several theories postulate such a syndrome and evidence to support them seems to be mounting. Given selenium's many important functions and uses, its deficiency may generate increases in many of the disease states that it can prevent and treat. With selenium deficiency, there may be increased risk and rates of certain cancers, cardiovascular disease, hypertension, strokes, myocardial infarction, and kidney disease—all heavyweights along death row. Other problems possibly associated with selenium deficiency include eczema, psoriasis, rheumatoid arthritis, cataracts, cervical dysplasia, alcoholism, and infections. As I have discussed, low soil selenium is related to higher cancer rates, and Keshan disease is likely a direct result of selenium deficiency.

Selenium deficiency is more common, of course, in areas of low soil selenium and also in infants fed cow's milk instead of breast milk. Selenium absorption may be reduced with aging; in addition, older people often consume less selenium-containing fresh and whole foods.

Cataracts have been shown to contain only about one-sixth as much selenium as a normal lens; research is needed to determine whether this is a cause or a result of the cataract. Many books describe more rapid aging and decreased tissue elasticity with selenium deficiency, but this has not been confirmed with solid evidence. Many other metals, including cadmium, arsenic, silver, copper, and mercury, are thought to be more toxic in the presence of selenium deficiency.

We need to find better ways to evaluate body levels of selenium. Blood levels are not easy to evaluate, as they are low and much of selenium is stored. Hair analysis is not very reliable for selenium. Until we find reasonably priced testing methods that correlate accurately with tissue levels and health status, it is wise to take additional selenium as outlined here, unless one lives in a selenium-rich area.

Requirements: Like many of the trace minerals, there is no specific RDA for selenium. The usual suggested intake is between 50 and 200 mcg., which is also the range provided by the average diet of wholesome foods and water. Selenium is increasingly available in vitamin-mineral supplements and is part of all nutritional antioxidant formulae.

The conservative safe amount of selenium is between 100–200 mcg. per day for adults and about 30–150 mcg. per day for children, depending on age. Men may need more selenium, especially when sexually active. I usually suggest no more than 200–400 mcg. per day in supplemental form, though some people do take more. Studies have used 1 mg. per day for extended periods without any adverse effects. It is likely that we need more than 100 mcg. daily to support some of selenium's functions, such as its antioxidant, anticarcinogenic, and immunostimulating effects, though further research is needed to confirm this.

Some of these functions may be best performed with the help of vitamin E; the antioxidant effects of selenium and E are synergistic. There is also a concern that vitamin C may inactivate selenium in the stomach or small intestine. This is not the case with organic selenium, selenocysteine or seleno-methione, but it seems that vitamin C combines with sodium selenite and may make the selenium formed by this interaction less absorbable and possibly more toxic. So for improved function, it is wise to take selenium in the absence of vitamin C and along with vitamin E.

Zinc Think zinc! This slogan comes to mind as I begin this section. Zinc has so many important functions and potential uses that both doctors and patients should think of zinc more often for handling many day-to-day problems. Zinc deficiency is fairly common now as a result of soil losses and losses in food processing, and this deficiency or depletion can produce a variety of symptoms.

More than 50 years ago, in 1934, zinc essentiality was first suggested. Not until the early 1960s, however, was it known that low intake or low body stores of zinc can cause deficiency symptoms. In recent years, since the discovery that this mineral is becoming less available in our soil and thus in our food chain, zinc has been given more attention, and increased research has produced much new information. We now know that zinc is needed in probably more than 100 enzymes and is probably involved in more body functions than any other mineral. It is important in normal growth and development, the maintenance of body tissues, sexual function, the immune system, and detoxification of chemicals and metabolic irritants. Carbohydrate metabolism is influenced by zinc, and zinc is needed in the synthesis of DNA, which aids our body's healing process. Zinc is often helpful in reducing healing time after surgery or burns, in many male prostate problems, in skin diseases, and in many other difficulties.

Zinc is found in the body in small amounts, only about 2–2.5 grams total. Of the trace minerals, it is second in concentration to iron, with 33 ppm to iron's 60 ppm. (Although fluoride is found at 37 ppm in the average human body, it is still questionable whether it is essential. This 37 ppm is also a result of the use of fluoridated water, vitamins, and stannous fluoride toothpaste.) Though zinc is the twenty-fifth most abundant element in the earth's crust, measuring about 0.01 percent, it is water soluble both in the soil and in food.

Rains can wash zinc (as well as iodine, sulfur, and selenium) from our farming soils, as can modern agricultural techniques. When we cook food, much of the zinc may go into the water, as do other minerals and vitamins, so the cooking liquids, especially from vegetables, should be consumed as well. More importantly, when foods are processed, as in the refining of grains, much of the zinc is lost, along with manganese, chromium, molybdenum, and B vitamins. Usually, only iron and sometimes vitamins B_1 and B_2 are added back in "enriched" foods (and this iron isn't even in the easily usable form). Adding zinc, manganese, chromium, and more B vitamins such as B_6, would be much better and help us avoid common deficiencies.

Zinc absorption may vary from about 20–40 percent of ingested zinc, depending mainly on body needs and stomach acid concentrations. Like iron, zinc from animal foods where it is bound with proteins has been shown to be better absorbed. When bound with the phytates or oxalates found in grains and vegetables, less zinc is absorbed. Calcium, phosphorus, copper, iron, lead, and cadmium all compete with zinc for absoprtion. Milk and eggs reduce zinc absorption. Fiber foods, bran, and phytates, found mainly in the outer covering of grains, may also inhibit zinc absorption. Phytic acid may combine with the zinc in the upper intestine before this mineral can be absorbed.

The zinc-cadmium relationship is interesting. Cadmium is considered a potentially toxic heavy metal. When it contaminates our food, it is found in the center of grain; zinc is found mainly in the grain covering. So eating whole grains, which have a higher amount of zinc than of cadmium, will reduce any possible absorption of cadmium. With refining of grains into flour, the zinc-cadmium ratio is decreased, and cadmium is more likely to be absorbed and cause problems.

In the human body, the 2.5 grams of zinc are stored in a variety of tissues. It is most concentrated in the prostate and semen, which suggests zinc's tie to male sexual function (impotence can be related to low zinc). The next most concentrated tissues are the retina of the eye, heart, spleen, lungs, brain, and adrenal glands. The skin contains a high amount of zinc, but it is less concentrated than in the organ tissues. Nails, hair, and teeth also have some zinc, and this mineral is important to those tissues as well.

Zinc is eliminated through the gastrointestinal tract in the feces. Some is also eliminated in the urine; alcohol use increases urinary losses of zinc. Zinc is also lost in the sweat, possibly as much as 2–3 mg. in a day. Stress, burns, surgery, and weight loss all seem to increase body losses of zinc.

In evaluating body zinc status, plasma or serum zinc levels may not reflect body stores; however, if they are low, zinc is likely deficient. Low hair levels appear to reflect zinc deficiency, which then should be substantiated through a blood test. High hair zinc levels may also be seen with zinc deficiency, though this is not as correlative as low hair levels. In general, the red blood cell (or white blood cell) measurement of zinc may be most indicative of the body's true status of zinc nutriture.

Sources: Most animal foods contain adequate amounts of zinc. Oysters are particularly high, with more than ten times as much as other sources (they are also high in copper and, possibly, in ocean-polluting chemicals and metals). Zinc is added to animal feeds to increase growth rates, so meat usually contains high amounts. Red meats (beef, lamb, and pork) and liver are fairly high; herring is good, as are egg yolks and milk products (though the zinc in eggs and milk products may not be as available to the body as that found in other sources). Other fish and poultry also contain fair zinc levels. As with iron, the zinc in animal foods seems to be better absorbed than that in the vegetable sources, but one can reduce meat foods and eat whole

217

grains and beans and still obtain adequate zinc. Overall, though, in my experience it is not easy for most people eating a relatively healthy diet to obtain the minimum requirement of 15 mg. daily unless they focus on zinc-containing foods.

Whole grains such as whole wheat, rye, and oats are rich in zinc and are good sources for vegetarians. Even though the mineral from these foods is utilized less well because the fiber and phytates in the grain covering bind some zinc in the gastrointestinal tract, much of the zinc in these foods is still available to the body. Nuts are fairly good sources, with pecans and Brazil nuts the highest. Pumpkin seeds contain zinc and are thought to be helpful to the prostate gland. Ginger root is a good zinc source, as are mustard, chili powder, and black pepper. In general, fruits and vegetables are not good zinc sources, although peas, carrots, beets, and cabbage contain some zinc.

The zinc in grains is found mainly in the germ and bran coverings, so refining them will lower the zinc content. Approximately 80 percent of zinc is lost in making white flour from whole wheat. Since zinc is soluble in water, canning foods or cooking in water can cause zinc losses. Zinc losses have also been prevalent in agricultural soils, and it is therefore less available in foods. Chemical fertilizers also decrease zinc soil levels. Many soils—nearly 30 states in the United States—are deficient in zinc. Water, especially from some wells, contains zinc. Water was a better source when some of the water pipes were galvanized (containing zinc), as were some cooking pots. Now, water pipes are more commonly made of copper, which can become toxic at higher levels.

Functions: Zinc is involved in a multitude of human body functions and is part of many enzyme systems. With regard to metabolism, zinc is part of *alcohol dehydrogenase*, which helps the liver detoxify alcohols, including ethanol (drinking alcohol), methanol, ethylene glycol, and retinol (vitamin A). Zinc is also thought to help utilize and maintain body levels of vitamin A. Through this action, zinc may help maintain healthy skin cells and thus may be helpful in generating new skin after burns or injury. By helping collagen formation, zinc may also improve wound healing. Zinc aids the skin's oil glands and so may help in acne problems.

Zinc is needed for *lactate* and *malate dehydrogenases*, both important in energy production. Zinc is a cofactor for the enzyme *alkaline phosphatase*, which helps contribute phosphates to bones. Zinc is also part of bone and tooth structure. Zinc is important to male sex organ function and reproductive fluids. It is in high concentration in the prostate gland as well as in the eye, liver, and muscle tissues suggesting its functions in those areas.

Zinc in *carboxypeptidase* (a digestive enzyme) helps in protein digestion. Zinc is important for synthesis of nucleic acids, both DNA and RNA. In fact, we are finding that zinc has some antioxidant function. As part of *superoxide dismutase* (SOD), it helps protect cells from free radicals. Through this antioxidant effect, zinc is also helpful in cell membrane structure and function.

Zinc has also been shown to support immune function. Zinc will improve antibody response to vaccines and can improve cell-mediated immunity by helping regulate the function of the white blood cells. A somewhat higher amount of zinc has caused an increase in production of T lymphocytes, important agents in cell-mediated immunity.

Zinc is important to normal insulin activity and seems related to normal taste sensation. Zinc may have an anti-inflammatory function, especially in the joints and artery linings. It may also be involved in brain function, in maintaining acid-alkaline balance through *carbonic anhydrase*, another zinc-containing enzyme, and in phosphorus metabolism.

More research is needed on this important mineral. As zinc, due to its function in many enzymes, is so important to chemical detoxi-

POSSIBLE USES FOR ZINC

Acne	Surgery recovery
Boils	Wound healing
Psoriasis	Skin ulcers
Gastric ulcers	Immune suppression
Sore throats	Prostate congestion
Colds	Benign prostatic
Anorexia nervosa	hypertrophy
Hypertension	Male sexual problems
Cataracts	Infertility
Infections	Pregnancy
Alcoholism	Decreased hearing
Schizophrenia	Fatigue
Environmental sensitivity	Weak muscles

fication and our ability to handle environmental chemicals and toxins, zinc deficiency may be an underlying factor in those people who become environmentally sensitive. This is just one example of where further zinc research may be valuable.

Uses: Just as it has many functions, zinc has a wide variety of clinical uses. Some of these regularly show very positive results; other uses have variable outcomes, and some new therapeutic trials are under way.

Zinc is used commonly to enhance wound healing. Taken before and after surgery, zinc has been shown in numerous studies to speed recovery time and reduce the incidence of postoperative complications, such as wound infections. This use has the potential to greatly cut down on hospital costs. In some studies, the hospital stay has been reduced by more than half. Zinc may be helpful in speeding healing after burns or injury as well. This wound-healing effect is a likely result of zinc's function in DNA synthesis. The results seem to be particularly pronounced when there is zinc deficiency prior to the treatment. In many of the wound-healing studies, zinc dosages of

150 mg. per day were used. It is possible that lower amounts, even 30–60 mg. per day, would produce these effects.

Zinc may be useful in treating such skin problems as boils, bedsores, general dermatitis, and acne. Research on zinc and acne shows variable results, but many teenagers and others have been helped, especially when zinc deficiency was present; it is likely that other factors and nutrients are also involved in acne. Leg ulcers have healed more rapidly with zinc treatment in a dose of 150 mg. per day. Internally, gastric ulcers have responded favorably to zinc in a similar dosage. Psoriasis is even occasionally responsive to zinc supplementation. White spots on the fingernails, which can be a result of zinc deficiency, may respond also to zinc treatment. Zinc may also be helpful to general nail health, as well as skin and hair health. Cataracts also seem to be associated with zinc deficiency and have been helped by treatment.

My friendly travel agent developed a case of hoarseness that persisted for more than a month. Her otolaryngologist diagnosed chronic inflammation and had suggested long-term quietude and learning to live with it—neither of which was a big hit. In passing (I was quite aware of the foibles of her diet), I suggested zinc lozenges. She began sucking on 3–4 daily and within a week her voice was back. In this case, the $5 bottle of zinc helped more than the $70 office visit. I believe that she was zinc deficient, and that the zinc supplement helped to heal her inflamed tissue.

Zinc is used in a variety of immune problems. It is one of the supportive nutrients used to treat lowered immunity. Zinc has been shown to increase T lymphocyte production and enhance other white blood cell functions.

219

Recent double-blind studies verify that zinc therapy is helpful in reducing the incidence and severity of colds and other infections. Also, infections such as herpes, trichomoniasis, or AIDS may be curtailed some with zinc, especially if it is deficient. Sucking a 25–50 mg. dissolvable zinc lozenge can provide dramatic relief in some cases of sore throat and has been shown to prevent the progression of viral flu symptoms. Individuals with allergies and environmental sensitivities may benefit from zinc supplementation. Measuring zinc status and following it during treatment may be useful in validating its positive effects.

For male prostate problems, there is no scientific evidence that zinc works, though there are a great many anecdotal accounts from men who claim to have been helped by zinc. Mild or persistent nonbacterial infections or congestion have commonly been helped by oral zinc treatments. Of course, when zinc deficiency produces such sexual symptoms as infertility, impotency, or poor sexual development, supplementation of this mineral may have great benefit. There is some suggestion that the prostate enlargement that comes with age, termed benign prostatic hypertrophy (BPH), is related to low zinc (and cadmium toxicity), and that regular zinc supplementation may prevent this common problem. More research is needed to clearly evaluate zinc's relationship to prostate and sexual health.

Zinc may also be beneficial in rheumatoid arthritis, for which it has been shown to reduce symptoms; in preventing dental caries by strengthening tooth enamel; and with symptoms of heart disease, where the zinc-copper ratio may be important. The use of zinc in cancer prevention and the support of patients with cancers such as Hodgkin's disease and leukemia has been the subject of some interest.

Zinc therapy can reduce cadmium toxicity from pollution or from cadmium in water or foods. Cadmium toxicity may aggravate hypertension, atherosclerosis, and heart disease and produce complications of hypertension or stroke.

Zinc with vitamin B_6 has also been used in the nutritional treatment of schizophrenia and, given along with manganese, has been helpful in some cases of senility. Zinc treatment may help with the loss of taste sensation that comes especially with aging, which is often due to zinc deficiency, and it may help stimulate the taste for food in patients with anorexia nervosa. Menstrual irregularity and female sexual organ difficulties may have some relationship to zinc levels and be helped by zinc therapy, though copper may be more important for these areas in women.

Deficiency and toxicity: Zinc is fairly nontoxic, especially in amounts of less than 100–150 mg. of elemental zinc daily, though this much zinc is probably not really needed and may interfere with the assimilation of other minerals. Zinc salts such as gluconate or sulfate are commonly available in 220 mg. tablets or capsules, each providing 55 mg. of elemental zinc. Taking one of these two or three times daily may cause some gastrointestinal irritation, nausea, or diarrhea but is more likely to have positive effects. Excessive supplementation may cause some immune suppression, premature heartbeats, dizziness, drowsiness, increased sweating, muscular incoordination, alcohol intolerance, hallucinations, and anemia, some of which is due to copper deficiency. More than 2 grams of zinc taken in one dose will usually produce vomiting. If not, it will likely lead to other symptoms until the body clears the excess zinc. Luckily, only a certain amount of it will be absorbed.

Zinc may interfere with copper absorption, so taking regular zinc supplements without copper can cause copper deficiency. This will interfere with iron metabolism and possibly cause anemia, as copper and iron are important in red blood cell formation. We usually need supplemental copper and vitamin A to balance the effect of extra zinc. Some formu-

FACTORS RELATED TO ZINC DEFICIENCY

- **Diet**—low in zinc or high in copper; high in fiber, phytates, clay, alcohol, or phosphates, all of which bind zinc in the intestines and reduce absorption; food grown in low-zinc soils.
- **Aging**—when zinc absorption and intake are often reduced.
- **Pregnancy**—when zinc needs are increased.
- **Growth periods**—infancy, especially with increased copper intake levels and for those on low-zinc formulas; puberty, especially in adolescent boys.
- **Birth control pills**—use of these increases copper levels and thus reduces zinc.
- **Premenstrual symptoms**—associated with low zinc.
- **Increased copper intake**—high copper intake in water, food, or supplements will reduce zinc.
- **Fasting or starvation**—causes zinc depletion and increases needs for zinc.
- **Serious illness or injury**—causes zinc depletion and increases needs due to tissue healing.
- **Hospitalization**—stress of illness or treatment, particularly intravenous therapy without zinc supplementation.
- **Stress**—increases zinc use and needs.
- **Burns**—increases needs for tissue healing and dealing with stress.
- **Acute or chronic infections**—greater requirements from stress and for healing.
- **Surgery**—increased requirements for dealing with stress and for healing.
- **Alcoholism**—often associated with low zinc intake and higher needs; alcohol flushes zinc from the liver, causing increased losses.
- **Diuretic therapy**—may cause extra zinc losses.
- **Psoriasis**—rapid skin activity may deplete zinc.
- **Parasites**—cause zinc depletion and poor absorption.
- **Malabsorption**—from pancreatic insufficiency or after gastrointestinal surgery.
- **Cirrhosis**—zinc levels may be half of normal.
- **Renal disease**—causes increased zinc
- **Chronic disease**—metabolic and debilitating disease such as cancer.
- **Athletics**—increased zinc losses in sweat.
- **Cadmium toxicity**—interferes with zinc absorption and utilization.

Other problems associated with low zinc levels are peptic ulcers, pernicious anemia, cystic fibrosis, and mongolism.

---

las, for example, Nutrilite's product, A plus Zinc, contain vitamin A and zinc together, which improves the effect of both; additional copper, about 2 mg., might also be supplemented daily, though at another time than the zinc.

Zinc deficiency is very likely more common and more complex than previously thought. It was first identified in Iran and Egypt in 1961, in male dwarfs with slow growth and poor sexual development. The unleavened bread that is a staple in the diet there is high in the phytates that bind zinc, and a type of clay used for cooking in Iran also ties up zinc. Zinc treatment was found to help these conditions, stimulating growth and sexual development.

Aging is one of the main factors in zinc deficiency. However, some recent environmental changes have also contributed to the deficiency problem. Soil losses and losses due to food processing are two of the main factors in zinc depletion in foods. With the change from iron- and zinc-containing water pipes to copper ones, not only is zinc intake de-

221

creased, but the additional copper interferes further with zinc absorption. The average diet, especially one with low protein intake, supplies only 8–11 mg. daily (the RDA for adults is 15 mg.).

In general, both infants and adolescents have more zinc deficiency, as do the elderly and women, often due to low intake. With the average American diet, we need to eat about 3,400 calories to obtain our 15 mg. of zinc, and most people do not eat that much. Good-quality food is needed, and therefore poor people are more likely to experience zinc shortages.

The subject of our diet and zinc deficiency is an important one. The all-too-typical advanced technology, antinature diet that is high in refined grains, fat, sugar, convenience foods, and fried meats, is often low in zinc and many other important trace minerals and B vitamins. Also, strict vegetarians and consumers of much grain and little animal protein may not obtain sufficient zinc.

SITUATIONS ASSOCIATED WITH ZINC DEFICIENCY

Acne	Prostatic hypertrophy
Alcohol use	Prostate cancer
Cataracts	Diabetes mellitus
Epilepsy	AIDS
Crohn's disease	Immune suppression
Ulcerative colitis	Infections
Anorexia nervosa	Male infertility
Psoriasis	Learning disabilities
Schizophrenia	Pregnancy
Dementia	Toxemia of pregnancy
Depression	Refined diet
Elderly	Teenagers
Diuretic therapy	Use of birth control pills
Vigorous exercise	Environmental sensitivity

There are many symptoms and decreased body functions due to zinc deficiency. It may cause slowed growth or slow sexual development in the pubertal years. Lowered resistance, fatigue, and increased susceptibility to infection may occur with zinc deficiency, which is related to a decreased cellular immune response. Sensitivity and reactions to environmental chemicals may be exaggerated in a state of zinc deficiency as many of the important detoxification enzyme functions may be impaired.

Children with zinc deficiency may show poor appetite and slow development, have learning disabilities or poor attention spans, and in later years have acne and decreased sexual development. Dwarfism and a total lack of sexual function may occur with serious zinc deficiency. Fatigue is common.

Acute deficiency may cause hair loss or thinning, dermatitis, and decreased growth. Both poor appetite and digestion are also experienced by adults with zinc deficiency. Loss of taste sensation may occur, as can brittleness of the nails or white spots on the nails, termed leukonykia. These and most other symptoms can be corrected with supplemental zinc. Sulfur may be helpful as well. Skin rashes, dry skin, and delayed healing of skin wounds or ulcers may result from zinc deficiency, and stretch marks, called striae, are also produced by this condition. Zinc and copper are both needed for cross-linking of collagen, and when they are low, the skin tissue may break down.

Zinc deficiency may cause delayed menstruation in teenage females or, in later years, cause menstrual problems. In addition to zinc, vitamin B_6 often also helps correct this. Females on birth control pills usually have elevated copper levels and need additional zinc and B_6. When zinc is further reduced by the increased copper, depression is more likely, a common side effect of birth control pill use. Morning sickness in pregnancy may result from low zinc and B_6 levels, and supplementing these nutrients may help reduce symptoms.

RDAS FOR ZINC

Under 1 year	3–5 mg.
1–10 years	10 mg.
11 years over	15 mg.
Pregnant women	20–25 mg.
Lactating women	25–30 mg.

Male teenagers with low zinc have delayed or absent sexual development. Sterility may result from zinc deficiency; when it is caused by testicular degeneration, it may be irreversible. Subtle zinc deficiencies may be responsible for male growth lag in puberty. Even in sexually developed males, low zinc levels have been correlated with a decrease in testosterone levels and a lower sperm count. Prostate problems are more prevalent with zinc deficiency.

Birth defects have been associated with zinc deficiency during pregnancy in experimental animals. The offspring showed reduced growth patterns and learning disabilities. In humans, children with zinc deficiency have decreased intelligence and erratic behavior. With zinc treatment, the IQ and behavior may both improve if the problem is related to zinc deficiency.

Requirements: The RDA for zinc in adults is 15 mg., with additional amounts needed during pregnancy and lactation. Yet the average diet contains only about 10 mg. of zinc. And when zinc needs are considered, we likely need even more than 15 mg. per day to be sure we are meeting our requirements. Adequate amounts can be met by a good diet, especially with good protein and calorie intake. Vegetarians can eat more whole grains; even with some of the zinc binding to grain phytate, we still get a fair share into our body from these zinc-rich foods. Since absorption is about 30–40 percent, our total zinc body tissue needs are about 4–6 mg. per day.

We probably need 15–30 mg. of available (elemental) zinc daily for maintenance and probably about 30–60 mg. for treatment, though more is sometimes used. Fifteen mg. of zinc is often included in general supplement formulas. Separately, zinc gluconate and sulfate in reasonable amounts are used commonly without any side effects, though zinc gluconate is usually a little better tolerated than zinc sulfate. The amino-acid-chelated zinc is probably the best tolerated and absorbed though it is more expensive. Zinc sulfate tablets or capsules of 220 mg. provide 55 mg. of elemental zinc. A supplement labeled "zinc 25 mg. as gluconate" should provide 25 mg. elemental zinc. In medical treatment or research, zinc sulfate 220 mg. may be used two to three times daily, supplying about 100–150 mg. of available zinc for absorption. This dosage is usually tolerated fairly well.

Although 30–60 mg. of elemental zinc per day is the usual therapeutic level, more may be needed to correct zinc deficiency. Taking zinc alone two hours after meals or first thing in the morning will increase absorption by reducing the competition with other nutrients, such as calcium and copper, or food constituents such as the phytates and fibers in grains. With infections, burns, before or after surgery, in pregnancy, or with aging (often accompanied with lower absorption), 50–75 mg. per day is suggested as a therapeutic dose.

When taking higher amounts of zinc, we must make sure we get adequate amounts of copper—at least 2–3 mg. supplemented, and possibly more with higher zinc intakes—so copper deficiency does not occur. The suggested zinc to copper ratio is about 15:1. About 200 mcg. per day of selenium should also be taken, to prevent depletion by supplemental zinc. Zinc may be taken with magnesium, vitamin C, and B complex vitamins, but it is best to take a regular vitamin-mineral combination with 15–30 mg. of zinc in proper proportion to other minerals, so that deficiencies of zinc or imbalances of the other minerals do not occur.

POSSIBLY ESSENTIAL TRACE MINERALS

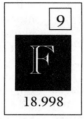

5

B

10.81

BORON

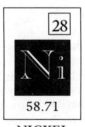

9

F

18.998

FLUORIDE

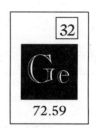

32

Ge

72.59

GERMANIUM

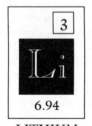

3

Li

6.94

LITHIUM

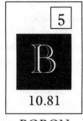

28

Ni

58.71

NICKEL

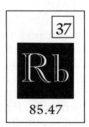

37

Rb

85.47

RUBIDIUM

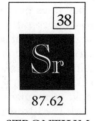

38

Sr

87.62

STRONTIUM

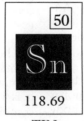

50

Sn

118.69

TIN

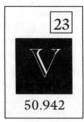

23

V

50.942

VANADIUM

The past two decades have brought a great deal of nutritional research. Seeking understanding and knowledge of the natural elements of the earth (of which little is known) has been part of this research. Though the initial studies began in animals, oftentimes the findings have applied to humans. Many of the currently known important trace minerals were discovered through this type of investigation during the twentieth century. We, of course, have much more to learn about mineral medicine.

Relatively recently, we have found valuable uses for such minerals as boron, fluoride, lithium, strontium, rubidium, and vanadium. Nickel and tin, though usually considered mildly toxic minerals, may be required in very small amounts. Arsenic, not mentioned here, is also possibly needed in modest amounts, though its toxicity is of concern (see discussion later). Germanium, an exciting mineral new to the nutritional scene, is not known to be essential, yet may be very valuable in the treatment of disease. It will be discussed mainly in the next Chapter 7, *Accessory Nutrients.*

Boron has been making nutritional medicine news very recently, and will likely be noted as the next essential trace mineral. It appears to help maintain calcium balance, keeping bones healthy and preventing osteoporosis. The most recent research has been government sponsored, and it looks favorable in regard to the positive effects from adequate boron nutriture. The level of boron needed in the diet is not known; it is probably between 3 and 5 mg. daily. The highest concentration of boron in the body is in the parathyroid glands, suggesting its tie to calcium metabolism and bone health.

Boric acid has been used for decades as an astringent and antiseptic for the skin and eyes. Boric acid eye wash is probably boron's most common medicinal use. However, boric acid use is not suggested for infants and small children, as many are sensitive. Excess use in anyone can lead to dry skin or gastrointestinal upset.

Sources: Boron is available in the soil and in many whole foods. Fruits, such as apples, pears, and grapes are high in boron. Leafy greens, legumes, and nuts also are good sources. A poor diet, high in refined foods and low in wholesome ones, will likely provide insufficient boron and may lead to deficiency problems, one of which may be osteoporosis in the elderly.

Functions: Boron physiology is not totally clear as yet. It possibly affects calcium, magnesium, and phosphorus balance and the mineral movement and makeup of the bones by regulating the hormones, mainly parathyroid, that control these functions. Boron's aid in preventing bone loss and osteoporosis is only projected at this date, and further study is needed to understand its relationship to the bones.

Boron may also play a role in hypertension and arthritis via its relationship to calcium metabolism. Both of these diseases, as well as atherosclerosis, are in part related to abnormal calcium metabolism and balance. Adequate calcium (and magnesium) may help maintain normal blood pressure, while abnormal calcium deposition may increase artery plaque and joint irritation. More research in these areas may prove very interesting.

Uses: The current suggestion is to provide adequate levels of boron (3–5 mg.) in the diet to maintain healthy bones. Boron is now used in more calcium/bone replenishing nutritional formulae. At this time, due to its low potential toxicity and possible necessity, elderly people and anyone at risk of osteoporosis should eat boron-rich foods and further supplement boron at a level of about 1–3 mg. daily. Whether boron is useful in the treatment of osteoporosis, arthritis, other bone diseases, or hypertension will need to be studied further.

Deficiency and Toxicity: Boron toxicity to date is associated with the excessive use or increased sensitivity to boric acid, as discussed earlier. The ingestion of boric acid can lead to immediate nausea and vomiting. Later problems could be anemia, hair loss, skin eruption, and seizures. Diborane inhalation or exposure to liquid boron hydride can adversely affect the lungs and nervous system.

Boron deficiency is apparently more of an everyday concern. It may be associated with an increased incidence of osteoporosis. Preliminary research of arthritis incidence suggests a correlation with soil boron levels. In Israel, where people have a very low rate of arthritis (less than 1 percent), there are high levels of boron in the soil, while Jamaica has the opposite situation; that is low boron soil levels and a high incidence of arthritis. Clearly, more epidemiological research is needed to isolate boron or boron deficiency as a factor in these diseases.

Requirements: There is no RDA for boron at this time. Probably about 1 mg. daily in the diet is sufficient to prevent deficiency. A healthy diet of wholesome foods probably provides 3 mg. or more daily. Drs. Neilson and Hung of the Department of Agriculture's Grand Forks, North Dakota, Human Nutrition Research say that 3–5 mg. of boron daily can improve calcium retention, based on a six-month study of postmenopausal women. After a low boron diet, 3 mg. daily were supplemented. These boron-supplemented subjects then showed lower daily losses, nearly 50 percent, for both calcium and magnesium than when on the boron deficient diet.

Currently, more multivitamin/minerals and bone supportive supplements are adding 1–2 mg. boron. It appears that this mineral will be part of our nutritional picture for the future.

Fluoride Though fluorine as fluoride has been shown to reduce dental cavities when added to toothpaste or drinking water, there is still some question as to whether it is an essential element. In other words, if we do not have fluoride, will we develop any problems? It is my feeling that eating a natural diet low in refined flours and sugars along with some basic oral hygiene will maintain healthy teeth and gums.

Fluorine itself is a poisonous gas, as are the related elements chlorine and bromine. Fluorine, as fluoride, is found in the earth's crust in combination with other minerals, and is also part of seawater. Fluoride is available naturally in the diet as calcium and sodium fluoride. It is sodium fluoride that is added to the drinking water of many cities to help reduce dental caries. There is some controversy as to whether fluoridation has some subtle poisoning effect or whether it is nontoxic and beneficial. In my opinion, fluoridated water is another example of technology's treating the effect instead of correcting the cause, which is primarily poor diet.

Fluoride is probably not essential to humans, though it is helpful in strengthening the bones and teeth. It is found only in trace amounts, about 2–3 grams, in the body, and most of that is in bones and teeth. The blood level of fluoride is about 0.3 mg. per 100 ml. Fluoride has no known function other than strengthening teeth and bones.

Intestinal absorption of fluoride, especially the more soluble sodium fluoride, is fairly good. Calcium, aluminum, and perhaps other minerals may interfere somewhat with absorption by making less soluble fluoride salts. About half of ingested fluoride, about 3 mg. per day, is eliminated through the kidneys and a little more through perspiration. The remainder is stored mainly in the bones.

Sources: Natural fluoride is present in the ocean as sodium fluoride, so most seafood contains some. People who eat large quantities of fish, such as the cultures of the Caribbean, have been shown to have stronger teeth and less incidence of dental cavities, the most common disease worldwide, than do others. This may also be related to other factors. Gelatin and tea also contain fluoride. In fact, a study showed that school children in England were obtaining over 1 mg. of fluoride daily from tea alone (that is black tea, with caffeinelike molecules theophylline or theobromine plus tannic acid, not herbal teas). Most plant-source foods contain some fluoride, though the amount can vary greatly depending on soil fluoride content. Soil deficiency of fluoride is fairly common.

Fluoride is added to the drinking water of many municipalities at the concentration of 1 ppm. More than 2 ppm can cause problems, so the concentration must be finely monitored. People drinking city water who also consume fluoride-containing foods or black teas can develop fluoride problems as well, though toxicity has not been found to be appreciable with moderate amounts.

Stannous (tin) fluoride was originally used in toothpaste for protection against tooth decay. But it has been found that fluoride is more effective in this area when provided internally by drinking water than when it is applied locally, and we probably do not want too much extra tin anyway (though tin may be an essential mineral in trace amounts as well). Overall, I do not advocate drinking fluoridated water—or any city water, for that matter (see Chapter 1, *Water*). It is better, I believe, to drink filtered water to be safe from chemical and toxic metal pollutants and to eat a more natural diet with some seafood, which is also thought to protect against atherosclerosis and heart disease as well as keep the teeth healthy.

Functions: Studies show that fluoride helps strengthen the crystalline structure of bones and teeth. The calcium fluoride salt forms a fluorapatite matrix, which is stronger and less soluble than other calcium salts and therefore is not as easily reabsorbed into circulation to supply calcium needs. In teeth, this fluoride salt reduces the potential for breakdown from acids in the mouth or from demineralization, minimizing tooth decay. In bones, fluoride reduces loss of calcium and thereby may reduce osteoporosis. No other functions of fluoride are presently known, though it has been suggested to have a role in growth, in iron absorption, and in the production of red blood cells. This needs further research.

Uses: Fluoride's main use is as an additive to drinking water as well as toothpaste and mouthwash for the prevention of tooth decay. When added to water at 1 ppm, it can reduce dental caries by 30–50 percent. Fluoridated water works best, however, when its use is begun in infancy or early childhood and continued throughout childhood. Fluoride-treated water does not decrease the gum disease that may also result from poor nutrition and poor hygiene. As is typical of Western medical thinking, we treat the result as if it were the problem itself, rather than correcting the cause—the overuse of sugar and poor dietary habits in general—which may be causing decay even deeper in the body, a process that may take us many more years to discover. I wonder what new xenon-coated bandage will be invented to patch that up.

On a more positive note, the use of sodium fluoride has been shown to be helpful in the treatment and possibly the prevention of osteoporosis, though the results from various studies are mixed. Epidemiologically, the incidence of osteoporosis is slightly reduced in fluoridated-water users. In older studies, bone density, as well as blood pressure, was improved by treatment with 50 mg. of sodium fluoride (NaF) and 900 mg. of calcium daily and 50,000 IUs of vitamin D twice weekly. There is concern, however, that fluoride-treated bones will not give up calcium easily to the body when needed, which may contribute to calcium deficiency. It is obviously much better to prevent osteoporosis by eating calcium-rich foods; supplementing calcium, magnesium, and vitamin D; maintaining overall mineral balance; eating a healthy diet; and exercising regularly.

There is some preliminary research evidence that fluoride may help in treating otosclerosis, a loss of hearing due to deposits in the ear. Hearing loss in later years, when it is due to osteoporosis, or loss of minerals from the tiny ear bones, may be reduced with fluoride treatment as well.

Fluoride is not generally used as a supplement in multivitamin/mineral formulas. It is added to some infants' and young children's vitamins to aid in the prevention of tooth decay. As sodium fluoride, it is occasionally prescribed medically in the prevention or treatment of dental disease.

Deficiency and toxicity: Toxicity from fluoride is definitely a potential problem. As stated, fluoridated water must be closely monitored to keep the concentration at about 1 ppm to effectively reduce dental decay without producing side effects. At concentrations greater than 2 ppm, fluoride can cause mottling, discoloration, and pitting of the teeth, though it will still maintain tooth strength and prevent cavities. At 8 to about 20 ppm, initial tissue sclerosis will occur, especially in the bones and joints, which can cause arthritic symptoms. At over 20 ppm, much damage can occur, including decreased growth and cellular changes, especially in the metabolically active organs such as the liver, kidneys, adrenal glands, and reproductive organs. More than 50 ppm of fluoride intake can be fatal. In terms of total fluoride intake, around 20 mg. per day will usually cause some tooth discoloration and bone problems. Animals eating extra fluoride in grains, vegetables, or in water have been shown to have tooth and bone lesions. Fat and carbohydrate metabolism has also been affected. There are many other concerns about fluoride toxicity, including bone malformations and cancer.

Sodium fluoride is less toxic than most other fluoride salts. In cases of toxicity, extra calcium will bind with the fluoride, making a less soluble and less active compound.

Fluoride deficiency is less of a concern. Low fluoride or lack of fluoride use does correlate with a higher number of dental caries, given a less stability and strength of the bones and teeth in general. It is possible, that traces of fluoride are essential, but it is not clear whether it is a natural component of our body tissues. Low fluoride levels may correlate with a higher amount of bone fractures in the elderly, but that is usually in the presence of osteoporosis.

Requirements: There is no specific RDA for fluoride. Nor is it mandatory to add fluoride to the water. Many cities do not follow this much-supported preventive measure. On a worldwide level, there has been a lot of disappointment with the use of fluoridated water. People who drink fluoridated city water get about 1 mg. per day from it. Research shows that the amount in the average diet varies widely, depending on choices of foods and water use. Nonfluoridated water users take in between .35 mg. and 1.5 mg. per day, while the average city diet with fluoridated water contains about 2–3 mg. The suggested safe intake of fluoride (not necessarily the optimum, which we really do not know) is between 1.5 and 4.0 mg. per day. Amounts up to 15–20 mg. per day are probably well tolerated, though we do not know the long-range effects. And until we do, I personally would discourage overuse of fluoride. A complete review of the fluoride controversy, written from a global viewpoint, appeared in the August 1988 issue of *Chemical Engineering*.

 Germanium, trace mineral 32, has recently become popular after being developed into an organic germanium compound in Japan. This organo-germanium, bis-carboxyethyl germanium sesquioxide (Ge-132), has been tested and used for the treatment of a variety of medical problems that require improved oxygenation and immune function, ranging from simple viral infections to cancer. Organo-germanium will be discussed in detail at the end of Chapter 7, *Accessory Nutrients.*

The trace mineral germanium itself may be needed in small amounts by the human body; however, research has not yet shown this. It is found in the soil, in foods, and in many healing plants, such as aloe vera, garlic, and ginseng. The organo-germanium currently used does not, however, release the mineral germanium to the tissues for specific action, but is absorbed, acts, and is eliminated as the entire compound, Ge-132. More research is needed to clearly understand the potential importance of both elemental germanium and the Ge-132 compound.

 Lithium is usually found in nature not as a metal but as lithium salts. Its name comes from *lithos,* the Greek word for "stone," as the lithium crystals are beautiful and very hard rocks. Aside from hydrogen, which is present in almost all of life, lithium is the lightest element in use. It is unique among the minerals in that it is used in medical treatment of manic-depressive disorders, commonly as lithium carbonate. It is chemically similar to sodium and can displace sodium (and vice versa) in many bodily reactions. Its involvement in sodium transport across cell membranes probably accounts for lithium's therapeutic support of people with manic disorders. Although it has been used in this area since about 1950, its acceptance has been slow, possibly because it is a natural mineral and not as profitable for the pharmaceutical companies as synthetic drugs. Recent evidence indicates that lithium may be an essential element, needed in trace amounts (minute in comparison to the high doses used in treatment).

We have in our body only about 2–3 mg. of lithium. Absorption from the intestine is good, about 70–90 percent. People with mania often have very good absorption of lithium. Excess lithium is eliminated in urine and feces.

Sources: We do not completely understand what effect lithium in foods has, or what particular foods are high in lithium. Some natural mineral waters are high in lithium, and these are said to calm the nerves, cheer the spirit, and soothe the digestion. Sugarcane and seaweed have been shown to contain lithium. Tobacco has some lithium, but the effect of inhaled lithium is not known.

Function: It is not yet known what particular function of lithium may make it an essential nutrient. It is thought to stabilize serotonin transmission in the nervous system; it influences sodium transport; and it may even increase lymphocytic (white blood cell) proliferation and depress the suppressor cell activity, thus strengthening the immune system. There is also speculation that lithium is in some way involved in cancer genesis or prevention.

Uses: Lithium's main use is in treating manic-depressive disorders, for which it is used in what could be considered megadosages. Certain depression problems, probably those sensitive to sodium transport difficulties, may be helped by lithium, even where there is little or no manic component. Manic symptoms of insomnia, hyperactivity, talkativeness, grandiose thinking, and delusions can usually be controlled with lithium therapy. Dosages of between 600 and 1000 mg. per day are needed to obtain the appropriate blood level to treat mania.

Lithium has occasionally been used in treating alcoholism, where it apparently decreased the taste for alcohol and generated a more cheerful attitude toward life. Lithium treatment does, however, produce some side effects, such as a metallic taste in the mouth, increased thirst, and more frequent urination. It is not routinely taken as a nutritional supplement but is used primarily as a medicinal drug.

Deficiency and toxicity: Deficiency of lithium is not really known. The theory that a deficiency of lithium can cause an increase in depression has not been adequately proved.

Lithium toxicity, however, is a very real possibility when it is used as a medicine. In the treatment of manic disorders, there is a fine line between therapeutic and toxic levels. Since it is cleared in the urine, anyone with kidney disease must take lithium with caution. It is given in therapeutic doses only by prescription, with blood levels followed closely by the doctor.

Lithium produces some of its symptoms by upsetting the fluid balance and mineral transport across cell membranes. Symptoms of lithium toxicity include nausea, vomiting, diarrhea, thirst, increased urination, tremors, drowsiness, confusion, delirium, and muscle weakness. Skin eruptions may also occur. With further toxicity, staggering, seizures, kidney damage, coma, and even death may occur.

Requirements: There is no specific RDA for lithium, nor is it known how much, if any, we need. Dietary studies estimate that we get about 2 mg. daily. A therapeutic intake can vary from 500–1,500 mg. daily, though usually 300 mg. of lithium carbonate three times daily will provide the blood levels needed to treat manic disorders, which may require long-term therapy. Under these circumstances, blood levels should be checked occasionally to make sure there are sufficient amounts present, and symptoms (side effects) of lithium toxicity should be watched for carefully.

Nickel has been considered as a possibly essential trace mineral for several decades. We have a total of about 10 mg. in our body, but we still do not know exactly what it does. Most of the nutritional research on nickel has been done with chicks and rats. It is an essential nutrient for these animals, and they suffer considerable problems with nickel deficiency.

Nickel is found in many foods and in all animal tissues. While it is found in most human tissues, so far as we know, it is not concentrated in any particular tissues. Since it occurs in food and is part of the earth's crust and not a contaminant, many scientists feel that it is probably essential to humans. But nickel is potentially toxic in its gaseous form, nickel carbonyl.

Nickel is rather poorly absorbed from the gastrointestinal tract, probably at less than 10 percent. It is carried in the body attached to a protein, forming a molecule called nickeloplasmin. Most nickel is eliminated in feces, some in urine, and a bit in perspiration. The kidneys can either clear excess nickel or retain it; such a control mechanism suggests essentiality.

Sources: Nickel is contained in many foods. Most beans, soybeans, lentils, and split and green peas have fairly high amounts. Nuts, such as walnuts and hazelnuts, are the best sources of nickel. Of the grains, oats have the highest content, followed by buckwheat, barley, and corn. Many vegetables and some fruits, such as bananas and pears, have moderate amounts. Animal products and fatty foods are fairly low in nickel; of these, herring and oysters are the highest. Refined foods are also low. It is possible that the nickel in grains forms a phytate, reducing the amount of nickel available.

There are external, nonfood sources of nickel also, but it is not clear how much nickel we actually absorb from these sources. Nickel is found in coins, costume jewelry, eyeglass frames, hair clips, pins, scissors, and some kitchen appliances. Regular contact with these nickel products may allow some absorption into the body. Allergic dermatitis from nickel products is not at all uncommon.

Functions: The biological function of nickel is still somewhat unclear. Nickel is found in the body in highest concentrations in the nucleic acids, particularly RNA, and is thought to be somehow involved in protein structure or function. It may activate certain enzymes related to the breakdown or utilization of glucose. Nickel may aid in prolactin production, and thus be involved in human breast milk production.

Most of the information about nickel comes from testing with animals, and its relevancy to humans is still not proven. More research is needed to reveal the properties of this interesting mineral in the human body.

Uses: There are presently no clear uses for nickel supplementation. Studies have shown that there are increased levels of nickel in patients following heart attacks, burns, and strokes, and with toxemia of pregnancy. Whether this is a partial cause or, as is more likely, a result of tissue metabolism or represents some other function of nickel is not as yet known. Decreased levels of nickel have been seen in psoriasis, in cirrhosis of the liver, and with kidney disease, but it has not been shown that nickel treatment helps any of these conditions.

Deficiency and toxicity: Toxicity is the main concern here—not from elemental nickel or the nickel found in foods but from inhaled nickel carbonyl, a carcinogenic gas that results from the reaction of nickel with heated carbon monoxide, from cigarette smoke, car exhaust, and some industrial wastes. Nickel carbonyl is toxic and can cause symptoms such as frontal headaches, nausea, vomiting, or vertigo with acute exposure. Inhaled nickel accumulates in the lungs and has been associated with increased rates of lung, nasal, and laryngeal cancers. Nickel allergy can also cause local skin or systemic reactions. The nickel in jewelry, dental materials, or prosthetic joints or heart valves may also be allergenic sources.

Nickel deficiency has not been shown to be a concern in humans, but it is definitely a problem in chicks and other small animals, where low nickel can lead to decreased growth, dermatitis, pigment changes, decreased reproduction capacities, and compromised liver function. In humans, increased sweating, such as from exercise, can cause nickel losses, and extra dietary nickel may be required to maintain its still mysterious functions.

Requirements: There is, of course, no RDA for nickel. About 500 mcg. is probably a safe daily intake; the average dietary intake is about 200–750 mcg. If nickel is clearly found to be essential, the minimum requirement would likely be 50–100 mcg. Nickel is easily obtainable in most diets and is not usually contained in any supplements, except for occasional trace mineral formulas.

 Rubidium is present in the earth's crust, in seawater, and in the human body. Our body contains about 350 mg. It has not yet been shown to be essential. Chemically, it is like potassium, and in some animals it can replace potassium in certain functions, though this does not seem to be the case in humans. Rubidium can possibly be a potassium antagonist in regard to absorption and utilization, though this needs further investigation.

Rubidium is absorbed easily from the gut, about 90 percent. It is found generally throughout the body, with the least in the bones and teeth; it is not known to concentrate in any particular tissue. Excess rubidium is eliminated mainly in the urine.

Sources: Food sources of rubidium have not been researched very well as yet. Some fruits and vegetables have been found to contain about 35 ppm. Rubidium may also be found in some water sources.

Functions: There are currently no known essential functions of rubidium. In studies with mice, rubidium has helped decrease tumor growth, possibly by replacing potassium in cell transport mechanisms or by rubidium ions attaching to the cancer cell membranes. Rubidium may have a tranquilizing or hypnotic effect in some animals, possibly including humans.

Uses: There are no clear uses for rubidium as yet. Because of its possible tranquilizing effect, it could help in the treatment of nervous disorders or epilepsy.

Deficiency and toxicity: There is no known deficiency or toxicity for rubidium.

Requirements: There is no RDA for rubidium. The average dietary intake may be about 1.5 mg. daily.

 Strontium There is no evidence yet that strontium is an essential mineral. Our body contains about 300–350 mg., nearly 99 percent of it in the bones and teeth. It closely resembles calcium chemically and can actually displace it. It forms strontium bone salts, which may actually be slightly stronger than those of calcium.

Radioactive strontium (Sr 90) is a hazardous by-product of nuclear fission. Taking trace amounts of strontium may possibly protect us from picking up the radioactive form when exposed to it. Generally, we do not need to worry about strontium, even if it is essential, because it is available in most diets, through the soil. This means that the strontium content in food will vary geographically.

Strontium absorption varies from about 20–40 percent. It is stable in the tissues, mainly the bones and teeth, and most extra strontium is eliminated in the feces.

Sources: Strontium is present in seawater and some other waters. Soil content may vary. Strontium is found, generally in low amounts, in most foods.

Function: Strontium may help improve the cell structure and mineral matrix of the bones and teeth, adding strength and helping to prevent tooth decay or soft bones, though it is not known if low body levels of strontium causes these problems.

Uses: There are no clear uses for supplemental strontium. The use of strontium to help bone metabolism and strength in osteoporosis has been investigated, but is still questionable. Whether strontium will prevent tooth decay has not been shown. As stated, trace amounts of nonradioactive strontium may be taken to reduce uptake of the radioactive form of this element.

Deficiency and toxicity: There have been no cases of known toxicity from natural strontium. Nor are there any deficiency symptoms related to humans, though in rat studies, strontium deficiency may correlate with decreased growth, poor calcification of the bones and teeth, and an increase in dental caries.

Requirements: There is no RDA for strontium. Food intake may supply us with about 2 mg. daily.

 Tin, or *stannum* in Latin, is essential in some mammals, including rats, but it has not been shown to be needed in humans. It is more often considered a mildly toxic mineral. One of the reasons its essentiality is questionable in humans is its absence in newborns and in many animals. It is present in the earth in very small amounts. Tin is most often thought of as an environmental contaminant, both as tin cans and as inhaled industrial pollution. Levels, especially in the lungs, increase with age.

Primitive humans had much less tin in their bodies than modern humans. Tin has been used since the Bronze Age began more than 3,500 years ago (bronze contains copper and tin). It has been used for food storage for more than 200 years. Food does absorb tin from cans, and so we ingest this tin. Luckily for us, it is poorly absorbed from the gastrointestinal tract, probably less than 5 percent, so this is not likely to cause toxicity. Most excess tin is excreted in the feces. Some is eliminated in sweat and even less in urine.

Sources: Tin is present in very low amounts in the soil and in foods. Canning, processing, and packaging often add some tin to food; the solder in iron or copper pipes contains tin; stannous flouride in toothpaste may add more. Since we consider tin primarily as a contaminant, though fairly nontoxic, we should try to avoid it. Using few canned foods and avoiding toothpaste with tin are some ways to do this.

Functions: There are no known functions for tin in humans. If it has a function, it may be related to protein structure or oxidation and reduction reactions, though tin is generally a poor catalyst. Tin may interact with iron and copper, particularly in the gut, and so inhibit absorption.

Uses: No uses for tin are presently known other than in food storage, in industrial processes, and as a fluoride carrier in toothpaste.

Deficiency and toxicity: Though tin is considered a mildly toxic mineral, there are no known chronic or serious diseases from tin exposure or ingestion. Studies in rats showed mainly a slightly shortened life span. I have found no cases of acute tin exposure; chronic low-level environmental and food contamination is more likely.

Avoiding eating too much food from tin cans is probably the best we can do (oily foods seem to pick up more tin than others). In the United States, tin cans are now lacquered, which prevents some food absorption. Lacquered cans have a slight yellow coloring, while the unlacquered cans, which are more common with imported foods, are brighter metal.

There are no known problems from tin deficiency in humans.

Requirements: There is currently no RDA or any known requirement for tin. We should avoid any large or long-term exposure. The average diet may contain about 2 mg. per day, but this can vary from about 2–20 mg. per day, depending on the foods ingested. Tin is not likely to be found in many supplements other than occasional trace mineral formulae, and there is no current reason to add tin to any nutritional program.

 Vanadium was classified as an essential trace mineral fairly recently, and it is still a little-known element. Our body contains about 20–25 mg., distributed in small amounts throughout, some being stored in the fat tissue.

Vanadium has been known to be essential in rats and chickens longer than it has in humans. Rats store vanadium primarily in their bones and teeth. Vanadium is needed by some bacteria and can occasionally substitute for molybdenum. The ascidian worms use vanadium in their blood cells as hemovanadium, which makes green-colored blood cells.

Vanadium is present in our soil, though the amount varies; its distribution is similar to that of selenium. Some studies have shown decreased rates of heart disease in vanadium- and selenium-rich areas, such as many South American countries. Modern humans get vanadium contamination through the air from burning petroleum. With age, it may accumulate somewhat in the lungs, though it seems to be fairly nontoxic.

Vanadium absorption is modest at best, probably about 5–10 percent of that ingested. It is, however, used fairly rapidly. Most of it is eliminated in the feces; whatever is absorbed and not used is eliminated in the urine. In humans, vanadium is stored mainly in fat.

Sources: Vanadium content in the vegetable kingdom varies, mostly according to soil differences. It is generally present in low amounts in foods, probably most available in fats and vegetable oils, especially the unsaturated variety. Soy, sunflower, safflower, corn, and olive oils and the foods these oils come from all contain fair amounts of vanadium. Buckwheat, parsley, oats, rice, green beans, carrots, and cabbage also contain vanadium. Dill and radish have fairly high concentrations, while eggs have a moderate amount. Most fish are low, though oysters and herring have good levels.

Functions: Not much is known about vanadium function. Vanadium seems to be involved in catecholamine and lipid metabolism. It has been shown to have an effect in reducing the production of cholesterol. This may be related to the cholesterol-lowering potential of polyunsaturated oils (good sources of vanadium). Other research involves its role in calcium metabolism, in growth, reproduction, blood sugar regulation, and red blood cell production. The enzyme-stimulation role of vanadium may involve it in bone and tooth formation and, through the production of coenzyme A, in fat metabolism.

Uses: Since vanadium has been shown to help reduce cholesterol levels in some people, it may be helpful in treating atherosclerosis and heart disease and could play a role in reducing incidence of heart attack. It may also help in lowering elevated blood sugar levels. The 1932 and 1957 editions of *Dorland's Medical Dictionary* recommended use of vanadium in the treatment of diabetes, of neurasthenia, and, with selenium, of cancer. In 1958, it was further recommended for the treatment of atherosclerosis.

Deficiency and toxicity: Vanadium has been thought to be essentially nontoxic in humans, possibly because of poor absorption. However, recent studies have revealed elevated levels of vanadium in patients with mania and depression. Some toxicity can occur in rats. Vanadium is more commonly an industrial and environmental pollutant, though this has not been shown to be a concern. There is some vanadium in the air, more in winter because of burning of petroleum. Workers who clean vanadium-containing petroleum storage tanks inhale and absorb additional vanadium. The dust can be a bit irritating to the lungs, and the tongue may become somewhat green, neither of which seems to be a serious problem.

Deficiency problems of vanadium have not been clearly shown in humans, though there is a suspicion that low vanadium can increase susceptibility to heart disease and cancer or lead to higher cholesterol and triglyceride levels. In chickens and rats, vanadium deficiency causes some problems with feather and fur growth, bone development, and reproduction.

Requirements: There is currently no RDA for vanadium. The average diet provides at least 2 mg. per day, which most likely meets anyone's needs, but some diets have been measured at higher amounts, such as 10–15 mg. per day.

Vanadium is not commonly supplemented or contained in many vitamin-mineral combinations. Some newer formulae may contain small amounts. Eating fish and using vegetable oils in the diet will usually supply sufficient vanadium.

TOXIC MINERALS AND HEAVY METALS

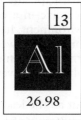

13
Al
26.98
ALUMINUM

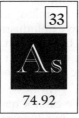

33
As
74.92
ARSENIC

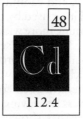

48
Cd
112.4
CADMIUM

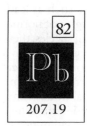

82
Pb
207.19
LEAD

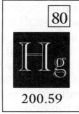

80
Hg
200.59
MERCURY

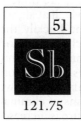

51
Sb
121.75
ANTIMONY

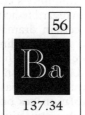

56
Ba
137.34
BARIUM

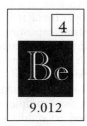

4
Be
9.012
BERYLLIUM

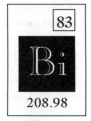

83
Bi
208.98
BISMUTH

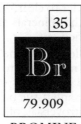

35
Br
79.909
BROMINE

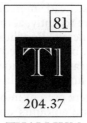

81
Tl
204.37
THALLIUM

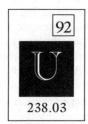

92
U
238.03
URANIUM

This is not a discussion of loud, electronic rock 'n' roll music, but one of impact to all people living in this day and age who are being exposed to heavy metals such as lead, mercury, and cadmium. Though not normally found in or used by the human species, they are becoming more widely present in our environment, leading to serious concerns. There are possibly more problems from these metals, which interfere with normal bodily function, than have been considered in most medical circles. Reviewing all of our vitamins and minerals has shown us that most every substance that is useful can be a toxin or poison, as well. The metals discussed in this section are known primarily—almost exclusively—for their potential toxicity in the body, though commerically they may have great advantages.

Previously, the medical community's concern over metal toxicity was in regard to acute industrial exposure, where certain dramatic measures were performed to stimulate elimination of those metals. More recently, there has been concern over lead intoxication in children from sucking or eating lead-based paint, for example, and legislation has been enacted to reduce this possible contamination, though these measures will probably have a greater effect on future generations.

For most of these potentially toxic minerals, there are many common uses and possible contamination sources throughout our society; our concern must be with more widespread and long-term observation of and protection from these dangers. Lead, mercury, cadmium, arsenic, and, more recently, aluminum are the main toxic minerals. Beryllium, bismuth, and bromine must be considered as well. And there are other heavy and radioactive metals that could bring future difficulties.

Most of these minerals were present in our environment only in minute amounts until recent centuries, when the orientation toward industrialization and production brought about our many technological advances. But technology, like medicine, has its side effects. Mining these metals from the earth and using them in society—as leaded gasoline or silver-mercury tooth amalgam, for example—have brought all of us into regular exposure with them—unless, of course, we live in a completely unindustrialized environment, harder and harder to find as we approach the twenty-first century. At present, these toxic metals have polluted our atmosphere, our waters, our soil, and food chain.

We cannot realistically put all the lead and cadmium for example, back into the earth and cover it up. We need to deal with their presence. At best, we can find better ways to evaluate them in our water, our air, our food, and our body; learn more about where we obtain them; and work preventively to avoid excessive exposure. Most of these heavier metals are quite stable and decompose fairly slowly, if at all, so they remain in the environment. Luckily, the human body is able to clear much of the modest amount we pick up by eliminating it through our urine, sweat, and feces. Absorption of these metals is usually pretty low as well. But when our natural means of elimination are reduced or our exposure is increased, we may run into trouble.

The basic way that these heavy metals cause problems is by displacing or replacing related minerals that are required for essential body functions. For example, cadmium can replace zinc, and lead displaces calcium; when this happens, the cadmium or lead is stored in the bones or other tissues and becomes harder to clear, while the important functions of the minerals that are replaced cannot be carried out.

Blood or urine analysis is not very reliable for measuring toxic levels of most of these heavy metals, especially with long-term exposure and tissue buildup. Hair analysis, though controversial, offers the best available evaluation for accumulation of heavy metals, and in many studies, hair levels do correlate fairly well with tissue stores. The heavier the element, the more reliable is the hair analysis. Measuring these toxic minerals is probably the most useful aspect of hair analysis. In the future, we may find even better ways to measure, treat, and prevent this dangerous heavy mineral contamination.

Most of the available information concerns the main heavy metals, aluminum, arsenic, cadmium, lead, and mercury. For each of these, I provide a general introduction to the history of the metal and how it is handled by the body.

Then, insofar as information is available, I discuss:

- Sources of contamination
- Methods of toxicity
- Symptoms of toxicity
- Amounts leading to toxicity
- Who is susceptible
- Treatment of toxicity
- Ways to prevent toxicity (exposure)

There are no known nutritional deficiencies or bodily uses of these metals, with the possible exception of arsenic, which may be both essential and toxic, so is it necessary to discuss requirements. The remaining heavy metals—antimony, beryllium, bismuth, bromine, thallium, and a few even more minor ones—less commonly produce toxicity problems, and they are described only generally.

 Aluminum has only recently been considered a problem mineral. Though it is not very toxic in normal levels, neither has it been found to be essential. Aluminum is very abundant in the earth and in the sea. It is present in only small amounts in animal and plant tissues. However, it is commonly ingested in foods and in medicines, such as antacids, and is used in cosmetics. Many scientists feel that, because of its prevalence in the earth and its common uses, it is not actually very toxic.

Aluminum is not really a heavy metal—that is, it is low (number 13 on the "periodic" table of elements) in molecular weight—so it does behave differently from metals such as lead or mercury. Recent investigations, however, implicate aluminum toxicity in Alzheimer's disease and other brain and senility syndromes. The evidence of aluminum's toxicity or essentiality is not conclusive as yet.

The amount of aluminum in the human body ranges between 50 and 150 mg., with an average of about 65 mg. Most of this mineral is found in the lungs, brain, kidneys, liver, and thyroid. Our daily intake of aluminum may range from 10–110 mg., but the body will eliminate most of this in the feces and urine and some in the sweat. With decreased kidney function, more aluminum will be stored, particularly in the bones.

Sources: For most people, the greatest aluminum intake comes from food additives. Sodium aluminum phosphate is an emulsifier in processed cheese, potassium alum is used to whiten flour, and sodium silicoaluminate and/or aluminum calcium silicate are added to common table salt to help it run freely and not cake. In the average diet, 40–50 mg. a day may come from foods.

With use of aluminum pots and pans and aluminum foil, some aluminum leaches into food, especially with acid foods such as tomatoes or rhubarb. Cooking with fluoridated water in aluminum cookware increases the aluminum in the water and the food; still, the amounts we obtain in this manner are small in comparison with those from additives. Aluminum salts used in antiperspirants are not a major contaminant either, unless these products are overused. (Aerosol sprays, however, should be avoided for environmental toxicity reasons.) Antacids containing aluminum hydroxide can be a big source if they are taken regularly or abused, as antacids sometimes are. Some children's aspirins have been found to contain aluminum as well.

Methods of toxicity: Aluminum is probably the least toxic of the minerals discussed in this section, although the concern is that it has become so pervasive and is now found in higher levels in human tissues. It is not clear how aluminum functions or interferes with activities in the human body, possibly through some magnesium functions. It may reduce vitamin levels or bind to DNA, and it has been correlated with weakened tissue of the gastrointestinal tract. In Alzheimer's disease, there are increased aluminum levels in the brain tissue and an increase in what are called "neurofibrillary tangles," which tend to reduce nerve synapses and conduction.

Oral aluminum, as obtained from antacids, can bind pepsin and weaken protein digestion. It also has astringent qualities, and thus can dry the tissues and mucous linings and contribute to constipation. Regular use of aluminum-containing deodorants may contribute to the clogging of underarm lymphatics and then to breast problems such as cystic disease. Ann Louise Gittleman, a prominent nutritionist, calls aluminum a "detrimental protoplasmic poison."

Symptoms of toxicity: Acute aluminum poisoning has been associated with constipation, colicky pain, anorexia, nausea and gastrointestinal irritation, skin problems, and lack of energy. Slower and longer-term increases in body aluminum may create muscle twitching, numbness, paralysis, and fatty degeneration of the liver and kidney.

Aluminum toxicity has been fairly recently described. It is worse with reduced renal function. Aluminum may reduce the absorption of selenium and phosphorus from the gastrointestinal tract. The loss of bone matrix from aluminum toxicity can lead to osteomalacia, a softening of the bone. Skin rashes have occurred with local irritation from aluminum antiperspirants.

Aluminum toxicity has been implicated in the brain aging disorders. Alzheimer's disease and parkinsonism have both become more prevalent as the incidence of aluminum toxicity has increased. Areas with high amounts of aluminum in the drinking water are showing an increase in the incidence of Alzheimer's disease (alum and aluminum sulfate are used to treat water in many cities). Nearly 100,000 people of the 1.5–2 million people with Alzheimer's are dying each year. Although increased aluminum has been measured in the brain and other body tissues in Alzheimer's diseases, other factors may be contributing as well. There seems to be a weakening of the blood-brain barrier in Alzheimer's disease, and this may allow a variety of brain toxins to reach the central nervous system. What is causing this breakdown of the barrier between the brain and the rest of the body is not yet clear. It is also important to examine aluminum toxicity in children with hyperactivity and learning disorders, as it has been implicated in these problems.

Amounts leading to toxicity: It is not known exactly what levels of aluminum or what other factors cause it to become a problem. With blood and hair analysis, normal ranges of aluminum may vary from lab to lab. Hair analysis is probably one of the better ways to measure body aluminum. The mineral analysis laboratory that I use, Doctor's Data in Chicago, suggests that a reading under 15–20 ppm in hair is considered normal, but less than that, say under 10–15 ppm, is probably ideal.

Who is susceptible? Everyone has contact with aluminum; it is present in most diets. However, why and how aluminum becomes a problem, if it truly does, we do not yet know. It appears that the elderly may have more of a problem with aluminum, if indeed it is a cause or part of the cause of Alzheimer's disease and other brain syndromes. Those who eat refined foods, refined flours, baked goods, processed cheeses, and common table salt are more likely to have higher aluminum levels in their bodies. Those who use antacids or antiperspirants that contain aluminum, or who cook with aluminum foil or kitchenware, will also have more contact with this potentially toxic mineral.

Treatment of toxicity: Decreasing contact with and use of aluminum-containing substances will reduce intake and allow more aluminum to leave the body. Oral chelating agents will also help clear aluminum more rapidly. Tetracycline is actually a mild chelator for aluminum. Calcium disodium edetate (EDTA) binds and clears aluminum from the body; this substance is fairly nontoxic and is used as the agent for "chelation therapy," an intravenous treatment used to pull metals such as lead from the body, and more recently used in the treatment of atherosclerosis and cardiovascular diseases. Deferoxamine, an iron chelator, also binds aluminum. In a study with Alzheimer's patients, nearly 40 percent of the patients showed an improvement in symptoms with deferoxamine treatment. There is some evidence that intravenous chelation with EDTA helps Alzheimer's patients. More research is needed to evaluate aluminum's involvement with this disease.

To evaluate toxic states of aluminum, the best testing we have is hair analysis, ideally used along with blood and urine analysis. The values can be followed during treatment by a doctor to see whether higher amounts are being eliminated and lesser amounts retained in body tissues.

Prevention: The best way to prevent aluminum buildup is to avoid the sources of aluminum. Eliminating foods that have aluminum additives is probably healthier overall. Not using common table salt is a positive health step as well. Some tap waters contain aluminum; this can be checked. Avoiding aluminum cookware and replacing it with stainless steel, ceramic, or glass is a good idea. Blocking skin and sweat pores with aluminum antiperspirants has always seemed strange to me; I would think it would be better to cleanse regularly, reduce stress, balance weight, and eat a wholesome diet that creates sweat that smells more like roses.

 Arsenic Despite arsenic's reputation as a poison, it actually has fairly low toxicity in comparison with some other metals, although with chronic exposure there is some concern about arsenic's effect on chromosomes and its carcinogenicity. In fact, arsenic may even be essential and functional in humans in very small amounts. It has been shown to be essential in rats and other animals, though it is found in higher concentrations in them than in humans.

Organic arsenic as arsenates (+5 form of arsenic) and elemental arsenic both found naturally in the earth and in foods do not readily produce toxicity. In fact, they are handled fairly easily by the body and eliminated by the kidneys. The inorganic arsenites or trivalent forms of arsenic, such as arsenic trioxide used industrially and found as a food contaminate, seem to create the problems. They accumulate in the body, particularly in the skin, hair, and nails, but also in internal organs. On the average, there is about 10–20 mg. of arsenic in the human body; higher levels may lead to problems. Arsenic can accumulate when kidney function is decreased. Luckily, absorption of arsenic is fairly low, usually less than 5 percent, so most is eliminated in the feces and some in the urine.

Hair and blood levels are currently the best way to evaluate arsenic levels. They will usually show increased levels when higher amounts are present in the body.

Sources: Arsenic is present in small amounts in soil and therefore is present in our food. It is present in the ocean, so there is some arsenic in most seafood, especially the filtering mollusks, such as clams and oysters. Some arsenic is present as a contaminant in meats as well.

Arsenic is also found in many fuel oils and coal, so it is added to the environment when these are burned. Weed killers and some insecticides (particularly the lead-arsenate sprays) are the main sources of contamination with arsenic. This use of arsenic is responsible for a twentyfold increase in the level found in humans since ancient times. Even so, this in itself is not a great cause for concern about wide-range toxicity.

Methods of toxicity: Though there is some suggestion that arsenic may be useful in the human body, no clear biological function has yet been proved. In some studies, arsenic has been shown to promote longevity in rats. The importance of arsenic in cardiac function in humans is being studied. Though arsenic can displace phosphorus and phosphates in some reactions in the body, this is not known to lead to any definite physiological change.

Symptoms of toxicity: These are not clearly known. The average intake of arsenic is estimated at 1 mg. per day, mainly from food, but this is not toxic arsenic; this organic arsenic bound in food is generally well tolerated. Elemental arsenic can accumulate in the body and be a problem, and the oxidized forms of arsenic are toxic in large amounts. Arsenic trioxide is used industrially and is the strongest poison of the arsenics. Below 7–10 ppm of arsenic in hair is a relatively safe level.

Amounts leading to toxicity: There is no clear picture of arsenic deficiency or toxicity in humans. Possible effects of arsenic toxicity include hair loss, dermatitis, diarrhea and other gastrointestinal symptoms, fatigue, headaches, confusion, muscle pains, red and white blood cell problems, neurologic symptoms, and liver and kidney damage. Acute arsenic exposure may cause a rapid series of symptoms. Arsine gas exposure is very toxic to the lungs and kidneys and is often fatal. Death from low-level, chronic arsenic exposure has the appearance of death from natural causes, very good for mystery books.

Who is susceptible? Exposure to insecticides, weed killers, contaminated meats, and fumes from the burning of arsenic-containing coals and oils may cause some toxicity problems. Miners, smelters, and vineyard workers may have a higher level of arsenic trioxide exposure and a higher incidence of lung can-

cer. The body does not clear trivalent arsenic as easily as it does some other toxic minerals, so buildup can occur with regular exposure, generating chronic problems.

Treatment: Chelation therapy with EDTA can clear some arsenic, but not as easily as it clears some of the other heavy metals. Dimercaprol is the treatment of choice for arsenic toxicity, but it should be given in the first 24 hours after exposure. Vitamin C protects the body somewhat from arsenic toxicity.

Prevention: Again, avoiding sources of contamination from arsenic is all we can do.

Cadmium has become a more prevalent cause for concern in recent years. Like lead, it is an underground mineral that did not enter our air, food, and water in significant amounts until it was mined as part of zinc deposits. Now there is widespread environmental contamination with cadmium.

As cadmium and zinc are found together in natural deposits, so are they similar in structure and function in the human body. Cadmium may actually displace zinc in some of its important enzymatic and organ functions; thus, it interferes with these functions or prevents them from being completed. The zinc-cadmium ratio is very important, as cadmium toxicity and storage are greatly increased with zinc deficiency, and good levels of zinc protect against tissue damage by cadmium. The refinement of grains reduces the zinc-cadmium ratio, so zinc deficiency and cadmium toxicity are more likely when the diet is high in refined grains and flours.

Cadmium levels in humans tend to increase with age (probably because of chronic subtle exposure), usually peaking at around age 50 and then levelling off. No cadmium is present in newborns. Interestingly, cadmium does not cross the placenta-fetal barrier or the blood-brain barrier as lead and mercury do, so it is not toxic to fetuses, nor does it cause the mental and brain symptoms of lead and mercury.

We may have as much as 40 mg. of cadmium in our body and probably consume at least 40 mcg. daily. Levels vary according to region, as we get most of it from soil by way of our food. There may be some in water from contamination and water pipes, and cigarette smoke plus industrial burning of metals puts some cadmium into the air. Cadmium levels in the atmosphere are much higher in industrial cities.

Cadmium is not very well absorbed, with a rate of about 20 percent, but this is still a higher rate than that of many other minerals. Cadmium is not particularly well eliminated. Besides fecal losses, it is excreted mainly by the kidneys. This mineral is stored primarily in the liver and kidneys. As zinc has an affinity for the testes, cadmium is also stored there in higher concentrations than in other tissues. With zinc deficiency, more cadmium is stored. With aging, cadmium accumulates in the kidneys and may predispose to hypertension. As I stated, it does not get into the brain, nor does it pass into the fetus during pregnancy or the breast milk with lactation.

Sources: There are many sources from which our environment and our bodies can be contaminated with cadmium. Cigarette smoke, refined foods, water pipes, coffee and tea, coal burning, and shellfish are all definite sources. Cadmium is also a component of alloys, used in electrical materials, and is present in ceramics, dental materials, and storage batteries.

During the growth of grains such as wheat and rice, cadmium (from the soil) is concentrated in the core of the kernel, while zinc is found mostly in the germ and bran coverings. With refinement, zinc is lost, increasing the cadmium ratio. Refined flours, rice, and sugar all have relatively higher ratios of cadmium to zinc than do the whole foods.

One pack of cigarettes contains about 20 mcg. of cadmium, or about 1 mcg. per cigarette. About 30 percent of that goes into the lungs and is absorbed, and the remaining 70 percent goes into the atmosphere to be inhaled by others or to contaminate the environment. With long-term smoking, the risk of cadmium toxicity is increased. Though most of it is eliminated, a little bit is stored every day. Marijuana may also concentrate cadmium, so regular smoking of cannabis may also be a risk factor for toxicity from this metal.

Water pipes can be a source of cadmium concentration. Cadmium is often used to protect metals from corrosion. Galvanized (zinc) pipes usually contain some cadmium, as does the solder used to hold them together. Soft or acid water is corrosive and causes the metals in the pipes to break down, releasing cadmium and other minerals from them. Hard water containing calcium and magnesium salts actually coats the pipes and protects against the leaching of other minerals.

Air pollution of cadmium comes from zinc mining and refining, and from the burning of coal. Cadmium is also an industrial contaminant from the steel-making process.

Soil levels of cadmium are increased by cadmium in water, by sewage contamination, by cadmium in the air, and by high-phosphate fertilizers. Coffee and tea may contain significant cadmium levels. Root vegetables such as potatoes may pick up more cadmium, and the grains can concentrate cadmium. Seafood, particularly crustaceans, such as crab and lobster, and mollusks, such as clams and oysters, have higher cadmium levels, though many are also higher in zinc, balancing the cadmium.

Methods of toxicity: Though cadmium has no known useful biological functions, it competes with zinc for binding sites and can therefore interfere with some of zinc's essential functions. In this way, it may inhibit enzyme reactions and utilization of nutrients. Cadmium may be a catalyst to oxidation reactions, which can generate free-radical tissue damage.

241

Symptoms of Toxicity: In his book *Trace Elements and Man*, the late expert in trace and toxic elements Henry Schroeder, M.D., described in detail cadmium's involvement in generating, or at least contributing to, high blood pressure. Cadmium concentrates in the kidney and can generate kidney tissue damage and hypertension, as well as an increased incidence of calcium kidney stones. Initially, protein and sugar may be spilled in the urine. Some patients with high blood pressure show elevated urine cadmium levels. This hypertension is likely related to the reduced zinc-cadmium ratio. The cadmium effect may contribute not only to hypertension but to heart disease as well. In rat studies, higher levels of cadmium are associated with an increase in heart size, higher blood pressure, progressive atherosclerosis, and reduced kidney function. And in rats as well as in humans, cadmium toxicity is worse with zinc deficiency and reduced with higher zinc intake.

Cadmium appears to depress some immune functions, mainly by reducing host resistance to bacteria and viruses. It may also increase cancer risk, possibly for the lungs and prostate. Cadmium toxicity has been implicated in generating prostate enlargement, possibly by interfering with zinc support.

Cadmium also affects the bones. It has been known to cause bone and joint aches and pains. This syndrome, first described in Japan, where it was termed the *itai-itai* ("ouch-ouch") disease, was caused by cadmium pollution there. It was also associated with weak bones that lead to deformities, especially of the spine, or to more easily broken bones. This disease was fatal in many cases.

We may be seeing an increase in emphysema due to cadmium exposure. Anemia also seems to be a problem. Most of these potential cadmium toxicity problems, including its immunosuppressant actions and its role in cancer, hypertension, and heart and kidney disease, need to be substantiated by more research.

Amounts leading to toxicity: What level of cadmium causes toxicity is not clear; zinc levels in the body play a role in determining this. Estimates of daily cadmium exposure range from 25 to more than 200 mcg., mostly from food. About 40–50 mcg. daily is probably a safe guess. This should be handled fairly well by a normally functioning body. Below 2 ppm in hair and .015 ppm in whole blood are considered current normal ranges for body cadmium levels.

Who is susceptible? People who have higher exposure to cadmium are at higher risk. Industrial workers, metal workers, zinc miners, and anyone who works with zinc galvanization may accumulate more cadmium. Those who drink soft water; those who smoke or whose friends, roommates, or coworkers smoke; coffee and tea drinkers; and those who eat refined flours, sugars, and white rice are also likely to receive greater exposure to cadmium.

Treatment: Intravenous EDTA chelation is effective in increasing cadmium elimination, though this is probably indicated only at more toxic levels. Avoiding further cadmium exposure is emphasized. High intake of zinc as well as of calcium and selenium will protect against further cadmium absorption, and adequate body levels of zinc may displace some tissue cadmium. Iron, copper, selenium, and vitamin C have been shown to increase cadmium elimination as well, as can be measured by urine levels. Hair analysis is a good way to follow cadmium levels.

Prevention: With good health, cadmium is probably not a problem unless there is increased exposure, zinc deficiency, or weakened kidney function. Cadmium toxicity also seems to be a little worse with lead intoxication. There are two good ways to protect against cadmium toxicity. The first is to avoid cadmium exposure and intake—primarily by minimizing smoking and exposure to cigarette smoke, avoiding refined foods, shellfish, coffee, tea, and soft water. Air contamination is usually minimal compared to that from food and water. The second way to protect against cadmium toxicity is to maintain good zinc levels by eating high-zinc foods, such as whole grains, legumes, and nuts (oysters are high in zinc but also high in cadmium). Taking additional zinc, 15–30 mg. daily in a supplement, will offer further protection against cadmium problems.

 Lead "Get the lead out!" is a common idiom referring to a heaviness of a body that cannot quite get moving. The heavy metal lead is the most common toxic mineral and the most abundant contaminant of our environment and our body. It is the worst and most widespread pollutant, though luckily not the most toxic; cadmium and mercury are worse. But when lead levels become too high, they can prove fatal, and this heavy metal will return our body to its origins in the earth.

Lead is found deep within the earth. Ancient civilizations had almost no exposure to it until four or five thousand years ago, when lead was found as a by-product of silver smelting. Since then, it has been used progressively throughout history. In the Roman Empire, lead was widely used in water pipes and drinking and storage vessels. Many scientists and historians now feel that lead led to the downfall of the Roman Empire, with the ruling classes suffering decreased mental capacities, decreased birthrate, and shortened life span.

In the twentieth century, lead has been widely used in paint, some containing a high percentage of lead. This has been a problem especially with children, who are more sensitive to lead than adults because of their better absorption and smaller bodies. Lead has a mildly sweet taste, and children often suck on or eat the paint chips off of houses or out of the dirt, leading to many cases of lead poisoning. In the 1920s, tetraethyl lead was added to gasoline as an antiknock, higher-octane additive. This has probably been the most widespread and pervasive source of environ-

mental contamination from lead to date. Other common uses for lead are as seals for tin cans, in pewter, in ceramics and pottery glazes, in insecticides, and more.

In recent years, however, there has been an attempt to decrease this environmental contamination. Cars are now using unleaded gasoline. This does not, of course, eliminate the problems of carbon monoxide and burned hydrocarbons, but it will help to decrease lead exposure in the future. In 1971, Congress passed the Lead Paint Act, limiting the use of lead in paints. This will also help, but not for many years to come, since many older homes still contain leaded paints. As they deteriorate, lead gets into the soil and does not degrade. In 1979, a law was passed decreasing the use of lead in food storage cans, though it is still present in some solders.

Bone analysis of very old skeletons indicates that modern humans have nearly 500–1,000 times more lead in our bones than did our ancient ancestors. Our total body content of lead nowadays is estimated at 125–200 mg. We can handle nearly 1–2 mg. daily with normal functioning, but the margin of safety is narrow. Luckily, most people's daily exposure is less than that, about 300–400 mcg.

Lead is a neurotoxin and commonly generates abnormal brain and nerve function. It passes into the brain and can also contaminate the in-utero fetus and breast milk. Most lead, though, is stored in the bones. With lead intoxication, "lead lines" are visible in the bones on X-rays. Some is also stored in the liver and soft tissues. Infants have very little lead, but our body concentrations usually increase with age.

Luckily, lead is not very well absorbed, usually less than 5 percent, though children absorb it at a higher rate. Many minerals, such as calcium and iron, interfere with further lead absorption. When lead gets into the blood, it does not stay long, either going into the bones and other tissues or being eliminated. Most ingested lead leaves via the feces; that which is absorbed or inhaled will usually be cleared by the kidneys, through perspiration.

Evaluating lead exposure and measuring lead levels in humans is not easy. Blood and urine tests are not very good indicators, because lead is cleared fairly rapidly. With acute toxicity, both of these body fluids may have high measurements, but most exposure is chronic. Hair analysis is the simplest and best test for evaluating chronic lead poisoning, which has become much more common with long-term exposure. Hair-test screening for lead is fairly reliable and can be done on both adults and children. Hair (and urine) levels can be remeasured to follow the progress of treatment. Increased body burdens of lead can be shown by testing with an intravenous dose of a chelating drug such as EDTA. A high level of urinary lead elimination suggests increased levels of body stores, especially in the bones. Also, since lead interferes with many red blood cell enzymes such as *delta-aminolevulinic acid dehydratase*, an increase in delta-aminolevulinic acid in the urine, as well as zinc protoporphyrin and erythrocyte protoporphyrin, suggests problems of lead toxicity. A blood level of zinc protoporphyrin is currently the best way to assess lead toxicity.

Sources: Lead exposure and body lead levels are higher in North America than anywhere else in the world. In the United States alone, it is estimated that approximately 1.3 million tons of lead are used yearly in batteries, solder, pottery, pigments, gasoline, paint, and many other useful substances. Somewhere between 400,000 and 600,000 tons per year go into our atmosphere, onto our earth, into our food, and into our body and tissues. So there is a lot of lead around. The following are some of the common contaminants:

Leaded gasoline. Tetraethyl lead was previously added to all gasoline; it is now used only for older vehicles. After combustion, this lead goes directly into the atmosphere as air pollution and is inhaled by us and other living, breathing entities. It also settles into the earth and its living vegetation; heavily traveled roadways show higher concentrations of lead in the air, soil, and nearby vegetation.

Paint. Though, by law, the amount of lead in paints must be reduced, some still contain lead. Many homes retain lead paints, so this change may not affect us in environmental lead exposure for a couple of decades.

Food. Lead is contained in many foods, especially in those grown near industrial areas or busy cities or roadways. Grains, legumes, commercial and garden fruit, and most meat products pick up some lead. Liver and lunch meats are usually higher. Liverwurst and other sausages may contain more lead than other foods. Roadside vegetation, such as herbs, fruits, and vegetables, has higher concentrations of lead than vegetation growing in more secluded areas. Measurements of lead in trees growing along roads show much more than was present in the 1930s. Bonemeal, a source of calcium and magnesium, is usually made from cattle bones and may contain high amounts of lead. Dolomite, an earth rock source of calcium and magnesium, is usually lower in lead. Pet foods may also be high.

Water. Drinking water may be contaminated with lead. Lead solder in pipes or lead plumbing in older homes and drinking fountains, can leach into the water, especially soft water. A more acid water will also pull lead and other toxic and nontoxic minerals from the piping.

Pottery. "Earthenware" in general has potential for lead exposure. Though some potters refrain from using much lead, it is hard to avoid. When the glazing is inefficient, lead containers can contaminate food stored in them. Fruit juices or acidic foods, such as tomatoes, will tend to pull out more minerals. Glazed coffee mugs should be avoided.

Cans. Solder in tin cans, usually used to hold the seam together, contains lead; some are nearly 100 percent lead. Some can manufacturers are changing this, but progress is slow. Avoid lead-lined containers or cans whose seams have a shiny, metallic solder appearance. Many imported cans contain lead. The leaded plugs in evaporated milk cans may contaminate the milk.

Cosmetics. Many pigments and other substances used for makeup and other cosmetics contain lead. Historically, lead has been part of face paints and other beauty creams.

Cigarettes. Lead is occasionally a contaminant in cigarettes. Lead arsenate may be used as an insecticide in tobacco growing.

Pesticides. Many pesticides and insecticides contain some lead, mainly as the lead-arsenate base.

Methods of toxicity: Though this is not completely clear, lead most likely interferes with functions performed by essential minerals such as calcium, iron, copper, and zinc. Lead does interrupt several red blood cell enzyme systems, including *delta-aminolevulinic dehydratase* and *ferrochelatase*. Especially in brain chemistry, lead may create abnormal function by inactivating important zinc-, copper-, and iron-dependent enzymes. (When body levels of these three minerals are high, there is first less absorption of lead and then more competition with lead for enzyme-binding sites.) Lead affects both the brain and the peripheral nerves. It may also diminish hemoglobin synthesis and can react with cell membranes. This may cause increased permeability of the cells and damage or even death of those cells. Lead can displace calcium in bone, deposit there, and form softer, denser spots that can be seen on X-rays as "lead lines." Lead also binds with the sulfhydryl bonds and inactivates the cysteine-containing enzymes, thus allowing more internal toxicity from free radicals, chemicals, and other heavy metals.

Lead is also an immunosuppressant; it lowers host resistance to bacteria and viruses, and thus allows an increase in infections. It may also influence our cancer risk. How lead affects the gastrointestinal tract causing symptoms, including a coliclike pain, is still uncertain.

Symptoms of toxicity: An estimated nearly 20 percent of men and 10 percent of women have problems with lead toxicity, though it is not clear what levels of chronic lead toxicity, which is most common, will produce symptoms. Lead in the body subtly interferes with optimum function and general health, and other toxicity factors may affect this. Lead accumulation may also cause shifts in important body minerals, such as zinc, calcium, and manganese.

Early signs of lead toxicity may be overlooked, as they are fairly vague: headache, fatigue, muscle pains, anorexia, constipation, vomiting, pallor, anemia. These can be followed by agitation, irritability, restlessness, memory loss, poor coordination and vertigo, and depression.

Acute lead toxicity symptoms include abdominal pain similar to colic, nausea and vomiting, anemia, muscle weakness, and encephalopathy. Lead encephalopathy is a brain syndrome that can arise also from advanced chronic toxicity. It is characterized by poor balance, confusion, vertigo, hallucinations, and speech and hearing problems.

A low level of lead intoxication may affect brain function and activity more subtly, influencing intelligence, attention span, language, and memory. Insomnia and nightmares may be experienced. Hyperactivity and even retardation and senility may also result. Moderate levels of lead may reduce immune and kidney function and increase risk of infection, and may be another factor in increasing blood pressure. There is some suggestion that lead intoxication may correlate with cancer rates. Further research is needed in this area. With heavy lead intoxication, death may result.

In children, lead is a special cause for concern. Hyperactivity and learning disorders have been correlated with lead intoxication; children with these problems should be checked. Several studies have shown a relationship between lead levels and learning defects, including daydreaming, being easily frustrated or distracted, a decreased ability to follow instruction or a low persistence in learning, and general excitability and hyperactivity. There is also a recent correlation between sudden infant death syndrome (SIDS) and increased lead levels. This needs further research to implicate lead intoxication as a cause of death.

Amounts leading to toxicity: The average daily intake of lead, as estimated by weveral researchers, ranges from 200–400 mcg. Most of that, 80–90 percent, comes from food or contamination from car exhaust. Average absorption is about 5–10 percent, so most of us should be able to eliminate most of what we get. Actually, with proper function we can excrete many times more lead than that daily.

It is not clear what exposures or body levels of lead will actually produce functional difficulties or specific symptoms; this probably varies from person to person. In measurements of any nutrient or chemical in the body, there is an estimated normal, or reference, range, above which some problems or symptoms may appear. For the level of lead in hair, the reference range of the lab that my office uses is 0–30 ppm. Many authorities set lower levels, perhaps below 15–20 ppm, as a concern; Doctor's Data in Chicago uses 10 ppm. Even lower amounts, especially in children, may be a body burden and interfere with optimum brain and metabolic functions. For whole blood measurements, below .40 ppm is usually considered within the normal range; less than .20 ppm is probably ideal. In children, lower levels than that, even .10 ppm may be a concern.

Who is susceptible? There is a long list (hundreds) of industrial and other workers who have a higher than average potential for exposure to lead. Obviously, anyone who works directly with lead has more exposure. Working in zinc or vanadium mining can also increase lead exposure.

As stated, children are especially at risk for lead toxicity. For instance, teething children

LEAD-SUSCEPTIBLE OCCUPATIONS

Lead miners and other lead workers
Insecticide makers and users
Glass makers and polishers
Dye makers and dyers
Vehicle tunnel workers
Police and fire fighters
Linoleum and tile makers
Solder makers and solderers
Shellac, varnish, and lacquer makers
Wood stainers
Pottery glaze workers
Paint makers and painters
Garage mechanics
Wallpaper makers and hangers
TV picture tube makers
Metal workers and refiners
Toll booth collectors
Dentists and dental technicians
Soap makers
Plumbers
Ink makers
Farmers
Bookbinders
Enamel workers
Canners
Printers
Bronzers
Battery makers
Crop dusters
Highway workers
Match makers
Rubber makers
Welders
Cable makers

may be exposed to lead; it is especially true for children living in older or low-income housing or who live and play near busy streets. Much less exposure than would affect adults can lead to problems in children, because their absorption is better and their bodies are smaller. A small amount of leaded paint can increase body levels enough to create symptoms of toxicity. Children showing signs of hyperactivity or poor learning should be screened for lead levels.

Pregnant women and even the fetus are at risk of lead exposure. Anyone who works around car exhaust or in any of the many industries in which lead is used, from printing to painting to plumbing, should be aware of lead problems and probably get checked for lead levels every few years, until we as a society are able to lower our lead use and environmental exposure.

Treatment: EDTA, a synthetic amino acid, is the standard intravenous medical treatment for lead poisoning. It is a strong chelating agent, as it "claws" or latches onto metals and increases their urinary excretion. This treatment for lead intoxication led to use of the newer "chelation therapy" for other problems as well, as some of the patients treated for lead poisoning also experienced improvement of cardiovascular symptoms. This benefit may be a result of pulling out extra calcium and other metals that may be clogging arteries. Though chelation therapy is a controversial treatment that warrants further research, EDTA does much for lead and most heavy metal intoxication. This intravenous treatment is administered by a doctor, often in a hospital setting. Other medical treatments for lead intoxication include Dimercaprol (British antilewisite, BAL), given intramuscularly, and oral D-penicillamine. Treatment by any of these pharmaceutical agents has risks, so the level of lead intoxication should be accurately assessed.

To reduce lead toxicity, a high-calcium diet or supplemental calcium will inhibit further lead absorption. Injections of calcium chloride and extra vitamin D will increase body levels of calcium, which may even displace some lead stored in the tissues, particularly the bones. Vitamin C also helps improve elimina-

tion of lead and other metals. The amino acids cysteine and methionine have some effect in detoxifying lead and other toxins, and foods such as eggs and beans, which contain these sulfhydryl-group amino acids, may also help bind and clear additional lead.

Prevention: Obviously, the number one prevention is to restrict lead exposure. That involves awareness of increased lead contamination potential. The following are some ways to practice this prevention:

- Do not exercise along freeways or in heavy traffic.
- Do not allow children to play near busy streets.
- Do not store food in pottery.
- Avoid soldered cans, which are mostly the tin cans.
- Evaluate for lead levels any questionable substances, such as water or bone meal, that are used regularly.

More positive things we can do to reduce lead problems in our body include eating a wholesome diet with plenty of fresh fruits, vegetables, and whole grains to obtain adequate minerals, avoiding refined foods, and possibly taking a mineral supplement so as to competitively reduce lead absorption. Calcium and magnesium do this well, so a good level of these minerals in our diet, as well as supplements, can reduce lead contamination. Iron, copper, and zinc also do this. With low mineral intake, lead absorption and potential toxicity are increased.

Algin in the diet, as from kelp (seaweed) or the supplement sodium alginate, helps to bind lead and other heavy metals in the gastrointestinal tract and carry them to elimination. Pectin and other fiber foods in the diet will also tend to bind the heavier metals and reduce absorption. With this, though, we need to take more of our essential vitamins and minerals, such as the Bs, vitamin C, iron, calcium, zinc, copper, and chromium, to help decrease lead absorption. As mentioned, L-cysteine, 250 mg. twice daily, is a sulfur-containing, detoxifying amino acid that will help bind and eliminate lead.

Children can be somewhat protected by getting adequate iron, calcium, and vitamins C and E in their diet and as supplements in appropriate amounts for their age. This program may also help get a little of that lead out and keep them clear thinking, more balanced, and active (but not hyperactive).

Our understanding of lead is just beginning. Better prevention and treatments for lead intoxication, along with reduced lead use by industry in fuels, cars, paints, and so on, should enable us to control the problems associated with this widespread contaminant.

Mercury, or "quicksilver," is a shiny liquid metal that is a widespread environmental contaminant. It is fairly toxic, though the metallic mercury is less so. Especially a problem is methyl or ethyl mercury, or mercuric chloride, which is very poisonous.

Modern humans have much higher body levels of mercury than did our ancestors, because of its greater use in recent times. It has been used for more than 2,000 years. Nowadays, mercury is employed daily by medical and dental practices in thermometers, drugs (more so in the past), and amalgam for fillings; by agriculture in fungicides and pesticides; and by the cosmetics industry. Mercury in industrial waste has polluted our waters and contaminated our fresh- and salt-water plants and fish.

In the 1950s, Minamata Bay in Japan was poisoned with industrial mercury; it was measured in the waters at between 5 and 15 ppm, about 20 times normal. Many people experienced serious nervous system symptoms, staggering, and even comas and death before the pollution was discovered. In the early 1970s,

the "mercury in the fish" scare spread across the United States. Swordfish, tuna, and other large fish were the subjects of concern, and, in some areas, were measured with higher than acceptable levels of mercury. Caused by industrial contamination, the problem was not as widespread as the concern. Currently, most fish do not contain toxic or problematic levels of mercury, though further contamination could certainly raise the possibility.

Today, the average person's body contains about 10–15 mg. of mercury. We obtain some daily from food, air, and water. Mercury is poorly absorbed from the intestinal tract, about 5–10 percent. Inhaled mercury fumes go into the blood, as mercury is soluble and passes through the lungs. Some mercury is retained in body tissues, mainly in the kidneys, which store about 50 percent of the body mercury. The blood, bones, liver, spleen, brain, and fat tissue also hold mercury. This potentially toxic metal does get into the brain and nerve tissue, so central nervous system symptoms may develop. Mercury can also get into a growing fetus and into breast milk. But mercury is also eliminated daily through the urine and feces. Hair tissue analysis is the best way to measure body stores of mercury, while urine levels will show whether the body is actively working to eliminate it.

Sources: Mercury is widely used in industry, agriculture, and health care. Even though hat makers are safer and saner these days since the mercury used for the felt linings of hats was reduced, there are still people walking about "mad as a hatter" from mercury. Common uses of mercury include:

Fungicides and pesticides. These are a large source, used worldwide to treat grains and seeds. Methyl mercury is the most common form here.

Cosmetics. Mercury is added to decrease bacterial growth.

Dental fillings. Mercury is widely used, though many dentists no longer employ the silver-mercury amalgam, as they feel that it leads to a variety of problems. The American Dental Association, however, still claims that there is no proven mercury toxicity due to dental amalgams.

Medicines. Organic mercurial diuretics have been the most common, though these are less used these days. Mercury-containing cathartics, anthelminetics, and teething powders were also employed in the past. Broken thermometers can increase mercury exposure, and mecurochrome also contains mercury.

Coal burning. This releases mercury into the atmosphere.

Fish. Fish may contain varying amounts of mercury. Ocean bacteria, algae, and small fish may all contain some; mercury concentrations usually increase with the size of the fish. An excessive intake of fish foods may lead to increased body levels of mercury.

Other sources of mercury are mirrors, latex paints, fabric softeners, felt, floor waxes and polishes, sewage sludge, laxatives containing calomel, cinnabar jewelry, tatoo dyes, and many others. Most of these are not specifically mercury toxic, as they do not give off high amounts of volatile mercury. Fungicides are the most widely used and probably the most potentially toxic.

Methods of toxicity: Mercury has no known essential functions, though it was at one time used to treat syphilis, with some success. Mercury probably affects the inherent protein structure which may interfere with functions relating to protein production. Mercury has a strong affinity for sulfhydryl, amine, phosphoryl, and carboxyl groups, and inactivates a wide range of enzyme systems, as well as causing injury to cell membranes. However, none of mercury's specific body interactions are clearly defined, though the main problems seem to result from its attack on the nervous system. Mercury may also interfere with some functions of selenium, and can be an immunosuppressant.

Symptoms of toxicity: There are many processes and symptoms of mercury toxicity. Poisoning can come from four categories of mercury: metallic or elemental mercury, which is relatively mild; inorganic mercury, such as mercury chlorides, which primarily affect the kidneys; organo-mercurials, such as mercury salts in diuretics or fungicides, which convert to inorganic mercury; and short chain alkyl mercury compounds, of which methyl mercury is the most toxic, more so than ethyl or diethyl mercury.

Acute symptoms are caused mainly by mercuric chloride or methyl mercury exposure. Chronic, lower level exposure may lead to specific acute symptoms or to subtle renal and nervous system problems. Inhaled mercury has a different effect differently than ingested mercury, for which most symptoms are related to the gastrointestinal tract and the nervous system. Inhaling high levels of metallic mercury (in an industrial setting or a dentist's office) can cause acute symptoms, such as fever, chills, coughing, and chest pain. With low, long-term exposure, more subtle symptoms such as fatigue, headache, insomnia, nervousness, impaired judgment and coordination, emotional lability, and loss of sex drive, may be experienced. Ingested mercury may cause stomatitis and gastrointestinal inflammation, with nausea, vomiting, abdominal pain, and bloody diarrhea, progressing to neurological problems. These symptoms, which are often confused with psychogenic causes, are referred to as "micromercurialism."

Mild or early symptoms of mercury intoxication include fatigue, insomnia, irritability, anorexia, loss of sex drive, headache, and forgetfulness or poor memory. This may lead to other nervous system symptoms, such as dizziness, tremors, incoordination, and depression; then progress to numbness and tingling, most commonly of the hands, feet, or lips; and to further weakness, worse memory and coordination, reduced hearing and speech, paralysis, and psychosis. Mercury toxicity may be a factor in multiple sclerosis. Other problems of severe mercury intoxication are kidney and brain damage, as well as birth defects in pregnant women. Luckily, these extreme symptoms are unusual. However, the subtle and nervous system symptoms from low-level chronic exposure may be more common than we realize.

Amounts leading to toxicity: The average intake of mercury varies with location and diet. It may range from 10 mcg. to more than 500 mcg., mainly depending on air contamination. Industrial cities and heavily sprayed farmland have the highest levels. The average overall daily intake is probably about 30–50 mcg. Most humans can process at least that much daily without any problems.

Blood levels of mercury should be below .02 ppm, while hair levels may be higher, up to about 3-5 ppm. More than 5 ppm becomes a concern. When these levels are exceeded, we should look for the sources of increased exposure and work toward avoiding or eliminating them.

Who is susceptible? Anyone working with mercury, especially methyl or ethyl mercury or mercuric chloride, is more likely to have problems of mercury toxicity. Farmers using mercury products should be very careful with them and should be aware of mercury toxicity symptoms or have mercury levels checked every couple of years.

Treatment of toxicity: Drinking milk helps reduce the acute effects of mercury, as the mercury will act on the protein in the milk instead of on the stomach and intestinal lining. This may prevent the acute symptoms of gastrointestinal tissue irritation, such as vomiting and bleeding.

Penicillamine is a chelating drug that can pull mercury out of the circulation. It works best when given soon after exposure, rather than after tissue storage occurs. Penicillamine itself, however, is potentially toxic. Dimercaprol (BAL) has also been used. EDTA, a

OCCUPATIONS WITH POTENTIAL MERCURY EXPOSURE

Barometer and thermometer makers
Ink makers
Dentists and dental workers
Paint makers
Dental amalgam makers
Neon light makers
Mirror makers
Paper makers
Insecticide makers
Dye makers
Pesticide workers
Embalmers
Explosives and fireworks makers
Jewelers
Wood preservative workers
Photographers

stronger chelating agent, can also be used to pull out body mercury. It usually has fewer side effects than penicillamine. Vitamin C, selenium, and the fibers pectin and algin may also reduce mercury levels and toxicity, though usually only in cases of less severity.

Prevention: Avoidance of mercury contamination is foremost in preventing mercury toxicity. Staying clear of mercury fungicides and avoiding fungicide-treated foods or eating only organically grown grains and produce may be helpful. Many health-oriented dentists now avoid mercury-containing amalgam to prevent further mercury exposure. Silver-mercury fillings during pregnancy, I believe, should be avoided.

Pectin and algin can decrease absorption of mercury, especially inorganic mercury. Selenium binds both inorganic and methyl mercury; mercury selenide is formed and excreted in fecal matter. Selenium is, for many reasons, an important nutrient for all of us, and in an amount of at least 100–200 mcg., it does seem to protect against heavy metal toxicity.

Other Metal Concerns

 Antimony is probably only slightly toxic in human beings, though in rats it affects the heart and reduces the life span. We obtain antimony mainly from food and water, with some from the air. Other sources are pottery glazes and cooking utensils. The approximately 100 mcg. consumed daily is poorly absorbed, and most is eliminated in the feces and urine. Our body stores some in the liver, spleen, kidneys, blood, and hair. Antimony is really only of mild concern in humans.

Industrial antimony toxicity from gaseous stibine (SbH_3) or ingestion of antimony materials is uncommon. High levels can cause acute symptoms of the gastrointestinal tract and cause damage to the kidneys, liver, and heart.

 Barium compounds are used in medical testing for X-ray evaluations; in printing, ceramics, plastics, textiles, and dyes; in fuel additives; in the production of glass, paints, paper, soap, and rubber; and in pesticides. Barium toxicity is relatively low unless there is ingestion of large amounts or aerosal exposure. Inhalation may cause short-term lung irritation. Accidental or intentional ingestion of barium may lead to vomiting, diarrhea, and abdominal pain. As barium becomes absorbed, it can displace potassium intracellularly and cause mild to severe effects in muscle tone, heart function, and the nervous system. Treatment with potassium and diuresis may reduce symptoms.

 Beryllium is very interesting as a metal; it is strong, light and heat resistant, and has a very high melting point. Thus, it is a good metal to use in airplanes and rockets. Its use has increased in recent years, and it is found in neon signs and some electrical devices. Beryllium is often part of an alloy used in bicycle wheels, fishing rods, and metal household gadgets.

However, this light metal is toxic in humans. Beryllium can reduce stores of magnesium and decrease organ function, possibly through interference with enzymes. Contamination with beryllium, primarily from its industrial uses, is becoming more widespread. Industrial smoke and rocket exhaust may contain higher than healthful levels of beryllium. Beryllium inhalation can cause shortness of breath, coughing, phlegm, and lujg inflammation, which can lead to chronic scarring and disability. There is some question as to whether airborne beryllium may accumulate in the lungs and create an increased risk of cancer. Though it is not very widely used, and its toxicity is fairly minor, more intense use could lead to further problems with people exposed to higher levels of beryllium dust.

 Bismuth is essentially nontoxic in ordinary amounts, but prolonged exposure or excessive use may lead to toxicity. This could cause mental confusion, memory loss, incoordination, slurred speech, joint pain, or muscle twitching and spasm.

The human body contains about 3 mg. of bismuth. Many people take in 20–30 mcg. per day, most of it in water, a minimal amount in food, and some from airborne contamination. Most bismuth is eliminated in the feces and urine. Some drugs, particularly remedies for the stomach, such as Pepto-Bismol, contain bismuth.

 Bromine like chlorine and fluorine is a poisonous gas. Bromine salts have been used to treat acid indigestion or for sedation. Bromine can displace chlorine in some body functions. Too much can cause toxicity. Mild symptoms may include fatigue, weakness, irritability, disturbed sleep, slow mental processes and poor memory. More severe toxicity can cause confusion and drowsiness, delirium, stupor, depression, hallucinations, and, in the extreme, psychosis.

 Thallium has again become a toxicity concern. Discovered in the 1800s by Sir William Crookes, it was used in medical treatments, for venereal diseases, gout, and tuberculosis. Its toxicity, however, caused it to fall into disuse, though thallium acetate continued to be employed for fungal skin infections for some time.

Industrial use of thallium has increased in recent years. It can form useful alloys with silver or lead and may be a byproduct of zinc and lead production. In electronics, thallium is used in power systems, such as batteries or semiconductors. It is also employed in optical lenses, photo film, jewelry, dyes and pigments, and fireworks. A bigger concern was its uses in pesticides and rodentocides, which were banned in 1975. Thallium sulfate was used with starch and glycerin to treat grains for poisoning squirrels and rodents. This led to some fatalities when humans mistakenly consumed some of that grain.

Thallium is in low concentration in the earth's crust. Humans cannot tolerate much thallium in their bodies. This mineral and its salts can enter our body through our skin, respiratory tract, or gastrointestinal route. It can be toxic in several ways. First, it can substitute for potassium in certain functions within the red blood cells, such as in the *sodium/ potassium ATPase*. Thallium also has a strong attraction to sulfhydryl groups and thus may interact with these active enzyme sites. Thallium can pass the placenta into the fetus. There is some suggestion that thallium has teratogenic effects.

Thallium has significant toxicity effects both with large acute exposure and lower-level, chronic intake. Acute ingestion can lead to nausea, vomiting, abdominal pain, bloody diarrhea, fatigue, and fever. This can be fatal through its secondary agitation state which can cause seizures and then coma and respiratory failure. If people survive this exposure, further problems can affect the kidneys, heart, and nervous system. Sensory and motor changes, peripheral neuropathy, loss of reflexes, hair loss, arrythmias, and renal disease may result. This may progress over several weeks. Most ingested thallium goes to and is excreted by the kidneys; the remainder is stored in many other tissues.

Chronic poisoning may cause polyneuritis with an inability to walk, fatigue, weight loss, and possibly reduced immunity. Thallium acetate has been used as a purposeful poison on several known occasions. Since it has no color or taste, it is well concealed in food and drinks; and it is not commonly looked for.

Thallium can be measured in the blood or urine. A 24-hour urine collection may reveal increased levels of this toxic mineral. A treatment with potassium chloride or EDTA may show increased levels of thallium in the urine.

Treatment for thallium poisoning is somewhat complex. Agents such as EDTA, dimercaprol, penicillamine, sodium iodide, and thiouracil have all been used with some benefit. Diuresis and potassium chloride are used more standardly to reduce thallium toxicity by increasing excretion levels. Prussian Blue (potassium ferric cyanoferrate) dye has been used to trap thallium in the gut after initial ingestion. Hemoperfusion or dialysis is used to reduce blood concentrations of thallium. Overall, we would be wise to avoid exposure to thallium.

Other New and Problematic Metals

Palladium, an old treatment for obesity, may be carcinogenic, but this needs further research. **Titanium**, once used to treat skin disorders and now made into beautiful jewelry, is not thought to be very toxic in the body, though there have been a few cases of high exposure causing problems.

Platinum may cause allergic pulmonary reactions in platinum workers. **Cesium** and **Tellurium** may also create some mild and infrequent toxicity. **Plutonium** is a potent carcinogen, and exposure, even small amounts in workers, is a concern.

Uranium is probably toxic, but there is little direct exposure to it. **Radon**, however, which comes from the radioactive decay of uranium, is a pollution concern in both air and water, and is probably an active carcinogen (see Chapter 11 for a more complete discussion). The government has become more concerned about radon exposure, and now there are new devices and organizations that will help us assess the levels of this radioactive element at home or at work. Some drinking waters, both city and well, also contain uranium. It is a radioactive element and, like most others, disintegrates eventually into lead. We have about 90 mcg. of uranium in our body. We obtain some in food and water, though it has low absorption and fair elimination. Toxicity, if it occurs, usually affects the kidneys.

For as long as these metals remain in common use by industry, they will continue to accumulate in our bodies. Further research is needed to better understand their effects on human health and well being.

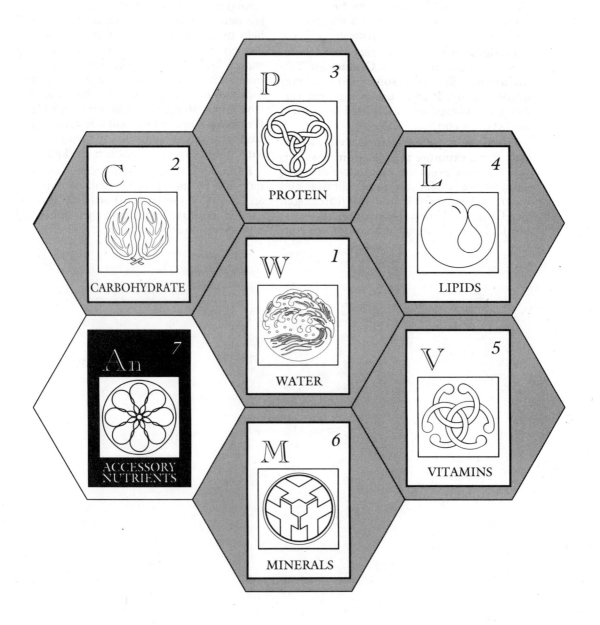

Chapter 7

Accessory Nutrients

In addition to the vitamins and minerals already discussed in detail, a number of other nutritional/biochemical supplements are in common use (many more than I will describe here). These might be prescribed by health practitioners, and various nutrients and dietary aids can be purchased in grocery stores, pharmacies, or health food stores or through the mail from many companies. Literally hundreds of new preparations are marketed each year. The supplement market has greatly improved and expanded in the last two decades, but the wide availability, heavy advertising, and variety of opinions about what is the best for us can make it very difficult for the individual to know or decide what he or she needs. And the literature from the manufacturers backing up their claims for these supplements ranges from common, promotional tales to good scientific research. Here I try to provide you with the most current, accurate information that is based on both science and experience.

This chapter deals with a variety of supplements, including digestive aids, oils, enzymes, nucleic acids, microorganisms such as bacteria and algae, herbs, glandulars, and more. Many of these are new on the market, others are as old as folklore itself. Often, new methods of production allow a nutrient to be more usable in the body. On the whole, the adventure that lies in deciding what medicinals and nutritional supplements we might take is another part of life's excitement.

O DIGESTIVE SUPPORT

A great many factors contribute to proper digestion, absorption, and utilization of the foods so needed to nourish our cells, tissues, and organs. The stomach, small intestine, liver, gallbladder, pancreas, and large intestine are primarily involved in the digestive

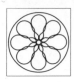

process. More subtly, the emotions, stress level, and balance within the endocrine and nervous systems also affect digestive functioning. A wide range of supplements support the digestive system. A healthy system does not need additional support. However, research shows that the natural level of hydrochloric acid (HCl) and digestive enzymes decrease as we age or if we abuse our gastrointestinal tracts and whole bodies through food excesses, chemical use, and stress. I have found that the elderly population and many younger people with digestive complaints do better with digestion-supporting nutrients. (Note that many of the special programs in Part Four suggest digestive enzymes, HCl, and other digestive aids.) I would think that most people older than 50 would have improved breakdown of foods and utilization of nutrients along with fewer gastrointestinal symptoms when supportive HCl supplements are taken with meals and additional digestive enzymes (usually pancreas extracts) are taken after eating. Occasionally, people have increased HCl secretion with acute stress; however, usually over time, chronic stress causes HCl production to decrease. The level of HCl can be measured easily, although most often an individual's symptoms will reveal if he or she is hyperacid. In that case, inappropriate supplements of HCl would create additional discomfort.

Hydrochloric Acid

[Note: People should use discretion in taking HCl, as its intake when there is already normal or excessive stomach acid production or gastritis may increase the risk of gastric irritation or ulcer development.]

The parietal cells of the stomach produce HCl and secrete it primarily in response to ingested protein or fat. Stress also may stimulate acid output. When we eat more frequently than required by the body or overconsume fats and proteins, acid production begins to decrease. Decreased HCl production may lead to poor digestion, with symptoms such as gas, bloating, and discomfort after rich meals. An HCl supplement may improve digestion of meals containing protein and/or fat, though not for foods such as rice and vegetables, which are largely carbohydrate and thus need less HCl for digestion.

Hydrochloric acid is available primarily as betaine hydrochloride. When a 5–10 grain (1 grain = 64 mg.) tablet is taken before, during, or after meals, it should help proteins break down into peptides and amino acids and fats into triglycerides. Glutamic acid hydrochloride is used sometimes in formulas, but this amino acid is only mildly acidic and does not work as well as betaine hydrochloride. Betaine may be used alone, in supplements, or along with pepsin or other digestive agents.

The use of HCl support is part of the antiaging process in this book, provided, of course, that HCl production is low. A Heidelberg capsule, gastric pH test (which directly measures stomach pH) can be done to verify a low or high acidity; then, a supplement can be administered to see what effect it has on stomach pH. One reason that stress can cause more rapid aging is that it diminishes HCl production and weakens digestion. It is the low-grade, long-term, emotionally oriented life stress that is more the culprit here. Stress in intense worriers or high-achieving businesspersons is associated more with HCl hypersecretion and peptic ulcer disease (at least initially).

Low HCl production is associated with many problems. Iron deficiency anemia, owing to poor iron absorption, and osteoporosis, resulting in part from decreased calcium absorption, are two important problems. General allergies and, specifically, food allergies are correlated with low HCl. Poor food breakdown and the "leaky gut" syndrome are associated with food allergies (see *Allergy* program in Chapter 17). More than half the people with gallstones show decreased HCl secretion compared with gallstone-free patients. Diabetics have lower secretion, as do people with eczema, psoriasis, seborrheic dermatitis, vitiligo, and tooth and periodontal disease. With low stomach acid levels, there can be an increase in bacteria, yeasts, and parasites growing in the intestines.

"But I don't want to take this forever," state many patients. We can correct our low stomach acid by eating a balanced diet of wholesome foods and by reducing our daily levels of stress. Niacin, vitamin B_3, stimulates HCl production. This can be taken before meals, as can magnesium chloride and pyridoxal-5-phosphate (the active form of vitamin B_6) to help stimulate the body's own HCl. I have suggested drinking the juice of half a lemon squeezed in water or a teaspoon of apple cider vinegar in a glass of warm water 20–30 minutes before meals with some success. Rosemary, ginger, cumin, or orange peel, used to make tea and drunk before meals, can also be helpful.

I have come to believe that the digestive tract and its function may be the single most important body component determining health and disease. Maintaining normal digestion, assimilation, and elimination is a necessity, and when these functions are faulty, we may not be aware that these dysfunctions are contributing to so many other problems. Another key digestive factor is that HCl is a stimulus to pancreatic secretions, containing the majority of enzymes that actively break down foods. The poor digestion of proteins, fats, and carbohydrates then further contributes to poor assimilation and nutritional problems. Thus, when they are needed, supplemental support of digestive enzymes may be even more important than HCl.

Digestive Enzymes

[Note: People should be aware that the use of digestive enzymes is not suggested when there is inflammation of the stomach lining.]

A number of digestive enzyme supplements are available. The simple ones are extracted from tropical fruits: bromelain from pineapple and papain from papayas. Papain has a mild, soothing effect on the stomach and aids in protein digestion. Bromelain is probably more important; it is an anti-inflammatory enzyme useful in posttraumatic responses and swelling and after surgery. It is also part of an antiaging program as it reduces tissue irritation. This proteolytic enzyme of pineapple also has

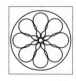

several actions that make it helpful in the prevention and treatment of cardiovascular disease. It reduces platelet aggregation, arterial plaqueing, and clot formation; 400–1,000 mg. daily has been shown to reduce the symptoms of angina pectoris. *Bromelain's* most popular use has been to reduce joint inflammation in rheumatoid arthritis. The ranges for *bromelain's* anti-inflammatory effects appear to be from 500–2,000 mg. daily, usually taken in two doses. More research is needed to clearly evaluate the potential medical uses of this enzyme as well as those secreted by the pancreas itself.

The pancreas secretes lipases, amylases, and proteases such as *trypsin* and *chymotrypsin*. Individual enzymes can be extracted and then added to nutritional formulas, but usually the best support is with the whole (glandular) pancreas, which will be discussed in the upcoming section on glandulars. Of all enzyme treatment, pancreatic enzyme support has the greatest potential in medicine. Preliminary research on pancreatic enzymes suggests a favorable response to all those problems mentioned as helped by *bromelain*. Furthermore, cancer may be influenced by high dosages of pancreatic enzymes. Many doctors believe that pancreatic insufficiency is at the root of many degenerative diseases, including cancer.

○ SUPPLEMENTAL OILS

Evening Primrose Oil (EPO) — Gamma-linolenic acid (GLA)

The oil that comes from the seeds of the evening primrose plant contains a high amount of its active ingredient, gamma-linolenic acid (GLA), an oil much like the essential fatty acids (EFA) of the omega-6 variety. In fact, GLA is a precursor of the EFA arachidonic acid, but even more important to its potential therapeutic benefits, GLA leads to the important prostaglandin E_1 series (PGE_1).

The use of evening primrose oil as a nontoxic source of GLA is a good mix of nutrition and herbal medicine. Actually, this night-blooming, bright yellow flowering plant is not a true primrose but is part of the willow family. The name comes from the fact that its flowers resemble those of the primrose plant. This herb has been used medicinally for centuries—externally, as a poultice for skin problems and internally to treat variety of complaints, such as asthma, gastrointestinal problems, gynecological problems, or to enhance wound healing. Native Americans used this plant and its seeds commonly, and in England it was known as "King's cure-all."

There has been a great deal of research with GLA in the last decade, much of it conducted in England where the majority of evening primrose oil is made. With close to 100 research papers published and many more in progress, the results are mixed. Most of the findings, though, are positive and promising, particularly in regard to clearing or reducing symptoms in arthritis, skin problems, and premenstrual syndrome, as well as for all kinds of inflammatory problems, cardiovascular disease, and immunodepression.

Our bodies can make some gamma-linolenic acid from one of the essential fatty acids, linoleic acid, and from this GLA, we form prostaglandin E_1 series. Many symptoms occur from deficiency of linoleic acid, and many of these may be contributed to by low PGE_1 levels, which also may arise from reduced or blocked steps in fatty acid metabolism. Many of these aspects are still unknown. When we take additional GLA, we encourage increased formation of PGE_1, which produces a variety of effects.

The prostaglandin E_1 series is probably the most important of the hormonelike prostaglandins. These substances help inhibit or reduce inflammation, platelet aggregation, thrombosis, cholesterol synthesis, blood vessel tone, and the formation of abnormal cells. PGE_1 is also thought to help lower blood pressure and protect the liver from the effects of alcohol and other irritating drugs. This prostaglandin also functions in maintaining the salt and water balance, insulin secretion, nerve conduction, and gastrointestinal function.

Other prostaglandins, such as series 2, have different functions; some, in fact, can stimulate inflammation. Series 3 prostaglandins are generated in part by the fish oils (discussed next) and have some anti-inflammatory status, but the GLA oils, which enhance PGE_1 formation and provide a good anti-inflammatory effect, have been more thoroughly evaluated in regard to their role in protecting us from cardiovascular disease. Gamma-linolenic acid may help reduce arterial spasm and clotting, two important factors besides vascular inflammation that may contribute to blood vessel disease and cardiac problems. GLA also seems to help the immune system. The following list outlines problems for which evening primrose oil (GLA) has been used with some success and the theoretical bases for its beneficial action.

- **Cardiovascular disease**—anti-inflammatory effect; reducing platelet aggregation, thereby reducing clotting; lowering blood pressure by decreasing vessel tone; cholesterol-lowering effect.
- **Arthritis** (rheumatoid arthritis and other inflammatory disorders)—anti-inflammatory effect; immune support; correcting possible EFA and GLA deficiency.
- **Skin disorders** (eczema, acne, dermatitis)—anti-inflammatory effect; EFA functions; immune support.
- **Allergies, asthma**—anti-inflammatory effect; EFA function; immune support.
- **Weight loss** (theoretical)—increased cellular metabolism; electrolyte and water balance.
- **Premenstrual syndrome** (theoretical)—electrolyte and water balance; EFA support (correction of possible deficiency).
- **Multiple sclerosis**—nerve conduction; correction of possible EFA and GLA deficiency; immune support; decreased platelet aggregation; balancing prostaglandins.
- **Benign (fibrocystic) breast disease** (theoretical)—correction of possible deficiency of PGE_1; possible anti-inflammatory effect.

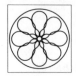

- **Hyperactivity in children**—unknown effect; GLA and EFA support; reduced allergies.
- **Schizophrenia**—correction of low omega-6 fatty acids, low PGE$_1$, and high PGE$_2$.
- **Alcohol protection**—reduced withdrawal symptoms, liver toxicity, and nervous system depression.
- **Depression**—correction of possible GLA deficiency.

The use of evening primrose oil is still experimental, but the research is very promising. It is not necessarily curative by any means, especially in diseases such as atherosclerosis, arthritis, and multiple sclerosis, but it may be helpful in reducing symptoms and/or in preventing further complications. I have recently become more enthusiastic about the use of gamma-linolenic acid because of the results my patients have been experiencing. Many people with arthritis pain, premenstural syndrome and breast symptoms, skin disorders, and some allergies have had a good response, especially when GLA is used in combination with vitamin E and beta-carotene.

Side effects from the use of evening primrose oil are almost nonexistent. Some nausea may be experienced initially because of the oils, but this can be avoided if it is taken with food. Mild skin rashes or acne can occur occasionally; otherwise, no problems have been noticed.

The recommended amount of evening primrose oil is between 500–1,000 mg., taken two or three times daily, with possibly higher doses (4–6 grams daily) in problems such as arthritis, asthma, or eczema. Most good primrose oils contain about 35–40 mg. of GLA per 500 mg. capsule; thus, we are using a therapeutic amount of 150–250 mg. GLA daily. Usually, I suggest a good-quality vitamin E, particularly for the premenstrual and breast problems, and specifically the active d-alpha tocopheral in one or two dosages of 400 IUs each to act with the GLA.

We should follow this interesting nutrient closely in the upcoming years. Other recently available sources of gamma-linoleic acid include black currant seed and borage seed oils, which can be even more concentrated in GLA than primrose, producing similar effects with less capsules and expense. Though these sources have not been evaluated as extensively as EPO, they may be good substitutes.

Eicosapentaenoic Acid and Decosahexaenoic Acid (EPA and DHA)

Eicosapentaenoic acid and decosahexaenoic acid are omega-3 long-chain (C$_{18}$), unsaturated fatty acids found in fish oils. EPA/DHA, which are usually found together, are exciting fatty acid nutrients that have become very popular recently in the literature and as supplements. Like GLA, EPA/DHA also seem to affect the synthesis of the prostaglandins series 1, but even more the series 3, and this may give them additional anti-inflammatory benefits. However, their main effect is to help lower blood fat levels. The intake of dietary EPA/DHA is enhanced by eating coldwater fish

FISH HIGH IN EPA/DHA

Salmon	Eel
Sardines	Trout
Mackeral	Bonita
Herring	Kippers
Butterfish	Bluefish
Pompano	

regularly, such as salmon, herring, mackerel, or sardines that feed on certain plankton, or by taking additional oil supplements. Increased intake of EPA/DHA has been shown in numerous studies to lower blood triglyceride and cholesterol levels, while raising the level of high-density lipoprotein (HDL), the "good" cholesterol.

These lipid-lowering effects, along with some benefits in reducing platelet aggregation and clotting potential, make the use of EPA/DHA very important in the treatment or prevention of cardiovascular disease or in anyone with high blood fats or low HDL. The decreased blood viscosity and lower fat levels help reduce the risk of heart attacks. The mild anti-inflammatory effects, possibly a result of increased PGE_1 and PGE_3 prostaglandins, may also be helpful and has suggested the possible use of EPA/DHA in arthritis and other inflammatory conditions. In rheumatoid arthritis, for example, EPA/DHA supplementation has been shown to reduce joint stiffness and soreness and to improve flexibility.

POSSIBLE USES OF EPA/DHA

Cardiovascular disease
   Atherosclerosis
   Hypertension
   Angina pectoris
Cerebrovascular disease
Rheumatoid arthritis
Migraine headaches
Bronchial asthma
Tinnitus
Lupus and other autoimmune diseases

There are no significant side effects from the use of EPA/DHA, except for mild nausea from taking oils that some people experience. Fish oils contain no vitamin C or E and are more likely to oxidize and go rancid. Therefore, many of the commercial

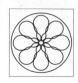

preparations have vitamin E added to prevent oxidation. Fish liver oils are not recommended, even though they contain some EPA and DHA, because they are too high in vitamins A and D, and because livers tend to concentrate any toxic materials the fish (or any animal) have absorbed.

In general, as a preventive for cardiovascular disease, it is recommended that we eat a portion of the oily fishes two or three times weekly. If we do have high blood fats, low HDL, or increased risk of cardiovascular disease, we can supplement 500 mg. of EPA/DHA twice daily to improve these conditions, though in my experience, it does not work that well to lower cholesterol. (Higher amounts may be needed for this effect.) Simple, moderate exercise works better, and as for nutritional supplements, it seems that other agents such as niacin or L-carnitine may be better at lowering lipids (see *Cardiovascular Program* in Chapter 16). Also, for supplying the valuable omega-3 fatty acids, cold-pressed flaxseed oil is a better and less expensive source. (EPA/DHA are also discussed in Chapter 4, *Lipids*, and under *Seafood* in Chapter 8, *Foods*.)

Wheat Germ Oil and Octacosanol

Wheat germ oil is very high in vitamin E and is often used as a source of vitamin E for internal use or for external application to burns, sores, and other skin problems. The antioxidant properties of vitamin E make wheat germ oil more stable to oxidation or rancidity than many other oils.

Octacosanol is another active ingredient of wheat germ oil. Many users and manufacturers of octacosanol capsules claim that it enhances endurance, reaction time, and general vitality, yet these effects may take several weeks to notice. Though scientific research has not completely verified all of the claims, octacosanol appears to improve oxygen utilization, and thereby performance, particularly at higher altitudes or when under stress. It also has a mild cholesterol-lowering effect.

Wheat germ itself is a good source of protein, B vitamins, vitamin E, and many minerals, particularly iron, calcium, copper, magnesium, manganese, zinc, phosphorus, and potassium. Nutritionally, it is more balanced overall than its isolated oil, which is almost exclusively vitamin E plus other oils and is more caloric. We do, however, need some oils for tissue health and to obtain natural vitamin E, so wheat germ oil supplements can be a good addition to a low-fat or low-vitamin-E diet.

○ AMINO ACIDS AND NUCLEIC ACIDS

Many people take supplemental amino acid powders, capsules, or tablets as insurance for obtaining all the essential and nonessential building blocks for protein. In my practice, I have found amino acid therapy, using both complete formulas and individual L-amino acids, to be very helpful for many patients' medical problems and concerns, including vegetarians or people with allergies, stress-related fatigue, or hypoglycemia.

In Chapter 3, *Proteins*, I discussed each amino acid and its application to nutritional medicine. Please refer to that section for current information on amino acid functions, metabolism, and therapy. However, the research and new findings in regard to amino acid use in medicine are moving very rapidly, so we might watch the medical literature and news for future applications.

The most common amino acids used in treating health conditions have been tryptophan, lysine, and phenylalanine. On the upswing are cysteine, carnitine, arginine, and tyrosine. All of these, except phenylalanine, are used in their L- form. (Both D- and DL-phenylalanine also have uses.) Each of the other individual amino acids have some possible uses as well. Their therapeutic amounts may range from 250 mg. to 5–10 grams daily.

I suggest that single L- amino acids not be used with regularity, as this may affect the balance and functions of the others. (This is also true when taking higher amounts of single B vitamins or minerals as well.) I would suggest two weeks as the limit for taking any single nutrient to the exclusion of the others of its family. After that time, either it should be stopped, or the other amino acids or B vitamins, as the case may be, should be taken at the same time.

Deoxyribonucleic and Ribonucleic Acids (DNA and RNA)

These nucleic acid polymers act as the genetic code and translators for the proteins, which in turn are the molecular building blocks of body tissues, and actually stipulate which amino acids go together to form body proteins. DNA is found mainly in the nuclei of cells and carries the genetic message; small amounts of DNA are also found in the mitochondria. RNA helps transfer this genetic message to guide the manufacture of proteins that use all the amino acids either created by the body or extracted from foods.

There are supplements containing good levels of nucleic acids, most commonly yeast or organ meats such as calf thymus, which have been recommended to retard aging, improve memory, or improve the immune or other protein functions. However, there is no proof that RNA or DNA, when taken orally, performs any of these fabulous feats. Most of the oral nucleic acid supplement is broken down into purines and pyrimidines, the basic components of RNA and DNA. These purines, such as adenine and guanine, and pyrimidines, such as cytosine, uracil, and thymine, may have some cellular regeneration functions and thus could help slow aging, improve immune functions, and so on. As these components are absorbed, they may aid the production of the body's RNA or DNA, though this has not been proved. Injectable nucleic acids may offer some benefit. These have been used to slow skin aging particularly.

Many foods contain good levels of these primordial nucleic acids. Brewer's yeast is probably the best source. Others include some fish, such as salmon, sardines, and herring, nuts, wheat germ, bran, oats, onions, spinach, and asparagus. Animal meats and eggs are rich in nucleic acids. Most glandular supplements also contain RNA and DNA.

Many nutrients support normal DNA/RNA synthesis. Folic acid is likely the most important. It may become known as a key antiaging nutrient, possibly through its nucleic acid support. One of the theories of aging suggests that distorted genetic messages generated by dysfunctional DNA and RNA allow communication breakdown, decreased cell division and duplication, and thus weakened tissue strength and life force. Other nutrients that contribute to DNA and RNA synthesis and health include the B vitamins pyridoxine, pantothenic acid, riboflavin, biotin, and choline, vitamin C, and the minerals zinc, magnesium, manganese, chromium, and selenium. Keeping all of these at adequate levels in the diet may be the best way to support healthy genes.

○ MICROORGANISMS

Immunizations

Many members of the microbial world have been used to prevent and treat illnesses and to stimulate various functions in the human body. Their most common use in twentieth-century medicine is for immunizations. This process involves either the injection or oral intake of live or inactivated microorganisms to stimulate immunity to those particular germs and is usually employed against microorganisms such as viruses or bacteria that produce some significant disease. Sometimes it means having a miniversion of that illness in order to activate an immune response for future protection.

Normally, our immune system makes antibodies to any germs, foods, or environmental agents with which we come in contact. These antibodies then create protection against these agents and prevent further infection. At times, when more antibodies are made, some allergic reaction may be generated. This is more common with frequently encountered substances such as pollens, molds, animal fur, and foods and less likely with microorganisms. With virus-caused diseases such as measles or mumps, once we have the infection or the immunization, we usually create lifelong antibodies and thus "immunity" to that disease.

Common immunizations include those for polio, diphtheria, pertussis (whooping cough), tetanus, measles, mumps, chicken pox, and rubella, also known as German measles—most of the childhood illnesses that might occur in this country. Smallpox vaccine is now rarely used, as the disease is nearly nonexistent. When traveling to other countries, we might obtain vaccines against diseases that could possibly be encountered abroad, such as cholera or typhoid fever. Many people use various vaccines against currently common influenza viruses to prevent getting stricken by the more severe disease. These "flu shots" are usually given to people who are sick or who have decreased resistance or to the elderly, for whom a severe case of flu might be fatal.

The use of immunizations has become a philosophical/moral/medical issue for many people in recent years, especially health-conscious parents who do not want to "mess around" with a healthy child's immune system or give them a little disease (and shots!) for illnesses they may or may not get. I tend to agree with the philosophy that healthy people do not acquire disease and, thus, it is silly to live in fear of infections that we likely will not contract. Although most of the infections for which we currently immunize are not very severe, serious or long-term problems may arise from such infections as polio, rubella, and mumps. Clearly, immunizations reduce the incidence of infectious diseases and can even eradicate some of them (but it appears that we are replacing many of our older infectious diseases with new ones); they also prevent the spread of disease by reducing the carrier state through enhanced immunologic protection. On the other hand, possible lifelong, adverse effects may occur from immunization, although recent research suggests there is less potential danger from immunizations than from acquiring these various infections, and, therefore, almost all doctors suggest immunization for children, and most people follow their advice. Flu vaccines and traveler's immunizations are questioned more.

As you can see, there is no clear answer as to whether we should immunize our children. Though there is much strong support for doing so, there is also a decent case against immunizing. Since individual immunizations protect other children from infections' spread, it is just about required for school children. Problems can spread very rapidly in a close setting such as school, so when children are going to attend public school, it is probably best that they be immunized, though parents who are strongly opposed to immunizing for moral or medical reasons can avoid this procedure.

Staphage Lysate (SPL)

Staphage lysate (Delmont Labs), a prescribed medication that can be used to stimulate the immune system, is a sterile solution of antigens made from parts of the common *Staphylococcus aureus* bacterium and a bacteriophage. These two components are recognized by our body as potential trouble. So when parts of the bacterial cell wall plus the bacteriophages are administered to us, our body responds as if fighting off a potentially serious infection.

265

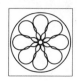

Its primary use is for treatment of chronic staphylococcal infections, such as serious cases of acne, boils, or other skin problems. But SPL appears to produce favorable results in a variety of other problems that seem to respond to increased cellular immunity, particularly the viral infections such as colds and flus, herpes, and illnesses resulting from Epstein-Barr virus (EBV) or cytomegalovirus (CMV). Some people with arthritis problems or allergies have also benefited from SPL injections.

I do not view treatment with SPL as curative, although I definitely have seen it be helpful in the healing and recovery process of many illnesses. I have found SPL most helpful for people in the early stages of viral infections or for whom fatigue remains after infectious illnesses—cases where I would rather not use an antibiotic, as it is not indicated, but where I want to speed recovery. SPL is very safe! I have seen very few, if any, side effects from its use in treatment over the last few years. There may be mild itching or swelling at the site of injections as the immune response to the SPL components is working; actually, we can base dosages on the size of the wheal (swelling at injection site) generated. Its primary use is by repeated intradermal injections of between 0.05 and 0.2 cc. (dependent on patient sensitivity), usually every other day for several weeks, then less frequently—perhaps twice weekly, then once weekly. Shorter courses are used, maybe one or two injections, at the onset of a cold or flu to prevent its progression.

Staphage lysate can also be used orally or topically or squirted into the ears or nose for mild infections or congestions there. Its use is not recommended for children or during pregnancy other than topically (mainly because it has not been studied, not because it isn't safe). I think doctors should become more aware of this pharmaceutical preparation and more research should be done to guide us in the best use of staphage lysate.

Intestinal Bacteria—Acidophilus and More

Several "friendly" intestinal bacteria perform many important bodily functions. There are actually a great many lactobacillus and other bacteria that can inhabit the human colon, but I will mention the three that seem to be most important. These are *Lactobacillus acidophilus* (the most famous), *Lactobacillus bifidus* (more common to the baby colon), and *Streptococcus faecium* (not *S. faecalis*, a possible pathogenic bacteria).

Various cultures of acidophilus are available in many stores, particularly health food stores, as powders, capsules, tablets, and liquids and measured by the amount of viable bacteria per dosage. There are many claims for the use of acidophilus, though it is best known for reimplanting friendly bacteria into the colon to assure return of bodily functions after a course of antibiotic drugs. Actually, acidophilus itself acts as a mild antibiotic—that is, it has antibacterial activity. With regular use, it may even replace harmful bacteria in the colon or vaginal tract of women, where acidophilus is also commonly used to treat yeast infections. It is further employed as part of the treatment for intestinal yeast overgrowth and the many symptoms that this may generate. These bacteria also help in the production of some B vitamins and vitamin K and in the breakdown of various foods.

Yogurt or acidophilus milk, sometimes with *L. bulgaricus* as well, is often used to provide some stimulus to the colon, though the live bacteria count is not very high in these products. Yogurt can also be used by people with lactose intolerance due to *lactase* enzyme deficiency, because the bacteria change or ferment the lactose sugar and produce lactic acid. Many people have also described yogurt or, more important, acidophilus as helpful for stomach and digestive upset, for intestinal gas, and even for inflammatory problems of the gastrointestinal tract, but these reports are more anecdotal than proved by research. The further suggestions that acidophilus improves immunity, produces its own antibiotics, helps allergies (particularly to foods), improves skin health, is a benefit in herpes infections, reduces cholesterol levels, and lessens cancer risk (especially colon cancer) are also yet unproved, though current research at several universities for one product looks very promising in regard to these possibilities.

Lactobacillus bifidus has become part of intestinal bioculture treatment, often along with acidophilus. The bifidus culture is more prevalent in infants, often as their first organism, but can also be an important part of the adult gastrointestinal tract. Like acidophilus, it helps in the synthesis of B vitamins, in food digestion, and in inhibiting the growth of the coliform bacteria and possibly more pathogenic colon bacteria, such as salmonellae.

Streptococcus faecium is another important colon bacterium that has received recent attention. Its actions are similar to those of acidophilus. It is important in B vitamin biosynthesis, aids the digestion of foods, likely by producing certain enzymes, and inhibits other, more toxic bacteria; thus supplementation with *S. faecium* may help in some cases of diarrhea. *Strep faecalis*, a potentially pathogenic bacterium, has been listed by mistake instead of *S. faecium* on some bacterial replacement products.

These three bacteria may be taken individually and alternated weekly or every couple of weeks. They can also be taken all together (there are some products that contain all three) on a regular basis when used to balance the effect of one or more courses of antibiotics. There is a possibility that the combination of bacteria works better to rebalance colon health than the individual organisms.

The count of live bacteria in products containing these bacteria is in the millions and billions daily per dose. There has been some question as to whether these bacteria are killed by the acidic stomach juices, but when taken in sufficient quantities, some organisms do make it down to the colon. I believe that these bacteria should not be taken regularly, but rather in specific courses to repopulate the colon with these "friendly" bacteria after antibiotic use or to treat intestinal yeast overgrowth; otherwise, I recommend them for one to two weeks once or twice a year, or when traveling to underdeveloped countries with higher risks of intestinal contamination from infectious organisms, for which the acidophilus bacteria offer some protection.

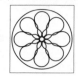

Algae

Algae are green, or "blue-green," freshwater, one-celled organisms that can be grown, dried, and safely used by our bodies. They have become available in the nutritional product arena as supplemental nutrients to enhance body functions only in the last couple of decades. Chlorella, spirulina, and blue-green manna are three of the main products produced from algae. Although they are not exactly the same, they are similar enough that I will discuss them together.

Spirulina made a big hit in the 1970s and has been the most popular algae product. Chlorella, however, was the first available to my knowledge and is still sold in many health food stores in a powdered or tablet form. Blue-green manna is more recent and usually harder to obtain.

All of these blue-green algae, or plankton products, have been used as "high-protein" nutrients that contain all the amino acids. They are considered a tonic and/or rejuvenator of the body and are used commonly during weight-loss programs or fasting. I have spoken with many people who have done a juice-spirulina powder fast and felt extremely well, with more energy than usual. Besides the high protein and low fat levels of these algae, they contain substantial amounts of vitamins and minerals and plant chlorophyll; spirulina was recently measured as rich in GLA, or gamma-linolenic acid, the oil found in the evening primrose plant.

It is possible that the GLA found in spirulina and possibly these other products accounts for some of the positive effects that people experience when using them, including decreased appetite, weight loss, and improved energy levels, especially mental energy. I personally have used all of these products and must say I have experienced a subtle increase in mental clarity and alertness (not like a nervous, caffeine-type stimulation). These algae must subtly stimulate our nervous systems or release certain internal neurochemicals that create this "up" feeling.

There has not been much medical research on any of these products, but I think there should be. When people find interesting substances from nature, I believe it is medicine's duty to investigate the activity of these products so we can apply them effectively in our lives. Such analysis with herbs has brought us the whole field of pharmacognosy/pharmaceutical medicine, and perhaps continued analysis of nature's potential remedies will bring useful new substances and help us to better integrate the drug and nondrug therapies.

○ ENZYMES AND CHEMICALS

Of the wide range of supplements in the chemical or enzyme categories, I will discuss only a few that have potential use and are somewhat popular in the nutritional world.

Butylated Hydroxyanisole and Butylated Hydroxytoluene (BHA and BHT)

These two chemicals are in common use as food additives/preservatives, especially for products containing oils, as they are good antioxidants—that is, they prevent the oxidation of fats. I personally avoid these chemicals in foods, and I suggest that others do as well, though they are definitely not the worst concerns.

Recent claims in Pearson's and Shaw's *Life Extension* and some other writings suggest that taking BHT as a drug in amounts of about 1 gram daily has positive effects in treating and preventing herpes infections, reducing cancer risks, especially those of a chemical cause, and reducing the aging process. However, this information is based almost exclusively on animal studies. There is decent evidence that it is a good antioxidant at these therapeutic levels, and we know that this antioxidant function is important in preventing a variety of diseases.

However, I have already described natural and safer antioxidant nutrients, and I believe the amino acid L-lysine is worth trying first for oral herpes problems. There is definite cause for concern about use of the possibly dangerous BHA and BHT, and the evidence is not very convincing that they are effective in the treatment of herpes and other lipid-containing viruses. Though use of BHT has not been shown to create specific toxicity in humans, there is a possibility that it may be carcinogenic in some situations or that it may aggravate existing cancers rather than helping to remedy them.

Overall, I do not advocate the use of BHA or BHT in treatment or for any reason. Until there is some very good evidence that it works safely in certain conditions, I would advise avoiding these substances.

Coenzyme Q_{10} (CoQ_{10})—Ubiquinone

Coenzyme Q_{10} is a substance made by our bodies and obtained in the diet, mainly in oily fish (that also contain EPA), organ meats, and whole grains. Ubiquinone may soon be called a fat-soluble vitamin as it is shown to be essential and also to create problems when deficient. There are ten types of CoQ; CoQ_{10} is the main active one in humans, which works along with certain enzymes to support the body's bioenergetic functions. CoQ_{10} is an electron carrier and is important to many body energy systems, particularly in the cell mitochondria, which are known as the energy factories, where it aids in generating ATP. CoQ_{10} acts as a mild metabolic stimulant and may facilitate

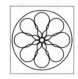

weight loss. It also appears to be a mild immune stimulant. This substance has been shown to help heart function by enhancing the pumping action and electrical functioning, as well as helping to lower blood pressure. CoQ_{10} seems to be related to vitamin E and is supportive of its functions, including those in the mitochondria.

Preliminary research regarding the use of coenzyme Q_{10} in patients with heart failure has produced very positive findings. Most of these patients describe some improvement; this supplement probably improves energy production in the heart muscle cells. It is possible that CoQ_{10} will be helpful in other cardiovascular functional problems, whether electrical arrhythmias or cardiac muscular dysfunction.

The amount of CoQ_{10} needed for effectiveness is approximately 10–20 mg. twice daily. Taking at least 600–800 IU of vitamin E daily, along with the basic nutrients, including vitamin C, niacin, and other cholesterol-lowering substances, such as EPA, is probably a good idea as well for cardiovascular problems. Look for more research and medical use for coenzyme Q_{10}.

Dimethyl Glycine (DMG)

DMG is a somewhat controversial substance. It is probably the active component of pangamic acid, or "vitamin B_{15}." Most of the positive claims for DMG are based on research conducted in the Soviet Union, where pangamic acid is considered a panacea, helping to oxygenate tissues, improve immunity, and enhance energy and physical stamina. Using it to increase endurance in exercise and to improve oxygenation of the brain in mental disorders were two primary areas of research. The negative comments come from this country, where it was suggested that DMG is either useless or possibly even carcinogenic. Though the preliminary research here has not verified the panacea benefits, the negative claims seem unfounded. Still, the FDA and AMA have worked to keep these products off the market and have succeeded with pangamic acid but not with DMG.

Functionally, DMG is an intermediary of many biochemical processes in our body, involving various enzymes, vitamins, neurotransmitters, and amino acids. For example, DMG is a precursor of the neuroinhibitory amino acid glycine, and thus may help calm excitable states such as in epilepsy or possibly in hyperactivity problems. It was suggested in an article entitled "Immunomodulatory Properties of Dimethyl Glycine in Humans" in a 1981 *Journal of Infectious Disease* that DMG in an oral dose of 125 mg. a day offers some immunological support, particularly in regard to infectious agents. It specifically increased the antibody and lymphocytic responses to a bacterial vaccine. DMG also may support more efficient use of oxygen, especially during the rapid oxygen use of exercise. During exercise, it may work also by reducing lactate production and by improving blood sugar metabolism. DMG has been shown in preliminary studies to improve oxygen utilization in exercise and thus endurance and strength as well as to lessen postexercise fatigue and soreness. This latter effect, of course, is more experiential and may also take higher amounts and several weeks of DMG use to be noticeable. DMG may also be helpful in conditions such as arthritis, where it should be part of an entire antioxidant program. DMG may also offer some tissue protection against various chemicals. Furthermore, DMG may help cardiovascular function by regulating heart rhythm through its support of efficient oxygenation. It also improves liver metabolism of fats and cholesterol and thus has a lipotrophic effect. In mental or memory disorders, DMG may help by its role in improving oxygenation. As an antistress nutrient, DMG may support adrenal function, improve energy levels, and protect the body from free radicals generated by stress.

DMG is not yet a primary treatment and still fits into one of the battlegrounds for nutritional "experiencers" versus medical and scientific "provers." With more research, this nutrient may find greater support, at least as an adjunct to some therapeutic programs. Also, the toxicity of DMG is very low, if any, especially in the usual amounts of 50–200 mg. daily. DMG is available in oral or sublingual tablets and is taken two or three times daily. Dissolving these tablets under the tongue is currently the simplest and most efficacious way to utilize DMG.

Dimethyl Sulfoxide and Methylsulfonyl Methane (DMSO and MSM)

DMSO, an industrial solvent, has been in use most recently in a pharmaceutically pure grade for its local anti-inflammatory action that reduces joint or soft tissue pain. It has been employed extensively by veterinarians and until recently when it was made illegal, has been available to the public for experimental use. There is a fair amount of experience and studies regarding the external use of DMSO for aches and pains from injury or arthritis. Results have been variable. DMSO may have some antioxidant effect, but this has not been shown clearly. Some government studies using DMSO both topically and intravenously for brain-injured patients have found it to be less toxic than was previously thought, though they have not shown it to be very helpful.

DMSO is easily absorbed through the skin and can be irritating to the eyes or may cause nausea or skin rash. It seems to be helpful for some arthritis symptoms but is definitely not curative. Although there are still some avid users, DMSO has fallen out of vogue and is probably best avoided.

A breakdown product of DMSO, methylsulfonyl methane (MSM), is a nontoxic, physiologically active sulfur compound that may possess some anti-inflammatory and antioxidant properties. Though more research is needed regarding its safety and actions, MSM has become available recently, and its future appears promising, possibly in treating problems such as arthritis or inhalant allergies.

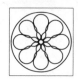

Quercetin and Other Bioflavonoids

We have previously discussed the bioflavonoids under *Vitamin P* (for permeability) in Chapter 5. They are ascorbic-acid-related substances, usually found in foods along with vitamin C, particularly in the white of the rind of citrus fruits, in buckwheat, and in vegetables such as green peppers and tomatoes. As a group, these bioflavonoids, including hesperidin, rutin, quercetin, and catechin, work to keep the capillary blood vessels strong and to reduce vascular fragility and subsequent bleeding and bruising, as well as to lower the microtrauma of tissue injuries. They have been used successfully in preventing injury and bruising in athletes and in speeding the recovery of acutely injured athletes and other performers. A mix of bioflavonoids containing hesperidin and ascorbic acid seems to have the best effect (including anti-inflammatory) in these injury conditions. Some bioflavonoids apparently act as immune supporters, antioxidants, and detoxifiers. There are a number of other uses of these interesting substances.

Catechin, one of the bioflavonoid components, appears to decrease histamine release in allergy and thus reduce symptoms. It also is a mild anti-inflammatory in rheumatoid arthritis. Furthermore, it has protective effects on the liver in response to alcohol and as a healing aid for people with hepatitis B.

Quercetin has been the subject of recent studies. It can decrease allergic reactions by several mechanisms. First, it helps to stabilize mast cells and basophils and inhibits their degranulation and subsequent release of histamine and other inflammatory chemicals. Quercetin also inhibits some inflammatory enzymes, such as lipid peroxidases, and decreases leukotriene (another inflammatory molecule) formation. Thus, quercetin may be helpful not only in allergies, but in all kinds of inflammatory responses, such as injury, bursitis, asthma, and arthritis. In rheumatoid arthritis, it has particular potential, since it decreases mast cell degranulation, one of the fundamental causes of inflammation within the joint spaces. Quercetin is further thought to decrease the infectiousness of certain RNA and DNA viruses, such as herpes, polio, and Epstein-Barr, by inhibiting their replication. It may also be helpful in preventing eye and nerve damage in diabetes by decreasing tissue irritation.

Usually, bioflavonoids are supplemented as a group in amounts of 250–500 mg., one to several times daily. Many vitamin C formulas contain bioflavonoids, particularly rutin and hesperidin. Quercetin is available in various strengths; supplementation of 100–250 mg. three times daily is probably an effective level.

Superoxide Dismutase (SOD)

SOD is a very interesting enzyme nutrient. In our body, it is usually coupled with zinc, copper, or manganese, and it acts within the cell to prevent oxygen free-radical damage. *Superoxide dismutase* is also a controversial nutrient, not because it does not have positive effects, but because taking it orally, as it is commonly practiced, provides questionable benefits.

On the positive side, SOD is considered an antiaging nutrient that acts as an antioxidant to protect us from free-radical damage. In this way, it is thought to help reduce the process involved in arthritis and protect us from radiation damage and cancer-causing substances, as well as cancer itself, and some of the inflammatory aspects of cardiovascular disease. Most of the research has been done with animals and is still preliminary. Injected intramuscularly, SOD has been shown to produce some positive effects with arthritis patients and in stimulating cellular immunity.

SOD is still experimental. As mentioned, there is no proof that oral supplements of SOD do anything systemically to warrant their use, though they may offer some help for the stomach or for gastrointestinal inflammation. They are easily digested. Unless a supplement company can show that oral intake of SOD will increase blood levels of that enzyme, it is probably not very helpful and likely a waste of money to use this nutrient. Sublingual tablets may offer some hope.

Gerovital (GH3)

This is another interesting nutrient that does not seem to have much medical backing. A derivative of the analgesic chemical procaine, it is claimed to be a great antiaging substance. This product is popular among the elderly population, but again, there is no good evidence as to what, if anything, it does.

○ PLANTS

The science of herbology is as old as medicine itself and is the people's healing system in nearly all cultures of the world. Plants and their specific parts—be it roots, leaves, flowers, or berries—have clear pharmacological activity in our bodies, ranging from very subtle to profound. The system of pharmaceutical medicine is based on the knowledge and effects of herbal medicine, where the active components discovered in the plants were concentrated or synthesized to make "patent medicines."

I have turned more to herbal medicine in the last decade and now use both herbs and pharmaceuticals in my practice. Overall, herbal remedies, individual and blended, tend to be more subtle in their effects than most drugs and are best used for mild problems or prevention. For chronic problems, herbs can be used to strengthen or detoxify specific organs or the entire body, but often must be employed for weeks or months to have an effect. For more acute or serious problems, when rapid relief is necessary, Western medicines clearly are very useful.

This discussion of plants is not intended to be a treatise on herbology, though some of the plants discussed are effective and very popular in herbal literature. Described below are some of the common plants often used as nutritional supplements. Some

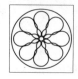

COMMON HERBAL SUPPLEMENTS

Alfalfa	Ginger
Aloe Vera	Ginkgo biloba
Cayenne	Ginseng
Echinacea	Goldenseal
Feverfew	Kelp
Garlic	Licorice

Wheatgrass and Barley Grass

popular herbs, such as peppermint (for nausea or headaches), chamomile (indigestion), raspberry (colds and uterine weakness), parsley (diuretic), and red clover (lung tonic and blood cleanser) will be left for herbal texts to explore.

Alfalfa

Those little green tablets come from the very green plants with the prolific and deep root system so loved by rabbits. Alfalfa is actually a legume plant and contains the eight essential amino acids. It is also high in chlorophyll, vitamins A, D, B_6, and E, and some calcium and phosphorus. Alfalfa is one of the few foods with good levels of vitamin K, the blood-clotting vitamin.

People who use alfalfa take it mainly as a natural supportive supplement for its nutrient content, much as they might take brewer's yeast or kelp. Alfalfa seeds are commonly sprouted, which are also highly nutritious. No grand claims are made for alfalfa, though recent research suggests that both the alfalfa plant and powdered alfalfa seed have a cholesterol-lowering and antiatherosclerotic effect. It is thought that the saponins contained in alfalfa help bind cholesterol and bile salts in the gut. High doses, 50 grams daily, of alfalfa were shown to reduce arterial plaques in monkeys. Some people are sensitive to alfalfa supplementation, and it has produced a lupuslike syndrome in monkeys. Overall, though, alfalfa is a safe and nutritious supplement.

Aloe Vera

The aloe "cactus," actually a desert succulent, has been touted as one of the "miracle" plants. The gel of the plant's leaves is used for treatment, both internally and externally. It contains some amino acids, vitamins, and minerals and a salicylate substance that may help reduce inflammation. Aloe vera has been used by many cultures for centuries as a healing plant. Though a number of studies have been performed worldwide, there is not much recent research evidence regarding its positive aspects, though a great deal of anecdotal evidence has come from the many users of aloe vera juice and gel.

The most common use of aloe vera is the application of its gel (the inside of the leaf) for burns. This is very soothing, and many people experience reduced inflammation and blistering and more rapid healing. Aloe concentrate or dried aloe gel powder is an intestinal purgative, that helps stimulate colon activity with less of the cramping that comes with many other herbal preparations. Aloe vera capsules are a useful remedy or preventive for constipation. The dried aloe gel is very bitter to the taste, so it must be either purified for oral use or dried and capped.

The use of aloe vera juice has been promoted with many claims of its miraculous effects. These include rapid healing of injuries, relief from arthritis, help in weight loss, alleviation of ulcers and gastrointestinal disease, and anticancer properties, to name a few. There is, however, no good research to substantiate these claims, but aloe vera juice seems to be completely nontoxic, and it is possible that there are some yet-undiscovered powerful healing agents within this plant (germanium is one possibility).

More recently, in 1984, a product trademarked Carrisyn was extracted from the leaf of the common plant, *Aloe barbadensis*. Carrington Laboratories has conducted research with carrisyn, a long-chain polysaccharide white powder, that appears to possess many of the healing properties attributed to aloe vera. Carrisyn has been shown to promote wound healing when applied topically, as well as aiding ulcer healing or providing tissue and ulcer protection in those sensitive to inflammation of the gastrointestinal mucosa. This aloe extract, in a 1 gram daily dosage, has also shown antiviral (and possibly anticancer) effects, helping clear the herpes and AIDS viruses, possibly by stimulating both interferon and macrophage and phagocytic white blood cell activity. Carrisyn is clearly nontoxic and very stable and may be available soon by prescription in tablets, capsules, gels, and injectables, pending FDA approval.

The common oral preparation of the aloe plant currently available is aloe vera juice, a partially refined and diluted extract of the active gel. This is sold in pints, quarts, and even gallons. Many people drink this solution beginning at 1 ounce twice daily and increasing to about 6 ounces per day. Many users describe positive health effects from drinking aloe vera juice regularly. I have taken this nutrient, and it seems at least to be very soothing and vitalizing if you can get past the taste (some preparations taste better than others).

Cayenne

If you like life a little spicy, try some cayenne pepper. Cayenne pepper can be taken in capsules or as powder in water or used in cooking. It is also called capsicum or African bird pepper. I think it is the cleanest of the red peppers and one of the true natural stimulants for both energy and metabolism. I personally think that cayenne pepper, when used regularly, has anticancer properties, which have not yet been studied other than epidemiologically in cayenne- and chili-using cultures. But some people do not like to get too hot!

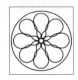

Cayenne pepper, actually a small red berry from the *Capsicum annum* or *frutescens* plants, creates heat when taken into the body, but it is not irritating or burning. The active oil, capsaicin, is now being studied in the treatment of some medical disorders. Cayenne pepper has been used to treat digestive disorders involving gas, nausea, or indigestion. It seems to stimulate gastric secretions and peristaltic activity and is actually thought to be soothing to the mucosal linings even though it is heating. It has been used herbally in the treatment of ulcers and for other gastrointestinal disease and, at diluted levels, even for eye irritation, though I do not recommend this use. As a throat lozenge ingredient, cayenne can help reduce soreness or inflammation. There is also belief that cayenne reduces clotting mechanisms, which may help reduce risk in cardiovascular diseases; for this reason it should be avoided by people on anticoagulant drugs. Cayenne is also used topically to provide local relief from joint pain or stiffness or sore muscles. It seems to enhance circulation and is sometimes helpful in treating certain headaches. For a therapeutic use in people who have weak circulation, such as cold extremities, atherosclerosis, or heart problems, taking one to two capsules twice daily is suggested. And feel that heat!

Echinacea

Echinacea root, most often as the species *Echinacea augustifolium* (Kansas snakeroot), has been a popular medicine with American herbalists for more than a century. They use it in the treatment of various infections, fevers, snake and insect bites, and many skin problems, such as acne, boils, abscesses, and ulcers. More recently, echinacea has become very popular with the American public, mostly for infections and to purify the blood and lymph. For treating skin problems, most natural practitioners feel that blood purification is important. Michael Tierra, in his popular book *The Way of Herbs* (Unity Press, 1980), calls echinacea the "king of blood purifiers." The availability of fine-quality tinctures and powdered root extracts has made the bitter echinacea more easily accessible.

Recent experiments have shown that echinacea root can increase the white blood count and thus our ability to handle bacteria and viruses, stimulate the important T lymphocytes' activity, and generally stimulate the lymphatic system to clear wastes. The immune-supporting aspects of this valuable herb makes it effective in the treatment of mild infections, such as vaginitis and prostatitis, poison oak and ivy, acne and boils, and respiratory infections. Although more research is needed to verify its effectiveness, many people describe a very good response to taking echinacea root products, either singularly or in combination with other purifying anti-infectious herbs and vitamins. Though echinacea use appears basically nontoxic, until more research can clarify its safety I do not advise extended use for more than three or four weeks due to possible effects such as liver irritation or changes in the normal intestinal flora.

Feverfew

Feverfew (*Chrysanthemum parthenium* and *Tanacetrum parthenium*) leaf has been more available recently as a supplement, and I have found it to be particularly effective in reducing the incidence and intensity of migraine headaches. Research tends to support this as well. Reports indicate that feverfew also has a moderate anti-inflammatory effect and inhibits platelet aggregation, suggesting possible use in circulatory disease and other pain problems.

At the first sign of a headache, one capsule is taken, and then another in 30 minutes. If this treatment is effective, another follow-up capsule should be taken in three or four hours. If the first two capsules do not work, a third might be attempted in an hour. If no therapeutic response is seen in two separate trials, feverfew herb will not likely be an effective migraine treatment. If it works, I then usually suggest one 500 mg. capsule once or twice daily for prevention. Though it appears fairly nontoxic, I suggest using it for only two to three weeks prophylactically and then stopping for a week. It can also be effective with no regular usage, taking it only when a headache begins.

Garlic

Garlic, or *Allium sativum*, is one of the bigshots in herbal lore. It has been used effectively through the centuries for a variety of concerns and is probably one of the best known herbs/foods. Many people use garlic regularly in their diets, easily identified by the telltale odor. In recent years, odorless garlic extracts have been used to treat a wide range of conditions without creating the bad breath, though many naturalists and scientists believe that this is not as beneficial as the pure garlic.

Garlic has always been thought to be a natural and broad-spectrum antibiotic. It may also have some immune-stimulating properties. Garlic may help prevent and/or treat some bacterial or fungal conditions, including the candida/yeast problem. And it has been used by many, either eaten or worn around the neck, to protect them from flus and colds caused by viruses. Garlic has also been used to kill some types of intestinal worms and parasites.

Garlic seems to be an energy stimulant, helps circulation, and has been touted as reducing blood pressure in hypertensive people (this has not yet been shown conclusively in research). More recently, garlic has been found to lower triglyceride and cholesterol levels and raise HDL cholesterol, which helps protect against atherosclerosis and coronary-artery disease; garlic's ability to reduce platelet aggregation may also contribute to this role. Recent evidence shows this to be true, but more research is needed to see how garlic may be used for cardiovascular disease and possibly protective against cancer development. Preliminary research also shows that oral garlic (and onion) can inhibit skin tumor incidence.

Other claims for garlic include its effectiveness in diabetes or hypoglycemia, arthritis, allergies, blood clotting problems, traveler's diarrhea, poor circulation, and, of course,

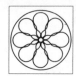

colds and flus. In higher amounts, garlic can be irritating to the gastrointestinal tract, and when applied to the skin as raw garlic, it can cause burns. Some women have used it intravaginally to treat infections; however, this is not recommended as it can cause more irritation if the shell coating of an individual clove is disrupted.

For internal use, fresh garlic is probably the best. The deodorized garlic used by researchers in Japan was prepared by an aging-fermentation process. This garlic seems to retain the natural effects, but not all deodorized garlic is prepared in this way, and it may or may not have the same benefits as fresh garlic.

Garlic oil capsules are commonly used as a therapeutic supplement. We can make our own garlic oil from chopped fresh garlic that is soaked a few days in olive oil. It can be used as an external or internal treatment, such as by applying it to the feet or chest during colds or taking it orally as a simple means of obtaining garlic. Garlic oil is good in salad dressings, too.

Ginger

The ginger used medicinally is from the root of the ginger plant, *Zingiber officinale*. Many of its properties and uses are described in the herbal literature. Recently, ginger root has received some medical attention as being useful in treating nausea and motion sickness. Ginger capsules or a cup of ginger root tea seems to allay nausea. Ginger has also been helpful for the nausea of pregnancy.

Ginger root in general seems to be a digestive stimulant and is used to improve weak digestion. A warm cup of tea made by boiling a few slices of root in a cup or two of water can be drunk about 30 minutes before meals. Ginger is also a diaphoretic (it causes sweating), and it seems to help in circulation and in warming the body when we feel cold, as can happen in winter. There is some preliminary research evidence that ginger acts as an antioxidant and that it can help lower cholesterol and prevent cardiovascular disease. It also inhibits platelet aggregation, a factor contributing to atherosclerosis and clotting problems. Ginger is both an energy and circulatory stimulant. Ginger root tea is also used as a compress for sore muscles or congested areas of the body. This is a common macrobiotic therapy.

Ginger root can be used in cooking, too, or as a tea with other herbs. It is a very helpful and safe herb. For improving body heat, one or two capsules of ginger root powder can be taken once or twice a day for about a month. Cayenne pepper can also be used in this way.

Ginkgo biloba

One of the oldest living plant species is the ginkgo tree. Estimated at well over 100 million years old, the leaves from this tree have a bilobal, brainlike appearance, hence the name, *Ginkgo biloba*. Though fairly new to the Western culture, the leaves of the gingko tree have been used for centuries in the Orient for complaints associated with aging.

An extract of the *Ginkgo biloba* leaves has been tested and reported to be effective at reducing ischemic symptoms—vascular insufficiency associated with aging and atherosclerosis. *Ginkgo biloba* appears to increase cerebral blood flow and thus help oxygenation; it also may inhibit platelet aggregation. In a study of geriatric patients, ginkgo was shown to reduce symptoms of vertigo, memory loss, tinnitus, and headache. In another study of lower limb claudication symptoms, ginkgo helped reduce pain and improve walking tolerance over the placebo group. Thus, the use of *Gingko biloba* extracts, which have been marketed in Europe for years, appears to help in both cerebral and peripheral arterial insufficiency.

Ginkgo biloba is easily absorbed and has no known toxicity. Either extracts or capsules can be used. Therapeutic amounts range from 40–200 mg. taken three times daily.

More research is needed to test the therapeutic value of *Gingko biloba*. Its use in Alzheimer's disease, other forms of dementia, neurological and cardiovascular diseases, as well as its potential antioxidant effects are some possible areas of investigation.

Ginseng

As with ginger, the root of the ginseng plant, usually *Panax ginseng*, is the active and commonly used part. It comes to us mainly from Asian cultures, where it is used extensively as a tonic, stimulant, and rejuvenator, especially for men. It is also used by women for fatigue and sexually related symptoms. It is often part of formulas used to balance the menstrual cycle, reduce premenstrual symptoms or hot flashes of menopause, or to improve the sex drive or enhance fertility. Probably the most common use of ginseng is to increase energy. Research is showing that it also reduces cholesterol and triglyceride levels, raises HDL, and stimulates the immune system. Its "rejuvenating" qualities may come from its stimulus to protein synthesis.

This herb is called the "man plant" because of the shape of the roots; its name *panax* refers to "all healing," as in "panacea." Other active ginsengs are *Panax quinquefolius*, or American ginseng, and *Eleutherococcus senticosus*, or Siberian ginseng. The ginsengs have a number of active ingredients, such as peptides, glycosides, and the more recently acknowledged trace mineral germanium (discussed shortly), which may turn out to be a very helpful and fascinating supplement. Yet we still do not know medically or pharmacologically what gives ginseng its powers.

Ginseng is used most commonly as a tonic and herb for longevity. It seems to contribute to general well-being and improved physical endurance. It is a stimulant but not an excitant like caffeine, and it is particularly useful for men with fatigue or sexual impotency. Ginseng root is drunk as a tea or is sometimes taken in capsules, though the brewed liquid seems to have a better effect. It is available in more forms

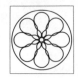

nowadays, in liquid elixirs, as a paste or powder used to make teas, or as the whole root. These roots, which come mainly from Korea and China, can be very beautiful and expensive. The cost is often based on the age of the root, older ones being more expensive as their power seems to improve with age. On traveling through China, I was impressed by the many displays of ginseng roots throughout stores, airports, and many other places. There is a wild American ginseng that can also be used, and some of it is thought to be very helpful, though it probably has somewhat different effects from those produced by the Asian plants.

A daily dose of ginseng root is usually about 500 mg. Larger amounts can cause overstimulation, which may result in increased blood pressure, diarrhea, skin eruptions, or insomnia. It may interact with the sensitive hormonal system and may also have some estrogenic activity; thus, it may aggravate fibrocystic breast disease in women. Any substance that has potential power and benefit obviously can also be misused. It you wish to try ginseng root as a tonic or remedy, obtain guidance from your physician, acupuncturist, or someone with experience in its use. (See my book *Staying Healthy with the Seasons* for a special preparation of ginseng root.) If there are any cardiac problems, ginseng should be used very carefully, and it should not be used by pregnant women.

Goldenseal

Goldenseal *(Hydrastis canadensis)* root has been a panacea and cure-all used by many herbalists and a very popular herb to the Native Americans. Its range of uses is probably as wide as that of any other herb. Goldenseal's active alkaloids, hydrastine and berberine, appear to have many body actions, and this bitter, tonifying herb is used as an antibacterial and antiparasitic, especially for giardia and amoebic infections, as well as other infections with yeast, worms, or other germs. Many people take goldenseal capsules at the first sign of a flu or other infection and claim good results. This golden powder has been used as a douche, gargle, or as a bitter tonic taken orally to strengthen the mucous membranes of the gastrointestinal tract, sinuses, eyes, and rectum. Goldenseal is also an antiseptic and detoxifier, possibly because of its liver-stimulating effect. It has mild laxative and vasoconstrictive actions, making it useful in the treatment of hemorrhoids, both applied externally and taken internally. Goldenseal has been used for skin problems such as acne or eczema, as a uterine tonic, and to stimulate glandular activity and strengthen the nervous system. Goldenseal may be helpful for many problems of the stomach and gastrointestinal tract, such as nausea, indigestion, infection, and constipation or diarrhea; here it can also reduce bacterial or parasitic proliferation, increase gastrointestinal tone, and stimulate bile secretion and digestion.

For most of these situations, goldenseal can usually be taken as one large or two small capsules (or 10–20 drops of an extract) twice daily for about two to three weeks. I do not recommend long continuous intake of this powerful herb because of possible liver irritation.

Kelp

Kelp seaweed is a common health food supplement. It is taken primarily for its iodine content by people who want to improve thyroid function, though there is no proof that kelp changes this function. The thyroid gland must, however, have sufficient iodine, and if we do not use iodized salt or eat a lot of fish and seaweed, kelp may be a helpful adjunct. It is also high in other vitamins and minerals, such as calcium, magnesium, potassium, niacin, riboflavin, and choline. Algin, which is helpful at pulling out intestinal toxins and heavy metals, is also found in kelp. Several tablets per day will usually supply the needed iodine; kelp powder used on food is a good salt substitute but should not be overused.

Licorice

Licorice *(Glycyrrhiza glabra)* likely has the most celebrated herbal past, extending thousands of years, beginning in the Orient and progressing around the world. It has many actions and clearly many uses. Also known as sweetwood or sweetroot, the "great detoxifier" and the "great peacemaker," this root contains many steroidlike chemicals related to adrenal and ovarian secretions. Historically, it was used for colds and coughs, and it has become popular as a laxative and for use in children, who tolerate its sweet flavor more readily than bitter herbs, with problems such as fevers, colds, and constipation.

Licorice root has many apparent actions. It is an antitussive and expectorant, anti-inflammatory and antiarthritic, antitoxic (through liver support and protection) and antibiotic, possibly anticancer (recent research has shown licorice's inhibitory effect in some tumor growth), and a laxative. It also acts as a demulcent and emollient, meaning it softens and soothes tissues and mucous membranes. Licorice further offers adrenal support with its mineralocorticoidlike substances and contains estrogenic chemicals such as beta-sitosterol and stigmasterol. Its adrenal stimulation allows it to be an antistress herb and to be helpful in inflammatory problems, such as arthritis, and in hypoglycemia, which is a problem related to weak adrenals. The estrogenic support allows its use in women as a sexual and uterine tonic and for problems of infertility. Licorice root has been used as a stomach and intestinal remedy for problems such as indigestion, nausea, and constipation; for infections of the respiratory tract, including colds and flus, and for hoarseness, sore throat, and wheezing; in hepatitis, ulcers, and hemorrhoids; for skin problems; for muscle spasms and fevers associated with sweating; and for general weakness. Licorice has also been suggested for people with high blood pressure, yet there is concern here since excessive intake can elevate blood pressure.

It appears that the whole root or deglycyrrhizinated licorice (DGL) is safe and has the positive attributes of licorice extract without side effects. DGL has been the subject of recent interest and research, and it apparently still helps in healing ulcers.

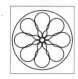

Usually, licorice root is used in herbal combinations and not by itself; it also balances the flavor of these formulas. In Chinese herbology, licorice is one of the most commonly used herbs, along with ginger. It is available in hard roots, soft ground roots, powdered in capsules, in elixirs, and as DGL. The dosage would be as recommended on the product or in an herbal text.

Wheatgrass and Barley Grass

These juice extracts of grain greens seem to offer an energy lift and act as a "purifier" and "rejuvenator," probably because of their chlorophyll and nutrient content. That, at least, is what users state. But these grasses may also help protect against cancer, and chlorophyll, as an antioxidant, can have an antiaging function. Barley grass has recently been studied in Japan and been shown to protect human cells and animal DNA from damage by X-rays and some cancer-causing chemicals. Of course, this effect was seen when the grass juice was given prior to exposure. This preliminary evidence suggests some possibilities. Along with the other nutrients available in wheatgrass or barley grass, these juices may be very useful in healing and disease prevention. There is a lot of enthusiasm about them in certain areas of the health community.

○ GLANDULARS

The use of animal tissues in treatment of disease and support of health is a controversial one in medicine, with opinions ranging from useless to miraculous. On the one hand, we have thyroid hormones, insulin, and estrogens, for example, which are used very commonly. On the other hand, we have what are called protomorphogens, or extracts of tissues from glands such as adrenal, pancreas, pituitary, thyroid, and ovary, which can be taken orally to help support those particular tissues in humans.

I used to feel that it was quite simplistic to think that eating an animal's glands would help strengthen my own like glands. Along with many other medical doctors, I also think we should be able to measure the hormone activity of many substances and monitor its effect in the body. The glandulars are usually measured by the amount of the actual glands present, but we do not really know what they do. Further, since these glands are broken down into their basic nutrients in the digestive tract, they would not necessarily go directly to improve my own glands. Previously, I was a strict vegetarian, so for that reason alone I did not want to consume animal glands, which might also have a buildup of toxins or chemicals.

Now I feel more open to the possibility that glandulars have some use in supporting and strengthening specific organ function. On the positive side, it is likely that the basic components of those gland tissues may offer the precursor substances that our own bodies and glands can use to enhance their functions. And there may be hidden factors that may offer some benefit. The glands, like foods, supply basic nutrients, such as amino acids, oils, vitamins, other active ingredients, and a potential "life force," where a drug will not. Some evidence from radioisotope studies suggests that glands, when eaten, do in fact get to the human glands and influence them.

In modern medicine, glandular therapy with the use of whole glands began in the late nineteenth century when doctors suggested that their patients eat the animal parts, usually from cows, that corresponded to the weak areas of their own bodies. So people began eating brains, hearts, kidneys, and so on as part of their medical treatment. Actually, the ancient Greeks and Egyptians used glandular therapy, following their basic premise that "like heals like." Technology and medical endocrinology evolved this therapy by isolating specific hormones at the source of the glands' activities (just as we extracted the active pharmaceutical drugs from whole plants). These new drugs are more potent, but they also have more potential for dangerous side effects than the whole glands.

For example, desiccated thyroid gland was first used in the late 1800s to help people with goiter and low thyroid function. Then thyroxine (T_4) was isolated and used, but many doctors still preferred the whole gland as it was felt to be better absorbed and utilized. Later, the other thyroid hormones, triiodothyronine (T_3) and calcitonin were discovered, but these were always part of the whole gland. Today, both individual synthetic hormones and measured active thyroid tissue are used to support or replace thyroid activity.

In the early 1920s, insulin was isolated by Sir Frederick Banting and Charles H. Best, who received the Nobel Prize for their discovery. Insulin has been a lifesaver for many diabetics, but it is also a very dangerous drug because it has such a narrow range of safe uses. Overdoses can cause very low blood sugar and shock. Insulin is destroyed in the gut, so it must be injected. It is possible that in the pancreas, as in other glands, certain molecules protect the active hormones from digestive juices, and some of these substances actually get into the body. The whole pancreas gland, which had previously been used, is definitely safer than insulin, but pancreas itself is not strong enough to treat diabetes once it is established.

Currently, opinion is split over the use of animal glands and hormones, separating those in the medical profession from other practitioners, such as naturopaths and chiropractors, who cannot write prescriptions. Allopathic medicine usually is not very supportive of the nondrug or natural approaches used by its professional competitors; however, glandular therapy is much more accepted by physicians in other countries, particularly in Europe. Currently in this country, there is not much definitive research to support those approaches, and the M.D.s might say those "doctors" are not trained to treat disease. Natural practitioners often feel that what they do is safe and effective for many people who do not have advanced disease; they work preventively. But the science and dollars are behind the medical profession, even though there is a lot of good experience with the more natural therapies. There does need to be more research

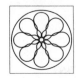

to show exactly what effects use of these glandulars has so that we can all better apply them to health.

Glandulars such as thyroid, ovary, adrenal, and thymus are not prescription items and can be purchased by anyone in health food stores. Practitioners such as chiropractors, naturopaths, and nutritionists often suggest certain glandular protomorphogens in an attempt to strengthen or balance the internal function and energies of their patients/clients.

I, personally, am not sure what to do with glandular therapy. It does not seem to cause harm, and it may do some good. As I said earlier, I am becoming more comfortable with this therapy, and I occasionally suggest adrenal, pancreas, thymus, or non-prescription thyroid for people who seem to need that support. I do not use these in medical conditions that I feel need actual hormone therapy. It is clear that more research and understanding are needed in this still-mysterious practice of using glandular substitutes.

Glandular supplements are made in a variety of ways. The best products are prepared from freeze-dried, defatted, fresh glands, as no heat or chemicals that can destroy the enzymes are used. A vacuum process is used to dry the glands after freezing. Because no chemical solvents are used to pull out the fat and potentially toxic chemicals stored in the glands, it is suggested that the glandular tissue be obtained from range-grazed cattle that have not been given chemicals, hormones, or antibiotics. Many companies use this type of processing, and the majority of these glandulars are imported from New Zealand. Some practitioners believe that removing the fat from the glands in the least toxic way is important, as the fat can contain any harmful residues of substances contacted by the animal, and is subject to oxidize and go rancid; the remaining protein tissues are stable. Another current safe method is by use of an organic, inert solvent in a low-temperature process termed "azeotrophic" extraction. As yet there is no clear answer to which process is best, but these two glandular preparations lead the way.

Adrenal

The adrenals are the glands that help us deal with stress, mineral balances, and inflammation. They release adrenaline into the body to increase activity and energy. They may be overworked these days in response to stress, caffeine, nicotine, and sugar. Adrenal glandulars are often suggested for people who experience fatigue, stress, environmental sensitivities or allergies, infections, and hypoglycemia. The symptoms that come from low blood sugar are probably more related to adrenal than to pancreas, and supporting the adrenals with freeze-dried adrenal at 50–100 mg. twice daily, along with other stress-supporting nutrients, such as the B vitamins, vitamins C and A, and zinc, may be helpful.

Pancreas

Pancreas is used mainly to support digestion by providing extra digestive enzymes. Lipases, proteases, and amylases are found in the pancreas gland. Taking digestive enzymes 30–60 minutes after meals often helps us to better utilize the meal's nutrition, especially for people whose digestion has been weakened by emotional stress, chemical irritants, or poor eating habits. I believe many people, particularly the elderly, need pancreatic enzyme support (and often hydrochloric acid as well) to properly digest and assimilate foods; this is part of many of the nutritional programs I propose in Part Four. There are those who suggest that pancreatic insufficiency is at the heart of aging and much disease, including allergies, weight problems, arthritis and other inflammatory problems, gastrointestinal problems, and cancer. Pancreatic support is important in cancer programs and the use of pork-derived pancreas for therapy is currently under investigation.

Thymus

The thymus is important to immunological activity. It contains the active hormone thymosin, which stimulates T lymphocyte (T cell) production and activity. T cells help the body defend itself against infection. Our thymus gland tends to weaken with age, and this may affect our defense system. If we experience fatigue, recurrent infections, or measurable immune deficiency, intake of oral thymus gland may be helpful. This is not well researched, but it most likely won't cause any problems. Injectable thymus has been definitely shown to stimulate immune activity.

Thyroid

Thyroid weakness can be caused by lack of iodine or too little protein in the diet and probably by emotional stress and blocked creativity as well. In such cases, thyroid glandular may be helpful in supporting the gland to work better. Nutrients that contain thyroid tissue and hormone precursors, such as iodine and tyrosine, seem to be helpful. Thyroid glandular has been used for fatigue and to support immune function.

Other Glandulars

Many other glandular tissues are available for support of body organs. Brain tissue has been used for ages to stimulate brain function. Likewise, heart or lung extracts have supported those organs. Stomach and duodenum, testicular and ovarian tissue, prostate, pituitary, and hypothalamus have all been employed to enhance body organ functions. Spleen glandular tissue has been popular for immunological support, to help boost lymphocyte activity, and to protect the body from infections. High-nutrient liver tissue is also part of many glandular programs to support this important metabolic

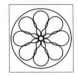

organ in our bodies. As many people describe, liver may help us energetically and functionally, but it should be good liver from healthy, nontoxic animals, as this organ in particular can have high concentrations of many toxins.

Live Cell Therapy

This advanced technique of glandular therapy was devised by the Swiss physician Paul Niehans in the 1930s. He initially injected a whole diced parathyroid gland from a sheep into a woman who had hers removed, and apparently she did remarkably well. This therapy has expanded to the use of all possible glandular tissues, from brain to lung to vertebral disks taken from freshly slaughtered fetal sheep. The fetus is used because of the early stage of cell development and patterning that theoretically helps most to restore our cellular pattern and stimulate the organ's regeneration and function. (The bone marrow transplant done in Western medicine is a specific, advanced technique analagous to glandular therapy.)

This glorified live cell glandular therapy is very popular in European countries and is available in Mexico; it is not currently legal in the United States. Health seekers as well as the rich and famous travel to experience this therapy proposed to extend youth and vitality, plus generate real healing. Whether this really works remains to be seen.

○ A FEW OTHERS

Chondroitin Sulfates—
Mucopolysaccharides and Glycosaminoglycans

There are substances present in the cartilaginous tissue between joints and concentrated in the artery walls. They are not essential nutritionally in that our body makes them. The commercially available mucopolysaccharide products are high in silicon, a mineral important to tissue strength and health. Mussels and oysters contain these chondroitin sulfates. A supplement extracted from green-lipped mussels, *Perna canaliculus*, is high in mucopolysaccharides and is currently available. It is theorized that taking oral chondroitin sulfates or products containing other mucopolysaccharides will help alleviate joint problems or rebuild degenerating cartilage. They may further help in maintaining strength and elasticity of the artery walls and in reducing potential inflammation and blood clotting time—all of which may help reduce cardiovascular disease potential. Mucopolysaccharides and collagen help hold our tissues together. Chondroitin sulfates may be an antiaging nutrient as well as support or increase production of seminal fluid in men, and may have mild aphrodisiac effects. These chondroitin sulfate/mucopolysaccharide products have been used in the treatment of various conditions, including headaches, arthritis, bursitis, ulcers, respiratory diseases, angina, and allergies. There is no hard evidence to date that these claims, often commercial, are accurate or that there is great therapeutic success in using the oral supplements (they may break down in the digestive tract), although bovine cartilage injections have been helpful in the treatment of arthritis and psoriasis. More research is needed to verify the potential for these very interesting molecules that are used in our body tissue.

Organo-Germanium

Germanium is a trace mineral that has recently come to the attention of the health world through some incredible work and results at a clinic in Japan. Germanium occurs naturally in very small amounts in the soil and in certain foods and herbs, such as shiitake mushrooms, ginseng root, garlic, shelf fungus, and aloe vera. It has been used for its semiconductor properties in making computer chips. Its possible medical value was discovered in the 1950s by Kazuhiko Asai when he noticed that fairly high amounts of germanium were present in coal, peat, and some of the more powerful and useful Oriental healing herbs. In 1967, Dr. Asai and his associates isolated an organo-germanium compound soluble in water and labeled it Ge-132 (bis-carboxyethyl germanium sesquioxide, the 132nd form they had synthesized). In 1968, Dr. Asai founded the Asai Germanium Research Institute to study the clinical application of Ge-132 further. Over the next 15 years, Dr. Asai and coresearchers found that germanium was essentially nontoxic and had an incredible effect on many pathological conditions, particularly in suppressing tumor activity in tumor-bearing animals. In 1980, Dr. Asai published a book very optimistically called *Miracle Cure: Organic Germanium.*

Germanium is trace element number 32 in the periodic table. It is twice as heavy as oxygen (16) and seems in some way related to it, as it supports cellular and tissue oxygenation. Research in Japan also verified a number of effects of Ge-132 on the immune systems of animals and humans. (This is not the effects of the trace mineral but of this special organo-germanium; see the discussion in Chapter 6, *Minerals.*) Ge-Oxy 132, as it is sometimes called, has been shown to have both antitumor and antiviral effects. These may be a result of its varying immunological actions, such as stimulating interferon production, stimulating macrophage ("Pac-man" white cells) and NK (natural killer) lymphocyte activity, and enhancing cell-mediated immunity. There is some suggestion that Ge-132 helps in pain relief; particularly dramatic relief has occurred in some cases of severe cancer pain.

Most of these effects are noted more in people who are immune suppressed than in normal individuals. Research on the topic has begun at the University of Texas. In an

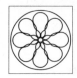

article published in the November 1984 issue of the *Journal of Interferon Research*, Fugio Suzulu and Richard B. Pollard commented, "Ge-132 belongs to a group of compounds capable of modulating immune response in hosts that have an alteration of immune homeostasis. Although there are a few reports describing enhancement of Ge-132 on natural killer cell activity in healthy subjects, studies in immune suppressed animals and patients with malignancies or rheumatoid arthritis suggest that Ge-132 restores the normal function of T-cell lymphocytes, B lymphocytes, antibody-dependent cellular cytotoxicity, natural killer cell activity, and numbers of antibody-forming cells, but does not enhance them above normal limits."

Interestingly, in both sick and normal animals and humans, Ge-132 is virtually nontoxic. Suzulu and Pollard's article continues, "Preliminary toxicological and pharmacological studies of this compound (Ge-132) indicate that it has several unique physiological activities without any significant toxic effects." Ge-132 really could be classified as a "highly safe drug" even though it is a trace mineral compound. It has practically no toxicity or influence on reproductive or other functions.

More research is needed on Ge-132. Organic germanium from Japan, as Ge-Oxy 132, has become available only recently in the United States as a pure white powder that can be made into tablets, capsules, or dissolved in water. It is still fairly expensive and will continue to be until it is produced in this country. Now, many companies are marketing germanium products; make sure that it is in this organo-germanium sesquioxide form. Amounts in supplements range from 25–150 mg. or are available as pure powder. Suggested dosages for treatment range from 50–100 mg. daily (probably the minimum needed for an effect), up to 3–6 grams daily (the doses used in Japan for cancer therapy). The level of germanium sesquioxide needed to induce interferon synthesis in humans is a daily intake of 50–75 mg./kg. body weight.

Ge-132 looks very promising, and I am quite excited about it. Its use in the treatment of viral disorders, especially Epstein-Barr, and other problems of immunological suppression appears helpful. Gastrointestinal diseases, such as diverticulitis, circulatory problems, mental symptoms, or really any problem that might be aided by improved oxygenation could be helped by organo-germanium (Ge-132) supplementation. In my clinical experience, I have found that allergies have also been reduced by the use of this nutrient, particularly those allergies that arise to foods based on weakening of the intestinal mucosa. Germanium's effect on cancer is probably due to its immunostimulating effects rather than a direct effect on cancer cells. Its current use by cancer patients may move it into the political arena soon, which will prompt the FDA and the medical establishment to set controls on its use.

Germanium is currently considered a food supplement. Since it is found in the soil and in many healing herbs, some levels of mineral germanium will always be available to us. More research into this fascinating, semiconductor trace element may help us to better understand the mysterious powers of some of our great, ancient healing plants.

Royal Jelly

Royal jelly is another panacea for health and longevity seekers. Worker bees make this exotic substance their queen bee. And all of us want to be queen or king bees, of course. Royal jelly is definitely an energizer. It is high in certain unique fatty acids, simple carbohydrates, and pantothenic acid, which is supportive of the adrenals. It also contains the other B vitamins, all of the essential amino acids, and many minerals, such as iron, calcium, silicon, sulfur, and potassium. Royal jelly has been used to support weight loss, as it is a rich and energizing nutrient yet low in calories (20 calories per teaspoon), and to treat problems such as fatigue, insomnia, digestive disorders, ulcers, and cardiovascular ailments. Whether this mysterious substance really is a great rejuvenator and supporter of youth and longevity will need to be studied. But many people, especially women, experience an uplifting feeling when they take either liquid or encapsulated royal jelly.

Propolis

Propolis is a resin obtained from the buds of some trees and flowers. This sap is rich in such nutrients as minerals and the B vitamins. Bees collect it along with pollen. Propolis is thought to contain a natural antibiotic, called galangin, and is used in a variety of remedies to treat or prevent low-grade infections, especially in people who do not want to take antibiotics. Many people have described to me positive results from using propolis products. Bees spread the propolis around their hives to protect them from bacteria and viruses. (The name "propolis" comes from Greek words meaning "defenses before a town.") Other theories suggest that propolis improves energy and endurance and helps immunity by stimulating thymus activity. All of these claims must be helpful in potentizing the placebo effect, but more research needs to be done before propolis is readily adopted by the scientific community.

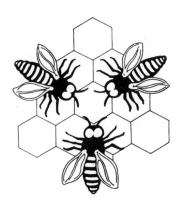

Royal Jelly

Propolis

PART TWO

FOODS, DIETS, AND THE ENVIRONMENT

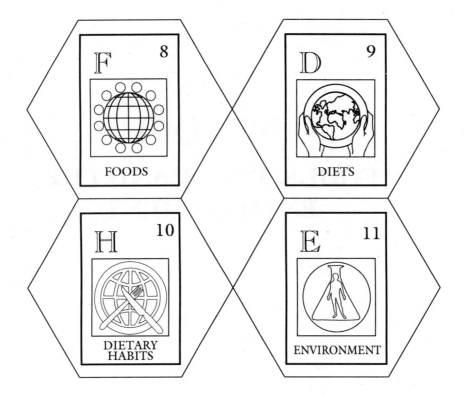

We had discussed the building blocks — the nutrients found in foods and other substances on our planet that make up our body tissues and guide body functions — now let us look at the many foods and diets that contain these important and essential nutrients. If we think of nutrition as a communication system, then the macro- and micronutrients discussed in Part One are the letters of our alphabet while the foods create the words to our language with their special mix of letters or nutrients, and the meals are the sentences or combination of words that bring together the multiple components of nutrition and allow us to communicate with one another.

After reviewing the various food groups and individual foods in Chapter 8, I will then discuss the various types of diets eaten in our culture as well as the many and varying cultural diets eaten throughout the world. Following that, I will elaborate on healthy and unhealthy dietary habits and then discuss some concerns about the state of our food and the use of chemicals, and the effects upon our planet's environment in Chapter 11. Following that, we will serve *Building a Healthy Diet* for Part Three and look at how to combine all the factors I have discussed in Parts One and Two into a healthy nutritional program.

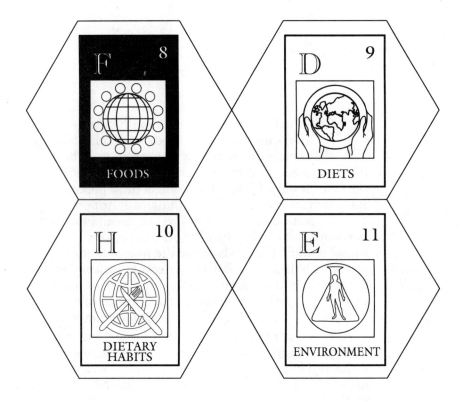

Chapter 8

Foods

This section provides an evaluation of the various food categories, such as fruits, vegetables, grains, and so on. This is not a discussion of the nutrient groups, such as protein or carbohydrates, which were previously reviewed, or the categories such as the four food groups classically used to describe a wholesome diet. These aspects of our diet, along with many other nutritional principles, will be discussed later in Part Three entitled *Building a Healthy Diet*.

Food availability varies around the world. Earth provides different plants according to climate. The peoples of our planet have also spread pleasurable and nutritious foods from culture to culture and country to country by carrying seeds or plants to cultivate in a new area. Many foods present in America, such as potatoes, rice, and even wheat, were not originally grown here.

One of the most natural concepts of eating is that of consuming primarily foods that are grown in the area in which we live, and consuming them near the time when they are grown—in other words, **seasonal eating of fresh foods**. Some foods, such as root vegetables, grains, nuts, and seeds, store better than others, and may be consumed in times, such as winter, when in many areas, most foods are not available in their fresh state.

Overall, it is important to eat a variety of foods. As we will see in the descriptions of specific categories of food, eating only one type will usually provide limited nutrition and an imbalanced diet. Also, in general, I advocate eating a predominantly natural diet containing fresh fruits and vegetables, whole grains, nuts, seeds, and beans, with only moderate amounts of the more concentrated proteins such as eggs, milk products, and flesh foods, rather than the opposite—one consisting mainly of meats, dairy products, and refined foods and only occasional fresh foods, a diet that is all too common in our society.

I will discuss the basic foods from the least concentrated to the most, basically, from fruits to animal meats. I actually begin with even higher octave or vibration foods, flowers and pollens, and move through the food chain to animal products, and then finish with seasonings and beverages. With each category, I will describe the basic nutrient makeup and vitamin and mineral content and give specific examples of foods that are part of that group. For the exact nutrient content of each food I refer you to food source books such as the *Nutrition Almanac*, where this information can be found in a section entitled "Table of Food Composition."

Using this information, we can analyze what we eat in regards to our exact nutrient intake. That, however, is a fairly complex and time-consuming process. I often suggest doing a diet survey to individuals wanting to see how their diet is balanced and what specific nutrients it contains. Appendix I has an example. A diet survey basically involves recording onto a special form all food consumed over a one-week period. This information is transferred into a computer programmed to analyze the daily intake of calories, fiber, cholesterol, and nutrients from vitamin A to Zinc. The percentages of fats, carbohydrates, and proteins are also important, as is the percentage of calories from various food groups. These all help us to see more clearly how the diet is balanced and how to shift to a potentially healthier one. This is a valuable exercise for anyone interested in personal nutrition.

Fiber

Before discussing the particular types of food, I want to say a few words about fiber, an important component of many of the "nature" foods. Fiber is basically the indigestible parts of plants, such as the skins of apples and other fruits and the coverings of wheat and rice. There are some nutrients contained in these fiber parts that may be extracted out for the body to use, but the basic fiber structure passes through our digestive tract to clean our intestines and give more bulk to our excrement. It actually helps the bowels function most efficiently.

Fiber is being found more and more to be important to health and prevention of many serious diseases. Our modern refined diet and fast food consciousness have taken many of us away from a fiber-rich diet composed of salads, fresh fruit, whole grains, and so on. This current inadequate diet is likely a big contributor to our main chronic diseases; specifically, the low-fiber component of the diet has been shown to be correlated with an increased level of heart disease, several gastrointestinal diseases, and cancer, particularly of the colon and rectum, one of the most common areas affected in both sexes. And when we avoid the fiber foods, we often replace them with higher fat or sugar ones, which have other disease associations. Some people eat a little daily bran with their "typical American" diet, and though this may help colon function somewhat, it is a poor substitute for eating more nutrient-rich fruits, vegetables, and whole grains.

Let's explore the foods in our diets so we can make more knowledgeable choices.

Flowers

This is a slightly eccentric category but one that is of import to those people interested in beautiful eating. I am referring here to colorful plant flowers and not to the fruits or vegetables of flowering plants, such as oranges, tomatoes, or zucchini. Those are discussed in upcoming sections. This section actually refers to those colorful flowers from the gardens or meadows.

Many flowers are edible and tasty. Many, however, are not, and some could make us sick. Really, there are only a few poisonous flowers. Many flowers have medicinal properties, and eating or using flowers in teas, poultices (compresses), or salves is often more a subject of herbology, the use of plants as medicines.

Flowers are the most subtle and often fragrant part of plants. They are not very concentrated in nutrition and are considered more a "food for the spirit," both as a delight to our mouths and in their appeal to our eyes and noses.

Commonly consumed edible flowers include nasturtiums, borage, and marigolds; there are also the many flowering seasoning herbs, such as basil and thyme, though we usually consume only the greenery of these. Mustard, radish, and watercress flowers are spicy additions to salads. Chrysanthemum petals are edible, as are squash blossoms (see recipe in *Spring* diet of Part Three). Flowers of many common herbs, such as rosemary, dill, oregano, chives, sage, and marjoram, are also edible.

Most of these flowers have a little carbohydrate, no fat, and not much protein. Many contain some vitamin C, and vitamin A is found in others. A few of the minerals, such as calcium, magnesium, and zinc, may also be found in certain flowers. However, we wouldn't really think of eating flowers for their nutrient content, which is low, but for the other subtle and lovely qualities they may offer. Borage is said to help us forget our troubles and marigolds or calendula flowers to fill us with happiness.

We should know which flowers are edible and be able to clearly identify them before consuming any to ensure against getting sick or poisoned from eating those delicacies.

Bee and Flower Pollen

Though allergists are not overly excited about the use of bee and flower pollens, the general public loves these forms of concentrated energy. Bee pollen is likely the first food supplement ever used. The common claim for bee pollen is that it improves energy and endurance in its users. Many athletes and health enthusiasts use bee pollen. There seems to be some scientific proof, scanty as it may be, that bee pollen does improve physical performance, but its many other claims for helping arthritis, heart disease, or bowel and prostate problems have not been verified. Many use it to enhance immunity, reduce allergy, lose weight, and relieve stress, but there is no evidence for these claims either.

Bee pollen is collected from bees' legs when special pollen scrapers and collectors are attached to their hive. It is essentially concentrated pollens from flowers, so its nutrient content may vary. There are usually some amino acids (protein), vitamins, and minerals in most pollens.

Because bee pollen is concentrated flower pollen, there is some theoretical concern about its use by people who have pollen allergies, though in practice there seems to be a big difference between the effects of inhaled and ingested pollens. The gastrointestinal action on the pollens, I am sure, changes their allergenicity. Theoretically as well, it would seem that pollens ingested might work to desensitize people who are environmentally allergic, but this has not been proved either.

There are some new flower pollen products on the market as well; these are different from bee pollen in that they are not collected from bees. The companies who promote them and people who use them speak very highly of their positive benefits to energy and health, but again more research is needed to actually show what these products do.

Suffice it to say bee and flower pollens are those extra products used more by personal choice than because they are a necessary part of the diet. They are more often recommended by friends or health enthusiasts than by medical practitioners. Many people realize some positive benefits from pollens; others may not notice much. Often the amounts used are begun at low levels and built up over days and weeks to a handful at a time to produce the desired effects. Physical energy and athletic performance probably are the reasons for most pollen use, rather than for disease or symptom treatment. Bee and flower pollen's effects may range from subtle for many to very strong for others, but most people claim that when they eat bee pollen, which has a slightly sweet and unique taste, they tend to "buzz" around with more life.

○ FRUITS

Fruits are considered nature's perfect foods. They are the only pure offering from nature, as a ripe fruit from the tree may actually drop into our hand. The fruit is the result of a healthy growing cycle of life for most plants and the bearer or potentiator of life, as it carries the seeds for the next generation of trees and plants.

Fruits have many positive qualities. They are natural and healthy (and best from organic sources), and they are juicy, with a very high water content, like the human body itself. Fruits are also well stocked in nutrients, par-

ticularly such important vitamins as A and C, a little of the Bs, and E in the seeds. Many minerals, such as calcium, magnesium, copper, and manganese, a little iron, and other trace minerals, are also present in fruits, especially when they are contained in the water and soil that nourishes the plants or trees. Fruits are low in fat and high in fiber, both very healthful attributes for our commonly high-fat, low-fiber culture. Fruits are also relatively low calorie and low sodium, two more helpful characteristics. Most are sweet, colorful, and cooling and can be crunchy too. Fruits' colors are some of the most beautiful in nature and cover the whole rainbow.

Fruits are high in natural sugars, thus making them a good substitute for those higher-calorie sugar treats when we feel we want something sweet. The sweet flavor is the most prevalent flavor in many diets. According to Chinese medical theory, too much sweet food may cause many problems. But eating whole fruits is the most natural way to obtain this sweet flavor.

Fruit juices are also an important beverage. Ideally consumed fresh, they are higher in vitamins and minerals than many other drinks. They are particularly a good replacement for sugary soda pops. Fruits and fruit juices without added sugars also tend to be purifying and help with our elimination. They are often part of a cleansing or detoxification program.

Fruits are also very easy to digest and utilize, and so they usually have low allergenic potential (allergy comes mainly from the protein components of food). Occasionally, someone is sensitive to such fruits as oranges or tomatoes, but this is less common than with other regularly used foods, such as milk, wheat, and other grains. Fruits may have a cooling and calming action for the body and nervous system and may be helpful in reducing body stress. Because of the natural nutrient content, fruit consumption may help strengthen our immune system as well.

It is most natural and economical to eat

298

fruits fresh in season. It is ideal to wash them to clean off any sprays, germs, and environmental contaminants and to eat organic fruits whenever possible. Eating fruit in its ripe state is probably best for our body, as the "green" or unripe fruits may be more irritating.

Also, fresh is best from a nutritional standpoint. Fresh frozen is next, as the fruits lose very little of their nutrients. Drying fruits for storage is probably a little better than canning, though fresh "canned," or, really, glass-jar-stored fruits in water that produce their own fruit juice, is much better than those with added sugars or syrups. Drying fruit pieces is more economical for storage purposes, and they will keep a long time if protected. Fruit is not usually cooked, though cooked fruits, such as stewed prunes, baked apples, and others are very tasty and can be eaten or used in some recipes; these may be easier to ingest for the elderly, who may not chew well, and are good for assisting normal intestinal activity. After cooking fruits, consuming the natural juices in which some of the fruits' nutrients are contained will make them more wholesome.

Fruits fall into such categories as citrus fruits, melons, berries, tropical fruits, dried fruits, and many common fruits such as apples and pears. Most fruits grow on trees, but some are found on bushes (berries) or on ground vines (melons). Most fruits follow the flower of the plant and are available during the summer, late summer, and autumn, though there are exceptions.

Fruits have also been categorized as sweet, subacid, and acid. The sweet fruits are mainly the dried fruits, such as raisins and figs, and some tropical ones, such as bananas. Most juicy fruits are considered subacid. These include peaches, plums, apples, pears, grapes, cherries, mangoes, papayas, and so on. Citrus fruits, some berries, pineapples, and pomegranates are examples of acid-tasting fruits. They have a higher level of acid, often ascorbic acid (vitamin C), and this may make them helpful in cutting fats or helping fat digestion.

When broken down in our body, though, fruits become more alkaline. (Cranberries, prunes, plums, and possibly strawberries and pomegranates are the main acid-forming fruits.) When fruits are utilized or burned, the minerals and ash that are left, even from lemons and pineapples, are alkaline, supporting our body's acid-alkaline balance. In regard to food combining (see Chapter 10), fruits are digested very easily and therefore best eaten by themselves, rather than with other more concentrated foods, which take longer to pass through our stomach and digestive tract.

Common Fruits

Apples	*Peaches*
Apricots	*Pears*
Cherries	*Plums*
Grapes	

These are the common tree fruits (except for grapes) of the United States and much of the world. Most of these are in the subacid variety of fruits. Apples and pears are similar in their growth and in the climates where they grow, as well as in their multiseeded cores. The single-seeded apricots, cherries, peaches, and plums each have their own unique flavor and avid followers. Grapes are our special vine fruit with many varieties used for eating, seasonal decor, and making wine.

All of these fruits are really tasty and juicy, and best eaten fresh; however, there is concern over the use of pesticides sprayed on them and the effects of these chemicals in our health, especially for our children. If possible, buying and consuming organically grown fruits is ideal.

Apples. Apple history is rich. From the Garden of Eden to Snow White and the Queen, the life of the apple had a questionable future. But Johnny Appleseed spread apples throughout the land and made them one of America's popular fruits. Now they help to keep doctors away and shine up our teacher. Apples are also a very nutritious fruit.

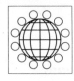

They are high in fiber, and apple pectin has a detoxifying quality and is used in many cleansing formulas. Eating apples also helps clean the teeth. Recent concerns over chemicals used in growing and harvesting apples has tainted the image of this "health" fruit, but organic apples or unsprayed apples are still one of the favorite fruits in our society.

One apple has about 100 calories, mainly from carbohydrate; nearly 2 grams of fiber; about 10 mg. vitamin C, 150 IUs of vitamin A, and some modest amounts of B vitamins—B_1, B_2, B_3, B_6, and biotin. Apples also contain various minerals—lots of potassium; over 15 mg. each of calcium, magnesium, and phosphorus; about a ½ mg. of iron; and traces of manganese, copper, selenium, and zinc. Apples even have some vitamin E, mostly in the seeds. Apples are like mini-multivitamins—they have a little of everything.

Apricots. Apricots have received recent notoriety about their laetrile-laden kernels. But the apricot fruit itself is very nutritious and tasty. It is high in vitamin A, mainly as beta-carotene, the vitamin A precursor. Each little apricot has nearly 1,000 IUs of vitamin A. The vitamin C content is fairly good, though lower than in some other fruits, as are the B vitamins. Potassium and other minerals, such as calcium and iron, are also contained in apricots. The trace minerals zinc, copper, and manganese are also present. Dried apricots may have even higher concentrations of vitamin A and minerals. Apricots are considered one of the longevity fruits contained in high amounts in the long-living Hunzas' diet.

Cherries. Cherries can be sweet or sour, red or black. They are good colon cleansers, as they enhance bowel motility. They are fairly high in vitamin C content, about 15 mg. per cup of cherries. Vitamin A content is good, the Bs are modest, and minerals are high. Potassium content is very high, calcium content is good, as is phosphorus content, and there are modest levels of magnesium and manganese, and fair amounts of copper and

iron, thus making this "bloody" fruit good for building our blood.

Grapes. There are many varieties of this fruit of the vine. Wines made from grapes are used in most cultures as part of both religious rites and secular celebrations. And many people celebrate daily.

Green Thompson seedless grapes are those most commonly consumed in our country, though red seedless, larger seeded Reiber (or Ribier) grapes, and other kinds are a real treat as well. Grapes have lots of nutrients and also help cleanse the bowels. Grape fasting—consuming only grapes and grape juice for days and weeks at a time—is a fairly popular therapeutic tool in the natural healing fields. Many anecdotal positive experiences have been described by those grape fasters, but, as with any kind of fasting, there is not very much research to demonstrate its value. Nor do grapes maintain a balanced diet.

Grapes are fairly high in fruit sugar, fructose, and are mainly carbohydrate foods. They contain no fat and minimum protein but a good amount of fiber. Grapes have about 100 calories per cup. They contain decent amounts of vitamin A; good vitamin C levels; some B vitamins; lots of potassium; some calcium, magnesium, and phosphorus; traces of iron and copper; and a fairly high level, for fruit, of the important mineral manganese.

Because bugs are very attracted to the sweet grapes, these fruits are often heavily sprayed. In fact, there have been recent grape boycotts by the Farm Workers Union to protest the use of dangerous pesticides that jeopardize the workers' health—and the consumers' as well.

Peaches. Peaches have very good press—they are sweet, fuzzy, and friendly, and when all is going well, it's "peachy." In season, peaches are usually so juicy that they should be eaten outdoors or with bibs.

Peaches have good levels of vitamins A and C, potassium, and phosphorus; fair amounts of calcium and magnesium; and traces of the important minerals zinc, selenium, manganese, iodine, sulfur, copper, and iron. The B vitamin content is modest, as in most fruits.

Pears. Pears are similar to apples in that they have modest to moderate amounts of many nutrients. There are many varieties, ranging from crunchy to very juicy. They are lower in vitamin A than other fruits but do contain good fiber. They have decent levels of vitamin C and folic acid and have high amounts of potassium and surprisingly good levels of manganese and selenium. Like apples, pears also have good cleansing and detoxification potential, probably related to their high fiber content.

Plums. Plums also come in many varieties and are one of our few purple foods. They range in flavor from sour to very sweet and are mildly acid-forming when broken down in our body. Plums are low in calories and have good levels of vitamin A and potassium. They contain a bit of calcium and magnesium, some iron and copper, vitamin C and phosphorous, and traces of B vitamins.

Citrus Fruits

Grapefruits	*Limes*
Lemons	*Oranges*

Citrus fruits are warm-climate fruits containing almost all juice. They seem to be available nearly year round in our hotter states, such as Florida, Texas, and California, but most citrus fruits are harvested mainly in late spring to early summer, with certain types, such as navel oranges, giving a winter crop.

Citrus fruits are known for their vitamin C content. An average orange, for example, contains about 65 mg. (about the RDA) of this important vitamin. Citruses are also high in potassium and other minerals. Like most other fruits, they are low in salt, or sodium.

Citrus fruits are used commonly for cleansing, as during colds and flus, and for cooling us down in the summertime. Citrus juice seems to help cut grease on the hands or dishes, and it likely has the same effect on the body, helping fat digestion and utilization. Citrus and vitamin C are thought to help reduce cholesterol. Gallbladder and liver function is thought to be supported by citrus fruits, especially lemons, and lemon water may help stimulate digestive juice secretions. More research is needed to evaluate the actions and effects of citrus juices in our body.

Grapefruits. Grapefruits are used in many diets to reduce the appetite and help digestion and utilization of foods. They are low in calories, and consuming them probably burns as many calories as they contain. Among the citrus fruits, grapefruits are an especially good weight-loss food.

One grapefruit contains about 75 mg. of vitamin C. Amounts of vitamin A and the Bs are fairly low, though there is some biotin. Potassium content is very good, and there is some calcium, magnesium, and phosphorus as well. Grapefruit juice straight or mixed with orange juice is a high-vitamin C meal.

Lemons. Lemons have been a very useful food in my life. Lemonade fasting has done wonders for me and thousands of others who have attempted the "master cleanse" described in my book *Staying Healthy with the Seasons* (Celestial Arts, 1981). Lemon water, as a half lemon in a glass of water, drunk 20–30 minutes before meals, seems to help stimulate gastric juices and help digestion. In general, liquids drunk a while before meals can reduce our appetite and thus help prevent overeating, and lemon water is a very good choice.

I consider lemons a cleanser, purifier, rejuvenator, and detoxifier, especially for the liver, as they help in fat metabolism. These functions come mainly from their astringent qualities, supported by high vitamin C and potassium levels. Like other citruses, lemons contain calcium, magnesium, and phosphorus, but most of these minerals are present more in the white part of the rind and in the pulp. Lemon juice is used in salads and, more for its biochemical behavior, in cutting fats and oils

301

(even in dishwashing liquid). It is more often used diluted in water as lemon water or lemonade (with sweeteners) than as a separate beverage, because its sour flavor limits its straight use. Lemon peel tea can be drunk after a meal as a digestive acid.

Limes. Limes are like minilemons in terms of nutritional content. Limes helped save the British sailors ("limeys") from scurvy by means of their vitamin C content. This little citrus is not as prevalent in our culture as many others; however, it is used commonly in alcoholic or refreshment drinks, as it is not quite as sour as lemon.

Oranges. Oranges are one of the most commonly used fruits in the United States. As orange juice (OJ), they are popular as a breakfast drink. One orange can give us our minimum vitamin C requirement of 65 mg., and one glass of OJ provides about 125 mg. Oranges' high potassium and good calcium levels are also helpful. Actually, oranges contain almost all the vitamins and minerals, at least in modest amounts. Since people can daily consume more oranges, as juice or fruit, than the other citruses, we are able to obtain higher vitamin C levels with OJ, often the drink for the common cold. Oranges also have more vitamin A, as beta-carotene, than other citruses, which may help fight infections and protect us from cancer by supporting our immune system.

Melons

Cantaloupes	*Honeydews*
Casabas	*Watermelons*

Melons are high-water-content fruits that grow on the ground in the heat of summer. Most are harvested in late summer; casaba and honeydew melons are more of an autumn/winter crop. When we are dry and thirsty in the summer, melons are a good answer. They are also high in calcium, potassium, vitamin C, and vitamin A as beta-carotene, especially cantaloupe and watermelon. Because of the high water and fruit sugar content of most melons, they are more easily digested than most any other food. For this reason, it is suggested that they be eaten by themselves to avoid abdominal gas and bloating, as fermentation may occur more easily when they are eaten with other, harder to digest foods. There are many varieties and colors of melons. I will discuss a few here—one red, one green, and a couple of orange ones.

Cantaloupes. Cantaloupes are very high in beta-carotene, a precursor of vitamin A. One-quarter of a cantaloupe may give up to 3000 IUs of A as well as about 30 mg. vitamin C; some Bs; potassium (about 250 mg.); a little calcium, magnesium, and phosphorus; and traces of iron, copper, manganese, and zinc.

Casabas. The casaba is a muskmelon that is higher in the minerals than in vitamins A and C. Potassium, calcium, and phosphorus are all found in good levels. The casaba-type melons are a little higher in sodium than other fruits.

Honeydews. Sweet, juicy, green melons, honeydews have a fairly good vitamin C content. The amounts of vitamin A and the Bs are lower, but potassium is high, as are calcium and phosphorus.

Watermelons. Eating watermelon can be quite an art. Red and juicy, watermelons are really America's national melon. They are almost all water and nutrients—high in beta-carotene, vitamin C, potassium, and magnesium. Watermelon is a great treat in the hot summer. Most people experience this fruit as a diuretic, stimulating urine flow. The ground seeds have been used as an herbal diuretic and kidney cleanser.

Berries

Blackberries	*Cranberries*
Blueberries	*Raspberries*
Boysenberries	*Strawberries*

There are many varieties of edible berries found all over the world. Discussed here are some more common berries available to us in both wild and cultivated forms. Berries usually can be found or harvested in later summer or early autumn, depending on the climate. Depending on ripeness, they may vary in flavor from very sour to very sweet.

Most berries have some vitamin C, about 20–30 mg. per cup. Vitamin A content varies, but at least 150–300 IUs can be found in a cup of berries. B vitamins are generally low, but minerals are fairly plentiful, with potassium content the best. Amounts of calcium, magnesium, silicon, and iron are actually pretty good. Most of the berries have a good fiber content as well.

Berries are a treat for young and old. Berry pie made with fresh-picked berries can be a flavorful and nutritious dessert, ideally consumed at least an hour or two after dinner. Berries with cream or a la mode can be a little heavy and harder to digest but definitely a taste treat. Berries with cereals are also fairly popular, but overall, berries are best by themselves.

Blackberries. Blackberries are almost exclusively wild and local, even to city folk. Come midsummer, we can stain our hands and get a few stickers pickin' and eatin' them blackberries. They need to be black and ripe to be sweet; otherwise they can make us pucker. They have pretty good amounts of calcium, magnesium, iron, and other minerals. Both vitamins A and C are found in blackberries.

Blueberries. Blueberries are sweeter and meatier and a little lower in vitamins A and C and minerals than the other berries, though they still have lots of nutrients.

Boysenberries. A really special treat, boysenberries may come earlier than the other dark bushberries. They are similar to blackberries in their nutrient content.

Cranberries. Cranberries are tart berries used mainly in their cooked and "sauced" form for celebration. Cranberry juice is commonly used to help acidify the urine to reduce

symptoms and clear mild urinary bladder infections. They are lower in vitamins A and C and minerals than the other berries but are still nutritious.

Raspberries. Both red and black raspberries are another summertime treat. They are fairly high in vitamin C and especially abundant in the minerals calcium, magnesium, and iron.

Strawberries. Our most popular American berry, strawberries grow in little ground bushes without prickers. Maybe their friendliness is what gives them top billing. But they are very tasty as well, and they are also highest in vitamin C, though a bit lower in vitamin A, and better in iron and potassium than the other berries. Strawberries are unique in that their seeds are on the outside. That trait, along with their red color, makes them the most yang, or activating, fruit from an Oriental perspective. I surely liked strawberries in my milk and cereal when I was growing up, especially drinking that pink, sweet milk at the end, with the extra white sugar, of course. Ooh!

Tropical Fruits

Bananas	*Papayas*
Guavas	*Pineapples*
Mangoes	

Tropical fruits are those that grow in a hot or tropical climate, usually one with lots of rain and sun—like Hawaii, Tahiti, the Caribbean, South America, or even Southern California or Florida. The tropical fruits vary in type of plants, fruits, and nutrients, but all are fairly exotic tasting. Each one is known for its unique taste and a particular nutrient in which it is high. Bananas are great in potassium and are likely the most popular fruit in our country, even though they are not grown here. Papayas are high in beta-carotene and the *papain* enzyme; guavas in vitamin C; pineapples in manganese and the digestive enzyme *bromelain*; while avocados, a tropical

303

and temperate fruit (will be discussed shortly under *Unusual Fruits*), have some protein and fat (they are really more like nuts in nutrient makeup). Some other less common varieties of tropical fruits are cherimoya, lychee, and zapote.

Bananas. Bananas have the number one vote as Americans' favorite fruit. They are commonly recommended as a potassium source in those patients on potassium-losing diuretic therapy. Bananas are almost completely carbohydrate. They contain many vitamins and minerals, including iron, selenium, and magnesium.

Bananas are used in flavoring for desserts, as in banana splits or banana bread, in breakfast cereals, or even in sandwiches. Most commonly, though, they are eaten after peeling the skin as a snack or dessert carried in lunch pails to work or school. As far as treats go, bananas are one of the healthiest. However, there is concern, since bananas are not indigenous in the States, over the pesticides that are used to fumigate these fruits when they come from Mexico or Hawaii. Also, some people do not digest bananas well, some are allergic, and others may become constipated from their use.

Guavas. A common tree fruit in tropical areas such as Hawaii, guavas taste similar to soft pears and have big seeds. Guavas are very high in vitamin C, with one medium-sized fruit having close to 200 mg. They are also good in fiber, are high in vitamin A and potassium, and have modest amounts of phosphorus, calcium, and magnesium. Though fairly popular in the tropics, they are not commonly imported.

Mangoes. Mangoes are a very tasty and juicy fruit that I first learned to eat in Mexico, peeled and eaten like a popsicle, using a fork stuck in the pit as a holder. Mangoes are fairly high in vitamin C and have some vitamin E but are extremely rich in vitamin A, with a high concentration of beta-carotene. One

mango may have nearly 10,000 IUs of vitamin A. Mangoes are also fairly rich in many minerals, including zinc, magnesium, and potassium.

Papayas. Papayas are best known for their digestive support, as they contain the enzyme papain. Their taste is delicious, rather like that of a melon. Papayas also may have a disinfectant property when used to clean wounds and skin or mouth sores. Papayas are rich in beta-carotene (and thus vitamin A activity) and vitamin C as well as potassium and other minerals. This is probably one fruit that can be used as an appetizer or dessert because of the digestive enzyme, *papain*, contained in it.

Pineapples. An interesting bush fruit most commonly grown in Hawaii, pineapples are very juicy and mildly acidic, more like a citrus fruit. They contain a digestive enzyme, *bromelain*, that allows for their easy digestion. Because of this, pineapples (a small amount) are one of the few fruits, papayas are another, that can be eaten following a meal. *Bromelain* may also have an antiinflammatory action in the body. Pineapples contain some vitamins A and C as well as potassium, calcium, and the trace minerals manganese and selenium. Manganese levels are in fact quite good; one cup of pineapple will supply our minimum daily needs, about 2.5 mg.

There is a concern that pineapples more easily accumulate chemicals from the fertilizers and pesticides commonly used in their cultivation, due to their very porous skins, whereas fruits such as oranges are more protected. For this reason, it is unwise to consume a great deal of pineapple or its juice unless organic fruits can be found. However, it is more difficult to find organic tropical fruits from Hawaii or Mexico, for example, than it is the more locally cultivated ones, such as apples or oranges, possibly because of the higher amounts of insects and germs that also thrive in those climates.

Unusual and Special Fruits

Avocados	*Persimmons*
Kiwis	*Pomegranates*
Olives	

These fruits—foods that grow on trees and that contain inner seeds, do not clearly fit into the other categories I have discussed. None of these are eaten commonly, other than olives possibly by some people. Olives, however, are unusual because they cannot be eaten fresh and also contain a high amount of oil, much like avocados. They are really more like a nut than a fruit. Kiwis have recently become more popular due to their unique taste, visual appeal, and modest caloric count. They are probably closest to grapes or the tropical guava; however, kiwis grow in more temperate climates including Northern California and New Zealand. Persimmons and pomegranates are also unusual in taste and appearance as well as in the adventure of eating them. These festive and seasonal bright orange or red fruits can be seen dangling from near-naked trees in autumn and early winter in the temperate climates in which they grow.

Avocados. Avocados are unique among the fruits in that they are a very concentrated food, more like a nut than a fruit. They are high in calories—one average avocado has about 300 calories and about 30 grams of fat, as well as 12 grams of carbohydrate and 4–5 grams of protein. They are fairly high in most of the B vitamins except B_{12}, being particularly good in folic acid, niacin, and pantothenic acid. They also have some vitamin C, good amounts of vitamin A, and contain a bit of vitamin E. Avocados are very rich in potassium and are also particularly good in many other minerals, including magnesium, iron, and manganese.

For vegetarians who do not eat a lot of fatty foods, avocados may be a good source of needed oils, but for those who consume more fat and calories, these fruits may add excess fat and weight. Avocados are commonly used in salads, dips such as guacamole, in sandwiches, or stuffed with seafood.

Kiwis. Little fruits with a tiny name, kiwis reveal a beautiful pattern when the green juicy fruit with furry skin is sliced. Kiwis are another fruit high in vitamin C and potassium and may contain an enzyme that helps reduce cholesterol and improve circulation.

Olives. Horticulturally, olives are considered a fruit, but in their nutritional makeup they are more like nuts, with a high oil content. In the fruit family, they are most like avocados. Olives grow in large quantities on small trees. They are most widely cultivated in the Mediterranean countries of Italy and Spain, though they are now being grown more in the United States, mainly in California.

The best use of olives is in the form of the clear, sweet oil pressed from their pulp. After the olives are harvested and cleaned, the first amounts of the oil are pressed out as "virgin" olive oil. This can be bright yellow to green-yellow in color and varies subtly in flavor. Fresh olive oil is used classically in salads and can be drunk in small amounts as a nutritive lubricant to the intestinal tract. Olive oil is one of our best oils for cooking, as it is mainly a monounsaturated fat, which is more stable to heat degradation than the common polyunsaturated oils. Olive oil also helps lower LDL cholesterol, which is implicated in heart disease.

Olives cannot be consumed just off the tree or even after ripening. They must be "pickled" or cooked in vinegar in order to be eaten. Stuffed (with pimento) green olives are familiar to the bartender for drinks. Black olives are more often used in cooking. Most table or dinner olives are much larger than the oil olives.

Olives are rich in oil (and calories) and the essential fatty acids, and generally have a good variety of vitamins and minerals, along with some protein. They contain vitamin E, vitamin A, and many of the B vitamins. They further contain many minerals, such as zinc, copper, iron, calcium, magnesium, and phosphorus. However, people avoiding salt or vinegar, or those on a low-fat, low-calorie diet, would best minimize their olive intake.

Persimmons. A seasonal (late autumn/winter) fruit, persimmons are common in the Orient, where they are associated with celebration. They also grow in the United States in temperate climates and are harvested here in the autumn/winter as well. A fully fruited persimmon tree that has lost its leaves and is left with many bright orange fruits is a beautiful sight. Persimmons must be eaten when very ripe. It is the cold weather or frost that aids the ripening process. If you buy them hard, you can freeze them overnight and they will ripen as they thaw. Persimmons have a unique, slightly acidic taste and are very messy to eat. They have some beta-carotene, as do most orange fruits and vegetables, and some vitamin C, as well as a little potassium, iron, and calcium. The fuju persimmon from Japan is ripe when still hard and has a texture more like an apple.

Pomegranates. Another autumn celebration fruit in our culture, pomegranates are eaten around Halloween on through the winter holidays. Parents may dread pomegranate season because they are not very easy to eat and the bright-red juice contained in their hundreds of little seed fruits stains clothes and skin. Pomegranates have some vitamin C and potassium but overall are not very nutrient rich.

Dried Fruits

Apples	*Figs*
Apricots	*Prunes*
Currants	*Raisins*
Dates	

Just about any fruit can be dried, but some are more typically eaten in their dried form. Drying fruits allows them greater longevity and shelf life. However, some of the vitamins, such as C, and minerals may be reduced with time. Also, many dried fruits may be preserved with sulfur dioxide, to which some people, particularly those with asthma or al-

lergies, may be sensitive. Generally, sulfur dioxide in small amounts is not too big a problem and may help maintain higher levels of vitamin C.

Since dried fruit has lost its water content, eating too much of it can make the intestinal matter drier, which may cause or worsen constipation. Rehydrating some of these dried fruits in filtered or spring water will make them juicy and more flavorful and prevent the problem of constipation.

Apples. Dried apples have only recently become popular commercially. Many of the trace minerals are lost in the drying process, but potassium and the apple pectin, which helps intestinal detoxification, are more concentrated in dried apples.

Apricots. Apricots are very tasty in their dried form. They usually have sulfur dioxide added to preserve their color, but organic, untreated dried apricots are also available. Dried apricots are very rich in vitamin A from beta-carotene and also contain a high concentration of potassium.

Currants. Black currants are tasty raisin-like fruits that contain very good amounts of vitamin C and decent levels of vitamin A, niacin, pantothenic acid, and biotin. They also contain good amounts of iron and potassium, as well as some calcium, phosphorus, magnesium, and manganese. Dried currants can be eaten alone or used on cereal or in baking. Recently, the seeds of the black currant have been used for their concentrated oil, gamma-linolenic acid (GLA), also found in evening primrose.

Dates. A very sweet, high-carbohydrate fruit harvested from the date palm trees, dates are found naturally in the "dried" state, though fresh dates may have a little more moisture. Date sugar extracted from dates is used as a sweetener. Dates are fairly rich in niacin, pantothenic acid, potassium, calcium, and magnesium. They are surprisingly concentrated in iron; about ten medium dates contain 3 mg. iron.

Figs. Figs can be eaten in the fresh or dried form, though packaged, dried figs are most common. Fresh figs, especially fresh picked, can be an exotic taste treat and great for cleansing the intestines. Dried figs in general are fairly rich in potassium, calcium, phosphorus, magnesium, iron, copper, and manganese. They are good energy foods, support blood formation, and, when soaked and rehydrated, figs are helpful to intestinal function.

Prunes. Prunes are best known for their laxative effect. A few prunes a day, especially soaked, rehydrated prunes, can keep us regular, and the elderly population favors them for this purpose. Prunes are essentially dried plums and are very rich in iron, with the highest amount of all the fruits. One cup of prunes may have 4–6 mg. of iron, and one cup of prune juice, the most common way prunes are used medicinally, contains nearly 10 mg. of iron. Prunes are also high in vitamin A, niacin, potassium, and phosphorus and have some calcium, magnesium, and copper as well.

Raisins. Dried seedless grapes, raisins are a common snack food or used in cereals, cookies, and puddings. They are fairly high in iron, with one cup of raisins containing nearly 6 mg. Raisins are also rich in potassium, calcium, magnesium, and phosphorus, and have traces of copper, zinc, and manganese. They have fair amounts of the B vitamins and are often helpful in providing quick energy.

○ VEGETABLES

Vegetables are another big topic, probably our most important one nutritionally. Health and vitality are dependent, I believe, on eating nutritious and vital foods, and vegetables are a major category here, especially the fresh-picked variety. Fresh vegetables have life force. The Latin word for vegetables means "to enliven or animate."

Most vegetables are very high in water and necessary vitamins and minerals and low in fat and protein. Thus, they are a perfect complement to animal protein meals to help supply the needed nutrients that aid the digestion and utilization of those concentrated foods. Most vegetables are predominantly carbohydrate, with important fiber bulk. Vitamins C and A, potassium, calcium, magnesium, and iron are the most commonly rich nutrients, along with some B vitamins and other trace minerals. The dark leafy greens, yellow or orange vegetables, such as squash and carrots, and red ones, such as peppers, are all high in beta-carotene, which produces vitamin A in our body. Many of the nutrients may be partially lost when cooking vegetables. Vitamin C and some minerals may dissolve in the water, and the B vitamins may be destroyed by heat and also lost in the water, yet, overall, the basic nutrition and fiber will still remain.

The positive flavors, many colors, and variety of textures of vegetables are a distinct advantage to those who enjoy natural tastes and aesthetic eating. However, the low salt and fat content tends to reduce interest for people who have developed a taste for those attractions. And many times children refrain, often passionately, from the pleasures of vegetables, as their tastes may tend toward sweet flavors and they may oppose the often slightly bitter flavors of the greenery.

The chlorophyll that is part of most plants, especially high in the green vegetables, has special properties. It is the basic component of the plants' blood, just as hemoglobin is in ours. Instead of iron as the focal part, as it is with our blood, magnesium is the center of the chlorophyll molecule, and thus many plants have a good magnesium level. Chlorophyll is produced as a result of the sun's effects on the plants, and it is known to have revitalizing and refreshing effects when used in humans. Many studies have been done with chlorophyll extracts. It seems to provide intestinal nourishment and has a soothing or healing effect on

307

the mucous linings, and it also has been used beneficially for skin ulcers and to help detoxify or purify our system, the liver in particular. Chlorophyll may even have antimutagenic potential, though this needs further study. Because of their beta-carotene and selenium levels, vegetables are thought to help reduce cancer rates. The cruciferous family vegetables, such as broccoli, brussels sprouts, and cauliflower, have a further anticancer effect, though the exact mechanism has not yet been determined.

The most nutritious way to eat vegetables is fresh and raw. But raw vegetables eaten in too much quantity are harder for some people to chew and digest and can produce intestinal gas. Light steaming of vegetables softens them without depleting much of their nutrients, and hot vegetables with a little seasoning may be more pleasing to the palate. Baked vegetables are also sound nutritionally. If we boil vegetables, many of the nutrients go into the water, so unless we plan to consume the water, by drinking it or making it into a sauce or soup, boiling is not ideal. Frozen vegetables, when they are frozen fresh, have not suffered much loss of nutrients and may keep for quite a long time, remaining nutritionally rich. Dried vegetables do tend to lose vitamins and minerals, and canned vegetables often lose the most, but this can vary depending on the additives canned with them. With water canning, many of the nutrients often dissolve into the liquid out of the vegetables. You can conserve water and gain nutrients by using left-over vegetable water for soup bases, gravies, or watering plants.

Many vegetables are sprayed or absorb some chemicals from the ground, water, or air. These are often most concentrated in the skin or on the surface. Washing or soaking the vegetables in water may help remove some of these chemicals. Many people even soak vegetables suspected to be contaminated in diluted bleach (Chlorox, sodium hypochlorite), then rinse them before preparing them for eating.

Fresh vegetable juices can be a very invigorating beverage. Their vitamins and minerals are concentrated in the juices. Many people have fasted on vegetable juices with positive effects, such as enhanced vitality and a diminishment of congestive-type symptoms. Vegetable juices are better the fresher they are. Carrot juice is probably the most common, though other veggies, such as beets, celery, or spinach, can be added for a mixed-vegetable cocktail. Really, almost any vegetable can be made into juice.

Leafy Greens

Cabbage	*Lettuce*
Chard	*Spinach*
Collards	*Watercress*
Kale	

The leafy greens are probably the richest in nutrients of any foods in the vegetable kingdom. And usually the greener they are, the more nutritious they are. They are very high in vitamins A and C and the minerals magnesium, potassium, and iron. The leafy greens are well known for their folic acid (name derived from "foliage") content. Calcium is also very high in the greens, though some of it gets bound up in certain ones, such as chard, spinach, and beet greens, that are high in oxalic acid. During cooking or in the intestines, calcium oxalate, which is not very soluble or absorbable, is formed. But an appreciable amount of calcium can still be obtained from the green leafy vegetables. Kale, collards, and mustard and turnip greens have a lower oxalic acid level and, thus, more available calcium. Dandelion greens are one of the richest sources of vitamin A.

To give an example of the rich nutrition of the leafy green vegetables, let's analyze a cup of cooked kale, which is a fairly large portion, requiring two to three cups of fresh kale. This has just over 50 calories, nearly 10 grams of carbohydrate, several grams of protein, 2–3 grams of fiber, and hardly any fat, less than 1 gram. The vitamin A activity is nearly 8,000 IUs, more than the RDA for A. Calcium content is between 150 and 200 mg., magnesium about 30 mg., iron 2 mg., potassium nearly 300 mg., and vitamin C 100–150 mg., and there are traces of manganese, copper, and zinc. Sodium is fairly low, less than 50 mg. There are also trace amounts of most of the amino acids. The vitamin B levels are fairly low except for important folic acid, about 40 mcg.

There are many edible leafy green vegetables. I give a few notes on some of the more common ones.

Cabbage. A nutritious anticancer cruciferous vegetable, cabbage is low in fat and may even help reduce body fat levels. Though not as high in nutrients as some of the other greens, cabbage is still rich in chlorophyll, folic acid, and vitamin C and especially good in that it contains some selenium, another known antioxidant/anticancer nutrient, and two detoxifying minerals, sulfur and chlorine. Red cabbage is higher than green in vitamins A and C, but lower in folic acid and chlorophyll. In longevity cultures, such as the Hunzas, cabbage is popular in the diets in both raw and cooked forms and as fermented sauerkraut (mostly in eastern Europe), which adds digestive enzymes.

Chard. Chard, mainly the Swiss variety, is a rich source of vitamin A; one cup of uncooked chard has about 1,200 IUs—and less than 10 calories. Chard is also about one-third protein and a good fiber food. It is fair in vitamin C, folic acid, calcium, magnesium, sodium, and potassium. Hot cooked chard served with a bit of melted butter or cold-pressed vegetable oil and a pinch of salt is a delicious vegetable.

Collards. Common to the Southern diet, these greens are one of the richer sources of vitamin A, with some protein and a good fiber content. Folic acid and vitamin C are also strong. The minerals calcium, potassium, iron, and zinc are plentiful—that's, of course, if you are eating those collard greens.

Kale. Kale, just described in the general discussion of leafy greens, is a fairly tasty vegetable with a special and rich array of nutrients, and especially a good source of calcium.

Lettuce. This is the common name for a number of related plants that grow in "heads." Head lettuce has been classically identified with the iceberg variety, which is a solid, round ball of lettuce leaves that stores longer than most other types, so that many restaurants and homes prefer it. Iceberg lettuce, though, tends to be less nutritious than some of the other lettuces, such as romaine, red leaf, green leaf, or butter lettuce, which are gaining in popularity. These are generally darker green in color and richer in chlorophyll, vitamin A, and folic acid. Lettuces also contain some calcium, potassium, and iron and are good fiber foods. They are low in sodium and calories as well.

Spinach. "Spinach makes ya strong!" That has been the Popeye tale for most of us, and that's because this dark leafy green food is rich in iron. One cup of uncooked spinach has nearly 2 mg. of iron—and for only 15 calories. It is also a good fiber food and has some protein. Vitamin A activity is very high, about 4,500 IUs for that one cup. B vitamins are low except for folic acid; vitamin C is good, and there is some vitamin E as well. Potassium, magnesium, and calcium are high, and copper, manganese, and zinc are also present. Raw spinach, however, contains oxalic acid, which may bind some of the calcium and other minerals. Spinach is a good substitute for lettuce in salads, and lightly cooked spinach is concentrated in nutrients. However, once fresh spinach is cooked or a can is opened it should be consumed within the day and not stored, especially in contact to a metal container, due to potential oxidation of iron.

Watercress. A special, spicy green from the mustard family, watercress is a nice addition to salads. It grows by or in streambeds in the early spring. Watercress is particularly high in vitamin A and calcium and also contains vitamin C, potassium, iron, magnesium, and traces of nearly all the B vitamins. Many herbalists claim that watercress is a good blood purifier.

Stems

Asparagus	*Leeks*
Celery	*Rhubarb*

The stem category is basically what is left after the roots, leaves, and flowers. Leeks are probably more similar to the bulb or root group, while asparagus is in a world of its own. Most of these plants are low in calories and very good in fiber content.

Asparagus. This is one of our spring vegetables, and the edible part is actually the young underground sprouts or shoots. The asparagus tips are actually little flowers. Asparagus spears are often more expensive than other vegetables, because of their short season and the work it takes to harvest them. Asparagus has very good amounts of vitamin C, vitamin A, sulfur, folic acid, and potassium. It has some iron, calcium, magnesium, iodine, and zinc as well. As an early sprout, it is relatively high in protein for a vegetable, and it is a good fiber food. Asparagus is also low in calories and sodium. The unusual smell that our urine may acquire after eating asparagus comes from the amino acid, asparagine, which actually acquired its name from this springtime plant.

Celery. A popular crunchy stem often used for oral gratification during weight-loss programs, celery is very low in calories (fewer than ten per stalk), though higher in sodium than other veggies. Celery is a good fiber and carbohydrate food with a high water content. It is also rich in potassium, with some calcium and folic acid, and celery is relatively high in vitamins A and C. This vegetable is thought to have a relaxing effect by calming the nerves.

Leeks. Leeks are a nutrient-rich, high-fiber food that are related to green onions. They are mainly carbohydrate and fiber, though they are rich in potassium, folic acid, iron, and calcium and fairly high in vitamin C, some Bs,

silicon, sulfur, magnesium, and phosphorus. They can be steamed or sauteed with other vegetables or used in soup.

Rhubarb. This is an interesting plant that comes from Tibet. The only edible part is the stem, which is actually an early sprout of the rhizome (large bulb) of the plant. The leaves are poisonous, and the stems, when eaten raw, may be toxic as well. When the stems are cooked or stewed, they can be eaten in a pie or sauce, usually with some sweetener to cover up the bitter taste. Rhubarb is a good fiber food and has some calcium and other minerals. Most of the vitamin C is lost with cooking.

Roots and Tubers

Beets	*Parsnips,*
Carrots	*Rutabagas,*
Garlic	*and Turnips*
Onions	*Radishes*
Potatoes	*Sweet Potatoes*
	and Yams

The root vegetables, which also include the tubers (potatoes) and bulbs (garlic and onions), are probably the most commonly consumed group of vegetables throughout the world. One of these root vegetables might be cooked along with the main meal or as a dish in itself, as part of a mixed vegetable dish, or as a seasoning for other dishes. Potatoes, carrots, and garlic and onions are the most popular. These vegetables vary in their nutrient content, though they all are "starchy"; that is, contain a high portion of complex carbohydrates. Carrots and sweet potatoes are both very high in beta-carotene, which generates vitamin A. Cooking potatoes are high in vitamin C and lots of other nutrients. Most of these root vegetables, especially yams, are rich in potassium.

Beets. Beets are those red-purple roots that stain the other vegetables red when cooked with them. Some people can have a scare after eating beets when they pass bloody-looking stools or see red water in the toilet after elimination. In fact, beets can be used to measure our intestinal transit time. Eat a couple of fresh raw beets, usually shredded in a salad, check the time, and watch when the first sign of them appears in the bowel movement. Canned beets will not work for this purpose, as much of the red pigment (and a lot of the nutrients as well) is lost in canning and storage.

Beet greens are particularly high in vitamin A, iron, and calcium, while beet roots are richest in iron, potassium, niacin, copper, and vitamin C. Folic acid, zinc, calcium, manganese, magnesium, and phosphorus are also present. Beet borscht is a classic Russian beet soup, but steamed, raw in salads, or cooked beets in soups are also simple ways to get these stimulating roots. A mixed carrot, beet, and parsley juice is supportive for women during their menstrual cycle.

Carrots. Carrots are one of the more commonly eaten vegetables. Children will often eat raw carrots when they will eat few others, but cooked carrots are another story. Carrots are amazing in their vitamin A content. One cup of carrots, with only 50 calories, contains over 20,000 IUs of vitamin A, mainly as beta-carotene. Folic acid, vitamin C, potassium, calcium, iron, and magnesium are also present. And carrots usually contain selenium, a hard-to-find important nutrient. Of course, the freshness and quality of a vegetable such as carrots determines its content. For example, carrots may range widely in their vitamin A value.

Carrots are most often eaten cleaned and raw, cooked in vegetable dishes (steamed is best for nutrition), or as part of soups or salads. Sliced, diced, shredded, or swirled, they all contain lots of vitamin A. An eight-ounce glass of carrot juice contains almost five times (25,000 IUs) the RDA for vitamin A and various concentrated minerals; it has the most nourishment when it is drunk within a short time of preparing it. With this vitamin A content, carrots and carrot juice are helpful in supporting skin health and providing immune protection.

Garlic. A whole book could be devoted to all the tales and remedies of which garlic has been a part for centuries. Its strong odor, from sulfur gas, accounts for the theory that garlic keeps away evil spirits—or any spirits, for that matter, other than other garlic-eating ones. But it is with good reason that garlic has been known as the "king of herbs"; it has been used for medicinal purposes including treatment of high blood pressure, atherosclerosis, worms and other parasites, the common cold and flu, and generally as the "poor person's antibiotic." It seems to help purify the body and may have immune-enhancing properties. The mineral sulfur promotes elimination of toxins from the blood, lymph, and body. Garlic has been shown to help lower fat levels and platelet aggregation, which can lower blood-clotting potential.

Garlic is actually a bulb made up of cloves, each of which is the seed for a future plant. In the low amounts usually used, it is not of high nutritional value. It is used raw in salads or in dressings or cooked with meats, fish, or poultry or with other vegetables. The hot or spicy nature of garlic gives it a stimulating action.

Onions. The effect of onions is similar to, though more subtle, than those of garlic. There are many varieties of these root bulbs. The standard yellow cooking onion is most common in our culture, though red onions, white onions, green onions, and chives are used frequently also. Onions can be eaten raw in salads or in dips, used as flavorings, or cooked in soups or in just about any kind of food dish. Liver and onions is a fairly popular (and unpopular) high-nutrient entree. Onion is a universal food and, like garlic, has a characteristic odor from the active sulfur bonds that release its purifying properties. Onions' antiseptic effects also come from its natural oils.

Onions are not high in nutrients, though they have a wide mix. They have some plant protein, calcium, iron, folic acid, and vitamins C, E, and A and are also a source of selenium and zinc, which they can pick up from the soil.

Green onions are higher in vitamins A and C and iron and are used most often fresh as chives in salads or with potatoes and sour cream.

Potatoes. Probably the most universal and highly consumed vegetable, potatoes are actually a tuber, like Jerusalem artichokes or taro root, meaning that they grow underground off the root after the plant has grown and flowered. I try to find organic, nongreen potatoes especially, as they can concentrate chemicals and produce their own toxicity when they turn color or are exposed to sunlight. The green color is actually chlorophyll, but it suggests that excessive solanine has been produced in the potato. In large amounts, solanine can produce symptoms such as headache, nausea, diarrhea, or fatigue. Potatoes that have sprouted should also be avoided.

Potatoes are very rich in nutrients, are low in sodium, fairly low in calories (one potato has between 100 and 150 calories), and negligible in fats. Potatoes are approximately two-thirds starch carbohydrate and about 10 percent protein. They contain a reasonable portion of vitamin C and B vitamins, especially folic acid, thiamine, niacin, and pantothenic acid, and are very high in potassium, with moderate amounts of magnesium, manganese, iron, and zinc.

Potatoes are very versatile in the kitchen as well. They can be baked, steamed, boiled, fried, cooked in soups or vegetable dishes, and more. They get costar billing in the standard poorly balanced meat-and-potatoes diet, but they are the least of any dietary problem, unless the diet is high in french fries or the potatoes are slathered in butter, sour cream, or highly chemical bacon bits. The basic potato, though, is really that—a basic nutritious food from the earth. Boiled potatoes can calm the intestines and reduce bloating. Externally, raw potato can draw out skin boils as well as reduce inflammation. Sliced raw potatoes on sunburns or other mild burns may help their healing.

Parsnips, Rutabagas, and Turnips. These three root vegetables are among our stranger and less consumed foods, unless they are passed on in a cultural diet.

They are mainly starchy vegetables, without a high amount of any one nutrient but a good mixture. They have some B vitamins, A, and C and are high in potassium, with a blend of other minerals. They are almost exclusively eaten cooked—steamed, baked, or in soups. Turnip greens are rich in vitamins A and C and folic acid.

Radishes. Those spicy, crunchy little red roots that grow very fast are really low calorie. They are nearly all water, with some vitamin C, folic acid, and most of the trace minerals, including iron, zinc, silicon, and selenium. The chlorine content may actually help in digestion. The spicier radishes can help clear the sinuses and any mucus in the upper airways. Wild radish flowers are also edible and can help spice up a salad. Radish sprouts make a good blend with the common alfalfa sprouts and are nice for those who like a little bite in their salads.

Sweet Potatoes and Yams. These two potato-related tubers are considered the celebration potatoes in our culture. Usually baked or steamed, they are a real taste treat. Sweet potato pie and candied yams are special holiday favorites. Sweet potatoes are very high in beta-carotene and fairly good in the B vitamins, vitamin C, potassium, and iron. Yams are very rich in potassium, folic acid, and magnesium but lower in vitamin A and some of the other nutrients.

Vegetable Flowers

Artichokes	*Brussels Sprouts*
Broccoli	*Cauliflower*

This group is different from both the flowers and the "flowering vegetables," such as tomatoes and squashes, that grow to replace the flower of the plant. Vegetable flowers are actually the early part of the potential flower of the plant, picked and eaten before they progress into a "real" flower.

These vegetables tend to be low in calories and high in carbohydrates but also have some protein and good fiber content. They are all good in vitamin C, folic acid, and potassium, and broccoli is very rich in vitamin A. Artichokes are actually the flower of a thistle plant that is very beautiful when left to fully flower, while cauliflower and broccoli are members of the highly nutritious cruciferous family, thought to help reduce the incidence of cancer.

Artichokes. These are a special treat and a meditation to eat, unless we gobble or add to our salad the oil-marinated artichoke hearts. Eating the fresh, steamed artichoke involves trimming the stickers and then peeling the tender leaves one by one to slide the edible parts through our teeth into our mouths; and then, we eventually get down to the hairy heart, which, after a shave, is a real delicacy. The whole experience can take half an hour or more, not counting steaming the artichoke for that long at least to make it tender and edible. Artichokes are good in fiber, low in calories (if not drenched in butter or mayonnaise), and pretty well endowed with folic acid and potassium. Some vitamin A and C, calcium and magnesium, phosphorus, and iron are part of the artichoke.

Broccoli. Sometimes eaten by children because they look like such cute little green trees, broccoli is also nutritious and very low in calories. The protein content is about one-third of its nourishment. Broccoli is a cruciferous vegetable that is thought to have anticancer properties and is rich in vitamins A, C, and folic acid. Some other B vitamins and most of the minerals are also present, being particularly best in potassium, along with calcium, phosphorus, magnesium, and iron. Broccoli should be eaten raw or lightly steamed, not boiled or overcooked, to maintain its nourishment.

Brussels Sprouts. These are one of the cruciferous vegetables recently known for their ability to reduce cancer potential. Even though they are not many people's favorite vegetable because of their peculiar taste (sulfur) and the fact that they seem to be gas producing, they are definitely loaded with nutrition. They were always fascinating to me in the way they grow and by their miniature replication of cabbage.

Brussels sprouts are high in vitamins A and C, folic acid, and fiber and fairly high in calcium, sulfur, phosphorus, potassium, magnesium, and iron. These little sprouts from Brussels are nearly half protein, though not completely balanced in their amino acid distribution. If we can get children to eat Brussels sprouts, that is a real victory on several levels.

Cauliflower. A cauliflower is really a little head of thousands of compact flowers. It is white because it contains no carotene pigment, and is thus low in vitamin A, but it is rich in potassium, folic acid, and vitamin C. It is also about 25 percent protein and one of the cancer-preventive* cruciferous vegetables. Cauliflower can be eaten raw with dips and steamed or cooked with other vegetables. Curried in eastern Indian cooking is a very tasty way to eat cauliflower.

Flowering Vegetables

Cucumbers	*Pumpkins*
Eggplants	*Squashes*
Peppers	*Tomatoes*

These plants are many, mainly growing on small bushes and vines. Each one that I will discuss here has many different varieties. The flowering vegetables are botanically like fruits in that they carry the plant's matured seeds for the next generation. These vegetables grow after and in replacement of the flowers, much like a citrus tree. And some, such as tomatoes and cucumbers, are as juicy and nutritious as many fruits.

Tomatoes are the very popular "fruit of the vine" that were once thought to be poison-

---

* See the *Cancer Prevention* program in Part Four for a further discussion of the cruciferous vegetables.

313

ous. There was also a question as to whether they were a fruit or a vegetable until the United States Supreme Court ruled that they are vegetables. Actually, tomatoes, eggplants, and peppers are all members of the nightshade family of plants, which are thought to be possible joint irritants in arthritis. Potatoes and tobacco are also in the nightshade family.

Squashes are multiple and vary from small, soft, high water content zucchini and summer squash to hard, starchy drier ones, such as acorn and hubbard squash. Even the pumpkin is in the squash family. Many beans, especially green peas and green beans, are also flowering vegetables, though these will be discussed in the section of legumes.

Cucumbers. The "coolest" of vegetables, cucumbers are actually used medicinally for burns or irritated tissues. Laying a slice of cucumber over each eye is a soothing treatment for stressed or inflamed eyes, or for hot or burned skin. Cucumbers are eaten in their unripe state and usually raw, though some cultures cook them. The smaller cucumbers may be "pickled" to make a fermented vinegary fruit, namely "pickles." Some people find cucumbers difficult to digest, in particular the skins, though they contain the cuke's folic acid. Cucumbers are not really high in any nutrients, but they are almost devoid of calories as well. They are, however, the best source of vitamin E (in the seeds) of the vegetables. Cucumbers also have some vitamins A and C, and contain potassium and other minerals as well. Cucumbers are commonly eaten raw in salads, as in cukes and sour cream, or as pickles.

Eggplant. Our main purple vegetable besides red cabbage, eggplant is usually eaten cooked. It is low in calories unless sauteed in oils; we must be careful with eggplant because it is like a sponge and can soak up large amounts of fats. Therefore, it is best to bake it first before cooking it in other recipes. Eggplant is used in many dishes throughout the world—in a Middle Eastern dip, in mixed cooked

vegetables, and as eggplant parmigiana, something like noodleless lasagna or moussaka, a Greek eggplant casserole. Eggplants are mainly carbohydrate and contain no fat. They are not particularly high in nutrients, except for niacin and potassium. Calcium, magnesium, iron, vitamins A and C, and folic acid are also present. Eggplant is also a member of the nightshade family, and thus may be avoided by people with concern about arthritis.

Peppers. Peppers are also grown and eaten throughout the world in a great many varieties, shapes, and flavors, from sweet to very hot. We are most familiar with red or green "bell" peppers and the hotter chili, cayenne, and jalapeño peppers. The bell peppers may be eaten fresh in salads or sliced with dips or stuffed with other foods, such as grains or meats, and baked. Some people have difficulty digesting peppers, especially the pepper's skin. The hot peppers are used to spice up salsas, cheeses, and in many other dishes of South America, where they originated. The chilis and cayenne peppers contain capsaicin, with medicinal properties in cleansing the blood and stimulating the circulation and perhaps in reducing cardiovascular disease and cancer. They also stimulate the gastric secretions and help digestion.

All peppers are very high in vitamin C, bioflavonoids, and vitamin A. One sweet pepper might have over 500 IUs of A and nearly 150 mg. of vitamin C. A smaller hot chili pepper is more concentrated and so may have similar levels. Folic acid, potassium, and niacin are also present in fairly good levels, as are some other minerals and B vitamins. The seeds surround the inner core of the peppers and often concentrate the hot nature.

Pumpkins. Another festive vegetable, pumpkins are used decoratively for Halloween and cooked for the tasty pumpkin pie dessert, eaten mainly around Thanksgiving and Christmas. Pumpkin seeds are also fairly popular. Some people eat baked pumpkin as they do other hard squashes, though it is more stringy, yet very high in fiber. Pumpkins are also high in vitamin A, as beta-carotene, the natural orange coloring. They are mainly a starchy carbohydrate with good water content. Pumpkins have some vitamin C, niacin, and pantothenic acid and are high in potassium. Other prevalent minerals include phosphorus, silicon, iron, magnesium, and calcium. Pumpkin seeds are high in zinc and other minerals (see the section on *Seeds*).

Squashes. These are also mainly autumn harvest vegetables. Many need to be cooked by baking or steaming, though the popular zucchini and yellow crookneck (both summer vegetables) can be sliced and eaten raw in salads or with dips. Most of the squashes are high in carbohydrates, mainly as starch, with a high fiber content. Many are high in vitamin A, especially the orange or yellow squashes. Vitamin C and potassium are also present in varying amounts, as are calcium, magnesium, and iron.

Zucchinis are probably the most commonly used squash in our culture because they are so easy to prepare. They are very juicy and flavorful after light steaming. The bigger ones can be stuffed and baked. Zucchinis can also be used raw in salads or for dips, or in soups or dipped in egg and breaded for deep frying. This vegetable seems to have a mild diuretic action and stimulates the intestines as well, probably because of its mucilage content.

Tomatoes. The vegetable mainstay of many Americans' diets and the diets of many cultures around the world, tomatoes have a wide variety of uses—juices, soups, raw in salads, stuffed, in sauces, in catsups and condiments, in salad dressings, in pizza and so many more. In 1980, it was estimated that nearly sixty pounds of tomatoes per person were consumed in the Unites States, though most of this was probably in catsup and sauces. The tomato, which is related to the belladona plant, was thought to be poisonous until one brave soul ate one in public and didn't die. Whether tomatoes are a fruit or vegetable doesn't really matter; they are a very delicious, mildly acidic food. The skins of the tomato are difficult to digest, and some people can suffer allergic reactions or irritation from too much tomato intake. Also, as a nightshade plant, they appear to be a joint irritant in some people with arthritis. Whether this is from allergy, acidity, or some other factor we do not know.

Tomatoes are not highly nutritious, though they are pretty well spiked with potassium, vitamin C, and vitamin A. They are low in calories and are mostly liquid and carbohydrate. Whole tomatoes contain some vitamin E, folic acid and other B vitamins, such as biotin and niacin, and a bit of iron, sodium, calcium, magnesium, and zinc. Tomato juice and tomato paste are more concentrated in some of the nutrients. Fresh-picked is the best and tastiest way to eat those red, ripe jewels of the garden.

Ocean Vegetables—Seaweed

Agar-agar	*Kelp*
Arame	*Kombu*
Dulse	*Nori*
Hijiki	*Wakame*

The vegetables that come from the sea are some of the most nutrient-rich foods we have, particularly in iodine, calcium, potassium, and iron, and some being very high in protein as well. Since these plants are constantly bathed in the mineral-rich ocean waters, they have a regular supply of nutrients. Sodium, however, can also be concentrated in these saltwater vegetables that supply food for many fishes.

Most seaweeds contain algin, a fiber molecule that binds minerals. When taken into our body, it can attract various metals within our digestive tract, possibly including heavy metals such as lead and mercury, and take them out of our system. It is further wise to include sea vegetables in our diets more regularly to provide good mineral nutrition and reduce possible absorption and utilization of

315

similar radioactive compounds, such as iodine 131, from environmental or medical sources.

The seaweeds are becoming more commonly used in our culture. They have been a traditional food in the Japanese culture for centuries. Sushi are rolls of rice (often with fish or vegetables) wrapped in a piece of nori seaweed. Kelp is a good high-mineral salt substitute, relatively low in sodium compared to regular salt, and may be useful for those with hypertension.

Agar-agar. Agar-agar is a seaweed combination that is used as a gelling agent in cooking and for desserts. It has no taste and no fishy smell and is healthier than gelatin made from animal byproducts. Agar is probably a good place to begin for children or people who want to bring these sea vegetables into their diet.

Arame. This is a dark, thin seaweed thread that can be used in soups or salads or mixed with rice. It is fairly rich in protein, iodine, calcium, and iron and is one of the tastier seaweeds.

Dulse. A red-purple leaf that is rich in iodine, iron, and calcium, dulse is a very tasty seaweed that can be used fresh in salads or cooked in soups. It is helpful to rinse the dulse prior to use to wash away some of the salt and the more fishy ocean flavor. Dulse powder, like kelp, is also available as a seasoning.

Hijiki. This is a very mineral-rich, high-fiber seaweed. Its dark, long strands look like thick hairs. Hijiki is about 10–20 percent protein, contains some vitamin A, and is richest in calcium, iron, and phosphorus. Soaked in water, it can be cooked in soup or is very good combined and eaten with rice. It is similar to arame.

Kelp. Kelp is usually used in smaller quantities than the other seaweeds, mostly as a seasoning. It has some protein and is very rich in iodine, calcium, and potassium, along with some of the B vitamins. Kelp is a common food supplement, used mainly for its iodine.

Kombu. A richer, meatier, higher-protein seaweed, kombu is most often used in soups—it adds minerals and flavor to the stock. Kombu contains vitamin A, some Bs, and lots of calcium and iron, yet is higher in sodium than most of the other seaweeds. One strip of kombu can also be added to the pot when cooking beans to reduce some of the potential gas-inducing qualities of the beans.

Nori. Nori is probably one of the most commonly used seaweeds. The dark sheets, as it is usually available, are very rich in protein, containing nearly 50 percent. Nori is high in fiber as well, and the sheets are used to wrap and hold rice, vegetables, and raw or cooked fish in small rolls that can be eaten with the hands. Nori is very high in vitamin A, calcium, iodine, iron, and phosphorus, and it has one of the sweeter flavors of the seaweeds.

Wakame. Another high-protein, flat and thinner seaweed, wakame is used mainly in soups. It contains some vitamin A, lots of calcium, iron, and sodium, and a bit of vitamin C as well.

Fungi
Mushrooms

Mushrooms, a type of edible fungus, are a fascinating species. Interestingly, when they are eaten, almost the entire plant is consumed. There are literally thousands of varieties, though probably only about twenty-five are consumed by humans. Most mushrooms are poisonous in varying degrees, with effects ranging from digestive upset to paralysis and death. It is very important, especially with wild mushrooms, to know the species that are edible and not make any mistakes. I remember a beautiful post–rain walk with herbalist Rob Menzies where we discovered nearly one hundred species of mushrooms.

White button, or field, mushrooms are found in most grocery stores and are the most commonly consumed. They may be the only variety known to most consumers, yet they have very little nutrition. Japanese shiitake mushrooms, boletus mushrooms, chanterelles, oyster mushrooms, and the tiny tree mushrooms are some other fairly common, more nutritious mushroom delicacies.

Most mushrooms have a fairly good protein content. I often describe them as the "meat" of the vegetable kingdom, especially some of those exotic forms found in Oriental cooking. The average button mushroom is low in calories and about one-third protein, while other varieties may have even more protein. Shiitake mushrooms are noted to have all eight essential amino acids, and are very nutritious. Many mushrooms are also high in two other, harder-to-find vegetable nutrients, iron and selenium. The B vitamins biotin, niacin, folic acid, and pantothenic acid are often found in good quantities. Potassium and phosphorus are usually the next most highly concentrated minerals, though other minerals are present in varying amounts, depending on the soil content.

Some people are allergic or sensitive to mushrooms. Also, people with intestinal yeast overgrowth, yeast sensitivities, or mold allergies may have crossover reactions to the fungi family.

Legumes

Peas and Beans

The legume vegetables are a special class of the pea and bean plants, which contain edible seeds inside pods that grow after the plant flowers. These include aduki beans, black beans, black-eyed peas, garbanzo beans, great northerns, kidney beans, lentils, lima beans, mung beans, navy beans, peanuts, green peas, pinto beans, and soybeans. There are also many other types of peas and beans. In fact, peanuts are actually a legume vegetable and not a true nut; however, since they are so commonly thought of as nuts, they will be discussed in the nut section.

The legumes are an interesting food, mainly a mixture of protein and starch, with many positive qualities as a food. They are low in calories, low in fat, a good complex carbohydrate, and fairly high in fiber, which may help intestinal action and even help to reduce cholesterol levels. Most important, though, especially for the vegetarian, the legumes are a good and inexpensive protein source. They cost on the average about 3 per pound of protein, whereas egg protein may cost about 6 and meat protein more like 12 per pound. And the extra advantage is that the beans have less than 10 percent fat content. So, though beans may be considered the poor people's meat, they might better be known as the healthy people's meat.

One concern, however, is that the protein in most of the peas and beans is not as complete as the animal proteins (though what protein is present is well utilized). In other words, all the essential amino acids are not contained in near-equal amounts. Tryptophan and methionine are the two amino acids most commonly low in the vegetable proteins. So we must eat more of these vegetable protein foods or mix them with different vegetable protein foods, such as grains (which are commonly higher than legumes in methionine but lower in lysine) to get all our essential amino acids at more optimum levels. This mixing of protein foods, called "protein complementarity," is discussed more in Chapter 2, *Protein*, and in Chapter 9 under *Lacto-ovo-Vegetarian*. Soybeans and peanuts are the most complete proteins of the legumes and of the vegetable kingdom, for that matter.

Another concern with legumes, especially beans, is that in many people they cause increased intestinal gas, which leads to burping, flatulence, or abdominal discomfort. This is caused mainly by the oligosaccharides in the beans fermenting in the lower intestines. Since these starch-type molecules are contained primarily in the coverings of the beans, we can soak the beans in water, usually overnight, and then discard that water first before cooking them in fresh water to help leach out some of their fermenting properties. This definitely reduces the gas-producing potential for which beans are notorious. Also, combining a bean such as mung, aduki, lentil or black bean with a grain such as rice or millet in a 1:3 (bean to grain) ratio will provide low gas but good fuel as a complete protein.

For this discussion, I have divided the legumes into three main categories: the *fresh beans*, the *fresh peas*, and the *dried beans*. In terms of nutrient content, the fresh peas and beans are more like the basic green vegetables, and the dried beans are more similar to the grains as starchier, protein-containing foods higher in B vitamins. The fresh beans, for example, include basic "green" beans and their many varieties, lima beans (also available dried), and yellow wax beans. These beans are usually higher in vitamins A and C than the dried varieties. Green beans are also usually good in folic acid and limas in potassium and iron, while yellow wax beans are lower in the supportive nutrients, though they have some vitamin A. These fresh beans are usually eaten steamed or cooked by themselves or with other vegetables.

The *fresh peas* include the standard green peas, as well as sweet, snap, snow, and sugar peas. When picked young, the whole pod and baby peas can be eaten fresh in salads or right off the bush, or they may be cooked. When more mature, the peas are bigger and the pods are stringier and less easy to chew and digest. This group is the highest in vitamin C of all the legumes, fairly high in the B vitamins, with some folic acid, high in vitamin A, and fairly well endowed with most of the minerals, including iron, potassium, calcium, and magnesium. Green peas even contain some vitamin E.

The *dried beans* are the category in which most of the legumes fall. There are many varieties, and their use tends to vary amongst the cultures. Lentils, often eaten with wheat or peas for complete protein, are very common in Middle Eastern diets, as are garbanzo beans, also known as chick peas. Hummus and falafel are two Middle Eastern foods based on this

bean. Pintos and black beans, usually eaten with rice or corn, are more common in Latin American countries. Kidney, navy, and great northern beans seem more Western–type beans—though most of the world's beans are consumed in the United States. Flavorful "baked beans" commonly use the red kidney bean. Soybeans have classically come from the Oriental cultures as tofu, or soybean curd, but in the last 20 years, soybean use has expanded rapidly worldwide.

Most of these dried and cooked beans contain some basic B vitamins, though the content is not really high. In general, the levels of thiamine, niacin, and pantothenic acid are best. There is a surprisingly high level of iron in most of these beans; calcium, potassium, and phosphorus are also abundant. Black beans, for example, are high in iron, calcium, potassium, and phosphorus; garbanzos are rich in those same minerals and good in vitamins B_1, B_2, and B_3; kidney beans are good in iron and potassium, as are navy beans and lentils; while soybeans are one of the better protein sources, they are a little less well endowed with the supportive vitamins and minerals, so eating them with more vegetables will help provide those nutrients. Soybeans do contain some A and C and some niacin and are actually fairly high in iron, calcium, potassium, and phosphorus.

Soybeans are a very important food. They are very versatile as well and could supply much of the world's hungry population with better protein and improved general nutrition. Growing soybeans for direct human consumption is a much more productive use of the land than raising meat. Raising soybeans can provide nearly 20 times the protein per acre that raising beef can. They contain complete protein as well, though not as concentrated as in beef. The amino acid balance of the soybeans is not perfect, being a little low in tryptophan and methionine, but a good intake of soybeans and soybean products can supply us with a fair amount of protein. Soybeans also contain very little if any saturated fat; most of their fat is the unsaturated variety. Soybean oil, commonly used, is high in linoleic acid and polyunsaturated fats and is more stable to oxidation and rancidification than some other oils because of its high content of lecithin and vitamin E, an important antioxidant.

Other soybean products that have hit the American scene in recent years include tempeh, or fermented soybean cakes, and soyburgers made from straight soybeans, tempeh, or tofu. Tofu is the classic soybean product made by fermenting the soybean and concentrating the curd, now used by many cultures. It has become known as the "food of 10,000 flavors" because it picks up the flavors from the other foods cooked with it. Tofu is a very versatile food. It can be used in salads, blended into dressings, eaten in sandwiches, or added to stir-fries or cooked vegetables. Tofu is not as high in protein and other nutrients as the whole soybean, though it retains fairly good levels of calcium, iron, and phosphorus. The sodium level is usually higher, though. Tofutti, or soybean-based ice cream, has also become popular as a low-cholesterol, lower-fat dessert treat. Ice Bean, another soybean dessert, contains more soybean and less sweetener than the Tofutti.

Sprouts will be discussed next, but I shall just mention here that soybean sprouts, as any of the legume sprouts, are very nutritious, vital foods. The vitamin C content, chlorophyll level, and protein level are all fairly good. The general protein concentration may go down when soybeans are sprouted, but protein is still found in good quantity, and the fiber content goes up. Anybody, anywhere can make and use these important sprouts as a healthful adjunct to their diet.

Overall, the legumes are a very important class of foods. They are especially important to the American diet, where we need to find lower-fat, lower-sodium, and lower-calorie (and lower cost) protein foods to substitute in the diets that are currently too high in meat, sodium, and fat and contribute so much to disease. The legumes are one of the best substitutes we have.

Sprouts

Aduki, alfalfa, buckwheat, clover, fenugreek, garbanzo, lentil, mung, radish, soybean, sunflower, wheat—these are only some of the protein- and vitamin-rich sprouts of many possible seeds, grains, and beans. Barley, corn, oats, green peas, and lima beans are a few others. Really, any "seed" that is endowed with the potential for the next generation of the plant life is sproutable. When a seed is sprouted into the first beginnings of the new plant, much of the stored nutrient potential bursts forth into the seedling, and these little sprouts, including the seed, grain, or bean with its shoot and greenery, become very wealthy with nutrients. Protein content increases by somewhere between 15 and 30 percent, depending on the plant, as the carbohydrate food source gets converted. Chlorophyll and fiber content also increase. The chlorophyll content can be very high when the sprout becomes green, as in sprouted wheat berries (wheat grass). Chlorophyll itself is rich in nutrients and has many health-giving properties. Also, sprouts are living foods that contain active enzymes which help our digestion and assimilation. With sprouting, most of the B vitamins are greatly increased, some over tenfold. Niacin and riboflavin are in particularly good amounts. The vitamin C level is greatly enhanced in sprouts compared to the dry seeds. Beta-carotene, the vitamin A precursor, increases with sprouting, as do vitamin E, K, calcium, phosphorus, and iron, though mineral content is not as greatly affected as that of the vitamins.

Many sprouts can now be purchased in grocery stores. Alfalfa sprouts, by far the most

319

common, are used in salads or sandwiches. They are very tasty but should be eaten fresh so that they do not ferment. Clover sprouts are bigger and have a fuller flavor than alfalfa; they are now more available in stores and can also be used fresh in salads or sandwiches. Mung bean sprouts have been used since ancient China, and are still popular in Oriental cooking. Mixed bean sprouts, with lentils, peas, and garbanzo beans, for example, are now more commonly available in little plastic bags. These can be eaten raw in salads or cooked in vegetable, grain, or even meat dishes or in soups. More and more people are coming to realize that the nutrient value and economical price of sprouts make them an ideal food.

Sprouting at home is very simple with a large glass jar or flat tray filled with soil. Most seeds, grains, or beans can be placed in a jar, rinsed, then covered with water for approximately 24 hours, being rinsed once or twice, then kept in the jar out of direct sunlight and rinsed two or three times a day, pouring off the water and letting the moist sprouts sit. I suggest using purified, chlorine-free water for soaking and rinsing sprouts. When they have sprouted, they can be placed in more light over the next day or two, again being rinsed two or three times daily to keep them clean and fresh. By this time, the amount of sprouts will have increased several times over the original volume. The sprouts and/or greenery are usually edible after a day or two in the light. Many types of sprouts, such as lentils, garbanzos, or alfalfa, can be eaten earlier than this and are very tasty along with being at peak protein levels at this time, day two or three.

Sunflower, wheat berry, and buckwheat sprouts all tend to grow better and healthier in a bed of soil. They are placed on top of the soil, watered well, covered with dark plastic or cloth, and left in a dark place for two to three days. Then they are uncovered and placed in

the light, being watered or sprayed as needed. The tall shoots with green tops can be trimmed and eaten fresh in salads, or they may continue to grow even further.

Lentils and garbanzos are very easy to sprout, may take only a couple of days, and are very rich in protein. Sprouted mung beans, the common "bean sprouts" used in Oriental cooking, can be used in salads or cooked into vegetable dishes. Fenugreek sprouts have a licorice flavor, while radish sprouts are more spicy. Soybean sprouting takes a little more care, as they must be rinsed more often to prevent fermentation.

Some practitioners feel that sprouts as the basic part of our diet can be very healthy and can, in fact, help heal a lot of medical problems. When the Hippocrates Health Institutes or the Optimum Health Institutes take people in for health care, they feed them mainly sprouts of various kinds, raw foods, and juices. These centers have been inspired by the work of Dr. Ann Wigmore, a well-known naturopathic doctor. Author Viktoras Kulvinskas, best known for his book *Survival into the Twenty-First Century* (Omango D'Press, 1975), has also published an entire book on sprouts, *Sprouts for the Love of Every Body*. These people feel, and I agree, that sprouts are likely the most vitally alive and nourishing foods we can eat. They are a great survival food, too. We can sprout these seeds, beans, and grains all year round. I believe that eating high amounts of sprouted foods, along with other vegetables and fruits, will promote health and vitality. Also, for overweight people, sprouts provide low-calorie, high-nutrient foods that also tend to support improved metabolism. Sprouts are also a good source of nutrients in the wintertime when there are less leafy greens and other vegetables available. And the amount of nourishment per dollar surpasses most any other food.

○ GRAINS

The grains are the most commonly consumed foods worldwide. Wheat, rice, and corn, in that order, are the three largest crops. They are also some of the oldest foods. Knowledge of their use goes back over 10,000 years. Grains are the main human fuel and are a good source of complex carbohydrate, which is slower burning and provides more sustained energy than the simple sugars. These rich sources of starch and fiber are also the cheapest caloric supply for the world masses. The whole (unprocessed) grains provide a healthy amount of B vitamins, vitamin E, and many minerals.

The grains, often known as the "cereal" grains, are the seeds of various grasses. There are three primary parts to each kernel, or seed, of the grains—the central core, or endosperm, which is about 80–85 percent of the grain; the germ and future sprout, about 3 percent; and the bran coverings of the grain, approximately 15 percent of the entire kernel. The endosperm, the bulk of the grain, is composed mainly of starch (and some protein) for energy to nourish the future seed. It has the nutrients to help the seed, and we humans, to grow. Though the major portion of the grain, however, it has less of the B vitamins and minerals than the germ and bran coverings, and less fiber as well. So when a grain is refined, most of these nutrients are lost along with the outer layers. The endosperm of wheat, for example, is what is contained in white flour.

The germ is only a small part of the grain, though the most essential part. It is the little embryo at the base of the kernel that is the future life. The rest of the grain is there to serve the germ; the coverings protect it, and the endosperm nourishes it in its new life. The germ actually is the part that grows, sprouts out through the bran covers when moisture and the sun bathe it. It will grow into leaves and continue as the roots go into the soil to gather more moisture and nutrients for continued growth. The germ is also the most concentrated part of the grain in nutrients. It contains protein, oils, and many vitamins and minerals. The germ is high in the B vitamins, particularly thiamine, riboflavin, niacin, and pyridoxine. Magnesium, zinc, potassium, and iron are some of the minerals contained in this part of the grain. Wheat germ particularly is high in vitamin E, and wheat germ oil is one of the richest sources. When the grain is broken apart, as in making flour, it is the germ content of the whole wheat flour that is less stable because of potential oxidation of the oils. This is a major reason for the wide use of white flour, which is devoid of the nutrient-rich wheat germ.

The bran of the grain consists of several protective coverings, which add most of the fiber and much of the nutrients as well. These include the B vitamins and some minerals, especially zinc. The outermost layers of the bran are mainly indigestible cellulose fiber and are not really high in nutrients. These layers also come off most grains more easily than the deeper layers, which contain more of the nutrients. Soft milling or hand milling can clean these outermost coverings and improve the digestibility and utilization of the protein and nutrients from the grain.

Another advantage in removing these outer bran coverings is that they also contain most of the phytic acid present in the grains. From our discussion on minerals, we learned that phytic acid can bind minerals such as calcium, iron, zinc, and magnesium in the gut and carry them out through the intestines so that they are not assimilated and utilized. This is not very helpful in people who are not obtaining sufficient nutrients, such as the elderly or younger people on poor diets. Even though bran, usually wheat or sometimes oat bran, is used by many people to add fiber content to the diet to help reduce or prevent constipation, and is known to reduce risks of colon and rectal cancer, I do not recommend its regular, long-term use because of the potential mineral depletion. Rather, I suggest eating more fiber-containing foods, such as the whole grains, vegetables, and most fresh fruits, plus drinking more water. Examples of other high-fiber foods include miller's bran, with about 40 percent fiber; high-fiber cereals, which may contain up to 30 percent fiber; and whole wheat bread, with about 10 percent fiber. This, particularly the use of high-fiber, whole foods, is overall a more healthful approach to bowel care, cancer prevention, and general nutrition.

Grains are the most basic whole foods of the Earth. The seeds of these grasses, or cereal grains, are a good source of complex carbohydrate, calories, energy, and fiber and a light source of protein. Vitamins B_1, B_2, and B_3 are the B vitamins most plentifully found in grains. Most grains are relatively low in vitamins A and C; however, these nutrients are prevalent in the vegetables, which go well with grains at meals. Vitamin E is found in the germ of the grain. The whole grains are rich in many minerals, especially magnesium, zinc, iron, and potassium, though calcium, phosphorus, and copper are often present. Rice and wheat are very good sources of hard-to-find selenium.

The fiber content of the whole grains is probably the biggest difference between the natural, or primitive, diet and the industrial, or Westernized, diet, and likely a big difference between poor health and good health.

The native diet averages several times more fiber than the modern, more refined way of eating. And lack of fiber may likely be the most significant cause in the advance of our chronic, serious, deadly diseases.

Medical research has shown that a low-fiber diet correlates with many diseases, and, conversely, an increase in fiber can reduce the risk of those same diseases. The increase in dietary fat and refined flours cannot easily be separated from the lowered dietary fiber, and all of these factors probably contribute to symptoms and diseases such as colon cancer (and possibly other cancers), constipation, hemorrhoids, diverticulitis, gallstones and gall bladder problems, high cholesterol, hypertensive heart disease, ulcers, varicose veins, and further problems whose correlations are yet to be discovered. As the fiber coverings of the grain are its vital life protection, the fiber content of our diet may protect us from many common problems. Just keeping our bowels moving regularly is an important daily step toward health. Eating more whole grains and vegetables as the mainstay of our diet is the best way to approach the fiber issue.

There are two main aspects to the topic of protein in the grains. The first is that they do not contain "complete proteins." This is a relative term since they contain all the essential amino acids, but the proportion of lysine is often low. In the legume section, we mentioned that most beans have a good level of lysine but are low in methionine. So when we eat the grains and legumes together, they complement each other and provide us with good levels of all the essential amino acids. Most cultures in the world have learned this important balance, sometimes painfully through deficiency diseases from not combining these foods. Recent thinking suggests that on the short term, such as a meal, this is not absolutely necessary, but over the day we need to get this variety of foods to maintain protein balance.

The second aspect of grain protein is that much of it is as gluten. Gluten is a protein-carbohydrate mixture that is contained in wheat, oats, barley, and rye. These glutenous grains tend to have a higher protein content than the nonglutenous ones, such as millet, corn, rice, and buckwheat. Some people have a sensitivity to gluten. This is most often intestinal, though a general allergy, most commonly to wheat or oats, may involve the body's interaction with the gluten protein. Celiac disease (a type of malabsorption) may in part be generated by an inability to handle gluten grains. Many intestinal symptoms, weight loss, and anemia may result. Usually, symptoms can be alleviated by avoiding the gluten grains and substituting others, such as corn, rice, and millet. However, certain nutritional deficiencies, psychological factors, and other aspects of diet, such as protein-fat ratios, may contribute as well to these intestinal symptoms of celiac disease.

Grain Allergenicity

Wheat	*most common*
Oats	↑
Rye	
Corn	
Barley	
Rice	
Buckwheat	
Millet	
Amaranth	↓
Quinoa	*least common*

Grains, though, are consumed without problems by most of the world's population. They are very versatile foods and are considered the "staff of life," a term often given to breads. Breads, the heated baked paste (flour) made from the grains, are in some form part of the diet of all populations in the world. From hand milling to using large machinery, breaking down the whole grains into fine powder, or flour, is the beginning process in making all kinds of edibles, such as breads, crackers, tortillas, cereals, pastas, pastries, and cookies. Wheat, of course, is the most commonly used grain, and most breads of the world, especially in our culture, contain wheat or refined wheat flour as the main ingredient. In 1977, it was estimated that nearly one-third of the world's population obtained at least half of their nutrition from wheat—that is, wheat was the main food in their diets. It is a good overall food, especially the whole wheat, but it must be balanced with other nutrients, protein, vitamin A, and vitamin C, for example, all of which may be consumed in amounts insufficient to sustain health. Another concern, especially in Western cultures, is that many people, children in particular, obtain many of their grains from packaged cereals and refined flour breads, which provide even less nutrition than the whole grain.

The refinement of grains and its contribution to nutrition and health is a very big topic, which I will discuss briefly. Refined grains and flours used to make breads, pastas, crackers, cookies, pastries, and so on have a couple of advantages over whole grains and flours. First, they are more stable in storage; there are no oils in them as there are in the grain germ, so they do not oxidize and rancidify as easily. Second, the refined grain products may be easier to digest and utilize in the body. They may also have somewhat less allergenic potential than the whole grains. The decrease in gluten in white flour, for example, reduces sensitivity to that protein.

On the other side of the coin, refining grains and flours creates a number of problems. The major one is the loss of nutrients that occurs from processing them, particularly the loss of most of the B vitamins, vitamin E, and the many minerals that are found naturally in whole grains. The protein content is only slightly decreased, the level of calories and the amount of starch content, which is found mainly in the inner kernel, remain the same, but just about everything else is greatly reduced. In the United States, by law, thiamine, riboflavin, niacin, and iron must be added back into the grain products, making the "enriched" breads, pastas, cereals, and so on. But other important nutrients are lost and not replaced. These include pyridoxine (B$_6$), pantothenic acid, chromium, zinc, manganese, folic acid, and vitamin E plus other trace minerals. And those are all essential to human health. Refined white flour contains about 75 percent of the whole wheat kernels but less than half of their nutrients.

Eating too much of refined grain products also increases consumption of the toxic mineral cadmium in relationship to zinc, as zinc is lost in the outer layers and cadmium, when it is present, is contained in the internal kernel, and so can lead to cadmium toxicity problems. (See discussion of *Zinc* and *Cadmium* in Chapter 6, *Minerals.*)

Here are a few suggestions for using the grains and their by-products. First, when using whole grain flours, it is best to refrigerate them so they do not rancidify. This will greatly increase their longevity. Also, most people are not allergic to whole grains, so these more wholesome and nourishing foods may be a good source of fuel. In regard to the whole grain-allergy issue, some allergists and other practitioners theorize that allergies to food may in part be generated by early and excessive intake of processed foods, sugars, refined flours, and pasteurized, homogenized milk.

It is wise to eat more whole grain products, if for no other reason than the increased fiber and nutrients. A taste for the richer and nuttier flavor of whole grains can be reacquired as well. For children, starting them early on whole grain cereal and such foods as cream of wheat or rice, cooked brown rice or oats, can get them started with a healthy base. Many natural foods stores carry all kinds of new, wholesome breakfast cereals in place of many of the high-sugar packaged cereals, to which kids easily become addicted. Some of the better big cereal company brands are the puffed grains, Cheerios, the various grain Chex, Kix, Grape Nuts, and bran cereals. Avoiding sugary foods and refined foods in the early years will help children maintain their taste for natural foods.

In review, the grain foods represent the bulk of the world's food supply, with wheat, rice, and corn being the three top crops. Whole grains are rich in energy-generating starch and complex carbohydrates, fiber, B vitamins, vitamin E, and lots of minerals. Each kernel of grain needs to have all of its parts intact to stay alive, or to keep the potential of life, which it can maintain for many years, perhaps hundreds or even thousands. Once the outer shell is disrupted or the grain is refined, it will slowly decay. But if nourished with water, sun, and good soil, it will generate new life and provide much nourishment for our new life for generations.

Specific Grains

Amaranth	*Oats*
Barley	*Quinoa*
Buckwheat	*Rice*
Corn	*Rye*
Millet	*Wheat*

Amaranth. Amaranth is a fairly new grain available in North American food stores (often pearled or polished), but is an ancient food to Central American cultures such as the Aztecs and Mayan Indians. This high-protein, high-iron grain can be cooked whole as a breakfast cereal or served along with vegetables or other foods for lunch or dinner. It is suggested to rinse first and then dry roast before cooking. Ideally, it is best used as a flour for baking, and can be found in breads, cookies, pastas, or tortillas. It is a substitute for wheat and other grains, though it is still a bit more expensive than the more common cereal grains. Besides iron and protein, amaranth is high in calcium, and it contains most of the B vitamins, as well as other minerals. Like most grains, amaranth is a good source of dietary fiber.

Barley. This glutenous grain is much used as cattle feed. It is also used to make beer and whiskey. As eaten by humans, barley is most commonly employed in making soups. Its gluten content gives it a pastalike consistency, and barley is a good heat-generating food. In ancient times, barley bread was very popular, especially in Egypt and the Far East. Barley grows well in cold climates, as do buckwheat and rye. Russia cultivates the most barley.

Sprouted barley is high in the sugar maltose, which can be extracted, and the remaining malt syrup can be used to make beer and to sweeten other foods. Barley water has been employed since ancient times for a variety of medicinal purposes.

Pearling is a refining process used to remove the barley's bran covering. The pearled barley is easier to cook but has less nutrient content than the whole barley. This whole grain contains about 10–15 percent protein, with the remainder being carbohydrate. Niacin and folic acid are the best represented of the B vitamins, while magnesium, calcium, iron, phosphorus, and potassium are barley's highest minerals.

Buckwheat. Buckwheat is not really a grass but a thistle plant that produces fragrant flowers, followed by the buckwheat groats, little fruits each covered by their own fibrous shell. Buckwheat does not have the bran and germ that characterize grains, but its flavor, consistency, and nutrient content are so much like those of the grains that it is essentially treated like one.

The use of the triangular buckwheat groats began in Russia and spread to the Orient and Western Europe, particularly as the mashed and cooked buckwheat dish called "kasha." Buckwheat can be mixed with other grains, and buckwheat flour can be used to make pancakes and other baked goods. This grain variant is about 15–20 percent protein. It contains a good amount of fiber, an assortment of B vitamins, lots of potassium, and some iron, calcium, manganese, and phosphorus.

Corn. Though a true grain, corn is different from the other grains in that its kernels are larger and softer, and they can be eaten fresh, like a vegetable. Dried corn can be ground into a flour or used to grow the next generation of corn stalks. Corn is a real American grain, possibly the only one that originated here, and was used as a primary food by the native American Indians. Corn spread easily to Mexico and South America and has also been grown in Europe and, more recently, in the Eastern world. Corn production has increased greatly in the last century and is now approaching that of wheat and rice. Formerly, it was grown primarily in the southeastern and northwestern United States, but now its cultivation is fairly widespread.

Corn, or maize, has many uses. Eaten fresh, usually steamed or boiled, corn is a delicious summer and autumn treat. Popcorn is a very popular and fairly healthy snack food, low in calories. Its high-fiber content helps intestinal activity. Cornmeal or corn flour can be made into cornbread or corn tortillas. Young corn is high in oil, and corn oil is commonly used in cooking, especially in baked goods, and in margarines. The mash left after the oil is pressed is made into a polenta that is much like cornmeal. Polenta can be mixed with beans to increase the total protein content or with leafy greens to improve the vitamin and mineral content of the meal.

Corn itself is fairly rich in vitamin A. It is about 10–20 percent protein, though mostly carbohydrate. Fresh corn has some vitamin C, folic acid, and other B vitamins, lots of potassium and magnesium, and some iron, zinc, and selenium as well. Actually, much of the manufactured vitamin C in this country is extracted primarily from corn. Cornmeal and corn flour lose the vitamin C and some of the Bs, but the minerals are fairly well retained. Corn oil is usually rich in vitamin E. The niacin in corn is not easily available unless the cornmeal is specially prepared. The American Indians, who used corn as the staple in their diet, were able to prevent pellagra, the vitamin B_3 deficiency disease, by pounding, soaking, and boiling the corn into a mineral ash (see *Niacin* discussion in Chapter 5). This sweet yellow grain, however, can provide a lot of nourishment, especially when combined properly with other foods.

Millet. Previously used here mainly as fodder and as birdfeed, millet, also known as sorghum, has recently become a more commonly eaten grain, though its food use goes back many thousands of years in China. A sweetener is extracted from the stalks of sorghum, and these stalks have also been used in making brooms. Millet is a nonglutenous grain. It is the most alkaline of the grains and thus is potentially the least congesting. It is tasty and a good nutrient grain, with nearly 15 percent protein, high amounts of fiber, good amounts of niacin, thiamine, and riboflavin, a little vitamin E, and particularly high amounts of iron, magnesium, and potassium. Millet is a warming grain, helping to heat the body in cold or rainy climates. It is a good winter grain and a healthy one to use more regularly.

Oats. Oats also have a growing role in feeding the world's population. It is fourth among the grains in production, following wheat, rice, and corn. It, like wheat, is a gluten grain, and should be avoided by those sensitive to gluten. Its primary use has traditionally been as a breakfast cereal, as in oatmeal, or porridge, and more recently granola. Oats are a soft grain; when rolled and flattened, they cook fairly easily. The nutritional level of the oats is much less affected by this process than is the case with other types of grain refinement. The harder whole oats take longer to cook and are richer in flavor and chewier than rolled or "steelcut" oats.

Oats have a great many uses. They have been commonly fed to cattle. Oatmeal is one of the healthier breakfast cereals; its high amount of complex carbohydrate provides sustained energy. Rolled oats can also be toasted to make a fairly healthy granola. This cereal is often sweetened with honey, maple syrup, brown sugar, or malt syrup and may have raisins, seeds, or nuts added to it. It is a nourishing snack but definitely still a sweet

treat and not a staple food. Oat flour can be used to make breads, oatmeal cookies, or biscuits. Oat bran is a good substitute for wheat bran, especially in those sensitive to wheat, and some preliminary research suggests that oat bran used regularly may help lower cholesterol levels. Recent cardiovascular research supports the use of oats and oat bran for heart health. In some ways, oats as an unrefined food are the most accepted whole grain in our American society. Oatmeal is the most available whole grain in restaurants across the United States.

Oats are about 10–15 percent protein and provide a source of fiber and a mixture of B vitamins. They have a modest level of folic acid, niacin, pyridoxine, and pantothenic acid, as well as decent amounts of iron, magnesium, zinc, potassium, manganese, calcium, and copper. Fortified oat cereals have a higher vitamin A content than natural oats. However, they usually also contain more sodium, as do most processed foods.

Quinoa. Quinoa is another new grain on the American scene that, like amaranth, is native to Central America. It can be cooked in a main or side dish, or in soups and puddings, or used as a flour in baking. Rinse quinoa thoroughly before cooking since it has a saponin (soaplike) coating. Quinoa is a quickcooking (20 minutes) whole grain and is high in protein, iron, and calcium, with a mix of the B vitamins and other minerals. It is still fairly expensive, and is available mainly in health food stores.

Rice. Rice is the second most highly consumed grain in the world; more than 200 million tons are produced each year. Rice is a staple food throughout much of Asia; in China, the same word, "fan," is used for rice and for food. In the United States, rice use has increased greatly in the last quarter century with the greater acceptance of the Oriental philosophies. Macrobiotic diets and many natural food diets use whole, or "brown," rice and its products as a main part of the diet.

Also, the concerns over wheat allergy and sensitivity have brought forth many new rice-based products as substitutes.

The primary place of origin of rice is Southeast Asia, where an average of more than 200 pounds per person a year are eaten. India, China, Japan, and Vietnam are some of the major rice-consuming countries. Warmer climates with abundant water are ideal for rice growth. Larger crops are now being cultivated in California and the southern United States.

A number of varieties of rice are commonly available. Sweet rice is more glutenous or gelatinous than other varieties and is used mostly for desserts such as rice pudding. Long- and short-grain brown rice are also commonly available, with many varieties providing different flavors. Besides just being boiled to be eaten with vegetables, tofu, fish, and so on, rice can be popped and used as a breakfast cereal; cream of rice, another breakfast cereal, is made from ground rice. Rice cakes are becoming very popular and can be found in most stores. They are a low-calorie, low-sodium, low-cholesterol, high-fiber snack and may be eaten plain, with butter, or with nut butters. Rice flour can be used in breads, cookies, and often in baked goods, and more of these products are available now for people who are moving away from wheat. Several recent rice products that are very good include mochi, a hard cake made from sweet rice that can be baked into crunchy and tasty rice balls; rice-based ice creams (Rice Dream) and crackers; and Amazake, a rich and sweet rice drink or nectar. Amazake is a tasty and nourishing milk substitute for diet-restricted people. The almond variety is very tasty and high in calcium as well. Children may love all these products.

However, especially in the Asian countries, most rice is refined, or polished. Although removing just the outer bran layers would still leave most of the nutrients, further milling takes place. The rice is bleached, cleaned, pearled (polished with talc), then often oiled and coated. This may make the rice more pleasing, even somewhat more digestible, but it unfortunately removes a great deal of the nutrients. The oils are lost, the protein decreases, and most (80 percent) of the thiamine (B_1) is removed, as well as other B vitamins, for example, 50 percent of the pyridoxine, B_6, and riboflavin, B_2, and two-thirds of the niacin, B_3, and some of the minerals. Polished or refined rice is easier for most people to digest owing to the increased starch level and loss of the outer hulls. Refined rice flour is also more stable because, as with wheat, the oils that can rancidify are lost. But what is the point if we lose the overall nutrition? People on a high polished-rice diet got into a great deal of trouble with a disease called beri-beri until it was learned that it came from a thiamine deficiency from eating refined rice. In China, the white rice was considered a more prestigious food than the whole, "dirty" rice that the peasants commonly ate.

Rice is not as high in protein as wheat and some other grains, about 10 percent, but the protein is very good quality and easily usable. Brown rice is better in thiamine, biotin, niacin, pyridoxine, and pantothenic and folic acids than it is in riboflavin and vitamin B_{12}. It has no vitamins A or C, but some vitamin E. Rice, if grown in selenium-rich soil, is very rich in selenium, a scarce but important trace mineral. Magnesium, manganese, potassium, zinc, and iron are all found in good amounts. Sodium is low, but phosphorus, copper, and calcium are all available. White rice, even when enriched, is lower in all of these minerals, yet, whole grain rice is one our more broad-based, nutrient-rich foods.

Wild rice is a special and more expensive type of rice (it is actually not rice, but a different grain plant). It has twice as much protein as regular rice, and more niacin, riboflavin, iron, and phosphorus than brown rice, though less of many other nutrients.

Rye. Rye grows best in a cold climate and is

much used in Russia, Scandinavia, and northern Europe. Rye is more resistant than wheat and will sustain itself in mountainous northern climates and sandy plains. Rye is often mixed with wheat to make what is called "rye" bread. Pure rye bread (not readily available) is a very nourishing black bread with a rich flavor. Light ryes are usually made with a refined rye flour. Dark rye breads are often made of wheat flour with some rye and dyes to darken the flour. Rye is also used to make whiskey but is not very often used as an animal feed. The rye stalks are very strong and are occasionally used in basket weaving.

Rye is also a gluten grain, though it is lower in gluten than wheat. It is nearly 20 percent protein and a good fiber food, with a mixture of the B vitamins. Iron, magnesium, and potassium are found in the greatest levels, though phosphorus, calcium, and copper are also present.

Wheat. The most important and oldest of the cereal grains, wheat feeds more people in the world than any other food and is now cultivated worldwide, with the exceptions of the colder climates and tropical areas. The Soviet Union, the United States, and China are the top three wheat-producing nations. Production has more than doubled in the twentieth century, and close to two billion people use wheat regularly in their diets. There are two basic varieties of wheat—"hard," or durum, wheat, and soft wheat. Hard wheat tends to have a little more protein and is often used to make macaroni and pasta. It also can be ground into flour to make bread, though the soft wheat is more commonly used for bread making. Wheat is the ideal grain for bread, not only because of its starch content but also because of its gluten protein. Gluten gives wheat its tenacious elasticity so characteristic of good dough, and it is primarily the gluten that responds and expands with yeast treatment. Refined soft wheat flour is used by most people to make pastries, cookies,

and cakes, though whole wheat flour can be used as well. When buying flours, get them fresh and store them in the freezer or fridge if possible to prevent oxidation and rancidity, or infestation with bugs.

The nutrient content of wheat may vary somewhat depending on the soil availability. The protein content may also vary between 10–20 percent of the wheat kernel. Wheat protein is of good quality and easily usable, but it does not contain high or equal amounts of all the essential amino acids. It is low in lysine and isoleucine. Gluten, the main wheat protein, can be concentrated by slowly running water over the flour dough to dissolve the starch. This leaves a gelatinous protein, which is the basis of a meatlike substitute, used in Oriental cooking, called seitan.

Wheat is also fairly high in the B vitamins except B_{12}. Vitamins C and A are not available, though vitamin E is present in whole wheat. Potassium, magnesium, iron, zinc, and phosphorus are all present in high amounts in whole wheat. Selenium is also very rich. Calcium and copper are found in wheat, but it contains very little sodium and no manganese.

Bulgur wheat is a special preparation of the wheat grain that is commonly used in the Middle Eastern countries, though its use has spread throughout the world, especially to Europe and the United States. The wheat kernels are washed, scrubbed, cracked, and then dried. These smaller grains can then be cooked or even just soaked in water, where they swell in size. This grain is most commonly used in a salad called tabouli or tabuleh.

Another variety of cracked wheat, smaller than the bulgur, is called couscous. It is also used commonly in the Middle Eastern diet— mutton and couscous is the traditional faire in those countries. Couscous is also very good with lentils or chickpeas, and this versatile grain can be used in a main dish, as a salad, or even in desserts. It is easily prepared by pouring boiling water over this soft grain or by light cooking.

○ **SEEDS**

Seeds are the potential for new life that are grown as part of a plant and in some way reach the earth to carry on their species. The long-lived plants, such as trees, may generate seeds of some kind at various intervals. The seeds discussed here are from annual plants and are contained within a hard shell that protects this potential for the next generation of life. These seeds are slightly different from the grains, which have softer shells and a different structural makeup, though they are very similar in many ways. Beans and peas are actually seeds as well, though contained in pods. Most seeds can be stored in their whole form. In fact, some seeds discovered from centuries past were still able to germinate.

Seeds were originally used in their ground form as seasonings or herbal flavorings for foods. Celery, cumin, mustard, cardamom, and coriander seeds, as well as many others, are still used in this way. But seeds are also very concentrated food. They are the initial source of the nutrition for the new plant.

The three main seeds discussed here—pumpkin, sesame, and sunflower—are high-protein foods, with more protein than the grains. Pumpkin seeds, for example, are more than 30 percent protein. High in vitamin E, these seeds are also a good source of fat, containing more than half by weight. Luckily, most (more than 80 percent) of that is poly-unsaturated fats, our essential fatty acids, and oil-soluble vitamins A, D, and E. So seeds can be rather high in calories, which is good for those few who are attempting to gain weight. There are some B vitamins in seeds, varying depending on the seed. They are rich in minerals; iron and zinc are plentiful. The amount of magnesium is good, especially in pumpkin seeds. Most seeds are a great source of copper. Calcium and potassium levels are also fairly good, yet there is very little sodium.

Phosphorus levels are high, especially compared to calcium, thus an excess of seed intake can throw off this important balance. Iodine is usually present in most seeds as well.

Seeds can be eaten raw after shelling and bought fresh either in shells or unshelled. They are a good protein addition to salads, can be cooked into grain or vegetable dishes, or can be blended to make a low-sodium protein sprinkle for food dishes. Unhulled seeds have a better shelf life than the hulled seeds, which should be kept refrigerated. Unhulled seeds can be stored in a cool, dry place. All seeds can be sprouted to make a highly nutritious seed-vegetable (green) combination. Sunflower and alfalfa are common and can be used in salads or sandwiches.

Most commonly, seeds are used to make oils. Sunflower, safflower, and sesame are very good ones among the seed oils. These can be used in cooking (sunflower is the most stable for storage and cooking) or to make margarines, but they are best used fresh on foods such as salads and cooked grains or vegetables. Usually, cold-processed oils (not heat-refined) give good nourishment, and using them uncooked is best, as discussed in Chapter 4, *Lipids*.

Seeds

Pumpkin	*Sunflower*
Sesame	

Pumpkin Seeds. These are best known for their concentration of zinc and their use in the treatment and prevention of male prostate problems. Pumpkin seeds have also been used in the treatment of intestinal worms. They are a good source of protein and contain a good balance of the amino acids, though tryptophan, methionine, and cysteine are a little lower in concentration than the others. Their fat content, mostly unsaturated, is over 50 percent of the seeds.

Pumpkin seeds are also very high in iron as well as calcium and phosphorus, with some magnesium and copper; they also contain vitamin E and essential fatty acids. There is a mix of B vitamins, with niacin being the richest. Pumpkin seeds are usually eaten raw, roasted, or blended into a seed meal and used on other foods. Like pumpkin seeds, most squash seeds are found within the hard vegetable and can be toasted and eaten as well. They have similar nutrient values.

Sesame Seeds. These seeds are probably the most commonly used worldwide, especially in the Middle East, where the sesame foods tahini (sesame mash) and halvah (a sesame candy) originated. These foods and other sesame products are used now in many countries. In the United States, sesame seeds are often used in breads or on bread crusts; as tahini or sesame butter to spread on bread or crackers or used in sauces; as halvah candy; and as a roasted, blended sesame salt called gomasio, which originated in Japan. Sesame seeds can be eaten raw, dried, or roasted or cooked with all kinds of foods. They are also great to add to other foods, such as grains and legumes, because they provide additional amino acids that may be low in those foods. Sesame can also be used with many seasonings, with other nuts or seeds, such as almonds or sunflower seeds, or blended with seasoning seeds such as caraway, poppy, dill, or anise, and used over various food dishes. Black sesame seeds, also very nourishing, can also be used in these seasonings. (Note: Sesame seeds, as do all seeds, and really all foods for that matter, need to be chewed well to help them be digested and assimilated; otherwise, many of these tiny seeds may pass through the intestinal tract unused.)

Sesame seeds come from little seed pods of one of the oldest of cultivated plants. In the Middle East, they are still called the "seed of immortality." The seeds are rich in oil, over 55 percent. Sesame oil is a very useful and common oil, especially in Oriental culture, where toasted and even hot-spiced sesame oil is used in cooking. Sesame seeds are also about 20 percent protein and contain some vitamins A and E and most of the B vitamins except B_{12} and folic acid. Minerals, however, are very abundant in sesame, as in most seeds. Zinc is high, as are calcium, copper, magnesium, phosphorus, and potassium. Sesame seeds are an excellent source of calcium for those avoiding cow's milk. However, the phosphorus content is much higher, as is true of most seeds, thus making it not quite as good for bone support. Iron is fairly high and sodium is fairly low, unless, of course, they are salted. Sesame seeds may also have a mild antioxidant effect, possibly because of their vitamin E content or some other factors.

Sunflower Seeds. Sunflowers are native to South and North America. These tall, strong flowers that open bright yellow to their sun, are filled tightly with hundreds of seeds to carry on life. Sunflower seeds have been used throughout history to enhance energy, and as a medicine as well. The Indians of the Americas and other herbalists have used sunflower seeds as a diuretic, for constipation, chest pain, or ulcers, to treat worms, and to improve eyesight. More recently, John Douglas, M.D., was quoted in *Food and Nutrition* (Rodale Press, 1983) as praising the medicinal powers of sunflower seeds. He recommends them to many patients with high blood pressure or cardiovascular problems and occasionally to help reduce allergic reactions, all with good success. He also suggests them as part of a stop-smoking program, having people in the program munch on raw, unshelled, unsalted sunflower seeds, which, in addition to their medicinal properties, gives them something to do with their hands and mouth.

Again, raw sunflower seeds are probably the best, higher in nutrition than roasted and definitely better than salted seeds. For people with blood pressure problems, sunflower seeds (unsalted!) are very high in potassium and low in sodium, a balance sorely needed by most of us these days with so many salty foods available. One cup of sunflower seeds contains more than 1,300 mg. of potassium and only 4 mg. of sodium. This is likely very helpful as a diuretic or for people who already take diuretics, to help replace some potassium. The high amount of oil in sunflower seeds as polyunsaturated fats, essential linoleic acid, and vitamin E is also helpful in reducing cholesterol levels and improving or preventing cardiovascular disease.

However, sunflower seeds are caloric; one half cup of hulled seeds is approximately 400 calories. If we are watching our figures, then we'll have to go a little easy on sunflower seeds, but from all other aspects of nutrition, they are a good food. For those who need to gain weight or substitute more vegetable oils for saturated fats, sunflower seeds can be very good. They are about 25 percent protein, have a good fiber content, the best of the seeds, and are richer in the B vitamins also, particularly in thiamine, pyridoxine, niacin, and pantothenic acid. With their high potassium and low sodium and with zinc, iron, and calcium all at good levels, sunflower seeds are a very mineral-rich food. The vitamin D that gets stored in these sun-filled seeds helps the utilization of calcium. Copper, manganese, and phosphorus levels are also relatively high; they are lower in magnesium than in calcium, which is different from other seeds.

Sunflower seed oil is a very good one. It is often used in margarines or cooking oils. It is rich in polyunsaturates and linoleic oil and has a fairly low rancidity level compared to other oils. This may be because of its vitamin E content. Cold-pressed sunflower oil is the best. It should also be refrigerated once opened to avoid spoilage. Cold storage of most nuts and seeds is generally suggested.

Sunflower seeds have many other uses besides as an oil or nutritious snack food. They can be sprinkled on salads, are used in baking breads and cookies, and can be baked in vegetable casseroles to add protein, flavor, and crunch. A ground or blended sunflower-sesame sprinkle with a bit of salt or other seasonings can be a nutrient-rich, low-sodium seasoning. Almond-sunflower blend is also good, and a spicy high-mineral protein blend includes ground sunflower and sesame seeds (either white or black), nori seaweed flakes, and cayenne pepper. If sunflower seeds are soaked overnight, it makes them more digestible and alkaline-forming. When added to green salads, they supply a tasty crunch, along with some protein and fatty acids. This is also true for nuts. A great combination is soaked almonds, sunflower seeds, and peanuts.

○ NUTS

Nuts are one of nature's richest foods. They have good-quality protein and are even higher in fats (as oils) than the seeds. Because of that, they are more caloric than other vegetable foods (remember, each gram of fat has nine calories, over twice that of protein or carbohydrate), so they are not a food that should be eaten in abundance unless we are trying to gain weight. For vegetarians, nuts may be the most concentrated foods they eat, and their main source of oil.

Like the seeds, nuts are bundles of potential, the part of the plant that feeds the future generations. The calories, proteins, fatty acids, and many vitamins and minerals are what provide the energy for the early growth of the next nut tree.

There are more than 300 types of nuts. Besides those discussed below, hickory nuts, macadamias, and pinenuts are also common. Most nuts are the fruit or seed that follows the blossoming of the tree. They are usually contained in a hard shell to protect them from birds, insects, and germs and also to keep them fresh, since the concentrated oils contained in nuts can easily rancidify and spoil in the air.

Because of the spoilage problem of these

oil-rich nuts, picking or buying the fresh, raw, unshelled (with shells) nuts are the best. They will store longer than any other. Once the shells are removed, nuts should be kept in closed containers or plastic bags in the refrigerator or even the freezer. If left out in containers or bags, they should be eaten within a month. Nuts will store longer in a cool, dry place in closed containers than left in the air or in damp areas. Roasted, salted nuts are best avoided. The salt is not needed, and roasting affects the oils and decreases the B vitamin and mineral content. Be aware of places that feed you free salted nuts, such as bars or airplanes, to increase your thirst, and your drink tab!

Sadly, most nuts in American society are eaten after they are roasted in even more oil and salted, and often with other additives or sugars. Raw nuts, especially almonds, walnuts, and hazelnuts, are probably the best. Peanuts, especially in peanut butter, are not easy to digest, and there is concern about potentially toxic molds containing aflatoxin, a potential carcinogen that grows on this leguminous nut/bean.

Many people have some trouble digesting nuts because of the high fat content, which is even worse after roasting. The nut foods are not the easiest to digest; this is true especially in people with low stomach acid or gallbladder problems. Overweight individuals with gallstone or gallbladder disease often have difficulty digesting fatty foods in general. To process the nuts in our body, we usually need a good level of hydrochloric acid, fat-digesting enzymes (*lipases*), and bile secreted by our gallbladder and liver.

Besides raw, fresh nuts and the roasted varieties, nuts can be cooked into foods such as grains and vegetable dishes. This will often add the other needed essential amino acids to make more complete proteins. A nut-seed blended mix such as almonds-sunflower-sesame with a little added sea salt can be kept in a jar in the refrigerator and used as a protein seasoning. Nuts can be blended into flours as well as used in baking with other flours. These also need refrigeration to keep the other, lighter flours from rancidifying. The use of nut butters as snack foods is growing. Peanut butter is, of course, the most common, but now many other butters are commercially available, such as almond, cashew, and even pistachio and macadamia nut butters, as many people move away from peanut butter. Nut milks are also becoming popular as nourishing milk substitutes and as wholesome drinks, especially for children. If we do not already have a high-fat diet, nuts and even a little bit of the nut butters are a much better snack than sugary foods, particularly in regard to nutrition and the sustained level of energy that comes from their metabolism.

In terms of nutrient content, nuts are among the best of the vegetable foods. Their fat content is, of course, fairly high, but it is mostly unsaturated fats, which are better for us than the saturated. The inner white meat of the dried coconut, however, is rich in saturated fats and thus more of a concern in regards to cardiovascular problems. The essential fatty acids and vitamin E are also part of the nut oils. Almonds, Brazil nuts, hazelnuts, and peanuts are the best in vitamin E content. Total fat content varies, from peanuts at 50 percent to pecans (and macadamias), the richest, at 70 percent fat.

The protein content of nuts is very good, with a fairly balanced amino acid distribution, which may be why the edible part of the nuts are termed "meats." They are the meat of the plant world. The nuts are somewhat lower in tryptophan and methionine, so the amino acid balance becomes more balanced when nuts are combined with a grain food at meals.

Most nuts have a general cross section of the B vitamins but are not real high in any, though peanuts are pretty rich in niacin. They are, however, very well endowed with the minerals, particularly potassium, magnesium, calcium, iron, zinc, and other trace minerals. Nuts are very low in sodium when unsalted, and some nuts, such as almonds, Brazil nuts, and pecans, even have some selenium.

In general, nuts can be used as a protein- and energy-rich snack food as a midmorning or midafternoon treat. Eaten alone in their raw state, and not much more than a handful, they should be fairly easily digested and assimilated by our bodies.

Nuts

Almonds	*Hazelnuts*
Brazil nuts	*Peanuts*
Cashews	*Pecans*
Chestnuts	*Pistachios*
Coconuts	*Walnuts*

Almonds. Almonds are probably the best all-around nut. Their fat content is less than most, about 60 percent, and the protein concentration is nearly 20 percent. The almond nuts are the fruits of a small tree that grows nearly thirty feet tall and is abundant in many areas of the world, including Asia, the Mediterranean, and North America. Almonds which are of the soft-shell variety possess a sweeter nut than those in hard shells, which may be slightly bitter. The presence of 2–4 percent amygdalin, commonly known as laetrile, has caused almonds to be considered as a cancer-preventing nut.

Most of the fats of the almond are polyunsaturated and are high in linoleic acid, our main essential oil. Almond oil is a very stable oil used in pharmaceutical preparations, to hold scents in fragrant oils, or for massage therapy. Almonds are very high in vitamin E, and contain some B vitamins. Calcium is also found in high amounts, and almonds or homemade almond milk (see recipes in Chapter 14) can be used as a tasty calcium source. Copper, iron, zinc, potassium, and phosphorus are also present in good amounts, as are magnesium and manganese. Sodium is very low. Some selenium is present.

Brazil Nuts. These are the very meaty and high-fat hard-shelled "seeds" of which about 10–20 are found in each big fruit of the very large (nearly 100 feet high) Brazil nut trees. Brazil nuts are a good-quality protein, yet are also about two-thirds fat, of which over 20 percent is saturated. The oil from this nut turns rancid easily and is not used commercially.

Brazil nuts are known to be rich in calcium, as well as magnesium, manganese, copper, phosphorus, potassium, and selenium. Zinc and iron are also found in good proportions in this high-mineral nut.

Cashews. Cashews are thought by some to be a toxic nut, probably because of the caustic oils found in the hard shell. Lightly roasting cashews may help to clear these oils. These sweet nuts are the real fruit of their 25- or 30-foot trees that grow best in tropical climates. These trees also provide another "fruit," the edible "cashew apple" that grows prior to the nut. Cashews are fairly rich in magnesium, potassium, iron, and zinc. Calcium is lower in cashews than in other nuts, as is manganese; cashews also have a lower fat and higher carbohydrate level than most other nuts. Some B vitamins are present, as is vitamin A, though very little vitamin E is found in cashews.

Chestnuts. These are the classic nut of the winter holidays throughout the world. Hot, roasted chestnuts can be a warming and nourishing snack for our innards. Chestnuts are very high in starch (carbohydrate) and low in protein and fats and therefore lower in calories (less than half) than other nuts. Chestnuts have lower levels of most minerals than other nuts, but they are still very good in manganese, potassium, magnesium, and iron.

Coconuts. The big nuts (fruits) of the common tropical palm tree, this large fruit has a thick husk covering, a very hard shell that surrounds the rich coconut meat. A nourishing liquid, called the coconut "milk" comes from the soft meat of the fresh green coconut. When the coconut dries or ripens, this "meat" becomes hard and much of the oils become saturated. The dried coconut meat contains about 65 percent oil, mainly as saturated fat which is solid or semisolid at room temperature. This oil, though, also has some nourishment and essential fatty acids and has been used in cooking and baking as well as in soaps, shampoos, and cosmetics. Coconut is used in cooking much more in the South Pacific and East Indian cultures than in ours, probably because they have fewer foods with good fat content. The fresh milk can be used as a marinade for fish, as salad dressing, or made into a yogurt-like dish. Coconut has a little protein, about 10 percent; some carbohydrate and fiber; and traces of the B vitamins, vitamin C, and vitamin E. It has some amounts of many minerals, with potassium, magnesium, manganese, copper, and iron being the best.

Hazelnuts. These are the fruits or seeds of a small shrub or tree that usually grows between six and twelve feet tall. They are also called filberts because they ripen about the time of St. Philibert's Day, August 20. The numerous varieties produce either round or elongated nuts. They are usually eaten raw or fried and are often used in confection making or as flavorings in sweet sauces.

Hazelnuts have one of the higher vitamin E levels of the nuts. Their protein content is about 15 percent, and they are nearly 65 percent fat, mostly unsaturated, being high in essential linoleic acid. Hazelnuts have a fairly good level of the B vitamins and are rich in most minerals such as calcium, magnesium, manganese, iron, copper, and potassium, as well as some trace minerals, including zinc and selenium.

Peanuts. The most peculiar of the nuts, and the most common in our culture, peanuts are not in fact a true nut but a legume or pea (thus "peanuts"), which grows on a small bush that yields small, soft, fibrous shells each containing usually two or three "nuts." Peanuts, or

"goobers," grow commonly in the southern United States but are now grown largely in China and India, where their oil is used widely in cooking. Peanuts are also called "monkey nuts" because monkeys love them, as do little human monkeys, especially as peanut butter here in the United States. In poorer, more populated countries, such as China, India, and Africa, peanuts are used in the daily diet in many vegetarian dishes, to which they add more complete proteins.

Peanuts probably have as good an amino acid balance as any vegetable food. They are about 25 percent protein and very rich in nutrients. Their fat content is about 50 percent of the nut, and three-fourths of it is unsaturated. The B vitamin content of peanuts is better than that of most nuts, probably because they are a bean. Niacin and biotin are best, but all B vitamins are represented except B_{12}. Potassium, magnesium, and phosphorus are highest of the minerals, while calcium, iron, zinc, copper, and manganese are also found in substantial amounts.

Stored peanuts may easily become moldy, a concern especially for those sensitive to molds. Peanuts have been known to become contaminated with molds containing aflatoxin, a substance that is thought to be carcinogenic. Also of concern is that much of the peanut butter consumed in this country is the processed variety, with not only the high fat and oil content of peanuts but additional hydrogenated fats, which are more toxic in the body. (See discussion of hydrogenated oils in Chapter 4, *Lipids*, and in the next section, *Oils*.) More additives—salt, sugar, dextrose, and others—make this manufactured peanut butter a poor quality food. Many companies now use ground peanuts only to make their butters; better yet, some stores have nut grinders where we can make our peanut butter right on the spot. It is best to refrigerate shelled peanuts and peanut butter to avoid rancidity.

Many people eat roasted and salted peanuts more than the fresh variety. Though a mild roasting of the peanut may make it a little easier to digest and not lower the nutrient value too much, the extra salt is not really needed. Some people do not do well on peanuts at all. Digestive problems, gallbladder irritation, or just plain allergy to these nuts are possible. Overall, they are still the most popular American nut and a good-quality food.

Pecans. Pecans are nuts for a special treat, such as for holidays or in the traditional pecan pie, usually sweetened with maple syrup. Pecans (and macadamias), however, contain the lowest protein (about 10 percent) and highest fat (over 70 percent) of all the nuts. They grow on large trees often taller than 100 feet; the nuts are about four to a pecan fruit, each nut protected by a hard, woodlike shell. In fact, pecan shells can be ground and used as wood sculpture material (I have a pecan shell lion in my collection).

Pecans contain some vitamins A, E, and C, niacin, and other B vitamins. They are low in sodium and high in most other minerals, including zinc, iron, potassium, selenium, and magnesium. Copper, calcium, and manganese are present in fairly good amounts as well.

Pistachios. Pistachios are those sweet and flavorful nuts of which it is "hard to eat just one." The pistachio nut or fruit grows on a small tree usually about 10–15 feet high and is very popular in the Mediterranean and middle Eastern countries. It is most commonly eaten in the shell but is also used in cooking, in making sauces, as flavoring in baking cakes, and in ice creams. It is best to avoid the less healthy salted and red-dyed pistachio nut and go with the natural variety.

Pistachios are about 20 percent protein and 50–55 percent fat and have good levels of thiamine, niacin, folic acid, and a little vitamin A. The potassium and iron levels are both very high; sodium is very low; phosphorus, magnesium, and calcium are all present in pretty fair amounts; while zinc, copper, and manganese are at modest levels.

Walnuts. Another of the great nuts, walnuts are a real brain food (they even look like little brains). The fatty acids and the 15–20 percent protein level nourish the nervous system, and the walnut when shelled looks remarkably like the human cerebral cortex. The walnut is about 65 percent fat. It can be eaten raw or used in baking, and the pressed walnut oil can be used in cooking or even for oiling wood. It should be used fresh, though, as it is not very resistant to spoilage.

Walnuts have a modest mix of vitamin A, the Bs (including biotin), C, and E. Their mix of minerals is similar to that of most of the other nuts, with many at good levels. Probably iron and potassium are the best in this very balanced nut, which grows on large trees as high as 40–50 feet in many parts of the world, including the United States.

O OILS

The edible oils are all liquid fats extracted from vegetable sources, with the exceptions of coconut, palm, and palm kernel oils. They are virtually 100 percent lipid, or fat, and most are high in unsaturated fat and low in the saturated component (10–20 percent). Commonly used oils include almond, avocado, corn, olive, peanut, safflower, sesame, soybean, and sunflower. Olive oil, a monounsaturated oil, is the main vegetable oil, possibly along with the newly available canola (rapeseed) oil, that should be used for cooking; most of the other oils contain more polyunsaturated fats and should not be heated. Polyunsaturated means that the oils have more than one unsaturated bond available in their carbon chain to which hydrogen atoms can be attached. These oils should be used on salads and other dishes in their cold-pressed form or consumed with extra vitamin E to prevent oxidation. The polyunsaturated fats may actually help to reduce blood cholesterol rather than raise it and, more importantly, can improve our ratios of LDL and HDL cholesterols to help reduce cardiovascular disease risk. These vegetable oils do not contain cholesterol.

All of the vegetable oils are liquid at room temperature except coconut oil, one of the few saturated vegetable oils. When the unsaturated vegetable oils are "hydrogenated" through a special industrial process, they become partially saturated, as in the solid vegetable margarines. These are usually fortified with vitamin A and have other additives, and they tend to function differently in the body. They may increase blood cholesterol and thus, the risk of cardiovascular problems; they have been associated with increased cancer risk as well. The animal fats—lard, butter, and chicken fat—have a much higher percentage of saturated fats and more cholesterol, and these fats are implicated as well in these chronic, serious cardiovascular diseases and cancer.

All of the vegetable oils contain nine calories per gram of pure fat, and one tablespoon of vegetable oil contains about 120 calories, so they should be used sparingly by people concerned about weight. These oils are rich in essential fatty acids, particularly linoleic acid, which is also present in the foods from which these oils are extracted. Linoleic and linolenic acids are needed for the growth and maintenance of our cells, tissues, and entire body. Other than vitamin E, which is found in these vegetable oils, they contain negligible amounts, if any, of other nutrients, such as the B vitamins and minerals. Some of the oils richer in vitamin E are soybean, safflower, cottonseed, corn, and wheat germ.

Oils can be used in salad dressings, in sauces, in baking, and in cooking food. To repeat the important point about cooking with oils, heating the polyunsaturated oils is not recommended, as heat may affect their chemical structures, making them less usable and more difficult for our body to process (they are also possibly carcinogenic). Overall, it is ideal not to fry foods but to add the uncooked oils after cooking the food. In general, the saturated fats are more stable when used in cooking, but are not the healthiest for us. I recommend either canola or olive oils, which are mono-unsaturated and more stable vegetable oils, or butter when cooking or sautéeing foods.

Though usually slightly more expensive, the least refined oils, most often called "cold-pressed," are the best. As heat and chemicals are not used in extracting them, they retain more vitamin E and are less likely to break down in the processing. For regular use, I do not recommend the refined or partially hydrogenated vegetable oils, the vegetable shortenings, or really very much margarine either.

Overall, the vegetable oils should contribute a higher percentage of the total fat in our diet than they currently do, as this would increase the proportion of polyunsaturated to saturated fats, which is helpful. But total blood cholesterol is influenced most by total fat intake, so for best health we should reduce our total fat intake. (The topic of fats in our diet is discussed in detail in Chapter 4, *Lipids.*)

○ DAIRY PRODUCTS

 With this food category, we enter into the animal kingdom and the foods made from and by animals and their products, such as eggs, milk, butter, cheese, and yogurt; and then the actual animal flesh—fish, poultry, and beef and other red meats. These are, in general, denser and higher-protein foods, more concentrated body-building foods, and also higher-fat foods. They are most important in growth years and during pregnancy and lactation, but because of their prevalence in our early years, many people, especially in Western cultures, continue to consume what turns out to be an excess of these protein and fatty foods. This may then contribute to the congestive problems and degenerative diseases that occur in later years. In general, other than for special therapeutic situations that will be described later, I believe that these animal-product foods should be consumed moderately in our diet, probably not more than 10–20 percent of our total intake, and can even be totally avoided with proper nutritional care to create a balanced strict vegetarian (vegan) diet.

Milk Products

Milk	*Cheeses*
Butter	*Processed cheeses*
Yogurt	*Cream cheese*
Kefir	*Cottage cheese*
Buttermilk	*Ice cream*

Milk is a special food—the primary baby food, the first food of most mammals. It is considered our basic food of life, the connection between mother and child. Milk is often associated in early years with survival, with our love from and for Mother—so it is no wonder that many develop a lifelong addiction to this sweet essence of life. Theoretically, the relationship to sweet food, of which milk is our first, may be the basis of so many people's acceptance and use of sugar and sweet foods throughout life. An excess of sweets in the diet creates all kinds of problems, from tooth decay to obesity to diabetes. (See more about sugar in Chapter 2, *Carbohydrates.*)

Lactose, a simple sugar, should be easy to digest and use in our body for energy, but some children may be unable to utilize this sugar; that is, they are lactose intolerant. Even more adults are sensitive to milk sugar; this is a separate (and major) issue from milk allergy. Nearly half of the world population is lactose intolerant, which may cause bloating, abdominal pain, and diarrhea after milk is consumed. Luckily, though, most children can handle at least mother's milk and do all right on milk products, at least in their early years.

When other milks, such as cow's or goat's milk, are substituted for mother's milk in infancy, milk allergy is very common. These milks are richer in proteins and have new protein molecules for the baby's system to handle. Lactalbumin and milk casein are two of the proteins to which people, especially children, may react. Milk is the most common food allergen. Milk allergies may manifest as skin rashes, eczema, chronic otitis media (fluid and/or infections in the ears), hyperactivity, and other problems. Taking a child off milk products for a three- to four-week trial period and seeing how he or she does and then retesting with a meal of milk products is probably the best way to evaluate whether milk is a problem. If there are mild allergies, it is still possible to bring milk products back into the diet later after eliminating them for a month or two, which reduces the allergic capacity, possibly to a degree that they can be tolerated in moderation. Then a rotating diet where they are consumed only every four days will often be better tolerated. Sometimes substituting goat's milk or, even better, soy milk or nut milks, will make a difference. (See more about this in the *Allergy* program in Part Four.)

(In the rest of this section, when discussing milk, I will be referring to cow's milk, which is by far the most commonly consumed.) Even for adults, cow's milk and its products are not ideal and really not even suggested, especially from factory-farmed cows. We know that when an upset mother nurses her infant, he or she may have intestinal difficulties; what can we expect from these mistreated animals?

On the more positive side, milk is a very good protein food and an important source of calcium. It has a better balance than vegetable foods in all the essential amino acids. Milk is considered a complete protein food from which we can build bodily tissue proteins. Milk also contains many of the B vitamins, including B_6 and B_{12}, has vitamins

A, D, and E, and contains most of the minerals, though mainly calcium and phosphorus, along with potassium and some sodium. It has traces of zinc, iron, selenium, manganese, and copper and a little vitamin C, but certainly not enough to meet daily needs for any of these essential nutrients.

One glass of milk contains about 300 mg. of calcium, a level hard to find in very many other foods, and it is also in balance with phosphorus, so good for bone health. Other foods, such as meats, nuts, and seeds, have a much higher proportion of phosphorus. Many cheeses made from milk are also concentrated in calcium. Some extra calcium is helpful for elderly individuals or people with high blood pressure, as it helps to relax the vascular tone and sometimes reduces muscle tension. However, research has recently shown that the actual calcium utilization is not that good from milk or meat, or when consuming a high protein diet. More important, though, the higher fat levels of milk may increase cholesterol and blood triglyceride levels, which increases the atherosclerosis risk and may create more long-range problems with

FAT AND CALORIE CONTENT OF MILK (one glass, 8 oz.)

	Whole milk	2% milk	Skim milk
Calories	150.0	120.0	85.0
Protein (g.)	8.0	8.1	8.4
Carbohydrates (g.)	11.3	11.7	11.8
Fiber (g.)	0.0	0.0	0.0
Total fat (g.)	**8.2**	**4.7**	**0.4**
Saturated (g.)	5.0	2.9	0.3
Unsaturated (g.)	2.7	1.5	0.1
Cholesterol (mg.)	33.0	18.0	0.4

Source: *Nutrition Almanac*, McGraw-Hill, 1984.

hypertension and other cardiovascular diseases. Thus, drinking milk or eating a lot of milk products is not generally recommended in the adult population.

A great concern with milk is its fat content. The regular drinking of whole milk and intake of dairy products leads to excess fat intake and all of its potential problems. Whole milk is described as 3.5 percent fat, but about half the 150 calories in a glass are from the 8–9 grams of fat (at nine calories per gram). Skim milk has most of the fat removed and has about half the calories of whole milk; low-fat, or 2 percent, milk is in between, with about 50 of the 120 calories coming from fat (two-thirds saturated). Yet whole, low-fat, and skim milks are very similar in their vitamin and mineral makeup, as well as their protein and carbohydrate levels. The only difference is the amount of fat. Another concern is that these milks are also processed products. This natural white substance that comes from cows is heated, treated, and diluted to make even the "normal" homogenized, pasteurized milk. It loses some vitamin E, biotin, B_{12}, and other vitamins with pasteurization; often, vitamin A and irradiated vitamin D are then added to "fortify" this food, which some erroneously consider a "drink." Homogenization is possibly the biggest concern in milk. It basically involves the blending of the milk fat into small globules so that it does not separate as it normally will do when it sits. It is possible that this process interferes with the body's ability to digest and utilize this fat in homogenized milk. The increase in cardiovascular disease has been correlated with the rise in the use of homogenized milk; however, further epidemiological study is needed to prove this relationship.

In general, I do not recommend the drinking of milk for adults. A warm glass before bed can be helpful for sleep, likely due to the tryptophan content. Generally, though, calcium and protein needs can be met with many other foods. Chamomile flower or valerian root tea may be helpful for sleep in nonmilk drinkers. For adults who seem to tolerate milk products well, are not overweight, and do not have high blood pressure, high blood fats, or a family history of heart disease, I would suggest moderate use of milk products, but not daily because of the possibility of developing milk sensitivities. I think that yogurt and kefir, the cultured milk products that get predigested by friendly bacteria, even though that may sound disgusting to some, are probably the best choices of the dairy family. Low-fat milk products and a low-fat diet in general are also wise guidelines to follow.

Butter. Butter, made from whole milk through a churning process, is mainly the milk fat. It is a high-fat (two-thirds saturated fats) and high-cholesterol food that is also high in vitamin A and added vitamin D. It has minimal amounts of some other vitamins and minerals, usually is salted so that it is high in sodium, and is fairly high in calories (100 per tablespoon). Because of its sweet flavor and the fact that it is saturated and so doesn't break down as easily as the unsaturated fats, it is used commonly in cooking and baking, and slathered on potatoes, noodles, vegetables, and other hot foods or poured over popcorn. A little butter is okay, but butter is one food that it is very easy to overuse.

Yogurt. Yogurt is considered the "health food" of the milk family. One of the foods thought to promote longevity, it is commonly consumed by those peoples who tend to live a long time. Yogurt is the end product of the fermentation process of either whole milk or low-fat or nonfat milk acted upon by bacteria and yeasts. The friendly human intestinal bacteria *Lactobacillus acidophilus* and the one originally used, *Lactobacillus bulgaricus,* are the common ones used to make yogurt, which resembles a milk custard. Yogurt is a form of soured milk that becomes reduced in fat and calories, usually with an increase in the B vitamin lev-

els. Many of the minerals become more concentrated as well. The calcium content of yogurt is very good. Yogurt, like the other cultured or soured milk products, is more stable and resistant to spoilage than fresh milk, and this can be helpful in many instances.

Yogurt is usually thought of in terms of its health or medicinal benefits. Many experience it as an aid to digestion. Acidophilus yogurt tends to help reimplant normal colon bacteria, which can then act more effectively in the complete digestion and utilization of high-fiber foods. Our friendly bacteria also aid in the production of many of our needed B vitamins.

Yogurt can be eaten alone as a snack or dessert, mixed with cereal, or made into sauces or dips. Lower fat yogurts are becoming more popular in recent years as people watch their fat intake. Frozen yogurt has also increased in use as a slight improvement over ice cream. Fruited and sugared yogurt is commonly available, but this is not recommended. Often, people who have a lactase deficiency do all right when eating yogurt because much of the lactose has already been acted on by the bacterial process and turned into lactic acid.

It is interesting that, on the one hand, we are trying to get rid of bacteria in milk products through pasteurization and on the other, we are trying to obtain more bacteria in yogurt and kefir. What we want to do is to keep our friendly colon bacteria *L. acidophilus*, *L. bifidis*, and *Strep. faecium* working for our benefit, not to obtain pathogenic organisms that can make us sick. People often eat yogurt after antibiotic therapy, which kills off some of their normal bacteria in the intestine or in a woman's vaginal tract. This may lead to an overgrowth of yeast organisms, such as *Candida albicans*, which may then need treatment to clear. (See discussion in the *Anti-Yeast* program in Part Four.) Yogurt or acidophilus culture douches or cultures of bacteria taken orally seem to be helpful clinically to prevent these

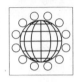

problems, though further research is needed to clarify what is really happening with this interplay of organisms. In some areas of Europe, acidophilus and vitamin B$_{12}$ are prescribed together with antibiotics.

Kefir. Another soured and fermented milk product, kefir is more of a drink than yogurt. It has similar properties, though most kefir available is flavored and sweetened with fruit. It is often a good nutritious substitute for milk, especially for children.

Buttermilk. Basically soured milk, buttermilk provides good nourishment with a reduced fat content while remaining high in calcium and protein, though its vitamin A content is lower (unless added) than that of whole milk. Buttermilk may be helpful for digestion, as are the other soured products, for those people who tolerate its fairly strong taste.

Cheeses. Cheeses have been made for centuries worldwide, directly from milk, by separating the curd, or milk solids, from the whey and then aging the curd. Cheese is a concentrated food; it takes about one gallon of milk to make a pound of cheese. In general, cheese is a high-protein, high-calcium food with good levels of vitamin A and an assortment of various vitamins and minerals.

Cheese has some of the problems of milk products in general—it is high in fats, mainly saturated fats, and high in cholesterol, and too much of it can cause the many problems that come from high-fat diets. Cheese is even more commonly abused in our adult population than milk. Sodium content is also usually higher in cheeses than in milk. There are some lower-fat cheeses available, such as mozzarella, farmer cheese, and cheeses made from skim milk. Recently, goat's milk cheese and fetas made from sheep or goats have become available, particularly helpful for people avoiding cow's milk products.

Most cultures around the world have their own cheeses, for which they may be famous throughout other countries. The French have brie, bleu, and Camembert; the Swiss have Swiss; Italians are known for mozzarella, Parmesan, and ricotta; Greeks for feta; and the Americans for cheddars, jacks, and colbys. On the negative side, the classic "American" sliced cheese is really a "junk" food and not part of the real cheese culture. It is often high in sodium and unnecessary additives. Cheeses are used in a great variety of food dishes, such as sauces, quiche, and omelettes.

Processed Cheeses. Processed cheeses and cheese spreads are often higher than natural cheeses in fat and sodium, neither of which is needed by most people. They are often fortified with vitamin A, but most of the B vitamins and minerals other than calcium and phosphorus are fairly low. Sodium levels are about 400–500 mg. per ounce. It is really a good idea to avoid these cheeses.

Cream Cheese. This mildly processed cheese is higher in fat and lower in protein and calcium than other cheeses. Other than vitamin A, its nutrient content is fairly scarce. However, children do like it, it is better than other cheese spreads, and many people feel they can't live without their Sunday cream cheese and bagels. But, overall, cream cheese should be used sparingly, if at all.

Cottage Cheese. Made from soured milk, cottage cheese is mainly the curd extracted from the whey. This curd is high in protein, and cottage cheese is somewhat lower in calories and fats than other cheeses. The low-fat cottage cheese is even better. Though the sodium content of most cottage cheeses is pretty high and the calcium content low, overall, cottage cheese is fairly good to use as the main part of an occasional meal.

Ice Cream. Ice cream is both the greatest joy and the greatest tragedy of our food culture, probably the biggest treat and the biggest threat to health of any food. The high-fat congesting nature of ice cream, along with the usual high-sugar content, makes it a food that should be eaten only infrequently and sparingly, if at all. Frozen yogurt and, more recently, Tofutti and Ice Bean made from soybeans or Rice Dream made from rice are tasty and lower in fat, and better nutritional treats than ice cream.

○ SEAFOOD

 Fish are really one of our most ideal foods. Seafood offers a good protein balance to a primarily vegetarian diet. I have eaten fresh ocean fish at least weekly over most of the last decade after many years of a completely vegetarian diet. Because I lived close to the ocean, I felt it natural to include it in my diet in moderation. And my body certainly felt a difference.

Fish is a very good quality protein, easily usable by our body, and a complete protein— that is, it contains all our essential amino acids. It is also low in fats, and the fat that is present in fish is very helpful. In fact, recent evidence suggests that the eicosapentaenoic acid (EPA) and docosahexaenoic acid (DHA) that are contained in many fish help to lower blood cholesterol and protect us from hardening of the arteries, or atherosclerosis. EPA and DHA also seem to reduce platelet stickiness, which then reduces clotting potential and increases clotting time. This effect then decreases the likelihood of arterial thrombosis, heart attacks, and strokes.

This information comes from an investigation of the reason why peoples in certain fishing villages in Japan and Alaska who eat a very high-fat diet, consisting mainly of fish oils and fats from animals who eat fish, had a very low incidence of heart disease. This seemed contrary to our knowledge that fat was tied into high cholesterol levels and heart disease. Yet the fish that these villagers eat are very high in EPA and DHA and, further, these fatty acids have a different and possibly

opposite effect from that of other animal fats. Many of the fish that contain EPA and DHA also contain cholesterol, though shrimp and lobster are the highest, but this cholesterol does not seem to be a problem when accompanied by these helpful fats. With further investigation, we are finding that some of those fats in fish that we thought were cholesterol are probably beneficial oils.

Examples of fish that are high in these special lipid-lowering fats, EPA and DHA, are salmon, mackerel, sardines, trout, and haddock. It is now suggested that eating these fish two or three times a week may help protect us from cardiovascular disease. A popular trend supported by both doctors and the vitamin industry is to supplement the diet with EPA and DHA oils in a dose of about 3 grams fish oil per day (e.g., 3 grams salmon oil may contain about 350–700 mg. EPA and 250–500 mg. DHA). This will help to lower blood cholesterol and triglyceride levels, especially if they are elevated, and reduce the risk of coronary artery disease.

Fish are also fairly low in fat, containing about 5–10 percent, in comparison to red meats, which are usually between 30 and 40 percent. And, as we just discussed, the types of fat present in fish are more health promoting than disease causing, unlike the saturated fats. Furthermore, besides being relatively low in calories, seafood is very rich in vitamins and minerals. The first few times I ate fish after five or six years of being a lacto-ovo vegetarian, vegan, and raw fooder, I could feel my body absorb and utilize this concentrated nourishment like a dry sponge soaking up water droplets. It was like the increased efficiency of food utilization after a period of fasting.

Fish liver is especially high in vitamins A and D. Cod liver oil is a common old-time supplement used mainly to obtain these two important fat-soluble vitamins. Most seafood contains some B vitamins, though usually in low amounts, but biotin, niacin, B_6, and especially vitamin B_{12} are often found in higher

341

amounts in nutritious fish such as salmon, halibut, herring, mackerel, crab, and oysters. Vitamin E is found in some of the oilier fishes, such as mackerel and herring.

Seafood is a very good source of minerals, especially some of those harder-to-get trace minerals such as iodine, selenium, and zinc. Oysters are especially high in zinc, while crab and lobster are also fairly high; selenium is present in high amounts in most of the shellfish and mollusks and in codfish. Most fish are high in potassium and phosphorus. Iron levels are usually very good, and calcium can be high, especially if bones are consumed, as in sardines, and in salmon, shrimp, and herring. Calcium is actually higher in the seaweeds or sea vegetation, which are ideal foods to eat with fish. This is done commonly in Japan, and it makes good sense.

A wide variety of fish are eaten throughout the world. I will briefly discuss some of the main categories and some specific fish that are common to our Western diets.

Shellfish consist of a variety of small meaty and mineral-rich fish from two families, the mollusks and the crustaceans. The **mollusks** animals that are the sea filterers, or "garbage eaters," as I call them. These include clams, oysters, mussels, and scallops. I usually suggest that people avoid eating much of these foods. Since these shellfish eat by pumping water through their bodies, they can easily concentrate pollutants from the ocean. Whenever there is water contamination, it is specifically suggested that these fish be avoided. They can pick up chemicals, heavy metals such as mercury, and germs from sewage, for example. The mollusks can be delicious and very high in nutrients, but unless they come from waters known to be very clear, they are risky foods to eat and can be toxic.

The **crustaceans** are of less concern. They are not sea filterers and live in deeper and usually cleaner waters than the mollusks. The major crustaceans, or soft-shelled fish, are crabs, lobsters, and shrimp. As mentioned

SEAFOOD SOURCES OF VITAMINS AND MINERALS

- **Vitamin A**—swordfish, whitefish, crab, halibut, salmon
- **B vitamins**—crab, salmon, trout, halibut, mackerel, oysters
- **Vitamin B$_{12}$**—herring, mackerel, salmon, oysters, trout, crab
- **Vitamin E**—herring, mackerel, haddock
- **Calcium**—salmon, sardines, shrimp, oysters, herring
- **Copper**—oysters, lobster, shrimp, crab, trout Iodine—most salt-water fish
- **Iron**—oysters, abalone, carp, perch, salmon, scallops, shrimp, trout
- **Magnesium**—mackerel, oysters, salmon, snails, shrimp, crab—generally low; some in snails and oysters
- **Phosphorus**—cod, trout, halibut, perch, scallops, snapper, salmon
- **Potassium**—cod, trout, halibut, perch, scallops, snapper, salmon
- **Selenium**—lobster, scallops, shrimp, oysters, cod
- **Sodium**—shrimp, lobster, mackerel, herring
- **Zinc**—oysters, lobster, crab, halibut

before, these shellfish had been avoided because they were thought to be too high in cholesterol, but it turns out that what they contain is not all cholesterol but a mixture of lipids. Crustaceans are also fairly low in calories and high in protein and are used commonly, as are most fish, by people who are trying to lose or maintain weight. However, some religions, such as Judaism, forbid the consumption of crustaceans.

The most nutritious fish overall I think are halibut, swordfish, and, probably, tuna, flounder, seabass, and cod from the sea, with some freshwater trout, whitefish, or perch and occasionally salmon or mackerel as the higher-fat, more caloric fish. Most of these fish are very high in protein, variable in fat, and low in carbohydrates. They vary in calories from about 400–800 per pound. The fattier fish, such as salmon, mackerel, eel, herring, and trout, often have twice the calories of the less fatty fish and the shellfish. So even though these are thought to be helpful fats, the calorie count can lead to increased weight.

There is a growing trend of eating raw fish, which is common in the Japanese culture. This is termed "sashimi" or "sushi," fish with white rice, usually eaten with salty (soy sauce) and spicy (horseradish) sauces. This can be a very nutritious and low-calorie meal, but the fish must be fresh and clean, as bacterial and parasitic contamination can lead to sickness in the consumer.

More commonly, baked or broiled fish with seasonings and lemons, often with some oil or butter and garlic or other herbs, is probably the overall best. Steamed or lightly sautéed fish can be very good. Fried fish and especially breaded fried fish should be avoided because of the high content of fat, calories, and salt, none of which are good for us in excess. Besides, the hydrogenated vegetable oils or polyunsaturated oils are difficult for our body to process, and this can lead to other problems.

For weight loss, fish and vegetable meals are ideal, without extra oils, carbohydrates, or breads, of course, and no dessert. Fish with rice or pasta and vegetables, often cooked with the special flavors of garlic or onions, is a good balanced meal. (For weight watching and proper food combining, have just the fish and vegetables.) Shrimp, tuna, or sardines added to a salad with lots of greens and other vegetables is a very wholesome, healthy, and filling meal. I'm hungry; I think I will go make dinner.

○ POULTRY AND EGGS

The raising and selling of poultry and eggs is a huge business worldwide. Some types of bird or fowl are consumed in most countries, chickens being far and away the most common. In the United States alone, more than four billion chickens are consumed each year; that is more than fifty pounds per person. The next most common bird is turkey, which has been associated with holiday celebrations and feasts. Like chicken, it is a fairly low-calorie, high-protein, moderate-fat meat. Ducks and geese are also eaten, but these birds have much more in fat in their skins and tissues (meat) and are therefore much higher in calories. Pheasant and quail are also eaten, and these birds are very high in protein. Yet, all of these birds other than chickens make up only a small percentage of the poultry business.

In general, chicken can be a high-protein (complete protein) food that is fairly low in fat. It contains about 11 percent fat, whereas beef may be more like 30–40 percent; and more of the chicken fat, about two-thirds, is polyunsaturated. Also, most of the fat in chickens is in the skin. Chicken eaten without skin is only about 4–5 percent fat, a better choice for a low-fat diet. These figures pertain to the entire bird, however, the protein and fat ratios vary among the parts. The light meat is lower in fat than the dark by about half. The backs and legs have the highest fat content, followed by the thigh and breast, but the breast also has the most protein. Eating just the meat of the chicken and especially avoiding any fried chicken is a way to reduce the fat and calorie content of this billion-seller bird.

Chickens are also very good in other nutrients, though not as concentrated as the vegetable foods, because most of the chicken is protein and fat and much of the vitamins and minerals are contained in the water and carbohydrate portions of foods. The dark meat

343

of chicken is a little higher in the vitamins and minerals. Overall, chickens have some vitamin A and a bit of the B vitamins, with niacin and pantothenic acid being the best. Some pyridoxine (B_6) and cobalamin (B_{12}) are present as well. There is some potassium, sodium, phosphorus, zinc, and iron. Calcium and magnesium and other trace minerals are fairly low.

In turkey, the light meat is richer in protein than the dark, with about the same amount of fat. As with chicken, about two-thirds of its fat is the unsaturated type, and the vitamin and mineral makeup is similar to that of chicken. Turkeys have a little more zinc, iron, potassium and phosphorus, with less vitamin A and some of the B vitamins. Ducks and geese have over four times the amount of fats and calories as do the leaner turkey and chicken.

There are so many recipes for cooking and eating chickens throughout the world, and even within each country, that we could likely travel our lifetime eating a different one daily. Baking, broiling, roasting, boiling, and frying are some methods of cooking, and each with its special spices or sauces. The Italians like chicken cacciatore, the French are known for coq au vin, and Asians for sautéed chicken and vegetables, and here in fat-fed America, fried chicken is the style. Baked or broiled is probably the best, and without the skin, if we are very fat conscious.

Many chickens are raised for the purpose of producing eggs. Chicken eggs are consumed in tremendous quantities worldwide, and many nutritional authorities suggest that eggs are one the best proteins available. The egg protein, which is about 50 percent of its makeup, contains all the essential amino acids to be readily used by our system. Other proteins are compared to eggs on a bioavailability basis. (See Chapter 3, *Protein.*)

Most of the rest of the egg is fat, about two-thirds of it unsaturated. Eggs also contain a fair amount of cholesterol, which has brought these little chickens to be under great

scrutiny in recent years. Two large eggs contain about 10 grams of fat and more than 500 mg. of cholesterol, which is a little higher than our suggested daily intake of cholesterol. However, recent research shows that the regular use of eggs alone when not associated with a high-fat diet does not raise the serum cholesterol. It is really the total fat eaten in our diet that more influences cholesterol. Thus, occasionally eating some eggs without much fried butter or oils, and especially in place of other fatty foods, such as meats, bacon, or sausage is probably a good choice. If there is a cholesterol problem or cardiovascular disease, however, eggs and all fat-containing foods should be consumed at a minimum.

Eggs are also fairly low in calories, each egg having about 75. Besides the fat and protein, eggs also have some vitamins and minerals. The white of the egg contains about half the protein, no fat, no vitamin A, about 20 percent of the calories, and less of the other nutrients except for sodium and potassium. The yolk is fairly high in vitamin A, has some B vitamins, vitamin D, and vitamin E, all the fat and cholesterol, and most of the calcium, iron, phosphorus, and zinc. Both yolk and white contain some selenium.

Eggs are used in a great variety of ways. They are eaten scrambled, boiled, fried, poached, and over-easy. They are used to make omelettes that can be filled with vegetables, such as onions or mushrooms, cheese, or herbs. Eggs can also be baked in the oven in casseroles or quiches or dropped into soups, such as Chinese "egg drop" soup. Eggs are occasionally eaten raw or blended into high-power drinks. Too many raw eggs should be avoided, as a part of the protein, avidin, can bind biotin, one of the B vitamins, in the intestines and cause a biotin deficiency. Fried eggs are best avoided because of the problem with fried fats.

However, on health and humanity levels, there is some concern over eating chicken and eggs. Mass production and turning the dollar have led to many "inchickene" (like inhumane) factories. Overcrowded housing with the use of antibiotics to prevent infections in those close quarters, lack of exercise, excessive feeding to increase size, and the use of stimulants or hormones such as estrogen (which has since been banned) to increase growth have made the poultry business more like a production line of processed food. We do not really know the long-range effects of eating chickens and eggs produced in this manner. For this and other reasons, I personally have chosen not to eat poultry or the red meats, which have a similar problem, during the last decade, even though I was a chicken-fed child. Anyone interested further in the economic, ecological, and health aspects of the poultry-egg agribusiness can review John Robbin's book, *Diet for a New America*.

One way to reduce the potential dangers of the mass chicken industry is to try to find the more "natural" or "organic" chickens and eggs for consumption. These can often be "free-range" chickens that have more room to roam and are fed nonchemical food with no added stimulants, antibiotics, or hormones. Eating eggs from these chickens or the chickens themselves is probably better for us, especially if we believe that the energy, experience, and consciousness of the food that we eat are passed on to us.

○ RED MEATS

The "red meats" are probably the most controversial of the food categories. It is very clear that an excess of meat in the diet can cause all kinds of problems from the high amounts of fat and sodium, and likely from excess protein as well. The saturated fat concentration is probably the worst aspect of meat. But many doctors and other people believe that they have to eat red meats for a balanced

diet—that without the protein and iron from meat, they will be undernourished. Eating meat does make it a little easier to obtain these nutrients, but the negative aspects of beef and other cultivated red meats, I believe, outweigh the positive, especially when meat is eaten at all regularly. I personally have chosen not to eat red meats, and many more health-oriented people are making that same choice.

Red Meats

Beef	***Pork***
Lamb	

Beef. The cow-steer-cattle family is what most people think when we say "meat." We will call this "beef," and most of our discussion refers to this flesh of the cattle, because that is the commonly consumed meat, though in some cultures lamb or pork is more common. Meat is basically the muscles of these animals. The organs such as the liver and heart are usually referred to by their specific name or as organ meats.

There are many parts of the steer that are commonly eaten. They all provide a high amount of complete protein, as these muscle meats are very close in makeup to human protein. Meats, then, probably supply the best mixture of the amino acids to build human tissues. But the different cuts of meat may vary greatly in their fat content, and this is, again, the greatest concern with meat. If eating meat, it is wise to eat more of the leaner cuts, such as flank or round steak, rump or chuck roasts, lean ground beef or stew meat, veal cutlets, or sirloin steaks, at the higher end. The richer and fattier meats also tend to have the richer flavor, as it is the fats, especially the saturated ones, that tend to add flavor to these foods. T-bone and porterhouse steaks, ribs, rib roast, brisket, pork chops, and ham are higher in fats, about 35–45 percent; this may vary somewhat depending on the grade of meat—choice, prime, or good. The good grades usually contain less fat, which

345

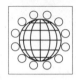

can make them a little less tender. The higher-grade meats are usually fattened on special foods just before they are slaughtered to make them more flavorful and tender, as well as higher priced. The highest-fat meats are the processed ones, such as bacon, lunch meat, canned hams, and salami. These "foods" also usually have very high sodium levels and chemical additives, such as nitrates, which may add further dangers.

Besides the protein, fat, and calories in the meats, there are many other nutrients. The iron content is very good and more usable by our body than iron from any other source. Zinc and selenium are found in some meats. The B vitamins are in fairly good levels, especially hard-to-get vitamin B_{12}. Niacin, folic acid, thiamine, and pantothenic acid are also found in most meats. Vitamin A levels are only moderate though very high in liver. Vitamin E and D are minimal. Potassium and phosphorus are the highest of the other minerals. The low amount of calcium makes the calcium-phosphorus ratio of meats another concern in terms of the health of our bones and kidneys. Sodium is also found in larger amounts than in other foods, but if meat is unsalted, it is not very high.

Beef or calf liver is known to be one of the most concentrated sources of nutrition available. The liver, though, may concentrate chemicals and other pollutants as well, since it handles much of the body's detoxification in humans and animals. Liver is fairly low in fat and high in protein. It is very high in preformed vitamin A—eight ounces of liver have 100,000 IUs, which may cause some side effects, though this is rare with infrequent intake. The vitamin B_{12} level is also the highest of any food. Other B vitamins, such as riboflavin (B_2), niacin (B_3), pyridoxine (B_6), biotin, and folic acid, are also high. Many of the minerals are very good, too, such as iron, zinc, copper, chromium, selenium, potassium, phosphorus, and sodium. Liver is often suggested as a medicinal food for anemia or fatigue because of its high iron and blood-building nutrients.

Other organs, such as tongue, heart, brains, and kidneys, are occasionally consumed by people with a taste for those things. These organs usually have a higher vitamin and mineral content than do the muscles, but they are not nearly as concentrated as liver.

Lamb. Another red meat consumed fairly commonly, especially in the Middle Eastern countries, lamb is similar to beef in its nutrient makeup and high protein content, and is said biblically to be the closest to human flesh. Its fat content is about midway between that of the richer and the leaner cuts of beef.

Pork. Pork comes from pigs and is eaten by many cultures since the first fragrant burnings of pigs caught in the barn fire. Pig muscles—that is, pork—are similar to beef and lamb in their content of protein, fat and other nutrients. However, the cured pork products, such as ham and bacon, have very high sodium levels and contain other additives, making them foods to be avoided. Also, pork may more easily become infected with bacteria and parasites. It should be refrigerated at all times until it is cooked very well before being eaten.

In general, all meats need to be refrigerated and cooked. The high amount of fats can rapidly lead to spoilage at room temperature. Steak tartare (raw), as served in some restaurants, should be very fresh. Uncooked meat should not even sit in the refrigerator for more than two days. It is best frozen until ready for use. The meats can be used in a variety of ways—roasted, baked, fried, broiled, made into stews with vegetables, in soups, and to flavor broth and sauces. There are many kinds of meat dishes, and different cultures use meats differently. In Western countries, large pieces of meat are eaten as the main part of a meal, while in Asian cultures, most meals contain some meat, but in a small portion compared to the vegetables and rice. Meat foods are really not meant to be a staple in the diet.

There are many philosophical and health reasons for not consuming modern meats, at least in large amounts. The main problem is that meat cultivated today is not like the wild animals on which our ancestors lived. First, they used meat for feasts and special occasions, not as a main food. Also, the free-ranging animals such as deer, moose, bison, and cattle had a much lower fat content than present-day animals. They lived naturally only on vegetation and were not force-fed on lots of grains with less activity. These practices have greatly increased the fat content of animals from about 5 percent with only 2–3 percent saturated fats (cattle have slightly more) to the modern-day levels of five or six times that. These extra amounts of fat in cultivated meats may make the difference, especially in a less active culture, between disease and health.

Also, like chicken, cattle nowadays live in close quarters and may be fed more food and more stimulants and antibiotics to prevent infection. Hormones were used commonly for many years, but they are hopefully being reduced due to new laws. And the meat we call veal comes from poor little imprisoned baby cows whose lack of activity keeps their muscles weak, undeveloped, and very tender. They are fed an iron-deficient slosh to keep them anemic, which also makes their muscles (meat) white.

Wild game, such as venison and rabbit, tend to be lower in fats and possibly more healthy to eat because they tend to graze and eat naturally. But then, if we want these we often need, as in olden times, to go out and hunt them.

This is not a serious attempt at building an emotional case against the eating of meat. I am trying to provide a logical understanding of eating in general from a sensible and balanced point of view—and to provide information to help make the right choices.

The medical concerns over beef include increased cholesterol levels, high blood pres-sure, and atherosclerosis. This may lead to coronary artery disease and heart attacks or strokes. Vegetarians usually have much lower levels of cholesterol and triglycerides than meat eaters and also have less atherosclerosis and heart disease. Circulating fats tend to increase arterial plaque formation. Vegetarians also tend to have lower blood pressure. In some epidemiological studies with Seventh-Day Adventists who eat a vegetarian diet, they show a decreased death rate from heart disease and an increased longevity. If they do develop heart disease, it is about ten years later than the average population. Other factors, such as exercise, stress, sugar, and salt in the diet or the eating of more natural foods may also affect these statistics.

Cancer rates are increased with the higher amounts of dietary fats, which many studies relate particularly to colon, rectal, and breast cancer, though the risk of other types of cancer is probably increased as well. The American diet averages over 40 percent fat, much of this the saturated variety. Dietary changes may reduce cancer risks. High-meat diets may also influence kidney disease and osteoporosis, two other very serious diseases of aging.

Overall, the best way to use meat in the diet is to apply the following principles.

1. **Eat meat only in moderation.** This means less meat than the average American now eats. Try more vegetarian dishes.
2. **When eating meats, try the leaner cuts.** For most cuts, trim the excess fat.
3. **Especially avoid all the cured meats,** such as bacon, ham, lunch meat, sausage, and franks, because of their higher fat content, high amounts of sodium, and cancer-causing chemicals such as nitrates. Chemical-free turkey franks and soy franks are now available as substitutes.
4. **When using meats, try them as smaller parts of other dishes,** such as casseroles and big salads, or cooked with vegetables such as onions, garlic, carrots,

or greens. This helps the meat go a long way in both cost and health.

5. **Add more fish to the diet** in place of red-meat dishes. This will help cut cholesterol and fats and protect us from cardiovascular diseases.

6. **Increase intake of some of the anticancer and disease-protecting nutrients,** such as zinc, vitamin E, vitamin C, beta-carotene, and selenium.

7. **Eat more fiber foods,** such as whole grains and vegetables. This also balances our diet and is protective against the degenerating diseases.

8. **Exercise regularly.**

9. **Do not use meat as a dietary staple.** If it is consumed, use it as a special treat or celebration.

10. **It is not necessary to eat meat at all.** Try going without it for a month and see how you feel.

○ SEASONINGS

A great number of seasonings are used in preparing food, to enhance or add flavor and not usually for their nutritional value, since such small amounts are generally eaten. But many of the herbs and spices, ginger, for example, are used for medicinal purposes, such as stimulating the appetite or aiding digestion. These seasonings vary throughout the world, each culture having its favorites and traditions, but the basic flavors—salty, sweet, spicy, sour, and bitter—seem to cover the common uses.

Seasonings

Salt	*Extracts*
Peppers	*Condiments*
Herbs and Spices	*Sweeteners*

Salt. As common table salt or as soy sauce, salt is definitely the most widely used seasoning. In fact, in many cultures, especially the Western ones, salt is much overused and may contribute to such problems as hypertension, fluid retention, electrolyte imbalance, and difficult pregnancies. Most salt is sodium chloride, though potassium chloride is also now common, as are other "salt" substitutes. Salt is mined from the earth or taken from the sea. Soy sauce is made through a fermentation process with soybeans. Salt is commonly used in cooking foods, adding flavor after preparation, or in preserving foods. (For more on salt, see the *Sodium* discussion in Chapter 6, *Minerals.*)

Peppers. Peppers seem to have a marriage to salt in many cultures. Black pepper is most frequently used, especially in our culture, in cooking, fresh ground in salads, or sprinkled with salt on eggs and other dishes. Even though black pepper has some good minerals, such as chromium, zinc, and selenium, it may be a little irritating to the digestive tract in many people. Red pepper or cayenne is a berry that is dried and ground and used on foods for a spicy taste. I feel that cayenne is a much healthier pepper, and it and chili peppers are much better for us to use, even though they are a bit spicier. The red peppers help the digestion, warm the body, and herbally act as a mild diuretic and are thought to cleanse the blood. Cayenne is one of the true natural stimulants and is also high in vitamin C and vitamin A.

Herbs and Spices. These seasonings come mostly from plants—from seeds (mustard, caraway, poppy), leaves (basil, oregano), tree bark (cinnamon), berries (cayenne, black pepper), roots (ginger, licorice), or bulbs (onion, garlic). These and many other herbs are best used fresh, and some of them can be easily grown at home. Their flavors vary widely, and the more aromatic, the less stable they are—that is, the more easily they lose their potency. Most herbal seasonings should be stored in tightly sealed jars or kept in the refrigerator and certainly out of direct sunlight.

Extracts. Flavorings come mostly from foods such as lemons, oranges, almonds, or vanilla beans. These concentrated liquid extracts have little nutritional value and are mostly employed in flavoring baked goods, drinks, or candies. These extracts also should be kept out of direct light in tightly sealed dark glass to prevent spoiling.

Condiments. Typically, in our culture, what is used most often for seasonings are some processed foods that have generally been well accepted as toppings or dressings for many dishes. Besides refined salt, which is used in great excess, and mustard, which is a more natural blend of the oily mustard seed, catsup, and mayonnaise, often called "salad dressing," are very common. Catsup is a tomato-based sauce often made with sweeteners, salt, and additives (though there are now more natural catsups) that goes with the highly eaten hamburger and french fries and, for some people, with eggs and other dishes. Mayonnaise is a gelatinous blend of eggs, vegetable oil, sugar, salt, lemon juice, flavorings, and additives as well. It is high in calories and fats, with some nutritional value. Mayonnaise is commonly used on sandwiches, as the basis of salad dressings and sauces, in salads such as potato salad and cole slaw, and mixed into other dishes for flavoring. Many people overuse this tasty dressing.

Then there are the real salad dressings—the liquid flavoring for salad that is composed of mixes of the vegetable oils, vinegars or lemon, the basic condiments, and/or the various seasonings. The manufactured varieties are usually high in chemical additives, and I recommend either purchasing natural dressings or making them at home fresh.

Sweeteners. Sweeteners are a large category of highly used flavorings for foods. We speak of a "sweet tooth," meaning a craving for sweets, but this is a strange term, since the eating of sugary foods is rather destructive to the tooth enamel because of its support for germ growth. All of these sweeteners other than the current chemical sweets are simple sugars or carbohydrate foods that provide quick energy. They are easily assimilated and converted into blood sugar, which is potential energy for the cells. However, a concern is that these sweeteners overstimulate the hormonal glands, the pancreas and adrenals, and cause problems in blood sugar, energy, and emotions. Most of these sweeteners are low in or devoid of nutrition.

White refined sugar, extracted from the sugar beet or sugarcane, is the prime example and the most used of these destructive sweeteners. Most things are tolerated in sensible quantities but the desire for sweet tastes has generated an excessive use by the food industry and by ourselves. There are literally tablespoonfuls of sugar in a can of soda pop. It is present in most of the aforementioned condiments, in baby foods, and in most pastries, candies, cookies, other baked goods, and syrups and jellies. The excessive use of sugar can deplete certain vitamins and minerals that are needed to metabolize it, and its use has been associated with dental caries, pyorrhea, diabetes, hypoglycemia, obesity, nervous system disorders, and mental illness. Obesity and diabetes are associated further with increases in atherosclerosis, heart disease, nerve disease, and cancer. More information on sugar is in Chapter 2, *Carbohydrates,* and in many other books, particularly *Sugar Blues* by William Dufty (Warner Books, 1976).

Natural fruit sugar, or fructose, can be used in place of sucrose (white sugar), but it still may overstimulate the hormonal system and irritate the teeth. Eating fruit is the best way to obtain this sweet, along with the bulk, fiber, and nutrients that probably even help digest and utilize the sugar as well.

Honey is a common sweetener that is considered by many to be a more healthful energy food. It may contain some B vitamins, vitamins C, D, and E, and traces of minerals. Honey is essentially a flower pollen extract digested and regurgitated by bees (sounds great), but it is clean, actually sterile. Germs do not really grow well in honey. Even this slightly more wholesome sweetener should be used in moderation. Overall, it is best to obtain our sweet flavor from foods. Most fruits, vegetables, and grains are considered sweet foods. This flavor is already overconsumed in our diet, so further sugar is best avoided.

Date sugar, an extract from dates, can be substituted for white sugar in baking or candies. Maple syrup is the partially refined sap of the maple tree. It has a unique flavor and is commonly used to top pancakes and waffles but can also be employed in baking, candies, and so on. The inexpensive, nonpure maple syrup is very high in white sugar water with a little maple flavor and often a few chemicals. It is best avoided.

Chocolate or cocoa by itself is more a bitter than a sweet, but it is often used in candy and as flavoring. Along with the added sweetness, "chocolate" has its own well-loved taste. The cocoa used to make chocolates comes from the cocoa bean, which has some caffeine-like substance, so it is a mild stimulant. Some people are sensitive, even allergic, to chocolate. It is one of the more common food cravings, and chocolate may even have antidepressant properties. Apparently it contains a substance, possibly beta-phenethylamine, a neurotransmitter and mood elevator, that is similar in chemical structure to a hormone secreted by women when sexually aroused.

Carob, another bean, tastes similar to chocolate; it is more naturally sweet and contains some protein, though mainly a carbohydrate food, along with calcium, phosphorus, and some B vitamins. The carob bean is also known as St. John's bread because of its biblical reference as an important food to John the Baptist's survival in the wilderness. Carob is now commonly used to flavor sweets, in baking, and as a drink, mainly as a substitute for chocolate, though some people prefer the carob flavor.

Stevia, or "sweetleaf," is an herb that is a fairly strong natural sweetener. It has no calories and can be used by people with diabetes, or hypoglycemia. This green leaf can be used straight or in cooking.

Artificial sweeteners, or chemical sweets, are not recommended. Cyclamate was popular for a while but has been since taken off the market because of cancer-producing tendencies. Saccharin has been around for a while and is still used, though there are long-range health concerns associated with its use. Aspartame, a new sweetener made from amino acids, aspartic acid and phenylalanine, is probably safer and more nutritious than saccharin, though aspartame is also under scrutiny. (See more about these sweeteners in Chapter 11, *Environmental Aspects of Nutrition*, in Part Two). Ideally, it is best to bring our cultural "sweet tooth" into balance.

○ BEVERAGES

 Beverages are those fluid substances that we drink for the primary reasons of satisfying thirst and maintaining our body's 65 percent water content. There are also further reasons for consuming different liquids, including body detoxification, energy stimulation, relaxation, nourishment, and merriment and celebration.

Favorite Beverages of Various Countries

United States—coffee, beer, sodas, milk, mineral water

Great Britain—tea, beer

China—tea

Japan—tea, wine (sake)

Germany—beer, schnapps

France—wine, coffee, mineral water

Russia—vodka

Italy—wine, coffee, mineral water

Australia—beer, milk

Different people and cultures have their favorite beverages. Many of the substances we drink have the potential for addiction and may produce certain problems when consumed in excess. Alcohol and caffeine, in our culture mainly as coffee, are two commonly abused ones. Milk use can create difficulties for many adults and children because of its calorie and fat levels, lactose intolerance, or allergy. Sugared soda pops, many of them containing caffeine, have become a common addictive problem in our culture, especially in young people.

We all need to consume liquids to maintain life. It is best for as much as possible of our liquid intake to be water and for the other beverages to be used only as special treats. In this way, along with a diet containing our essential nutrients, we will more easily provide our body and cells with what they need rather than make it harder for our digestive and other systems to obtain the replenishment they require.

Beverages

Water	*Teas*
Fruit juices	*Coffee*
Vegetable juices	*Sodas*
Milk	*Alcohol*

Water. Water has been discussed rather thoroughly in the beginning of this book. Ideally, we should consume about six to eight glasses of water daily with average activity and a fairly balanced diet, consuming a fair portion of water-content fruits and vegetables. If we are more active and sweat, or if we consume a higher portion of richer or fattier foods, we usually need more water.

The water that I believe is best for us is not city-processed tap water but well water, spring water, or home-purified water. Any water can be checked for basic minerals, toxic minerals, or chemical contamination. This is suggested when there is any concern about the water that we use for regular consumption.

Solid-carbon-block water filtration, reverse osmosis, and distillation are the predominant water purification processes. Each has its advantages and disadvantages, but all are effective and helpful systems for home water use. (See discussion in Chapter 1, *Water.*)

All living things need water to thrive and survive. Animals, both domestic and wild, the plants of nature, our garden, trees, and the grass on our front lawns—all require water to stay alive and grow. All of the other substances discussed here are basically water with some other nutrients or chemicals added, for which the water is the vehicle that carries them to the appropriate areas of our body.

Fruit Juices. The extracted liquids from fruits are particularly high in fructose, or fruit sugar, so they provide calories and energy. They also contain some vitamins and minerals, most commonly vitamin C and potassium. Other B vitamins, some vitamin A, and other minerals, such as calcium and magnesium, may be found in various fruit juices.

Orange juice and apple juice are the most consumed of the fruit juices. Grape juice, grapefruit juice, and prune juice are also used, most often as breakfast drinks. The nectars of pears, peaches, or apricots may be special treats as well. Some juices are used therapeutically, such as papaya or pineapple for digestion or cranberry juice for soothing urinary tract irritations.

Children may drink a lot of fruit juice, more than adults, who are more given to coffee, tea, or alcoholic beverages, though soda pops have replaced some of the more natural fruit juices in young people as well. Fruit juices are still useful, nourishing, and often a good way to obtain the concentrated juice of several pieces of fruit at one sitting.

Vegetable Juices. These are similar to fruit juices except that they are, of course, the extracted liquids of various vegetables. These are also liquids with concentrated nourishment, even more than the fruit juices. Vitamins A and C may be high, with some B

351

vitamins also. The mineral content is usually fairly rich in potassium, calcium, magnesium, and phosphorus.

Tomato juice is the most commonly consumed vegetable juice, though other juices from carrots, beets, celery, and greens are also used. Fresh vegetable juices are available in health food stores more frequently now. Making vegetable juices at home requires rather complex equipment, though there are some simple, relatively inexpensive juicers to accomplish this.

More and more people are going back to juice fasting or cleansing for brief or extended periods of time as part of their yearly dietary program. Juice or liquid fasting is a traditional part of many cultures, both human and animal, and may be a very beneficial process to clear the body of maladies and revitalize the life force.

Milk. Milk is really more a food than a beverage. Its high fat, protein, calorie, and vitamin and mineral content, in fact, makes it a very nourishing food. And at mealtime, it should be considered a food and not something to be drunk along with meals.

Even though it is such a nourishing food, milk can pose problems. As discussed more thoroughly in *Dairy*, a previous section, milk can provide excessive fat and lead to cardiovascular problems in those who consume it in excess. And many people are allergic to milk or lactose intolerant, not possessing the enzyme lactase to metabolize the milk sugar.

Teas. Teas are classified as the basic commercial tea, or black tea, and the herbal teas. Tea is essentially a drink, usually hot, made from soaking various plants in boiling water. Teas, like coffee, really should be considered more as drugs or medicinals than just as liquid beverages. The commercial teas contain theobromine, a central nervous system stimulant like caffeine, and tannin, or tannic acid, which can be an irritant to the intestinal mucous linings and kidneys. Other than fairly high amounts of fluoride, common tea provides little nutrition. It is used commonly in our culture, the Orient, and the British nations as a social beverage. "Tea time" is an afternoon relaxation period, often concluding in caffeine restimulation.

Herbal teas are better overall than the caffeine-tannic acid teas and are becoming more popular. The berries, barks, flowers, leaves, stems, and roots of all kinds of plants have specific therapeutic actions when consumed in sufficient dosages. The knowledge of these medicinal properties has been passed down through the ages and can be found in a variety of texts. The science of the use of herbs is termed "herbology."

Coffee. Coffee is probably the most commonly used and abused drug (caffeine) in our society—and in many other cultures, for that matter. The caffeine-containing coffee bean is roasted and ground and then "brewed" by passing boiling water through the coffee grounds.

Caffeine has a number of metabolic effects as a central nervous system stimulant. It increases the heart rate, blood pressure, respiration, gastrointestinal activity, stomach acid output, kidney function, and mental activity. Some people use it to relieve fatigue, though many develop a taste and love for the unusual, slightly bitter flavor. Coffee abuse is very common, with regular drinking of it throughout the day, especially in the 9–to–5 work force. This may create cardiac sensitivity, with abnormal heartbeats, anxiety and irritability, stomach and intestinal irritation, insomnia, and withdrawal symptoms such as fatigue or headaches. Coffee can also interfere with the absorption of many vitamins and minerals, such as calcium and iron.

Caffeine addiction can be a problem, though usually not a major one, and withdrawal from coffee may be very difficult. Many coffee substitutes are available, and decaffeinated coffee is used much more commonly by those who like the flavor and social scene of coffee drinking but do not like the caffeine stimulation. There are some concerns over the chemicals used to decaffeinate coffee and about coffee in general. It is wise to reduce and minimize the regular intake of coffee. (See more about coffee in the *Caffeine* program in Part Four.)

Sodas. Sodas are carbonated (with carbon dioxide gas) beverages whose use has increased greatly in the last 25 years. I believe that these "beverages" have a fairly destructive nutritional pattern and are greatly abused. They have no nutritional value, contain high amounts of phosphates, which can influence calcium and bone metabolism, and often contain tremendous amounts of white sugar or chemicals that may rot the teeth—and the body, too, for that matter. The cola drinks often contain high amounts of caffeine as well, which prepare the children who often drink them for later coffee abuse. I have seen people completely addicted to colas, drinking 10–12 bottles or cans a day. These drinks can deplete the body of nutrients as well as overstimulate. Most of the noncola drinks are also high in sugar or chemicals. If these beverages are used regularly or in excess, it is wise to replace them with good, clean water or other more nutritious drinks, and use these "soda pops" only as an occasional treat. Though the huge industry that promotes the use of these drinks and their availability in all stores and restaurants make this more difficult, as with other tantalizing treats of our society, our will power and discipline to avoid or replace these sugars or drugs that can hurt us with more healthful habits or substances is one of our challenges of life.

Alcohol. This is another commonly used and abused "drug," and even more so by our younger population in recent years. Alcoholic beverages come in many varieties, such as beer, wine, and more alcohol-concentrated liquors. These are produced by means of fermentation (usually by yeasts) and/or distilla-tion. They have little nutritive value but a fair amount of calories. The gut or "beer belly" is characteristic of the regular beer drinker who must consume higher amounts of liquid and calories to obtain the drug effect of alcohol.

Alcohol is different from caffeine; it is a central nervous system depressant, or sedative. Even though it seems to "loosen people up," it does so by sedating the usual inhibitory mechanisms. Alcohol slows the brain actions and affects physical coordination and reaction time. It is also irritating to the gastrointestinal tract and liver, which handles the detoxification of this drug. Furthermore, the chemicals used in alcohol beverage production are a big concern. Often grapes and grains are heavily sprayed with pesticides, and sulfites and heavy metals may also be contaminants.

Many people drink too much and too often; some become addicted to alcohol and are then known as "alcoholics." This disease can be devastating to them and their families. Usually, there is an underlying emotional problem (possibly a genetic predisposition as well) or inability to make contact with and express the emotions. Drinking alcohol in excess is greatly influenced by social and peer pressure as well.

In general, alcohol is not something that is particularly beneficial to health. Though some medical articles suggest that moderate alcohol consumption (one or two drinks a day) may be helpful to cardiovascular health, this is most likely through its action as a mild stress reducer. Other forms of stress management, such as exercise and a variety of relaxation techniques, are much better, though they may take more work. Occasional drinking as a social sharing or for celebration may be beneficial in some ways. However, if we are drinking daily or in regular excess, it is wise to reduce or even eliminate this potentially addicting drug. If it is not possible by oneself, it is wise then to seek help. (A complete discussion of alcohol and its problems can be found in Part Four.)

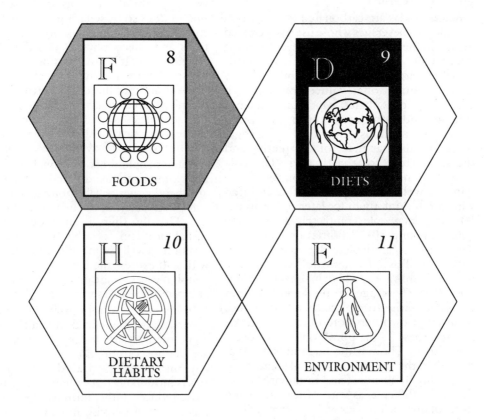

Chapter 9

Diets

Adiet is whatever we eat, and there are literally millions of them. What each one of us eats is our individualized diet. When we say this word "diet," many of us may think of a particular time when we might try to lose or gain weight before going back to what we usually eat. Who we are, how we feel, and how we look in size and shape are the results of what we eat, our eating habits, and all that we do and think. **So, if we wish to change in any way, we probably need to *change our diet*—that is, what and how we eat—rather than *go on a diet*.**

In this chapter, I discuss the variations in diets, their different classifications, such as vegetarian or omnivorous diets, and the common cultural diets throughout the world. I define each one and then discuss its strengths and weaknesses, along with ways to modify it or additional supplements needed to make it healthier. In the next chapter, I review the various eating habits—both health-supporting and not—on our way to the culmination in Part Three, entitled *Building a Healthy Diet*, where we will use much of the information already discussed—that is, all the basics of nutrition.

Diets are influenced by a number of factors. First, the classification of the diet is based on its content. This initially was based on availability of foods indigenous to locale—what could be grown or hunted, gathered or caught. Nowadays, it is even wiser to eat locally and minimize imported foods, which often are heavily treated to protect them from decay and germ and insect infestation, as well as to meet government regulations. However, eating locally obviously has its limitations as our foods are subject to seasonal and climatic influences.

Each culture has its own dietary patterns regarding what is eaten and how it is prepared. These patterns are very strong, as are our tastes and food conditioning. Even stronger are family influences. Thus, both our culture and our environment affect our eating patterns. Specifically, diets and habits seem to run in families, as do many of the problems that cause them. I believe that in many cases, such diseases as hypertension, heart disease, adult diabetes, obesity, and even cancer are related more to familial influences, both psychological and nutritional, than to a genetic predisposition.

Our genetics may also play a factor in our diet. Over generations, our bodies adapt to the foods we eat and our physical well-being is influenced by our ability to digest, assimilate, and utilize any food. Although the human species is adaptable, genetic mutation is a slow process. When we shift cultures or markedly change diets, we may consume foods that our body will react to rather than receive easily. Digestive problems, other sensitivities, and allergies may occur from this. We should pay close attention to how our body handles new foods and new recipes.

Our general eating patterns and habits are greatly influenced by our upbringing. Such preferences as when we eat, whether we snack, or whether we like to eat quietly or very socially may have their origins in childhood. The emotional ties between love and food or between love and cleaning our plate are deep-seated and influence our whole life. Sweets such as ice cream or milk and cookies after dinner or before bed or sweets and treats as rewards may create lifelong problems with our relationship to food. These eating patterns, likes and dislikes, develop early and are very difficult to change. (I will discuss these aspects more in the next chapter, *Dietary Habits*.) Each of our individual constitutions affects how we respond to these influences and how we grow on the diet fed to us. As we age, our individuality usually creates a new diet that fills our own needs; occasionally, though not often, this varies a fair amount from our family's diet.

The increased availability of foods due to the industrialization of our world has influenced dietary changes more than any other factor in the last fifty years. Technology has led to food refinement, increased storage, and flavor control. Salt, sugar, and fried foods have never been so prevalent. Diets have shifted from more natural ones to fast and snack foods. The working class has always looked for ways to save time and effort in food preparation. Even in the last decade or two, we have seen a shift from TV dinners and other frozen foods to the huge "fast-food" restaurant business and microwave meals. The influence of technology on our food chain, though it has helped somewhat in food shelf life, has had a very bad effect overall on general nutrition. The Western or American diet has been the most shaped by these industrial changes, which are spreading rapidly to other nations.

These technological influences have definitely played a major role in the field of nutritional medicine. Our main concern in the past was deficiency disease, caused by not getting enough of certain important nutrients. Though this still occurs in some people, we now have the added concerns about problems that arise from excesses found in the new world diet.

There is no longer any doubt that there is an important relationship between diet and disease. Even the federal government has recently acknowledged this relationship. The U.S. Department of Health and Human Services published in 1988 *The Surgeon*

General's Report on Nutrition and Health. Dr. C. Everett Koop and other contributors discuss the dietary aspects of the most common diseases that plague our society, including high blood pressure, coronary artery disease, cancer, diabetes, obesity, dental diseases, behavior, and many others.

Probably the most significant aspects of diet are the fat and fiber content. Protein sources are a concern, and vitamin and mineral levels are also important. But overall, it is the high amount of fat, specifically saturated fat, that is associated with the major diseases cancer, cardiovascular disease and hypertension and their secondary problems.

Though the high-fat (and high-protein) diet has made Americans and others consuming this diet bigger in stature and weight than most of the more vegetarian cultures, it is not necessarily healthier. Cancer and cardiovascular disease, both nutritionally related, are the two biggest killers of our adult population and the two greatest costs to society, in terms of direct medical costs and lost work. But these diseases can be changed, and they are changing, because more doctors and the public are responding to the suggestions contained in this book and many other good nutrition texts.

There are usually big differences between the diets of rural and urban families. The availability of restaurants, fast-food outlets, and giant supermarkets have become obstacles to good nutrition for many people. Growing our food, either as our means of making a living or in our own gardens, brings us back into contact with the earth and provides us with the freshest, most vital nutrition on the planet. This influence often will affect the rest of our diet for the better. And it has! Words such as _natural_ (as nature provides), _organic_ (chemical free), and _fresh_ (just picked) are becoming more popular again in societies that have moved far from these qualities.

Each of us needs eventually to find our own balance in diet. Through knowledge and experimentation, we can learn what works best for us. Each culture must find this balance as well. Each has its basic natural diet, as well as extremes or abuses that may undermine health. For example, the Oriental diet is high in fiber and complex carbohydrate, with a good balance of fat and protein. But it uses a lot of salted or pickled, preserved, foods which influences the incidence of stomach cancer. Those Western cultures that consume more fat and less fiber have a much higher incidence of colon cancer.

Balancing the diet is what is needed. This often requires developing new tastes. And sometimes it involves taking some supplements to assure that we consume some hard-to-get nutrients or those that may be deficient in our soil or foods, as well as more of those nutrients that help protect us against cancer and atherosclerosis, such as the fish oils and the antioxidant nutrients vitamin C, vitamin E, beta-carotene, zinc, and selenium.

Historically, the evolution of our diet began with the nomadic tribes who moved with the seasons, eating those foods available through hunting and gathering. With more stable village life, we had to learn anew to feed ourselves, to cultivate, to store, and to prepare foods to feed the growing numbers of people. Both farming and hunting were necessary for survival. And these were influenced by the climates and the spirits. Droughts or floods affected feasts or famines and health and disease.

Different areas of the world had different foods available, and this led to the cultural-type diets. Knowledge and recipes to nourish the family were passed from generation to generation. Each generation usually added something new. And the increase in food cultivation and industrialization went hand in hand with the rise in the population and urban living. More food was needed to feed the masses.

Survival was dependent on the food supply. We had to become more adaptable and learn to eat new foods and even change our diet. And we still do and we still can. Adaptability is the key to survival. Even if we have eaten a similar diet for 40 years, we can still change if we feel that shifts may be helpful. Such change is often very important for continued health or to reduce the level or incidence of many diseases. And it is even more important as we age. Changing our diet or lifestyle is not necessarily easy, but it can be done, and it may influence many other aspects of our life for the better.

○ TYPES OF DIETS

Omnivorous

An omnivorous diet is one in which both animal and vegetable foods are eaten. Most people of the world are omnivorous, and this is the type of diet that is the easiest to balance, as there are no limitations. Of course, the knowledge of how much and what specific foods to eat is needed. These types of diets will be discussed more in the sections on the specific cultural diets. In the animal kingdom, though, many species are either vegetarian or carnivorous; some, such as bears and crows, are omnivorous.

Carnivorous

A carnivorous diet is one that contains animal flesh—that is, meat. From a vegetarian viewpoint, anyone who eats meat is a carnivore, but truly most people who eat meat are omnivores. True carnivores who eat only meat are hard to find; in the animal kingdom, they include the wolf and cat families, which naturally subsist on the flesh of other animals. These animals are naturally adapted to hunt and consume flesh. Their speed, power, pointed teeth and sharp claws help them a great deal. They have no molars and cannot really chew; they rip the flesh from their prey and swallow it. And their digestive tracts are specifically designed to process the high-protein, sometimes fatty meals. They only eat vegetables, local greens, when they are sick.

The human, on the other hand, has different characteristics and a longer digestive tract, designed more to process the vegetable foods. We are adaptable and most likely can function as omnivores, though there are varying opinions on this question. One theory suggests that the eating of meat creates the desire and aggressiveness to acquire more, which initially resulted in further hunting. Nowadays, we find members of our culture hunting in the stores and in the streets and sometimes for each other.

Meats are a concentrated food, high in protein, with varying degrees of fat, only certain vitamins and minerals, and almost no fiber. The protein helps in growth and many other functions such as tissue repair, and the iron content is very good. Without the proper balance of fiber, a high meat diet will increase the risk of disease of the colon and other organs. The high-fat types of meat increase the risk of cancer, atherosclerosis, heart disease, and other problems. To balance the meat in our diet, we need supplementary fiber and more of the B vitamins, vitamins C and E, and the many minerals found in the vegetable foods.

Lacto-ovo-vegetarian

This is the most common of the vegetarian diets, one that does not include animal flesh but does use the by-products of the chicken and/or cow—eggs and milk products (vegans, or strict vegetarians, do not eat these foods). Some vegetarians are lacto and not ovo, because of a moral aversion to eating unborn chickens. And some may be sensitive to milk but find eggs okay. However, usually the vegetable foods are the largest part of the diet, which consists mainly of fruits, vegetables, grains, legumes, nuts, and seeds.

Throughout history, most people's diets have been primarily vegetarian, with meats eaten only occasionally. This is still true today throughout much of the world. It is just in the last century that the meat foods have been so heavily consumed in the Westernized cultures, such as North America, Australia, and the European countries. This is due mainly to the commercial herding, slaughtering, and packaging of flesh foods to make them readily available at the corner store.

This book and, of course, I myself lean strongly to a more natural and vegetarian-type diet as one that is more healthful, especially as compared with a typical American diet. The suggestion is not that people become vegetarians, which is a very scary proposition to many (What? Give up my meat?!), but that people become more vegetarian, eating less meat and animal fats. Moving toward meatless meals is a beginning step. A more vegetarian diet clearly reduces our risk of many common chronic diseases, and as long as we consume adequate protein, we are safe from deficiency problems.

The most common reason for not giving up meat, besides people being used to the taste, is the fear of not getting enough protein. I believe the protein concepts perpetrated by American nutritionists to be one of the biggest fallacies about our diet. We do not really need as much protein as we might think, and it is likely that excess protein is a bigger concern than protein deficiency, at least in Westernized cultures. On the other hand, vegetarians need to be aware of obtaining adequate protein, and maintaining efficient digestion and assimilation; I have seen many people with problems in these areas.

A mixed vegetarian diet with or without eggs or dairy products can theoretically supply adequate protein, though it may take more effort than with the omnivorous diet. As long as the diet is not filled with a lot of sugars and other empty calories, the protein content is usually adequate. Protein combination, or complementarity, suggests (this is a theory) that we mix two or more vegetable protein foods at a meal so as to provide sufficient levels of all the essential amino acids. Usually one or two of these amino acids may be low in each food, and mixing them at the same meal will mean that our body has what it needs to make new proteins. However, it is important that the vegetarian eats sufficient calories so that the body does not use the proteins for fuel instead of its many other functions.

FOOD COMPLEMENTARITY

Complete Proteins	Incomplete Proteins
Milk	Grains (low in lysine, isoleucine)
Eggs	Legumes (low in tryptophan, methionine)
Fish	Seeds and Nuts (low in lysine, isoleucine)
Poultry	Vegetables (vary—most low in methionine, isoleucine)
Red Meats	

Food Complements for a Vegetarian Diet

To obtain complete proteins combine:

Grains + Legumes—(main combination)
    e.g., Rice and lentils, wheat and peas, bean burritos.

Seeds or Nuts + Legumes
    e.g., Garbanzo and sesame (hummus), tofu and sesame.

Grains + Milk or Eggs*
    e.g., Quiche, rice and eggs, French toast, lasagna.

Vegetables + Milk or Eggs
    e.g., cream soups; vegetables with eggs or cheese sauce;
    salad with sliced eggs, omelette, eggplant parmesan.

---

*Not if following food combining

Carbohydrates and fats are more readily used for fuel, and it is they, not protein, that actually nourish the active muscles. Protein (amino acids) builds the tissue during growth, though, and this may come from dietary protein of either animal or vegetable origin. Another fallacy in many people's concepts about protein is that animal proteins are needed for strength and endurance, or athletic prowess. Although the percentage of vegetarians in our culture is generally very low compared to omnivores, there have been some outstanding athletes and record setters through the years who were vegetarians.

The human body is really more adapted to eating as vegetarians. Our long and convoluted intestinal tubing is very different from the carnivore's short system, where the meats can move through rapidly before they putrify. Our digestive tracts are more like those of the herbivores, where the length allows increased absorption area to help break down the plant fibers and utilize the nutrients.

The strengths of the lacto-ovo-vegetarian diet are many and the weaknesses few. Both are more pronounced for the strict vegan diet, but here we focus on the lacto-ovo diet, which usually provides sufficient protein, calcium, iron, and vitamin B_{12}, all of which are concerns for any vegetarian. If eggs or milk products are eaten once a day along with other wholesome foods, the diet should be fairly balanced in all respects.

Vegetarians have in general lower blood pressure and weight than their meat-eating companions. Their incidence of hypertension, obesity, high cholesterol, athero-sclerosis, heart disease, osteoporosis, and cancer are all reduced. Studies of the Seventh Day Adventists, a large vegetarian population, shows their incidence of coronary artery disease about half that of the average population. The incidence of coronary artery and heart disease correlates with each country's intake of meat throughout the world.

The high amount of fiber and lower amount of fat in the vegetarian diet are also very helpful in keeping cholesterol down and digestive tract diseases at a minimum. The high amounts of vitamins and minerals present in vegetables, especially, are also an advantage. Many vegetarians find that they have a higher level of energy. I certainly did when I changed to vegetarianism, and this has continued through the years. My diet has been re-created numerous times to suit my lifestyle and the changing seasons. It is still primarily vegetarian, with occasional fresh fish or organic poultry.

Potential problems for vegetarians include a reduced iron and vitamin B_{12} intake and thus a higher incidence of anemia. As stated earlier, this is less a concern for the lacto-ovo-vegetarian than for the strict vegan, but it is still something of which to be aware. Oral iron and vitamin B_{12}, or even B_{12} injections, could be needed to fulfill the body's needs (more likely with poor digestion and low hydrochloric acid output) and maintain the tissue stores of these important nutrients.

There is some concern that infants, growing children, and women who are pregnant or lactating should avoid vegetarianism. This is unfounded, particularly for the lacto-ovo diet. Pure veganism, in these cases, I think, should be avoided. If children can eat a wholesome diet with a good protein balance, they can grow well and be healthy on a lacto-ovo-vegetarian diet, as can pregnant women. Sometimes they may be even healthier, perhaps because vegetarians tend to have better food habits and less abusive tendencies in general than the average population.

Vegan

This is the strict, or pure, form of vegetarianism. No animal products are consumed, only fruits, vegetables, legumes, grains, nuts, and seeds. No eggs, cheese, yogurt, ice cream, butter, or other milk products are eaten.

This diet is not suggested for children unless the parents can painstakingly oversee it and select the right foods. It is difficult with this diet to obtain a balanced intake of all the nutrients that are needed during growth; however, it can be done. This is true also in pregnancy and lactation, where higher intakes of most nutrients are needed. I am not suggesting that this cannot be done; it just is more dangerous in its risk of creating deficiencies and subsequent health problems.

Overall, the vegan is often of a lower than average weight, even underweight for his or her size, and usually has a low cholesterol level. Many of the advantages of the lacto-ovo-vegetarian diet are even truer of the vegan diet. There is a much lower incidence of hypertension, obesity, heart disease, and some cancers, most notably of the colon, breast, uterus, and prostate. The fiber content of the diet is usually very good.

However, the potential nutrient deficiencies are a concern. Vitamin B_{12} is the main one. Iron and calcium may also be low. Protein levels may be all right if the person is very conscious of protein intake and complementing food. Vitamin A may be low unless a high amount of the orange, yellow, and green vegetables is consumed. Vitamin D is often low; some sunshine will help. Zinc may also be low unless seeds and nuts are consumed regularly.

In general, though, I suggest a good supplement program for vegans, including those above-mentioned nutrients. A vitamin B_{12} level and general biochemical profile every few years will help reassure us that the diet is providing adequately for bodily functions. As with any type of diet, if health is faltering or sickness is recurring, an investigation should be made. Overall, though, with the right intention and knowledge, the vegan diet may be a very healthy one.

Macrobiotic

Macrobiotics is a philosophy of life centered around a diet originally brought to this country from Japan by George Osawa. It has been expanded upon and shared with many by teachers and authors Michio and Aveline Kushi, a Japanese couple living in the Boston area, and by the magazine *East West Journal.* Macrobiotic diets, either very strict or more liberal, have been adopted by a great many young people in this country and throughout the world.

A macrobiotic diet consists almost exclusively of cooked foods. Raw foods are felt to be difficult to digest and too cooling for our system. A minimum of fruits is consumed, less than 5 percent of the diet, and most of those should be cooked. Dairy foods and eggs are usually avoided; the only animal products recommended are whitefish such as halibut, trout, and sole, and these are also kept to less than 5 percent of the diet. Thus, it is primarily a vegetarian, almost vegan, diet, but it seems to contain more protein and nutrients than the standard vegetarian cuisine.

The macrobiotic meal includes between 50 and 60 percent whole cereal grains, such as brown rice, whole oats, millet, barley, corn, wheat berries, rye, and buckwheat. Flour products and baked goodies are avoided, and pastas and breads are eaten only occasionally. Vegetables make up about 20–25 percent of the meal; members of the nightshade family, such as potatoes, peppers, tomatoes, and eggplant, as well as avocados, spinach, yams, and sweet potatoes, are all avoided. Beans and sea vegetables (seaweeds) are suggested to complement the meal, making up 5–10 percent of its quantity. The primary beans eaten are azukis, lentils, and garbanzos, along with fermented soybean products such as tofu, tempeh, and miso. Most other beans can be eaten occasionally in this diet. Some seeds, nuts, and vegetable oils may be used. Soups and salads can also be eaten, constituting about 5 percent of the meal. Such other exotic foods as umeboshi plums (and other pickled foods, such as daikon radish and ginger, usually eaten at the end of a meal to aid digestion), tamari soy sauce, sesame salt (gomasio), and bancha twig tea are also included.

Overall, these are very basic and wholesome foods, but the diet is somewhat controversial. On the positive side, this diet is considered to be very balanced. It provides a lot of vitamins and minerals and is very good in complex carbohydrates and fiber. The protein content is usually adequate, and the fat content is low. By balanced, I mean that a majority of the foods are from the center of the food spectrum, such as vegetables and whole grains, with a minimum of foods from the extremes, such as fruits and sugars, which are more cooling, and the meat and dairy foods, more stimulating. Also, herbs and spices, such as garlic, onions, and cayenne are considered too stimulating. From the viewpoint of Eastern philosophy, this diet is felt to be a good balance of yin and yang and to be stabilizing, nourishing, and healing. With the avoidances of chemicals, sugars, refined foods, and high-fat foods, it is a good step, I believe, toward a more balanced and healthful diet for many Americans. With a variety of foods eaten, there is not a great deal of concern over malnutrition, though many practicing macrobiotics appear very trim by American standards.

MACROBIOTIC DIET

Includes	*Avoids*
Cooked whole grains	Meats
Cooked vegetables	Poultry
Legumes	Eggs
Soybean products	Dairy foods
Cooked beans	Sugar
Tofu	Nightshade vegetables
Tempeh	Yams and Sweet Potatoes
Pickled vegetables	Spinach
Sea vegetables	Avocado
Soups	Fruit juices
Bancha twig tea	Baked goods
White fish (< 5 percent)	
Cooked fruit (< 5 percent)	

My first book, *Staying Healthy With the Seasons*, was felt by many to recommend a macrobiotic diet, but it was very liberal macrobiotics at most. Whole grains and vegetables, I feel, are the mainstay of a healthy diet. They provide wholesome fuel without being too rich and clogging for our finely tuned body machine. But I think that fruits, salads, and more raw foods can be tolerated well, especially in warmer climates or in late spring and summer, and these are often richer in many nutrients that might be lost during cooking and other preparations. Also, many of the special foods recommended are not available locally, and this, I think, is a weakness in suggesting that macrobiotic practitioners everywhere eat a similar diet. Furthermore, I am an advocate of juice fasting, a process that macrobiotics does not support; fasting may be an extreme practice, but I feel it is a useful therapeutic tool in many situations.

Another drawback to macrobiotics, especially for Americans, is that it is served with a whole philosophy—near religion, if you will—but at the least a way of life that goes along with the diet. I will not get into a discussion of this philosophy, but for many people it can, as can the often radical change suggested in the diet, become a psychological barrier against acceptance of the dietary principles. With some of its proponents and in much of its literature, there is almost a fanaticism that this system will solve many problems and difficulties in the world. Though much has been written about the theory that a macrobiotic diet can help cure many diseases, including cancer, there is no good evidence for this, only some anecdotal experience. Maybe some further research will provide more useful information, especially in regard to the fatty acid effects on cells. The omnivorous diet generates more arachidonic acid, which cancer cells need to thrive, while a vegetarian and macrobiotic diet reduce production of arachidonic acid, a possible reason for the benefit it may provide.

Overall, I am much more supportive than otherwise of the macrobiotic-type diet. Except for my period as a raw-fooder, my own diet through the years has been closer to a macrobiotic one than to any other type, though I usually eat more raw vegetables and fruits than suggested. I feel that it has a lot to offer, including some sound, wholesome information, that may provide many Westerners with an improved sense of health, peace, and well-being.

Noodletarian

by Bethany ArgIsle

[*Author's note:* Noodletarian is a term coined by Bethany ArgIsle for people who love noodles; i.e., pasta, as a main part of their diets. Her upcoming book, *The Neon Noodle*, will tell much about her noodle concepts and provide many of her favorite noodle recipes, anecdotes, and reviews.]

For me, eating has been an adventure, a joy. In my lifetime, I have investigated many styles of appetite fulfillment, from pablum to school cafeteria food, from steak tartare to caviar, from MacDonald's to Julia Child's—to now, a healthy, natural food, low-fat diet. From eating many meals a day with family and friends to fasting, to starving—it all became a way of life, an adventure.

Recently, however, my busy lifestyle has made it more and more difficult to allow me the time to do the gourmet cooking I once did. For a decade now, I have given up Campbell's Soup, MSG, tap water, and processed sugar in exchange for a raw food diet and even periods of fasting—and this evolved to cooked grains and vegetables and simple eating. I found that this diet left a hole in my soul and I had memories of being a young child and my mother serving me elbow marcaroni with melted butter, salt and pepper and a little sprinkle of parmesan cheese. This lacto-ovo cuisine led me to realize that well-informed, sincere, earnest food combining techniques coupled with soul satisfaction were the keys to my now evolved noodletarian diet.

Hence, I became nicknamed "The Neon Noodle" as I began to share this joyous means of noodle communication with my friends and supporters. My adventures have led me to do two *Neon Noodle* cable TV spots on Dr. Haas' show "To Health," as well as to be a collection center for seemingly unrelated Noodleology Anthology tidbits.

The noodle, through history and myriad cultures has become a universal means of food communication and is included in all types of diets, even wheat-free diets, as there are now many products available for people with an allergy to wheat. Fresh-made noodles are delightful, yet in the cupboard, well-sealed packages seem to have a shelf life which future archaeologists may find themselves researching and cataloging.

There are oat bran noodles, rice sticks, black squid noodles, beet red noodles and my all time favorite, chocolate noodles. There are many, many shapes and textures. Noodles are high performance food and in many cultures are responsible for the very survival of a people. Noodles can be eaten as leftovers, served in the best restaurants, used as a side dish, or endurance meal. In fact, I have never met a person who didn't like noodles in some form.

The elements for Noodletarians are basic. First, the choice is made for the type of noodles. With all I have collected, including packages of pasta made of apples, this in itself can be quite an adventure. Then, good water, a bit of sea salt or a splash of oil in the water to keep the noodles from sticking...the water is boiled (one of the most basic elements of food preparation worldwide since cave dwellers), then the noodles are added, or in some cultures, grain, corn meal or gruel is used.

When the noodles are al dente, the flame is turned off, the noodles are drained and washed when appropriate, and other ingredients can be added for flavour, for perfect food combining and ultimate digestion. If you're organized, it doesn't mess up your kitchen much to make a one-dish meal.

Noodles are around the world—from Soken Ramen in the Bay Area to Fara San Martin in the Italian countryside, noodles seem to be a part of a universal food language. The places where noodles are not plentiful, either fresh or packaged, have revealed another layer of ethnic staples, such as rice for the Chinese, potatoes for the Irish and Europeans, breads for the American Indians, and corn, tortillas, and rice for the Mexicans.

There are many foods I enjoy because of their immediacy and their accessability right out of the package into my mouth, or as we call "instant gratification." Well, noodles are quite the opposite. Unlike chips or sauces, noodles must be boiled. You don't see people sitting around at lunch time eating raw noodles out of the package. However, noodle salads are a booming deli business for nine to fivers.

With the growing craze over physical fitness begun in the 1980s (however, much,

much earlier by Jack LaLanne and Olympians)—noodles became more highlighted in our culture. Why, you ask? Noodles are a top performance fuel.

There are as many methods of eating them as there are shapes and types of noodles—some swear by the fork, others add a spoon, some use a wedge of bread to push with, and others delve deftly with chopsticks.

Noodles seem to be available for all types of budgets and can be eaten at any meal of the day. I have had noodle pancakes.

Noodles are an emotional food with savorability enhanced by many other ingredients. Whoever invented noodles hit upon another food language. Noodles are the glue (the paste, quite literally) that holds the bones of the soul together, while chocolate, another food language component, is the putty (often quite nutty) that seeps into the crack of the heart and seals it.

Whereas lamb, beef, or chicken, or even tofu used to be in the center of my plate, now noodles sit in an ArgIsle Pile in front of me with salad or a vegetable on the side. As history changes, it appears our diets do, too. We have come a long way from food gathering in the forests and fields, to pushing our carts down the aisle—or have we?

"No Noodles, No Wonder" — *Bethany ArgIsle*

Raw Foods

A raw food diet is a very interesting one and potentially very healthy or healing for those who have congestive maladies. It basically consists of uncooked whole foods. Foods are eaten in their uncooked, most potentially nutritious state, with the vital elements of nature still contained in them. The sun's energy, water, and nutrients from the earth invigorate fruits, vegetables, legumes, nuts, and seeds. Sprouted beans and seeds are often a very nutritious component of the diet. Sprouted grains can be made into breads and wafers. Raw (unpasteurized) milk products may be used. Water, fresh juices, and sun teas are the main drinks in this diet. All stimulants, chemicals, and alcoholic beverages are avoided.

Though this diet can be a very healthy and adventurous one, I believe that unless it is very astutely balanced, it is not a good one for very long. It can provide good vitality and nutrient content, however, it is usually low in protein, calcium and iron, all of which could lead to problems in the long run. Also, with no heat added to the foods and an avoidance of the more concentrated and heat-producing foods, the body could become cold. People in warmer climates, those who are overweight, or those with good body heat are more likely to do well on this diet. Many people lose weight on a raw foods diet. Proper chewing and good digestion help with this diet; some people experience more difficulty in their digestive tract than on a more cooked diet.

For one spring and summer, I ate a completely raw food diet—lots of fresh fruit and vegetable juices, blended fruit shakes, sprouts and vegetable salads, nuts and seeds, and a special treat I used to call "nice cream," made solely from frozen fruit, such as bananas or berries, put through a Champion juicer. My neighbor kids used to come running to see me when they heard Dr. Elson was making "nice cream." During that particular dietary experience, I felt great, very light and more open spiritually. I weighed the least I have in my adult life, though I definitely felt less grounded—more spacey—than when on a more cooked diet, and my intestines were very active and somewhat gassy. I guess they had a little less to hold onto and felt a bit insecure.

In lecturing about nutrition and fasting, I have talked to many people who eat a raw food diet, often for a period of from one to three years. They speak very highly of their experiences and especially how healthy and alive they feel. The raw foods diet is really the "living food" diet. It definitely goes against the flow of the Western dietary tradition, but it is something to try for those with an adventurous spirit who want to lighten up and cleanse themselves on deeper levels. Many of the same concerns must be watched for as on the vegan diet.

Natural Hygiene

The "natural hygiene" diet is not a New Age fad, but an ancient system of a raw foods diet supported by cleansing the colon and occasional fasting. This program and philosophy began with the Essenes, an ancient tribe of Jewish scholars. They believed in preparation for the "messiah" via detoxification of their bodies, minds, and spirits through clean living and keeping the body free of waste. This pure diet and evolved lifestyle is written about in the *Essene Gospel of Peace* by Edmond Bordeaux Szekely and in other texts.

The natural hygiene diet was repopularized in the 1930s in Germany, and has had its followers in Europe and America since that time. Aspects of it have been discussed as part of the *Fit for Life* book by Harvey and Marilyn Diamond. I will review more of the Essenes concepts and practices of natural hygiene in the last part of this book in the *Detoxification*, *Fasting*, and *Immortality* programs.

Fruitarian

There are some people who attempt to subsist solely on nature's true gift of nourishment—fruits. However, fruits do not contain all the nutrients that human beings need to live, at least not on a long-term basis. Protein content is very low, and many of the B vitamins, iron, calcium, magnesium, and other minerals are scarce in fruits. They are also deficient in fats, though if the seeds of the fruits are eaten, the essential fatty acids, the only fats that are truly needed, can be obtained.

Overall, a fruitarian diet is a limited one and it is generally considered poor nutrition. It can be invigorating and purifying on a short-term basis, a couple of weeks at the most; staying on such a diet any longer than that could be dangerous.

Fasting

True fasting is consuming only water—and air, of course. This provides a strong inner experience; I believe that it should be done only under certain circumstances and ideally with the guidance and supervision of a physician or experienced nutritionist. However, a surprising number of people have done water fasting successfully for short periods of time on their own. It is undertaken basically as a detoxification-cleansing-purifying process. It is not really a diet, since it provides no nutrients.

Juice fasting is more common, provides more nutrients, and can be undertaken for a much longer period than water fasting, but it is still deficient in total nutrition. Drinking only fruit and vegetable juices can be done for several days, a week or two, or even longer; the longer fasting is done, the more problems (called "cleansing reactions" by those experiencing them) and deficiencies may be experienced. I have known people who have fasted for longer than two months and have personally monitored some patients through thirty-day fasts, most often on the "Master Cleanser," or lemonade, diet. This fast and others, as well as the how-to's of fasting, are discussed in many books on the subject, including my first one, *Staying Healthy With the Seasons*. It will also be discussed in Chapter 18 of this book, entitled *Detoxification and Healing Programs*.

The fasting process is best used as a means of transformation to enhance the potential for change in habits and lifestyle during the reevaluation, detoxification period. Weight is usually lost during the process, though I do not suggest fasting as a weight-loss diet. I do feel that it is one of the best natural therapeutic tools available to the healing arts, given the right situation. Resting from foods and letting the body process what is already stored is the perfect balance to our typical excessive and congesting way of eating. (Body-organ-cell congestion comes from eating more fat and protein foods than we need.) I have called fasting, or the cleansing process, the "missing link in the American diet."

Weight Reduction

Weight-loss diets come and go by the hundreds. Every year at least half a dozen new diets become popular with Americans, who are always looking for the latest, greatest, shortest route to that trim figure. There is usually at least one diet book on the best-seller list, while publishers are always on the lookout for a hot new book that can take a few million dollars out of the American people's wallets.

Thus, there is no one specific type of reducing diet but a whole collection of diets that either reduce calories, restructure eating habits, or add a special food that cuts fat. I will not discuss all of them here; several are described in some of the therapeutic diets in Part Four, and most specifically in the *Weight Loss* program in Chapter 17. Overall, we who are overweight or who easily put on extra pounds need to think of "diet" as our basic wholesome daily food intake, rather than a special project that we struggle through on occasion so we can return to the enjoyable habitual way of eating that creates the body that necessitated the original struggle.

Very simply, for the average overweight person, the best diet to reduce weight is one that provides fewer calories and burns more with exercise: less intake plus more output equals decreased mass, or as one ArgIslizm ends, "sweat equity." Eating small meals and drinking lots of water helps. Avoiding breads, sweets, dairy foods, and excess fats and oils will greatly reduce calories. Low-calorie fruit or vegetable snacks are best. Importantly though, simple meals of lean proteins and lots of vegetables provide a good level of nutrients, enhance digestion and metabolism, and, if not overdone, will cause us to burn more calories and stored fat and thus reduce our weight. Developing good eating habits to change our basic diet is the only way to create the body we want in the long run.

Warrior's

The "warrior's diet" is a term that I have used to describe the way I often eat, especially on the days when I am busy and want to be productive. This diet consists of small meals or snacks eaten every two to three hours throughout the day. These are simple meals and often only simple foods, such as a handful of almonds or sunflower seeds, an apple or two, carrot or celery sticks, crackers with avocado, or a bowl of rice with sprouts or cooked beans. Consuming the contents of one small to medium bowl should generate sufficient fuel to continue energetically along the day's path.

A warrior is always ready for action, with energy available whenever he or she is called. Big meals or lots of different foods can act as a mental and physical sedative, as they cause a lot of our energy and blood to be shunted to to our abdomen (liver, stomach, intestines) to digest and assimilate our food. The warrior eats large meals only in celebration or ritual, or given our modern society, at the end of a workday to relax at home alone or with friends or family. At this time, we can let go more of our physical concerns and tensions, be more aware of inner levels, and digest our meal and the day's experiences.

The warrior's concept is that food is our fuel; we give our body what it needs for continued combustion of energy. When I refer to being a warrior, I am talking about embracing the challenges of life with some feeling or passion. Food nourishment should support this and not devitalize us or generate excess aggressiveness or moodiness. Since I am a strong supporter of peace and positive action, I think of the warrior as one who does battle not with others but rather with life, the main struggle being to conquer our own weaknesses. Illness is, in a sense, succumbing to that battle; from a nutritional standpoint, when we take in too much, we may block the energy that is needed to cope with stress, and then we get stuck in the specifics of the battle, such as conflict with a person or job. Keeping ourselves clear through light and simple eating will allow our full energy to be available to us so that we can be the true "spiritual warriors" or "spiritual athletes" we were intended to be.

Natural Food

The natural or whole foods diet is really the original native or tribal diet intrinsic to all cultures before the industrial age. What was available from nature varied according to the area of the world, but all people cultivated their own food or gathered or captured wild vegetable and animal foods. Whatever the culture—North or South American Indian, Mexican, African, Mediterranean and European, or Asian —the diets consisted of very similar food components. The foods that nature provided were used directly and in a multitude of ways to feed all these people. And nature can still provide all the people of the world with the best possible diet if we use our land harmoniously and productively, as caretakers cultivating respect for Earth's resources.

The whole grain cereals, such as wheat, rice, and corn, have been and still are the predominant foods on Earth. Fruits and nuts can be cultivated and gathered from the trees. Fruits were often a special treat, eaten freshly picked, ripe and juicy. Vegetables could be grown in abundance—the greens, legumes, and root vegetables alike. Most native cultures knew to mix their grains and legumes or seeds together for complete protein nourishment. Most of these cultures, however, were not vegetarian, although their diets consisted largely of vegetable nutrition. Fish was a good source of protein for the tribes who lived near big lakes or streams or by the ocean. The wild birds or animals, when they could be found, provided an important source of food for some people, according to the skills of their hunters. Water or brews from their foods were drunk freely. And there was occasional fasting from foods, either voluntarily or because availability was low. This may have helped keep the people in balance—and most definitely sustained their reverence and appreciation of food.

Nowadays, a "natural food" diet is followed by more and more people. The health food industry has grown greatly, and many stores provide the wholesome or basic foods as nature provides them; if we look, we may find bags, boxes, or bins containing a variety of grains, beans, nuts, seeds, and so on at most markets. Fruits and vegetables are usually widely available, though some natural food stores attempt to find or specialize in "organic" produce, as the natural foods diet is as low as possible in chemical sprays. It also avoids food additives and prefabricated and refined foods with extra sugars, salts, flavorings, and chemicals added to increase shelf life and to appeal to the addicted taste buds of the industrial-age consumer. The natural food diet is rich in natural flavors. Foods are prepared so that the flavor of each food can be tasted, and that usually means with the least amount of tampering. Herbs and spices may be used to enhance flavoring if desired.

I'm particularly enthusiastic about this topic, because these are the dietary principles that I follow and advocate to others—***eating foods as wholesome, as chemical-free, and as much from our local environment as possible***. Foods are obtained for their quality, even though the more wholesome foods may be slightly more expensive. When we prepare our own foods and eat the more vegetarian diet that we all were intended to eat, the average cost is usually less than that of the typical American diet.

If a minimum of animal foods are eaten, we should take special care to get sufficient protein, calcium, iron, zinc, and vitamin B_{12}. A natural food diet can be omnivorous or vegetarian; if properly balanced, it will provide a good level of all the nutrients we need for our body to function optimally.

Paleolithic (Hunter-Gatherer)

This is one of the more fascinating of the diet plans to come forth in recent years. And yet, it is based on some of our most ancient, evolutionary eating patterns—the "caveman" or "caveperson" diet. (This is not to be confused with the dinosaur era, which was some 70 million years ago.) Actually, these peoples belonged to nomadic tribes and mainly used caves for winter shelter.

This hunter-gatherer diet of the Paleolithic humans, our ancestors who inhabited Earth some 40,000 years ago, has been carried on in many tribal cultures. Nowadays, however, it is essentially an extinct species of humankind that continues to hunt wild game and gather their foods such as fruits, vegetables, nuts, and seeds as available on a seasonal basis.

Recent archeological findings suggest that these ancient ancestors of ours were a healthy bunch—tall, strong bones, and body structures like modern-day athletes —they appear to be most similar to ours in regard to stature, and as long as they survived accidents, infections, and childbirth, their longevity was similar to ours, but with much less chronic degenerative disease. Further anthropological studies suggest some of the food and life habits of these early human beings. They had regular vigorous exercise applied to hunting and gathering their food for survival. Flesh foods provided their proteins; seeds and nuts their oils; fruits and berries were available for quick energy; and some starchy vegetable tubers provided more complex carbohydrate fuel.

The theory behind the health benefits of this hunter-gatherer diet, called the "Paleolithic Prescription" in the book of the same name by Dr. S. Boyd Eaton, Dr. Melvin Konner, and Marjorie Shostak, is that our modern diet should be adapted more to that of our ancestors than to the current one commonly consumed. The grains, eggs, and dairy foods, though wholesome in many ways, are the most common allergenic ones, and create both evident and hidden problems in many people. A big reason for much of the chronic disease in our culture involves the large amounts of fats, especially saturated fats, which were nearly nonexistent in ancient times (free-running animals had a much lower fat level, and most of the fats were of the polyunsaturated variety). The high intake of refined foods and grains in general also may be problematic in modern humans. The *Paleolithic Prescription* suggests an avoidance of refined foods and recommends that the main animal foods be closer to the wild game of ancient times. It includes fish and free-range poultry, obviously with low chemical application to the raising, cultivating, and preparation of these foods.

The average tribe's food consisted of about one-third hunted food to two-thirds gathered, so it was a primarily vegetarian diet that varied seasonally and had added high-protein, low-fat meats based on hunting success. The Paleolithic diet was estimated to be roughly 60 percent carbohydrate, 20 percent protein, and 20 percent fats with a calcium intake often over 1000 mg. daily, and that is without milk products. As compared to the modern diet, the hunter-gatherer diet, as outlined in *The Well Adult* by Nancy Samuels and Mike Samuels, M.D., consisted of:

Half the fat	Twice the calcium
Two to three times the protein	One-sixth the salt
Low grain consumption	Two to three times the potassium
No refined sugar	Four times the vitamin C
No refined flour	Twice the fiber
No or low alcohol	Higher B vitamins
No tobacco	Higher minerals

Besides the various wild game available at that time, the majority of the food consumed consisted of the following uncultivated vegetable foods:

fruits	nuts	leaves
berries	seeds	stalks
melons	beans	bulbs
flowers	tubers	fungi
	roots	gums

For most tribes, 10–20 common foods made up the diet staples with possibly up to 50 other foods eaten less frequently. Herbs were also used, more as medicinals, often with different parts of the same plant gathered or used at different times of the year.

Interestingly, the evolution of our current diet began with the Neolithic revolution some 10,000 years ago. In the following 2,000 years, the population became more settled and began to increase rapidly. Organized agriculture began then, along with the increase in whole grain foods, especially wheat. Animals were domesticated and sheep, goats, pigs, and cattle provided various meats and milks that have been used throughout the centuries. Chickens and their eggs were also eaten. These new and richer, fattier foods are thought to be at the source of many of our chronic degenerative diseases. The whole grain foods are also the more common allergenic foods, as are cow's milk and chicken eggs. This suggests that evolutionarywise, many of us have not even yet adapted to these foods genetically. The Industrial Revolution is only 200 years old and added another dimension to our new modern diet—that of refined foods and the use of chemicals in our foods. This is a big problem which we will discuss in greater detail next in the *Industrialized Diet* as well as later in Chapter 11.

In *Paleolithic Prescription*, the authors suggest that "modern disease is a result of a mismatch of our genetic makeup and our lifestyle." Dr. Eaton calls our twentieth century diseases "afflictions of affluence" or "diseases of civilization." These include atherosclerosis, hypertension and heart disease, heart attacks and strokes, adult-onset diabetes and cancer.

Following a hunter-gatherer diet is not an easy task in this day and age. Grains, both whole and refined, and milk products are readily available, and the two very common foods, wheat and cow's milk get into a great variety of foods found in our commercial stores. The wild game and uncultivated vegetable foods are not found in our supermarkets. Meats are domesticated and high in fats and potential chemicals. Most all grains and vegetables are cultivated and sprayed with pesticides and other chemicals. More organic foods and meats with lower concentrations of chemicals are available but these are not always easy to find, and they are still not as clean as foods were in regard to chemicals and heavy metals of the preindustrial cuisine. So, it is a chore to adapt our diet and eat in a way that's close to our Paleolithic, Stone-Age, Cro-Magnon ancestors.

Some suggestions for eating this more natural diet will blend together Paleolithic nutrition with some more modern foods. This will clearly reduce fat intake and reduce the incidences of many of our "diseases of civilization." We should bake, roast, and steam our foods instead of frying or sautéing them. Eating more raw, organic foods is helpful. We need to reduce the fatty meats and all processed meats as well as most of the whole milk products. We can eat a good breakfast of whole grain, fruit and juice, or skim milk. Lunch is a good meal that we prepare and eat at home or carry to work or school. It may include a protein like fish or poultry with vegetables or a sandwich and soup. Dinner is a lighter meal of raw salad and soup. Late eating is minimal and our main beverage is water. Many of these suggestions will be incorporated into my *Ideal Diet* of Part Three.

Exercise is as key an issue for good health as is diet. Our Paleolithic brethren had a good level of physical activity incorporated into their daily lives. If we are tilling, planting, growing, and harvesting our own foods full time, we all experience that similar benefit, especially if we did a little distance running as the ancient hunters did. Construction workers probably have that level of physical labor though they are possibly not as aerobically active and are exposed to more pollution in regard to noise, dust, and chemicals.

Most of us need to develop and maintain a lifelong exercise plan that will blend with our more sedentary work lifestyles. This should include a natural seasonal variance that ideally coincides with the cycles of light and darkness in our area. Our activity should be outdoors and energy expending during the warmer, lighter months; energy-gathering exercise, such as yoga, done indoors is best in the colder, darker times. Our exercise program should provide a balance that leads us to our optimum weight, good strength, and adequate endurance—and should be an integral part of our life—as it was with most of our ancestors.

Industrialized

The industrialized diet is very different from the natural foods and Paleolithic diets. By *industrialized*, I am referring not to the foods eaten by people who work in industry but to the trend of our times toward mass production and factory processing. The industrialized diet contains a large proportion of refined foods. Many of the basic grains and sugar containing plants are stripped of their fiber and nutrients, leaving the concentrated sweet or starch powder that can be used to make or flavor other foods. Refined white flour and white sugar are the two basic components. These "new" foods often have additives and preservatives to allow for packaging, shipping, and "shelf life." They fit in with the mass production ideology and fast-paced lifestyles of not only the American culture but many other technological and urban cultures of the world. Rural peoples still tend to eat more basically and naturally.

An interesting fact is that when the industrial or refined foods diet was introduced to different tribal cultures throughout the world, a general degradation of their health followed, usually within one generation. Tooth decay and diseases such as diabetes, cardiovascular disease, and cancer increased to levels that correlated with those in industrialized societies. One of the people who had observed and described this phenomenon was Dr. Weston Price, a dentist, who studied native cultures eating such diets and compared them to like tribes who were still eating their classical diet. Dr. Price has reported on the descriptions of the tribal people themselves regarding the changes they have experienced, as well as his own observations. This whole story is contained in his book *Nutrition and Physical Degeneration: A Comparison of Primitive Diets and Their Effects* (Price-Pottenger Nutrition Foundation, 1948).

Modern medicine and technology have made some fantastic advances that have affected the lives of almost every being on Earth, but the greatest dilemma now is how to balance these industrial changes with a healthier diet. The refined and fast food diet has been one of the greatest economic supporters of our currently expensive medical system and has made medical doctors one of the richest professions because of all the acute and chronic disease that this technological diet generates. And herein, I believe, lies the dilemma. The Western economic structure is dependent on mass production, corporations, fast food restaurant chains, and refined, packaged foods. The American consumer must consume them in even greater quantities, as more are being produced all the time. It is very possible that if more people cultivate foods and go back (or ahead) to eating more natural, chemical-free foods, it will either bankrupt or totally transform our current big business economy and health care system, instead of so many farms going bankrupt. But there is a lot of resistance and dollars preventing that from happening. Billions are poured into advertising to brainwash people into buying and eating these nonfoods. Also, sweet and salty flavors are addicting, making it harder for the people eating all those premade snack foods to eat more naturally and enjoy it. I do not have the answer to this dilemma (maybe more advertising for apples and sunflower seeds) other than writing this book. Time will tell. Change is usually slow, and adaptability and survival are timeless. It is ultimately an individual choice. As more of us choose to eat more healthfully, more new and natural products will be developed and made available. Good luck to all of us.

○ CULTURAL DIETS

In my recent quest for books that deal with the different types of diets and dietary patterns of the many and varying cultures around the globe, I have found very little contemporary information. I would like to see more research into cultural diets, especially their relationship to diseases within a culture so that we can attain a more global knowledge of diet and health. Here I will share with you my knowledge of these diets and some theories as to their strengths and weaknesses, related deficiency problems, and supportive nutrients that might make them more complete. Obviously I cannot discuss each and every culture around the world; that would require a whole book in itself (which I hope someone will write). But I will dicuss some commonly encountered and intriguing "ethnic" diets. Please realize that my nutritional portrayals will be rather broad and generalized, because even within each country a diet may vary greatly from north to south or from province to province based on the climate, local nationalities living within that region, and available foods. For example, in China, the northern provinces tend toward a diet containing spicier foods, more meat products, and more wheat, than in the southern provinces, where a milder diet is consumed with more rice, greens and other vegetables, special fruits, and generally less meat. Also, within each nation, the diet of poorer people is usually healthier than that of the middle or wealthier classes. Rather than the richer diet of affluence, which may include more meat, dairy foods, coffee, and sugar, the poorer rural populations (the city poor may consume highly refined and malnourished diet) still consume the more traditional and natural foods—local grains, vegetables, and fruits—in a generally healthy balance. This factor is less apparent in the United States where the poor quality and refined foods so readily available in our local stores and supermarkets are accessible to nearly the entire population. Happily though, in most cultures there is an improved nutritional awareness with a return, even in the affluent population, to a more wholesome, balanced, and natural diet. Let us hope that this continues.

WESTERN DIETS

The "Western" diet is that of the Westernized cultures (not the cowboy diet), including many European countries, Canada, Australia, and New Zealand, as well as the United States. Although the diets of these cultures are all similar, I will first take on the current American diet.

Many of the concerns about this North American diet and the problems that arise from its consumption also plague other Westernized countries. Many European populations eat a diet similar to the American one, though shaped around their basic cultural practices; those "down under" in Australia and New Zealand probably consume even more meat and milk products than we do in the United States. Most have a high intake of red meat and fat and a very high sodium intake, as well as regular alcohol use. The meat consumption rates in New Zealand and Australia, the Scandinavian countries, as well as some South American countries, such as Argentina and Venezuela, are among the highest in the world. The incidence of the diseases generated by this food component correlates with its intake. Many Europeans consume less meat and fats but sometimes more sugar, alcohol, and tobacco, which all generate their own diseases.

The Western dietary influence affects many cultures. Technological advances can bring benefits to everyone, but sometimes the time-saving, mass-processing preservation of food is not in the best interest of nutrition. People of all cultures can be influenced by sweeter or saltier foods or new and different foods altogether. We all like change, especially if it appears to be a "step up." But often it isn't (see previous discussion of *Industrialized Diet*). Eating refined flour or sugar products may be all right occasionally, but the natural, wholesome and homemade foods are better. And whether these refined foods are tastier, easier to chew, or a status symbol, when they replace the basic staples of the diet, that is when trouble may begin.

North American

Though the North American diet (South Americans have a very different diet) varies regionally and culturally, I will focus here on the common trends that cross over and influence so much of the population. The Canadian diet, in my understanding, is very similar to that of the United States. Diet-linked diseases that are common in both countries similarly affect immigrants, even though those diseases may be rare in their native lands. This has been demonstrated in studies of the incidence of breast cancer among Japanese women living in the United States, of colon cancer among Asians, and of diabetes.

All the factors that were discussed in the *Industrialized Diet* apply particularly to the American diet, which has been most affected by technology in our food industry. The evolution in the tastes of the average food consumer of today has involved a significant desensitization to the natural flavors in food. The modern consumer is attracted to the rich taste of fatty meats and fried oily foods, salty and sugary snacks, artificial flavorings and additives, and coffee, colas, and other stimulating soda pops. To speak of the refined food diet is actually a contradiction in terms, as this does not represent a "refined" taste at all, but taste buds that need to be knocked with a sledge hammer to wake up. Many nutritionists consider those refined flour products such as breads, pastries, and doughnuts and the refined sugary goodies from cereals to sodas as hardly "foods" at all. It is difficult for people used to these "processed" foods to experience much enjoyment or psychological satisfaction from a simple meal of rice and vegetables, with or without some animal protein. The diet of our culture has become an "anticultural" diet, definitely not one that our ancestors would have approved.

Nutritional Problems associated with the Standard American Diet	**Problems and Diseases** correlated with the Standard American Diet
High calorie	Obesity
Low nutrient	Tooth Decay
Low fiber	Atherosclerosis
High fat	Coronary artery disease
Excess saturated fat	High blood pressure
Excess hydrogenated oils	Heart attacks
High protein	Strokes
Excess salt	Vascular insufficiency
Excess sugar	Diabetes
Excess alcohol	Breast cancer
Excess milk foods	Colon cancer
Excess meats	Prostate cancer
High vitamin D	Other cancers
Excess phosphorus	Arthritis
	Behavior problems / Crime

How processed the diet is varies according to the quantities of fast foods, junk foods, sweets, sodas, and other "dead" foods consumed. Teenagers can be the worst offenders, eating too much of these foods and very little of anything else. Some refined breads and pastas or occasional sodas, sweets, or fatty meats will not hurt most people, but when they become predominant in the diet, it is very poor nutrition. I believe that it is one of the greatest sins of our health care system that doctors so readily accept and support (often simply by not condemning) the industrial-age American diet. Many of the potential problems of our diet, such as the lack of fiber and excessive fat, sugar, and sodium, have been and will be discussed throughout this book. With awareness of and attention to these areas, we can make our diet a healthier one.

There are also some positive aspects of the American diet. There are many wonderful foods available to nourish us. We grow all types of grains, vegetables, legumes, nuts, and fruits and raise cattle and other animals for milk, eggs, and meats. (The main concern with all of these foods is the chemicals used in growing and raising them.) We can certainly choose most of our foods in their more nourishing untreated and unprocessed state. Another positive aspect is the growth patterns that our children develop from eating the typical protein- and calcium-rich diet. Our race is growing bigger and stronger with each generation. The average height of our population continues to rise. The downside of this is that how we learn to eat as young people affects our eating patterns throughout life. As children are usually much more active than adults, obesity and chronic disease result from eating this rich diet, high in protein and fats, throughout life.

With the change in our taste for foods that has occurred over the last ten decades, there has been a decrease in consumption of fresh fruits and vegetables and the complex carbohydrates, with an accompanying decrease in fiber intake, and an increase in consumption of salt, sugars, and fat. This eating pattern, with its overall increase in calories and decrease in nutrition, is associated with many chronic diseases, such as obesity, diabetes, atherosclerosis, cardiac disease, and a variety of cancers, as well as liver disease and nervous system problems from alcohol abuse.

More specifically, each of these potentially negative dietary choices contributes to specific pathogenic processes. First, the standard American diet provides less nutrition per calorie consumed than does our true cultural diet of natural foods. Our body needs a certain amount of nourishment to function. The high amounts of white sugar and refined flour foods in the current American diet provide useless calories with few nutrients. Therefore we require more food on this diet to obtain all our needed nutrients. This is a crucial aspect underlying one of America's biggest problems, obesity. I have already discussed obesity (also see *Weight Loss* program in Chapter 17) and its effect on other diseases, especially cardiovascular disease and many types of cancers.

The decreased consumption of vegetable and complex carbohydrates foods, means a lower intake of vitamins, minerals, and fiber. The lack of fiber has significant adverse effects on digestive function, which may lead to colon diseases such as diverticulitis and cancer. The decrease in nutrient intake resulting from an unbalanced diet with a lot of empty-calorie foods may lead to a wide variety of depletion and deficiency symptoms and diseases. This may occur in the diets of both the poor and the rich of our population.

Higher protein levels, especially from the protein-concentrated meat foods, may contribute to kidney problems, hypertension, and an increased risk for certain cancers, although this has not been well documented. The dairy foods may also cause digestive problems because of many adults' inability to properly utilize them (lactose intolerance), as well as common allergy or hypersensitivity reactions to milk. Another concern is with the chemicals fed to dairy cows that may then end up in our milk. Dairy foods also add more saturated fats to the diet unless only nonfat products are used. The higher calcium content of milk can be helpful, but the extra vitamin D intake can cause problems when combined with even higher phosphorus ingestion from more meats and carbonated beverages. This mixture of nutrients affects bone metabolism and may be a major factor in osteoporosis. Maintaining adequate calcium intake while keeping it in balance with phosphorus is probably important in this regard.

The three aspects of the American diet that have received the most attention in the last decade are salt, red meats, and fats. Salt restriction is often suggested for people only after they have high blood pressure, but there should be attention to avoiding high-salt foods and reducing total sodium intake (and raising potassium intake) before this problem arises. Salt contributes not only to high blood pressure but also to kidney disease and to heart disease as well. Salt is contained in so many foods, often hidden, that we may need to read labels and avoid certain restaurant foods to really reduce our intake of sodium.

Eating red meat, the cooked muscles (and organs) of dead cattle, sheep, or pigs, is both a nutritional and a philosophical issue. Nutritionally, these meats, especially the domesticated, overfed animals, contain a high amount of fat, and regular consumption of meats may add to an already fatty diet. Meats are also high in protein, phosphorus, and usually sodium, and are low in fiber, all of which may contribute to other difficulties. Meats, of course, do provide nourishment; we just need to moderate their intake.

The idea of an association between meat eating and war is an interesting one. Throughout history, meat eating has been correlated with hunting, fighting, conquering, and a desire for power. Eating meats seems to stimulate aggressiveness, hostility, and competitive feelings. Now that most people do not hunt for food, meat consumption may stimulate these same feelings of aggressiveness, which we now take to the streets, to our jobs, or home to our families. In contrast, the vegetarian diet has always been associated with peace and nonresistance and a general respect for life, as manifested in a spiritual sense of our connection to all living beings. This is seen in the peoples of India and exemplified by the life of Mahatma Gandhi. While many people are reducing their meat consumption for health reasons, this may have the fortunate secondary effect of improving the relationships between people and among nations, increasing the chances for peace.

Meats, as I said, also contribute to our total fat intake, as do milk products. Vegetable oils, of course, are all fat, but of greater concern are the hydrogenated fats, which may contribute more specifically to disease. The use of these fats as magarines, in cooked or fried foods, and in baked goods has greatly increased; the trend should be in the other direction. Fats in the diet contribute specifically to increased cholesterol levels, atherosclerosis, cardiovascular disease, and many types of cancer, particularly cancer of the breast, colon, prostate, and uterus. Atherosclerosis, or clogging of the arteries with fatty plaque, is the basic process that contributes to all kinds of cardiovascular diseases. Reducing total fat intake is probably the most important step to creating a healthier diet.

Overall, we need to ask how can we make the American diet better so that it will nourish a healthy and long-lived race of people? What can we do with this diet based on quick eating, fast preparation, microwave meals, stop-and-go diets; the diet we can fit between two pieces of white bread; the diet we can eat with one hand while driving our car or working at our desk; this processed, refined, junk food, high-sodium, high-fat diet; this diet that generates death more than life? Generally, we need to reevolve back to the basics, back to nature, back to the garden.

SUGGESTIONS FOR MAKING THE
AMERICAN DIET HEALTHIER

1. Consume less fat via

2. Consuming less red meat, lunch meat, bacon, ham, and so on and

3. Consuming less milk and milk products.

4. Consume less fried foods and

5. Less hydrogenated oils.

6. Eat less refined flour products,

7. Less white sugar and simple sugars, and

8. Less salt and salty foods, such as crackers, pretzels, chips, and pickled foods.

9. Consume fewer calories.

10. Consume less coffee and alcohol.

11. Smoke less or not at all.

12. Eat more fresh fruit and

13. Fresh vegetables.

14. Eat more whole grain cereals, such as rice, whole wheat, oats, and so on.

15. Eat more fiber foods—the fruits, vegetables, and grains.

16. Eat more fresh fish and poultry to replace red meats and

17. More vegetable protein, such as nuts, seeds, and beans and the sprouts of these foods to replace animal proteins.

18. Drink more filtered or spring water.

19. Drink more fruit and vegetable juices and herbal teas to replace coffee, black teas, soda pops, and other stimulating beverages.

20. Get more regular, preferably daily exercise with some aerobics—that is, more vigorous exercise. In other words, let's get in physical shape.

21. Take better care of our air.

22. Keep our waters free of pollution.

Getting back to the basics means learning to take the time again to shop for, prepare, and sit down to eat wholesome, nourishing meals—to generally be more conscious and conscientious with our diet. This is a tough request for a very busy population always trying to catch up with their bills and credit cards. Believe me, it is worth the price, because we will feel better longer and be more productive.

New Healthy American

The new healthy American diet is basically what I am clarifying in this book. It is what many of us have turned to as we realize the consequences of this refined, processed, and chemicalized American diet. The new "health food" industry and health or natural food stores are providing us with the ingredients needed to create our new diet. Hopefully our own garden will also help. More supermarkets and chain stores are supplying many of the new, more natural, less processed "health foods." Furthermore, the use of chemical farming (see Chapter 11) brings the term "organic," grown without chemicals, to national attention. Even animals are considered "chemical" when they are factory farmed, treated with antibiotics or hormones, and fed chemically-treated foods, or "natural" when they are fed well without chemicals and drugs and given space to live.

This "new American diet" is thus more natural and really a traditional diet, but with the advantage of industrialization where we have many well-made and tasty packaged foods. However, the basis of our new diet is a return to whole, unprocessed foods—fruits, vegetables, nuts, seeds, legumes, and whole grains. With this diet, there is an avoidance of refined flour products, refined sugar, red meats, lunch meats and sausages, high fat and high salt foods, and the regular use of dairy products and alcohol. More and more people are turning to a vegan or lacto-ovo-vegetarian diet, or to one that I have followed for a few years, the "pesca-vegan" diet, which is fish added to the vegan diet. In this diet, milk and egg products are avoided as are poultry and meats. All the foods eaten are high in nutrients, and fish protein (and oils) is chosen over milk and eggs, which, in many people, are not handled as well.

My personal diet has shifted over the last two decades from standard American to this new American diet. It recently has ranged from strict vegetarianism to pesca-veganism, even with occasional organic or free-range poultry, mostly at holidays. Because my weight rises so easily when I eat with my usual love for foods, I focus my diet on vegetables and add other foods as needed—seeds and nuts, legumes or fish when I feel I need more protein and fuel, or fruits and juices (even to fasting) when I feel I need to lighten up and clean out.

As an example, over the winter of 1989, I was working hard, exercising less, more stressed, and consuming more foods, especially grains, which put weight on me. I organized a ten-day fast for myself and patients in my office, which we began in early spring. It felt so good, so right for me that I continued for 16 days; I felt great, light, and productive with lots of energy on my lemonade diet, the "Master Cleanser" (see my first book, *Staying Healthy With the Seasons*). Though cleansing like this is not for everyone, it certainly works for me. (For more specifics, see the *Detoxification* programs and *Fasting* in Part Four.) Now my diet is moving slowly back into a strict vegan diet for the spring and summer and I will maintain a high-alkaline diet, consisting of green salads, fruits, sprouts, millet, soybean products, and some soaked nuts and seeds. Meals are protein/vegetable or starch/vegetable, described in the *Ideal Diet* of Part Three, and this spring will include a lot of green salads. I will avoid all animal products, refined foods, and wheat and other gluten grains (oats, barley and rye) as well as minimize rice and corn, which I so love. This will clearly be more strict than I have been in years, but my body and energy is already knowing the benefits, and I look forward to the final production and publishing of this monumental undertaking you now hold in your hands.

Australian/New Zealand

As well as a great deal of meat, the people of the down under countries eat large amounts of milk, cheese, and other dairy products. These two food categories mean a diet high in saturated fat and protein, which contribute to high blood fats and the higher incidence of atherosclerosis, high blood pressure, heart disease, and cancer. Skin cancer is very prevalent in the hotter, northern climates of Australia. The high beer consumption may undermine the liver and general health of the inhabitant. Luckily, vegetables are grown by many of people and eaten in good quantities along with the other, richer foods.

British Isles

The diet in Great Britain is notorious in Europe as one of the worst. The diets of surrounding Scotland and Ireland, which make up the British Isles, are very similar. Overall, there is a high amount of industrialized, processed foods consumed in England along with their classic meat-and-potatoes diet. And some claim that, unlike many cultures, the poorer people often have the worst diet with a lot of refined and fried foods.

In general, this northern, cold climate island does not have much agriculture, and therefore does not provide many fresh foods most of the year. Most of their fresh fruits, vegetables, grains and nuts must be imported, and this is usually expensive and seasonal. It is known to be very difficult to find fresh fruits and vegetables in Great Britain; a raw green salad is a rare treat. Often, visitors from Europe will carry fresh food with them. With this situation, the British have a low intake of high-nutrient, whole foods that are so important to health.

In the British Isles, the consumption of red meat is high, with pork and mutton eaten as much as beef. Raising sheep for food is very common in the countryside. Fish is readily available for those that live near the sea, but most often it is eaten fried, with fried potatoes, a meal called fish and chips. Butter is the main cooking fat, and milk, cheese, and butter are also regularly consumed. All of these animal foods provide a high-fat diet, and since this is generally not an exercise-oriented culture, but does have a lot of smokers, cardiovascular diseases are a prevalent process of aging. With its industry-oriented culture, chemical carcinogenesis is another big concern in Great Britain.

Other aspects of the diet include refined flour products, with a lot of bread, pies, cakes, and pudding. Whole grain products are low in consumption, save a bit o' porridge for some in the morning. Sugar is eaten regularly in desserts, along with sugar in tea. The British drink a lot of black tea, with its caffeinelike agents and tannic acid, contributing to teeth stains and stomach ulcers. Also, beer and ales are drunk throughout the British Isles, with many local brews.

Overall, the British are waiting for their health and nutrition wave. It would be wise for them, as for all of us, to reduce their intake of animal foods, refined flour and sugar products, alcohol, and nicotine. Obtaining more fresh foods via agriculture and importation, and storage for the colder, wetter months would also help. Dehydrating vegetables and making sprouts are a couple of ways to obtain these important foods, and eating more whole grains and the products made from them will improve this diet as well.

Western and Eastern European

The Germanic diet (Austria, Germany [until recently, West Germany], Switzerland) is a little spicier and even sweeter than the British diet, with more breads, cakes and other sweets, potatoes, and meats (beef, venison, and pork), and especially the sausage-type meats. Each region of West Germany has its own type of sausage. Butter and lard are used as the main cooking fats. Baked goods are a staple of the German diet. In Switzerland, chocolate and cheese are very popular. Austria is known for its sweets and cakes. Hot chocolate and pastries are a favorite late afternoon tradition, followed by a light dinner. Fermented foods, such as sauerkraut and sour cream, may help the intestinal tract handle this higher-fat, low-fiber diet. Fresh fruits are less available, and the colder-climate vegetables, such as cabbage, cauliflower, and potatoes, are used more than others. Beer consumption is very high, leading to more weight problems than in many other cultures.

The Eastern European countries (Hungary, Poland, Czechoslovakia, and former East Germany) are basically poor and consume a less industrial diet with less sugar and fewer desserts. They still use more natural food preparation and preservation, such as pickling foods for the colder winters. Western Europeans ate this healthier, more natural diet before industrialization. The people of Hungary and Poland consume more rye bread, cabbage, potatoes and other root vegetables, buckwheat, paprika, onions, peppers, pork, pickled fish, and cottage cheese. Food is expensive and not always readily available. More fresh vegetables, fruits, and whole grains could be added, but overall, this is a poorer, yet healthier diet than many of the more Westernized nations.

Balkan

The diet of the Balkan countries (Romania, Bulgaria, and Yugoslavia) is similar to that of their neighbor, Hungary, and other Eastern European countries. Thanks to a warmer, more agriculturally favorable climate, there are more fresh foods available. Fish is plentiful from the surrounding seas and meats are grilled or roasted, even on open fires. Fewer sauces and fermented foods are used than in other Eastern European countries.

Russian

The Russian diet is usually higher in complex carbohydrates and lower in protein, especially animal protein, than most other European diets—and the Russian people have better longevity than most other cultures. There are more centenarians there than anywhere in the world.

The Russian diet includes dark bread, buckwheat (kasha), wheat, goat's milk and yogurt, potatoes, other root vegetables, cabbage, beet borscht, and some meats. The grain and vegetable basis of the diet, with less consumption of refined flours and sugars, makes it one of the healthier diets in Europe. Concerns may include the high consumption of vodka and the animal fats used for cooking. Also, because there is less variety of available foods, vitamin and mineral deficiencies may pose a problem.

Scandinavian

The Nordic diet of Sweden, Norway, and Finland has many healthy aspects for such a low agricultural area, and certainly produces people of strong constitution; however, there are several types of food that are overconsumed, thus increasing the potential for and incidence of a number of chronic degenerative diseases. Because of the cold climate, a higher fat diet is the common faire and is probably handled better than in most other areas of the world. This would be more actualized if they ate less animal foods and more cold water fish (freshly cooked) from the surrounding seas. Cod and herring are very popular, but these are often pickled or smoked. Fish is widely consumed, but other meats and milk products are as well. Finland's high animal food consumption gives it the distinction of having the highest average blood cholesterol level of any place on Earth. The high-salt Scandanavian diet also increases incidence of hypertension and other cardiovascular problems. Alcohol use, particularly beer and schnapps consumption, adds another health concern; black teas are also very popular.

Some wholesome traits of the Scandinavian diet include the regular use of rye as crackers and whole grain breads, which add fiber and important nutrients. Sweets are not common and pastries tend to be light. Fresh fruits and vegetables are available during the three to four warmer months of the year. Nordic peoples would be wise to dry and store more wholesome fruits, vegetables, nuts, seeds, and legumes, to use through their long winters. Sprouted foods are ideal for cold climates or areas of low agriculture. Scandinavians would benefit by foregoing their "smorgasbord" style of eating (with too many choices and poor food combining), in favor of simpler meals.

MEDITERRANEAN DIETS

This area includes a cross section of Greece, Spain, Portugal, Italy, and Southern France. Morocco offers a mix of Mediterranean and mid-Eastern cuisine. The Mediterranean diet is similar to the nearby Turkish and Middle Eastern diets, with wheat, rice, lamb (and goat), cheeses, yogurt, olives, and olive oil as major components. Due to the lower animal (saturated) fat intake and more olive oil used as the main cooking fat, the risk of cardiovascular disease is relatively low in these countries. Fresh fruits and vegetables are more plentiful in these warm coastal areas than anywhere else in Europe. Daily shopping in outdoor markets is a Mediterranean tradition. Fish and seafood, tomatoes, peppers, citrus fruits, nuts, and fresh and dried herbs give this diet great variety. Wine and coffee (espresso) are in high consumption. Fruits such as apples, pears, cherries, and apricots may be eaten fresh or cooked. Negative aspects of the Mediterranean diets include excessive use of coffee, cigarettes, and sweets.

Italian

The Italian diet contains more breads, pastas, and cheeses than that of other European countries. Italians drink more wine than beer. In many regions of this coastal country, they produce local wines, cheeses, and prosciutto (cured ham). In general though, dairy product consumption is low, primarily as cheeses such as mozarella and Parmesan. Spaghetti is classically Italian, as is a thin-crusted pizza (nothing like heavy American pizza). Meats, such as prosciutto, veal, chicken, and the fatty processed spicy meats, such as salami and pepperoni, are popular. Vegetables are usually well consumed, especially tomatoes, as are fresh herbs such as basil, oregano, thyme, and marjoram. Minestrone is the common soup. Olive oil is used regularly as the main cooking fat and on salads and other foods; even though it is better than other fats, it is high in calories when used in quantity. Other foods prominent in the Italian diet include garlic, hot peppers, wild local greens, white breads and breadsticks, and fresh figs and melons in the summer.

A typical Italian meal is served in several courses, as is true in much of Europe. Breakfast is light if at all, consisting of coffee, juice, and croissants. Lunch is the main meal, with most businesses closed between one and four p.m. The first course is pasta, followed by meat or fish with vegetables and a green salad. Dessert is often fruit, followed by an espresso, which has a stronger taste but less caffeine than a typical American cup of coffee. After a rest, people go back to work. Dinner is generally light or just a social time, with some soup, bread, and wine. Luckily, the portions in Italian meals are modest; thus, there is less overeating than is typically stereotyped in the Italian-Americans.

Some concerns of the Italian diet include recent increases in refined and processed foods. As elsewhere in Europe, the heavy consumption of alcoholic beverages, cigarettes, caffeine, and sweets may lead to health problems.

French

In this large European country (as is true in many larger countries), the diet may vary widely from north to south with climate, cultural differences, and available foods. The mid-Europe northern area consumes more meat and a generally heavier diet, while the southern, Mediterranean regions eat more fish, local vegetables, and a lighter diet overall. In most countries of the world, especially the European ones, the native, rural, or peasant-type diet contains a higher amount of natural foods than the urban diet. For example, a typical meal served in American "French" restaurants is rich in creamy sauces, gravies, pastries, sweets, fats, cheeses, bread, pates, and, of course, wine. This type of food is also consumed by the wealthier classes and in the fancier restaurants in France.

In general, the French are very involved with food, and often consume multiple course meals as is true in much of Europe. There are local street markets that provide fresh seasonal foods and their special cheeses and sausages. The French tend to shop often, preparing their meals to suit the locally available foods. The more rural or peasant diet in France consists of potatoes, some meats and "charcuterie" (sausages and cold cuts), poultry, breads and cheeses, and vegetables. Meals often include a small green salad, and finish with cheese as "dessert." Breads, croissants, and pastries, are often consumed daily. Wine and very strong coffee are the national beverages. Overall, the French diet is richer and higher in fats and refined flours than many other European countries.

Spanish

The Spanish diet is similar to the Italian, at least along the coastal regions. Having more inland terrain, Spain's beef production and consumption is higher than in other Mediterranean countries. The Spanish enjoy a wide variety of foods, including fish and meats, olive oil, tomatoes, greens, wine, white breads, figs, and citrus and other fruits. Paella is a common dish that combines rice and seasonings, especially saffron, with seafood and shellfish, chicken, or sausage. Wine is consumed regularly with meals. Problems with refined foods and animal fats are beginning to appear in Spain. Coffee consumption and cigarette smoking are also high.

The Portuguese consume a similar diet to the Spaniards, yet, being a poorer nation, the people tend to eat simpler, more natural meals of locally available foods. Wine is also consumed regularly.

Greek

This southern, coastal mecca provides a relatively simple diet, mostly cultivated from its own land. Goats and sheep are raised for milk and meats. Goat milk cheeses, such as feta, and yogurt are eaten regularly, as is lamb meat. Fish is very popular. Moussaka is a popular local dish—a layered, baked "casserole" with lamb, eggplant, feta, tomatoes, and onions. "Greek" salads are eaten almost daily, made of tomatoes, black olives, red onions, cucumber, feta cheese, and dressed with olive oil and herbs. A yogurt and cucumber appetizer dip for pita bread is also common. Greece is less industrially developed than the other Mediterranean countries and thus, has probably one of the healthier diets in Europe.

ASIAN DIETS

In most Asian countries people are poor and must cultivate their own food and, thus, their diet from the land around them; and these hard-working peoples do a very good job of it. These cultures are basically non-carnivorous, though not strictly vegetarian either. However, their diets are vegetarian based, focusing on grains and fresh vegetables, usually with some meat, poultry, or fish cooked into one of the dishes. Eggs and milk products, mainly as yogurt, are occasionally consumed by adults.

Due to this generally healthy—more natural, local, and seasonal—diet, there is a reduced incidence of many of the chronic degenerative diseases that are nutritionally related. Thus, the elderly population is healthier and more active in these cultures, and is less plagued by atheroscleroses, high blood pressure, heart disease and their consequences, such as heart attacks and strokes. However, with the increasing use of refined sugar products, especially in China and Japan, combined with other factors, possibly even food and environmental chemicals, adult diabetes and cancer are on the rise.

With the following examples from China, Japan, and India, please realize that as times change and there is more industrialization and "Americanization" of these countries, the general diet, nutritional adequacy, and basic health and longevity of their populations will be affected.

Chinese

When we consider that China contains more than one billion people, about a quarter of the Earth's population, what the Chinese people eat is the major diet of the world. That diet is primarily vegetarian, with usually only small amounts of animal foods consumed.

When I visited China in late 1984, I was most impressed with the agriculture—the incredible use of the land and the masses of people working it. Crops were planted in huge fields, on hillsides, along riverbanks, around houses, literally everywhere. It is a very green and fruitful country. Rice is the main crop, although more wheat is used in the north. The northerners also eat more meat and spicier foods, to keep them in balance with the colder climate, though people throughout China make spicy dishes using tiny, hot red peppers; and chili oil, vinegar, and soy sauce are on most tables.

The basic Chinese diet is fairly consistent, containing polished white rice, cooked vegetables, mushrooms, tofu, and small amounts of meat, pork, or fish, with occasional poultry and eggs (a luxury). Large amounts of meat are rarely consumed at one meal. Fruits are eaten as they are available. Soybeans are used in a variety of ways—as tofu (soybean curd) or as soy sauce, a favorite flavoring. Milk products are consumed infrequently, mostly as yogurt, which spoils less easily. Pickled, smoked, and salted foods, usually fish or meats, are also common to the culture. There is some concern that these pickled and smoked foods may irritate the gastrointestinal mucosa and, when consumed excessively, may increase the risk of stomach cancer.

This diet is lower overall in fat and higher in magnesium than the Western diet, which helps to reduce the risk and incidence of cardiovascular disease. With the high fiber and complex carbohydrate, moderate protein, and low fat levels, there is very little obesity and less degenerative disease in general. These people are very hard working, especially on the land, and being outdoors cultivating food also contributes to good health. The elderly poplulation seem healthier and more capable because, I believe, they have eaten well and been more connected to the earth. They are usually more involved in family care than in Westernized countries, which gives them a sense of purpose and a positive self-image.

Rice is the staple of the diet. In Chinese, the word for rice, *fan* (pronounced "fahn"), means "food." White, polished rice does lose some of its nutrients, but in China, it represents status and success. It is considered a little easier to digest and utilize in the body. Peasants still consume a less refined rice with more nutrition.

Most Chinese live in rural areas and work the land. In the larger cities, where people have access to refined foods such as sugars and flour products, sugar abuse and poor nutrition from consumption of candy, sodas, and other junk foods are causing concern. But the basic diet is a fairly sound and healthy one, the product of a culture thousands of years old.

Japanese

The Japanese diet is similar to the Chinese, with the basic rice, cooked vegetables, pickled vegetables and meats, and a modest amount of animal products. Since Japan is actually a group of islands, seafood is consumed in much higher quantities than in other Asian countries. Raw fish, or *sashimi*, is characteristic of the Japanese cuisine. Tofu, a soybean curd, and other beans such as aduki are also used. *Miso*, a fermented soybean paste, is a common salty soup base. Milk products are eaten minimally, and fruits are consumed as available. Raw, fresh vegetables are consumed rarely, as is true throughout the Asian countries. Most everything is cooked (or pickled or smoked), except for raw fish. This practice may have evolved because of concern over spoilage and contamination. Japan is more westernized than other Asian countries, so concerns over an industrialized diet are present there as well. Also, the higher use of condiments, pickled, and fermented foods may offer some concerns in terms of health.

East Indian

The Indian diet is similar to the other Asian diets with its basic cooked rice and vegetables. However, in India, the major legume is lentils, rather than the soybean. *Dahl* is the main East Indian lentil dish. Wheat is used to make various flat and pocket breads. Curry flavoring, a hot mixed spice, is used throughout India, and fermented milk products, mainly yogurt, are also consumed regularly, often to cool down the spicy foods. Lahsi is a yogurt drink taken with meals. A more common beverage is chai, a black tea served hot or cold with added milk and sugar. White sugar is used all too commonly in India. A fair amount of fried dishes are popular. Due to heat, hygiene, and concern over food poisoning, few raw foods other than peeled fruits are eaten; most are cooked. The main cooking fat is *ghee*, a clarified butter. Coconut oil and coconut meat are also used in cooking in some East Indian recipes.

The cow is considered the sacred animal of India, and vegetarianism is much more common there than anywhere else in the world. However, the Hindu people tend to maintain their lactase enzyme function and thus can handle eating cow's milk products, such as milk, yogurt and paneer, a fermented cheesecake curd made from milk. The main concern in this populated country is basic shortages of food and subsequent malnourishment.

Thai

Thai cuisine is becoming increasingly popular in the United States. This diet is very close to that of Southern China, which Thailand borders. This food can range from mild to very spicy, and the Thai people are quite artful in their use of special spices and flavors. Meals consist of white rice and mixed vegetables, along with tofu or an animal protein such as fish, chicken, pork, or beef. Since Thailand is so fertile, the fresh food, especially green vegetables, are readily available much of the year.

OTHER COUNTRIES

Middle Eastern *(Morocco, North Africa, Arabian Countries)*

The Arabian nations consume a variant of the Indian diet, though wheat is used more than rice, eaten both as breads and crackers and as cooked wheat grain (couscous), often with peas or lentils. More types of legumes are used, including lentils, peas, and garbanzo beans. Meat, mainly lamb, is eaten regularly; with yogurt and some cheeses are an important part of the diet as well. Vegetables are usually cooked with meats. Olives are also eaten. Few fruit trees (other than date and occasionally fig) grow in these desert climes. Alcohol is forbidden by Moslem law, as is pork. Sweets are very popular, such as halvah, a sweetened sesame seed candy, as well as sugared fruits.

African *(South Africa)*

The diet of the white population of South Africa is similar to that of Australia and England, with the same high consumption of meat and dairy products that leads to an increase in disease. There is also an acceptance of many of the refined foods. The traditional diet of the native black Africans is closer to the "natural" (cultural) food diet. Cultivated and gathered grains and vegetables with some hunted meats (for rural tribes) and fish for coastal tribes make up the basic diet that has supported this culture for many generations. But the acceptance of more refined foods and sugars has been to the detriment of these already malnourished people.

Mexican

The staples of this Central American country are rice, beans, and corn, with a bit of shredded beef or chicken. Tomatoes and chili peppers are particularly common, as Mexican people like their food spicy. Chili con carne is a popular dish, made with meat, chili peppers, and perhaps some vegetables. The spicy chilis stimulate the digestive function, clean the blood, and may help prevent certain degenerative diseases.

Corn is used in a variety of ways, mainly ground for tortillas or corn bread. Red beans are the most commonly used legumes. The rice used varies in its degree of refinement. The high amounts of starches in the diet, along with cerveza (beer) and tequila, makes many Mexican people fairly heavy around the waistline, although usually strong in constitution. *Burritos, tostadas, tamales,* and *enchiladas* are Mexican names for a variety of dishes, rather like sandwiches, made of meat, beans, cheese, or vegetables and corn or flour tortillas.

Refined foods have become more common in the Mexican diet. Breads, sugars, cookies, and candies are eaten more and more by young children. Hydrogenated oils and lard for cooking may be a problem too, related to obesity and atherosclerosis.

The Mexican people would do better with less refined foods and more whole grains and vegetables for fiber. Fruits are plentiful and should be eaten more. Excessive alcohol intake should, of course, be avoided. Because water and food contamination is common, most foods are well cooked before eating, though eating more fresh fruits and vegetables for their cooling effect would probably be more healthy for a hot climate.

South American

The South American diet varies a bit from country to country. Most are similar to the Mexican diet, with a fair amount of corn, rice, and beans. In the wealthier countries such as Argentina and Venezuela, where cattle are raised on a large scale, beef consumption is very high. Fresh vegetables are not consumed often, though fruits are available. More dairy foods are eaten than in Mexico, but really the basic diet is meat, grains, beans, and fruit. A more natural diet with less beef consumption, both in South America and elsewhere internationally, would reduce the necessity to use rain forests as cattle feed and save these beautiful environments.

Tropical

The diet of the tropical locales such as Hawaii, the Caribbean, and other ocean islands seems to be potentially very healthful. Fruit and fish are both very plentiful, though they are not usually eaten together. Some vegetables are grown and eaten, especially the sweet potato, taro root, the banana-like plantain, and breadfruit. The coconut is also popular; its inner water is drunk for nourishment by many natives before eating its meat. Coconut milk and meat are used in many tropical dishes. The island diet is generally a light one, often with more raw foods than cooked ones, appropriate for keeping energy up in these humid climates.

However, problems of malnourishment, obesity, loss of teeth, diabetes, and other diseases have increased since the islanders have adopted a more Westernized diet, consuming more refined, canned, and fried foods, sodas and other sugar products. This trend, occurring within native cultures around the world, must be addressed and changed for the peoples of this Earth to be healthier.

Jewish

Let us look at the Jewish diet, not just as an example of a special cultural diet that exists within the state of Israel, but also as an ancient ancestral diet that has been passed down through generations and across national boundaries. The Jewish people are very involved with food, and can be classic overeaters, often associating food with love and safety. Italians, other Europeans, and Mexican people also seem to share these attitudes toward food. Often, these are people who have known poverty or starvation, for whom eating to satiation represents security, contentment, and even wealth.

Most of the food eaten is cooked, often involving complex preparations. More flour products than whole grains are eaten, though buckwheat may be more common than in other cultural diets. Vegetables are eaten either in soups or with meats. Tomato soup, beet borscht, and the famous chicken noodle soup are common. Fruits are often eaten cooked, such as baked apples, stewed prunes, compotes (mixed stewed fruit), or fruit soups.

The Jewish diet usually includes only one animal protein at a meal, and, for religious reasons, the traditional menu does not include meat and milk foods at the same meal. Of the red meats, only those of cud-chewing animals, such as cattle, goats, or lambs, are eaten; pork is avoided. Roasts and beef brisket are popular cuts of beef. Chicken is eaten regularly, most often baked, broiled, or boiled for soup. Fish, usually whitefish, is consumed fairly often. Gefilte fish—balls of grain meal and whitefish—are a Kosher classic. Shellfish are usually avoided. Other common foods are potato flour pancakes (latkes), matzoh balls, kreplach, blintzes, and flour pastries, such as apple streudel.

The Jewish diet may cause weight problems. Including more natural foods, such as fresh fruit, vegetables, and whole grain products, would increase fiber, decrease calories and sweet cravings, and help to prevent some chronic disease problems. Learning not to overeat and avoiding too many sweets are important habits to develop not just for this diet, but for any diet.

Enough Food?

Many cultures of the Western world have plenty of available food and have a tendency to excesses and the many congestive and degenerative problems that this creates. But many of the densely populated areas of the world, such as the African countries, India, and China, do not have advanced agricultural technology, and still count on manual labor. Many do not have enough resources or enough usable agricultural land to feed their ever-growing populations. Even if they can grow enough food (which is often not the case), slow or nonexistent transportation may not be available to distribute food, and thus, many people are underfed. Often, they do not get enough nutritious food to support normal growth and development in young people or maintenance for adults. Malnourishment and starvation are among the greatest diseases we confront on a global basis. The high consumption of animals, who eat half of the world's grain before they themselves are eaten, is considered a poor use of energy, poor economics, and poor sense. We need to change this focus from the excessive amounts of meat we eat to a more healthy, vegetarian-based diet; this will help reduce the destruction of our Earth, the only home we have.

Keeping people healthy enough to recultivate the earth and teaching and inspiring them to do so will go a long way toward solving one of humanity's greatest challenges—malnourishment and starvation. Feeding the hungry babies, adults, and elderly of the world is a growing and vital concern of everyone.

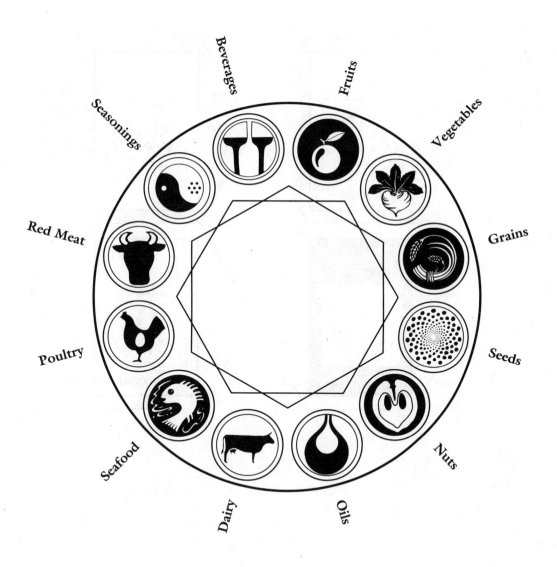

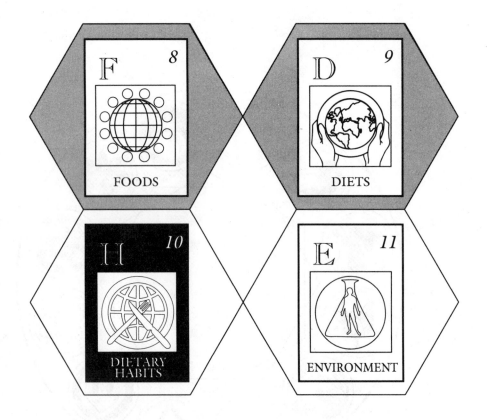

FOODS 8

DIETS 9

DIETARY HABITS 10

ENVIRONMENT 11

Chapter 10

Dietary Habits

O ur dietary habits—that is, the way we eat—probably influence our health even more than the foods we choose to eat. Developing good dietary habits should begin as early as possible, because these habits will help or hinder us for life. Once they are "under our belt," so to speak, they are very difficult to change. For example, obesity is as much a result of *how* we eat as it is of *what* we eat. Overeating, eating late at night, or eating too many different foods at a meal can weaken our digestive functions and make it much easier to gain weight. Overeating at meals and snacking between meals are common eating problems, and often these habits are picked up from other family members during our developmental years. The focus on food and the socialization around eating are family dynamics that become deep-seated very early. Our psychological and emotional states are often tied into habits such as these. Equating food with love or prosperity, and eating for emotional satisfaction or security, are powerful psychological factors which are influenced by eating patterns and problems. Thus, weight reduction is a significant challenge that encompasses major shifts in our psyche, attitudes, emotions, and, hopefully, our physique.

Specific food attractions are also part of our personal eating pattern. These likes and dislikes often develop when we are children and are usually difficult to change. They also influence our health and weight. Breads, pastas, meats, peanut butter, chips, ice cream, fried foods, sugars, hot dogs, hamburgers, and french fries are not our most healthful foods, but these are surely in greater demand than carrots, celery, and apples. The Western family's attraction to fatty foods continues to influence children, teenagers, and young adults, toward the trend of obesity and cardiovascular disease.

Tastes for specific flavors, such as for salty or sweet foods, also develop when we are young, and are accordingly difficult to change. Occasionally, people become attracted to sour or spicy foods, to bitter foods, such as leafy greens, or to other, less common, flavors. In our culture, abuse of or addiction to sugar and salt is very widespread and influences health significantly. From sugar added to baby food, cereal, coffee or tea, and salt added to almost everything else, to further hidden salt and sugar in most restaurant or fast foods, we are constantly bombarded with these two flavors. The Chinese consider that there are five flavors—sweet, salty, sour, spicy, and bitter—all of which must be balanced to create a healthy diet (see further discussion in Chapter 12, under *Flavors* [*Balance*]).

The abuse of sugar and salt in America and even worldwide is significantly influencing the types of diseases seen. Too much sugar affects the teeth, contributes to obesity, and may be an important factor in the development of adult diabetes. Extra salt affects the body's water balance, thereby affecting the kidneys, blood pressure, and, eventually, the entire cardiovascular system. Most of these problems could be greatly reduced with a more balanced diet.

During the last quarter century, we have seen a dramatic increase in fast foods, snack foods, artificial foods, and foods containing excessive amounts of sugar, salt, or fats. Though these foods may be less expensive for the consumer, the overall costs are more than just what it takes to pay for big factories, expensive equipment, and many employees; it affects the health of our internal and external environment, and that's a high price to pay! Nowadays, nearly 40 percent of the food dollar is spent in restaurants. Fat intake is more than 40 percent of the average diet. A large portion of the American diet consists of those poor-nutrition foods with their empty calories and excess fat, salt, and sugar—hamburgers, french fries, soft drinks, pizza, hot dogs, fried chicken, bacon, potato chips, candy, pastries, and so on. The attraction to and regular intake of these foods because of their flavors, consistency, availability, or social acceptance easily become "habits"—we seek them out without thinking, and they become a regular part of our diet, often in place of more nutritious foods.

Luckily, we can change these habits. We can change what we eat, how we eat, and when we eat. We can shed addictions to sugar, salt, or other specific foods. We can gain new attractions to more wholesome foods, and lose weight, allowing our body to find its more optimal shape and metabolism. Any change, however, does require motivation and time to allow for physiological readjustments and even withdrawal to take place; this usually takes at least a few weeks. But more and more people are choosing natural foods and losing their tastes for unnatural, oversweetened, salty, greasy, meaty foods. Preparing simpler meals with simpler foods in modest quantities spread out through the day is a healthful way of eating that has come back into vogue.

○ FOOD HABIT INTERVIEW

Who, What, When, Where, Why, and How

There are many factors involved in eating to achieve a balance of physical nourishment, mental relaxation, and emotional harmony. These goals are easily undermined when we let certain patterns develop and lose our sense of eating as a way of nourishing body, mind, and spirit. When we do not take the time to prepare wholesome food, or if we hurry our meal or eat in unpeaceful settings, we risk creating difficulties in digestion and assimilation and losing the basic nurturing potential of our food. Let us take a brief look at a healthful way to approach food and our relationship to it.

Who is it that is eating? Of course, it is each of us that is ultimately responsible for our nutrition, except when we are babies or young children. However, many of us never grow up when it comes to being responsible for what we consume and learning about healthful nutrition—how to shop, how to store food, and especially how to prepare it. It is not the responsibility of our spouse or the cook at the local restaurant; we all need to learn the art of food preparation so that we can ultimately nourish ourselves and others. Anyone who feels that their only role is to go out into the world and make money is selling himself or herself short as complete human beings. I am not suggesting that we all become gourmet chefs, but I would urge everyone to learn the basics of meal preparation so that when left to our own devices we will not just survive, but thrive. As we grow, we need to develop our sense of what is the best diet for each of us, and not live by the needs of our housemates, spouse, parents, or children. This individual process is an essential part of good nutrition throughout life.

With whom we eat is also important. Creating a peaceful setting around food preparation and food consumption is a vital part of the nutrition process. "What goes in is what comes out" is a wise saying regarding the transformative powers of energy— and if love and a nourishing spirit go into food while it is being prepared, it is likely that the person eating it will experience those qualities. When a meal is prepared by someone who is frustrated or angry, it may take on a whole different nature. That is why loving mothers and grandmas are often the best family cooks—they put their love into everything they make.

This leads to another important aspect of eating—the social setting in which we eat. The family meal, with its members sitting around the table sharing the day's experiences, is potentially wholesome and relaxing. But if there is more stress than peace, more argument than discussion, or too much coming and going, digestion and nourishment can be negatively affected. If we are particularly sensitive to others or easily upset, it might be best to eat in peace by ourselves or with another who likes to eat quietly. But many families and cultures use mealtimes to socialize, and I believe that we can adapt to this with the right attitudes. Everyone should make the time to relax and breathe before eating—before receiving new energy. To receive nourishment, we must be receptive. Eating on the run or while doing other things, even having an intense conversation during a meal, does not really allow us to pay attention to the whole process of eating—chewing, tasting, and swallowing our food. Overeating is common in these situations. I believe that when individuals, couples, or families have their main or primary contact around the dinner table, inappropriate attitudes toward food can be created—associating being social or close to others while eating, or even using food as a barrier against social interactions and closeness, are some resulting problems.

It is a good idea to ask ourselves with whom and in what kind of setting we like to eat—quietly alone, with a certain friend over an intimate dinner, or in a quick, move-'em-through meal. When we tune into our own preferences, we can nourish ourselves to the fullest potential.

What we eat is probably the most important factor. (However, even the healthiest diet will not be utilized properly if we are stressed, upset, or eat on the run.) A balanced diet is, of course, what we all need. What this actually is may vary from person to person. Our diet is ultimately based upon our individual needs, our cultural background, and our current knowledge and tastes. At best, we should eat moderately and eat a variety of foods.

A balanced diet in my "book" contains lots of fresh foods—fruits, vegetables, whole grains, seeds, and nuts. More concentrated foods such as eggs, milk products, and animal meats, can be added as desired and tolerated, though they should make up a much smaller percentage of the diet than the vegetable source foods. An even smaller amount of manufactured, processed, or baked foods should be included—these are really not needed at all.

Food combining and rotating our foods so as not to eat the same things every day, may help alleviate or prevent such problems as poor digestion or allergies. We may find that certain foods feel very good in our body both short and long term, while others do not resonate very well.

The topic of "what to eat" is really what a good part of this book is about. Also, see Part Three, *Building a Healthy Diet*.

When we eat is a fairly controversial concept in nutrition. Though most cultures have regular mealtimes, this is ultimately an individual choice based on body cycles, work, energy levels, and sleep patterns.

The first rule of eating is to eat when we are hungry. The message of hunger tells us that our body has digested and used the last food we consumed and is ready for more. Many people, especially those who are overweight, experience more emotional or psychological hunger than the physical feeling we are talking about here.

We need to balance this hunger response with regular eating patterns, as it is also important to plan meals and have food available when we are hungry. If our schedule is such that we have specific times for breakfast, lunch, and dinner, we need to eat sufficiently but not excessively, so that we are feeling some hunger at the time of our next meal. There are many people in the world, especially in Western cultures, who rarely experience hunger. There are also millions of impoverished people on this earth who rarely experience nutritional satisfaction.

When to eat what kinds of foods and how much food to eat are nutritional issues about which there have been a variety of theories. That we should not eat too much too late in the day is a pretty unanimous viewpoint. Eating a wholesome, well-balanced dinner in the late afternoon or early evening is a fairly well-accepted activity. Dinner tends to be the most social meal, a time to relax after a hard day at work, school, or home. In many parts of the world, particularly Europe, people tend to eat lightly in the morning, and then eat their main meal in the early afternoon. Dinner is usually light with soup and bread or salad, and often a social time with friends or family. See Chapter 9, the *Italian* diet, as an example.

Breakfast is a more open question. The word breakfast means to "break the fast" after not eating overnight, often for nearly twelve hours. Some traditional schools of thought feel that breakfast is the most important meal of the day—that a big breakfast consisting of fruit, starch, protein, fats, muffins, and so on is what gets us going. Clearly, if we finish eating for the day by 6:00 or 7:00 P.M., the next morning we should be hungry again and need a wholesome, nourishing breakfast. However, many adults eat later in the evening. Thus, there are many, myself included, who think that our fast should be broken in the morning very lightly, with fruit, for example, and that we should progress through the day with more concentrated foods. The best-selling nutrition book, *Fit for Life*, suggests that the "natural hygiene" of our body cycle wants to cleanse the previous day's food from 4:00 A.M. until noon and to want only cleansing fruits in the morning. At noon, we may begin to eat vegetables and use more concentrated starch, protein, or fat food per meal. We consume most of our food from midday until 8:00 P.M. If we are early risers and workers, our food intake cycle can begin earlier, though it should probably end earlier as well. When it is very cold, or if we do a lot of physical work, we may need a more warming and fuel-oriented breakfast, though many people can do very well on fruit alone in the morning. With this system, fruit is eaten by itself, not with or after other foods (see the section on *Food Combining* later in this chapter).

Often, we do not know our own needs unless we experiment. By eating different amounts at different times of the day, we can see what will work best for our work and energy schedules. If we get very fatigued in the afternoon after lunch, we may need to shift things around. A big dinner and light breakfast may be best for us, or it may be the other way around. We won't know unless we try it. Just because we have been doing things one way for a long time does not mean that it is the best way.

Where we eat can be particularly important for people who are overweight because of poor eating habits. With our concerns about time, convenience, and comfort, it is easy to find places to eat or snack away from our usual ones, such as the dinner table. Eating in front of the television, in the car, or while walking around leads to an increased intake of food, especially of the more highly caloric snack foods. This can become an extra assault on our digestive tract, which gets no chance to rest. While eating, avoid "techno-traps," such as telephones, television, and computers. Choose foods which will reduce electrical interference in our digestive, assimilative, and mental abilities (see *Electropollution* in Chapter 11).

I suggest to people on weight-loss programs or to those who have developed poor eating habits that they pick one or two places to consume their food, usually one indoors and the other out. Eating outdoors, especially in a natural setting, can contribute to the relaxation and enjoyment of the meal. The dining room table is usually the best indoor spot, so that eating is mainly centered around meals instead of snacks. Restaurant eating involves another place we may need to include, but, for a variety of reasons, restaurant eating is best done only occasionally.

People who are overweight tend to snack or eat while watching television or become "prowlers" in their own home, checking the refrigerator and cupboards for treats even after a good-sized meal. Retraining ourself to eat in a limited number of places, those that are in our best health interest, may be difficult, but it is a good habit to develop. Where do you usually eat? Do you like quiet meals, with nice music, or social meals?

Why we eat is definitely an interesting question. We should basically eat to nourish our being—our organs, our tissues, every cell in our body. Food is the main human fuel for life; it provides heat and all of the specific nutrients that we have discussed so far in this book. It helps the body function. For a period of time when we rest or fast, our body can use stored nutrients to run itself, but eventually we need to refuel.

As my associate Bethany ArgIsle suggests, we have many more mouths to feed other than just our oral cavity. Our eyes need to be nourished with color and beauty, our ears with music and the sounds of nature, our nose with the natural fragrances of the world, our hands and body with the touch of another, and, of course, our heart and spirit with the love and friendship of other living beings. Nourishment comes in many forms and on many levels. Many people feed their bellies but not their souls, and this will not lead us where we are meant to go.

There are, of course, many other reasons why we eat—loneliness, frustration, reward, and punishment to name a few. Some of us use food like a drug to sedate or numb ourselves to our life situation. We should be aware of this aspect of eating.

Most of us at some times eat for social reasons. Sharing food is a custom of friendship. When we are asked to join someone in their creative cuisine or for a drink or snack, it is often taken as a rejection or even an insult if we decline. I have learned through the years, especially since my diet has usually been so different from those around me, to share what I was or wasn't doing and why, as a means to educate or inspire friends or relatives to other possibilities. But it is often difficult not to succumb to their temptations. If we are planning to go to a social gathering for eating, it would be wise to eat lightly in the hours prior to your arrival; the extra hunger will allow us to really enjoy the meal, though we must be careful not to overeat. We all, on some level, want our friends or family to be like us. Still, individuality is the beauty of our species and one of the most important aspects of nutrition.

How we eat can also make a big difference in our nutrition. Eating slowly and chewing our food well are very important. Starting the digestive process in the mouth saves a lot of wear and tear on the stomach (which does not have teeth) and digestive tract. We can then more easily break down the food and utilize the nutrients contained in it. When we rush through meals, we are doing our body and digestion a disservice. Our emotions influence our digestive functions as much as any system in our body, so getting into a peaceful and receptive state is important to healthy food consumption. Allotting enough time to nourish ourselves is also helpful.

How we get the food from the plate or bowl to our mouth—what utensils we use— is also an interesting topic. The choice of the Western world is silverware (or other metalware). Personally I do not like to eat with metals. (Forks are sharp and hard, and if the metal hits the metal fillings in our mouth, well, that's no fun.) Those of us who enjoy Eastern influences prefer chopsticks, especially the wooden (not plastic) variety. My favorite utensils, though, are my God-given chopsticks called fingers. My mother and my more "proper" friends have never been very supportive of this habit. Whether with fingers or chopsticks, eating can be a very primal and personal experience. Many foods, such as fruits, vegetables, nuts, and seeds, adapt easily to hand- or finger-eating. Soup may be drunk, and soft foods such as mashed potatoes or oatmeal may need a little creativity and practice. If we adapt to the individual characteristics of the food and the individual dietary needs of our body, we should do well.

○ HABITS TO CHANGE

Overeating

Overeating is one of the most common and dangerous dietary habits. It is natural, on festive occasions such as holidays or parties, to eat more than usual, but many of us have turned up the level of our satiation state so that we need to eat a large amount of food to feel satisfied all the time. This is contributed to by a great many emotional and psychological factors that may have started in our early years. It is often influenced by our parents and family members and by our own insecurities and self-image.

Overeating often leads to obesity, which is a factor in many other diseases. The overconsumption of food also causes stress to the digestive tract and other organs and can lead to the overworking and weakening of those areas. Congestion or stagnation occurs more easily with overeating.

These problems need to be dealt with at the level from which they arise. If they stem from a nutritional deficiency, so that the body is craving missing nutrients, that should be discovered and corrected. If they are of recent onset, stress may be the source. More often, though, overeating is a long-term and deep-seated problem that needs to be dealt with on both the psychological and nutritional levels.

Moderation in eating is a very important habit to develop. Eating small meals several times a day instead of one or two large meals is probably better for most people. Balancing flavors as well as types of food will help satisfy us and may lessen our desire to eat more.

Undereating

In recent years, there has been growing concern over problems associated with undereating, such as the medical conditions known as anorexia nervosa and bulimia. Undereating usually has a strong stress or psychological component, which can range from being too nervous or concerned about an upcoming event or relationship, to part of a full-blown psychosis.

All forms of undereating, skipping meals, or eating only limited foods will lead to poor nutrition and eventually, to problems from protein, calorie, vitamin, or mineral deficiencies. Other symptoms include lack of energy and subsequent weakness, malnourishment of internal organs, skin problems, and hair loss. Severe weight loss in spite of regular eating may indicate an underlying medical condition and warrants an evaluation by a doctor.

People who undereat are often overly concerned about obesity or have a distorted self-image. This is more common in women and in teenage girls who become very body conscious or are concerned about becoming too shapely. Often, being very thin is similar to being fat in that it makes us less attractive and is a protection against intimacy with others. These issues may come up during sexual development—that is, in adolescence.

Anorexia means "loss of appetite," and anorexia nervosa means not eating because of "nervous" or psychological problems. The majority of people with that condition are young females who want to be trim, or to be models or ballerinas, which require a long and lean body. This may not be the natural body shape of many people, who literally need to starve themselves to maintain that weight or shape. Bulimia is voluntary vomiting by people who wish to get rid of food just eaten so as not to absorb the calories and add weight. Many "bulimics" and "anorexics" also use laxative pills or take regular enemas to clear out the intestines more rapidly. All of these problems have strong psychological bases and usually require counseling as well as a lot of support from loved ones. Occasionally, these situations become extreme and, as with overeating, can be fatal. Fortunately, these conditions are often short-lived, and those troubled by them see their way clear to begin a new balanced diet and create a newly shaped body and self-image.

Eating Late

This is a common problem among people with busy daily schedules. Food often acts as a sedative and helps us to physically relax. After a meal, more blood goes to our digestive organs and away from our areas of physical and mental activity. So eating lightly during the day, getting hungry at night after work, and then eating our main meal in the evening is a convenient pattern for most schedules. However, going to bed on a full stomach is not necessarily helpful for digestion or sleep. The food may just sit there, undigested through the night, so that we wake up full and sluggish. Eating late can become a habit that robs us of our vitality.

It is best to try to eat earlier in the evening, ideally before dark, and not too heavily; to engage in some activity, both mental and physical, after dinner; and to eat very little in the two or three hours before bedtime. When we have not eaten enough through the day, it is wise to eat lightly in the evening also and sleep well to awaken energized for some exercise and a good, hearty breakfast.

Rigid Diet

Many people develop rigid eating patterns and consume only a limited selection of foods. This inflexibility is often based on a preference for certain tastes or just a discriminating personality. Teenagers and elderly people are subject to this lack of flexibility (as are some health food fanatics) more often than other areas of the population. Sometimes this is based on fear, rebellion, lack of adventure, or just being stuck in an attitude that will not allow them to be open to other ideas. They just maintain themselves on a few foods, such as hamburgers, hot dogs, french fries, and sodas for the younger crowd, or eggs, toast, potatoes, and meat in the older group. All lack the freshness and vitality found in natural foods.

There are people who develop what I would call positive restrictions in their diet. We all have certain foods we do not like because of their flavor or past experience with them. Specific allergic foods are clearly best avoided. Restricting foods such as meats, milk, or chemical-containing foods may be based on certain philosophical or health choices. However, being too rigid in our diet is usually not in our best interest.

It is difficult to get people to change when they do not wish to, especially in regard to what they eat. They already know that they won't like it before they even try. Sometimes, consulting with a nutritionist and doing a diet analysis by evaluation or computer can show people the excess or lack of nutrients in their diet, and this may educate and influence them to make some changes.

Ideally, we should eat a variety of foods, from all the groups that I have discussed previously, unless there is a particular sensitivity to certain ones. This gives us the opportunity to absorb the nutrients that nature and our world provide. Eating them in moderation while introducing new ones daily is a healthful path to follow.

Emotional Eating

We have already discussed overeating and undereating, but there are other issues surrounding the use of food in dealing with stress and psychological troubles. Some people eat when upset or depressed; others cannot eat at all in this condition. Our emotions strongly influence our eating behavior, so if we want to maintain a more balanced diet, and thus a more balanced life, we need to learn to deal with our emotional states in ways other than with food.

Using hunger as a guide, integrated with a regular eating plan, we create our basic diet. If we are overweight, we need to plan our meals to include less food; if underweight, we will include more food and calories and then maintain a balanced diet when we are at a better weight.

We can learn to deal with stress, sadness, frustration, depression, and so on through self-development techniques, through counseling, or through mental affirmations and visualization, all good ways to clear these problems—or at least not let them take hold of us and run our lives. There are very few issues that are important enough to take precedence over our health. And not using food to cover up these important feelings, thoughts, and issues is crucial to maintaining our health.

Liquids and Eating

Many of us drink liquids with our meals. This is not really a good practice, since extra fluids can dilute the digestive juices, making it more difficult to break down food. Drinking water before meals or sometime after them is much better. A small amount (less than a cup) of water with meals may help dissolve the food and stimulate digestive juices.

Water is generally our best beverage, and consuming about eight to ten glasses a day (most of us will need less when we consume a higher amount of fruits and vegetables), is very helpful for weight loss and keeping the body functioning. It is best to drink two or three glasses first thing in the morning, several glasses between meals, and then a couple of glasses about 30–60 minutes before dinner to reduce the appetite a bit. Sweetened soda pops should be avoided. Milk is a food (to be used sparingly by adults), not a beverage to be drunk with meals. Many people feel that a bit of alcohol before a meal stimulates the appetite and the digestion of food. Coffee or tea following a meal is enjoyed by many people, and is probably not too detrimental when done occasionally. Overall, it is wise to be aware of needs and drink when thirsty, and it is best to drink only between meals, giving our digestive tract the best shot at getting those nutrients ready for our cells.

Additional Habits to Cultivate

Preparation of both ourselves and our food is helpful. Food made with awareness and love adds that little extra, and when we take the time to prepare ourselves to receive nourishment, such as with a little prayer or some quiet time, we also give ourselves the chance to get the most out of our meal.

Relaxation around eating is a good habit to develop. This is part of preparation and digestion. After a fair-sized meal, it is important to take some time to let digestion begin. After about an hour, we can begin some light activity. A walk is ideal. However, most of us cannot afford the luxury of taking this time around meals. When I cannot, I try to follow the *Warrior's Diet* (see Chapter 9) of frequent small snacks, through the day, until I can take more time to prepare and eat a proper meal.

Exercise is very important to keeping our body healthy and to utilize the nutrients that we consume. I do not recommend exercising for at least an hour, or longer, after eating. It is usually several hours after a meal before my body feels right doing any vigorous activity. Often, I exercise first and use eating as a reward for doing the physical activity that I feel is needed. Early in the day before breakfast, and after work before dinner, are the two best times for exercising.

○ FOOD MIXING

There are three important factors which will help us choose what foods to eat in combination and when to eat them. These are acid-alkaline balance, food combining, and food rotation. I will discuss them briefly here, as they are useful in developing ways to improve our general health or digestion or to reduce food allergies. They are discussed more fully in Part Three, *Building a Healthy Diet*.

Acid-Alkaline Balance

Since our body tissues and blood are slightly alkaline, we need to eat more foods that break down into alkaline elements. The ash or residue that remains when a food is metabolized influences our body's pH, or acidity. The foods that generate an alkaline ash are the fruits and vegetables (even the acid fruits, such as lemons), except for cranberries and most dried fruits. The whole grains, nuts, and seeds are slightly acid in our body, though millet, buckwheat, corn, almonds, and all sprouted seeds tend more toward the alkaline side. The cereal grains tend to be more acid-alkaline balanced than the more acidic nuts, milk products, meats, and refined flour and sugar products.

For a system that does not get too acidic, congested, or mucusy, the diet should contain about 70 percent alkaline foods. This means the type of diet that I have been talking about throughout this book—one that focuses on fruits and vegetables, with some whole grains, more sprouts, and smaller amounts of animal foods and refined treats. This will keep our system functioning optimally, provided we get the balance of vitamins and minerals we need, as well as the essential fatty acids and amino acids to perform the required fat and protein functions.

Food Combining

Food combining is a somewhat complex issue—and a revolutionary idea in terms of the standard diet. The basic theory is that for best digestion and utilization of our food, we need to observe certain rules for the way we combine foods within a meal.

Fruits are eaten alone, as they are more easily digested than other foods. We eat lots of vegetables and combine them with either starch or protein foods—protein foods, such as meats and milk products, are not eaten with starches, such as potatoes and breads. So meat and potatoes are out, as are cheese sandwiches. The reason for this is that, for best digestion, proteins require an acid digestive medium and starches an alkaline one. When eaten together, they interfere with each other's utilization, so that digestion takes longer and is inefficient.

Fruits and simple sugars are not eaten along with or after other foods, because doing so would cause them to be delayed in the stomach juices and begin a fermentation process, allowing gas to go through the intestines. Milk is not drunk as a beverage but used as a food. The fruits of the melon family are eaten alone, not even with other fruits.

Fruit is usually eaten in the morning or several hours after other foods. Meals are simpler than is usual in the American culture, consisting of lots of vegetables with either a protein food, such as dairy products, eggs, or meats, or a starch food, such as grains, pasta, or potatoes. This type of diet, I believe, generates less stress on the intestinal tract and creates overall better health, both immediately and on a long-range basis. In *Fit for Life*, the authors stress the principles of food combining and the need for a more alkaline diet in their program. I feel that it can be a healthy one provided we balance our diet properly and obtain all of our necessary nutrients.

Food Rotation

Rotating our foods is a common method for discovering or diminishing the effects of allergies or hypersensitivities. It also may be helpful in preventing the development of many food allergies in the first place. When we overconsume a food, our body can become sensitized to it and make antibodies that will react with it when it is absorbed into our system. The most common allergens are protein foods, including milk, wheat gluten, eggs, beef, yeast, soybeans, and corn, though most any food can generate allergic reactions.

Food allergy is fairly common and can be short- or long-lived. Some people who are allergic to certain foods as children may remain allergic to them for most of their lives, while for others, sensitivities to certain foods may come and go.

The physiology of food allergy is somewhat complex and still mostly theoretical. It involves both our cellular system and our immune system. Keeping stress to a minimum, reducing incidence of infections and colds, and maintaining basic health and digestive tract ecology all seem to minimize food reactions. If we do have problems with certain foods or wish to prevent such problems, food rotation is a good idea. The theory is that it takes about four days for the body to entirely process a food and clear it from our system. Thus, each food in the diet is consumed only in one day out of every four, so as to minimize the potential allergic stimulus of each food. Following this program also allows us to isolate foods more easily should we have any reactions. It is not a simple process, but it can be very helpful, and it is probably a good habit to develop. It provides us with a variety of foods and brings a certain discipline to our diet, which is positive practice for developing other useful habits.*

---

*For more information on acid-alkaline foods, food combining, and general nutrition, see Dr. Haas's *Seasonal Food Guide* poster and booklet (Celestial Arts, 1990).

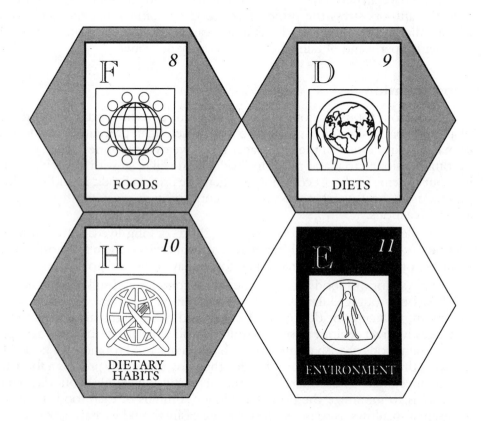

Chapter 11

Environmental Aspects of Nutrition

Although I am generally an optimistic person, thinking about the chemical pollution of our beautiful planet makes me sad. Actually, unconscious pollution, even smoking cigarettes, makes me more angry than sad, and when I see people smoking around their children or in a closed car, I become even more upset.

What can we do? Is it too late? We live in a world plagued by industrial chemicals. Pollution is really a side effect of our technological age. There are now so many new substances, some highly toxic in nature, which are proving difficult for both Earth and our bodies to handle. We do not have enzymes to metabolize them.

Besides the growth of technology as a cause of increased chemical pollution, a greater difficulty is generated by the capitalistic viewpoint—concern for profits often outweighs concern for people, health, and the state of Earth. This problem is worsened by the fact that those creating or allowing the pollution are not willing to clean up their own mess. This is both shortsighted and irresponsible; these continuing problems may take us many years, even centuries, to heal, if this is indeed possible.

There is also a state of consciousness, a belief or approach to life, that is also responsible for our environmental pollution. This attitude is aligned with the "magic bullet," "attack and conquer" approach of Western medicine—kill the germs, spray the bugs, add more chemicals to the soil to stimulate growth. If things get worse or side effects develop, we will use a different or stronger chemical. There is no end to the cycle because this approach is continually reaching for a new series of effects rather than addressing the causes. The condition that was originally identified as the problem will never be corrected this way. There have always been germs and insects; they also inhabit the Earth. Yet, we found that if we spray the whole field to kill them and those pesky weeds, we have a better crop yield and more profits. Everything still looked the same, with no apparent side effects. Later, we found that if we preserved foods or added new chemicals or colors, the foods would last longer or look better, even if we used cheaper ingredients.

This shortsightedness is a result of our concern with just this year's crop or one particular germ, and lacks the vision to see what might happen to the "host"—Earth or our very own bodies. When the concentration of chemicals used in our food chain, at home, or in industry rises to a certain level, there are side effects, everything from mild irritations to blood and immunological disorders. Our body may be stressed by chemical insults, whether we breathe them, drink them, or eat them, and this stress may increase our potential for disease. Indeed, many radiation and air-borne chemicals, are well-known causes of many specific diseases and cancers. Often, however, we do not find out that these chemicals are dangerous to humans until they have been in use for many years. For instance, chemically-induced cancers often take many years, even decades, to develop.

This topic could easily fill many volumes; with chemical testing, reported experiences, new drugs put on the market, and old ones taken off, new knowledge comes to light every day. I will try here to provide basic information on the subject and look at ways to survive our "New Age of Industrial Chemistry," with a focus on chemicals in foods. I first explore the theories about how chemicals may endanger our health and then look at how we can avoid or at least balance out their effects and survive into the twenty-first century.

○ GENERAL CONCERNS

What Is the Danger?

The health of Earth and the health of our bodies are aligned—if Earth is sick, we cannot be entirely healthy. Pollution in many forms occurs alone, upon, and within our planet and in every person's body. Industrial chemicals have surrounded and invaded our entire world.

Of course, these chemicals also have a beneficial role in our current consumer-oriented society. The human species has worked diligently to develop ways to make life easier (though really more complex—nature herself is simple!), to make new products, to improve worldwide communications systems, and theoretically to improve agriculture and crop yields as well as develop new foods. Most of these developments could not happen without creative new discoveries in the field of chemistry and the use of chemicals. But there is a price! Everyone needs to be aware of and concerned about the impact of industrial chemicals on our personal health and the health of our children, as well as the impact on our local and global environments.

Our societies' leaders and developers would like us to believe that exposure to tiny amounts of toxic materials poses little or no risk. This is not true! Chemicals are tested for their effect on small laboratory animals in both small doses and larger than "safe" or usual doses. We must believe that a chemical or drug may be dangerous to humans if it causes problems for rats or mice, but we must also consider that a substance could cause serious problems in humans even if it seems safe for these laboratory animals. The hidden danger is in the repeated small exposures over time with regular use. Partly because of many chemicals do not break down (and therefore accumulate), their presence in the body can cause repeated insults or lead to chronic diseases. Nature does not provide the enzymes necessary to break down all of these synthetic chemicals, nor can our body readily metabolize and excrete them.

As Earth becomes more and more polluted, so do our bodies. Today, most of our common diseases are environmental in nature, involving our interaction with our surroundings—contact with viruses, bacteria, fungi, and other parasites; food intake; and exposure to chemicals and wastes in the air and water. These exposures can occur at home, at work, while traveling or shopping, or on vacation. Some of this we can do something about, but in most cases of chemical exposure we are at the mercy and conscience (and unconsciousness) of others—past, present, and future.

There are several factors that influence the potential dangers of chemicals. First is repeated insults from the same or similar chemicals; the more exposures to a potentially toxic synthetic chemical, the greater the danger to our health. The condition of the host is also very important. Are we in generally good health, or is our body already stressed or dealing with other chemical insults, such as smoking ciga-rettes, drinking alcohol or caffeine, or eating highly processed or fatty foods? The process is similar to that with germs: some microorganisms are strong enough to cause problems even in the healthiest person, but most germs and parasites need a weakened host or weakened immune system in order to take hold and multiply in the body.

The third factor is that chemicals can interact with each other. Various industrial chemicals may combine in nature, in products, or in our body to make new chemicals, which may be more toxic than the original. A good example of this is the formation of trihalomethanes (THMs), many of which are carcinogenic. These chemicals are formed when a halogen, such as chlorine or fluorine, combines with an organic hydrocarbon (gasoline and petroleum products). Another example is the nitrosamines, which are also carcinogenic. These are formed when nitrites and nitrates in foods or in the soil react with other organic acids in our body or in the foods we eat. There are potentially many chemical interactions occuring within our body, though much of this is beyond the scope of our current knowledge.

Obviously, our greatest concern individually and as a species regarding environ-mental chemical contamination is cancer, the feared, growing "twentieth-century" disease. The carcinogenicity of many chemicals is well documented; there are many other cancer-causing chemicals that have not been confirmed by research studies. Cancer is the worst possible outcome, but chemical exposure may also result in weakened immune function with increased susceptibility to germs and allergens, disruption of cell integrity and possible changes in DNA, and ultimately, increased sensitivity to other chemicals in the environment. Cancer itself is, in part, the inability of our body to process chemical agents that have carcinogenic potential to cells and tissues, or, as Bethany ArgIsle suggests, it may result from the "confused digestion of the indigestible."

How Chemicals Cause Damage

Industrial chemicals both contaminate and interact with life. Some can even destroy life when they become concentrated enough. Many pesticides, fungicides, herbicides, and preservative chemicals can cause liver disease, cancer, and death. Radioactive fallout and air pollution also affects us. But our focus here is on food, both processing additives and the contaminants that get into our food.

Food and water are the main vehicles whereby we receive the chemicals that get into our body. Air pollution and car exhaust, for example, are a real concern but less so nutritionally in comparison to food and water pollution, though some air contamination may settle onto our food. Industrial and agricultural chemicals that contaminate our soil, our water, and our food are our greatest concerns. Local areas may have an emphasis on a particular type of pollution, such as Los Angeles or Gary, Indiana, with air pollution, New Orleans with water contamination, or active agricultural areas with chemical sprays. Ironically, the government agencies charged with insuring the health of the nation and the safety of our air, food, and water refer to these unsafe industrial and agricultural chemicals as "economic poisons."

There are two levels to the process whereby chemicals cause disease, particularly cancer. The first is by direct irritation, causing change at the cellular and DNA level. A chemical that is a potential carcinogen may actually bind to the DNA in the cell nucleus and/or in the mitochondria, thereby altering its structure and potential for normal duplication. It may also make the DNA more vulnerable to the same or other carcinogens. Further generations of the cell with damaged or transmuted DNA may be either metaplastic or malignant. Our bodies have remarkable capabilities when it comes to the repair and even elimination of any abnormal DNA and malignant cells; however, when our immune system is weakened, or there are just too many chemical insults for our body to handle, chronic inflammation and cancer may develop. Cancer, or malignancy, is a mass of rapidly dividing, undifferentiated cells that takes the body's energy without using it creatively.

The condition of the host's immune system is another important aspect in regard to potential carcinogenesis, and indeed, is a contributing factor in a wide variety of diseases. Chemical damage is largely due to the generation of free radicals, unstable molecules that can cause irritation and breakdown of tissues unless they are countered by antioxidants in our body. This oxidation of natural biochemical molecules in the cells and tissues may be a process of degeneration of the body leading to inflammatory probems, allergies, and cardiovascular disease. Stress of all kinds, including aerobic exercise, increases free-radical formation in the body. It is also likely that some environmental chemicals and food additives cause increased free-radical generation. Potentially, these are the same kinds of problems caused by radiation, including tissue damage, abnormal effects on cell division (most noticeable in the rapidly dividing cells of the skin, mucous membranes, and gastrointestinal tract), and the production of mutated cells. The antioxidant system is a series of enzymes and essential nutrients within the body that protects us from these chemically-induced free radicals, just as a fine-mesh screen protects us and our home from the shooting sparks generated by burning wood in the fireplace.

Free radicals are a normal product of metabolism; in the body they are generated by both enzymatic and chemical reactions, including the metabolism of fats. Peroxides, epoxides, and superoxides are examples of free radicals. The *glutathione peroxidase* and *superoxide dismutase* enzyme systems neutralize some of these potentially damaging free-radical molecules. Vitamin A and beta-carotene, vitamins C and E, glutathione, and selenium are all important antioxidants that help protect us from disease. For example, a recent study revealed, that smokers who were low in beta-carotene had an increased lung cancer rate than those with higher or supplemented levels.

Cigarette smoke is a complex mixture including chemical carcinogens known to everyone. Although exposure to cigarette smoke does not invariably cause cancer, it is irritating to everyone. Smoking is a good example of the factors we discussed earlier: repeated chemical insults over time make a mild carcinogen into a progressively stronger one. The condition of the smoker and his or her nutrient status and lifestyle are also important. Nicotine and tars in cigarettes, may interact with other environmental or body chemicals to increase the risk of cancer. This is an area we do not know much about; indeed, there is a lot more to discover regarding the world of chemicals in general, their effect on the human species, and how best to protect ourselves when necessary. Until then, common sense is our most important ally.

Exposure to chemicals, free-radical damage, and immunological changes probably affect us in other ways as well. Chemical sensitivity and food allergy often go hand in hand. Allergies in general are becoming more common with increased environmental chemical exposure. With the effects of the environment and our emotional stress upon our immune system, we can become weaker and more environmentally sensitive overall. Concerns over these interactions have generated a whole new field in medicine, that of clinical ecology.

The two main components of environmental disease, food allergy and chemical susceptibility, come together in the chemical pollution of foods. Many chemicals are present in food as both additives and contaminants. Contaminants accidentally get into food as residues of fertilizers, pesticides, or pollutants in the water or air. Additives are deliberately "added" to food, both in processing and as ingredients to improve flavor, color, or shelf life. Only those additives mixed into foods need be listed on the label; neither those used in the various steps of processing nor any contaminants are required to be identified on the label. This is a big problem in our food industry and of concern to the chemically conscious consumer. Most foods have some additives and contaminants, and the problem is getting worse, not better. Even organic produce has some extraneous chemical contamination from the soil, water, and air; however, "certified organic" foods should have little or no added chemicals.

Industry also contaminates our water and air. The millions of people driving cars around our major cities increase the density of air pollution, which is causing more environmental illness in urban regions. Areas with the worst air pollution have higher incidences of rhinitis, bronchitis, asthma, headaches, allergies, and general irritability, and who knows what the long-term effects will be!

Pollution within the work environment is caused by the manufacture of specific goods as well as by chemicals in the furniture, carpeting, insulation, and chemical cleaners found in the workplace. Industrial chemical pollution is a major side effect of technology. This affects us individually and as a species who must breathe the air, drink the water, and eat the food.

The dumping of chemical wastes needs immediate attention. There are now countless incidents of chemical pollution causing disease in local citizens—from deadly mercury poisoning in Minimata Bay in Japan to the Love Canal in the United States where homes were built on top of a dump site. Industry, of course, claimed that this site was safe, but evidence was found of increased miscarriages, birth defects, and liver cancer in the local populations; further research revealed many carcinogenic chemicals at the site, including dioxins, probably the most toxic chemicals ever made by humans.

There are many instances where profits speak louder than people. This often seems true in agriculture. The sale of chemicals to farmers is a huge business, based on profits, not knowledge of what these chemicals ultimately do to humans. Forests are sprayed with herbicides such as 2,4-D and 2,4,5-T, which can cause miscarriages and birth defects. Farmers spray their fields with thousands of different herbicides, insecticides, and fungicides. Many of these chemicals kill natural pests and their predators, throwing off the ecological balance of nature. The result is that even more potent chemicals are needed to eradicate the pests, which developed a resistance to the earlier chemicals used.

In our culture, it is possible that indoor chemical pollution is an even bigger concern. Some estimates suggest that pollution is 5–10 times more damaging indoors than outdoors. This is because there are so many sources of it—gas heaters and ranges; insulation; carpets and carpet padding; adhesives; aerosols, such as hair sprays and deodorants; insect sprays, pesticide powders, and pest strips; synthetic carpets, drapes, and clothes; cleaning compounds, detergents, deodorizers, and disinfectants; and cosmetics, perfumes, and colognes—to name a few. It is difficult to know or evaluate what effects various combinations of specific chemicals will have on us. If we want to reduce chemical exposure, the home is a good place to begin.

416

Chemicals in Foods

The food industry uses about 3,000 different food additives in a wide variety of packaged and preserved foods. These range from added vitamins and minerals to emulsifiers, buffers, natural and artificial flavoring and coloring, and large amounts of salt and sugar. The average American consumes nearly 150 pounds of food additives per year, supporting a multi-billion-dollar food processing industry, about 130 pounds of sugar and sweeteners, along with 10–15 pounds of salt, and 5–10 pounds of "enriched" vitamins, flavors, preservatives, and colored dyes. Some people on our planet do not consume that much food in one year.

Besides the acknowledged additives, there are about 12,000 other chemicals that contaminate our food during the various stages of propagation, growth, harvesting, packing, shipping, and preparation. These chemicals include sprays and pesticides, many of which are more dangerous than most food additives. Plastics are another example of contamination. Plastic wrap contains polyvinyl chloride (PVC), a potentially carcinogenic chemical. Many grocery stores seal meats, poultry, fish, and other foods in this plastic wrap using heat, which releases PVC as a gas. This threatens the consumer with free-radical formation, cellular irritation, increased allergies, and the potential for the genesis of cancer cells. Should our immune system not be functioning properly, we could be in danger of actually developing cancer from this type of exposure over time.

Why, then, are chemicals used in foods? Originally, foods were grown and eaten directly from a relatively unpolluted Earth. Wild foods were sought and gathered. The oceans and other waters fed us nutritious fish. Animals in the wild provided food to hunters. As the human population multiplied, the world expanded, farming progressed, trade specialties developed, and town markets shared a variety of goods among a diversity of people. Techniques for preparation and preservation, such as pickling, salting, and smoking, were developed to deal with the new problems of storage, waste, and food-borne illnesses.

As technology developed, we learned to create new chemicals to manipulate, preserve, and transform foods—and life changed. The subtle balance of nature shifted with each new assault on our body's unique biochemical balance. Foods and food processing also changed. Scientists were able to mimic natural flavors, to color foods to make them look more "natural," and to aid in the creation and preservation of breads, crackers, and many more commonly used foods. Now there are even "foods" that are made entirely from chemicals. Coffee creamers, sugar substitutes, and candies are made of completely processed ingredients.

But there is a method to this madness. There are actually reasons (or rationalizations) put forth by the food industry for using these chemicals besides the fact that processed foods are usually more profitable. The following are six "reasons" why we have processed foods:

417

1. ***To improve shelf life or storage time.*** This was, I believe, the original reason for using additives. It allowed more food to get to more people and prevented waste and spoilage. Most canned foods are heat treated and vacuum packed so that they can be preserved and stored for years. Many fruits, especially dried fruits, are treated with sulfur dioxide or sprayed with chemicals to prevent their destruction by the air or bugs. Many breads and baked goods are treated or "embalmed" with chemicals to improve shelf life. This may be helpful to the manufacturer, but not necessarily beneficial to the health and longevity of the consumer.

2. ***To make food more available.*** This is achieved not only by improving shelf life, but also through the use of specific types of packaging: separate dishes or entire meals boxed or frozen, such as TV dinners, cake mixes, and microwave meals.. This technique of food processing has brought thousands of new products to grocery stores and demonstrates the convenience of modern food technology. Just walk down any grocery aisle; these products are everywhere!

3. ***To increase the nutritional value.*** Many foods have synthetic vitamins added to them. This can be of moderate benefit to people who consume these "enriched" foods. Often these added vitamins are the same ones that were removed during processing. The great flaw here, though, is that many important vitamins and minerals are processed out of whole foods and not added back into them. Vitamin B_6, chromium, and zinc are a few examples of important nutrients that are lost during the processing of grains and flours and not replaced. For that reason, it is better to eat whole grains. Occasionally foods are "fortified," which means that they have an added nutrient that is not normally found in the original food. Cow's milk fortified with vitamin D is the most common example.

4. ***To improve the flavor of foods.*** Many flavorings, both natural and artificial, are used in an attempt to create greater consumer appeal. Making foods sweeter, saltier, or spicier often tantalizes the taste buds and creates a certain identity and desire for repeated use of those foods. The unique flavor of many processed and packaged foods is created through much time and expense on the part of the manufacturer. Salt and sugar are the two most common flavorings. Monosodium glutamate is another common "flavor enhancer."

5. ***To make foods easier to prepare.*** These days, people take less time with food preparation. Family orientation has changed through the years, and many wives and mothers no longer spend their days at the supermarket or in the kitchen. So, the manufacturers prepare the foods for us and package them in boxes or cans, freeze them, or make them "instant" so that we can add water, heat, microwave, or otherwise take very little effort to get them ready to eat. Mashed potatoes, breakfast cereals, instant oatmeal, cookies, cake mixes, hot dogs, lunch meats, and thousands of other products fit into this category.

6. ***To improve consumer acceptance.*** This is a scary one, because the chemicals used to maintain a food's color or prevent it from being discolored are often the more

potentially toxic substances. Even our natural produce, the fruits and vegetables, are exposed to these chemicals. Oranges are dipped in dyes to keep their "orangeness." Chickens may be treated with yellow dyes to keep their skin looking "healthy." Sprays are used on produce to prevent insects and micro-organisms from moving in or consuming them before the consumer. Bananas are gassed, many fruits and vegetables are sprayed with fungicides, and breads have added mold inhibitors. What increases the selling power of many items, in the eyes of the consumer, may not benefit other parts of the body.

It is obvious from my writings that I am not a big supporter of food processing, chemical sprays, and food additives. I know there is definite value to both manufactur-ers and consumers of "modern foods." Luckily, many of them are safe, and more research is allocated to food additives than to any other areas of industrial chemical use.

Our ignorance regarding both food and environmental chemical interactions is still an important issue. Individual chemicals that are nontoxic alone may be combined to form new chemicals. There are literally millions of possibilities that could cause serious problems before they are discovered. Overall, I believe that we should do everything in our personal power to avoid or minimize the use of chemicals and processed foods. Cultivating and consuming wholesome, natural, and organic foods, ideally grown locally and eaten fresh, has long-range benefits for our environment, our bodies, and our health.

People using chemicalized foods take a risk. The chemical companies and the food processors make a lot of money, most assuredly at our expense, both in terms of our health care costs as well as money spent on their products. The health of our planet Earth is also at stake. It is in our personal health interest to avoid chemical additives and processed foods, and to eat naturally. However, even in natural foods such as fruits, vegetables, and grains, there is a great deal of potential contamination when these foods and the land on which they are grown are chemically treated. For this reason, we can try to eat "organic," but this is not easy, especially in some areas of the country and at certain times of the year. Even organic foods can have small amounts of unavoidable environmental contamination, such as acid rain, contaminated water, chemical residue in soil, and nuclear fallout.

With all of this, we need to try to maintain an optimistic attitude and pray a lot. An otherwise healthy lifestyle of exercise, stress management, and good dietary habits will reduce the risks that chemical food additives pose to our health.

Who Is Responsible for Food Safety?

In the United States, the Food and Drug Administration (FDA) is the government agency responsible to the consumer in assuring the safety of foods. The FDA decides whether a certain food additive is allowable to what degree, and for what specific uses.

It oversees food sanitation and quality, acceptable manufacturing procedures, nutrition and nutrition labeling ("truth in packaging" laws), interstate shipping of foods, and additive usage rules. This is an enormous undertaking for one government organization, and with all the red tape, there is no doubt that any changes in food guidelines will take some time. The FDA is assisted by the Public Health Service (PHS), U.S. Department of Agriculture (USDA), Federal Trade Commission (FTC), and National Bureau of Standards (NBS).

Food labeling is important to the conscientious consumer. The FDA is also responsible for overseeing proper labeling, standards of quality and quantity, enriched product standards, nutritional misinformation, enforcing compliance, researching and accepting new foods, and educating consumers. For certain food creations, such as catsup, mayonnaise, and jam, there are standards of identity required—they must contain certain ingredients to be called by those names. (In the next section, we will see how chemicals covertly get into our foods, without showing up on the label.)

Everyone who touches food is responsible for consumer safety—the farmer, picker, shipper, manufacturer, grocery store, and cook. Chemical additive manufacturers are only responsible for proving that a new additive is safe for human consumption. If it generates cancer in any animals, it will not be accepted. However, these companies have a vested interest in new products appearing to be safe.

Reading Food Labels

Packaging information laws are slowly changing to help consumers learn more about what they are buying. If we choose to purchase packaged foods this chapter provides information to help us make conscientious, healthy, and environmentally sound choices.

- *Minimize the purchase* of plastics, styrofoam, and other nonbiodegradable products. Precycle means not buying products you cannot recycle. This will create a demand for the production of environmentally sound packaging.
- *Additives to avoid* include the artificial colors, excess sugars, and salt, BHA and BHT, nitrites and sulfites (see following chart).
- *A shopping guideline to follow is:* "If you can't pronounce it, don't buy it."

○ TOXIC PROBLEMS IN OUR FOOD CHAIN

How Do Chemicals Get into Our Foods?

In this section, I discuss the contaminants and chemical additives that may enter our food—from the elements that help it through its growing cycle, harvest, and processing until it reaches our tables and mouths. This involves the following areas: air, water, soil, cultivation, processing, storage, preparation.

AIR

In regard to food, air pollution is probably the least of our concerns. It contributes very little, if any, contamination, unless certain chemicals, gases, or metal molecules are present where the food is grown. Some airborne contamination may get into water, which may in turn pass into food. Food grown in fields near industrial plants or along heavily traveled roads may pick up more chemicals, lead, or other auto and truck pollutants.

Air pollution is of greater concern in regard to general health. There are higher levels of chemical irritants in the air in smoggy, heavily populated, or industrial areas. Although I know of no specific studies associating air pollution with weakened immunity, increased infection, or a higher incidence of cancer, I believe that such studies would establish a relationship, as is certainly the case with air pollution and respiratory illnesses.

Indoor air pollution at work, at home, in stores, or at the hair salon may be much worse than outdoor air pollution because there is more contamination with less dilution. More chemicals are used in everyday work and home life than most of us imagine. This means that a great deal of pollution occurs virtually unnoticed. (See the section on *Pollutants in the Home and Office* ahead for further details on this topic.)

The following list shows some common air pollutants. Many are released directly into the atmosphere by industry or the discharge of industrial waste. It would be best, to reduce air pollution as much as possible by enforcing stricter industrial controls and reducing the manufacture of unnecessary products, such as styrofoam, that may generate more severe pollution.

COMMON AIR POLLUTANTS

Carbon monoxide	Ethylene
Ozone	Acetylene
Nitrogen dioxide	Tetraethyl-lead
Sulfur dioxide	Beryllium
Hydrogen sulfide	Cadmium
Ammonia	Methyl chloride
Butane	Vinyl chloride
Propane	Fluoromethanes
Methane	Benzopyrenes
Ethane	Cis-2-butane
Cigarette smoke	Trans-2-butane
Formaldehyde	

421

WATER

While Chapter 1 reviewed the subject of water in relationship to many topics, especially bodily requirements, types of water to drink, and home purification, it only touched on the major problem of water pollution. This section deals with its effects on us and on Earth and some ideas on how to help clean it up.

Water is probably our biggest area of concern in regard to chemical pollution. Undrinkable water was thought to be a problem only in Third World countries, but it is a major problem in the United States and the rest of the Western world as well. Bacterial contamination is a problem in poor nations without proper water-treatment plants and sewage systems. For most tourists and many natives, the water in such areas can cause illness with immediate gastrointestinal symptoms, such as diarrhea and abdominal cramps; a severe case can even be fatal. However, while the problem with infectious microorganisms in water is obvious and usually immediate, our problem is more subtle, invisible, and long range and may even be more dangerous.

The industrial productivity of Western societies has been accompanied by the accumulation of vast quantities of waste, especially chemical waste. Billions of pounds per year are dumped into waters, soil, hundreds of thousands of landfills, and city dumps. This chemical waste is polluting underground water, termed "groundwater." Groundwater feeds wells supplying many people, probably about 90 percent of this country's rural population; current estimates are that between 30 and 50 percent of groundwater is contaminated. Surface waters, such as our lakes, streams, and rivers, often connect with groundwater sources where chemicals can cross contaminate.

Both groundwater and surface-water chemical pollution have become serious problems. This is both a political and an economic issue, involving industry, agriculture, and, of course, you and me, the water drinkers. Here is another example of Western nearsightedness—kill the immediate problem (such as bacteria or bugs) or make the quick buck without a serious thought of the consequences to Earth or its inhabitants in years to come. The consequences of drinking water contamination by pathogenic microorganisms must be dealt with by everyone; the less visible problems of organic, industrial, and agricultural chemical contamination and their potential toxicity and carcinogenesis have been overlooked until recently, but clearly are a serious concern for today and the future. Some particularly toxic chemicals found in groundwater include vinyl chloride, methylene chloride, carbon tetrachloride, trichloroethylene (TCE), benzene, xylenes, and petroleum byproducts. Groundwater contamination is currently irreversible; it is estimated that it would take billions of dollars to even begin to clean up our groundwater, rivers, and lakes, and we do not yet really have the technology to do this, even if the money were allocated. I have a few ideas; see *Can We Really Heal Earth?* ahead.

The Environmental Protection Agency (EPA) is the governmental agency responsible for keeping our water clean. That is an almost impossible task, especially given the fact that other political agencies and lobbyists currently support the interests of big business. During the early 1970s, the EPA was quite productive. The Clean Water Act, passed in 1972, helped regulate industrial dumping of chemicals into the environment. However, the problem was so prevalent and the potential fines were so much less than the costs of changing business practices or the profits to be made, that controlling industrial pollution was never accomplished. In 1974, the Safe Drinking Water Act (SDWA) was passed. This set a standard for any water system serving more than 15 homes. Water treatment plants were required to test periodically for certain bacteria, as well as specified organic and inorganic substances. But this requirement covered only the EPA-regulated substances—ten metals, six pesticides, and the total level of trihalomethanes (THMs). There are literally thousands of other possible chemical contaminants; this is also a very tough job to oversee, so this law was not well enforced. In 1975, the EPA found chloroform in all of 80 municipal waters tested. (Chloroform, one of the THMs known to cause cancer in lab animals, is made when chlorine interacts with other organic matter, such as rotting leaves.)

In 1980, the new Reagan administration took the side of industry and has since worked to lower pollution standards as well as to cut the EPA budget. Luckily, people are concerned about water pollution, and almost every bill calling for the regulation of industrial waste or for cleaner water has been passed. But much remains to be done in both cleaning up water supplies and preventing further pollution. In 1982, for example, nearly half of the large public water systems were shown to be contaminated with some organic chemical, and many of the chemicals found have been shown to be carcinogenic.

Water can be polluted in a variety of ways and by a wide range of substances. In *The Nontoxic Home* (Tarcher, 1986), a very helpful book on reducing chemical exposure in our home and environment, Debra Lynn Dadd groups these water-contaminating substances into the following categories. Microorganisms, such as bacteria and viruses, are one form of contamination. (Chlorine is usually added to water to reduce these organisms.) Dissolved solids are the second group. These are materials that dissolve in the water, many of which come from the soil. Included in this group are the nitrates, the sulfates, fluoride, and various mineral salts. These are relatively safe. The third group contains the particulates, undissolved materials such as dirt, rust, asbestos, or heavy metals—lead, mercury, cadmium, silver, aluminum, cobalt, and so on. These are relatively safe unless they are found in high concentrations. The fourth group, volatile chemicals, is the biggest concern, because many of these are unsafe even in small amounts. These include pesticides, such as DDT and lindane, chlorinated hydrocarbons, chloroform and other THMs, trichloroethylene (TCE), and many more. Chemical water pollutants include both inorganic and organic substances. (See chart page 428.)

Water Contamination Occurs in a Variety of Ways, Including:

- **Agricultural activities.** Pesticides, herbicides, selenium, and the nitrates in fertilizers are some examples of substances used as sprays. These accumulate in run-off waters and end up in underground aquifers or in lakes and rivers.
- **Industrial wastes.** These are very common as production by-products dumped into local rivers or lakes, or buried underground if very toxic.
- **Chemical dumping and waste sites.** Common outlets for industrial waste, these include the multitude of municipal landfills, many of which may be contaminated, while other chemicals, radioactive wastes, or sewage are injected directly into the earth. Some chemicals affecting water found near waste dumps include DDT, vinyl chloride, benzene, carbon tetrachloride, TCE, PCBs, and metals such as lead and mercury. Land disposal of wastes is a very inefficient way of storing pollutants, but it is less expensive than other more responsible solutions, and changing established ways of doing things is always difficult. The reason given for these this is the business/bureaucratic rationalization used to sweep major problems under the rug.
- **Underground storage tanks.** Gasoline, probably the most common substance stored in this way, may leak into groundwater.
- **Mining of metals and radioactive materials.**
- **Leaking septic tanks.** These may contaminate water with bacteria and other waste products.

There are many chemical contamination problem areas in the United States, often in areas with large industrial facilities. In New Orleans, which is surrounded by the Mississippi River on one side and Lake Pontchartrain on the other, chemical dumping by industry has been going on for some time. Possibly as a result of this dumping, New Orleans has a higher cancer rate than many other cities. In 1974, the EPA analyzed over sixty different organic chemicals found in the New Orleans drinking water supply. On a recent trip there, I found that Lake Pontchartrain is considered "dead," with swimming and fishing considered to be a high risk. The Mississippi River is also very polluted.

A patient of mine who grew up in New Orleans told me, "It is very polluted. My mother died of a brain tumor last year. I believe it was from drinking the water. Also last year, six people on the block on which I lived died of cancer. The people are not even aware of the water. You can hardly even buy good water."

California's Santa Clara Valley, also known as Silicon Valley because it is a major center of the computer industry, is also a troubled area when it comes to water. In 1980, for example, one local company discovered that over a one-year period they had leaked nearly 60,000 gallons of trichloroethane (TCA), a toxic waste that can cause damage to the nervous system or birth defects in animals, into the Santa Clara Valley groundwater. Preliminary research suggests that there is a higher incidence of birth defects in infants of women who drank the contaminated water. The EPA estimates that approximately 300 leaks and spills from high-tech manufacturers have contaminated groundwater in that area alone.

The military is probably the biggest polluter in the United States. An estimated one billion pounds of hazardous wastes is disposed of yearly, much of this as a result of nuclear weapons development and manufacture. New Mexico, Colorado, and California, are among the affected areas. The beautiful Snake River in Idaho has been found to have a low level of some radioactive compounds.

Ethylene dibromide (EDB), a pesticide commonly sprayed on citrus trees and other crops, has been found as a water contaminant in Florida and many other states. It has been shown to cause male sterility and cancer.

The pesticide concern grows progressively worse over time, as these chemicals accumulate in the soil and are very slow to break down. Rains and storms that appear to clean everything actually worsen pesticide pollution, as these chemicals are washed into streams, contaminate larger waters, and reach the groundwater, which eventually reaches us.

Many of these anecdotes and others regarding water problems are taken from the fascinating book *Troubled Water* by Jonathon King (Rodale Press, Emaus, PA, 1985) with research assistance by Matt Rothman. I recommend it as one of the most complete books about water contamination problems and solutions. Another recent book, *Save Our Planet*, by Diane MacEachern, points out many problems of pollution in our waters as well as the rest of the environment, outdoors and indoors. In the introduction, she reports that "between 1971 and 1985, over 100,000 cases of disease in the United States were attributed to drinking water, representing more outbreaks in any 15 year period since 1920." We clearly have a water problem.

If you live in a dense city or industrial area, you should be wary of your tap water. If your water has a funny taste or odor or stains your tub or sink, have it checked. It is fairly inexpensive to have the bacteria count verified. With all the chlorine added to the city waters, most microorganisms will not grow very well. Analyzing the water for chemicals can be much more difficult and costly. There are very few companies that perform this service and it can cost hundreds of dollars just to check for the more toxic chemical contaminants, such as the organic halides—trihalomethanes (THMs), vinyl chloride (VC), trichloroethylene (TCE), ethylene dibromide (EDB), and dibromochloropropane (DBCD). There are many others.

Well water is not necessarily safe, either. It usually comes from groundwater, the underground reservoirs also known as aquifers, which may be contaminated. In recent years, many thousands of wells have been closed in over half of our states throughout this country because of contamination, and those are only the ones that have been discovered; there may be many more. Even living in the country does not totally protect us if there is much local agriculture. If you are going to use a particular well for a number of years, it is now necessary to check the water for chemicals; your life could depend on it.

Lake Pontchartrain

They plot with no thought
the drought has been bought
with the money for the children's future
only thing to do for you for me
is to go beyond economy
we know the flow must flow free
beyond the shit we drown in—
our own toxic waste/toxic haste
Lake Pontchartrain
what have you done
to create such disdain
filled to the brim
you let them all in
fish and fowl
families at the bow
ships on the prowl
majestic space
Now you've been bought
caught on the lie
They let you die
Treasure undulating
up against the sky
We let you die
With no fight to right the plight.

—*Bethany ArgIsle*

Can We Really Heal Earth?

Humankind has not yet reached the evolutionary state whereby we can move from our focus of fear and desire for money and power (which clearly have led to technological progress along with pollution and warfare), toward love and trust and a desire to heal and purify our planet. Our ingenuity and technology, I believe, can be applied to discover ways to clean up our water and air. There must be some process, such as using solid carbon and volcanic ash systems, through which we can run our polluted rivers, lakes, and ocean waters, allowing these filtering factories to remove heavy metals and toxic chemicals and turn out mineral-rich, clean water. Large air filtering factories could be set up around cities to purify the air. If we use only a tenth of the monies that we put into nuclear power and weapons, we can do it. These new high-tech buildings and underground sites can replace our nuclear power plants and chemical producing, smoke-spewing factories that now hasten Earth's demise. Cleaning the air will allow the sun to function for us, as it once did, and not become a danger. We can also harness solar, wind, and water power to further supply our living needs, so that Earth can continue to survive for many centuries even after the cosmos shifts or the sun itself weakens. I believe that the real answer to disease, and specifically to the increasing cancer problems, will not be chemical warfare on the body, but learning to reharmonize and support the body's natural healing forces. So will the healing of Earth result from our reattunement to its ecosystem.

It is also worthwhile and fairly inexpensive to use a home filter system to protect ourselves and our families. Most are reasonably priced and will remove most of the chemical contamination. Solid carbon block filtration is a good basic system; avoid granulated carbon filters. Reverse osmosis filters are also a good choice; however, these systems usually have three different filters and are usually more expensive. Reverse osmosis also needs good water pressure and can waste water. (Water filters are discussed in more detail in Chapter 1, *Water.*) Bottled water is usually free of toxic chemicals, but it too can come from contaminated groundwater. Polyethylene, a soft plastic commonly used for water containers, can contaminate water, though the level of this toxicity is low.

For various reasons, I recommend that people not drink city or tap waters. Public water treatment leaves much to be desired. Chlorine has become a panacea to treat and prevent microbial contamination. Although such treatment has helped clean up our water, chlorine can interact with organic wastes, such as dead leaves, and form the carcinogenic trihalomethane (THM) chemicals. Chloroform is commonly found in city waters. In 1979, the EPA set the limit for THMs to be 100 parts per billion (ppb) in water. They estimated that this level would add only 200 cancer deaths per year. Several studies have shown an increased incidence of cancer, especially of the gastrointestinal tract and rectum, in people who drink chlorinated water.

WATER CHEMICALS*

Common Dangerous Drinking Water Pollutants	Chemicals Found in Ground Water	Chemicals Found in Waste Dumps That Affect Water
Lead	Petroleum by-products	Carbon tetrachloride
Mercury	TCE	DDT
DDT	Vinyl chloride	Vinyl chloride
PCBs	Methylene chloride	TCE
PAHs	Carbon tetrachloride	Benzene
Chloroform	Tetrachloroethylene	PCBs
Vinyl chloride	Cis-dichloroethylene	Lead
Trichloroethylene (TCE)	Trans-dichloroethylene	Mercury
EDB	1,1 di-chloroethylene	
Organophosphate pesticides such as Aldicarb	1,1,1, tri-chloroethylene	
Gasoline		
Xylene		
Toluene		
Benzene		
DBCP		
Herbicides like 2,4-D		

Inorganic Water Pollutants	Organic Chemical Water Pollutants	
Lead	Chloroform	Toluene
Nitrates	Trichloroethylene (TCE)	Xylene
Mercury	Trichloroethane (TCA)	DDT
Nitrosamines	Polychlorinated biphenyls (PCB)	2,4-D
Cadmium	Carbon tetrachloride	2,4,5-T
Cyanide	Tetrachloroethylene	Benzene
Arsenic	Vinyl chloride	Toxaphene
Silver	Methoxychlor	Endrin
Asbestos	Dichlorobenzene	Lindane
Chromium	1,2 Dichloroethane	Dioxin
Selenium	Dibromo-chloropropane (DBCP)	Aldicarb
	Ethylene dibromide (EDB)	Gasoline
	Polynuclear aromatic hydrocarbons (PAH)	

* This table was compiled with the help of *Well Body, Well Earth* (Sierra Club Books, San Francisco, 1983) by Mike Samuels, M.D. and Hal Zina Bennett, plus other book sources.

There are other problems with tap water. Plastic pipes more easily leak or interact with industrial solvents, pesticides, or gasoline. Polyvinyl chloride (PVC), polybutylene (PB), and polyethylene (PE) are three common pipe plastics; the first two are mild carcinogens.

Lead leaks occur in certain pipes. Old asbestos cement (AC) pipes, of which some 200,000 miles were laid after World War II, can leak asbestos and may be associated with an increase in gastrointestinal cancer. Copper pipes may add excess copper to our bodies, and often have lead solder lines, which adds to lead contamination. Fluoridation of water is also of concern to many people. Although no definite short-term dangers have been found to be associated with it, other than toxicity from excessive intake levels, the long-range effects of drinking fluoridated water are not yet known.

Most inorganic pollutants are safe at low concentrations, although lead and mercury can be neurotoxic, and nitrosamines are carcinogenic.

Almost all of the organic chemical water pollutants in the accompanying table have been shown to cause cancer or to be toxic to the nervous system.

Controlling chemical pollution and polluters at the state level is a problem since most states do not have the financial resources to clean up contaminated waters. In most cases, this pollution is often not detected, or only when it is too late. Low-level contamination creates long-range problems, nothing that we notice immediately unless very widespread and expensive testing is done routinely. Cancer, birth defects, reproductive problems, miscarriages, and liver and kidney disease are some of the health problems we will have to look for. Immune weakness that could allow more infection and cancer may be an earlier sign of pollution. **We must prevent further pollution!** California, Florida, and New Jersey have recently enacted legislation giving individuals greater power to pursue and legally stop industrial polluters. It remains to be seen what effect such laws will have. In the meantime, here are ten things that can be done to reduce water pollution.

1. Do not use toxic agricultural or industrial chemicals.
2. Recycle wastes safely. Find ways to deactivate or recycle dangerous chemicals.
3. Foster awareness of local problems, including water status, common pesticide use, and industrial waste dumping.
4. Find better ways than the use of chlorine to disinfect water. Ozone can be used to disinfect water without causing a change in taste or increasing toxicity.
5. Enact, support, and enforce better standards and limits for industrial and agricultural contamination.
6. Make examples of polluters (or officials who allow pollution) with more lawsuits, stiffer fines, and even threat of plant closure or jail sentences. It is not acceptable that the negligence of so few can affect the health of so many.
7. Support the EPA in doing its job of monitoring industry, agriculture, and water treatment facilities.

8. Test water to make sure of its safety.
9. Use water filters for drinking and cooking water.
10. Foster heightened concern about ecological and futuristic issues and take action to further natural harmony on Earth.

SOIL

Almost anything in the soil can get into food while it is growing. Plants absorb chemicals and minerals from the soil. Water is one way some of the chemicals keep recycling back into the soil and food. Since Earth and our body do not break down most of the new chemicals used, they accumulate and last a long time.

Nitrogen-based fertilizers are commonly used to stimulate plant growth and create bigger crop yields. These fertilizers can create some imbalances in the soil and produce depletion of other important minerals, such as chromium, selenium, and iodine. Heavy metals such as lead and mercury can also contaminate soil.

Herbicides such as 2,4,5-T and 2,4-D are used on the soil in the preplanting period and in the early stages of plant growth to kill weeds so that there will be less growth competition and easier harvesting. Most of these herbicides are fairly toxic and potentially carcinogenic. These are also sprayed over forests and along highways to reduce foliage and allow easier clearing of timber.

Pesticides are applied primarily during food cultivation, and these are discussed in the next section. Of course, pesticides from previous applications to crops may linger in the soil for years. For example, DDT, which has not been used (legally) for over ten years, still contaminates most soil, plants, animals, and humans. A 1983 Natural Resource Defense Counsel study found DDT residues in more produce samples than any other pesticide.

In California, one of the few states that have legislated "certified organic" standards, crops cannot be considered officially organic (grown without chemicals) until no chemicals have been used for several years. Even then, these foods may still contain traces of long-lived chemicals.

FOOD CULTIVATION

Much of the chemical contamination that gets into our foods comes from pesticide sprays used during the subclassifications of pesticides. The three main classes of chemical pesticides are organochlorides, organophosphates, and carbamates.

Organochlorides. This is a very toxic class of chemicals; they kill pests by attacking their central nervous systems. Most of them have been shown to cause cancer, birth defects, and genetic changes in animals. They are also stored in the body fat when absorbed and accumulate there.

Organochlorides were commonly used as pesticides in the 1940s, 1950s, and 1960s. They are used less commonly in the United States now but are still shipped to other countries, so they may return to us in imported foods such as bananas, coffee, sugar, tea, rice, cocoa, or chocolate.

Three of these common organochlorides were banned—DDT in 1972, Aldrin in 1974, and Endrin in 1979. These poisons and their relatives still remain in the soil after many years of spraying, but they no longer kill the pests, just the people. Most of these chemicals have a half-life of about 50–100 years.

ORGANOCHLORIDES

DDT	Aldrin
Dieldrin	Heptachlor
2,4-D	2,4,5-T
Chlordane	Endrin

Organophosphates. These are the most common pesticides used today, with malathione and parathione leading the group. They are less dangerous than the organochlorines, since they break down into less harmful chemicals within weeks of their use. In pests, organophosphates interfere with nerve conduction and can lead to convulsions and death. The human concern is that the organophosphate pesticides may have a genetic effect that could generate cancer or birth defects, or that they may directly cause allergic reactions or neurochemical abberations in the brains of those exposed. However, they do seem to be much safer than the organochloride pesticides.

Carbamates. This variety of chemical pesticides are in fairly wide use today. The toxicity of these chemicals is somewhere between the organochlorides and the organophosphates. They may also cause birth defects.

Pesticides and their residues in food are a growing problem. Each year in California alone, more than 200 million tons of pesticides are dumped on fields and crops, and most of it never reaches the pests. These pesticide products contain more than 1,000 active ingredients. Nationwide, over half of the produce measured has been found to contain detectable residues of about 20 pesticides.

Pesticides are used because they are toxic to pest life; unfortunately, they are also toxic to wildlife and people. Many of these chemicals become more concentrated as they move up the food chain. Eagles and other large birds that eat insects and rodents contaminated with DDT acquire huge and sometimes fatal levels of that chemical. High concentrations of certain chemicals can have serious consequences for humans as well.

431

The industrial chemical and agriculture businesses work together. Agribusiness is highly oriented toward use of chemical fertilizers and pesticides. Often salespeople are out on the farms selling new chemicals before there have been thorough studies to prove their safety. The EPA was created in 1970 partly to control the use and abuse of these pesticides; unfortunately, they often find out that a pesticide is unsafe after it has been used for years. For example, Dibromo-chloropropane (DBCP), which was sprayed on Hawaiian pineapples for years and contaminated the waters there, was banned in 1979 because of its toxicity, but it will remain in the environment for decades to come.

Many imported foods, particularly tropical fruits, are sprayed or fumigated to keep bugs away during shipping. Spraying with pesticides is not uncommon for fruits such as papayas, mangoes, and pineapples. Bananas are less likely to be sprayed but may be gassed or fumigated before they are shipped.

Spraying after harvesting is of concern because of the high concentrations of the chemicals on the foods when they get to the consumer. Dieldrin, a toxic organochloride pesticide that was banned in 1974, used to be sprayed on produce after harvesting to prevent insect infestation. Now other chemicals and sulfurs are used, most of which are not as toxic as Dieldrin, but they may still create some problems.

Many people become sensitive to one or more of these chemicals and may experience symptoms after consuming chemically treated produce; some very sensitive people may get sick just from being around the fruits or vegetables or their boxes. People who become chemically sensitive must often avoid a great number of foods and products that are sprayed or grown with chemicals. Even soaking the fruits in bleach, for example, or washing them with soap may not remove enough spray residue for the fruit to be tolerated. Pesticide spray residues in foods are not only a problem for the chemically sensitive person but are of long-range concern to the general public because of their potential for promoting cancer.

Many chemical sprays are used on cultivated vegetables. In some ways the cruciferous vegetables may be the biggest problem in this regard, because they absorb the chemicals so well. Cabbage, broccoli, cauliflower, and brussels sprouts may be eaten more now because of their alleged reduction of cancer potential, but if they are sprayed with subtle carcinogens, that potential may actually be increased. Certified organic produce may be helpful in this regard, especially with vegetables without any skin to protect them.

Meat and poultry can also be contaminated by sprays. Much of the feed for these animals has been sprayed or may have pesticide residues. The animals themselves may be sprayed on occasion. The fat of animals is where the chemicals become most concentrated, so for that reason and to avoid increased saturated fats, I recommend that nearly everyone minimize consumption of animal fats.

Fruits, especially dried fruits such as dates and figs, as well as many grains and legumes, may be fumigated with chemicals such as methyl bromide to protect them from insects and molds. Bananas are gassed with ethylene to help them ripen. Sulfuring foods by treating them with sulfur dioxide helps keep them looking "fresher" and may keep dried fruits brighter and moister. Corn, for example, may be soaked in sulfur dioxide, and wine may have excess residues of sulfur dioxide. Sulfured foods are fairly common. Dried fruits such as apricots, raisins, and peaches are often sulfured. But even if dried fruits are unsulfured, they may be fumigated, and many of those chemicals may cause irritations or allergic symptoms.

FOOD PROCESSING AND STORAGE

This section discusses many of the chemicals that are used by the food manufacturers. Fruits, vegetables, and whole grains, are ground, mashed, boiled, and taken through many processes to create the multitude of boxed, canned, packaged, and plastic wrapped "foods" that we find in our stores.

Chemicals are added to foods in three ways. First, there are the intentional additives that become ingredients in our foods. These chemicals are the only ones we will see listed on the packages, but sadly, there are many hidden additives that never appear on our "truth-in-packaging" labels; these are classified as "contaminants." Chemicals that are used during processing may contaminate the foods without being direct additives. Chemicals used in packaging may get into foods as well. Plastics, cans, and boxes may all pose a danger, since various chemicals and metals are used in their production. Finally, there are the "silent additives," which are of most concern—the pesticides; chemicals in water and air; antibiotics, hormones, and other medicines given to animals; and ubiquitous industrial chemical pollutants. The best way to prevent harm from these "economic poisons" is to prohibit their use in the first place.

It sometimes seems that there is more concern about chemical exposures in the home or at work, where very little regulation protects us from toxic substances, than about chemical dangers in food. Food additives, in particular, are more closely regulated by the FDA, so that these chemicals pose less short-term risk. However, we do not really know the risks posed by long-term use of most chemicals, especially since we are exposed to so many that if we do develop some health problems, it would be difficult to isolate which specific chemical(s) or other factors may have generated them.

Just because certain food additives are used today and deemed "safe," that does not mean that they are, in fact, safe. The FDA must be constantly aware of possible long-range effects. It is currently conducting or overseeing a great deal of research regarding both chemicals in use and potential new ones. The FDA can change the status of any chemical used in food, removing old ones from use or approving new ones. Some additives that were found to be unsafe and removed after years of use include Red Dye #2, cyclamates, and cobalt sulfate. Currently under investigation as suspicious are sodium nitrite, most artificial coloring agents, and caffeine.

There are currently about 3,000 food additives approved for use in the foods we eat or the beverages we drink. As mentioned earlier, the average American consumes nearly 150 pounds of additives each year, nearly 90 percent of it sugar. In 1980, almost 30 billion pounds of sweeteners were consumed by the public. Salt intake is about 15 pounds per year per person, while various other food additives account for another 5–10 pounds. Additives have really helped the success of both the "junk food" and "fast food" markets, where a great deal of that 150 pounds of additives is consumed.

In 1958, the U.S. Congress approved the FDA's "Generally Recognized as Safe" (GRAS) list when it enacted the Delaney Clause, which also required rigid testing for any new food additives. Some several thousand additives that were already in use were reviewed by a number of scientists, and those that were felt to be safe were placed on the GRAS list. This meant that they were accepted without further testing. The accepted list also included several thousand substances, such as salt, sugar, spices, vitamins, minerals, flavorings, preservatives, emulsifiers, and so on. With some of these, levels or application to certain foods are restricted; they are classified as "for intended use based on standard manufacturing processes." Other additives can be used freely.

One of the problems with the GRAS list is lack of knowledge regarding many of the additives. With better testing, some of them have been shown to be unsafe, particularly when increased consumption causes intake to exceed "intended exposure" levels. In 1977, a fairly extensive review of the GRAS list was undertaken; many of the additives are still being investigated.

As noted in *A Consumer's Dictionary of Food Additives* (Crown Publishers, 1984), Ruth Winter clarifies a 1980 report of the FDA's ten-year evaluation of 415 common additives (some evaluated as groups). Only 305 were considered safe, a Class I rating, for their current and projected uses. Another 68 were given Class II ratings—that is, they were deemed safe as currently used, but it was felt that more research was needed to evaluate their effects at higher levels. These included some of the basic vitamins and minerals, such as vitamins A and D, iron, and zinc salts. Class III included 19 substances, such as BHA, BHT, and caffeine, where further research brought up more questions; their use was approved until further testing showed them to be unsafe. Could the FDA's motto be "better sorry than safe"? Class IV included five items that were generally safe but that required some use restrictions, due to sensitivities in certain individuals. These included salt, modified starches used as thickening agents, and lactic acid and calcium lactate used in infant formulas. Another 18 items, rated as Class V, were taken off the list until sufficient data could be gathered to prove them safe. These include some glycerides and specific iron salts.

Types of Additives

Sweeteners. There are many sweeteners used in processed foods in addition to all of the natural sweet flavor from fructose in fruits, lactose in milk, and maltose in breads. Sweeteners are the most common additive and they are consumed in the largest volume.

Natural or nutritional sweeteners are extracts of real food. These sweeteners, as pure carbohydrate and simple sugar, contain four calories per gram. For example, one tablespoon of cane sugar contains 50 calories but no other nutrition. Honey has about 64 calories, maple syrup about 50, and raw sugar about 15 per tablespoon. Other nutritional sweeteners include beet sugar, brown sugar, molasses, fructose, corn syrup, barley malt, and rice syrup.

The nonnutritional, or chemical, sweeteners are also very popular, especially in our overweight culture. There are currently two common artificial sweeteners, saccharin and aspartame. Cyclamate was banned in 1969 but is still legal in some countries that feel that the results of cancer studies in rats are not a cause of concern for humans. The FDA has been trying to ban saccharin, but the public continues to demand it. Aspartame is somewhat controversial; as Nutrasweet or Equal, it is now the most common artificial sweetener.

These chemicals are supposedly used to minimize obesity, but many people use them merely as an opportunity to eat other, more caloric foods and desserts. Studies show that artificial sweeteners do not really help weight loss in the majority of people unless they are already eating a low-calorie diet. It is better to eat the naturally sweet foods, such as the whole grains, fruits, and vegetables, to obtain an adequate level of fiber, vitamins, and minerals along with that sweet flavor, and to reduce intake of the processed, more heavily sweetened foods.

Flavorings. Flavorings constitute the largest group of all the additives, with sweeteners being the biggest portion. There are over 2,000 different flavorings, 500 natural and more than 1,500 synthetic. Flavor additives are used to attain a certain taste in foods, and this taste needs to be consistent, persistent (last with time), and uniform throughout the food item. Since many ingredients used in preparing foods may vary in flavor, these additives are used to ensure that the consumer's expectations are met.

The natural flavors, which are basically concentrated extracts, include the essential oils, various spices, and oleoresins. Most of these are considered safe and in my opinion are more acceptable for use in foods than are the synthetic versions. A few natural flavors, such as nutmeg and safrole, the oil from saffron, may be toxic.

The synthetic versions of natural flavors are made from a great number of chemicals. Current FDA regulations state that any of these chemicals need be listed on packaging only as "artificial flavor" or "imitation flavor." If there is only one chemical used, it might be listed, but to simulate a particular flavor, a chemist must often use a sensitive mixture of a number of chemicals

Most of the artificial flavors are on the GRAS list. Although they are not as dangerous as the food colors, they are much more widely used. Some of them can be toxic to the nervous system, the kidneys, or liver, but in the amounts in which they are commonly used, they are usually fairly safe. They are not known to be carcinogenic.

Flavorings are used in a wide variety of foods. Soft drinks, chewing gum, confections, ice creams, baked goods, puddings, gelatins, and other desserts are some

NATURAL FLAVORINGS

vanilla	licorice	cocoa	garlic
kola nut	mustard	cassia	clove
fenugreek	peppermint	anise	lemon oil
fennel	orange oil	ginger	other fruit oils

examples. Most of these flavorings are considered fairly safe in modest amounts. There are also "flavor enhancers," substances that seem to bring out or improve the flavors of the foods in which they are used. Salt is probably the most common, though monosodium glutamate (MSG) is also used frequently. Maltol is another example of a flavoring agent.

Most labeling on packages will not specify whether flavorings are artificial or natural; they usually just state "natural" or "artificial flavoring." So if we want to avoid the 1,500 or so chemicals used as artificial flavors we had better start reading labels.

SOME CHEMICALS* USED AS ARTIFICIAL FLAVORS

Amyl alcohol	Isoamyl alcohol and acid
Amyl salts	Linalol
Benzaldehyde	Linalyl salts
Benzyl acetate	Nonyl alcohol
Benzyl alcohol	Nonyl salts
Butyl acetate and salts	Octyl alcohol and salts
Diacetyl	Phenethyl alcohol and salts
Ethyl acetate	Pinenes
Ethyl butyrate	Propyl alcohol and salts
Ethyl formate	Rhodinol
Formic acid	Salicylaldehyde
Geraniol	Valeric acid
Geramyl acids	

* Many of these chemicals can be found naturally in some foods, such as fruits or nuts, but most of those used to flavor foods are prepared synthetically.

Coloring agents. As a general category, this one is probably of most concern. Natural colors include carotene, caramel, annatto, beet red (powdered beets), saffron, turmeric, paprika, grapes, vegetable and fruit juices, and titanium dioxide. All of these are considered safe in the usual amounts used to color foods, though there is some concern about extracts such as safrole and turmeric.

COMMON FOODS THAT CONTAIN
ARTIFICIAL FLAVORS

Alcoholic beverages	Ices	Sauces
Baked goods	Icings	Seasonings
Candy	Jams	Shortening
Cereals	Jellies	Soda pop
Cordials	Liquors	Soups
Desserts	Maple syrup	Spices
Gelatins	Margarine	Syrups
Gum	Meats	Yogurts
Ice cream	Puddings	

However, most coloring agents are synthetic and potentially toxic. These synthetics are a fake substitute for the natural, fresh color of foods. Artificial colors are chemicals synthesized from petroleum and coal-tar products. Many of these chemicals have been used by the food industry as experiments on human beings, and some have been withdrawn because of studies showing toxicity or carcinogenicity.

Colors derived for food, drugs, and cosmetics (labeled FDC colors by the Food and Drug Administration) have been used for many years. Many of the same dyes and pigments are used to color clothing. In 1938, about 15 dyes were certified for use in foods. Through the years, many have been eliminated from food use. In 1950, FDC Orange #1 and #2 and Red #32 were withdrawn because they caused illness in children. More were removed in 1973 for various reasons (hyperactivity, allergy, general toxicity, carcinogenicity); these included Red #1 and #4, Yellow #1, #2, #3, and #4 and Violet #1. In 1976, Red #2 was removed (except for use in coloring orange skins), because of its carcinogenicity in rats. More recently, Orange B (used in casings for frankfurters and sausage) was withdrawn because of cancer links. Those in current use include:

- *Citrus Red #2*—withdrawn in 1976, except for use in coloring oranges, because it was shown to cause cancer in animals. It had been widely used in desserts, cereal, and maraschino cherries.

- *Red #3 (erythrosine)*—used in cherries, cherry pie, gelatins, ice cream, fruit cocktail, candy, sherbet, pudding, cereals, and baked goods. It is on the safe list, but it has been suggested that this coal-tar derivative is harmful, possibly causing gene mutations, cancers, or changes in brain chemistry. Clear evidence is lacking, so FDC Red #3 stays on the safe list and does not have to be listed on labels except as "artificial color."

- *Red #40 (Allura Red AC)*—took the place of banned Red #2 and is used in foods, drugs, and cosmetics. It may cause cancer in animals.

- *Blue #1*—a coal-tar derivative used in soft drinks, candy, ice cream, cereals, and puddings. It is on the permanent safe list. It is a possible allergen, and it can cause tumors in animals at the site of injection.

- *Blue #2*—used the same way as Blue #1 and is on the permanent FDA list. The World Health Organization rates it in category B—questionable for use in food.

- *Green #3*—this color is used for green foods such as mint jelly, gelatins, candy, frozen desserts, and cereals. It is classified as safe but is a potential allergen and is tumorigenic upon injection.

- *Yellow #5 (tartrazine)*—this is the most notable color agent, partly because it causes the most immediate allergic reactions in people sensitive to salicylates, such as aspirins (to which it is related), and because, by law, it is the only artificial color that must be listed by name on packaging. Tartrazine is used in yellow-colored foods such as spaghetti, puddings, gelatin, soft drink, sherbets, ice cream, cereals, and candy. Attempts to ban it have not succeeded. Most people can tolerate some Yellow #5 in foods, but those with sensitivity may develop skin reactions or asthma symptoms (problems are worst in sensitive asthmatics).

- *Yellow #6*—another coal-tar color, it is used in many foods, such as candies, baked goods, carbonated beverages, and gelatins. It is considered safe, though there is also some concern about allergy.

There are several major concerns with colored foods. The first is potential toxicity, including allergic reactions, liver stress from metabolizing these chemicals, and potential carcinogenicity. Another problem is that they may cause behavior problems in children. Benjamin Feingold, M.D., has shown that hyperactivity in children is related to food colorings. Many kids with short attention spans and learning disabilities improved on a diet without food coloring. Still another concern is that the FDA does not even require food manufacturers to list the specific agents used in their foods; they need only be designated as "artificial colors," so we cannot differentiate between those that are classified safe and those in question. As stated, yellow #5 is the only one that must be listed, because of possibly allergic reactions.

On the basis of all the currently available information, my advice is to avoid all foods that have artificial colors listed on their labels. Many children's (and adult's) drugs have added food coloring, and we must be careful with these as well. If it is necessary to take medications, I advise taking the pure pharmaceutical preparations as white tablets or clear fluids if available. In that way, we are most likely to get the effect we want and avoid other, undesired ones. It is possible that some side effects from drugs are caused by ingredients other than the active ones, such as these coloring agents.

Preservatives. This group of about 100 different chemicals is used to prevent spoilage. Each of these is specifically mentioned on the label when added to food. There are three main types of preservatives: antioxidants, mold inhibitors, and sequestrants.

- *Antioxidants*, such as BHA, BHT, and benzoic acid, are used to prevent oxidation of the fats within foods. Oxidation leads to a change in the flavor and odor of certain ingredients, which essentially spoils the whole food. These additives are used commonly in many packaged and bottled foods that contain fats, such as shortening and vegetable oils. Cereals and crackers commonly contain BHA or BHT.

- *Mold inhibitors*, also termed "antimycotics," are used commonly in breads and baked goods to prevent or retard the growth of yeasts and molds. Cheeses, syrups, and other foods might also contain mold inhibitors. Some common ones are sodium or calcium proprionate, sodium diacetate, sorbic acid, acetic acid, lactic acid, and various sodium and potassium salts. When these are used, they are specifically listed on the label. Most of these are fairly safe.

- *Sequestrants* are substances that prevent physical and/or chemical changes to the color, odor, flavor, or appearance of a food. These are commonly used in dairy foods as sodium, potassium, or calcium salts of citric, tartaric, or pyrophosphoric acids—for example, sodium citrate. EDTA, a sequestrant that binds metals, is used mainly in liquids, such as soda pops and salad dressings.

There are other common preservatives—salt, vinegar, and sugar are the main ones. Sulfur dioxide is used often to preserve dried fruits. Propyl gallate is an antioxidant used in fats and oils.

Acids, alkalis, buffers, and neutralizers. Many of these are common mineral acids and/or salts that help adjust or balance the pH (acid-alkaline condition) of foods. These items may or may not be listed on the package label. Acids are used in baking to help make the dough rise and in soft drinks (as phosphoric acid or phosphates) for a tangy taste. Citric acid (from citrus fruits), malic acid (from apples), and tartaric acid (from grapes) are other mild acids used in foods. Alkalis, or bases, are substances that reduce the acidity of foods. Some examples are baking powder, baking soda, aluminum hydroxide in cocoa, and aluminum carbonate in various crackers, cookies, and candy. Buffers and neutralizers help to adjust or maintain the acid-base balance of foods. Calcium carbonate, sodium aluminum phosphate, potassium tartrate, and ammonium bicarbonate are some examples.

Bleaching and maturing agents. Most of these are used in flour products and sometimes in cheeses. Bleaching agents such as benzoyl peroxide and chlorine dioxide are used to help oxidation and speed the whitening of fresh-ground flour. These chemicals also act as maturing agents and are sometimes called "bread improvers." Chlorine, nitrosyl chloride, and oxide of nitrogen are some other food bleaches. Milder ones that are used to aid in yeast and dough conditioning include mineral salts, potassium bromate or iodate, and ammonium sulfate or phosphate. Most of these are used in small quantities and are listed on the labels.

439

Moisture controls. These chemicals help prevent foods from drying out or from getting too moist. Calcium silicate is used in salt to prevent caking; it attracts the moisture instead of the salt. Moisture controllers are also termed "humectants." Other examples include propylene glycol, glycerine, and sorbitol. These additives are not always listed on the label.

Activity controls. These agents either slow down or speed up the ripening or aging of foods. They are most often used on fruits or vegetables and so would not be listed on any labels. Ethylene gas is sprayed on bananas to speed ripening. Potatoes and onions may be prevented from sprouting by application of maleic hydrazide. This is a potentially toxic chemical that is also sprayed on most tobacco crops in the U.S. Some enzymes such as amylase may be used to stimulate food reactions such as the digestion of starch or the fermentation of sugar. This is helpful in brewing alcoholic beverages and making bread, candy, or certain milk concentrates.

Emulsifiers. Emulsifiers help to blend water and oils together to maintain the consistency and homogeneity of such products as mayonnaise and salad dressings. These additives are in part stabilizers and thickeners. They help keep the fineness of the grain and uniformity of the material, which allows cake mixes, for example, to work so well. Lecithin, mono- and diglycerides, and propylene glycol alginate are some examples. These are fairly safe and are listed on labels. Sorbitan and the "polysorbates" are also useful emulsifiers.

Texturizers. Texturizers are stabilizers and processing aids that give body and texture to food. These additives are mostly safe, natural ones that are usually listed on the label. Agar-agar, gelatin, and cellulose and other gums are some texturizers. They may be used in ice cream for consistency and to maintain the size of the ice crystals. Some gums or carageenans are used in chocolate milk to thicken it and prevent the cocoa from settling out. Pectin, starch, and gelatin are used in confections, and thickeners such as the alginates might be used in soft drinks. To keep canned tomatoes and potatoes from breaking apart in the fluid, calcium chloride or other calcium salts are used to maintain texture. Nitrites and nitrates are used in curing meats to maintain pink color and texture. These nitrogenous additives and the foods that they are used in are best avoided for a variety of health reasons.

Other processing aids and clarifying agents. Sanitizing agents help to clear bacteria and debris from foods. Gelatin and albumin help to remove small particles of copper or iron from liquids such as beer and vinegar. Tannin from teas can be used to clarify liquids such as beer and wine. These agents may or may not be listed on food labels.

Nutritional supplements. This category includes a long list of both natural and synthetic vitamins and minerals used to both enrich foods (add what was depleted during processing) or fortify them (add more than was there or something totally new). The B vitamins are commonly added back into grain and cereal products, as is iron. Vitamin A is used in margarine, D in milk, and C in fruit drinks, while iodine is added to table salt. Some of these additions are helpful, but eating the whole food is a better way to get the nourishment. The supplements most commonly added to foods are thiamine (B_1), riboflavin (B_2), and iron. Next in use are niacin (B_3), calcium salts, and vitamins D and A. According to what is lost during food processing, more pyridoxine (B_6), magnesium, chromium, manganese, and others should be added back to foods.

○ WHAT IS OUR BEST APPROACH TO FOOD ADDITIVES?

First, we must try to reorient ourselves to the natural diet of our ancestors and eat more wholesome foods, such as fresh fruits and vegetables, whole grains, nuts, seeds, beans, and range-fed animals. To find and purchase the organic produce and organically fed poultry and beef, and thus support those farmers and ranchers (and our own health) who raise them, will make these foods more available and at a better price. And whenever possible, we should grow our own foods, plant more fruit and nut trees, and share or barter our harvest with our friends and neighbors.

It is also very important to buy and eat less of the packaged foods that contain additives. We should definitely avoid the nitrates and nitrites, as they can form carcinogenic nitrosamines in the food and in our body. The sulfites, such as sulfur dioxide, sodium sulfite, bisulfite, and metabisulfite, which are commonly used to prevent or reduce spoilage or discoloration, are best avoided, particularly by people with allergies. BHA and BHT, as well as EDTA, should be consumed minimally, as should the flavor enhancer MSG. Artificial colors should definitely be left out of our diet; artificial flavors should be minimized also. See the accompanying chart for a list of common additives that are best avoided, those that should be used with caution, and those that are probably safe.

Food Shopping

The following chart is a brief summary of my understanding of the safety of food additives. All of these substances are discussed in the next section.

Please copy this list and take it with you if you need it as a shopping guide for the more healthful packaged products. Add any of your own concerns to the list, in case you have any allergies, digestive problems, or follow a low-salt, low-sugar, or low-fat diet.

The Center for Science in the Public Interest (CSPI) produces a very helpful, large and colorful chart, "Chemical Cuisine." CSPI can be contacted at 1501 16th St. NW, Washington, DC 20036.

FOOD ADDITIVE CHART

Additives to Avoid

Artificial colors (FD&C colors)
Sodium nitrite and nitrate
BHT (butylated hydroxytoluene)
Saccharin
Sulfites (especially sodium bisulfite)
Sulfur dioxide
BVO (Brominated Vegetable Oil)

Additives to Limit (use with caution)

BHA (butylated hydroxyanisole)
MSG (monosodium glutamate)
Sugars (sucrose, dextrose, corn syrup)
Artificial flavorings
THBQ
Propyl gallate
EDTA
Hydrogenated vegetable oils
Salt
Aspartame
Caffeine
Propylene glycol
Gums
Xylitol
Aluminum salts

Probably Safe Additives

Vitamins A, C, and E
Beta-carotene or Carotene
Carrageenan
Annatto
Acids—citric, sorbic, lactic
Alginates
Minerals—iron, zinc, and others
Glycerin—mono- and diglycerides
Gelatin
Pectin
Natural flavoring
Calcium proprionate
Polysorbate 60, 65, 80
Sorbitol
Sodium benzoate
Lecithin
Casein and lactose
Vanillin
Potassium sorbate

○ COMMON FOOD ADDITIVES

This section provides more specific information about individual food additives—what each is used for, in what common foods, and whether it is safe (or its safety is unknown). Of the more than 3,000 different chemicals that are used in preparing foods for sale to consumers, only some are true "food additives"— agents actually added to the foods and listed on the ingredient label, such as the just desribed emulsifiers, sweeteners, or preservatives. Many other additives are not listed but are used in various stages of processing; a few of these will also be mentioned in my list. Some of these are GRAS list additives, while others are not meant to be consumed at all. These latter chemicals include solvents such as formaldehyde, benzene, and carbon tetrachloride—all carcinogens—used to extract "salad oils," for example. Some of these oils may also be heated up to 400 degrees Fahrenheit which may change their molecular structure. Lye may even be used to extract the fatty acids. That is why many people use "cold-pressed" oils, because they are not made with solvents or by heating. Different detergents and bleaching agents may also be used in processing without being listed on the label.

Although here we are talking about "food" additives, many of these synthetic chemicals are used in the preparation of pharmaceutical drugs, both prescription and over the counter. None appear on the labels. Large amounts of FD&C colors are used in drugs, and these are often potentially as toxic as the active ingredients. In his book *How to Survive Modern Technology* (Ecology Press, 1979), Charles T. McGee, M.D. describes an analysis of a common female hormone product, Premarin. This is a conjugated estrogen drug made from pregnant mare's urine (sounds great!) used most commonly in menopausal women. Estrogens are, of course, very helpful in relieving menopausal symptoms, but they can also cause other symptoms and may play a role in carcinogenesis. Besides a little bit of estrogen, an analysis of Premarin shows more than twenty-five other chemicals, including talc, polyethylene glycol, shellac, edible black ink, carnauba wax, sucrose, corn starch, propyl paraben, Yellow Dye #5 (tartrazine), sodium benzoate, and more. Most pharmaceutical drugs, especially children's flavorful liquid preparations, contain many chemicals besides those we think we are getting; and many of these additives can cause problems.

There is also a long list of contaminants that we will never see on food labels. All the pesticides, herbicides, and toxic environmental chemicals from dumps or from the water can get into our food. Closest to the consumer are the fungicides that are often sprayed on crops after they are harvested. These may still be concentrated on crops, in the produce boxes, or in the papers wrapping the foods. Some people may be sensitive to these substances; in addition, the effects of long-term intake of small amounts of these toxic chemicals is not yet known.

The best we can do is to be aware of what is known and demand that the government and food growers give us complete information. Then, we can either push for change or find alternatives that will meet our needs.

INDIVIDUAL FOOD ADDITIVES

Acacia (*gum arabic*) is a vegetable gum, a thick excretion that comes from many species of acacia tree found in Africa and the southern United States. It has been used for many thousands of years, especially in the Middle East. Acacia gum is a complex polysaccharide that is soluble in water and in foods; it tends to blend mixtures together, retards sugar crystallization, and acts as a thickener. For these reasons, it is used in the confection industry for candies, jellies and glazes, and chewing gum. It is also used as a stabilizer in soft drinks and beer.

443

Gum arabic has been on the GRAS list since 1976 and is actually pretty safe, according to most studies. The acacia tree is a fairly common allergen, however, and there are some people who also have allergic responses to oral ingestion of acacia, with possible skin, sinus, or asthmatic reactions. Anyone who is allergic, especially to acacia, should avoid gum arabic. Although most of the foods that contain this additive are overly processed or sweet, acacia gum itself seems safe in modest amounts.

Acetic acid (also *sodium acetate* and *sodium diacetate*). Acetic acid is another ancient food additive; it is the acid in vinegar and is found naturally in apples, cocoa, coffee, wine, aged cheeses, grapes, and other fruits. Acetic acid is used as an acidic flavoring agent for catsup, pickles, mayonnaise, wine, and some cheeses. It is found in any foods that are preserved in vinegar. Acetic acid also used as a synthetic flavoring agent (possibly as ethyl acetate) in many beverages, processed cheese, cheese spreads, cottage cheese, baked goods, confections, pickles, and vinegar foods. Though its vapors can be irritating to the bronchial tubes, it is on the GRAS list and seems to be safe as currently used. A 1980 review maintained its GRAS status.

Agar-agar (*seaweed extract*) is a polysaccharide that comes from several varieties of red algae. In liquid, it has the ability to swell and gel. Agar is used in making ice creams, jellies, icings, preserves, and for thickening milk and cream. It can be used as a substitute for gelatin, which is an extract of animal proteins. Agar also acts as a mild bulk laxative. It is used by the food industry and is also sold in stores for home use. Agar-agar is a safe, even beneficial, food additive that is on the GRAS list. Though in rare situations it can be a mild allergen, it is otherwise completely safe.

Alginates—*alginic acid; algin gum; ammonium, calcium, potassium, and sodium alginate; propylene glycol alginate.*

These are all (except for propylene glycol alginate) natural extracts of various seaweeds. They are used in the food industry primarily as thickening and stabilizing agents. Alginates are also water retainers, prevent ice crystal formation, and help uniform distribution of flavors through foods. As a clarifying agent, they add smoothness to mixtures. The alginates are used in ice creams, custards, ices, chocolate milk, cheeses, cheese spreads, salad dressings, jams, jellies, confections, baked goods, toppings, and beverages.

All of these alginates are on the GRAS list and were reapproved in 1980. Propylene glycol or antifreeze, a fairly safe solvent, does pose a little more cause for concern; the propylene glycol alginate salt is used fairly often in food processing.

Aluminum salts—*alum (aluminum potassium sulfate); sodium aluminum phosphate; aluminum ammonium sulfate; aluminum calcium silicate; aluminum hydroxide; and others.* Since aluminum is found abundantly in the earth's crust, we all ingest it daily. However, in recent years, there have been concerns about accumulation of aluminum in the body and its effect on brain chemistry and health. (See *Aluminum* discussion in Chapter 6, *Minerals*.) Other than this, most of these compounds are well handled by the body and considered safe, and all are on the GRAS list.

Aluminum compounds are used to adjust acidity (that is, as a buffer), as an astringent, to keep canned produce firm, to lighten food texture, and as anticaking agents. Sodium aluminum phosphate, the most commonly used, is found in baking powder and self-rising flours. Alum is used as a clarifier for sugar and as a hardening agent; aluminum calcium silicate is used as an anticaking agent in salt and other powders. Aluminum hydroxide is a strong alkali agent that can be toxic but is safe in small amounts, as a leavening agent in baked goods, for example. It is also used in antiperspirants and antacids. Aluminum ammonium sulfate is used as an astringent, buffer, and neutralizing agent by the cereal industry; it is also used in baking powder. By itself, it can be burning to the mucous membranes. In small amounts most of these aluminum salts seem to be well tolerated in food. Overuse of aluminum products, including cookware, deodorant sprays, and antacids, may lead to aluminum toxicity; however, this is not very likely from moderate food use.

Ammonium salts—*ammonium bicarbonate, ammonium chloride, ammonium phosphate, ammonium sulfate.* Ammonium salts occur naturally in foods when ammonia (as in proteins) combines with acids. Ammonium ions are important in the body for acid-base balance, in amino acid metabolism, and in the urinary tract. Ammonium salts are used in foods as leavening agents, dough conditioners, and buffers to lighten texture; to create uniformity within a food mixture; and occasionally as flavor enhancers. Ammonium bicarbonate is most often used as a leavening agent for baked goods and confections. Ammonium chloride is used as a dough conditioner and a nutrient for yeast in breads and baked goods. It is also used in making batteries and dyes. Ammonium phosphate is used in baking powder, as a buffer and leavening agent in breads, rolls, and other baked goods, and in the brewing industry. Ammonium sulfate is also used, mainly as a buffer and dough conditioner.

All of these ammonium salts are generally recognized as safe (all are on the GRAS list). Ammonia by itself can be toxic in large amounts, as it affects basic biochemistry and kidney function, but as salts in small amounts, it seems to be okay.

Annatto is a natural coloring agent extracted from the seeds of a tropical tree, *Bixa orellano.* It is a yellow to light orange vegetable dye that is used commonly in dairy products such as butter, buttermilk, cottage cheese, and other cheeses. Annatto is also used to color margarine, ice cream, cake mixes, baked goods, and the casings of hot dogs. Annatto is on the GRAS list and really has no known toxicity. Research, which is still going on, has not yet shown any ill effects.

Ascorbic acid (vitamin C)—*ascorbate salts: sodium ascorbate, ascorbyl palmitate.* Ascorbic acid, either natural or synthetic, is a very popular vitamin supplement. It is found naturally in many fruits and vegetables, such as citrus fruits and green and red peppers. It is also used in food processing as an antioxidant and preservative; vitamin C, as ascorbyl palmitate, prevents oxidation and rancidity, especially in fats, and can help preserve the flavor, color, and aroma of the foods in which it is used. Vitamin C is also used as a nutritive additive for artificial fruit drinks and has recently been added to cured meats to prevent the formation of carcinogenic nitrosamines from their added nitrites. Ascorbic acids or ascorbates are also used in soft drinks, alcoholic beverages such as beer and ale, juices, candies, dry milk, and dips.

Ascorbic acid is basically nontoxic even in high doses. Its use in food is often beneficial, as vitamin C is a required nutrient, and a deficiency can cause serious problems. Vitamin C is the most commonly used vitamin supplement in our culture.

Aspartame—*Nutrasweet, Equal.* Aspartame is the latest of the artificial sweeteners. Actually, it is somewhat more natural than the previously discovered cyclamates and saccharin, and probably safer. Aspartame is a mixture of two amino acids, aspartic acid and phenylalanine, which are both found in foods and used by the body as building blocks for proteins. It was accidentally discovered by a researcher who tasted the result of a chemical reaction and found it very sweet. Aspartame is about 200 times sweeter than sugar; since it is so much sweeter than sugar, very little is needed, so it is much less caloric. Cyclamate is 30 times sweeter than sugar but was banned in 1970 as a possible

445

carcinogen. Saccharin is 300 times sweeter; it, too, is close to being banned.

The huge "world of dieting" needs a low-calorie sweetener, and right now aspartame is its main product. It was approved by the FDA in 1974 and has become the big favorite. Nearly 70 percent of American households use it in some form, and 70–80 million Americans use artificial sweeteners. In 1980, aspartame, as Equal, was accepted as a tabletop sweetener to be added to foods and beverages by the general public. In 1983, it was approved for use in soft drinks. Under the brand name Nutrasweet, aspartame is used in candies, diet foods, soft drinks, and chewing gums.

There are some potential problems, especially for people with phenylketonuria (PKU), a genetic disease that affects about 1 in 15,000 people. Lacking the enzyme to metabolize phenylalanine, people with PKU cannot handle large amounts of phenylalanine, either as it occurs naturally in foods or in aspartame, which breaks down into aspartic acid and phenylalanine. With increased levels, these individuals may experience headache, dizziness, sleeping problems, and other behavioral changes. A study by R. Wurtman, M.D. and the Community Nutrition Institute reported in 1984 that people without PKU could also be sensitive to increased levels of phenylalanine and might exhibit the same symptoms of headaches, dizziness, mood swings, insomnia, and possibly increased blood pressure. Aspartame should also probably not be used by pregnant women, since high phenylalanine levels might affect the baby's intelligence. Further research is needed on this, but occasional small amounts are probably "safe."

In sum, aspartame is not completely safe, and some people may be sensitive to it, but it is probably better than any other artificial sweetener. Even so I recommend that people eat a low-calorie diet including foods that are naturally sweet.

Benzoic acid—*sodium benzoate (benzoate of sodium)*. Benzoic acid or its sodium salt is commonly used as a preservative in food processing. Benzoic acid is also found naturally in many berries, cherry bark, prunes, anise, cloves, cassia bark or cinnamon, and tea. It was first found in gum benzoin in the 1600s.

Benzoic acid is used as a flavoring agent in chocolate, orange, lemon, nut, and other flavors in candies, beverages, baked goods, ice cream, and chewing gums. As a preservative, it is used in a wide variety of processed foods, including margarine, soft drinks, juices, pickles, condiments, jellies, and jams. In perfumes and cosmetics it prevents spoilage by microorganisms. Benzoic acid is also a mild antifungal agent. In medicine, sodium benzoate is occasionally used in testing liver function, as it is metabolized by the liver.

Benzoic acid and sodium benzoate are probably the safest of the chemical preservatives, certainly much safer than BHA and BHT. Tests have not shown the benzoin derivatives to be carcinogenic. Occasionally, larger amounts can cause intestinal upset, especially with weakened liver function. Benzoic acid can also be slightly irritating to the skin, eyes, and mucous membranes, and both it and sodium benzoate can cause allergic reactions, though these are rare. Overall, small amounts of these additives seem to be safe.

BHA (butylated hydroxyanisole). BHA and BHT (see below) are very interesting chemicals. They are both petroleum by-products used in preserving foods. BHA acts as a preservative and an antioxidant to prevent the rancidity of fats and fat-containing foods and thus prevent spoilage that causes a change in taste, odor, or appearance. BHA is used commonly in many packaged and processed foods, probably more than BHT, and is a little easier for the human liver and kidneys to metabolize. Further studies are being done.

BHA is used in such foods as dry cereals, crackers, instant potatoes or potato flakes, soup bases, seasonings, dry mixes for desserts or beverages, canned or bottled beverages, lard, shortening, baked goods, ice cream, candy, and more. It is almost always listed on the label, but it may not be when it has been added to lard or shortening that is an ingredient of the food product.

BHA is still on the GRAS list; during the 1980 review, additional studies were recommended, though previous studies had revealed no major hazards to public health. The FDA has set limits on the amount of BHA that particular foods may contain, such as 50 ppm (parts per million) in dry cereals or 200 ppm in shortenings. Allergies to BHA and BHT have been known. Liver toxicity is possible but is unlikely from the small amounts used in food. There is some suggestion that both these antioxidants may be helpful in preventing disease and aging, as they reduce oxidative and free-radical irritation of the tissues. This has not been scientifically proven, and my advice is to avoid any regular use of the chemical BHA.

BHT (butylated hydroxytoluene). BHT is another common antioxidant. It is not used as frequently as BHA, probably because it may be a little more toxic. BHT has a mild preservative effect as well. It has a faint odor, and rancidity.

Common foods that contain BHT include enriched rice, breakfast cereals, shortenings, animal fats, dog and cat foods, potato flakes, chewing gum, and cake mixes. BHT may also be a cancer preventive; it has recently been used by some people in the treatment of herpes viral infections. If it is helpful in such cases, it is probably because of its antioxidant properties, but there is no good evidence that it works, and the doses that are needed for such treatment have not been established.

BHT can be irritating to the liver and kidneys, especially when there is decreased function of these organs. Allergic reactions have been known. There is also some concern that BHT may convert to other substances in the human body that may be carcinogenic. The use of BHT is prohibited in England. In the United States, it is on the GRAS list, with further research pending. I suggest avoiding foods with BHT, partly because most of them are prefabricated food-industry creations and also because we do not really know whether BHT is safe.

Bromines—*calcium bromate, potassium bromate, brominated vegetable oil (BVO).* The bromates are used in flours and breads as dough conditioners and maturing agents. Since they are used during processing, these ingredients may not be listed on the label. Bromination makes oils heavier so that they can evenly distribute flavoring in soft drinks, especially citrus and fruit-flavored beverages, as well as in ices, ice cream, and some baked goods. BVO also gives drinks a cloudy appearance, so it may make those artificial fruit drinks resemble natural fruit juice.

The bromines and BVO are not considered safe, and the FDA limits their use. They have been known to cause allergic reactions, with high amounts causing intestinal irritation and food-poisoning symptoms as well as kidney or central nervous system problems. High doses may even be fatal. Small amounts of most of these chemicals can be tolerated, but the FDA currently has them, especially BVO, on the "suspect" list.

Caffeine is found naturally in coffee, tea, mate leaves, guarana root, and kola nuts. As part of coffee, tea, and cola, it is one of the world's big drugs. Caffeine is a stimulant to the heart, central nervous system, and respiratory system. It gives people "energy."

Caffeine is currently used as a flavoring in cola and root beer; by regulation, this chemical must be present in any beverage termed "cola" or "pepper." For any food in which it is naturally found, such as coffee, tea, or cocoa, caffeine need not be listed on the label. Much of the caffeine added to other foods is extracted in making decaffeinated coffee (and that has often been chemically treated with such solvents as formaldehyde, although I hear this usage is declining). Decaf has become more popular in recent years among those who do not want the caffeine effect. But there are also many people who still like their caffeine fix. On a trip to the supermarket to research food additives, I found "Jolt" cola, for those who want "all the sugar, and twice the caffeine"—fine if you like drinking caffeinated syrup.

Caffeine use is only questionably safe. It is on the GRAS list, but the 1980 review suggested further testing. One big concern is that caffeine passes the placental barrier, so it can affect the growing fetus; therefore, it is not recommended during pregnancy—or during nursing, since it also gets into mother's milk. Young children or anyone with cardiovascular disease or ulcer problems should avoid caffeine. In general, caffeine should be considered a psychoactive, potentially addictive drug and should be used intermittently and with caution. Regular or excessive use should clearly be avoided. (See the *Caffeine* program in Part Four.)

Calcium proprionate—*proprionic acid, sodium proprionate*. The proprionates are naturally found in dairy products such as butter and cheese. They are used as preservatives and mold inhibitors, as they reduce the growth of most fungi and some bacteria. Proprionic acid and its salts are used as mold inhibitors in baked goods, breads, rolls, cakes, and cupcakes and as preservatives in natural and processed cheeses, chocolate products, jelly, and preserves. Calcium proprionate, proprionic acid, and sodium proprionate are all safe. Studies in animals revealed no problems even with levels higher than are usually consumed. They have all been reapproved by the FDA and remain on the GRAS list.

Calcium salts—*calcium carbonate, chloride, citrate, gluconate, hydroxide, lactate, oxide, phosphate, and sulfate*. The various calcium salts are helpful in providing important

mineral calcium, which the body needs in significant quantity for many functions, especially healthy bones. Various calcium formulae, such as calcium carbonate and calcium gluconate, are taken commonly as dietary supplements to attain adequate calcium levels. Many calcium salts are used as nutrient additives in enriched foods, especially grain products—cereals, flours, infant formulas, cornmeal, farina, noodles, and breads.

Calcium salts are also used as emulsifiers in evaporated milk, frozen desserts, and breads; as dough conditioners in baked goods; and as clarifying agents in sweets. Some calcium salts, such as calcium carbonate, oxide, and hydroxide, are used as antacids and as buffering agents in milk products, for example, to help control acidity. Calcium lactate is used as a buffer in baking powder. Some salts, such as calcium chloride, gluconate, and hydroxide, act as firming agents. These may be used in jellies or in canned fruits, tomatoes, or potatoes. Calcium sulfate can act as a carrier for bleaches and is used in the brewing industry. Problems from use of the many calcium salts are very unlikely. High amounts of any of them could cause shifting of the body's acid-base balance. Their basic use in foods, however, is considered safe.

Caramel is made by heating sugar, giving it a burnt, slightly bittersweet taste. It is used both as a coloring for soft drinks such as colas and root beer, candies, ice cream, and baked goods—and in many different flavorings, such as butterscotch, chocolate, cola, caramel flavor, ginger ale, brandy, vanilla, and cream soda. Caramel is used mostly in beverages but also in ice cream, candy, and baked goods.

There is some question about the safety of caramel. The heating process uses ammonia, which may be toxic, and the nitrogen going into the caramelized sugar produces compounds which may be harmful. Studies regarding possible carcinogenesis have been negative so far; caramel in modest doses is still considered safe.

Carob (St. John's bread)—*locust bean gum*. Carob, or locust bean, is a natural flavoring that has seen increased use in the last decade as a healthier substitute for chocolate and sugar. Carob powder is an extract from the bean pods of the carob tree. It is more nutritious than other flavorings; it is termed St. John's bread because it is said that it sustained John the Baptist in the wilderness.

As a flavoring, it is part of caramel, butterscotch, chocolate, cherry, maple, and root beer flavors in beverages, ice cream, candies, baked goods, gelatin desserts, and toppings. Carob is used as a thickener and stabilizer as the gum extract added to foods such as chocolate milk, syrups, gassed whipped cream, cheeses, ice cream, and sherbert.

Carob is on the GRAS list. There have been some recent studies to see whether it is mutagenic, with particular concern for pregnant women; so far, nothing has been found. In fact, it is possible that locust bean gum in significant nontoxic doses may lower cholesterol. Overall, this food additive is considered safe.

Carotenes—*beta-carotene, provitamin A*. Carotenes are found naturally in many vegetables and fruits; for example, carrots, sweet potatoes, spinach, apricots, papaya, and cantaloupe. In the body it is converted to vitamin A. Carotene is a yellow-orange pigment that is used primarily as a natural coloring agent in food manufacturing. It is employed to color butter, buttermilk, margarine, and cottage cheese. Carotene, mostly as beta-carotene, is a useful additive. It is known to be a helpful antioxidant, possibly a cancer-preventing nutrient. It is a safe additive or supplement even in high dosages, where its only side effect is yellowish pigmentation of the skin.

Carrageenan (Irish moss extract)—*ammonium, calcium, potassium, and sodium carrageenan*. Carrageenan is a useful seaweed extract. This gluey and salty substance is used as a natural stabilizer and emulsifier in food processing, in such foods as French dressings, ice cream, cheese spreads, chocolate milk,

evaporated milk, puddings, sherbet, candies, and jellies. As an herb, Irish moss is used as a demulcent and emollient to soothe and soften irritated tissues such as the skin and mucous membranes. It has also been known to be helpful in lung conditions.

Carrageenan is basically thought to be safe though there has been some concern about its effect on reproductive function. Studies have been inconclusive. To date, it is still being used, and at the current levels of use, it is probably safe. Its GRAS status continues.

Caseinates—*sodium, potassium, calcium, and ammonium*. Casein is one of two major proteins in cow's milk (lactalbumin is the other). It is used as a texturizer in ice cream, ice milk, sherbet, and frozen custard. Casein is a nutritive protein source in many "protein" powders. Calcium caseinate is probably the most useful here. Caseinates are also used as binders or extenders in some lunchmeats and soups and as a clarifying agent in wine. Casein is essentially nontoxic and is on the GRAS list. However, many people are allergic to milk and specifically to the casein molecule. Those people should avoid foods with added caseinates.

Cellulose derivatives—*carboxymethylcellulose, cellulose gum, methyl cellulose, and others*. Cellulose is the basic structure of plant tissues. The cellulose used in food processing as a thickener or stabilizer and emulsifier is extracted from plants, cotton, or even wood. It can help in the blending of ingredients, aiding gel formation and preventing ingredient caking. Cellulose products are used both in foods, such as ice cream, icings, fillings, candies, and jellies, and in toiletries and cosmetics, such as hair gels, shaving creams, shampoos, beauty masks, and dentifrices. They are also used in some medicines, such as laxatives and antacids, as stabilizers.

There is some concern about many of the products that contain cellulose, more from the chemical extraction process than the cellulose itself, which is inert. Carcinogenicity of some of the cellulose derivatives is being studied, but they are still accepted as safe and remain on the GRAS list.

Citric acid and its salts—*calcium, potassium, and sodium citrate*. Citric acid is an old and versatile food additive. It and its salts are found naturally in citrus fruits, tomatoes, coffee, apricots, peaches, pineapples, and some berries. Commercially, citric acid is usually either extracted from citrus fruit or made by fermenting crude sugar.

In food processing, citric acid or, occasionally, its salts are used as a flavoring agent or enhancer to impart a tangy, tart, or sour taste to foods, including beverages, candy, ice cream, baked goods, and chewing gum. Citric acid is also used as a buffer, being a mild acid, to maintain acidity in foods such as fruit juices, carbonated beverages, wines, jellies, and sherbet. As a sequestrant, it removes metal contaminants from food and allows preservatives to work better, maintaining food flavor. Calcium citrate is used as a firming agent in canned tomatoes, and the citrate salts, such as calcium, are a vehicle for adding various mineral nutrients.

Citric acid and its salts are safe food additives, secure on the GRAS list. They are normal constituents of foods and are easily metabolized in the body at levels much higher than those used in foods. These are very useful and safe additives.

Cornstarch is mainly used to coat foods or containers to prevent sticking. It is also used in home cooking and as a medicinal for irritated mucous membranes or colons. It is basically a safe additive, not always listed on the label, but it may cause mild allergic symptoms of the skin, eyes, or nose in people sensitive to corn.

Corn sweeteners—*corn syrup and corn sugar*. (Note: Sugar, in the form of dextrose, may also be extracted from corn.) Corn syrup, the most commonly used corn sweetener, is made by chemically splitting cornstarch with a weak acid. Corn sweeteners are fairly prevalent in the food industry, used for flavoring in various beverages, candies, baked products, and ice cream. Corn syrup is used in a wide variety of products, including the adhesive on postage stamps, envelopes, and various tapes. It is also eaten commonly in catsup, dressings, Chinese foods, cereals, carbonated beverages, candies, jellies, peanut butter, and processed meats.

Corn sweeteners are on the GRAS list with no limitations, and they seem to be safe overall, though they are caloric sugars that may help create tooth decay and obesity if overused, as well as possible emotional or mental ups and downs. Occasional allergic reactions may occur, though this is much less likely with corn sweeteners than with corn itself or cornstarch, both of which contain some of the corn protein, which is the actual allergen. We may also wonder how much of the pesticide commonly sprayed on the cornfields ends up in the corn syrup. The majority of the population tolerates corn syrup and other sweeteners fairly well in moderation.

Cyclamate (Sucaryl). The cyclamates, sodium and calcium, were the diet sweeteners of the 1960s. More than 30 times sweeter than sugar, they were used freely. When research showed that high amounts of cyclamates caused bladder cancer in lab animals, they were removed from the food market by the FDA in 1969. There is a theory that cyclamate is converted in the body to cyclohexylamine (CHA), which may cause chromosomal changes and damage in embryos, though this has not yet been clearly shown.

Cyclamates were used mainly in soft drinks, chewing gums, and diet candies. In fact, these "artificial" or "nonnutritional" sweeteners are still used in Canada and other countries. In 1984 the FDA reviewed the research and considered reinstating cyclamates for food use, but the results and long-term effects are still unclear. More investigation is being done. The cyclamates were once a very popular noncaloric sweetener, and with saccharin possibly going out again, the diet-conscious population wants other choices besides aspartame.

DES—*diethylstilbestrol, stilbestrol.* This synthetic estrogen has been used commercially to fatten cattle and poultry. It has been found to be carcinogenic, specifically in daughters of women who have used the drug medically. Its use in animals was recently banned in the the United States, but it is still used in other countries. It is wise to purchase meats and poultry that have not been treated with this or other hormones or antibiotics.

Dextran is a polysaccharide produced by bacteria growing on sugar; it is used as a plasma expander in medicine, a foam stabilizer in beer, and a mild sweetener as a substitute for barley malt. There is some concern about the safety of dextran, though no proof shows it to be dangerous. It is still on the GRAS list.

Dextrin (starch gum). Dextrins are carbohydrate chains of glucose molecules prepared by heating starches such as cornstarch, potato starch, or tapioca. Dextrin has a variety of uses in food processing. It holds water and is used as a thickener in many sauces and gravies and as an expander in bakery goods. Dextrin is also used in pill coatings, as a diluting agent, and as a foam stabilizer in brewing. It can also be used as a mildly sweet sugar substitute. Nonfood uses include thickening industrial solutions and in flammables such as matches and firecrackers.

Dextrin is considered safe, is on the GRAS list, and is basically metabolized easily as starch is in the body. Studies have shown no problems with dextrin.

Dextrose is the dextrorotary form of glucose and is used as a sweetener in many beverages and packaged foods. It can be extracted from corn, sugar cane, or sugar beets, and like all sugars, its use should be limited or avoided.

DHC (dihydrochalcone). This is possibly an upcoming chemical sweetener. It is made by a chemical modification of naturally occurring bioflavonoids. It is about 1,500 times sweeter than sugar, but the sweet flavor takes longer to be released and tasted than other sugars, so use might be limited. Dihydrochalcone is thought to be safe, but further testing is being done before it will be available for use.

Diacetyl, an ingredient with a flavor and odor like butter, is found naturally in some cheeses, cocoa, coffee, berries, and pears. It can be made chemically or by fermenting glucose. Diacetyl is the primary component of starter distillates used to culture flours and milk products. It is used predominately, however, as a flavoring agent in margarines, candies, and chewing gum and to help carry a buttery or coffee taste in foods. Many flavors might contain diacetyl, including strawberry and other berries, chocolate, coffee, butterscotch, caramel, rum, nut, and butter. These flavorings may be used in making baked goods, gelatin desserts, ice cream, beverages, gum, and candy.

Diacetyl may be listed on the label as such or merely as "artificial flavor." Diacetyl is considered a safe ingredient. Studies have shown no significant problem, and it remains on the GRAS list.

EDTA (ethylenediaminetetraacetic acid, calcium disodium). EDTA is a mineral chelator that binds metals and takes them out of a solution. In medicine, it is used, mainly as EDTA-calcium disodium, to treat lead poisoning, and in "chelation" therapy. In food processing, EDTA and its acetate salts are used as chelating agents to decrease metals in food mixtures. EDTA is used even more commonly as a preservative in salad dressings, mayonnaise, sandwich spreads, condiments, margarines, juices, and drinks. The sequestering action is a result of its chelating effect, which allows EDTA to prevent changes in the color or flavor of foods, particularly from metals.

EDTA is on the safe list even though it is under further study. Results of research for any harmful effects or tumorigenic properties have not been conclusive. It is possible that EDTA has some modest positive effects when metal toxicity is a problem.

Ethyl alcohol (*ethanol*), or grain (drinking) alcohol, is used as a solvent in a variety of foods, such as candy, beverages, ice cream, baked goods, pizza crusts, liquors, gelatin desserts, and many medicinals (tinctures and elixirs). Since it is used mostly during processing ethyl alcohol is not always listed on the packaging label. It is basically a safe additive in small amounts, although, as we know, higher dosages can be toxic, or even fatal.

Fructose is a natural sugar found in many fruits and in honey. It is twice as sweet as sucrose, or cane sugar, and fructose is being used more frequently used as a sweetener. It is available in bulk as well as being used in candies, preserves, ice cream, and "natural" beverage drinks and ices. The health food industry often uses fructose instead of sucrose. It seems to stimulate blood sugar and pancreatic insulin less rapidly than glucose (part of sucrose) and is absorbed more slowly.

Fructose is basically safe in small amounts, as are most of the simple sugars. When used in excess, however, all sugars seem to affect the emotional, mental, and physical states of the user. It is best to use fructose and other sugars moderately and to consume more natural fruits and vegetables to obtain the simple carbohydrates.

Gelatin is a protein made from collagen, animal connective tissue. It can be extracted from hooves, skin, snouts, tendons, or ligaments and is used commonly in the food industry. In the vitamin supplement and pharmaceutical industries, gelatin is an important ingredient for making capsules and pill coverings. In foods, it functions as a thickener or stabilizer by absorbing as much as five to ten times its weight in water. Gelatin itself is tasteless and colorless. It is employed as a base in gelatin desserts, pudding, chocolate milk, whipped cream, and marshmallows and is also used in ice cream, sherbet, custard, cheeses, and cheese spreads. It has been used as well as a medicinal to treat weak fingernails.

Gelatin is basically safe, and according to research, there seems to be no toxicity. Some strict vegetarians avoid gelatin because of its animal origin. It does contain most amino acids but is somewhat low in tryptophan.

Glycerides—mono- and diglycerides. The glycerides are used commonly as emulsifiers to maintain softness and consistency in dressings, gum, milk, ice milk, ice cream, toppings, shortening, chocolates, lard, margarines, shortenings, confections, and baked goods. The basic mono- and diglycerides are naturally occurring fats (more specifically, alcohol-fats) and are easily metabolized in the body. Triglycerides are one of the more predominate body fats. These are all basically safe. However, there are a number of chemically synthesized glycerides currently being used. Oxystearin is the one of most concern. Fats in general should not be used in high amounts; they do seem to correlate with increased incidence of cancer and cardiovascular disease, though clearly some glycerides in foods would add very little to this risk.

Glycerin (*glycerol*) is an alcohol that is part of all fats, about 10 percent by weight of both animal and vegetable fats. Most of the glycerin used in food processing is made from animal oils and fats. It is a mildly sweet agent that has many functions. Glycerin is a solvent that helps carry food colors and flavors. It absorbs water, and so is used as a humectant. It is also used as a thickener in gelatin desserts and chewing gums. Glycerin is also a plasticizer used in the coverings for meats and cheeses, providing a waxy protection when mixed with other ingredients. It is also added to some baked goods, fillings, beverages, and gelatinous meats. In medicines and cosmetics, it is used in suppositories and a wide range of skin products.

Glycerin is on the GRAS list and is basically safe. It causes occasional irritation to mucous membranes in some people, but it can also be a soothing emollient (softener).

Guar gum is a complex carbohydrate, soluble fiber extracted from the guar plant grown in the Middle East. It acts as a stabilizer, thickener, and binder of foods, as it easily absorbs cold water, forming a thick, pastelike substance. It helps to stabilize and add texture to foods such as ice cream, ices, cheese spreads, dressings, and some meat products. Guar gum is also used in baked goods, fruit drinks, frozen fruits, and bakery glazes. It is on the GRAS list, though there is some concern about its use by pregnant women. Research to date has not shown any specific problems with guar gum, especially in the amounts commonly used.

Gum arabic—*see Acacia*

Honey is being used more commonly as a sweetener by food manufacturers. Many new natural, preservative-free beverages, cereals, ice creams, and candies contain honey instead of cane sugar. Honey contains both glucose and fructose and has less dramatic effects on blood sugar levels than cane sugar. It can be used directly from nature instead of being chemically extracted and processed.

Honey is a safe food additive and actually has some preservative action. Of course, it is caloric and, if used in excess, can cause dental cavities and weight gain. It is best used in moderation, as are all sugars.

HVP (hydrolyzed vegetable protein). HVP is used occasionally as a flavor enhancer in soups, gravies, and meats. It is also used in baby foods, although there is some concern about this, as HVP may affect certain growth-related proteins. Certain types of HVP are produced by extraction with petroleum distillates; these petroleum residues are a cause for concern, though studies have been inconclusive in regard to specific hazard. HVP is still considered safe.

Hydrogen peroxide—*calcium and benzoyl peroxide.* Hydrogen peroxide is a commonly used antiseptic that works by releasing oxygen, thus, its bubbling action. It is also used in food processing, although it is not directly added to food, and therefore it is usually not listed on the labels. The peroxides are mild preservative and antibacterial agents used in processing milk and making cheese. They are even more commonly employed as bleaching and oxidizing agents in butter, cheese, and powdered eggs. The Japanese have used hydrogen peroxide to disinfect fish and noodles before they are eaten. Benzoyl peroxide is sometimes used as a bleaching agent for milk, cheeses, and flours.

Hydrogen peroxide is safe when used in food processing but not when added to food. Studies for carcinogenicity did not reveal any positive findings. The peroxides can be an irritant to the skin and eyes and have a mild allergenic potential. Some people use oral food grade hydrogen peroxide (H_2O_2) for treatment of a variety of ailments.

Iodine salts—*calcium iodate, cuprous iodide, potassium iodate, and potassium iodide.* Iodine is a mineral that occurs naturally in the earth and sea and is needed by our body for proper thyroid function. It is sometimes found in foods grown in iodine-rich soil and foods harvested from the ocean, such as fish and sea vegetation. Because iodine deficiency is common, potassium iodide is added to table salt to ensure that we receive our daily requirement. Calcium or potassium iodate is added to breads as a nutrient and as a dough conditioner to improve texture. Potassium iodide is also used in drinking water.

Iodine is basically safe and is essential for life. Pregnant or lactating women usually require extra dietary iodine. Occasionally, susceptible people may have mild allergic skin reactions to iodine, but this is not very likely with the small amounts used in foods.

Lactic acid—*calcium lactate, butyl lactate, ethyl lactate.* Lactic acid is produced naturally in our body as a result of metabolism and exercise, and by bacterial fermentation of milk.

453

Some lactic acid is found in tomatoes, apples, molasses, beer, and wine. It can also be made by fermenting molasses, whey, cornstarch, and potato starch.

Lactic acid is used to give flavor and tartness to carbonated juices and other beverages and to some desserts. Its acidity reduces spoilage in such foods as cheeses, olives, breads, butter, and candy. Lactic acid helps condition dough and stabilize wine as well. Calcium lactate helps to firm some processed foods, to inhibit discoloration in processed fruits and vegetables, and to stabilize powdered milk and some baked goods.

Lactic acid is safe and on the GRAS list. Research shows no deleterious effects, though it is not used in infant formulas.

Lactose (milk sugar) occurs naturally in milk and can be extracted from whey or during cheese making. Lactose represents about 7 percent of human milk and 5 percent of cow's milk. It is made up of one molecule each of galactose and glucose. Lactose is much less sweet than sucrose (about one-sixth as sweet). In the food industry, it is used in powdered formulas, such as infant formulas and protein powders for weight loss, weight gain, or body building. Lactose also helps carry flavors and aromas in foods and can improve the texture and flavor of baked goods.

Lactose is quite safe except for people who are sensitive to milk or who are lactose intolerant—that is, they do not have the enzyme, *lactase*, needed to metabolize lactose. Gastrointestinal symptoms, such as nausea, diarrhea, and bloating, or a variety of other symptoms may occur in the lactose intolerant person. Lactose may help absorption of some nutrients, most notably calcium.

Lard and animal fats—*pork fat, beef fat (tallow), cheese fat.* Fats extracted from animals are commonly used in preparing soups. Saturated fats are also used in various ointments, salves, and lubricants. In food, their main purpose is flavoring, giving a richer taste. These fats, especially lard, may be treated with preservatives such as BHT, which may not be listed on the package label. If lard or shortening is listed, it probably contains other additives as well.

In small quantities, these animal fats are safe, but we know the consequences of too much fat, and these saturated, sometimes processed fats are the worst. Animal fats can store environmentally harmful chemicals; however, the usually small amounts used as food flavoring are safe and the least of our fat worries. In general though, I suggest avoiding most lard products.

Lecithin—*soy lecithin.* This nutrient is an oil found in most living tissues and is important to many body functions, particularly healthy nerves and cell membranes. Commercially, it is extracted from eggs, soybeans, or corn. In food processing, lecithin is used mainly as an emulsifier and stabilizer in oil-containing foods, such as salad dressings, mayonnaise, margarine, chocolate, frozen desserts, cereals, and baked goods. Lecithin also acts as a mild antioxidant, preventing changes in flavor and fragrance of oil-containing products. It is also used in paints.

Lecithin is safe and may even have some beneficial effects. Certain chemically prepared lecithins, such as hydroxylated lecithin synthesized with hydrogen or benzoyl peroxide, may be a little more risky, but these too have been found to be basically safe.

Locust bean gum—*see Carob*

Maleic hydrazide is a dangerous chemical that we will not find listed on food labels. It is sprayed on most tobacco leaves, making tobacco smoke even more dangerous. Maleic hydrazide is sometimes sprayed on potatoes and onions to prevent sprouting, but may cause the sprouting to occur inside the vegetables, which is probably worse.

Maleic hydrazide is very toxic to humans. Animal studies have shown carcinogenicity and damage to the liver and central nervous system. Some studies have denied this cancer-causing potential. Until the use of maleic hydrazide as a pesticide is discontinued, we should avoid it, if possible, by buying organic produce or by making sure it is not used on the products we buy. Also, by not smoking, we will avoid it and the other toxins in cigarettes.

Malic acid occurs naturally in many fruits and vegetables, including apples, cherries, peaches, tomatoes, rhubarb, pears, plums, and berries. It is used provide a tart taste to various sweets. Malic acid is used in wines, jellies, jams, sherbet, candies, beverages, and frozen milk products. It is basically safe, and studies show no potential hazards.

Malt—*malt syrup, malt extract, Maltol.* Malt is basically an extract from barley. It is a mildly sweet substance that is used commonly in the brewing industry. It is also used as a sweetener in foods, such as ice cream, flavored milk, candy, cereals, and dressings, and is occasionally used to flavor meat and poultry products. Malt is safe, with no known toxicity, and is on the GRAS list.

Maltol, which is not malt but an extract from larch trees and pine needles, is also used to flavor foods and give them a fresh-baked smell. Ethyl maltol is the synthetic maltol. Both of these are used in flavorings for frozen desserts, gelatins, soft drinks, ice creams, candy, baked goods, and gums. Maltol is also known to be safe.

Maple syrup, a natural extract from maple trees, is a flavorful sweetener. It is now commonly used in place of sugar in many "health" foods, such as baked goods and cereals. Pure maple syrup is also used commonly on pancakes and waffles. Many maple syrup manufacturers in the United States use formaldehyde, a toxic chemical, on their trees to improve the syrup production, which also contaminates them. Canada does not allow formaldehyde use on its maples. Many maple syrups are "imitations" and not pure. They contain a high amount of corn syrup and

artificial flavors and maybe a small percentage of actual maple syrup. These types of syrup are best avoided. Genuine maple syrup is a safe food, although excessive use should be avoided, as with all sweeteners.

MSG (*Monosodium glutamate*) is a fairly controversial food additive. It is used both in food processing and in restaurant and home cooking. It is basically a flavor enhancer that is commerically extracted from molasses which is derived from cane or beet sugar. MSG is the monosodium salt of glutamic acid, an essential amino acid. It is used commonly in seasoning salts, soups, spices, condiments, meats, some baked goods, and candies. Other fermented and Oriental food preparations contain MSG, as do most food dishes served in Chinese restaurants.

It might appear that MSG should not be a problem. After all, it is found naturally in foods such as soybeans, beets, and seaweeds. However, glutamic acid seems to affect brain chemistry, and certain tests in rats suggest that high amounts of MSG can cause brain damage. There was more concern in the past about its use in infants, as it was added to many baby foods for flavor, but that practice was stopped in 1969.

More recently, "Chinese restaurant syndrome" has become associated with the use of MSG. Symptoms occur after eating foods high in MSG and include headaches, tingling, numbness, and chest pains. These effects have been confirmed by some studies but not by others, though it seems that many people are sensitive to MSG and experience some untoward reactions when using it, especially at the high levels added to Chinese food. Some theorize that it may be the various mushrooms, sprouts, teas, soy, mustards, fish, or sauces used in Oriental cooking; either these foods themselves or their interactions with MSG may cause the aforementioned symptoms.

More research on MSG is needed, and studies are being done. In 1980, the FDA evaluated the research findings that were available and decided that MSG could be left on the GRAS list. I avoid foods with MSG or restaurants that use it because I do have unpleasant reactions to it. I suggest that, until further research clears it as being safe, foods containing monosodium glutamate should not be eaten.

Nitrates—*sodium nitrate, potassium nitrate (saltpeter).* Nitrates, in relatively low amounts, are found naturally in many vegetables and in most water supplies. The prolonged use of nitrate fertilizers has increased these levels in food and water. Vegetables that are high in nitrates include spinach, beets, celery, radishes, lettuce, and other greens.

Nitrates, particularly potassium nitrate, have also been used in curing meats, acting as a color fixative. The nitrates are not as stable as the nitrites (see below), and therefore sodium nitrite is the main meat-curing chemical used. In fact, nitrate converts easily to nitrite can interact with amines in the digestive juices or tissues to form nitrosamines, which are highly carcinogenic chemicals.

Nitrates have been used for decades to cure hams, bacon, sausage, hot dogs, corned beef, lunch meats, and some fish products. They were thought to be safe until recent years; now they are considered unsafe. They are safer when used with vitamin C, which prevents nitrosamine production. But still the nitrates and nitrites have not been banned, and they are still in use in the $100 billion processed-meat industry. Manufacturers claim that there is no good substitute for the nitrates and nitrites. My suggestion is to avoid all foods, especially bacon and cured meats, containing these substances for obvious health reasons.

Nitrites—*sodium nitrite, potassium nitrite.* Sodium nitrite is used primarily to cure meats in that megabusiness. This chemical is a color fixative that works by reacting with the muscle myoglobin to create a red color like that of blood. Sodium nitrite also protects against the growth of the bacterium *Clostridium botu-*

linum, which causes botulism. It adds a tangy taste to the meats treated with it. These meats include hams, bacon, lunch meats, bologna, frankfurters, meat spreads, some smoke-cured fishes, and corned beef. Sodium nitrite is also combined with salt, their characteristic flavor and color and helps prolong their shelf life.

There are many problems associated with eating these processed meats. First, they are usually high in both sodium and fats, which endanger the cardiovascular system. The chemicals used in raising animals and found in their meat are also a cause for concern. The biggest health hazard, however, is the direct carcinogenic effect of nitrosamines, which are formed when nitrite interacts with amines (parts of proteins) in the digestive fluids or in the foods eaten. Nitrosamines have been shown to be potent carcinogens in animals, producing increased amounts of cancer in the liver, lungs, and pancreas—all usually fatal. Also, the nitrites can form amyl and butyl nitrites, which are suspected of being carcinogenic as well.

It has been demonstrated that vitamin C reduces the production of nitrosamines. More recently, vitamin E has been shown to help as well. In lieu of banning the use of nitrites, for which the cured-meat industry claims there is no effective substitute, the FDA has asked processors to at least add vitamin C and, more recently, vitamin E to the brines used to cure meats. If you do happen to indulge in any of these fatty, chemical meats, take additional vitamin C and vitamin E when you do.

Further research needs to be done to substantiate the clear dangers of nitrite use in human foods. For the many reasons mentioned, it is wise to eliminate all nitrite-containing foods from the diet and substitute more healthful foods.

Oleic acid, one of the fatty acids, can be obtained from various animal and vegetable fats, most notably safflower and olive oils. Pure oleic acid is slightly sensitive to oxidation, but less so than the polyunsaturated fatty acids. Impure oil can more easily become rancid. Oleic acid is used in food processing in making fake butter, as a defoaming agent, and as part of some flavorings for beverages, candy, ice cream, and bakery products. It can also be used as a lubricant and binder in foods. Oleic acid is basically nontoxic in moderate oral doses; it is on the GRAS list. However, when it is hydrogenated, it poses more of a problem. Processed fats are best avoided as much as possible.

Oxystearin occurs in animal fat as a blend of glyceride and stearic acid; it is usually hydrogenated commercially. It is used for many nonfood products needing a waxy consistency, such as soap, candles, cosmetics, and medicines. It has also been used in salad oils to reduce crystallization and in the preparation of sugars and yeasts. Oxystearin is usually not listed on food labels. Though it is on the FDA GRAS list, the safety of this additive is still being researched; to date, there are no clear data to show danger.

Palmitic acid is another of the fats found naturally in many animal and vegetable sources, such as butter, celery seed, palm oil, coffee and tea, anise seed, and other herb seeds. Palmitic acid is used occasionally to create butter or cheese flavorings to season foods. It is basically nontoxic and is on the GRAS list.

Parabens—*methyl, butyl, and propyl paraben.* Paraben, or parahydroxybenzoic acid, is closely related to benzoic acid and sodium benzoate, both common food preservatives.

Methyl and propyl paraben are synthetic compounds that are esters of paraben and also act as preservatives, preventing the growth of molds and yeasts, as well as other microbes. They are used commonly in the cosmetics industry and are useful in both liquids and solids. They are also protective in alkaline products. In the food industry, the parabens are used in baked goods, some milk products, frozen desserts, and sugar substitutes and the artificially sweetened foods that contain them, such as jellies, jams, and dietic foods and beverages.

The paraben esters are basically nontoxic. Their desirability for use in cosmetics is partly because they are nonirritating and nonallergenic. These preservatives are considered safe. Though some birth defects were noted in rats and hamsters fed high amounts of propyl paraben, the current level of use does not warrant concern. However, there are those who wish to avoid synthetic chemicals with unknown effects, and I would put the parabens in that class.

Pectin is a binding agent found in most plants, particularly in fruits and vegetables, such as apples and citrus fruits. It is a polysaccharide consisting of many simple sugars, and is extracted for food use from the rinds and pressings of apples, oranges, and lemons after they have been squeezed for their juice. Pectin is used in foods as a stabilizer and thickener; it helps food to blend and gel. It is a common ingredient in jams, jellies and preserves, ice cream, chocolate milk, sherbet, beverages and juices, and French dressing. Pectin can also be used as an antidiarrheal agent. It is a safe and even helpful food additive.

Polysorbate 60 and 80—*polyoxyethylene (20), sorbitan monostearate; sorbitan monooleate.* Polysorbate 60 and 80 are sorbitan derivatives made from sorbitol (see below), a sugar-alcohol that is sweet, and that is produced by converting glucose. Polysorbate 60 is made by chemically combining palmitate and stearic acids with sorbitol and sterilizing it with 20 parts of ethylene oxide, a toxic gas.

Polysorbate 60 is an emulsifier that helps blend oil and water together and also aids in spreading flavor through the various mixtures to which it is added. Polysorbate 60 is used in many processed foods, including salad dressings, bakery products, dairy products, gelatin desserts, shortenings, cake mixes, whipped vegetable toppings, candy and sugar toppings, and vitamin supplements.

Although there are other polyoxyethylene derivatives besides polysorbate 60 and 80, such as sorbitan monostearate, tristearate, and palmitate, polysorbate 60 is used most com-

457

monly. It has been classified as safe, but the FDA wants further study. The effects of the ethylene gas are unknown, and polysorbate 60 is a little questionable as well. I would recommend avoiding it when possible until further information is available.

Polysorbate 80 is very similar to 60 except that it contains oleic acid instead of stearic acid. It can be used as an emulsifier and flavor carrier in the same foods and dietary products as polysorbate 60. It is also employed as a defoaming agent in brewing and yeast production and in chewing gum. It also appears to be basically nontoxic and is on the GRAS list. Studies with it and polysorbate 60 have not revealed specific problems, but further studies are being done. I also recommend avoiding polysorbate 80 whenever possible.

Propyl gallate is a synthetic chemical that is added to foods for its antioxidant effect. It reduces rancidity and prevents changes in color, taste, and odor in foods containing fats and oils. Propyl gallate is often combined with other antioxidants, such as BHA and BHT, to reduce the level of each used. It might be added to foods such as meats, shortenings, vegetable oils, candy, snack foods, nuts, baked goods, and frozen dairy foods. It has also been used as part of fruit or spice flavorings in beverages, ice cream, candy, and bottled goods.

Propyl gallate is on the GRAS list. It has been studied fairly thoroughly, and no research has revealed any carcinogenic or toxic effects. It is considered a safe additive; however, it is a synthetic chemical.

Propylene glycol—*propylene glycol monostearate and alginate*. Propylene glycol is a blending agent used in food processing. It is made from propylene gas (a by-product of petroleum refining) and glycerol. It is a solvent that attracts water and improves the flexibility and spreadability of the products in which it is used. These include confections, ice cream, beverages, toppings, icings, chocolate, shredded coconut, and baked goods. In meats, it helps prevent discoloring. Propylene glycol is also used in a variety of cosmetics, as it promotes absorption through the skin.

Propylene glycol alginate is extracted from seaweed with propylene gas. It is a defoamer and stabilizer used in some salad dressings, ice creams, and sherbets.

Propylene glycol monostearate acts as an emulsifier, texturizer, and dough conditioner in baked goods, puddings, and toppings. Butylene glycol and polyethylene glycol are related compounds produced with different gases.

These products, especially propylene glycol, have been studied fairly well and have shown to have very low toxicity. The 1980 review by the FDA substantiated their safety and it remains on the GRAS list. I would be wary of using these products, because of their chemical nature and because the foods in which they are used are not always the healthiest; however, there are apparently worse additives than these.

PVC (Polyvinyl chloride). This is a potentially toxic plastic (a polymer of vinyl chloride) when it releases vinyl chloride on exposure to heat, light, or chemical solvents. It is more a food contaminant than an additive. Plastic wrap contains polyvinyl chloride and other chemicals that leach into foods, especially meat, when they come in contact with them. Heat increases the release of vinyl chloride into the food which then fixes with the tissues. PVC, which is derived from vinyl chloride, is a very stable material, resistant to environmental breakdown. That is why it is used so widely in industry, as in pipes, records, containers, linings, film, toys, and so on.

There is a suspicion that PVC causes lung damage and may be a carcinogen. If possible avoid prepackaged plastic-wrapped animal foods. PVC will not be listed on food labels.

Quinine—*quinine hydrochloride, quinine sulfate*. Quinine is a bitter extract from the bark of the cinchona tree. It is used as a flavoring to impart a refreshing bitter taste to carbonated beverages such as tonic water, bitter lemon, and quinine water. It is also used in some over-the-counter medicines and in the treatment of malaria. Quinine hydrochloride and sulfates are synthetic variations used as flavoring agents in various bitters and citrus beverages.

Quinine can cause some problems. While it is generally safe, it is not recommended for use by pregnant women. Some people are allergic to quinine and can have skin reactions or a syndrome named cinchonism, consisting of flushing, nausea, vomiting, visual disturbance, and hearing changes. This is usually a result of an overdose of quinine, though sensitive people may experience some symptoms with low intake.

Rennet (rennin) is an enzyme extracted from the linings of cow's stomachs that is used to make cheese, as it helps to curdle milk. It has been found to be safe in the small amounts used. However, many vegetarians and health-conscious people prefer rennetless cheeses, which are made with various vegetable enzymes.

Saccharin (sodium saccharin) has been a very popular artificial sweetener, in use for nearly 100 years. It contains no calories and is several hundred times sweeter than sugar, though it has a slightly bitter aftertaste. The FDA and many consumer advocates, however, have been pushing for a ban on saccharin use because of studies that suggest that it is a mild carcinogen. In 1969, it was studied along with cyclamates, which were subsequently banned. In 1977, the FDA tried to ban the use of saccharin in foods, but the public resisted the ban, claiming that it had been used for many years with no apparent problems. Many studies suggest that it can cause bladder cancer in laboratory animals and their offspring; other studies fail to show this. The FDA currently plans to remove it from the market, and at present a warning label must be placed on all food products containing saccharin. With the increasing use of aspartame, the FDA now feels that it can eliminate saccharin.

Previously, nearly five million pounds of saccharin were used yearly—about 75 percent in diet drinks, 15 percent in other diet foods, such as canned fruits and ice cream, and about 10 percent as a table sweetener. One advantage of saccharin is that it does not convert to glucose in the body, so it is popular among diabetics. However, it is a chemical that must be metabolized and eliminated from the body.

Saccharin is not considered safe. It may be mildly to moderately carcinogenic, depending on the level of use and the health of the consumer. There is special risk to children, teenagers, and pregnant women. More studies are needed, but my current suggestion is not to use saccharin. It might be helpful in certain medical conditions, such as diabetes or for low-calorie or weight-loss diets, and it probably would be best to make saccharin available only by prescription.

Salicylic acid and salicylates—*amyl, phenyl, benzyl, and methyl salicylate*. A number of foods, including apples, almonds, apricots, berries, plums, prunes, raisins, cucumbers, cloves, wintergreen, and tomatoes, naturally contain salicylates. Salicylic acid, made synthetically by heating phenol with carbon dioxide, is the basis of aspirin, acetylsalicylic acid. Aspirin is a commonly used anti-inflammatory and pain reliever. White willow bark contains a natural salicylate that has similar effects. Tartrazine, FDC Yellow 5, is a salicylate used as a food dye. The salicylates are also used in a variety of flavorings, such as strawberry, root beer, sarsaparilla, spice, walnut, peach, and mint, in some beverages, candies, baking goods, chewing gum, and ice cream.

The salicylates are known to cause symptoms when consumed in higher doses. Ringing of the ears (tinnitus), gastrointestinal irritation, nausea, vomiting, increased respiration, acidosis, and skin rash may occur with salicylate intoxication. Only a small amount is used in foods, so except for those with allergic sensitivity to the salicylate products, they are basically safe. Because of the phenol derivation and possible side effects, salicylic acid and aspirin are substances of which to be wary.

SAP (*Sodium acid pyrophosphate*)—*sodium pyrophosphate*. SAP is a diphosphoric acid (pyrophosphate) of sodium used in processing, so it will usually not be listed on the label. It is a mild buffer and acid constituent of self-rising leavening mixtures for cakes, pancakes, doughnuts, waffles, and other baked goods, flours, and mixes. SAP and sodium pyrophosphate are added to lunch meats, hot dogs, and sausages to accelerate the development of their red color and to reduce the amount of nitrites needed. They also help hold in the juices of cooked pork.

SAP is basically safe; studies have shown no toxicity. Often the foods that it is used in are more a health risk than sodium acid pyrophosphate itself.

Silicates—*silicon dioxide, sodium aluminosilicate, calcium and mangesium silicate, sodium calcium aluminosilicate, talc*. The silicates are salts of silica oxides, which is found in rocks and sand, in gems such as quartz, amethyst, and agate, and in flint. Silica is related to silicon, an important element in the earth and probably essential to humans for bone calcification and connective tissue strength. The various silicates are used infrequently in food processing as defoaming agents in beer production or as anticaking agents in powders such as salt, dry mixes, and baking powder. These silica salts absorb water and prevent the powders from sticking together. Silicon dioxide may also be used in vitamin tablets, BHT, sodium proprionate, and other food additives.

There are some concerns about health hazards from the aluminum-containing silicates, and talc may contain asbestos (see Talc, below); otherwise, the silicates are safe in the usually small amounts used.

Smoke flavoring—*liquid smoke, char-smoke flavor*. Liquid smoke flavorings are manufactured by burning various types of hardwoods, maple and hickory most commonly. They are used for flavoring foods,

particularly meats and cheeses. They are also mild antioxidants, protecting against fatty changes and helping to reduce bacterial contamination. Smoked yeast can be made by exposing yeast to the smoke. It may be used in cheese, pizza, soups, crackers, and dips.

Smoke flavorings have been studied fairly extensively and seem to be free of at least short-range risks, possibly other than allergic symptoms. However, dangerous long-range effects have not been excluded. One concern is the benzopyrenes, suspected carcinogens, that are produced from the burning of the tars and resins in the wood. During processing, most of these benzopyrenes can be eliminated. So cooking with charcoal may be even more dangerous than the use of these flavors in regard to benzopyrenes. Fire starters are also hazardous chemicals to breathe or to consume in foods. Until there is more research clearly proving the safety of smoke flavorings, I recommend avoiding these food additives.

Sodium benzoate—*see Benzoic acid*

Sodium bicarbonate—*baking soda, bicarbonate of soda*. Sodium bicarbonate is an alkaline powder that is used to balance acid products and as a leavening agent to lighten and help raise dough. It is found in many biscuit, muffin, and pancake mixes; in baking powders; in many crackers; in self-rising flours; and in other foods. Baking soda is also used as an antacid for stomach acidity, topically for insect bites or poison oak, and to absorb odors and freshen refrigerators. This useful substance can be further used to clean our teeth as well as remove the acid-chemical residue found on the surface of foods (see *88 Survival Suggestions* at the end of this chapter).

Sodium bicarbonate is a safe product. Bicarbonate is used by the body as a buffer to help maintain acid-base balance. Excess baking soda could affect this balance, but the amount used in foods poses no real problem.

Sodium bisulfite—*see Sulfites*

Sodium caseinate—*see Caseinates*

Sodium chloride (common table salt). One of the most widely employed food additives in both processing and preparation and at the table, sodium chloride has a number of valuable uses. It is found naturally in small amounts in many foods but is much more concentrated in processed and restaurant foods. Sodium chloride can be used as a pickling and curing agent, by soaking foods in the salty brine. It acts as a mild preservative in foods such as vegetables, meats, and butter. It is also used as a dough conditioner and occasionally as a nutritional supplement, though most people acquire plenty of salt without even trying. Sodium chloride can be commercially extracted from salt mines or seawater, or through brine evaporation.

Salt is basically safe when used in modest amounts. Some people with salt-sensitive, high blood pressure must avoid it. As a factor in causing high blood pressure, it is implicated in heart disease, as well as in kidney disease. Though salt is safe, it is unwise to consume high-salt-content foods. (See the Sodium discussion in Chapter 6, *Minerals.*)

Sodium hydroxide (lye, caustic soda). Sodium hydroxide is a strong alkali used in food processing, so that it will not usually appear on labels. By itself, it is very caustic and dangerous. It is used in the refining of vegetable oils and animal fats, in modifying food starch, in glazes, cocoa products, and some curdled milk products, and as an acid neutralizer in some canned vegetables. Sodium hydroxide has also been used in liquid drain cleaners, but that use has been limited.

When ingested, lye causes internal burns, nausea, and vomiting; it can irritate the lungs when inhaled. In food use with the small amounts ingested, which are usually balanced by other acid products, sodium hydroxide is basically safe and innocuous.

Sodium nitrate and nitrite—*see Nitrates; Nitrites*

Sorbic acid—*potassium sorbate*. Sorbic acid is found naturally in the berries of the mountain ash. For use in food processing, it and its salt, potassium sorbate, are made synthetically. Sorbic acid is a mild preservative and is used to inhibit yeast and mold growth, especially in beverages and cheeses. It also reduces bacterial growth and works best in acidic foods. It is used in wine, many cheeses, cheesecakes, chocolates, syrups, fruit juices, baked goods, margarine, premade salads, pie fillings, and artificially sweetened preserves and jellies.

Sorbic acid is basically safe and nontoxic. It can cause some skin irritation with contact, but it is one of the safer food preservatives.

Sorbitan derivatives—*see Polysorbate 60 and 80*

Sorbitol is a natural sugar found in berries and other fruits, including pears, plums, apples, and cherries, as well as in sea vegetation. It can also be made chemically by modifying corn sugar (dextrose). In food processing, sorbitol helps control crystallization and viscosity of foods such as candy, frozen desserts, and dietetic fruits and soft drinks. Sorbitol has many functions. It is a thickener, humectant, texturizer, sequestrant, stabilizer, and sweetener and can be used as a sugar substitute by diabetics. It does not act as a sugar metabolically and has minimum potential for causing tooth decay or diabetic problems. Sorbitol is commonly used in chewing gums. It is also the basis of the emulsifiers polysorbate 60 and 80 and other sorbitan derivatives.

Sorbitol is thought to be safe, though it can be irritating to the intestinal tract when taken in larger quantities. Further studies are being done on sorbitol to prove its safety. Although its use in moderation is probably safe, I believe that it should be limited.

Soy protein isolate—*texturized vegetable protein (TVP)*. Soybeans have become a major commercial crop. When soybean oil is extracted, what is left is a high-protein residue that can be processed to make soy protein isolate. This protein powder can be used in milk-free formulas for infants and in protein-powder formulas for weight loss, weight gain, or body building. Soy isolate may also be used in soups, sauces, gravies, flavorings, seasonings, artificial bacon bits, cereals, frozen desserts, and meat substitutes. Other soy products are used in soy sauce, salad dressings, Worcestershire sauce, lunch meats, and candies.

Soy proteins are basically safe, especially if they are prepared with minimal chemical processing and without dangerous chemicals such as formaldehyde. In people who are allergic to soy products, their use could cause intestinal upset, bloating, headache, or skin rashes. Heat treatment of the powders reduces allergenic potential. Soy protein may contain a small level of nitrites formed in processing, and these could generate carcinogenic nitrosamines. Soy protein is not a complete food and should not be consumed exclusively. Diet powders usually have added amino acids and vitamins and minerals. Consult a doctor or nutritionist for weight-loss programs with soy protein. In general, moderate amounts of the soy protein isolates are safe.

Soy sauce—*hydrolyzed and fermented soybeans.* This is a salty food flavoring prepared by acid hydrolysis and mold fermentation of soybeans. Usually, the Aspergillus mold species are used. Soy sauce contains some amino acids, carbohydrates, a few other nutrients, and about 20 percent salt. It is used in some food preparations, such as soups or crackers, but is added in cooking, especially in Oriental restaurants, or as a tabletop seasoning.

Soy sauce is safe and on the GRAS list. Its salt content may be a disadvantage to those with high blood pressure, and some people are sensitive to mold-fermented products. Soy sauce, like all salt products, should be used sparingly.

Starches—*acid-modified, modified, unmodified, gelatinized.* Starch is a complex carbohydrate found in whole grains, such as rice, wheat, and corn, and in vegetables such as squashes, potatoes, and tapioca. It can be chemically separated from the proteins and other nutrients in these foods so that the pure

starch can be used in food processing as a thickening or gelling agent. After extraction, it can be further chemically "modified" to make it "easier to digest." To modify starch, it is bleached, oxidized, and treated with such chemicals as aluminum sulfate, sodium hydroxide, and propylene oxide. When the starch molecules are left to swell and burst, they form a gel—gelatinized starch. Starches are used to thicken foods such as baby foods, gelatins, and cake mixes, and sometimes to prevent caking or to dust baked goods to prevent sticking. Often, neither the type of starch used nor the chemicals employed to make the starches are listed on labels.

These starches are on the GRAS list. Some of them have been studied and shown to pose no hazards, but there is concern about the chemical modification, extraction, and treatment processes. Starch is basically easy for the body to digest and metabolize. It is best to get our starches from whole foods and avoid, as much as possible, starch-added foods.

Stearic acid—*calcium stearate.* This is a saturated fatty acid that occurs naturally in animal fats and some vegetable oils. It is prepared synthetically through hydrogenating vegetable oils such as cottonseed oil, and is used in foods to lubricate or help blend them. Synthetic stearic acid is also used in some flavorings, such as butter and vanilla, which may be used in candies, chewing gum, beverages, or bakery products. Calcium stearate is often the form of stearic acid used. It is also employed in cosmetics and medicinals, such as ointments and suppositories.

Stearic acid is basically safe and is a by-product of fat-containing foods. Some people are slightly allergic to it, and overall, I think we should avoid much use of foods containing added stearic acid or calcium stearate. Further research is pending regarding possible dangers from the use of these additives.

Succinic acid is found naturally in meats, cheese, fungi, and many vegetables with its distinct tart, acid taste, such as asparagus, broccoli, beets, and rhubarb. Succinic acid is involved in carbohydrate metabolism and can be made synthetically for food processing by chemically changing acetic acid or maleic acid. Succinic acid can be used as a buffering or neutralizing agent. It is added to some foods to give an acid taste. It is also used by the perfume industry.

Succinic acid has been rated as safe. Studies have shown that, in amounts thousands of times higher than the quantities used in food, succinic acid creates no problems. It is, however, only infrequently used in food processing.

Sucrose (cane or beet sugar)—*white sugar, refined sugar.* Sucrose, or "sugar," is the primary food sweetener and the common table sugar. Sucrose (a dissaccharide) is a carbohydrate, each molecule being composed of glucose and fructose. It is obtained mainly from sugarcane and sugar beets. These crops are now grown plentifully throughout the world as the sources of refined sugar.

Sugar is used throughout the food manufacturing industry and is found in a great variety of foods. Condiments, dressings, candy, cereals, baby food, and beverages are some common examples. It can also be the starting substance in the fermentation process and is used widely in pharmaceuticals as a preservative, coating for tablets, or sweetener in syrups and children's formulas. Table sugar is used freely by many adults and children to sweeten coffee or tea, cereals, and fruit dishes and is liberally added in cooking and canning. Bakery products may contain high amounts of sucrose, and the soft drink industry uses millions of pounds.

Sucrose is probably the most commonly abused substance on Earth and the number-one food additive, both before and after processing. The average American consumes more than 125 pounds per year—that's billions of pounds just in the United States. Sucrose is on the GRAS list, and studies show that it is generally safe—unless, of course, it is overused or there is individual sensitivity.

Sucrose is not safe for diabetics, and sugar use is implicated in causing adult-onset diabetes. It is highly caloric and contributes greatly to obesity, which increases the risk of diabetes and many other diseases. Tooth decay is much higher in people, especially children, who consume lots of sugar and practice poor oral hygiene. In addition, the pesticides and chemicals sprayed on cane and beet sugar and the chemical bleaching process used to make "white" sugar are potentially hazardous; we are not advised about this on sugar packages or food labels. Many people become hypersensitive to sugar, either because of repeated insults or weakened body condition. Sucrose use may affect activity levels, physical energy, and emotional and mental states. It is a substance that should be avoided or used in moderation. It is better to get our natural sugars from the many wholesome foods that contain them.

Sulfites—*sodium sulfite, sodium and potassium bisulfite, sodium and potassium metabisulfite.* These sulfiting agents, which can release sulfur dioxide (see below) are used in food processing as preservatives and sanitizing agents. They prevent bacterial growth and the browning of exposed foods. They are antispoilants and actually prevent undesirable microorganisms from growing during fermentation and food processing, thus preventing food discoloration. They have been used for this purpose in many processed foods, such as syrups and condiments, as well as in preserving fruits and vegetables, in wine making, and as a spray on restaurant salad bars. This latter use, fortunately, has recently been banned. Now sulfites must be listed on packaging labels, including alcoholic beverages.

These sulfites are on the GRAS list and thus considered safe, though they are under review. In the body, they are oxygenated and changed to harmless sulfates. But many people seem to react to sulfites, especially those sprayed on foods or added in restaurants. Allergic reactions are worse in asthmatics, whose condi-

463

tion, wheezing and shortness of breath, can be exacerbated by sulfites. Sulfite reactions, including diarrhea, nausea, and headaches, also occur in nonasthmatic people as well. All of the sulfites are on my personal "avoid" list.

Sulfur dioxide, the gas that is formed when sulfur is burned, is used in food processing for a variety of purposes. It is sprayed on many fruits and vegetables to preserve their color and protect against attacks from microorganisms. Many grapes are so treated, and thus much wine contains this gas or other chemical by-products. Raisins, particularly golden raisins, and many other dried fruits are treated with sulfur dioxide. It is used as a disinfectant in food manufacturing; a bleaching agent; an antioxidant and preservative; and an antibrowning agent. Other foods that may contain sulfur dioxide include beet sugar, corn syrup, jellies, soups, fresh and dehydrated potatoes, condiments, fruits, and beverages.

Sulfur dioxide gas is highly irritating and a strong oxidant. It also destroys vitamin A and some B vitamins, such as thiamine. Its use is not allowed in treatment of meats. It is on the GRAS list, and reviews have found no apparent hazard. The healthy body can metabolize the reaction products of sulfur dioxide contained in foods. Even so, I recommend avoiding sulfur dioxide as much as possible.

Talc (*magnesium silicate*)—*talcum powder.* Talc is a silica chalk (see *Silicates*) that is used in coating and polishing rice and as an anticaking agent. It is also used externally to help dry the skin and genital areas.

Talc is thought to be carcinogenic; it may contain asbestos fibers. The substance itself is chemically very similar to asbestos. We have so trustingly used it on babies' bottoms for decades, but is it really safe? The FDA has asked that only talc free of asbestos be used in food processing, but at this time, there is no good way to determine the presence of asbestos. I recommend avoiding talc in food, talcum powder, and white rice that is polished and coated with it.

Tannic acid is found naturally in coffee and tea, wine, and the barks of some trees, including oak, cherry, and sumac. Commercial tannic acid is derived from the seed pods of palms or ferns or from oak nutgalls, little growths on the twigs. Tannic acid is used as a clarifier in brewing, filtering out proteins, and as a refining agent for fats. Its main use is in flavorings, where it provides its enjoyable astringent taste. Some of these are caramel, nut, maple, butter, brandy, and fruit, which may be used in beverages, candy, bakery goods, ice cream, and liquors.

Tannic acid is on the GRAS list, and studies show it to be safe. It can stain the skin or irritate the stomach with higher doses, as with high intake of coffee or tea. In food use, where it is probably safe, it is not usually listed on the label.

Tartaric acid is found in grapes, wine, and a few other fruits, and a little is present in coffee; it is also formed as a product of grape fermentation. In food processing, tartaric acid is used to augment flavoring and to adjust acidity in beverages, candy, jelly, baked goods, and frozen dairy products. It also acts as a stabilizing agent to prevent color or flavor changes due to rancidity. It is sometimes the acid component of baking powder.

Tartaric acid may be a bit irritating to the gastrointestinal tract in large doses; in food use, however, it is safe. Studies show no toxicity, and it is on the GRAS list.

TBHQ (*tertiary butylhydroquinone*) is a butane gas derivative of petroleum and is fairly new in food processing, where it is used as an antioxidant. It is often used along with BHA or BHT, but it may work alone to prevent rancidity of fatty foods, oils, and even low-fat products. It works best on unsaturated fats, particularly the vegetable oils, such as soy and safflower.

TBHQ is the most recent antioxidant to be approved by the FDA. It is very toxic in even modest amounts if ingested, but it is limited in foods to 0.02 percent of the fat and oil content (0.02 percent is the maximum content for antioxidant combinations as well). In small amounts in food, it is apparently not dangerous. However, I would suggest avoiding this additive.

TCE (Trichloroethylene) is a chlorinated hydrocarbon related to vinyl chloride, a strong carcinogen. Trichloroethylene is also a degreasing solvent. It is used in the process for decaffeinating coffee and in some spice preparations. It is not directly added to food, but it might be a contaminant; it will not be listed on the label. TCE has also been used in medicine as an analgesic and anesthetic.

TCE, like other chlorinated hydrocarbons, is dangerous in any concentration when taken into the body. Since it and other solvents are used to make decaffeinated coffees and teas, it is wise to avoid these products. Water-processed decaf, even made from organic coffee beans, is available.

Vanilla—*vanillin, ethyl vanillin*. The aromatic and flavorful substance vanilla is naturally found in the vanilla bean as well as in some other foods, such as potatoes. Vanillin and ethyl vanillin are stronger, synthetic analogues of vanilla, made from eugenol (an oil from cinnamon or clove). When natural vanilla is used as a food flavoring, it is listed as such. When the synthetic vanillas are used, they are probably listed only as artificial or imitation flavors. Vanilla and its analogues may be used in caramel, chocolate, root beer, butterscotch, butter, and some fruit flavorings for foods such as candy, ice cream, beverages, puddings, gelatin desserts, toppings, frostings, and even margarine.

Vanilla, vanillin, and ethyl vanillin seem to be very safe flavorings. Even when used in much higher amounts than they would be in foods, studies showed no adverse effects. All are on the GRAS list.

Whey—*whey protein concentrate, milk serum*. Whey is the liquid part of milk left after the casein is removed, such as in cheese making. Whey contains the lactalbumin protein and the lactose, or milk sugar. Whey can be dried to yield a mildly sweet, high-lactose powder containing minerals, such as calcium, phosphorus, and potassium. Whey can be used complete, demineralized, or delactosed for certain purposes.

Whey is used in a variety of foods, such as ice cream, candies, imitation breakfast cereals, baked goods, and eggnog. Whey solids have been used as an extender and binder for meats, meat loaf, and sausage products. Whey protein may be used in powdered formulas for breakfast, weight-control programs, or body building.

All of these products are basically safe. People allergic to milk or with a lactose intolerance may have reactions to whey. Otherwise, they are well tolerated.

Xanthan gum is a complex carbohydrate made commercially by fermenting corn sugar with *Xanthomonas campestris* bacteria. The gum formed is used commonly in food processing as an emulsifier and thickener, particularly in salad dressings to create a viscous, thick-pouring substance and to keep oil and water together in suspension. Xanthan gum is also used in dairy products and in low-calorie foods such as puddings, as a starch replacement.

Xanthan gum in itself is safe. Tests show no hazards at very high levels. Often, however, the foods in which it is used are artificial and contain unnecessary chemicals, so I recommend avoiding them for that reason.

Xylitol is a simple carbohydrate alcohol, similar to sorbitol, that is found naturally in some berries, fruits, and wood. Wood sugar, or xylose, is used to produce xylitol, a waste product of the wood-pulp industry. Finland is the main producer of this sugar.

Xylitol is not a true sugar (hexose). It is metabolized differently and therefore is usable for diabetics. It is caloric like sugar, however, although it does not seem to promote dental decay (it may even help reduce cavities), so it is popular for use in chewing gums. It is found in many dietary foods and beverages.

Xylitol has not been used as a food additive for long, and it is currently under review. It appears safe in the amounts used in foods, but studies have suggested some long-term tumorigenic effects from regular use. For now, I suggest that this additive should be used only in moderation, not on a daily basis in gum, drinks, or foods.

Yeast—*baker's, brewer's, dried, torula yeast.* Yeasts are unicellular fungi that are grown by fermentation of carbohydrates. Yeasts have a wide variety of uses in food processing and preparation and have been used for centuries. Enzymes in yeast help convert simple sugars to alcohol and carbon dioxide.

Baker's yeast is used for making breads and baked goods. Brewer's yeast generates an alcoholic fermentation in making beer, ale, wine, and some whiskeys. Brewer's yeast is also high in vitamins and minerals and may be used for vitamin supplements, usually to pro-

vide the B vitamins, such as folic acid. Dried yeast is rich in protein and nutrients. Torula yeast is a different fungus, Candida, and is grown on molasses or, more recently, on petroleum by-products. Yeasts are also used to enrich refined flour products. Some foods that contain yeast are breads and other baked goods (as leavening and dough conditioners), including crackers, bread crumbs, and pretzels; alcoholic beverages; soup mixes and gravies; vinegars, catsup, barbecue sauce, and other condiments; mushrooms; many vitamin preparations; and some dried fruits and herbs (as a contaminant).

Nutritional yeasts are basically safe. Smoked yeast used as seasoning should be avoided because of the smoking process. Some people are allergic to yeast or may experience intestinal gas, bloating, or indigestion with its use. People with overgrowth of intestinal yeast (*Candida albicans* or *rhodotorula* yeast) should avoid all yeast-containing foods. Otherwise, yeast can be a nutritious, safe, and very useful food additive.

FOOD PREPARATION

What kinds of problems come up during food preparation and/or while it is stored? All food in cans, boxes, plastic bags and containers, jars, and bottles have a particular shelf life, which may vary from a few hours to several years.

Foods can spoil. Most of the fresh fruits and vegetables, depending on their ripeness and refrigeration, must be used within a few days to a week or two. Fresh-cut meats, poultry, and fish, which are most easily contaminated by microbes or insect larvae, must be refrigerated. Wrapping may give some protection, but these foods should be eaten as soon as possible. The whole grains and beans store well because of their protective coverings, although bug infestation can be a problem, especially with organic foods. Storing grains and flours in the refrigerator will often help prevent this. Nuts and seeds are definitely best refrigerated to prevent these oily foods from going rancid. Most foods which are prepackaged in boxes, cans and jars contain some kind of spoilage retardants and do well when stored in cupboards. Often, open packages of cereals, crackers, and other grain products must be used rapidly or be refrigerated to protect them from insect infestation, especially in the warmer months (assuming that the house is not sprayed regularly with pesticides, an area of concern we will discuss later).

Food preparation presents several other possible problems besides food spoilage. The main one is food contamination by microorganisms such as bacteria, viruses, or molds. Other concerns are the use of chemicals in cooking or seasoning and the hazards involved in the various cooking processes.

Food contamination may occur at any step, from the time the food is grown to the time it reaches the plate and palate of the consumer. Molds are the most common microbes that contaminate foods; they may grow on cheeses, nuts, breads, meats, herbs, and grains. In general, most molds are fairly well tolerated when consumed in small amounts. Some people, however, are allergic or sensitive to molds. Certain molds and foods may produce specific toxins that can be dangerous. Aflatoxin, produced by the molds *Aspergillus flavus* and *parasiticus*, is one such substance that is potentially harmful, especially to the liver, where it can cause a type of hepatitis or even cancer. It has been associated most commonly with peanuts but may also contaminate other nuts as well as corn, wheat, and barley. Many bacteria produce toxins while most mushrooms contain toxic chemicals that could cause problems ranging from intestinal upset to fatal neurotoxicity. The chemical cycasin is produced by certain nuts grown in Japan; the bracken fern, also found in Japan, may cause stomach cancer; and the betel nut leaf chewed as a tobacco in India has been shown to cause mouth cancer.

Another source of food contamination is produced by the widespread use of antibiotics in animals. Statistics published in 1978 suggested that nearly 50 percent of all antibiotics produced in the United States were used in animals, either in their feed or administered by injection. Approximately 90 percent of pigs, 60 percent of beef cattle, and more than 90 percent of poultry were treated with antibiotics; however, these were most commonly used over extended periods at low levels to reduce infection and to increase weight, in addition to their use in the treatment of specific diseases. This type of antibiotic use may lead to the development of resistant, harder-to-treat organisms and toxic residues or antibiotic breakdown products, often stored in the animals' livers and fatty tissues. Most ranchers and farmers allow a drug-withdrawal period before they slaughter their livestock in order to reduce the drug levels in the edible tissues. However, this is not always done, and even after a two-week withdrawal period, antibiotic levels in tissues may still be high enough that a penicillin or sulfa-sensitive person may have an allergic reaction to the drug residue in the meats.

There are also weight-promoting drugs used, especially in beef. Various hormones have been and are still used to increase weight and reduce the estrous cycle in animals. Some cancer-producing steroids, such as diethylstilbesterol (DES), an estrogen hormone, have been used. DES was banned from use in livestock to be consumed by the public in 1979, but that does not mean that it is no longer used. Most of these estrogenic hormones are potentially carcinogenic in humans, particularly in women.

Food poisoning refers mainly to illness caused by bacterial or viral contamination of food that occurs during food shipping, as a result of improper refrigeration, or during preparation. Foods, such as meats, may be infectious even before the animals are slaughtered.

Contamination of the human intestinal tract with pathogenic bacteria and viruses is the cause for most cases of acute diarrhea. The FDA has estimated that somewhere between 100 million and 300 million cases of diarrhea occur yearly and nearly one-third of those are caused by contaminated foods. (Other causes include food allergy, absorption problems, emotional stress, and intestinal diseases.)

A 1982 study of traceable cases of food poisoning found that more than half were caused by contaminated poultry and fish, about 20 percent chicken and 40 percent fish, mainly shellfish. Most of these cases involved contamination by bacteria, such as the Salmonella bacteria, which can contaminate the intestinal tract of animals (especially affecting poultry and red meat); only a small percentage, 10 percent, involved viruses. Salmonella is the most common bacterium to cause food poisoning; Campylobacter species are also becoming common. Certain strains of Staphylococcus may cause intestinal problems. Botulism, a result of a toxin released by the *Clostridium botulinum* bacterium, is not really very common, but it can be fatal, as the toxin affects the nervous system and can cause changes in vision and speech, then breathing problems, and finally paralysis.

There are an estimated two to three million cases of diagnosed Salmonella food poisoning yearly, commonly from contaminated raw meats, milk, poultry, eggs, mayonnaise, and fish. This infection produces fever, chills, diarrhea, abdominal pain, sometimes vomiting, and often a severe headache—definitely not a pleasant experience. Luckily, it is rarely fatal and will respond to treatment with an antibiotic such as ampicillin. Symptoms usually clear in one to two days. Even when acute, this infection and other food poisonings are usually mild to moderate problems, though they can be severe or even fatal in infants, the elderly, or already debilitated people. About 9,000 people per year die from food poisoning.

Food can be contaminated in several ways. Contamination can occur before a food is packaged if the cans, jars, or packages already contain microorganisms. The occurrence of this seems to be decreasing as packaging conditions become safer and more sanitary. Food can also be contaminated by nature; microorganisms are everywhere, and if food is not properly protected or stored, these germs may multiply and cause disease.

People also contaminate food, either those working in factories helping to process or package it or, more commonly, those who prepare foods at home or in restaurants. Some viruses, such as those that cause hepatitis, may be transmitted in this way, but luckily, this is not common. Most intestinal viruses are not thought to be very contagious by respiratory transfer. However, staphylococcal germs may get into foods from either the skin or the respiratory tract of the food preparer, and this occasionally causes food poisoning. The symptoms are similar to Salmonella poisoning, occurring within several hours of exposure and usually lasting a day or two. If the diarrhea is not too severe, food poisoning can even be a good means of purging, of cleaning out the intestines. People often feel better than ever, and a little lighter, after experiencing it; still I do not recommend this as a new weight-loss program.

How can we avoid the spread of infections through food? First, it is important that the food preparer, whether at home or in a restaurant, be responsible for keeping their hands clean and avoid handling foods when he or she is sick. If there are cuts or open sores on the hands, rubber gloves will reduce the spread of any bacteria. We should make sure to wash our hands before handling food, especially after handling money or animals. It is important to wash while caring for children, particularly after wiping noses or changing diapers. Food-preparation surfaces, such as countertops and cutting boards, should be cleaned after each use so that organisms do not grow. Cutting utensils should also be kept clean.

Foods can be contaminated before they are purchased as well. Avoid buying overripe produce; also, do not buy or use bulging cans, outdated foods, or packaged foods with broken seals. If a food smells or tastes funny or spoiled, take it back or throw it out. Meats and poultry should always be kept refrigerated and used within a day or else they should be frozen when you get home from shopping. Frozen foods should be kept frozen, or used very soon after thawing.

Care must also be taken to avoid contamination after food is cooked. Bacteria grow rapidly at room temperature but very slowly when cold. Cooked foods should not be left sitting out overnight; if they are, they should be thoroughly recooked to kill any bacteria they may have grown. Home "canning" or jarring should be done very carefully in sterile conditions; if done improperly, this is probably the most common cause of botulism (meats and green beans being the worst culprits).

When eating out, make sure that the restaurant is clean and the foods used are fresh if that is possible. If you can see the chef, make sure that he or she looks healthy. When the food is served, smell it and taste it first before gobbling it down so you can more easily tell whether it is of good quality. Watch for heavily salty tastes or extra additives in the food—even ask whether such additives as MSG or sulfites are used. Nowadays, more Chinese restaurants advertise that they use no MSG, or will at least avoid using it in your food if you ask.

○ A NEW CONCERN: FOOD IRRADIATION

Is gamma radiation of food with nuclear waste products the greatest food preservative we have? Many in the government, such as the FDA and the Department of Energy, would like us to think so; actually, they would just like to irradiate foods and not have us know anything about it. There is definite support from the food industry, the nuclear industry, and the U.S. Army to irradiate a wide range of foods. Currently, there is justification for demanding at least that irradiated food be labeled so the consumer can choose whether to eat it or not. Politically, we need to question whether we want to begin a food irradiation industry with the use of recycled nuclear wastes to achieve social justification for nuclear weapons production.

The army originally began using irradiated foods in the early 1960s, serving such foods as irradiated bacon, ham, potatoes, and strawberries to personnel on 12 military bases. The FDA later repealed their use after cellular studies suggested that irradiated sugar affected cell growth and produced damaged chromosomes. But food irradiation has come back strong in recent years. As with many low-level radiation studies, it causes no obvious immediate effects on the consumer. Many spices and herbs have been irradiated for years, as has pork, with which there is always a danger of contamination. It is now likely that some grains (irradiated grains have been shipped abroad), fresh fruits and vegetables, and frozen foods are irradiated.

Foods are irradiated, ostensibly, to improve their shelf life and prevent microbial and insect contamination, so that there is less waste and more profits. It can also mean a reduction in the use of toxic chemicals that are now used to preserve these foods. Irradiation is done by exposing foods to gamma rays emitted from a nuclear source, such as cobalt 60, as they pass on a conveyor belt. It is claimed that the irradiated foods do not themselves become radioactive and thus are not introducing radiation to the consumer.

The concern with food irradiation is that it may produce by-products that are carcinogenic and increase the incidence of leukemia and other types of cancer or disease of the liver and kidneys. These health problems may not become evident for 20 to 30 years. Most of us are very skeptical about radiation in general, whether it be X-rays or even microwaves, let alone gamma radiation of our food. It is also possible that irradiation may affect the nutritional content of the foods treated, by altering protein structure, reducing vitamin levels, or deactivating sensitive enzymes.

The Western "attack and conquer" approach is to find stronger and more potent forces to kill germs or cancer cells. In cancer treatment, if chemicals and surgery do not work, we can try radiation. Obviously, radiation affects cellular growth—it can kill cancer and can cause cancer. We must be very careful about food irradiation, because it can affect a lot of people in a very short time, and the effects are probably not reversible.

Another way of irradiating food is the use of microwave ovens. Instead of gamma waves, these ovens use pico waves, which have a much less toxic effect. These waves penetrate tissue deeply and rapidly, and increase the vibrational rate of the water and tissue molecules, which generates the heat and cooks the food. It is suggested, however, that people avoid being near their microwaves while food is cooking. With increased exposure, as with restaurant workers using microwave ovens regularly, there is also an increase in symptoms such as headaches, fatigue, irritability, sleeping problems, and deep tissue burns. Microwave exposure may cause hormonal changes and affect our immune defenses. Long-term effects are really not known. Microwave ovens are a great convenience, but we must use them sparingly, I believe, and not get too far away from natural cooking methods.

○ ANOTHER CONCERN: ELECTRICITY AND ELECTROPOLLUTION

It may be hard to accept that something we cannot sense, something that all of us depend on daily at home and work, might be a significant problem in our modern lives—yet electricity may fit into this category. I have been concerned for more than a decade that excessive exposure to environmental electricity, electromagnetic radiation (EMR), is possibly a danger to our health, and may even be a factor in carcinogenesis. Foresighted scientists throughout the world are now beginning to show us that EMR may indeed be one of the newest threats of our modern age.

After all, our body is an electromagnetic generator; its electrical potential can be measured in the cells, nerves, and our heart and all muscles. In fact, many vital functions in our body depend on the electrical energy generated by ionic movement of minerals across cell membranes. An electromagnetic force field can also be measured around our body, and our life force or vitality influences the strength of this field. In fact, we vibrate with direct, not altering, current, and at very specific frequencies, or hertz. Why then, wouldn't it make sense that certain machines, wires, homes, and businesses could vibrate or contain EMR at levels that are either harmonious or discordant with our own vibration levels. Machines and power lines all have fields of electricity surrounding them which could be hazardous to our biological force. Overhead powerlines, especially high-voltage ones, have been one of the main concerns of EMR that may be negatively affecting those who live close to them. The higher frequency radiations, from X-rays to nuclear radiation, are clearly dangerous.

Electromagnetic radiation can be divided into two categories. The first is *ionizing radiation* and includes X-rays, gamma rays, and nuclear radiation. Exposing our body to these highly reactive ions at certain levels can dramatically affect our atomic structure. Ionizing radiation can actually rip electrons from atoms and molecules and directly affect cell division and cell structure. It causes problems initially in areas of our bodies which have a rapid cellular turnover, such as the skin, gastrointestinal tract, and blood.

Nonionizing radiation includes the forms of EMR below 300 hertz, or cycles per second (cps), and notably the 60 hertz alternating currents that power our homes and offices. This form of energy does not clearly destroy the cellular function, but it can "shake" the micromatter, and at higher frequences, this shaking generates both vibrational changes and heat. This is how microwaves work, by increasing the vibration of the water and other molecules in the food, which then generates heat. At the lower end of the nonionizing radiation frequencies, ranging from 30–100 hertz, this effect is less, and the consequences are not known. However, the supposition here and in current research is that exaggerated or regular exposure, such as many hours per day surrounded by or working with electrical objects or wires, to this extremely low frequency (ELF) level of electricity is hazardous to our health.

Electropollution is generated by the constant use and wide variety of electronic instruments and lines. Electricity and other forms of radio waves are how we connect and communicate with each other. Common electropollution components include computers, underground radio transmitter grids, medical imaging, and high-voltage power lines. Home devices that may affect us include hair dryers and electric blankets. Some common avenues of electrical exposure are seen in the following chart.

ELECTRICAL EXPOSURE

Electrical outlets	Power lines
Electrical wires	Metal detectors in airports
Lamps	Antitheft systems in stores
Televisions	and libraries
Radios	Medical equipment/monitors
Tape players	Dental equipment
Telephones	Computers
Electric heaters	Underground radio
Electric blankets	transmitter grids
Clothes dryers	Microwaves

Earth's vibration is approximately 10 cps (hertz) which is in the alpha, or resting, range of our brain. The ELF common range of 45–70 hertz of most machinery and power lines is close enough to ours and to Earth's vibration that it influences us, mainly in the sense of agitation or stimulation. The most general effect of this is probably in our biocycles and in increasing stress and fatigue, as well as in lowering resistance to disease. I am sure that it also may affect our ability to sleep and rest deeply.

The subtle vibrations of Earth most assuredly influence our biocycles, and clearly, changes in magnetic energy must alter us as well. Research has shown that our pineal gland, which produces serotonin and melatonin and may be at the core of our entire endocrine system, is affected not only by light, but also by magnetic fields. The seasonal light and dark cycles of each day appear to regulate our psycho-emotional being through our pineal gland. Many birds, insects, and reptiles daily use Earth's natural magnetic influence of 10 hertz (this is the primary frequency of the brain in most animals) for their movement and instructural sense of direction. Subtle changes in magnetism will alter their behavior. Research with homing pigeons has clearly shown this. Even the growing patterns and movements of bacteria are influenced by their magnetic fields. Atmospheric ionic gases, solar and lunar influences, and the metallic core of Earth all affect its electromagnetic vibration. Electromagnetic energy changes in Earth's field seem to affect responses in animals, as observed in their behavior prior to earthquakes and dramatic weather shifts; clearly, they sense these changes.

More specific effects of electromagnetic fields (EMF), in addition to the aforementioned activation of our stress response, include most vital body systems, particularly the central nervous system (CNS), as well as the cardiovascular, endocrine, and immune systems. Similar effects and changes occur with microwaves, radio waves, and electrical and magnetic fields. Clearly, for all of these, as the exposure increases their potential effects become more deleterious. In the CNS, brain chemistry may be altered, particularly in the hypothalamus and cerebral cortex. Microwave exposure clearly affects stress levels and mood shifts. Possible changes in electron transfer in cellular mitochondria may also occur and thus reduce general energy levels. Research into depression and suicide shows a relationship to EMR exposure. In the cardiovascular systems, heart efficiency, oxygen capacity, and hemoglobin and red blood cell levels are all reduced, as is the sodium-potassium response which is at the base of body electricity (membrane electrical potentials). Immunologically, there is a decreased response. This "electrical" system leaves a large area open for exploration and some researchers theorize that our increase in infectious diseases such as herpes, AIDS, and Lyme's disease is correlated with changes in EMF. Cancer and leukemias may also be associated with more specific exposures, which I will discuss shortly. The endocrine system is probably influenced by EMR, though research is needed to verify this; thyroid and pituitary functions are additional concerns.

Magnetic fields are measured in gauss. The level found near high-voltage power lines and many high-current appliances is one gauss. Government research has revealed that humans, in the presence of a one-gauss field, demonstrate reduced performance in adding sets of numbers and in short-term memory than when not surrounded by this type of electromagnetic field. Specifically, these high-voltage power lines, which generate a constant irritating hum, have been studied more than other EMF effects in regard to their influence on human behavior and disease. Intially, concerned residents living near powerlines complained of an increase in headaches, lethargy, memory loss, and the recurrence of illness. Local farmers observed that their vegetable growth and crop production were reduced. Cattle that grazed by the power lines showed lower milk production and more birth defects. In 1979, researchers Edward Leeper and Nancy Wertheimer reported increased cancer and leukemia rates in children who lived near high-voltage power lines. Other researchers in this country and Sweden have had similar findings. An increase in the incidence of brain tumors in electricians, electronic technicians, and utility linemen has also been shown. Pregnant women who sleep under electric blankets have a higher incidence of miscarriages than other pregnant women. EMFs appear to stimulate microbial growth and cell division; this is possibly related to an increased incidence of infections in people who have high exposure. In the last 30 years there has been a higher incidence of birth defects, infertility, and cancer; this may be related to higher levels of electrical exposure.

Other than some specific electrical concerns, I believe we are dealing with a total body electrical load, or exposure, in regard to these health effects. Making a drink in a blender, cooking on an electric stove, or even using a microwave on occasion are probably minimal risks unless we are particularly sensitive. However, I see a lot of businesspeople, office workers, airline and medical workers in my practice who receive regular exposure, such as 10–12 hours daily, to electrical machinery, computers, and hospital equipment. (Potential hazards of computers, or VDTs, will be discussed further in the next section.) Most seem to get sick or burned out more easily, are less able to handle stress, and, generally, do not appear as vital as those people who work in more natural environments. Both in my practice and in teaching courses, I have become aware of the high level of stress and burnout among nurses; fatigue and recurrent infectious illnesses were most common.

Most people who work around electrical machinery, such as nurses, wear rubber-soled shoes. This may reduce the risk of electrocution, but it also does not allow them to clear (ground) the electromagnetism they pick up from their surroundings. When I do some form of massage on my patients, I feel uncomfortable whenever I wear my rubber-soled shoes, for example, because I cannot easily clear the energy I pick up from them. Some body workers are adversely affected because they get congested or weakened when they work on others. If we remove our shoes, our body is then a conduit for electromagnetic energy, and we can clear ourselves of electricity or another's magnetic energy more easily.

The earth and water are very useful to help balance electromagnetism and electropollution after working around electrical devices. Showering, bathing, or swimming help. Instead of, or in addition to bathing, we can go outdoors and put our bare feet on Mother Earth (grass or dirt) for a few minutes to help ground ourselves and clear body electricity.

In *The Body Electric*, Robert O. Becker, M.D. discussed many of the current theories and research about EMR as well as our internal electrical vibration, external electricity and electropollution, and the use of electricity in medicine and healing. The right vibration of electrical energy used correctly may increase our healing forces. Electricity can also be used to stimulate regrowth and regeneration. The body's ability to regenerate and heal may be even more profound than we have thought, especially with the right bioelectrical support. Dr. Becker describes many cases of this in animal studies, and, most spectacularly, in children under 12 years of age having the ability to grow back a normal fingertip if it is severed above the first crease. In these cases, when surgeons attempted to repair the wound or to sew the finger back, it did not heal as well as when left alone to regenerate anew.

Clearly, electropollution is a controversial topic. It has wide political and economic concerns, and it is unlikely that either the government or electric companies would admit to much danger after more than 50 years of use. Yet, research may show that certain frequencies may be disruptive to cellular resonance. It is possible that these rates of extremely low electrical frequencies (30–100 hertz) that are in common use interfere more with biochemical impulses or the cell rate for release and absorption of calcium, for example, than might a higher frequency, such as 400 hertz. More research will help with this. Burying the big power lines may help reduce some electropollution, but could cause other problems as well.

We do not really know the safe level of EMR exposure. With the increased use of EMR and subsequent electropollution ranging from hairdryers to power lines to nuclear radiation, our concerns should grow; continuous or regular high exposure of any type of EMR seems to create problems. From stress activation to impaired cellular growth processes and immune response to increased cancer rates and reproductive problems, there is also a wide range of potential effects. The combined concerns of EMR and toxic chemical exposure may be an even greater dilemma in upcoming decades. Our government and, indeed, all governments have their work ahead of them. We need more regulation in regard to pollution of all sorts, and maybe even electropollution in particular.

The art and science of geomancy, carried on over centuries, studies Earth's forces and energy lines and may provide insight for those people who want to live in areas of lower geopathic stress and avoid areas of electropollution and negative influences from the earth. Home planning and building with this in mind, and clearing negative forces from existing homes and workplaces are part of our future. Learning to live in harmony with the earth's electromagnetic fields is a part of living in harmony with nature and her laws.

○ POLLUTANTS IN THE HOME AND OFFICE

Our immediate environment, our home and our workplace, are major contributors to our chemical exposure, and in my opinion, are a major health concern. Indoor pollution is much worse than outdoor pollution for most people; outdoors, pollution has room to spread and dissipate, but when chemicals are used indoors or the indoor air is contaminated, the contaminants are easily concentrated and potentially more hazardous. Chemicals in the air from aerosol sprays, cleaning agents, perfumes, synthetic rugs and furniture, industrial solvents, and pesticides, to the surrounding fluorescent lighting, electricity, and noise, places we may visit. The following lists some specific areas of concern.

INDOOR POLLUTANTS

- *Hydrocarbon fuel combustion*—the burning of coal, gasoline, natural gas, wax candles
- *Pesticide sprays*—used on insects and rodents
- *Cleaning fluids*—cleansers, soaps, bleach, detergents, ammonia, window cleaners
- *Paints, adhesives, glues, and solvents*—used in housework and hobbies, for example
- *Plastics*—used in many areas
- *Heating systems*—which can spread toxins
- *Smoke*—(secondary, or side-stream, smoke is now clearly a big problem), fireplace smoke or barbecue chemicals can also be hazardous
- *Aerosol sprays*—hairsprays, antiperspirants, disinfectants, and cleaners—mostly propellants, which may be fluorocarbons or hydrocarbons, neither of which are good
- *Dust*—which can carry sensitizing or toxic materials, including mites, molds, bacteria, pollens, carbon monoxide, asbestos, pesticides, solvents, sulfur dioxide, lead, smoke, and vinyl chloride

Indoor air pollution is a large and important topic; however, since it is not directly related to nutrition (unless we consider everything we see, breathe, hear, and contact to be part of our nutrition), I will just summarize the general concerns and give examples of specific risks. Useful references that treat the subject more fully include *Office Hazards*, by Joel Makower (Tilden Press, 1981); *The Nontoxic Home*, by Debra Lynn Dadd (Tarcher, 1986); and *The Household Pollutants Guide*, by the Center for Science in the Public Interest (Anchor Books, 1978). *Detox*, by Phyllis Saifer, M.D., and Mella Zellerbach (Tarcher, 1984), contains a more general discussion of the various areas of potential toxicity, such as foods, drugs, environment, and home and office pollutants, and offers specific suggestions on how to handle these concerns. A new book, *Save Our Planet* (Dell Publishing,1990) by Diane MacEachern, has many organized lists of chemical pollutants in the home and office. Yes, it is time to save our planet, and the 1990s is the time to do it!

Problems of chemical sensitivity affecting our ability to work and function in life are becoming more common. Episodes of strong chemical exposure or infection may weaken our body's ability to defend itself or may create allergy or hyperreactivity to the environment. This becomes a complex problem that must be dealt with very carefully, and invariably includes the avoidance of all industrial chemical and air pollution exposure.

We are exposed to chemical toxins through three main routes—**ingestants**, **inhalants**, and **contactants**. (A fourth route, injectants, is minor in occurrence compared to the others; however, this very direct form of body contamination by these chemicals occurs in medical practice or by insect bites and stings, and can create problems ranging from minor itching to death.) The ingestants include food, drink, and drugs. Food may contain both intentional (food additives) and unintentional (contaminant) chemicals, as well as the individual protein allergens within the food. Water may, and often does, contain some chemicals, even dangerous ones. Beverages such as alcoholic and caffeinic drinks can cause toxic reactions. Ingested drugs, both prescription and over the counter, take effort for the body to metabolize and eliminate. The inhalants are transported by the air, through which toxic substances can be carried both indoors and outdoors. Dust can carry all kinds of things, from mites to molds as well as many chemicals. These can create allergies, sinus congestion, and lung irritation. Contactants, another large class, include cosmetics and cleaning supplies. Skin rashes are the most common problem caused by contactants. Pesticides can be spread by all three methods: When sprayed, they are carried by the air; they get into water; and they contaminate food.

There are many symptoms of chemical toxicity, affecting nearly every system of the body. Some of these symptoms are headache, fatigue, behavior changes, mood swings, nervousness, confusion, depression, loss of sex drive, skin rashes, coughing, wheezing, anorexia, nausea, and edema. A careful personal history may help isolate and correlate specific chemical exposures or environments that precipitate the symptoms. Then, the solution often involves avoiding the chemicals, changing jobs or making changes within the work environment, and learning less toxic ways to work, clean, and live.

Chemicals are ubiquitous and invade our lives more and more. Some are needed and helpful, but many are now created to support the huge chemical and home products industry with the manufacture and marketing of faster and more powerful cleansers, stronger and lighter plastics, denser insulation, or stronger pesticides. I do not believe that this is what we need. Of course, it is beneficial if the new products are safer and less toxic than what was previously used, but often they are not. We need to allocate more effort and money toward cleaning up our contaminated environment, homes, work-places, and bodies.

Pollutants in the Workplace

While some environmental problems can affect us anywhere, in the work environment there is a much wider range of potential pollutants, depending on the type of job. People work in a great variety of situations—indoors and out; cities, suburbs, farms, and industrial locations; small and large offices; big factories; and so on. The types and degree of chemical exposure vary with the situation. The following list shows people whose jobs put them at particularly high risk.

HIGH-RISK OCCUPATIONS

Airline flight crews	Janitors
Anesthesiologists	Leather workers
Auto mechanics	Manicurists
Chemical researchers	Miners
Chemical workers	Painters
Clerical workers	Pharmacists
Computer chip factory workers	Photocopy workers
Dental hygenists	Plastic workers
Dentists	Printers
Dry cleaners	Radiologists
Electronic assemblers	Radiology technicians
Explosives workers	Soldiers
Farmers	Steelworkers
Firefighters	Tanners
Grape workers	Textile workers
Hairdressers	Welders
Insulation workers	

Many of these occupations have above-average risks of cancer, and all of them have more chemical exposure than the average population.

Women of childbearing ages (usually defined as 15–44 years) who work in these jobs are especially at risk. They should familiarize themselves with particular dangers in their workplace and do their best to minimize their exposures. If this is not possible, it may be worth considering a change in job or occupation. Many of these lead to create exposure to substances on the following list, which could be harmful to a fetus.

Concern about links between occupational hazards and cancer began in the early 1900s with the increased incidence of genital cancer in chimney sweeps, thought to be caused by the benzopyrenes in the soot created from burning coal. Throughout this century, occupational and environmental cancer has become a major problem. The environment, including nutrition, influences cancer rates more than any other factor. Petroleum and its by-products are the major industrial chemical problem of the twentieth century, not specifically with regard to cancer, but because of general contamination as a result of their wide use.

SOME OCCUPATIONAL AND CHEMICAL HAZARDS

Acrylonitrile	Dyes	Photocopier gases
Aerosols	Ethanol (alcohol)	Silver nitrate
Anesthetic gases	Fibers/dust	Soaps
Antimony	Flame retardants	Solvents
Asbestos	Formaldehyde	Tin
Benzene	Hair spray resins	Toluene
Bromides	Industrial chemicals	Trichloroethane
Carbon monoxide	Inks	Trichloroethylene
Carbon tetrachloride	Lead	Vinyl chloride
Caustics	Mercury	X-rays
Cigarette smoke	Methylene chloride	Xylene
Detergents	Microwaves	
Dry cleaning solvents	Noise	

Tobacco, asbestos, and alcohol also affect both health and cancer rates. For example, people who drink alcohol and smoke cigarettes have a higher incidence of cancer—specifically, cancer of the esophagus—than those who have just one of those habits. People with certain nutrient deficiencies, such as beta-carotene, folic acid, or selenium, usually from poor nutrition, are also predisposed to higher incidences of cancer.

Most studies of chemical carcinogenesis are done with animals. Although there may be close correlation between humans and animals in regard to tumor production caused by chemical irritation, it is not exact. For most chemicals, we do not really know the safe level of exposure; for some sensitive people, any contact has adverse health effects. We must assume that there is no really safe level, or else rely on animal studies, as they are currently the best predictors we have.

Though cancer is the most serious outcome of chemical exposure, it is probably not the most frequent; general chemical sensitivity, which can create a great number of symptoms and illnesses, is most prevalent. We might suspect we are sensitive to chemicals if our contact with them causes any of these symptoms: headaches, dizziness, burning eyes or nose, stuffy nose, confusion, light-headedness, inability to concentrate, sore throat or cough, wheezing, slurred speech, blurry vision, itching, or rashes. Some of these symptoms may result from irritations caused by the chemical inhalants.

CHEMICAL IRRITANTS

Art supplies	Nail polish remover	Photographic supplies
Car exhaust	Natural gas	Room deodorizers
Carpets	Newspapers	Scented detergents
Deodorants	Oven cleaners	Smog
Gasoline	Paint removers	Synthetic clothes
Glues	Paints	Toilet paper
Nail polish	Perfumes	Typewriter correction fluids

In addition to chemicals, the average office setting of today may pose dangers from fluorescent lights, computer screen radiations (and other electrical equipment), and even noise in some jobs. Of course, people who work directly with chemicals, especially in closed settings, are at greatest risk, but we must recognize the wide variety of dangerous exposure in the typical work environment.

Lighting is much more a cause for concern than most people, especially employers, would believe, not so much by posing a grave danger as by affecting how we feel from day to day. Fluorescent lighting has been shown to increase illness and absenteeism, reduce productivity, and diminish morale. On the other hand, natural lighting or full-spectrum lights to replace fluorescent ones at work will reduce illness and improve attitude and productivity, as you will find if you sit and work under fluorescent lights for six to eight hours and then try full-spectrum bulbs. Their use is increasing, and their price has been reduced in recent years, now making them a wise business and health investment. However, some very sensitive individuals may not even tolerate full-spectrum tubes and must use the incandescent bulbs.

With the use of computers so widespread in this technological age, I am concerned about the effects of sitting at a video display terminal (VDT) for eight hours; people I see in my practice who spend much of their time working at VDTs often have a variety of symptoms. I still write primarily longhand on yellow pads because I do not want excessive exposure to the electricity, noise, or other hazards of VDTs.

In *Office Hazards*, Makower devotes a whole chapter, entitled, "Terminal Illnesses," to the problems of VDTs. Results of research done by the National Institute for Occupational Safety and Health are compiled in a chart showing the "health complaints of VDT users," which reveals a long list of symptoms that occur at a much higher rate (two to five times as often) among VDT users than others. Many eye problems, including strain and color-perception changes, sore wrists, back and neck aches, stiff shoulders, arm pains, numbness, fatigue, and irritability are just some of the problems. It is best to vary our time at work, to take breaks from the VDT, rest our eyes, drink lots of water, and follow the other suggestions given at the end of this chapter.

Noise, even inaudible sounds, can also affect mental and physical health. Both office and factory jobs with high levels of noise definitely affect not only our hearing but our general disposition as well. Typewriters, tabulating machines, computers, and conversation all combine to increase the decibels in the office. Insulation is not always effective; and in large, open offices with many workers, it is difficult to concentrate and "hear ourselves think." The spread of disease is also easier in such settings. Outdoor work in construction or with jackhammers or near a busy airport can be the noisiest. If we have this type of job, it is wise to protect our ears, but the sound vibrations also penetrate our body and influence our organs, tissues, and cells. We need some peace and quiet to balance us.

We all have a right to work in a safe location. Noise reduction and protection, good lighting, and, especially, clean air, are part of a healthy work environment. Let us educate industry and our employers toward the realization that a safe, healthy work environment provides greater health, success, productivity, and prosperity for all concerned.

Pollutants in the Home

Most of us are exposed to more chemicals in the home than anywhere else, mainly because there are so many possible uses for chemicals and also because we spend more of our time in our own or friends' homes. The use of chemicals in the home affects everyone there, and this is particular cause for concern when there are small children in the household.

It is wise to minimize chemical use at home as much as possible. Besides irritations from contact and inhaling them, generalized chemical sensitivity and allergy can result from recurrent chemical aggravation. I believe that regular contact with various chemicals weakens us immunologically and makes us more susceptible to disease in general. In her book, *The Nontoxic Home*, Debra Dadd does a wonderful job of outlining the types of toxic products that are available and, in many cases, the possible exposure we have by using them. I referred to her work and other sources to create the following general list of home chemical dangers. All of those listed are, of course, a greater danger to those who are chemically sensitive. Children, the elderly, and invalids may also experience more serious reactions. And all of these products are much worse when ingested, so childproof your chemicals; put them out of reach.

Most cleaning supplies, cosmetics, and toiletries have a dual route to irritation and toxicity—by contact and by inhalation of the fumes. Of course, if ingested, most of these products may be very dangerous, even deadly. In recent years, more and more new products that are less toxic or nontoxic have been created or old ones redis-covered. Safe cleaners, for example, include lemon, baking soda, vinegar, salt, and trisodium phosphate. Check at local health food or environmentally conscious stores for the safer products.

Plastics have become extremely pervasive in our society, with a great many uses. They are a variety of synthetic materials made from coal or petroleum. Some of them, such as nylon and polyester, are relatively safe; others, such as polyethylene, acrylics, and polyurethane are less safe; and some, such as polyvinyl chloride and those which contain formaldehyde, are toxic. These last should be avoided. I think it best not to store or microwave food in plastics in order to avoid outgassing of the soft plastic resins into the food and air. I do not keep water or juices in polyethylene unless they are refrigerated because these "thermoplastics" tend to soften with heat and release more chemicals. Cooling keeps these plastics more stable.

There are many alternatives to the chemical-based home pesticides and other toxic products. Often, they are not as strong or fast acting, just as natural remedies may take more time and effort than strong pharmaceuticals in the treatment of illness. Check health food stores, books, and suppliers' catalogues for less toxic products to use in place of more harmful chemicals.

HOME CLEANING SUPPLIES

Detergents—may cause eye irritation.

Fabric softeners—residues on clothes can be irritating or allergenic.

Spray Starch—phenol, formaldehyde (aerosol).

Mothballs—paradichlorobenzene—toxic to the liver and kidney, irritating to mucous membranes.

Dry cleaning spot removers—perchloroethylene—a solvent that when inhaled can irritate the liver and nervous system.

Chlorine bleach—should not be mixed with ammonia or vinegar, as the resulting chloramines can be toxic fumes.

Ammonia—may cause rash or irritate eyes and skin, especially in aerosols.

Drain cleaners—lye, caustic sodium hydroxide—very toxic to skin and when ingested.

Oven cleaner—lye aerosols are the most dangerous.

Furniture and floor polish—nitrobenzene, napthalene, and phenols.

Silver polish—ammonia, petroleum products.

Glass cleaners—ammonia, blue dye—aerosols worse than spray pumps.

Air fresheners—phenol, cresol, ethanol, xylene.

Germ-killing disinfectants—cresol, phenol, ethanol, formaldehyde—very irritating.

Mold cleaners—phenol, kerosene, formaldehyde—irritating, especially to eyes.

Carpet shampoo and upholstery cleaner—perchloroethylene, ethanol, ammonia, detergents.

Dishwasher detergents—chlorine, detergents—should not be mixed with ammonia or ingested.

TOILETRIES

Toothpaste—phenol, cresol, ethanol, artificial color and flavor.

Mouthwash—hydrogen peroxide, phenol, cresol, ethanol, ammonia, formaldehyde, artificial color and flavor.

Cosmetics and mascara—polyvinylpyrrolidine plastic (PVP), artificial colors, plastic resins, alcohol formaldehyde.

Talcum powder—may contain asbestos.

Perfume and aftershave—alcohol, phenol, cresol, trichloroethylene, formaldehyde, artificial colors and fragrance.

Aerosol hairspray—PVP, formaldehyde, artificial color and fragrance.

Antiperspirants and deodorants—aluminum chlorohydrate, ammonia, alcohol, formaldehyde, artificial fragrance.

Dandruff shampoo—PVP, formaldehyde, detergents, artificial colors and fragrance.

Hair color—coal tar dyes, ammonia, detergents.

Hair removers—ammonium thioglycolate.

Bubblebath—detergent, artificial color and fragrance.

Nail polish and remover—acetone, phenol, toluene, xylene.

Denture cleaners—many salts with artificial colors, fragrance, and preservatives.

Disposable diapers—synthetic fibers, various deodorizing chemicals.

Spermicides—methylbenzethonium (benzene) chloride, alcohol, formaldehyde, perfumes, preservatives.

Feminine douches and sprays—ammonia, phenol, detergents, artificial fragrance, talc (may contain asbestos).

CLOTHES

Permanent Press—resins, formaldehyde.

Fabric dyes—dichlorobenzene, benzidine.

Flame-resistant fabrics—TRIS—now banned in children's sleepwear because of carcinogenicity.

Synthetic fibers—nylon, polyester, acrylic—which are all plastics.

ART AND HOME OFFICE SUPPLIES

Glues—epoxy contains vinyl chloride, formaldehyde, and ethanol; "super glue" has acrylonitrile, phenol, napthalene—all are toxic.

Permanent ink markers—acetone, toluene, xylene, ethanol, cresol.

Typewriter correction fluid—cresol, trichloroethylene, naphthalene, ethanol.

Computer terminals—may cause eye irritation, headache, fatigue, and neck, shoulder, and back pains.

Television—may cause eye irritation, headache, fatigue.

PLASTICS

Polyurethane foam—beds, cushions, pillows—lung, skin, and eye irritants.

Polyester—clothing, bedding, diapers, tampons, upholstery—may cause irritation, allergy, skin rash.

Nylon—clothing, toothbrushes, other brushes, upholstery and carpets, and so on (probably safe).

Acrylics—made from acrylonitriles—acrylic fiber, waxes, paint, plexiglass.

Polyethylene—containers, wrappers, kitchenware, plastic bags, squeeze bottles—possibly carcinogenic.

Vinyl chloride—worst of the plastics—carcinogenic.

Polyvinyl chloride—adhesives, containers, records, tapes, toys, beach balls, pacifiers, raincoats, boots—can release vinyl chloride, which can cause cancer, liver disease, birth defects, and more.

Urea-formaldehyde plastic resins—particleboard, plywood, insulation, tissues and towels—outgas formaldehyde, a suspected carcinogen.

Fluorocarbon plastic—tetrafluoroethylene—Teflon, nonstick coating, ironing board covers; irritant to skin, eyes, respiratory tract.

OTHER HOME TOXINS

Smoke—96 percent of cigarette smoke pollutes the air and increases carbon monoxide levels. It is also an irritant and secondary smoking is becoming more of a concern.

Garbage—can bring insects and rodents. Keep the house clean and recycle wastes.

Gas appliances—emit gas fumes, carbon monoxide.

Kerosene lamps and heaters—kerosene fumes, carbon monoxide.

Fireplaces and woodstoves—emit chemicals in wood, carbon monoxide.

Particleboard—urea-formaldehyde—possibly carcinogenic.

Foam insulation—urea-formaldehyde foam insulator (UFFI)—carcinogenic, banned in 1982 but later reapproved.

HOME PESTICIDES

These range from mildly dangerous to very dangerous.

Rodent killers—mousetraps, arsenic, strychnine, phosphorus—deadly if eaten.

Insecticides—all kinds, for various bugs. Pyrethrum, a plant extract, is useful. Most other chemicals, even "inert ingredients," may be dangerous.

Lice shampoos—lindane (Kwell)—when used on body, may be carcinogenic. They are used for lice and crabs and also as an insecticide. Pyrethrin powders and sprays may be helpful; useful for animals too, but not for humans.

Suggestions for Reducing Waste and the Use of Toxic Products

- *Avoid Chlorofluorocarbon (CFO) products*, such as polystyrene (Styrofoam) containers and packaging protectors, whose production and breakdown are polluting the atmosphere and destroying the ozone layer.
- *Avoid aerosol sprays*, such as deodorants, hairsprays, and cleaners.
- *Avoid plastic containers* or use products with comparably minimal waste, for example bulk cheese instead of individually wrapped slices.
- *Use biodegradable products*, such as paper, not plastic; waterbased soaps; eggs packed in cardboard, products; waxed paper rather than plastic wrap.
- *Purchase reusable products*, such as cloth napkins and towels, returnable bottles, and rechargable batteries.
- *Support legislation for deposits on bottles, cans, and plastic containers*.
- *Recycle everything possible*, such as glass, cans, paper, cardboard, plastics.
- *Reuse as much as possible*, such as paper bags, plastic bags, cardboard boxes, bottles, Styrofoam packing pellets.
- *Buy more durable products*.
- *Buy less whenever possible*.
- *Shop at coops* and farmer's markets where products are available in bulk, there is less fancy and costly packaging, and they support using recycled plastic and paper bags.
- *Buy in bulk*, for example, larger bottles in place of six-packs, or large containers of regularly used products, such as soaps, detergents, shampoos, and cleansers.
- *Voice your objections* to stores and manufacturers when you first see new throwaway, nonrecyclable products; the plastic can and the throwaway camera are two recent examples.
- *Ask for more biodegradable products*.
- *Borrow or rent items* that you only need infrequently, and keep other items in good repair; loan them to neighbors, also. (Make responsible agreements for shared maintenance and repairs if you do.)

Some Facts on Waste*

- Twenty-five million tons of acid rain is generated each year from sulfur dioxide and nitrogen oxides spewed from factories.
- Packaging costs about 10 percent of total product cost.
- The average American produces about 4 pounds of garbage daily.
- Americans go through 2.5 million plastic bottles every hour.
- We throw away enough glass bottles and jars to fill the 1,350-foot twin towers of New York's Trade Center every two weeks.
- We throw away enough iron and steel every day to supply all the nation's automakers daily needs.
- Consumers and industry in the United States throw away enough aluminum to rebuild our entire commercial air fleet every three months.
- Recycled paper takes 60 percent less energy and 15 percent less water. One ton of recycled paper saves: 17 trees, 7000 gallons of water, 4200 kilowatts of energy, 3 cubic yards of landfill.

What Can I Due?

What can I due? I mean it's so massive—I stooped over & picked up another heap Sumone tried 2 sweep aneath. What can I due? demonstrate? try 2 relate? wipe the slate? Headlines advertising divine decadence at a price. What & how then, Paradise? Zenith tidal wave surfers who prefer peace. What can I due to guarantee release? Keep my hands in my pockets & ignore the score? Force the issue & insist? Hang my head over in remiss? This life slips away quickly. There is no after or before.... Love is the door.

—Bethany ArgIsle

---

*Sources include the Environmental Defense Fund and the book *Save Our Planet* (New York: Dell Publishing, 1990), especially "Can You Believe It?" on page 119.

○ PERSONAL AND PLANETARY SURVIVAL

The use of certain chemicals has been a great boon to the technological age; it has also been a great detriment to the ecology and health of Earth and her people. Chemistry has changed the balance of life. I am a naturalist at heart and appreciate the beauty and purity of nature more than almost anything else. It is sad to think that Earth has been violated and to sense the hidden dangers in much of her water, soil, air, and now the food that we eat. The previous sections of this chapter have been devoted to revealing these problems; this final section suggests ways to avoid or counteract them. I again refer you to *Save Our Planet* by Diane MacEachern for a more indepth look at all the things you can do personally—at home, at work, in your community, and globally.

The chemistry of today involves a large amount of both safe and harmful substances. Food additives, for instance, range from natural vitamins, minerals, and salts to more disturbing preservatives and artificial colors and flavors. But, as I have shown, our chemical concerns are not all related to food. Occupational and industrial uses of chemicals, most of them affecting the food chain in some way, pose additional problems as well. Home use of potentially toxic chemicals increases yearly and is a large part of total chemical exposure.

From one perspective, it may seem harmless to spray some bugs or kill some weeds to make our home "safer" or more beautiful or, more commonly, to improve the yield of commercial crops. Chemicals in food help protect it and usually lengthen its storage time or shelf life. These factors figure into the profit motive of the agricultural and chemical industries and are affected by the politics of our society. A side effect of laissez-faire capitalism is that the emphasis on profits and return on the dollar invested may supersede any concerns for the health and well-being of the people and the environment. In the United States up until a few years ago, it appeared that only a few alarmed citizens and government employees had been looking at the global cost of pollution. Today, each of us must face our responsibility, which, inevitably, will require cleaning up our mess; this will probably cost more than the profits that were made in the first place. And, as always, you and I will pay for it, possibly with our lives. More citizens now show concern about the pollution of our planet than ever before; however, the problem has escalated and will continue to worsen unless stronger measures are taken to stop it.

Chemicals are both an outcome of technology and a factor contributing to its development; and chemistry has made life easier in many ways. New products and plastics facilitate basic daily tasks, creating less expensive and more durable toys and kitchenware, for example. Some impressive medical advances have resulted from applied chemistry. Foods can be processed more simply in the factory and the kitchen, and we have new taste treats and more edible products every year.

In the terms of testing and use, I believe the government underplays potential toxicity, especially immediate effects, not the results of long-term exposure or ingestion, possible interaction with the environment or other chemicals in use, or Mother Earth's reactions to chemical dumping or underground weapons testing. Synthetic chemicals are used that are not found naturally anywhere on Earth, and neither Earth nor our human body knows how to break them down. The organochloride pesticides such as Aldrin and Dieldrin are examples.

The latency period between exposure to carcinogenic industrial chemicals and cancer may be as long as 20–30 years. Realistically, it is difficult to test for carcinogenicity unless we postpone the use of various chemicals for decades of testing or find more sophisticated methods of predictive testing. Often it is an increased cancer rate in a certain population exposed to a carcinogen, such as asbestos, that alerts us to its danger. Since chemical use is expanding so rapidly, it is unlikely that everything can be studied thoroughly (or that the integrity of the chemical industry executives can be trusted), so life experience must ultimately be our teacher on what works safely. Industrial and home use of chemicals has increased nearly 10,000 times in the last 60 years. More than 33,000 chemicals are in use, and nearly 1,000 are added yearly out of the many thousands presented to the EPA and other government agencies.

Currently, there are several hundred chemicals on the EPA's hazardous list. These either cause cancer or are poisonous in some other way or both. Most of these are hydrocarbon petrochemicals, made through chemical processing of petroleum. They include the aromatic amines, such as dyes and epoxies, the chlorinated olefins (hydrocarbons), such as many plastics and pesticides, and the alkyl halide solvents, such as trichloroethylene (TCE).

What makes these industrial chemicals so harmful is the damage or irritation they can cause on a cellular level, whether immediate or over time. Many of these toxic chemicals seek out free electrons, which are plentiful within the DNA of the cell nucleus. Molecular damage of the DNA can generate birth defects or cancer, with cell growth either aberrant or out of control. Cancer potential seems to increase with certain chemicals and with increased exposure. We must avoid these chemical "time bombs" whenever possible, even though research might not yet show them to be dangerous. In many cases, we are not sure of the long-term effects; I would not bet my life on the safety of most industrial chemicals. I believe that the widespread use of these chemicals is a substantial detriment to human health and contributes greatly to the weakness in the individual and collective human immune system. Ironically and sadly, we are often turning to chemical therapies that may further alter our immune response as well as add more pollution to our environment.

Chemical use is now part of all aspects of life; chemistry is here to stay. The question is, "Do we have better living through chemistry?" Learning to live with chemicals and to use them appropriately so that they do not destroy us before our time is my fervent hope. This involves maintaining a healthy immune system, a positive attitude, and a high purpose. Protecting ourselves by reducing chemical usage and exposure, I believe, will greatly reduce our chances of disease, cancer, and early death. This is important for everyone, but especially for the chemically sensitive, our infants and small children, the elderly, and invalids, all of whom are more susceptible to chemical toxicity. Making changes and a commitment to living as chemically-free as possible is, I believe, a strong investment in our personal and collective life insurance plan.

The following *88 Survival Suggestions* include activities, ideas, and changes that each of us can implement to benefit ourselves, our families, and friends. Further suggestions are offered by Charles T. McGee, M.D., in *How To Survive Modern Technology*. Dr. McGee also cites *Closing Circle* by Barry Commoner, in which Dr. Commoner discusses his four "laws of ecology." They are:

1. *Everything is connected to everything else.* We cannot do something in one area of the environment without affecting the rest of it.
2. *Everything must go somewhere.* In nature, all waste products nourish something else. We now use materials that nature has no mechanisms to break down.
3. *Nature knows best.* Human advances that violate nature are detrimental to us all.
4. *There is no such thing as a free lunch.* Many of the gains in productivity are achieved at the expense of the ecosystem in the form of pollution. A price will be paid for this somewhere down the line. Many people are paying the price now in the form of chronic illness caused by artificially synthesized new chemicals.

Don't give me anything for free, I can't afford it.
—Edward Spritzer

Not just Survive, live life Alive.
—Bethany ArgIsle

---

88 SURVIVAL SUGGESTIONS

DIETARY

1   *Eat* moderately on a regular basis. Overeating stresses the body, and being overweight or obese may result in further health complications.

2   *Avoid* processed foods, particularly those that contain highly refined ingredients.

3   *Reduce* or eliminate food additives, particularly preservatives, artificial flavors, and artificial sweeteners.

4   *Read* package labels to learn about what additives the foods contain. Do not be confused by "natural" or "no preservatives" on the label.

5   *Eat* more high-fiber foods, particularly whole grains, vegetables, and fruits.

6   *Eat* more wholesome, natural foods, as they come from nature—primarily fruits, vegetables, and whole grains, plus some nuts, seeds, and beans.

7   *Buy* and use organic foods, those that are grown without chemical fertilizers and pesticides; this action supports the organic food industry and the consciousness of cleaner food. Much produce is contaminated with fumigants and fungicides even after it is harvested.

8   *Wash* appropriate foods—know how to clear contaminated foods, with baking soda or bleach.

9   *Buy* more foods at local farmer's markets, where you can find out directly how the food is grown. This supports small or family farms. Also, the food sold at such markets is probably fresher, less expensive, and less chemically treated.

10 *Refrigerate* or store food appropriately as soon as possible to prevent spoilage.

11 *Drink* clean water. Use a water filter, buy purified water, or drink well water that has been analyzed and shown to be free of chemicals and germs. Avoid tap water!

12 *Avoid* red meats—beef, pork, and lamb. Raising livestock on a vast scale is destructive to any natural environment. Overconsumption of these products is unhealthy.

13   ***Especially*** avoid chemically treated red meats. Whenever possible, buy the meats of range-fed animals, free of antibiotics and hormones. Do not consume lunch meats or other nitrate- or nitrite-cured meats.

14   ***Reduce*** total saturated fat intake, to a maximum of 5–10 percent of total calories in the diet. Consumption of saturated fat is related to increased incidence of cardiovascular disease and cancer.

15   ***Limit*** total fat intake to 15–25 percent of dietary calories. This range is based on climate and personal needs, and includes saturated (animal, dairy products, and eggs), monounsaturated (such as olive oil), and polyunsaturated (vegetable oils) fats.

16   ***Increase*** the dietary ratio of polyunsaturated to saturated fats. This reduces the risk of cardiovascular disease.

17   ***Use*** cold-pressed vegetable oils. These are not extracted with chemical solvents. Olive oil, a monounsaturated fat, may be the best for cooking.

18   ***Avoid*** all organ meats, such as liver, heart, and brain. These can be high in accumulated chemicals.

19   ***Buy*** organic poultry and eggs from range-fed chickens, if you eat such foods. These are not treated with antibiotics or hormones or fed highly chemical feeds.

20   ***Eat*** deep-sea fish. Of the animal foods, fish may be the best. Avoid shellfish, cod, and many freshwater fish, as they are more easily contaminated. The fattier fish, such as salmon, sardines, and mackerel, actually help reduce cholesterol and risk of heart disease.

21   ***Use*** low-fat or nonfat milk products if you use milk at all. It is not recommended that milk be consumed either regularly or in large amounts; goat milk products, plain yogurt, kefir, or some cheeses are probably better.

22   ***Minimize*** soft-drink use. Substitute water or a combination of fruit juice and carbonated mineral water.

23   ***Minimize*** use of sugar, particularly sucrose, or "white sugar." Try natural sweeteners, such as date sugar, rice or malt syrup, honey, maple syrup, or fructose, probably in that order of preference.

24   ***Avoid*** waxed fruits and vegetables. The paraffin covering is potentially harmful.

25   *Avoid* aluminum and Teflon cookware; use glass, Pyrex, iron, or stainless steel.

26   *Eat* more cruciferous vegetables (organically grown is preferable). Cabbage, broccoli, cauliflower, and brussels

27   *Rotate* foods to avoid allergic/sensitivity reactions. Eating most foods only every three or four days helps reduce this potential.

28   *Eat* simple meals. This allows better digestion and utilization and makes it easier to isolate any food reactions. Food-combining is a beneficial practice.

29   *Use* a pulse test to see whether food reactions occur. Check the pulse before eating and again ten and twenty minutes afterward. If the pulse rate increases by more than ten beats per minute, one of the foods eaten may be causing a reaction.

30   *Eliminate* any reactive food completely for one month, then reintroduce it, eating it no more than once in every four days; if there is a repeated reaction, avoid it.

31   *Do* occasional cleansing or fasting, as appropriate to the season or your health condition.

32   *Use* an additive-free general nutritional supplement and even a hypoallergic one if you are sensitive.

33   *Avoid* cheap, colored vitamin pills, as they may contain petroleum products, hydrocarbons, artificial colors or flavors, BHA, BHT, or sugars—all potentially toxic chemicals.

34   *Take* additional antioxidant nutrients, which may help minimize chemical irritations. These include beta-carotene and vitamin A, vitamin C, vitamin E, zinc, and selenium.

35   *Minimize* consumption of microwave-cooked foods. We do not really know what the long-term effects are.

36   *Don't* use irradiated foods. Effects are unknown. These may include pork, some herbs, and now possibly various fruits and vegetables. Keep your eyes and ears open to the progress, or, actually, regress of food irradiation.

37   *Minimize* barbequing or broiling with gas, as the benzopyrenes created may be hazardous.

LIFESTYLE HABITS

38   *Avoid* smoking, both primary and secondary smoking. If you do not smoke, ask others to refrain. If you do smoke, try to stop—and succeed!

39   *Reduce* or avoid alcohol use. Alcohol depresses the senses and reduces immune resistance. In addition, chemicals are used in processing most alcohol products.

40   *Use* organic wines or beers if drinking for social celebration. This may help avoid the common sulfites, solvents, defoamers, and chemical pesticides found in many alcohol products.

41   *Create* a good exercise program. This includes regular exercise, stretching, and at least 30 minutes of vigorous activity several times a week.

42   *Avoid* excessive sun exposure. With the depletion of the ozone layer and the effect of ultraviolet light, risks outweigh benefits.

43   *Practice* some form of stress reduction daily. Meditate, lie down without sleeping, or just sit with eyes closed, breathe deeply, and relax for at least 15–20 minutes. There are many teachers and tapes to help.

44   *Minimize* overall use of drugs, particularly over-the-counter drugs and unnecessary prescription drugs.

45   *Reduce* use of carcinogenic drugs, such as the antiparasitic drugs lindane (Kwell) and metronidazole (Flagyl); estrogens; and the antifungal griseofulvin.

46   *Try* alternatives to drugs and surgery whenever possible. These include herbalism, homeopathy, acupuncture, and chiropractic, to name a few.

47   *Avoid* habitual drug use, such as consumption of caffeine in coffee, tea, or colas and regular sugar use.

48   *Minimize* use of recreational drugs, such as cocaine, sedatives, alcohol, and marijuana. They all have negative effects, especially in the long term.

49   *Avoid* cosmetics with warnings of certain dangerous ingredients, such as antiperspirant sprays containing aluminum. Also, if you believe in animal rights, avoid using products from companies who conduct experimental testing on animals.

50   ***Drink*** more clean water and less soda, coffee, juice, and alcoholic beverages.

51   ***Wear*** more natural-fiber clothes, especially if you are sensitive to synthetic materials. Cotton, rayon, and silk are more comfortable to many people and do not hold and conduct static electricity.

52   ***Avoid*** X-rays whenever possible. They may weaken tissues and increase cancer risk.

POSITIVE CHANGES AT HOME

53   ***Keep*** all chemicals and toxic products away from children, and keep children away from them.

54   ***Keep*** the house clean and put food away to avoid unwanted pests and the growth of infectious microorganisms.

55   ***Try*** more natural pest-control practices. There are many substances, such as herbs, powders, and fragrant oils that help fight insects and rodents. Avoid using pesticides at home whenever possible.

56   ***Avoid*** chemical cleaning agents whenever possible. Use more natural products, such as low-phosphate and unscented soaps, baking soda, borax, vinegar, and lemon. Do not replace dirt with chemicals.

57   ***Avoid*** using aerosols, artificial scents, and toilet colorings. Use herbs and naturally fragrant oils instead.

58   ***Use*** unscented and uncolored paper products, such as toilet paper, paper towels, and napkins, to avoid unnecessary chemicals.

59   ***Try*** natural drain cleaners, such as hot water with vinegar or baking soda.

60   ***Wash*** fruits and vegetables with soap and water. Especially for store-bought, nonorganic produce, diluted clear liquid kitchen detergent can remove about half of the pesticides. All produce should be rinsed and scrubbed with a brush. Also, remove the outer leaves of vegetables when appropriate.

61   ***Recycle*** waste products whenever possible. Organic waste, such as food scraps, can be used in the garden as compost. Glass can be reused or recycled, and so can aluminum and newspaper. All this saves energy and materials.

62   *Avoid* living near toxic industry, such as chemical plants, refineries, toxic dump sites, or water- treatment plants.

63   *Avoid* living near power lines and electrical plants, and any escessive electrical exposure, all of which may pose some health risks. Remember, our bodies are electromagnetic in nature.

POSITIVE CHANGES AT WORK

64   *Avoid* traveling in rush-hour traffic, if possible, or behind buses and trucks to reduce carbon monoxide and hydrocarbon gas exposure.

65   *Obtain* natural lighting or full-spectrum lights at work. If possible work by a window; if not, full-spectrum fluorescent lighting is worth the small investment.

66   *Create* good air circulation. Try to get a desk by an operable window or invest in an air purifier for your area. Circulation of good-quality air is vital to health.

67   *Avoid* tobacco smoke around you. Put a sign on your door or desk and demand a smoke-free area at work.

68   *Have* good drinking water available in the office. If there is no purified water cooler, bring your own water.

69   *Minimize* synthetic fibers at work—in rugs and furniture, for example. Hardwood floors are better, especially for the chemically sensitive person.

70   *Avoid* chemical use at your desk. This involves typewriter correction fluid, glue, and toxic art supplies. Use nontoxic supplies such as staples or paper clips, erasers, or a self-correcting typewriter.

71   *Take* regular breaks from a computer if you use one. Walk and stretch, drink water, and get fresh air.

72   *Avoid* occupational carcinogenic and/or hazardous chemicals at work. Learn more about what substances you use and their potential effects on you.

LEARNING NEW ACTIVITIES

73   *Really* think about the previous suggestions and decide whether there are any you can initiate in your life.

74   *Make* a list of foods that you have in your refrigerator and cupboards, and the specific chemicals they contain. See if any of them can be or should be avoided; then eliminate foods containing them and find more healthful substitutes.

75 *Learn* to listen to your body's messages so you become more adaptable and sensitive to your true nature. This is a very important part of staying healthy.

76 *Consult* a stress counselor if you experience anxiety or emotional difficulties or are unable to decide what to do regarding any area of your life.

77 *Learn* to meditate so that you can become your own stress counselor and can be more attuned to your inner nature.

78 *Have* faith and a positive image about life. Often what you see is what you get. The more you visualize what is right for you, the more it becomes part of your life.

79 *Learn* to prepare healthy foods and to be able to nourish yourself and others.

80 *Carry* your own food and water with you if you have special requirements so that you need not accept whatever is around. Make choices in your best health interest.

81 *Discipline* yourself to put into effect what you need, desire, and visualize.

82 *Learn* some healing arts, such as massage, herbal therapy, and nutrition for yourself and others.

83 *Learn* about local healing plants for use in day-to-day care and nourishment and for future survival should you need them.

84 *Learn* to sprout and eat seeds and beans. These are very nutritious and wonderful survival foods.

PREPARING FOR THE FUTURE

85 *Plant* a garden and grow your own food. This will give you the freshest, chemical-free foods. If you own land, plant fruit and nut trees, which can provide food for many years. Even in cities, flower and vegetable boxes can surround your home.

86 *Prepare* home and family for disaster. Whether it be for flood, snow, or earthquakes, gather the essentials. Know where the gas and electric lines are and how to turn them off.

87   **Store** water, food, and supplies. Keep extra water in durable containers. Store extra nonperishable food, such as grains, beans, dried fruits, and vegetables. Refrigerate nuts and seeds for best storage. Keep extra supplies like rain gear, warm clothes, flashlights, life raft, and so on, depending on the requirements of your area.

88   **Join** with neighbors for preparation and planning. Know what to do. Believe in survival. Love one another.

PART THREE

BUILDING A HEALTHY DIET

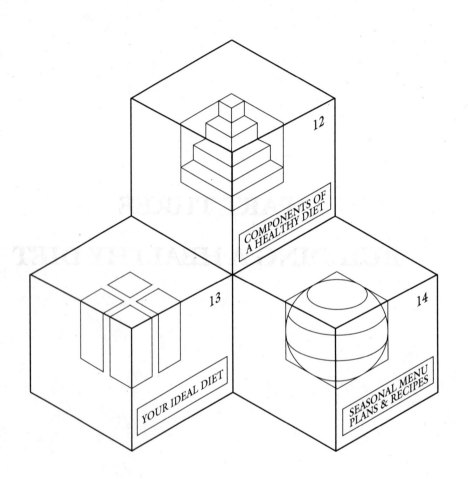

COMPONENTS OF
A HEALTHY DIET

12

YOUR IDEAL DIET

13

SEASONAL MENU
PLANS & RECIPES

14

In previous chapters, I discussed many aspects of a healthy diet—the macronutrients (proteins, fats, carbohydrates), the micronutrients (vitamins and minerals), and various food groups, possible diets, and habits including drinking uncontaminated water and breathing clean air. Now, let us put all of this together into a healthy diet using the positive information and philosophy emphasized throughout this book. Chapter 12 explores *The Components of a Healthy Diet* including food groups and proper dietary balance.

I gave Chapter 13 the optimistic title *Your Ideal Diet*. Based on diets of simple, natural cultures of the world—a cross-cultural "natural diet"—the Ideal Diet is oriented to the highest good of the individual, the population of Earth as a whole, and of Earth itself. Nowadays, there is often a great difference between a culture's rural and urban diets, especially in highly industrialized societies. One of our biggest needs in this technological age is to learn to change our focus from processed food, the supermarket, and quick meals to the garden and family-oriented, home-cooked meals. Really, God and Nature have already provided our Ideal Diet.

The diet also needs to be individual and intuitive. Our cultural upbringing and individual needs are important influences, and learning to listen to our bodies from day to day and season to season is a crucial aspect of creating and maintaining a healthy diet. This Ideal Diet is based on our current knowledge about foods and their positive and negative effects on humans, beyond a moral judgment as to eating animals or being vegetarian. The Ideal Diet is primarily vegetarian with some low-fat, good quality protein foods such as fish and consciously raised poultry for those interested, and a low intake of milk products for adults. Currently, less than 1 percent (but growing) of our population is vegetarian, so we must be realistic to find the proper balance and use of all foods.

This is not another of the multitude of fad diet books. What we really need to create is a long-term, even lifelong, diet, which will keep our bodies in their optimum state. I plan to provide you with the knowledge to be able to make proper choices and create a healthy diet and way of life. The idea is to transform our diet and eating habits so they work, not just go on a "diet" to improve health or lose a few pounds and then return to our old habits. That doesn't work; we want a diet that nourishes us optimally for life. So our main question is, "What are the basic components that provide the needed nutrients, and how can these foods be prepared and combined to make the best possible diet for us?"

Building a healthy diet is like creating a meal. As we might choose a number of particular foods to make a meal, so too we mix many foods and food groups together over days, weeks, and months to create our diet. And we apply the basic concepts and knowledge of what will be discussed here to put it all together.

As I have said, no one diet is perfect for everyone. Each of us has likes and dislikes, often based on our body's chemistry and needs. We have genetic and family backgrounds, our basic foods, and our special "feast" or celebration foods. We have our own particular eating patterns and habits regarding foods and even chemicals. These are what we begin with. Then we must sort out what works and what we need to change in order to improve our diet.

Sometimes we must change totally. I know many people who have completely transformed their ways of eating and have made big improvements in their health. I for one used to eat a basic American diet—lots of hamburgers, french fries, and Cokes; milk, ice cream, and cookies; peanut butter and jelly on white bread; more meats and chicken, and a sparse amount of fresh fruits and vegetables. I was overweight and congested in a lot of ways as a result of this very rich, unbalanced diet. I used fasting as a means to clear old patterns, and then began eating a more natural and vegetarian diet, continuing this process of slow detoxification, much of which I discussed in my first book, *Staying Healthy With the Seasons*. For more than a decade now, I have continued to adapt my diet to the seasons and my personal needs, maintaining a natural, primarily vegetarian diet.

In Chapter 14, I have acquired the excellent, efficient, and healthful assistance of international cuisine artist Eleonora Manzolini to provide you with specific seasonal menu plans and simple, yet tasty, recipes to exemplify the basic concepts and

502

foods that I have emphasized in Part Three and throughout this book. I know you will enjoy what you create from these foods and recipes, and I know it will energize you with optimum health.

In summary, Part Three is oriented to finding the nourishing foods and diet that will work for each of us. Part Four, *Nutritional Application—Special Diets and Supplement Programs*, deals more specifically with needs for individual age groups and conditions (such as pregnancy), optimum health states, special diet-nutrient plans for certain symptoms and diseases, and programs for clearing abusive substances from our life and healing our bodies.

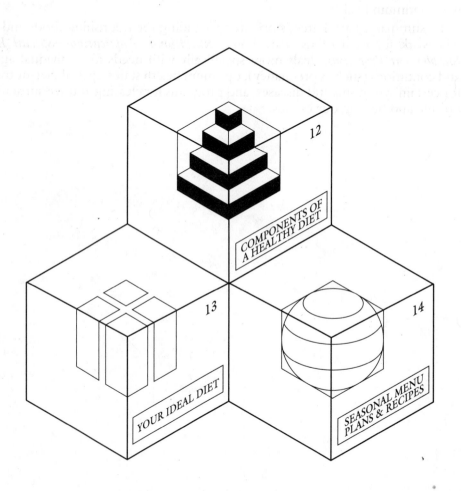

COMPONENTS OF
A HEALTHY DIET

12

YOUR IDEAL DIET

13

SEASONAL MENU
PLANS & RECIPES

14

Chapter 12

The Components of a Healthy Diet

There are many components involved in a healthful diet. Yet we need to make it simple. Nutrition has gotten very complex, and there is a continual flood of new information, both insightful truth as well as propaganda, surfacing daily in the news and various publications. Even though this book provides an immense amount of information, we have attempted to make it simple and easily accessible—easy to digest, assimilate, and utilize. Basically, though, we need to return to our own instincts of proper nutrition.

Our natural locale provides our best and most wholesome foods available to us. Our local stores, however, much like the complex and unusable information that is provided by technological manipulation, have a continuing fancy array of new packages, boxes, and cans hyped by equally flashy advertising to entice us to buy these products. Profitability is the key motivation in the food industry, and much of what we are buying is the packaging and advertising, which often costs more than the actual food in the product. If we took some of this big business money and paid all the mothers (and fathers, brothers) to grow food and prepare wholesome, natural meals, we would take a big step in the health and well-being of all of us and our planet. Though this may sound revolutionary if done on a mass level, that is exactly what we need to do individually—go back to the basics and redevelop our nutrition. To do this, we need to change our thinking and the conditioning of an entire century of misguided advertising that has so strongly influenced and molded many generations of Americans' diets, and, really, worldwide nutrition. To begin with, let us first look at one of the earlier misconceptions still taught in most schools of our nation—"four-food-group" nutrition.

○ FOOD GROUPS—OLD AND NEW

This complex, important concept regarding the basics of our diet is a challenging area of nutrition. For nearly a century, mainstream nutritional thought has centered on the "Basic Four" food groups—meats, dairy products, cereal grains, and fruits and vegetables. But there are many of us who feel that this approach, the result of a large advertising campaign that has been perpetrated and perpetuated through this highly industrialized twentieth century, is archaic, unhealthy, and part of the reason for the large increase in the chronic degenerative diseases.

BASIC FOUR FOOD GROUPS

Meats
Dairy products
Cereal grains
Fruits and vegetables

There are some good reasons why the "basic four" approach is difficult to change. The main reason is that people have been conditioned to believe that these are equally important categories of foods, and that animal, bird, or fish meats, as well as milk, butter, and eggs, are crucial parts of a good meal. This belief is taught in school and exemplified in the cafeteria diet. All of these foods, of course, can be used and are nutritionally helpful, but only in modest amounts, not as two out of four of the main food groups and not at the level currently consumed by the average person (and clearly not at 50 percent of the diet, which does occur). Actually, if these meats and dairy foods were all removed from the diets of anyone older than eighteen years of age, our society would be much healthier. Even younger children need far less of these high-protein, high-fat foods than we think, even though these foods do stimulate growth. Protein deficiency is highly unlikely in a balanced diet, as are most mineral and vitamin deficits, and we need less protein to maintain health than most people assume.

Another area of resistance to changing the "basic four" is the food industry. Billions have been spent in creating and advertising products that are less healthy for us than the basic foods that nature provides. And many of the high-fat, high-salt, and high-sugar foods are so intensely promoted that our profit-oriented industry often has more influence on our diet and health than do informed parents and nutritionists. We are convinced by distorted advertising to try these new boxes, cans, and frozen treats that imitate our natural wholesome foods, and create refuse for the earth, as well as for our bodies. Thus, this concept of the "basic four," created by the power and advertising of the food industry giants—the dairy, meat, and breakfast cereal industries—and supported by the medical kingdom and educational system, leaves the farmer with only one category to cover all the nourishing fruits and vegetables.

Finding the proper balance and mix of these foods is our first important step in creating a healthy diet. A starch-centered, that is, a complex-carbohydrate-oriented, diet is the native or traditional diet throughout the world during the last ten centuries. This allows our main foods to be high in nutrients and low in calories, with a substantial fiber intake. The high fiber content of the vegetables and whole grains allows them to be less caloric, as the vegetable fiber material is not used as energy. It is the fat in our foods that contributes the most calories. The simple sugars and refined sugars also add up.

This starch-centered diet, as I said, is the typical native diet. Which carbohydrate is used, however, may vary with the culture. Traditional Asian cultures used mainly rice, with some wheat; the East Indian diet was similar, with more wheat; in the Middle East, the staple was wheat; Europeans ate wheat and potatoes; and the Native Americans used a large amount of corn. These cultures also used some peas or beans to balance the grains and make complete proteins, and then many local vegetables were added. This main diet was usually supplemented with smaller amounts of seasonal fruits, milk products, and animal foods.

As technology developed and humans moved up the ladder of success, richer living meant richer foods. Meats, eggs, cheeses, and milk became associated with success. No longer did we need to hunt and move with the seasons. We could pen animals and milk or slaughter them for food. With more technology, shelf life replaced health life. A rejection of the "peasants'" diet went hand in hand with this high-fat diet. The refinement of foods was also part of this move up. As I have discussed, none of these factors has improved nutrition. In fact, they have been steps backward in terms of nutritional health. What we need is a "New Basic Four" Food Groups.

Our new "basics" start with ten basic food groups, the foods nature provides—the whole food ingredients of our diet: fruits, vegetables, whole grains, legumes, nuts, seeds, dairy products and eggs, fish, fowl, and meats.

NEW BASIC FOUR

Fruits
Vegetables
Whole grains and Legumes (beans and peas)
Proteins and Fats/Oils:
Vegetarian—nuts and seeds
Omnivore—milk, eggs, and meats

This is really not very different from the old basic four, but I believe it is the first step in a transition to a healthier diet. The main thrust is the de-emphasis on the meats and dairy products, which need to be combined into one category. The vegetables and the whole grains and legumes are the most significant groups and should be the largest part of the diet. The protein and fat foods are really secondary groups, and combined into one, though they also are very important to balance out the diet.

The specific individual proportions of these groups vary somewhat from person to person and season to season, as we will discuss more fully later. Let us now look at the different components that, I believe, we should bring together to make up our new, healthy diet.

○ TEN KEY COMPONENTS OF A HEALTHY DIET

Natural foods	Tasty and appealing foods
Seasonal foods	Variety and rotation
Fresh foods	Food combining
Nutritious foods	Moderation
Clean foods	Balance

These are not necessarily listed in order of importance. A balanced diet and moderate consumption of foods, without regular overeating, are likely the most important components of a healthy diet, especially on a long-term basis. Other aspects, such as food combining or rotating foods, may be more important in the fine-tuning of our diet or in treatment of special problems, such as poor digestion or food allergies. However, following these ten guidelines preventively will assure us of keeping our digestion, immune system, and entire body functioning at their optimum capacity.

Some of these "components" may also overlap. Freshness and nutritiousness or seasonality and variety may often include the same characteristics and choices in foods.

Which foods are tasty and appealing is a more personal thing—to some this may mean a beautiful, colorful salad and to others a burger and fries. This has a lot to do with the conditioning of our taste buds and brains, which may be the most difficult aspects to change in order to create a healthier diet.

NATURAL FOODS

It is my personal feeling that natural foods are the best. The closer our foods are to the garden, fields, and orchards, the more energy, vitality, and nutrients we will obtain per calorie of food consumed. I do not believe that the human species has improved upon our food other than in the artistry of the culinary chef who makes appealing and very tasty cuisine with fresh, natural foods. Though the food processing and manufacturing industries have improved somewhat on shelf life and the ease of shipping foods, processed foods in cans, boxes, and various packages are a distant second to the foods that nature has provided us. And many packages themselves contain chemicals or metals that pose toxicity concerns; in addition, the packaging is often a costly waste product that may not be recyclable, and thus, creates digestive problems for Earth.

Fruits, nuts, seeds, vegetables, whole grains, and legumes should constitute the majority of our diet, at least 80–90 percent. People eating much more than 10–15 percent of their diet in the form of animal foods should reevaluate their choices, as the high-fat and low-fiber content of these foods can be detrimental to health in the long run. The only times I might suggest a diet higher than this amount in animal products (mainly fish or poultry with vegetables) would be for weight loss or in the treatment of intestinal yeast overgrowth, where it is important to temporarily reduce the foods high in natural sugars. In these two situations, the main foods are vegetables and fish and poultry, with a modest amount of whole grains.

Part Two and especially Chapter 11, *Environmental Aspects of Nutrition*, provide more lengthly discussions of chemical versus natural foods. Here I say simply, natural foods are best!

SEASONAL FOODS (INDIGENOUS DIET)

Eating seasonally—eating foods that are available and grown in our own area—keeps us attuned to the Earth, its elements, and the cycles of nature. This also supports eating naturally of God's bounty of fresh foods. It gets us thinking about gardens and being able to pick our own food. Eating seasonally is also a most economical dietary pattern and gives us potentially the cleanest foods, as less chemicals are needed to store or ship them.

My first book, *Staying Healthy With the Seasons*, focused on nutrition through the seasons, with many concepts and practical suggestions about seasonal awareness and diet. Since I still feel strongly about seasonal eating, I want to describe what this basically means.

Eating seasonally is important first for providing the right type of fuel to protect us from the climates as our environment provides the best foods to support our health and keep us in balance. For example, in summer's hottest months, the juiciest of fruits are available. Fruits and fruit juices help to cool the body. In contrast, in cold and wet winter, the foods that require most cooking are the most prevalent. In pretechnology time, these were foods that stored well and were protected by shells or hard skins. These are the grains, nuts, seeds, and the hard squashes, tubers, or root vegetables—foods that are either higher in protein and fats or that need to be cooked well to make them ready to eat. The fresh, juicier foods are not available then. We often eat somewhat heavier or richer foods when it is colder and may easily gain a few pounds to better protect our body from the cold. Be aware that food availability may vary somewhat, even by a couple of months, around the normal harvest time, due to weather differences, crop timing, and refrigeration.

Being aware of and using the foods as they are available will help reattune us to nature and, most importantly, to our own body cycles. This is an essential step in attaining and maintaining health. It is very difficult to stay healthy year around without being sensitive to our inner needs and taking extra measures and time to care for ourselves during times of stress and change. Our personal challenges may be emphasized around the two to three weeks of seasonal changes that occur at the equinoxes and solstices, the demarcation days of change. Here's a summary of some seasonal nutritional advice.

Spring is a time of purification, healing, and rejuvenation. It is the time I most often suggest for a period of cleansing or fasting. In nature, the greens are growing freely, and these chlorophyll-rich foods are the body's best cleansers. In many climates, citrus fruits or apples also help in the purification process. I usually do ten days of the "Master Cleanser," or lemonade diet (see *Fasting* program in Chapter 18) at the beginning of spring.

As spring progresses, the amount of fresh fruits and vegetables in the diet usually increases in proportion to the other foods, such as whole grains and legumes. The heavier protein and fat foods, which were likely at their peak intake in winter, are now eaten less. Sprouted seeds and beans are a helpful addition to meals.

Spring is a great season to do a whole reevaluation of our health program and create a new one, incorporating whatever changes seem necessary. Spring is the most creative and fertile time in nature. That is why we should get our body ready by cleaning out the unnecessary past, that which no longer serves us, and planting new seeds and nourishing them to fruition at a later time.

Summer is a time of growth and activity, when things are expanding. The warmth of summer requires both a lighter diet and fresher, higher-water-content foods. And isn't it amazing that those are exactly the foods that nature provides? After the greens of spring blossom into fruit, many more succulent fruits and vegetables can be harvested to feed us in summer. More raw salads of these available foods can be used, with a reduction of cooked foods in hotter times. The juicy fruits and especially the melons can be eaten, though usually not mixed with other foods (see the section on *Food Combining*, ahead).

Summer is also a time of more activity, so it is an easier time to slim ourselves, though we may need a fair amount of good foods to support our increased energy output. Our protein and heavier cooked fats are best reduced to allow the simpler fuels to run our body at this time. If a heavier meal is eaten, it is best done in the cooler parts of the day. Drinking more water, juices, and herbal teas will keep us hydrated, especially when we are active in hot weather.

Autumn is a time of a big shift in energy, climate, and diet. It is the official harvest time of nature, and we are provided with an abundance of nourishing foods. First the remaining fruits and watery vegetables are harvested, and then the harder root vegetables and squashes come in, most of which require more heat to prepare. Whole grains, legumes, seeds, and nuts also are harvested in this season. Our diet thus shifts to more cooked foods, whole grains, and the richer protein-fat foods as the weather cools and the days shorten. Fewer raw fruits and vegetables and more complex carbohydrates are now the mainstay of our diet, especially from later autumn into spring. More indoor-focused activity and exercise need to be developed as well to be in harmony with autumn.

Winter has us craving richer, more warming foods. Foods requiring more preparation are part of our cuisine, and hopefully we can be at home more, resting and recharging, cooking, and, of course, eating. We often need more fuel to feed our furnace to generate more energy to keep us warm. However, we do not want to overeat, especially the sweets and fatty foods, as the usually decreased activity level can cause us to gain too much weight during this season.

As in autumn, the mainstay of our diet is the complex carbohydrates found in the whole grains, squashes, and root vegetables, such as carrots, beets, potatoes, onions, and garlic. Dairy foods and meats might be consumed more during winter but should never be a large portion of our diet. More fish and the high-mineral seaweeds are good in the winter, and poultry may be eaten more if it is desired.

Seasonal eating really involves a number of the other components of a healthy diet. The earth-grown foods are natural, usually fresh and appealing, definitely nutritious, and often clean, especially if grown organically, and give us a wide variety of foods over the year. We will emphasize the seasonal diet in other sections to follow; it is an essential part of the Ideal Diet. Also, for more specifics on seasonally available foods, see another of my projects, *The Seasonal Food Guide* poster and booklet, also published by Celestial Arts (Berkeley, California).

FRESH FOODS

Eating fresh foods is one of the healthiest aspects of a diet. This applies obviously to the natural foods, or foods from nature—the fruits, vegetables, grains, nuts, beans, and seeds. It also applies to most milk and animal products, which can cause more problems if they are old. Spoilage or rancidity of the animal foods can more easily cause microbial diseases, since bacteria, viruses, and parasites, for example, grow very well in these substances. Fruits and vegetables are best eaten as fresh as possible, but most of these foods store well for several weeks. Many of the whole grains and legumes keep for years after harvesting. The nuts and seeds must be more carefully stored (closed containers in a cool, dark place, or refrigerated), as they may easily go rancid because of their oil content.

Mostly, we just need to be aware of the different foods, how they store, and how to use them appropriately (see Chapter 14). As previously noted, eating seasonally allows us to get the freshest produce. When we say fresh, we usually think of fruits or vegetables, not a fresh can of spinach or a fresh box of Wheaties; even though prepackaged foods often have a long shelf life, they are often better when eaten soon after packaging. What I mean by fresh eating, however, is specifically as close to the garden, field, or orchard as possible, such as eating an apple or apricot off a tree, gathering a salad from the garden, or cooking some "just picked" sweet corn—all examples of "really fresh."

NUTRITIOUS FOODS

Eating a nutritious diet primarily means acquiring all the vitamins, minerals, amino acids, and fatty acids that our body needs to function optimally. It also means eating specific foods that contain good levels of many nutrients. These, once again, include those natural fresh foods such as fruits, vegetables, whole grains, legumes, nuts, and seeds. The animal foods, though not as balanced, can be high in certain important nutrients, such as protein, iron, calcium, or vitamin B_{12}, but they are often high in fats as well. Also, the fresher the foods are, the higher in potential nutrients they are, as they lose certain vitamins, minerals, and especially enzymes when they sit around or when cooked, which usually reduces some of the nutrient content. The industrial processing of foods greatly diminishes the level of nourishment.

When I speak of a nutritious diet, I am referring to the focus throughout this book— the consumption of a high percentage of whole foods, as fresh as possible. Also eating a variety of foods allows a greater balance of nutrients. Many processed and refined foods are enriched or fortified to make them more "nutritious." This does help some but is a distant second to the nourishment received from natural, fresh foods.

CLEAN FOODS

Eating a clean diet refers to two important areas. The first level regards consuming chemical-free foods as much as possible. This specifically means avoiding chemical additives and chemically treated foods, as well as refined sugar and flour foods. Finding organically grown produce and organic (untreated) poultry, beef, and eggs is becoming even more important as pollution worsens in our world. Buying organic foods grown by farmers and ranchers who raise fruits, vegetables, and nuts, or cattle, chicken, and other animals will let them know there is a market that will support them, in contrast to unconscious, high-chemical-using producers.

Clean also refers to washing and storing food properly to avoid spoilage and contamination. Washing fresh produce with water and even soap or Clorox bleach (which can remove more germs and pesticides) before eating or cooking is helpful to clean off the dirt, bugs, or chemicals. Packing food properly for storage in plastic bags or containers will protect it longer as well. Keeping ourselves and our homes, kitchen counters, and utensils clean also protects us and others from spreading disease. Drinking clean, filtered, chemical-free water is very important as well.

TASTY AND APPEALING FOODS

Eating a diet that is tasty and appealing satisfies our senses, and that is important, too. The more we make each meal a feast for our eyes and mouths, the more it nourishes the deeper levels of our being. It is necessary that our diet be gratifying, and if we do not eat foods we enjoy, it will not completely satisfy us. Food that is visually appealing and colorful is as important to many people as the taste, because this improves the appetite and the enjoyment of the foods. And often the food tastes especially good when someone has taken the special time to prepare a beautiful meal.

All foods have their characteristic flavors. Our attraction to some of these flavors, and thus to certain foods, is inherent in our natures, while other tastes are learned or conditioned. Often, to change our diet more positively, we need to work at changing our tastes, or, really, developing new tastes. (This was discussed more thoroughly in Chapter 10, *Dietary Habits*.) A lot of unnatural or concentrated sweet and salty flavors in foods, as well as chemical tastes, have taken people away from simple, natural eating. To return to or support the many components of the healthy diet discussed here, we may need to recondition ourselves to enjoy the true natural flavors of the real foods of Earth.

VARIETY AND ROTATION

Eating a variety of foods provides us with a variety of nutrients, thus preventing any marked deficiencies. That is, of course, if the variety of foods we choose is mainly a nutritious one. If we vary pizza, franks, and hamburgers from day to day, our diet is not going to be very balanced. Eating and varying many of the whole foods will assure a proper amount of nutrients without excesses of potentially harmful levels of sugars, fats, or even protein.

Rotating our diet means eating different foods from day to day and not repeating the same foods every day. This reduces the potential to become allergic or sensitive to particular foods, which can result from repeatedly stimulating our body's immune and cellular systems with the same nutritional biochemistry. The protein molecular parts of a food are usually what we become sensitive to; we build up antibodies against these antigens, and then, whenever we eat the food, we may get a reactive immune response. Common foods that may generate allergies include cow's milk, wheat, eggs, soybeans, corn, beef, coffee, chocolate, tomatoes, yeast, shellfish, and mushrooms.

We may also be genetically sensitive or allergic to foods or have developed allergies through other stresses or illnesses we have experienced. If we are very reactive to foods—if we do not feel well after we eat, with fatigue, irritability, or specific symptoms such as nasal congestion, itching, or skin rashes—we might want to find out what foods may be causing this. We may then wish to eliminate those foods for a while and go on a very specific four-day rotation diet, with any specific food consumed on one day not again consumed in the next three following days, thereby allowing our body to deal with it and clear it completely, reducing the constant stimulation to our immune system that can occur when we consume a food daily. (This will be discussed in more detail in the *Allergy* program in Part Four.)

We reduce our potential for food reactions by avoiding repetitive consumption of the same foods, especially the commonly allergenic ones. For this reason, and to obtain all of the important food nutrients, it is wise not to limit our food choices or eat the same foods consistently but to consume a wide range of foods from all the various groups on a daily as well as a seasonal basis.

FOOD COMBINING

Food combining (also discussed in Chapter 10), I believe, is a basic component to good nutrition. It allows us to digest and utilize the foods and their inherent nutrients optimally. Many people overstress their digestive tracts by eating a large number of foods at each meal. Our culture has been conditioned more to the balanced meal than to the balanced diet, and people may eat foods from all the different groups at each sitting. This, as I have stated, is very taxing on the body, and may in part be why, in our culture, there is so much digestive disease from stomach to colon. Simple meals of a few ingredients each, using a variety of foods over time, with concern about balancing our diet over the day or week, is a more healthful overall approach to eating.

The basic principles of food combining are as follows:

1. *Fruits are eaten by themselves or with other fruits.* Fruits are high-water-content, simple-sugar foods. They digest very easily and may move through our digestive tract rapidly. When eaten with other foods, they tend to remain and ferment in the stomach acid. The only exception is that citrus fruit and nuts seem to be handled well together, possibly because the citric acid assists in the digestion of the nuts. Subclasses of fruits include acid, subacid, and sweet. Ideally, we should eat only fruits from the same class at any one meal. This seems to be of only subtle importance, though the very watery and sweet melons seem to be digested best when eaten alone.

2. *Proteins and starches are not eaten together.* Basic proteins such as meats, poultry, fish, eggs, and milk products require maximum stomach acid levels for best digestion, mainly because of their high fat content. Nuts and seeds are also better digested with good hydrochloric acid production. Starches, or complex carbo-hydrates, are digested best in a relatively more alkaline stomach. These foods include whole grains, pastas, potatoes, and breads. When proteins and starches are combined, their stimulation to the digestive juices generates a conflictual response and a medium that digests neither food very well. This may lead to indigestion, gas, bloating, abdominal discomfort, and a poor utilization of nutrients. Most of the starch foods contain some protein, but their basic component is the complex carbohydrate. Beans, however, have a good level of both protein and starch, which offers some insight as to why many people have difficulty digesting them. They are notorious for causing intestinal gas, which may also be related to the difficult-to-digest poly-saccharides in the bean coverings.

3. *Combine protein and vegetables or starch and vegetables.* With the first two rules, this leaves meals that concentrate on vegetables with either a protein or starch complement. Some legumes may be combined with the starch, particularly the whole grains, to provide all the essential amino acids. These meals allow the body to best digest the foods and utilize their nutrients. This is a difficult step to make in meals, as it conflicts with a lot of basic nutritional concepts and many of the meals that people commonly eat, such as meat and potatoes, fish and pasta, cheese or lunch meat sandwiches, pizza, and even the basic hamburger or hotdog on a bun. So, food combining can be a major undertaking, though a positive one for many people by aiding digestion of meals and keeping excess weight off.

4. *Do not eat more than one protein per meal.* Mixing more that one protein, such as eggs and ham or cheese and meat, can be a little taxing on the digestive tract and often provides an excessive amount of fat and protein. Most people in our culture eat too much fat and protein, and this is one way to reduce this.

Food combining is especially important for any of us who have sensitive digestive tracts or intestinal problems. It is also a preventive, I believe, to wearing out our digestive organs too early. Many people consider food combining an extreme that is too difficult to carry out. However, if we do not try it out to see how we feel, we will never know.

MODERATION

Eating moderately, not overeating or undereating, is probably the basic first habit of good nutrition. Many nutritionists feel that overeating, especially on a regular basis, is the worst thing we can do to our body. Overeating applies to not only the total amount of food consumed but also, as we will see in the next section, to the overconsumption of specific foods leading to improper dietary balance. Over-consumption or abuse of sugars, fats, protein, salt, and chemicals can lead to the most disastrous results. We must be careful to control the intake of foods that contain large amounts of these ingredients.

Eating too much food at any time, as most of us have experienced, causes great stress on the body. After a meal, much more blood is sent to our digestive organs, and we are often sedated and unable to move very well until digestion is completed many hours later. Regular overeating also tends to reduce our exercise potential, and this, along with the increased calorie intake, contributes to weight increase. Almost all obesity, other than from hormonal imbalance, is caused by overconsumption of calories along with physical underactivity. Obesity, as I have discussed, leads to an increase in most of the serious and chronic diseases, such as hypertension, heart disease, diabetes, and cancer.

When we follow the other "components of a healthy diet," we will nourish our body in the best way. This will reduce the nutritional reasons for overeating, where the body craves more and more food to satisfy its malnourishment. This happens most often when foods low in nourishment, such as processed foods or foods high in fat, protein, or sugar, are eaten as a major part of the diet. The craving for food will not be diminished until the cells and tissues are nourished.

There are also many common psychological factors that cause overeating. These can be specific short-term stresses or more long-range problems. Early conditioning can cause patterns of overeating to cover up emotional pain or insecurity. These issues must be dealt with also. (More about overeating was discussed in Chapter 10, *Dietary Habits*.) Whatever the reason, it is wise to do what is needed, even counseling and hypnosis, to learn to eat moderately and focus on the most nourishing foods. This will contribute to our health, both daily and lifelong.

BALANCE

Eating a balanced diet is probably the most important aspect of nutrition in regard to long-term health. However, the concept of a balanced diet is one of the most controversial topics in the nutritional field. Very few authorities agree on the specifics of this balance, though there seems to be general agreement on the basic trends. In this section, I will discuss the following five aspects of balance:

- **Macronutrients**—proteins, fats, and carbohydrates.
- **Micronutrients**—vitamins, minerals, amino acids, and fatty acids.
- **Food groups**—fruits, vegetables, grains, legumes, nuts, seeds, dairy products, eggs, fish, poultry, and meats.
- **Flavors**—sour, bitter, sweet, spicy, and salty
  and Colors—red, orange, yellow, green, blue, purple.
- **Acid-alkaline**—acid-forming and alkalizing foods.

Balance—Macronutrients

How much of each of the carbohydrates, fats, and proteins we need will be discussed further in later sections; also, Chapters 2–4 discuss the three macronutrients in detail. Here I review specifically the basics of these important nutrients and give my suggestions for the right balance. Carbohydrates, which include simple sugars and starches, provide our body and cells with easily usable energy. Proteins provide amino acids, the building blocks of body tissues, and many active biochemicals. The fats provide lubrication and protection, as well as fuel for our body.

An excess or deficiency of any of the macronutrients can generate problems, so the art of nutrition is to create a diet with the right balance. The biggest concern, of course, is with the excessive amount of fats, particularly saturated fats, consumed by many people. Second is the high amount of refined sugar eaten. Excessive protein intake may contribute to some congestive, degenerative problems as well. On the deficiency side, the most important is the low amount of complex carbohydrates and fiber eaten in our diet. Deficient intake of usable protein, though less a concern in our culture, is still a factor for many people. If we can balance these key areas, we can greatly enhance our nutrition and prevent future problems.

FOOD SOURCES OF THE MACRONUTRIENTS

Proteins	Fats		Carbohydrates		
	Saturated	*Unsaturated*	*Complex*	*Simple*	*Refined*
eggs	coconut or	vegetable oils	grains	fruit	pastry
milk	palm oil	mayonnaise	legumes	honey	refined flour
cheese	animal fat	nuts	hard squash	maple syrup	bread
nuts	butter	seeds	whole grains	other	cookies
seeds	mayonnaise		breads	sweeteners	donuts
legumes	whole milk		and pasta		candy
fish	cheese				soft drinks
poultry	eggs				sugar
meats	meats				
	lard				
	bacon				

MACRONUTRIENTS IN THE DIET—OLD BALANCE AND NEW GOALS

	Average American Diet	*New Goals**
Carbohydrates	46%	60%
	22% complex	45% complex
	6% natural sugars	10% natural sugars
	18% refined sugars	5% refined sugars
Protein	12%	15%
Fat	42%	25%
	7% polyunsaturated	8% polyunsaturated
	19% monosaturated	10% monounsaturated
	16% saturated	7% saturated

*may range from 60–70% carbohydrates, 10–20% protein, 20–30% fat

The average American diet contains 46 percent carbohydrates, 12 percent protein, and 42 percent fat, as shown in the above table. The table also suggests a healthier balance among these macronutrients, with 60 percent carbohydrate, 15 percent protein, and 25 percent fat. The staples of this type of diet are the vegetables and grains, with some fruits and protein-fat foods. The traditional diets of many cultures of the world may have contained approximately a 60–20–20 percent balance among carbohydrates, protein, and fat, with some meat, milk, nuts, and seeds consumed to provide a higher protein level. The naturally hunted range animals and fish eaten in these cultures had a much lower fat content than today's heavily fed, penned animals. Oils and fatty processed foods such as bacon and potato chips were not available either, so the protein level could be increased without adding much fat. Today, that is more difficult to do.

Fat has more than twice the calories of protein and carbohydrates, so a little can greatly increase its percentage of the diet. In my analyses of people's diets, 40–50 percent dietary fat is not uncommon. Decreasing fat consumption to between 25–30 percent fat may be one of the hardest goals to attain for many people. But if we follow the guidelines outlined in this chapter, we can attain a healthy balance.

Balance—Micronutrients

There are about 52 essential nutrients—those substances that our body needs in order to carry out its many functions but that it does not make, at least in sufficient amounts to provide for our needs—in other words, substances that we need to obtain from food or additional supplements. These include the vitamins and minerals—the other micronutrients—as well as the essential amino acids from protein foods and the essential fatty acids from oils.

To obtain all of these nutrients from food, we need to eat a variety of natural, fresh, tasty, and nutritious foods as mentioned throughout this book. Still it is not easy in this day and age, with the diminishing nutrients in the soil and the high amount of food processing, to obtain all of our nutrients from food. That is why I often suggest a general supplement for those who are not eating a completely balanced and wholesome diet or who have any signs or symptoms of a possible deficiency. Many people choose to take a general vitamin-mineral supplement and even additional amino acid formulas or essential fatty acids as insurance that they are obtaining all of these needed nutrients.

Balance—Food Groups

Food groups is a very broad term that can mean many different things, such as the basic food groups discussed earlier in this chapter or specific classifications of foods, such as the cruciferous vegetables (broccoli, cauliflower, Brussels sprouts, and cabbage), discussed in Chapter 8. We use the term here to refer to the larger categories of food, such as fruits, vegetables, grains, and legumes, also discussed in Chapter 8. We need to obtain a proper balance among these foods to support the other components of this healthy diet.

ESSENTIAL NUTRIENTS

Amino Acids
Isoleucine
Leucine
Lysine
Methionine
Phenylalanine
Threonine
Tryptophan
Valine
Arginine**
Histidine**

Vitamins
A—retinol and carotene
B_1—thiamine
B_2—riboflavin
B_3—niacin
B_5—pantothenic acid
B_6—pyridoxine
B_{12}—cobalamin
Biotin
C—ascorbic acid
Choline
D—calciferol
E—tocopherol
Folic acid
Inositol
K—quinones
P—bioflavonoids
PABA—Para-amino-benzoic acid

Fatty Acids
Linoleic acid
Linolenic acid

Minerals
Calcium
Chloride
Chromium
Cobalt
Copper
Fluoride
Iodine
Iron
Lithium*
Magnesium
Manganese
Molybdenum
Nickel*
Phosphorus
Potassium
Rubidium*
Selenium
Silicon
Sodium
Strontium*
Sulfur
Tin*
Vanadium
Zinc

*may not be essential
**These are "semiessential," needed in special times of growth and development

As I mentioned in the earlier discussion of seasonal eating, our ideal food group balance will not be the same all year round; even the proportions of the different macronutrients will vary with the seasons. But the following list provides a good general guideline, ranking the groups from those we should consume most to those we should eat least. (This ranking does not necessarily indicate the relative importance of the food groups, because many foods that may not be eaten in great quantity are needed to make our bodies work or to provide vital nutrients.)

FOOD GROUP PRIORITIES: OMNIVOROUS

1. Vegetables	9. Eggs
2. Whole grains	10. Dairy products
3. Fruits	11. Fish, freshwater
4. Legumes	12. Poultry, nonorganic
5. Fish, salt water	13. Shellfish
6. Poultry, organic	14. Meats
7. Seeds	15. Processed meats
8. Nuts	

For vegetarians, the ranking is as follows (with the exception of eggs and dairy products, this also applies to vegans):

FOOD GROUP PRIORITIES: VEGETARIAN

1. Vegetables	5. Eggs
2. Whole grains	6. Dairy products
3. Legumes	7. Nuts
4. Fruits	8. Seeds

Balance—Flavors and Colors

The concept of the five flavors of food representing a balanced diet comes from the Laws of the Five Elements in traditional Oriental practice. According to this philosophy, each of the five flavors is associated with a different element and supports different organs and functions of our body.

In the Chinese philosophy, eating a variety of foods that contain these different flavors is an important part of a balanced diet. An excess or deficiency of a certain flavor can cause an imbalance of energy in the body and thus lead to specific symptoms and diseases. Excesses of salt and of sweet are two common examples; low intakes of bitter or sour foods may lead to other difficulties.

All the flavors are not necessarily eaten in equal proportions. The flavor focus may vary from season to season, as the elemental dominance changes, and according to our individual balance. There are many naturally sweet foods available, and these are consumed more plentifully than sour, salty, bitter, or spicy ones. Making a meal that contains all the five flavors is a challenge for any artful chef. The following table provides examples of foods associated with the different flavors.

Another way of viewing this balance is in terms of the colors of the foods, with a different element associated with each color. These colors may act like the flavors in stimulating certain organs and functions. Thus, the red foods, such as meats, cayenne, and tomatoes, may stimulate blood and circulation; green foods, such as many vegetables, may help purify us and support metabolism or strengthen the liver. This view actually seems to have a physiological basis in many instances.

ELEMENTAL NUTRITION

Element	Wood	Fire	Earth	Metal	Water
Organs	Liver Gall Bladder	Heart Small Intestine	Spleen Stomach	Lungs Large Intestine	Kidneys Bladder
Color	Green	Red	Yellow	White	Blue/Black
Functions	Purification Metabolism	Circulation Vitalization	Digestion Distribution	Elimination Mental Circulation	Storage Emotional Circulation
Flavor	Sour	Bitter	Sweet	Spicy/pungent	Salty
Foods	Lemons Other citrus Sauerkraut Pickles Vinegars Buttermilk Yogurt Preserved foods	Lettuce Spinach Chard Other greens Celery Asparagus Eggplant Some nuts Herbs	Grains Potatoes Carrots Beets Squash Peas Corn Yams Sweet potatoes Most fruits Sugar cane Honey Maple syrup Milk	Onions Garlic Radish Mustard Cayenne Chili pepper Horseradish Chives	Seaweed Ocean fish Celery Olives Salted foods Miso Capers Soy sauce Brine foods

A more common approach to dietary color balance is the "rainbow diet" approach: eating foods from all colors of the rainbow—red, orange, yellow, green, blue, indigo, and violet. This makes for very beautiful and colorful meals, and when we look at the various foods that fit into this color spectrum, we can see that this can be a way of balancing nutrients in the diet. Gabriel Cousens, M.D., has specifically addressed this diet in his recent book, *Spiritual Nutrition and the Rainbow Diet*.

There is also a whole system of nutrition based on the Chinese concept of the Five Elements. In this system, all the foods are associated with specific elements, and each individual is evaluated in terms of his or her elemental balance. Then a diet is designed that contains a certain percentage of each element to help correct or support the energy state of the person. For example, the various grains, vegetables, or meats may be split up so that each element contains a wide mix of all the food groups. This interesting yet subtle system of nutrition is described by John W. Garvy, Jr., in a booklet called *The Five Phases of Food: How to Begin* (Wellbeing Books).

Balance—Acid-Alkaline

This concept, which I discussed briefly in Chapter 10 and more thoroughly in my first book *Staying Healthy With the Seasons*, fits in well with many of the other aspects of a healthy diet. To put it simply, foods are classified as basically acid or alkaline, not according to their taste but to the residue left after they have been metabolized in the body. If the human body is decomposed or burned, the final ashes are slightly alkaline—that is, they have a pH of above 7.0, the neutral pH of pure water. When foods are completely combusted, they are broken down into an alkaline or acid ash.

Our blood has a normal pH of 7.41 that is fairly stable. When this shifts, because of respiratory changes or metabolic changes via the kidneys, our body goes through further metabolic and respiratory responses to try to correct our acid-alkaline balance. A diet that is too acidic affects our blood and tissues, and our body will try to clear unwanted elements through enhanced elimination via the colon and kidneys and secondarily through the skin, sinuses, or other mucous membranes. The congestion of mucus we experience in different body areas may often be caused in part by this acid-alkaline imbalance, usually because of too much acid food intake.

This is a difficult concept for many people to accept, because it is just that—a concept or theory. However, based on my experience and on good sense, I encourage people to eat more alkaline foods and reduce very acid ones because, on many levels, this fits into a more balanced diet. It is also consistent with my basic belief that we need to consume more vegetables and fruits (all more alkaline foods), with some whole grains (more midrange foods) and smaller amounts of the meats and milks or refined sugar and flour products (the main acid foods). The list on the following page gives examples of alkaline, balanced, and acid foods.

Usually I suggest 70–80 percent alkaline and balanced foods in spring and summer months. During later autumn and winter, at least 65–70 percent alkaline and balanced foods would be all right. In very cold climates, a higher percentage of richer acid-forming foods may be tolerated, as these foods are higher in fats and burn hotter as body fuel. Also, fewer vegetables and far fewer fruits are available at these times. By and large, whenever possible, we need lots of vegetables and whole grains to keep the body balanced.

ACID-ALKALINE FOODS

Alkaline	*Balanced*	*Acid*
all vegetables	brown rice	wheat
most fruits	corn	oats
millet	soybeans	white rice
buckwheat	lima beans	pomegranates
sprouted beans	almonds	strawberries
sprouted seeds	sunflower seeds	cranberries
olive oil	Brazil nuts	breads
soaked almonds	honey	refined flour
	most dried beans	refined sugar
	and peas	cashews, pecans,
	tofu	and peanuts
	nonfat milk	butter*
	vegetable oils	milk*
		cheeses*
		eggs
		meats
		fish
		poultry

*Some authors place milk products in the balanced area; I don't.

○ A REVIEW OF RECOMMENDED DIETARY CHANGES

We know that we have our work cut out for us when we consider that it is very likely that the poor farming people of the "backward" nations have a better diet than we do. The American diet is far from the local seasonal vegetable-grain diet of most poorer cultures. Instead of the traditional fare, many of us dine regularly on prefabricated, processed, or treated foods with increased amounts of meat, fats, sugar, salt, and the many additives that help to flavor the refined foods.

With this all too popular American diet, there has been a huge decrease in the complex-carbohydrate fiber foods and in the natural high-vitamin/mineral whole foods, as well as deficiencies of the essential fatty acids while intake of many unnecessary and damaging fats have increased. The high amounts of refined oils and saturated fats can cause much disease. The decrease in the nutrition per calorie ratio with the increase in simple sugar and refined food intake has led to a strange combination of obesity and malnutrition. Many of our vital nutrients, such as vitamins A, C, and E, the B vitamins, calcium, magnesium, chromium, and zinc, may be missing from our diet. This is of special concern in teenagers and the elderly who tend to limit their diet more than other segments of the population.

A primary focus of this book is to help the reader shift his or her diet from the Standard American Diet (SAD) to a healthier one. For this we first need to reject the processed foods, high fat foods, lunch meats, and high-sugar foods that are so prevalent. For example, many Americans are consuming close to half of their dietary calories as fats, nearly twice the level that is healthy. Jane Brody points out that additives, as well, are a dominant part of our consumption. The average American in recent years annually consumed 128 pounds of sugar, 15 pounds of salt, 9 pounds of 33 common additives, and 1 pound of the other 2,600 food additives, for a total of 153 pounds—yes, the average human weight—consumed yearly in mostly unnecessary, possibly harmful ingredients.

Changing our diet may be a difficult task. It takes guts and a lot of work. Our taste for fats, sweets, and processed foods is so ingrained. And our image is at stake. The meat and potatoes, beer and pretzel man could not possibly eat those sissy salads and wholesome natural foods such as rice and vegetables. Some of us still think we need our hunk of protein, but evidence to the contrary is building. Any of us who are reading or listening know that we have to get more basic and natural and less salty and sweet or fatty foods into our diet.

We need to begin by selecting healthful foods, as Dr. Ballentine points out in *Diet and Nutrition*, when shopping, when cooking, and in restaurants. We should not shop when hungry. When we do shop, we could skip many of the aisles with those fancy, colorful boxes and cans. This will help to get rid of many of our unnecessary and unwholesome foods. We want to choose foods as close to their natural state as possible.

Jane Brody and many other authors suggest that these changes may decrease the death rates from cardiovascular disease and diabetes by 25–30 percent and also reduce the cancer rate. A diet such as this will most assuredly affect both the vitality of newborn babies and our longevity, let alone how much better we will feel in our later years. The increase in chronic disease is primarily related to diet, and with more farsighted vision, we can be growing both older and healthier simultaneously.

ADDITIONAL RECOMMENDED READING*

1. *The Airola Diet Cookbook* by Paavo Airola.
2. *Diet and Nutrition* by Rudolph Ballentine, M.D.
3. *Jane Brody's Nutrition Book* by Jane Brody.
4. *Food and Healing* by Annemarie Colbin.
5. *Spiritual Nutrition and the Rainbow Diet* by Gabriel Cousens, M.D.
6. *Fit for Life* by Marilyn and Harvey Diamond.
7. *Nutrition Desk Reference* by Elizabeth Somer and Robert Garrison Jr.
8. *Nutrition Concepts and Controversies* by Eva Hamilton and Eleanor Whitney.
9. *Mega-Nutrition* by Richard Kunin, M.D.
10. *The McDougall Plan* by Mary and John McDougall.

---

*This selection of nutrition books gives a variety of ideas about what constitutes a healthy, balanced diet.

SUGGESTED DIETARY CHANGES

Decrease	*Increase*
Calories	Fresh vegetables
Fats	Fresh fruits
Saturated fats	Sprouts
Cholesterol	Drinking water
Red meats	Exercise
Dairy foods	Love
Refined sugar	Complex carbohydrates
Refined flour	Fiber
Salt	Whole grains
Processed foods	Legumes
Soda pop	Vegetable oils
Ice cream	

Unhealthy	*Healthier*	*Ideal*
Sodas	Fruit juice	Water, mineral water
Refined sugar	Honey, raw sugar	Small amounts of honey, molasses, date sugar
Saturated fat	Unsaturated fat	Low-fat diet
Refined oils	Vegetable oils	Cold-pressed olive oil
Shortening and margarine	Butter or chemical-free margarine	Other cold-pressed vegetable oils, such as flaxseed, canola, or sunflower
Refined flour	Whole grain flour	Home-ground flour
Refined grains	Whole grains	Organic whole grains
Processed foods	Naturally prepared foods	Whole foods
Additives and preservatives	Natural foods	Whole foods
Enriched or fortified products	Natural nutrients	Whole foods

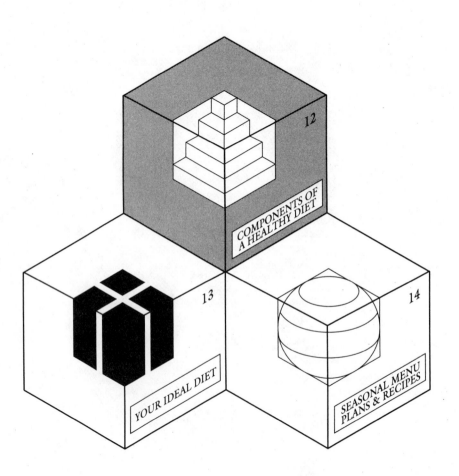

12 COMPONENTS OF A HEALTHY DIET

13 YOUR IDEAL DIET

14 SEASONAL MENU PLANS & RECIPES

Chapter 13

Your Ideal Diet

D are I even attempt to discuss "the ideal diet"? To call any one diet "the diet" is to misunderstand the basic aspects of nutrition and to mislead ourselves that we can find a diet, stick with it forever, and not worry about anything. We need here to deal with principles first and then lay out the basic foods that we can apply to these patterns.

The Ideal Diet is the individual diet that adapts and fluctuates with our needs. It will correlate with our activity level, our state of health, where we live, the time of the year, and even the daily weather. Let us assume that we are healthy and we expect this diet to maintain our good health. (Programs for illnesses and special needs are discussed in Part Four.) Learning to listen to our individual needs, or, better stated, keeping alive our basic ability to sense what our body needs through our inherent intuitive knowledge, is vital to both maintaining and adapting our own correct diet. The biggest problem in this, of course, is that our current lifestyle and busy environment take us out of this sensitive mode, and most of us get caught up in what the technological society has to offer instead of creating what we need to nourish ourselves and our families. The essential food is already available, but it takes time to gather (shop) and prepare it, and we may not wish or choose to take this time when we could be working or doing other things to support ourselves. We must realize that to create our Ideal Diet, we need to make nourishing ourselves a high priority, because without that basic support (good nutrition) for health and vitality, the rest of our life has less meaning. If we can momentarily step back from our day-to-day existence and take an honest look at our lives, we will realize that simply dragging ourselves around to a job and working by caffeine stimulation lacks quite a bit. Learning to nourish the body to give it the best possible chance for optimum energy makes sense from the standpoint of physical productivity, mental clarity, and emotional contentment, and of religious-spiritual well-being, as the body is a holy temple to house the spirit.

Our best diet, as Daniel Reuben, M.D., points out in his book *Everything You Always Wanted to Know About Nutrition* (Avon Books, 1978), begins with mother's milk. Since mother is the sole source of nourishment to her baby, she has the responsibility to also take the best possible care of herself. I do notice that many mothers make a real effort to cultivate better habits during pregnancy and lactation, often eating home-prepared nourishing foods more regularly and eliminating harmful habits, such as drinking alcohol or coffee or smoking cigarettes. We should all nourish ourselves as if our life, activity, and purpose here on Earth were important not only to our immediate friends and family but to the entire world. I believe we have that responsibility. If we can move beyond our own individual scope and dilemmas to a more cosmic reality, we will realize that each of us is an important and necessary cog in the giant wheel that turns the universe—and we cannot break down, because it affects everyone else.

Listening to and supporting our individual needs in regard to nourishment is no more difficult than it is in regard to our life, work, relationships, and so on. Some of us make an effort to keep this inherent ability alive, and some of us rediscipline ourselves to redevelop this quality (so easily lost in our technological age) through a variety of individual processes, which might include relaxation exercises, meditation, dream awareness, or planting a garden, working the earth, and watching nature. Following these natural practices will allow our true nature to resurface.

The beginning years of our nutrition are very significant in affecting our lifelong eating patterns and particular likes and dislikes for food. Our early family relationships and parental examples may set us up for potential addictions to particular foods or flavors. These factors definitely influence us and often may interfere with healthier eating patterns or restrict us from developing better eating habits in later years.

Babies begin to eat some solid or pureed foods somewhere around four to six months of age. It is best, in my opinion, to feed them initially the fresh fruits, vegetables, and whole grains in the right form for an infant, to provide them with both good nourishment and a basic sense of the natural and wonderful flavors of food. Avoiding cans, boxes, and jars of special baby foods that may have additives or extra sweet or salty flavoring is essential so as to not desensitize their very alive taste buds to simple, less concentrated flavors! Avoiding cow's milk and formulas, as Dr. Reuben suggests, is helpful in the first year to reduce the potential problems, such as allergy and digestive difficulties, that these more complex protein foods can generate. Other proteins, such as eggs and animal meats, might also be withheld for a few months to allow the baby's digestive tract to mature. Babies need simple foods first, and chemical-free foods at that. When these new protein foods are used, buy organic poultry, deep-sea fish, chemical-free eggs, and, if red meat is used, organic, range-fed beef. All of these can be prepared so that baby can handle them. As much as possible, grow or purchase organic produce and wash it well to minimize pesticide exposure. It is likely that the cancer potential of chemicals is increased in infants with their undeveloped immune systems, so we should be even more careful about chemicals in foods and environmental exposure than usual. Be aware of the environmental and home chemicals that are so commonly used nowadays. This is not meant to instill fear; the healthy baby or child is very durable and can handle most of what society has to offer, but overall it is best to reduce the exposure to potential toxins as much as possible.

As children grow, it is wise to continue to nourish them with wholesome foods and not create patterns of candy, cookies, and ice cream rewards for being good. This leads to a confused relationship to these foods. Remember, as-close-to-nature-as-possible is a priority in our diet. Protecting our children from the processed and fast-food industry pushed by street advertisements and television is next to impossible, but we must find this balance. Keep emphasizing the basic foods and the fact that these fruits, vegetables (the most difficult parental task), grains, legumes, and simple protein meals are essential. Occasionally the less wholesome foods may be consumed, but they should never become a regular part of the basic diet.

As children begin school, it is best, given the current state of public nutrition, to create their menu as much as possible. Packed lunches, if they are not swapped for less nutritious foods, can provide a varied diet and the continued support of parental nutritional guidance. Home cooking is an essential part of nutrition. Restaurant meals should be limited and considered as special dietary treats, though now there seem to be more restaurants offering natural and wholesome food from which to choose.

If we ever become sick, it is a wise idea to avoid hospital meals. One of the basic conundrums in Western medicine is why hospitals feed people as if they want them to remain ill. I guess it makes economic sense, but it sure does not make health sense. If we need to spend time in a hospital, we would best make sure to have water and food (in harmony, of course, with the recommended diet) brought in unless we can get fresh and vital foods from the hospital, which fortunately is becoming more possible. We need the vitality of good nourishment to help heal our body. (In Part Four we will look more at detoxification and the high fruit and vegetable and fasting diets that might be beneficial in treating a large number of illnesses.) And again, when we are sick, even more than when healthy, we need to stop and listen to our body's needs for the best advice on how to move us along the path of health.

So, of what might our ideal diet consist? When we talk about a diet or anything as "ideal," we seem to place it a little out of our reach, as if we were seeking to attain perfection. And even then, the "ideal" may be only a momentary experience. There is really no universal perfect or ideal diet, but individually, we can come as close as possible to our optimum diet by following some important guidelines.

Ideally, we want to obtain and consume (and even grow) the most wholesome, fresh, and organic (chemical-free) foods. Our meals should be simple in the number of foods, the amount consumed, and the way we combine them. Our diet also needs to vary with our activity level (usually in quantity and type of foods) and with the local climate and the time of year and, of course, with the best foods available. Finding the best and freshest foods at our stores or local farmers' markets and creating our meals around them is a much better plan than the opposite approach of planning a meal and then searching for the appropriate foods.

Preparing more natural foods and redeveloping our taste for the basic food flavors while avoiding the more processed foods and minimizing the amount of cans, boxes, and already prepared meals is a good beginning. Fresh-frozen foods, especially vegetables, are the most acceptable second choice over fresh ingredients. Rich meals with fatty foods or sauces can be reduced. Many other positive changes that can be made were discussed in the previous section.

As I have emphasized throughout this book, in the long run, a diet centered around whole grains and vegetables would best serve us individually as well as contribute to greater planetary harmony. The whole grain-legume mixture with abundant vegetables, both cooked and raw, is the main diet of the majority of Earth's people and, I think, the necessary beginning of our Ideal Diet. We must assume that following our instincts to nourish ourselves with what is available on our planet makes for the best diet. There is some order, I believe, to this universe, and we will have a lot less difficulty if we attune ourselves to that, as well as to our own individual participation in it.

In *The Complete Book of Natural Foods* (Boulder, CO: Shambhala Publications, 1983) Fred Rohé affirms this basic whole-grain-oriented diet. Though his approach has a macrobiotic focus, it makes sense when we think of the amount of the earth covered by the "staff of life" and the amount of grains already consumed.

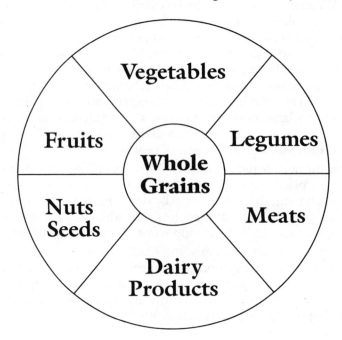

**A GENERAL GUIDELINE FOR THE
PROPORTIONS OF FOODS IN DIFFERENT TYPES OF DIETS**

	Omnivore	Lacto-ovo-Vegetarian	Vegan
Whole grains	25–30%	25–35%	30–40%
Vegetables	25–35	25–35	30–40
Legumes	5–10	10–15	10–15
Fruit	10–15	10–15	10–20
Nuts and seeds	5–10	5–10	10–15
Dairy products, eggs	5–10	10–15	
Meats, poultry, fish	10–15		

The Ideal Diet will vary somewhat with the seasons, so that, for example, our fruit intake may rise in the summer, with lesser amounts of meats and possibly even fewer whole grains and beans. In winter, we need warmer foods, and there are not many fresh vegetables available, although the hard, starchy squashes and the cold-weather cruciferous vegetables are good choices in this season. Fruit intake in winter is usually also at a minimum. Sprouted grains, seeds, and beans can bring a few more fresh and vital foods into the winter diet. Mr. Rohé uses the term "omnivarian" to describe this new diet, which is primarily vegetable based, in contrast to the more typical carnivorous/omnivorous diet. I am currently eating this omnivarian diet, with small amounts of dairy products, mainly as yogurt, butter, or cheese (less than 5 percent of the diet), and a bit of the animal meats, solely as fresh fish and organic poultry, not more than three or four times per week. We may feel comfortable to move anywhere along the spectrum from the omnivorous plan to the pure vegan diet. Our Ideal Diet for the modified omnivore also has a new organization of food groups:

1. **Produce**—5 or more servings per day of vegetables and fruits. Fresh is best.

2. **Starches**—4 or more servings per day of whole grains, potatoes, hard squashes.

3. **Proteins**—2–3 servings per day of sprouted legumes or seeds, cooked legumes, fish, eggs, seeds, nuts, poultry, lamb, beef, or pork—pretty much in that order of preference, in my opinion.

4. **Calcium foods**—2 or more servings per day but no more than two of the dairy foods if tolerated, and fewer are probably best. These calcium foods include nuts, seeds, and green leafy vegetables for any diet; milk, cheese, and yogurt for lacto-ovo or omnivore diets.

5. **Oils**—1 or 2 servings per day of vegetable oils. Olive, safflower, flaxseed, canola, and sunflower oils are the best choices. Nuts and seeds will also provide some vitamin E and the essential fatty acids.

○ INDIVIDUAL NEEDS

How can we decide what our individual dietary needs are? First and foremost, we can always attempt to listen to our body. If we have forgotten how to do this, we can relearn. But many people cannot or will not take the time or change their lives in order to reconnect with this instinctual process, so we need to have some basic knowledge, which these hundreds of pages are hopefully providing. If we get the basic concepts down, the fine tuning of our diet then really becomes the art and adventure of nutrition.

Besides listening to ourselves, it will do us well to listen to Nature. She is a great teacher and will provide us with the information and nourishment as we need it. Watching the seasons and the growing cycles of plants is obviously the beginning and basis. Working in a garden or planting our own food with family or friends is the best way to stay connected to Earth and her secrets of health. When we do not eat from our garden, we should be aware of where and how these foods are produced, as well as how our body uses and recycles them (digestion, assimilation, elimination). Another way to support our individual needs is to be aware of our own state of health. Part Four of this book suggests specific programs for various problems and stages of life; the Ideal Diet discussed here is for those of us in basically good health who wish to maintain that state. Yet this Ideal Diet is usually a marked improvement over what we have been eating. This will often make a difference in our health and reduce the incidence of many degenerative disease processes.

In *The Complete Book of Natural Food*, Mr. Rohé offers a method of choosing which foods are best for us on the basis of our metabolic type. This metabolic typing program is based on the work of William Donald Kelley, a dentist who has done fairly deep investigations into nutrition. According to Dr. Kelley, there are three types of people or, more accurately, states of being, based on previous diet, activity, and life experience atop our basic nature. Each of us fits into one of these types according to whether we are dominated by one or the other of the two branches of our nervous system—the sympathetic and the parasympathetic—or are in balance between them. Certain types of body chemistry are also associated with these states.

Most people are balanced types and need to create a balance between alkaline and acid foods. If we are healthy, our diet is usually more alkaline in spring and summer and slightly more acid in autumn and winter. Overall, the balanced healthy person needs to eat broadly from the wide range of natural foods. I believe, however, that we need to consume more alkaline-forming foods, at least 60 percent of the diet, all year around.

If we seem to be more the acid, or sympathetic, type, we are likely to have a more acid biochemistry, prone not only to subtle congestive problems, such as tension, constipation, or insomnia, but also to long-term degenerative diseases, such as atherosclerosis or hypertension. People with this biochemistry or temporary state of being would do better on a more vegetarian or alkaline diet, which is also lower in protein and fat foods. Lots of fruits and vegetables can be consumed. Lighter eating and even fasting would probably be helpful for this metabolic type.

The following chart lists characteristics of the "sympathetic" and "parasympathetic" metabolic types.

SYMPATHETIC *(Acid Body Chemistry)*	PARASYMPATHETIC *(Alkaline Body Chemistry)*
Action-oriented	Inaction-oriented

More nerve energy into
  energy production
	More nerve energy into
	  digestion and internal function

Intellectual	Intuitive
Fast or catabolic metabolism	Slower, anabolic metabolism

Lose weight easily, gain
  with difficulty
	Gain weight easily, lose
	  with difficulty

Prone to tension,
  constipation or insomnia
	Prone to lethargy or
	  diarrhea or insomnia

Exercise-oriented	Exercise-avoidant
Energy improves with vitamin C	Little effect on energy with vitamin C
Minimum niacin reaction*	Big niacin reaction
Do better on alkaline diet	Need more acid diet

* The niacin reaction mainly involves heat flushing and tingling of the skin.

Which type we are determines the relative amounts of acid and alkaline foods we need in our diet. The chart below lists foods according to these types.

Alkaline	*Neutral*	*Acid*
Fruits	Vegetable oils	Meat
Vegetables	Milk*	Fish
Sea vegetables	Cream*	Eggs
Millet	Butter*	Beans
Seeds	Cheese*	Grains (except millet)
Salt	Honey	Nuts
Herbs		Food additives and drugs
Spices		Beer, whiskey
Wine		

*Based on Donald Kelley's plan as reviewed in *The Complete Book of Natural Foods* by Fred Rohé. This is slightly different from acid-alkaline foods as discussed in other areas of this book and by other authors. The main difference is that dairy products are considered more acid and mucus-forming, which I believe they are.

The alkaline, or parasympathetic-dominant, people need just the opposite type of diet to bring them back into balance. For these individuals, fasting could be disastrous, often causing a worsening of fatigue and other symptoms. Eating a more acid diet, even meats and fish, will often help. A diet with higher levels of protein (and usually a little more fat) and even more food will help the energy level and with it the metabolism to handle this food.

This metabolic typing reminds me very specifically of the basic Chinese principle of duality, or yin and yang. These two states are reflected in the human condition and in our health. All illness can be seen as an imbalance of this yin-yang equilibrium, which fluctuates throughout the day and year. This cycle is discussed very thoroughly in my first book, *Staying Healthy With the Seasons*.

SEASONAL DIET CYCLE

Climate

Yang Weather			*Yin Weather*
Hot/dry	Wind/transition	Inward/dampening	Cold/wet
Summer	*Spring*	*Autumn*	*Winter*
Heat		Cold	

←———————————   ———————————→

Lighter Cooling Diet	Richer Heating Diet
More Fluids	Concentrated Foods
More Raw Foods	More Cooked Foods
Lower Fat	More Oils and Protein

Diet

Cooling	*Cleansing*	*Balancing*	*Building*	*Warming*
Liquids	Greens	Grains	Roots	Fish
Fruits	Vegetables	Legumes	Sprouts	Seaweed
Salads	Citrus	Soups	Yogurt	Seeds/Nuts

People who are more yang dominant (acid, sympathetic) are action-oriented and prone to symptoms and diseases of tension and congestion, such as musculoskeletal pains, headaches, constipation, high blood pressure, and cardiovascular disease. They would do better on a more yin (alkaline) diet, higher in fruits and vegetables. These people also do very well with juice fasts, an extreme alkaline program. Yin people tend to be slower and reflective, more likely to be engaged in the arts and other sensitive fields of work than in physical labor or financial business (more yang activities). Yin-dominant people need a more heat-producing, yang diet, richer in protein and fat foods, with less of the raw and cooling fruits and vegetables, as well as minimal sweet and refined flour foods.

In summary, then, we can adapt our basic diet of whole grains (slightly more acid) and vegetables (more alkaline) by using the other foods to shift to either a more acid or alkaline diet. With this knowledge, if we are balanced, the time of year and our climate will suggest the predominant focus of our food choices.

If we are an acid, or yang, type, and our diet tends toward more alkaline or cooling foods, we may still eat our richest foods in the winter. In the summer, however, we may fast occasionally or consume a much higher percentage of fruits and vegetables and juices. If we are a more alkaline, or yin, type, we need a more acid diet to fuel our body. Our shifting with the seasons may allow us more fruits and vegetables in the spring and summer as the warm sun and weather strengthen our yang energy, while in the winter we need to get that warmth from the richer fuel of the meats, dairy products, beans, and nuts.

If we follow this plan, our health will improve, and we will move toward a balanced chemistry. Then we will need to shift our diet again to meet our new needs and to support our new energy state. Being healthy then becomes a process of continued awareness and adaptation to our ever-changing state of being. And that's when the fun begins!

○ CHANGING YOUR DIET

Eating seasonally provides us with foods from nature close to the time they are available, which gives us the most nourishment and subsequent vitality from our foods. Ideally, the natural flavors of the wholesome foods will be what appeals and to and satisfies our palate and body. From day to day and season to season, the diet described here will also provide us with a variety of foods and nutrients. It contains a balance of the food groups just discussed—protein foods, calcium foods, essential oils, produce, and starches—with the latter two the dominant groups. In our new diet, meals and snacks are simple, not combining a wide range of foods. There is a balance through the day, rather than at each meal, as many people eat now. Not eating fruits or the many sweet foods that contain simple sugars at the same time as more complex-to-digest foods, as well as minimizing the combinations of starches and protein, will aid our digestion and allow the best utilization of the nutrients coming from our wide variety of foods.

I suggest that we organize our daily diet according to the food groups that we will consume at certain times, also taking into account our day's activities, including exercise, work, and relaxation. A sample day's plan is presented below. Those with special work or sleep schedules or with varying types of productivity or cycles will have to adapt this plan to meet their schedules.

YOUR IDEAL DIET

Natural
Seasonal
Rotational
Balanced
Moderate
Well Combined

Obviously, this diet will vary with the seasons and climate as well as our activity level and individual needs and metabolism. If we are trying to gain or lose weight, we will have to make modifications. If we are weight training, for example, and trying to increase our bulk and muscle mass, we will need bigger meals and more protein for dinner. If we want to drop some weight, eating a light dinner is probably the key (without later snacks), as well as eating moderately at all meals and increasing our physical activity. No kidding! It works if we actually do it.

Depending on our work schedules and specific metabolisms, we may want to switch the lunch and dinner meals (see menus in next chapter) and have our main meals at dinner instead of lunch. This will be discussed later in regard to the specific menu plans and recipes. Overall though, it is generally healthier to consume more of our food earlier when it can be digested and assimilated more completely, and to eat very lightly if at all after nightfall.

Now, I will go through a more complete example of a day's schedule for liquid and food intake, general activities, and other healthful tips.

SAMPLE DIET

Time of Day	Food	Examples	Portion	Reason
A.M. 6:00– 7:30 A.M.	Fruit	Orange or grapes	½–1 piece 10–20 grapes	A simple carbohydrate to break-our-fast and kick-start our engine/digestive tract.
Breakfast 7:00– 8:30 A.M.	Starch	Whole grain cereal or hard squash	unlimited 1–2 bowls ½–whole	A complex carbohydrate breakfast is our time-release energy capsule.
Snack 10:00– 11:00 A.M.	Nuts or seeds	Almonds or sunflower seeds	our own handful	This fat/oil primes our engine and stimulates HCL and pancreatic enzymes, such as *lipase*.
Lunch 11:30– 1:00 P.M.	Protein and green vegetable	chicken w/ broccoli or spinach salad w/tomato and garbanzo sprouts	moderation to satisfaction	This combination offers more nutrient/fuel intake and chlorophyll to further support digestion.
Snack 3:00– 4:00 P.M.	Fruit, vegetable, or starch	apples, carrot sticks, or rice cakes	1 portion	A simple food to provide some energy lift for late afternoon.
Dinner 5:30– 7:30 P.M.	Starch and vegetable	brown rice w/mixed vegetable or pasta primavera	moderation to satisfaction	A basic complex carbohydrate meal to provide energy and nourishment, and light enough to allow proper digestion before bed.
Optional Snack 7:30– 9:00 P.M.	Fruit, vegetable, or starch	apple and dates, celery, or popcorn	1 portion	A light snack if needed, depending on other foods consumed and individual metabolism.

○ SCHEDULE

Morning

- Arise from sleep with the sun. Go to sleep early enough to awaken without an alarm. Try to arise at least one hour before you must leave home.
- Sit quietly or lie propped up in bed and meditate and/or plan your day. Let any concerns or frustrations settle and visualize clearly how you would like to see your day.
- Drink two cups of purified or spring water. One may have a quarter or half of a fresh lemon squeezed into it to help with morning purification.
- Do some stretches and light exercise.
- Eat a piece or two of fruit.
- A more vigorous exercise period may be included in this time period as well, either before or after fruit, depending upon your needs.
- Shower or bathe, and get ready for the day.
- A whole grain or starch breakfast (single or double portion) can be consumed within 30–60 minutes after the fruit. Some tea can be taken at this time or even with the fruit earlier.
- If supplements are taken, this can be done now.
- In an hour or two (midmorning, or 10:00–11:00 A.M.), a handful of one type of nut or seed may be consumed.
- More water or tea can follow, up to about half an hour before lunch.

Morning note—You have started your body slowly and moved into a work pace. You have taken several cups of liquids (not caffeine), done some exercise, cleaned and nourished your body, first with simple fruits, then more complex carbohydrates, followed with fat/oil-containing protein food. This allows early light eating and allows your digestive tract time to "break fast."

Afternoon

- The midday meal can be a substantial one to nourish you for the afternoon and may consist of a protein food and vegetables, including at least one green vegetable.
- A brief period (15–20 minutes) of relaxation and recharging may follow lunch. A short walk outdoors would be helpful as well to air out the brain, especially for indoor workers.

- Supplements can be taken at this time.
- A midafternoon snack may consist of a fruit, vegetable, or starch, or even a protein food, depending upon your needs and food organization plan.
- Later afternoon might include another cup of tea or a glass or two of water, in preparation for exercise.
- After-work exercise or relaxation, also depending on needs and previous activities. Your main exercise may be at this time, as it is for many individuals.

Evening

- Dinner may consist of a starch and vegetables or a protein and vegetables.
- It is best to follow a good meal with a relaxation period.
- Supplements can also be taken at this time.
- Then some type of mild activity may aid digestion and assimilation. A short walk with the kids, the dog, a friend, or by yourself is a good idea.
- The evening brings relaxation through reading, viewing a square box with moving, talking figures, working, or romancing, depending on your wishes. The evening is a good time to nourish yourself in other ways besides eating food.
- A light evening snack of a fruit, vegetable, or starch may be consumed. This is optional. Fruit may be preferred as it is sweet, a common flavor choice after dinner, and simple to digest.
- Some relaxing tea, warm lemon water, or a glass of plain water can be imbibed in the evening.
- Certain before-bed supplements, such as calcium/magnesium, can also be taken.
- A good night's sleep is now in order.
- Be aware of your dreams and open to remembering them in the morning to learn a little more about yourself.

DAILY DIETARY SCHEDULE

Diet Activity	Possible Time	Food Choice
Preparation	6:00–7:00 A.M.	water
Breakfast	6:30–7:30 A.M.	fruit
Breakfast	7:30–8:30 A.M.	starch
Snack	10:00–11:00 A.M.	nut or seed
Lunch	12:00–1:00 P.M.	protein/vegetable
Snack	3:00–4:00 P.M.	fruit, vegetable, or starch
Dinner	5:30–7:00 P.M.	starch/vegetable or protein/vegetable
Snack	8:00–9:00 P.M.	fruit, vegetable, or starch

In food groups this is broken down into the following, depending, of course, on the size of portions consumed:

Breakfast	1–2 fruits, 1–2 starches
Morning snack	1 nut or seed (1 protein, 1 calcium, and 1 oil food)
Lunch*	1–2 protein, 2–3 vegetables
Afternoon snack	1–2 vegetables or 1 fruit
Dinner*	1–2 starch or 1–2 protein, and 2–3 vegetables
Evening Snack	1 fruit, 1 vegetable, or 1 starch

The breakdown of our "new" food groups gives us the following totals:

Produce	6–8 servings on the average
Starches	4–6 servings
Proteins	2–3 servings
Calcium foods	2–3 servings, includes green vegetables, nuts or seeds, and some protein foods
Oil foods	1–2 servings nuts/seeds and/or vegetable oil

*Fresh cold-pressed vegetable oil might also be consumed with lunch or dinner; in that case add one oil food.

○ SUPPLEMENTS TO THE DIET

Even if we eat the Ideal Diet for an extended period of time, it is hard to maintain an entire balance of nutrients from day to day, and our utilization of the nutrients from these wholesome foods is dependent upon a generally healthy digestion and absorption and a minimum of stress or special, extra needs.

If we are healthy, with strong, consistent energy, and we sleep well, live in an unpolluted natural environment, do not hustle and bustle about to work and play, eat a variety of wholesome foods from the earth, and have good digestion and assimilation, we probably need very little, if any, additional supplements. If anything, some extra minerals may be required, particularly those that might be deficient in the soils where we live.

However, most of us living in the latter twentieth century do not live or eat in this ideal fashion. We may eat on the run, drive on freeways, breathe in polluted air, drink contaminated water, come in contact with various chemicals, and have a lot on our minds. In other words, we have a lot of stimuli, stress, and energy needs.

Those of us who fit into this more realistic lifestyle category of today, I believe, need a stabilizing, nourishing program of vitamins, minerals, and other supplements. Throughout this book, I have discussed most of the nutrients we could possibly take, why they are needed, by whom, in what special situation, and how to take them. In this brief section, I suggest an optimum supplement plan to accompany a basically healthy diet for the average adult male or female with a mild amount of activity and stress. There are two columns in the accompanying chart: one for the suggested supportive intake level to supplement the basic diet, and the other to offer a possible daily intake range to take into account the various supplement preparations and individual variances. In Part Four, entitled *Nutritional Application,* there will be a series of programs for increased stress situations, different people and life stages, and various medical conditions. At the end of each of those programs, there will be more specific supplement suggestions for that particular situation.

The following table lists the basic essential nutrients. There are, of course, many more vitamins, minerals, amino acids, fatty acids, herbs, and so on that could go into a general formula. Hydrochloric acid as betaine HCL is often added to help digestion and utilization of many of the minerals, in particular. Many formulas contain other products, such as acidophilus culture, tryptophan, ginseng, different glandulars, more phosphorus, various bioflavonoids, RNA, superoxide dismutase, inositol, or glutamic acid. Not all of these have been clearly shown to do all they are claimed to do, which is the case even for some of those listed in the table, though almost all are at least known to be essential to life. Some of the B vitamins are also usually manufactured in the healthy human colon.

GENERAL ADULT INSURANCE DAILY SUPPLEMENT PROGRAM

Vitamins	Form	Suggested Daily Amount	Possible Range
Vitamin A	palmitate	5,000 IU	5,000–10,000 IU
Beta-carotene	vegetable	15,000 IU	10,000–25,000 IU
Vitamin B_1	thiamine-HCL	10 mg.	10–50 mg.
Vitamin B_2	riboflavin	10 mg.	10–50 mg.
Vitamin B_3	niacin or	10 mg.	10–100 mg.
	niacinamide	50 mg.	10–100 mg.
Vitamin B_5	calcium pantothenate	100 mg.	50–100 mg.
Vitamin B_6	pyridoxine-HCL or pyridoxal-5-phosphate	25 mg.	10–100 mg.
Vitamin B_{12}	cyanocobalamin or cobalamin	100 mcg.	50–500 mcg.
Folic acid	folacin	400 mcg.	400–1000 mcg.
Biotin	biotin	250 mcg.	150–500 mcg.
PABA	para-aminobenzoic acid	50 mg.	25–100 mg.
Choline	choline bitartrate	500 mg.	100–1000 mg.
Bioflavonoids	mixed complex	250 mg.	100–500 mg.
Vitamin C	ascorbic acid	2000 mg.	500–3000 mg.
Vitamin D	D_3-ergocalciferol	400 IU	200–600 IU
Vitamin E	d-alpha tocopherol with mixed tocopherols	400 IU	200–600 IU
Vitamin K	phylloquinone	100 mcg.	50–200 mcg.

The amounts suggested are usually at or above the RDA but not at the much higher levels that might be suggested for a more stressed or imbalanced, symptomatic individual or that might be used in specific therapeutic situations. Remember, this insurance formula is for the basically healthy man or woman. There are some slight variations between the RDAs for men and women; these are discussed in Part Four (*Adult Men* and *Adult Women*), along with recommendations for other life stages, as well as special programs for the prevention and treatment of many medical conditions.

Minerals	Form	Suggested Daily Amount	Possible Range
Calcium	dicalcium phosphate or calcium aspartate or citrate	650 mg.	500–1200 mg.
Magnesium	oxide, citrate, or aspartate	350 mg.	300–750 mg.
Potassium	chloride	400 mg.	100–1000 mg.
Iron	citrate or chelate	15 mg.	10–18 mg.
Zinc	sulfate, gluconate, or picolinate	30 mg.	15–45 mg.
Copper	sulfate or chelate, such as gluconate	2 mg.	1–3 mg.
Iodine	potassium iodide	150 mcg.	50–200 mcg.
Manganese	sulfate or chelate	10 mg.	2–10 mg.
Selenium	selenomethionine or sodium selenite	200 mcg.	50–200 mcg.
Chromium	amino acid chelate or picolinate	200 mcg.	50–500 mcg.
Silicon	equisetum-horsetail	20 mg.	10–50 mg.
Molybdenum	sodium molybdate or chelate	200 mcg.	50–200 mcg.
Vanadium	pentoxide or chelate	200 mcg.	50–200 mcg.

Other possibilities:

Minerals	Form	Suggested Daily Amount	Possible Range
Flaxseed oil	Balanced omega-3 and omega-6 combination	2 tsp. or 4 capsules	1–3 tsp. 3–6 caps.
Omega-3 fatty acids	EPA and DHA oil capsules	1000 mg.	500–1500 mg.
Lactobacilli cultures	powder or capsules	1 billion count	50 million to 10 billion organisms per dose

Note: Supplements should be hypoallergenic—not made from milk, yeast, wheat, corn, or soy—and contain no sugar, preservatives, or artificial colors.

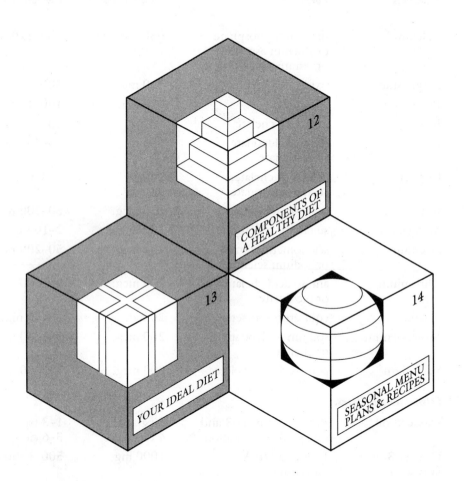

12 COMPONENTS OF A HEALTHY DIET

13 YOUR IDEAL DIET

14 SEASONAL MENU PLANS & RECIPES

Chapter 14

Seasonal Menu Plans and Recipes

with Eleonora Manzolini

Our Ideal Diet menu plans in this chapter will consist of four 4-day rotation diets, one for each season. This diet/eating plan may require some adaptation from our usual way of eating, and may not necessarily be an easy diet plan to follow. For many people, it could be a very difficult shift, because it essentially includes no already prepared foods, such as pizza or sandwiches. Others will feel limited because they are used to more foods per meal, more variety, and especially the commonly consumed protein-starch meals, which personally I find the most challenging change to make in my diet. However, this diet is also potentially highly therapeutic for a variety of food-generated and digestive problems. It is also very helpful in normalizing weight and for the average person with some food reactions or allergies. Those who have usually eaten a variety of foods and who are healthy with good digestive function will probably not need to follow strict food combining or a strict rotation diet. This is to say that in order to make them more realistic to the average consumer the following diets and recipes are not exact to some of my previous rules of rotation and food combining. The recipe variances we have made in our food combining are usually minor, such as dried fruits or nuts with a grain breakfast. It is wise, though, to continue to eat simply of a variety of foods and to avoid the daily eating of specific foods, especially commonly allergenic ones such as milk, eggs, wheat, corn, soy, tomatoes, and oats.

The food charts shown later offer four days of sample meals for each season. With my guidance, Eleonora Manzolini has put together these seasonal menu plans and many delicious, yet simple, recipes. Even so, our suggestions may not all be to the liking of everyone. There are, of course, many other possibilities; feel free to adapt them to feed your heart, mind, soul, and of course, body. Creativity is an important part of nutrition. The sample menu plans and recipes are offered primarily to educate and inspire you to follow the principles of simple, regular, wholesome meals combined so as to best promote digestion and utilization.

For example, in reviewing the meal guidelines of the previous chapter, we see that breakfast is a meal composed of a simple carbohydrate (fruit) followed by a complex carbohydrate, such as whole grains. Some of our breakfast recipes are even a little more involved, with some fruit, grain, and even nuts combined. Often we may give more than one breakfast suggestion, and those wanting to follow stricter guidelines and eat lighter can just consume fruit in the morning, which may be followed in an hour or two by some starchy food. In the summer, this may be even more apropos. Even our complex breakfasts are still simpler than many people may currently eat, containing much less protein or fat, and allow our body to prepare for those heavier foods later. However, if our jobs require strenuous physical effort or we feel our bodies require more substantial foods earlier in the day (this may be true when we do not eat anything after dark), some proteins can be used for breakfast. Eggs (poached or soft-boiled are best; over-easy with a small amount of butter is okay) can be eaten with toast or tortillas and some vegetables. One of my favorite (and heavier) breakfasts is two eggs over easy served on tortillas with alfalfa sprouts, diced tomatoes, a slice of avocado, and some salsa. However, I definitely do not support the typical American breakfast of bacon or sausage (no cured or lunchmeats ever) and eggs, potatoes, toast, and juice; it is excessive in food, fats, and protein.

Overall, these menu plans provide a modified, not strict, rotation diet; our suggestions and recipes may overlap some of the common foods. If a strict rotation diet is desired to help with food allergies, it will only take a little more discipline and adaptation from the provided plans. Clearly though, no foods are suggested at all meals, or even daily.

With the common American eight-to-five lifestyle, it may be difficult to have our main meal at lunchtime. Our business schedule does not allow us a 1:00–4:00 P.M. break for lunch and siesta time as in many other countries. Since this is the case, some of the menu plans can allow switches between lunch and dinner; yet, they will still be written as the main meal at midday because this we believe is best nutritionally. As an example, on Day 3 of Spring, the fish lunch would need to be prepared the night before and taken to work. If this is not practical, the couscous dish can be eaten at lunch and the fish and vegetables prepared fresh for dinner.

Following the sample menus and recipes are seasonal food lists. These seasonal foods are primarily from the vegetable kingdom. Most animal foods are available year round, and in many parts of the world, with modern technology and improved storage, a lot of fruits and vegetables can be found outside their season. If we can consume about 50–75 percent of our foods as fresh and seasonal–that is, near the area where they are grown and at the time when they are naturally harvested—that will be a good beginning.

I am very supportive of vegetarianism, yet I realize that most people in our culture

548

and the world do not choose to eat this way. To be realistic and also supportive of the omnivorous diet, some of the meals in the menu plans contain fish and poultry; I have included no red meats. I believe that if we keep our priorities and food groups in the right perspective, an omnivorous diet can be equal to or healthier than a vegetarian one, and often easier to follow as well as easier from which to acquire all the essential nutrients. Our menu plans and recipes are also low in milk products and eggs, foods that are best eaten only moderately by most adults. At the end of each season, following the menu plan and its specific recipes, I've included a few extra vegetarian recipes to replace omnivorous ones, a couple of fish recipes, and some that include eggs and dairy products to provide more choices. These extra recipes are either very unique ones, have special healing properties, or are good ones from books no longer in print. Otherwise, I will provide references for suggested recipes from other popular books.

It is more common now for both vegetarians and omnivores to be finding a new balance that combines many of the wholesome foods of the strict vegetarian with the avoidance of land animals and their by-products milk and eggs. Instead they consume the nourishing water animals, both fresh water and ocean fish. The quality of usable protein in fish is excellent, the nutrient content is high and the digestability is very good for most people. I have termed this diet "pescaveganism"—fish and strict vegetarianism— and it is the main diet I have followed for many years.

Seasonal food lists follow the recipes to help you with shopping and food awareness. These lists are taken from another project, *The Seasonal Food Guide* poster and booklet, also published by Celestial Arts. Our menu plans and recipes are not taken exclusively from these seasonal food lists; that would be too difficult nowadays, and unrealistic. Many foods, such as the grains, legumes, nuts, and seeds store relatively well and are used commonly throughout the year by most people. Mainly, it is the fruits and vegetables that should bring out our seasonal awareness, and our recipes will give the suggestion that we are shopping for fresh, local produce as we hope you will. Many of our recipes will cross over seasonally, depending on the climate in which we live, and some of the additional recipes taken from other books, since they often provide a combination of foods, may likewise be used in other seasons if you wish.

In *Staying Healthy With the Seasons*, based on the Oriental Five Element Theory, five seasons are discussed. Yet here we have only four seasonal menu plans. The "fifth" season the Chinese call the "doyo," meaning transition. It relates both to late summer as well as to the two to three weeks of seasonal change around the solstices and equinoxes. These are the times that I make some shifts in my diet—at least I take a closer look at it and ask myself whether it needs any changes to best support my energy and health and adaptation to the next season. Often I will write down a plan encompassing what I am doing and outlining the changes I wish to make. The equinoxes—moving into spring and autumn—appear to be the most significant shift periods of the year. At these times I usually will do a cleansing diet to rest from food and lighten myself up so I can be more aware of shifts happening in my life. In spring,

I do a ten-day Master Cleanser fast and then, in autumn, I usually take a few days or a week for a fast or cleansing diet of fruits and vegetables. Most people, unless they are too nutrient deficient, weak, or ill, can follow this type of program. It is outlined in Chapter 18 in some of the later programs, specifically *Fasting* and *General Detoxification*.

Prior to the menu plans, recipes, and seasonal food lists, "some basics" will be provided by Ms. Manzolini and myself to help in creating our healthy diet. Simple utensil and shopping lists, basic cooking and storing ideas, and some general tips and shortcuts will also be included. A specific nutritional assessment will follow our seasonal menu plans, generated by recording each diet as it might be eaten over a seven-day period, and then entering it into a computer to quantify the nutrient values. It then will print out the daily levels of fat, protein, and many vitamins and minerals, which I have summarized in the chart. This chapter ends with a glossary of new and unusual foods that may be found in some supermarkets and most health food stores. Natural food products have grown by leaps and bounds in recent years, and there are some very good products available (also some "junk").

We hope all of this information will help you on your path to a new way of eating, or will allow you to fine tune your already health-oriented diet. Enjoy!

○ INTRODUCTION

by Eleonora Manzolini

In today's industrialized countries, people are eating more than ever before, yet most are receiving less nourishment. Real food, for the most part, is virtually unknown; yet fortunately, more and more people are becoming conscious that both shelved and perishable products in supermarkets contain a wide array of chemical additives and contaminants, and that their food choices have an impact not only on their health, but on that of the entire planet.

Food is the earliest form of addiction; it may be more controversial than sex, politics, religion, or drugs. People in general have become out of touch with nature and have very little instinctual or rational basis for their diet, and as a result they can become very emotional about it; thus, they may defend their diet and resist suggestions for change. The average person is not familiar with natural foods and doesn't know how to maintain good health; doctors in general may know a lot about disease, but very little about health-promoting factors such as nutrition.

"You are what you eat." Today there are many philosophies around diet and many choices of food and its preparation. I have examined the diets from many perspectives and have come to the conclusion that we are all different; this predisposes our body to choose certain foods. In a natural setting we would instinctually choose foods that provide just the right amount of energy and nutrients for our needs and for the level of consciousness and life adventure we would like to experience.

I would like to stress the point that there are no good and bad foods per se, just as there are no correct and incorrect ways of preparing them (though definitely some foods and preparations may support health more than others); it is a matter of personal choice that has to do with our very unique make up and way of being in the world. Moderation and balance are the keys. Our bodies are perfectly well-equipped to handle everything in small amounts, and if we understand that we are part of Earth just like the plants and animals, we will naturally have more respect for these other creatures and gravitate toward a more frugal and simple lifestyle, which will not only protect our health but also our entire ecosystem.

My advice then, to you and to myself, is: Don't fight your vices; be kind to yourself, and they will eventually fall away. Don't make food an end in itself. Construct a diet as good as your head can tolerate without losing the joy of living. And remember, everyone's needs are different.

I am happy to have had the opportunity to cooperate with Dr. Elson Haas because I feel in alignment with his philosophy and like his direct and practical way of explaining things. In keeping with this simplicity, prior to the seasonal menu plans and recipes, I will provide you with a few time-saving tips for the busy person, as well as basic shopping and utensil lists.

I also wish to achnowledge Michel Stroot of the Golden Door of Escondido, CA, who does wonderful creative work with food and from whom I have learned a great deal, and Annemarie Colbin, whose books have been an inspiration to me. I offer to you a few adaptations of their recipes together with some of my own.

As you will see the recipes are all very simple and quick to prepare. I believe it is important to eat well on a daily basis, and in order to be able to do this realistically in our busy lives, cooking cannot be an ordeal. We have to learn to put together a healthy, well-balanced meal in a half hour with a few fresh ingredients, and without having to give up taste or resort to lifeless, chemical, or processed foods. I hope my contribution to this book will help you accomplish this.

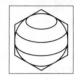

Basic Utensils

The size and number of pots and pans you need depend upon how many people you are serving. The following basic collection should take care of up to 12 people. The materials I prefer are stainless steel (Durotherm), cast iron, glass, Corningware, and enamel.

- one 1-quart saucepan
- one 2-quart saucepan
- two 3-quart saucepans
- one 9-inch skillet
- one soup pot
- one pressure cooker (could be same as soup pot)
- one 3- or 4-quart covered, ovenproof baking dish
- two shallow lasagna-style baking dishes
- two glass pie plates
- one cookie sheet
- six wooden stirring spoons of various sizes
- one set of measuring cups
- one set of measuring spoons
- two rubber spatulas
- one grater
- one hard brush for scrubbing vegetables
- one wire whisk
- two paring knives
- one good knife for chopping vegetables. *This is the most important purchase of all.* Make sure that the weight is comfortably distributed and that the blade is thin so that it cuts easily. It may take several purchases to find "your" knife. My favorite is a Mac knife.

Shopping List For The Beginner

Grains: Short grain brown rice, millet, wild rice.

Quick cooking grains: Couscous, polenta, rolled oats.

Noodles: Whole wheat veggie spirals or other noodles; wheat-free alternatives include corn elbows, quinoa pasta, or soba noodles.

Breads and flours: Sprouted whole grain breads and tortillas, unyeasted breads, wasa crackers, Essene or manna bread, whole wheat pastry flour.

Beans: Pinto, aduki, mung, garbanzo, navy beans.

Quick cooking beans: Lentils, red lentils, split peas.

Soybean products: Tofu—plain and marinated; tempeh—plain, marinated, and tempeh/grain mixtures; tofu and tempeh burgers.

Sea vegetables: Kombu, agar-agar, nori, arame or hijiki.

Oils: Extra virgin olive oil, toasted sesame oil, safflower oil, corn oil. Brands of known quality include Spectrum, Eden, and Sciabica olive oil.

Condiments: Tamari, miso, brown rice or other vinegars, mustard, soy mayonnaise or a tofu or eggless mayonnaise, tahini, gomasio, kuzu, miso.

Herbs and Spices: Thyme, marjoram, basil, oregano, parsley, garlic, ginger, cayenne, scallion (green onion), cilantro (coriander), chili pepper, garlic, cumin, curry powder.

Sweeteners: Maple syrup, date sugar, honey, apple butter, rice syrup.

Snack foods: Mochi, rice cakes, various rice crackers, dried fruit, grain-sweetened cookies, apples, carrots, celery, raw nuts (especially almonds or walnuts).

Dairy substitutes: Soy milk, amazake, nut milks, nutritional yeast.

Fresh Foods: Fruits, vegetables, nuts, seeds; alfalfa seeds, lentils, garbanzos, and green peas for sprouting.

Kitchen Basics

Washing grains: I like the swirling method I learned from Annemarie Colbin. It is more effective than running water over the grains in a colander. Put the grains in a bowl and cover with twice the amount of water. Swirl thoroughly and pour off all the floating debris and stray grains. Catch the rest in a colander. If the water is very dirty, repeat the procedure. Quinoa, amaranth, and millet need to be washed more carefully, several times at least.

Cooking grains: The following are some cooking times and grain-to-water ratios for the more commonly utilized grains.

Brown rice: Combine 1 cup rice to 2 cups cold water and a pinch of salt. The salt is important even if you are on a salt-free diet because it brings out the full flavor of the grain. Bring to a boil, adjust the flame to low, and cook the rice in 50–60 minutes. If you are making rice with steamed vegetables, you can lay the cut up vegetables on top of the rice during the last 10 minutes and they will cook with the steam from the rice. Rice connoisseurs suggest cooking the rice undisturbed for 1 hour over a low heat. The pot must have a tight seal so the steam does not escape, and to tell it's done, listen to the pot; it will stop bubbling and you will hear a slight crackling or popping sound of rice toasting. Many rice lovers will also prepare the rice with more salt, about ¼–½ teaspoon per cup of uncooked rice, and ½–1 Tablespoon of oil or butter.

553

Barley: Cook with the same amount of water as you would rice. I have found it takes slightly longer, 60 to 70 minutes.

Quinoa: 1 cup of quinoa to 2 cups of water and a pinch of salt. Cover, bring to a boil, and simmer 15 minutes.

Millet: Another trick I learned from Annemarie Colbin is to dry roast this grain in a cast iron or stainless steel skillet until a few grains begin to pop, about 5–10 minutes. Then add 2 cups of water for each cup of millet and the usual pinch of salt. Cover, bring to a boil, lower the heat and simmer for about 30–40 minutes. Fluff with fork before serving. If just cooking millet in water, rinse it well to remove any unseen dirt.

Kasha: Bring 2 cups of water and a pinch of salt to a boil. Add 1 cup of kasha, lower the flame, and simmer for 15–20 minutes.

You may wish to use a pressure cooker for some grains in order to shorten the cooking time. In that case add less water, about 1½ cups of water to 1 cup grain. Also do not cook any cracked grain in the pressure cooker since it may clog up the escape valve and cause an explosion. Pressure-cooked grains have a totally different texture and taste, especially rice, which tends to stick together. It is wonderful for making sushi, but not appropriate for a rice salad or pilaf.

GRAIN/WATER
PROPORTIONS AND COOKING TIMES

Brown rice	1:2	50–60 minutes
Millet	1:2–2½	30–40 minutes
Oats	1:2	15–20 minutes
Kasha	1:2–2½	15–20 minutes
Barley	1:2½	1 hour
Couscous	1:1½–2	10 minutes

Washing and soaking beans: Beans that are bought in bulk need picking over since they often contain stones. The worst are red lentils and I suggest that you do not buy them in bulk, but get the already cleaned and packaged ones.

The following beans do not need soaking: all kinds of lentils, split peas, and aduki beans. All other beans are best soaked overnight in twice the amount of water. Throw away the soaking water. This will shorten the cooking time and also reduce the gas-producing effects. If you do not have time to soak the beans overnight, you can use a quick method. Boil them in twice the amount of water for 5 minutes and then let them sit covered for 1 hour; then change water for further cooking.

Cooking beans: Black-eyed peas, lima beans, small white/navy beans and aduki beans can be cooked together with rice in the same pot since they have similar cooking times. Just add more water.

Pressure cooking reduces the time to about one half of the above, but be careful not to cook lentils and split peas in a pressure cooker since they may clog the escape valve and cause the pressure cooker to explode.

BEANS/WATER
PROPORTIONS AND COOKING TIMES

Red lentils	1:2	15–20 minutes
Lentils and split peas	1:2–2½	½ hour
Black-eyed peas, lima beans, small white/navy beans, mung beans, aduki beans	1:3	1 hour
Kidney beans, pinto beans, soybeans, black beans	1:3½	1½ hour
Garbanzo beans	1:4	2 hours

Always salt your beans at the end, about 10 minutes before they are done. This is important since adding salt at the beginning will cause the beans to remain tough. If you prefer not to use salt, remember that beans cooked with no salt at all tend to disintegrate. This may be okay for soups and stews, but not if you are making a bean salad.

Beans, like grains, can be slow cooked in an oven or crockpot. Place beans and water (add additional cup of water per additional cup of beans) in ovenproof bean pot or casserole dish. Put covered dish in oven and cook overnight or all day at low setting, 200°–220°. The beans will be more tasty, tender, and thicker than if you use the quicker cooking method.

For more flavorful, spicy beans, cook with lightly sautéed onion and garlic. Dice a large onion and a few cloves of garlic and lightly sauté with 2 teaspoons of canola or other light oil in the cooking pot. Add 2 cups of beans and about 6 cups of water, and simmer until the beans are tender. Optionally, to avoid the oil sauté, just add all the ingredients to the pot and cook.

To enhance and vary the flavor of beans, a variety of herbs and spices can be added to the cooking pot at the start or midway. If beginning with 2 cups of beans, try one or more of the following at your inspiration and taste:

Vegetables	*Dried Herbs*	*Fresh Herbs*
garlic, 2–4 cloves	bay leaf, 1 or 2	cilantro, 4–6 teaspoons
onion, 1 medium or large	oregano, ½ teaspoon	parsley, 2–3 sprigs
carrot, 1 or 2 chopped	basil, ½–1 teaspoon	sage, 2–3 leaves
bell pepper, 1 chopped	cumin, 1–2 teaspoon	rosemary, 1 sprig
jalapeño, 1 sliced, seeded	cayenne, ¼ teaspoon	thyme, 2 sprigs
tomatoes, 2 fresh chopped	chili powder, ½–1 teaspoon	
	sage, pinch	
	rosemary, ¼ teaspoon	
	thyme, ¼–½ teaspoon	

Cleaning vegetables: If you buy your root vegetables, such as carrots, radishes, turnips, etc. from organic sources there is no need to peel them; just scrub them with a stiff brush. Vegetables from commercial sources most of the time have been treated with chemical pesticides and waxed and therefore need peeling.

To peel tomatoes, drop them in boiling water for 10–15 seconds. Allow to cool and the skin will come off very easily.

To peel garlic, place your knife flat on the garlic clove and whack with your other hand. The covering will burst open and the clove can be easily removed.

For leafy greens, cut off the root end and plunge into a sink full of cold water. Swirl around a few times and let sit for awhile. The sand, dirt, and other debris will settle to the bottom, and the leaves will float to the top and can be removed. Repeat the procedure if the greens such as spinach are very dirty.

Some tips about fish: When buying a whole fish, make sure it has firm flesh, red gills, and bright eyes. Steaks or fillets should be moist and not flaky. Also it is a good idea to get your fish from a dependable source, not a supermarket, since it is often dipped in a solution of nitrites and nitrates to cover up any smell. Also many stores use paper that is saturated with chemicals to lay the fish on so as to preserve the color. Before cooking it is best to rinse the fish under cold running water. Also do not use a wooden cutting board for chopping up fish or meat, since the wood absorbs the juices and becomes a breeding ground for bacteria.

Seasoning: By seasoning I don't mean just salt, even if that is a very important ingredient. I like to use sea salt, which is free of additives, and use it only in cooking, not at the table.

Herbs and spices can lend a great deal of taste to even the simplest dish, but it is important to use just the right amount that will enhance and not overpower the flavor of the food. This is especially true for strong tasting ones such as garlic, cayenne, sage, and tarragon. It is best to start with a little and add more if necessary. For best results, fresh herbs should be added at the end of the cooking time, while dried ones should be added at the beginning. Cayenne and freshly ground black pepper can be added individually at the table, since not everybody likes a very hot taste.

Here are some suggestions if you end up with too much of anything.

too salty: Wash off the salt, or add oil or butter. When cooking grains or pasta, if the water is too salty, add a whole potato.

too sweet: Add salt, or increase the liquid.

too bitter: Avoid salt, and add something sweet.

too spicy: Add potato or grain, or something sweet.

too sour: Add salt or liquid.

For giving basic dishes like rice, vegetables, or chicken an international flavor, a simple seasoning list might include the following:

Italian: basil, oregano, thyme, marjoram, garlic, olive oil

Chinese: ginger, soy sauce, cayenne or chili oil, scallions, toasted sesame oil

Mexican: cumin, cilantro, cayenne and chili pepper, garlic, salsa

Indian: curry, coriander, cumin, saffron, cardamom, ghee (clarified butter)

French: dill, tarragon, thyme, rosemary, mustard, butter, wine.

East European: paprika, poppy seed, caraway, dill, onion, sour cream.

SEASONING MIX

A general seasoning mixture can be made from your own favorite choices or from the following recipe of dried ingredients:

1–2 teaspoons sea salt	2 teaspoons basil flakes
1–2 teaspoons onion powder	1 teaspoon parsley flakes
½ teaspoon garlic powder	½ teaspoon thyme
½–1 teaspoon mustard	½ teaspoon marjoram
¼–½ teaspoon cayenne powder	½ teaspoon celery seeds
1 teaspoon paprika	½ teaspoon curry (optional)
½ teaspoon kelp (optional)	

O A FEW TIPS AND SHORTCUTS

- Soak beans overnight to cut cooking time; throw away soaking water.
- Soak nuts and seeds overnight, and they will become crunchier and easier to digest because the fats in them become more available as fatty acids. Soaked nuts and seeds also make wonderful additions to salads and can be stored in the refrigerator for a few days.
- Pressure cooking beans and grains cuts the cooking time by approximately one third. I like to pressure cook a big batch of beans at a time and then store them in the freezer in small containers, just about enough for two people. In this way I can prepare a bean dish in no time at all, and besides, freezing helps get rid of the agents that cause flatulence in many people.
- Wash salad and other leafy greens when you buy them; let them dry, and then keep them in plastic bags in the vegetable compartment of the refrigerator so you do not have to waste a lot of time when you want to use them. I also like to keep the basic vegetables, like chopped onions, garlic, carrots, celery, parsley all ready to use.
- Keep a few basic sauces ready in the refrigerator, such as tomato sauce. Just simmer fresh or canned peeled tomatoes for about 20 minutes with a little salt. For a quick tomato sauce you can then sauté onion, garlic, celery, carrot, and parsley and a little chili pepper in a small amount of olive oil, and add it to the tomatoes. It takes about 5 minutes to put the whole thing together. Store in plastic or stainless steel, not in aluminum or pottery ware.
- Miso/tahini is also a basic condiment that keeps well. Just blend miso and tahini with a little rice vinegar and water. You can add garlic, ginger, or mustard to it to make it different every time, and use it as a salad dressing by adding more water, and as a dip or creamy sauce over grains if you keep it thicker.
- Flavored oils add zest to any dish. Being Italian, I am partial to olive oil, but you can use any oil you like. Make small bottles and add a different herb to each, i.e. garlic, hot chili pepper, tarragon, sage, rosemary, thyme, etc.
- If you do not have time to marinate things, here is a way to quick marinate. Bring your marinade to a boil and drop whatever you want to marinate into it for a few minutes.
- Instant pizza can be made by using tortillas or pita bread. Place them in the oven for a few minutes to crisp, spoon on some tomato sauce, your favorite toppings, and a little grated cheese, and put them into the oven again for a few minutes until the cheese melts.
- Quick-cooking grains are couscous, millet, quinoa, and polenta.
- Frozen grapes and cherries make wonderful alternatives to candy, or as "ice cubes" for drinks.

- Almost any juices, fresh or bottled, can be placed in popsicle containers and frozen to make warm weather treats for children of all ages.
- For thickening sauces and gravies, there are many substitutes for wheat flour. Equivalents to one tablespoon of wheat flour include half tablespoons of arrow root powder, rice or potato flour, or cornstarch.
- For those avoiding salt, lower sodium substitutes include kelp, regular or low sodium tamari, light miso, lemon juice, ume vinegar, celery salt, various vegetable "salts," and the seasoning mix just mentioned in Kitchen Basics.

For Those Who Wish to Avoid Fats

- Substitute fish, chicken, or vegetable stock for half or for the whole amount of oil called for in a recipe.
- Water-sauté food instead of stir-frying it in oil. Put about ½ to 1 cup of water or stock into a wok or skillet and bring it to a rapid boil. Quickly add vegetables and keep stirring over a high flame until done.
- Onions sautéed in their own juice and pureed with light miso make a wonderful onion butter which is great on toast or bread instead of using real butter. The same thing can be done with most vegetables.
- Apple butter is a great no-fat spread for those with a sweet tooth.
- Puree a very loose oatmeal (about 1 cup of rolled oats to 4 cups of water). Use instead of milk to make cream soups, gravies, and any dish which calls for milk.
- Tofu pureed with lemon juice makes a great mock sour cream.

About Storing

- Cooked grains may be kept in a porcelain or wooden bowl in a cool place but out of the refrigerator. Covered with a napkin, they will keep for about 3 days. In the refrigerator they should be stored in airtight containers or they will absorb the flavor of other foods.
- Beans can be kept in jars on shelves or inside a cupboard. Cooked beans are best stored in the freezer in small containers.
- Mushrooms should be kept in a brown paper bag in the vegetable compartment of the refrigerator.
- Fresh herbs keep best in a glass of water in the refrigerator.
- Oils once opened should be refrigerated. The only exception is olive oil which should be kept in a dark place.
- Nuts and seeds are best refrigerated or even frozen.
- Flour should be kept in the refrigerator or freezer.
- Fruits, potatoes, tomatoes, onions, and garlic are best not refrigerated, but kept in a basket in a shady place or in a pantry.

559

○ RECIPE TABLE OF CONTENTS

SAUCES

SIDE DISHES

DESSERTS

BAKED GOODS

KEY

Sp, Su, Au, Wi: following a recipe
title indicates the seasonal menu
plan in which that recipe is listed.

○ SOME BASIC RECIPES

Here are a few simple recipes to follow our basic rice and beans discussion and the food preparation tips. With all the diet and recipe books, once you learn to cook, you may use these basic ideas to create your own recipes in the kitchen. For many people, grains, beans, and vegetables, both raw and cooked, make up the major part of their diet; recipes are often used to learn new preparations or dishes, or for special occasions.

General Salad Ingredients

Limit to 4–6 choices

mixed lettuce, i.e., red or green leaf, romaine, or butter

head lettuce, shredded

spinach, broken

green or red bell pepper, diced

carrots, sliced or grated

cabbage, red or green, shredded

mushrooms, wiped and sliced

green onions, sliced

alfalfa sprouts

bean sprouts, i.e., mung, green peas, garbanzo, or aduki

sunflower seeds

Any green should be washed carefully and dried. Remove spinach stems. The sprouts, sunflower seeds, and mushrooms add some protein to the vegetable salad. Toss with a salad dressing of your choice.

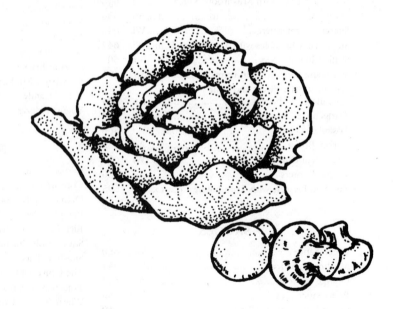

Mixed Sprout Salad

—Serves 4–6

1 cup each very fresh
   alfalfa, lentil, and
   mung bean sprouts

½ cup aduki, green pea,
   or garbanzo sprouts
   or a mixed bean
   preparation

2 Tablespoons
   sunflower seeds

½ cup chopped green
   onions

½ cup diced green
   pepper or cucumber

1–2 Tablespoons chopped
   fresh herbs (optional),
   or 1 Tablespoon dried
   salad herbs

2 ripe tomatoes or
   12 cherry tomatoes

Toss ingredients together and then decorate with tomatoes. Serve with a dressing of olive oil, lemon juice, and salad herbs, or a dressing of your choice. This high-protein, nutritious salad is very filling.

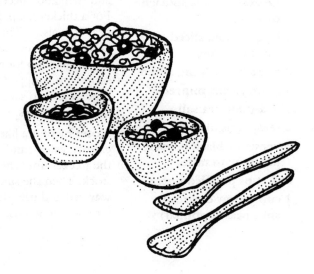

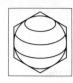

Vegetable Broth

—Serves 6–8

**2 cups potatoes,
 cut in small chunks**

1–2 zucchinis, sliced

**2 cups green cabbage,
 sliced (and/or other
 greens, such as spinach
 or kale)**

**1 large onion, sliced
 top to bottom**

2 carrots, medium, sliced

1 clove garlic, minced

½ teaspoon sea salt

2 teaspoons olive oil

**cayenne or black pepper,
 pinch or to taste**

6–8 cups purified water

**1 cup yellow or green
 split peas (optional)**

Slowly simmer all ingredients in a covered pot more than 2–3 hours, adding water if necessary. Mushrooms, especially shiitake mushrooms (4–6 for this recipe), will give a richer broth flavor.

For vegetable soup, cook the harder vegetables first, and then add zucchini, cabbage and/or greens, if used. For a thicker soup, add a cup of yellow or green split peas (see also, "Thick (Spicy) Vegetable Soup"). Other herbs and spices can be used if desired. Blend part or all of cooled soup for a thicker broth or a rich soup. Serve soup with chopped green onion or cilantro, or eat vegetables and save broth for other recipes, such as for sauces or gravies.

Note: Eleonora likes to keep the scraps from onions, carrots, celery, and other vegetables in a plastic bag in the freezer until she has enough to make a vegetable stock. Then she simmers all of it with a strip of kombu seaweed and uses this broth as a base for other soups or for cooking grains.

Low-fat, Low-salt Vinaigrette

—Makes about 1 cup

2 Tablespoons oil,
  safflower, sunflower,
  or olive

1–2 ounces vinegar, rice,
  or apple cider, or
  ½–1 lemon, juiced

1–2 cloves garlic, minced
  or pressed

½ teaspoon dried mustard

¼ teaspoon dried tarragon,
  ½ teaspoon salad herbs,
  or 1 teaspoon chopped
  fresh herbs

¼ teaspoon dried basil
  or marjoram

½ cup nonfat yogurt,
  unsalted tomato juice,
  or water

pepper to taste

This variation of a recipe from Dean Ornish's Stress, Diet, and Your Heart *is a healthy and tasty vinaigrette. There are even some decent oil-free dressings available in most stores.*

Mix the ingredients together well, or place in blender for a short blend (15–30 seconds) on low speed. Achieve desired thickness with water.

Joe Terry's Miso Magic Dressing

–Makes about 2 cups

3–4 cloves garlic

¾ cup balsamic vinegar

½ cup water

6 ounces white miso,
  unpasteurized

1 teaspoon prepared
  mustard

⅛ cup olive oil

This is also a low fat, cholesterol-free yet spicy, flavorful dressing for salads or other dishes, such as grains or vegetables. It needs a long, slow blender ride to make it really creamy and mix all the flavors.

Blend garlic cloves in vinegar and water. Slowly add miso, mustard, and olive oil.

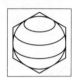

Guacamole   —Serves 4

3 medium avocados

1 small tomato, chopped
   and drained (optional)

2 green onions,
   chopped fine (optional)

¼ cup of Spanish,
   Bermuda, or yellow
   onion, diced (optional)

2 cloves garlic, minced

½ lemon or 1 lime, juiced

¼ teaspoon cayenne or
   chili powder, or to
   taste, or small jalapeño
   pepper, chopped finely,
   seeds removed

¼–½ teaspoon salt, or
   to taste

Mash avocados in a bowl, and mix in other ingredients. Serve cold with chips and salsa or with vegetables. Add water and lemon to make avocado salad dressing in blender. Add miso paste to taste for miso-avocado dressing. Blend in a block of tofu (with more water) for avocado-tofu dip or dressing. A simple guacamole will use only avocados, lemon, and salt. For a creamy version, add yogurt or sour cream.

Tostadas *(tortilla meals)*

tortillas, corn or wheat

grains

refried beans

cheese, grated (jack,
   cheddar, cottage,
   or soy)

chopped onion

sprouts or iceberg
   lettuce, shredded

avocado slices or
   guacamole

black olives

salsa

sour cream
   (optional)

Oil skillet and heat (on low) one side of tortilla. Turn and lay in grain or refried beans, sprinkle with cheese, and cover to melt. Serve with toppings. For a taco, fold in half and heat, flipping to other half if necessary. Remove and add vegetable ingredients of choice, and seasonings.

Salsa

—Makes 3–4 cups

3 cups chopped tomatoes, ripe

½ small onion, chopped

1 small jalapeño or chili pepper (¼ cup chopped bell pepper for milder salsa)

2 cloves garlic, minced

½ teaspoon chili powder or ¼ teaspoon cayenne

2 teaspoons fresh lemon or lime juice

2 Tablespoons chopped cilantro (optional)

¼–½ teaspoon cumin (optional)

¼ teaspoon salt (optional)

½ teaspoon oregano (optional)

Chop everything and mix. Remove seeds from hot peppers. If put in blender or food processor, will make a creamier salsa.

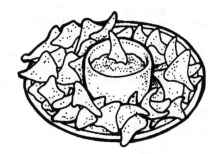

Steamed Veggie Platter

Use several or all of the following vegetables:

new potatoes, unpeeled

carrots, half-length strips

beets, quartered

broccoli florets with a little stem

cauliflower florets

zucchini, steam whole, then slice lengthwise

Steam vegetables until only slightly soft, about 10–15 minutes (zucchini, 5 minutes). Arrange all on a platter and season with melted butter or olive oil, lemon juice, and salt or herb seasoning. Garnish with cherry tomatoes if available. May also serve around a bowl with an herbal butter or any dip of your choice. Raw celery sticks, carrot sticks, and tomatoes can be used as well. In summer, a lightly steamed vegetable platter really brings out the natural flavors.

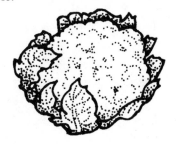

567

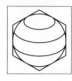

Thick (Spicy) Vegetable Soup
—Makes 5–6 cups

1 pound small or
 medium potatoes,
 or cauliflower pieces

4 cups water

¼ teaspoon cayenne
 or to taste (optional
 for spicy)

½ teaspoon dried basil

½ teaspoon cumin

3 Tablespoons sesame oil
 or corn oil (for a
 buttery flavor)

½–1 teaspoon sea salt

1 small onion, chopped

2 cloves garlic, chopped
 (optional)

½ cup tomato, diced

½ cup of several of the
 following vegetables:
 carrot, celery, green
 pepper, zucchini,
 broccoli, cauliflower,
 beets (for pink soup)

½ cup green onions,
 chopped

Scrub and wash potatoes or cauliflower and boil in 4
cups water in a medium-sized pot or sauce pan for 15–20
minutes. Allow to cool a bit, and blend with the water in
which they were cooked, adding the seasonings, the oil,
and the salt. Rinse vegetables, and chop into bite-sized
pieces. Place the blended mixture and chopped vegetables
into the pot or saucepan, cover, and cook over a low heat
for 10–15 minutes. Top with green onions and serve.

For a specific vegetable soup, such as potato or broccoli,
use primarily that vegetable. For a cream soup, use milk
(preferably low-fat), or for a milk-free cream soup, blend
in an appropriate amount (1 cup in this recipe) of well-
cooked, moist oatmeal.

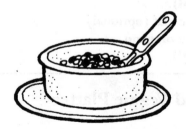

Here are three basic recipes for some common tomato sauces from a very useful recipe book, *The New Laurel's Kitchen*, by Laurel Robertson, Carol Flinders, and Brian Ruppenthal, published by Ten Speed Press.*

Homemade Ketchup
—Makes 1¾ cups

1 12-ounce can tomato
  paste
½ cup cider vinegar
½ cup water
½ teaspoon salt
1 teaspoon oregano
⅛ teaspoon cumin
⅛ teaspoon nutmeg
⅛ teaspoon pepper
½ teaspoon
  mustard powder
squeeze of garlic
  from press

We like this version better than store-bought. It's free of additives and sugar, and much lower in salt—and cheap.

Mix all ingredients together. Store in a jar in the refrigerator.

Quick Spicy Tomato Sauce
—Makes 2 cups

½ cup chopped shallot
  or red onion
2 cloves garlic
1 Tablespoon oil (olive)
1 Tablespoon
  coriander powder
1 teaspoon cumin
¼ teaspoon turmeric
½ teaspoon salt
3 cups chopped tomatoes

In oil, sauté shallot or onion with whole garlic cloves until soft. Add spices and continue cooking and stirring for a minute or so, until spices are fragrant and onion begins to brown. Stir in the tomatoes, cover, and cook gently at least until tomatoes have turned to liquid. Force through food mill or sieve.

*Another nice "Italian Tomato Sauce" can be found in *The Moosewood Cookbook* (page 66) by Mollie Katzen, also from Ten Speed Press.

Tomato Sauce

—*Makes about 3 cups*

½ onion, chopped

1 clove garlic

2 Tablespoons oil (olive)

1 small carrot, grated

2 Tablespoons chopped
green pepper

1 bay leaf

½ teaspoon oregano

½ teaspoon thyme

1 teaspoon basil

2 Tablespoons chopped
fresh parsley

2 cups tomatoes,
coarsely chopped

1 6-ounce can
tomato paste

¼ teaspoon honey

1 teaspoon salt

⅛ teaspoon pepper

One of our most praised recipes. Use vegetable broth or water to thin it to the right consistency for spaghetti, or use it "as is" for dishes like pizza.

Fresh tomatoes are wonderful, of course, but if they aren't in season, use canned. (Check the label to avoid added salt and sugar.)

Sauté onion and garlic clove in oil until onion is soft. Crush garlic with a fork.

Add carrot, green pepper, bay leaf, and herbs. Stir well, then add the tomatoes, tomato paste, honey, salt, and pepper. Simmer 15 minutes. Remove the bay leaf.

VARIATIONS

Mexican Sauce: When onion is nearly done, stir in 1 teaspoon cumin and 1 teaspoon chili powder, or to taste. Increase oregano to 1 teaspoon.

Italian Sauce: Add a pinch of fennel. Increase oregano to 1 teaspoon.

Dr. Sun's Granola

—*Makes 12 cups*

6 cups rolled oats

2 cups almonds, chopped

1 cup chopped walnuts or peanuts (optional)

2 cups sunflower seeds

1 cup safflower or soy oil

½–¾ cup maple syrup or honey

1–1½ Tablespoons vanilla

1 Tablespoon cinnamon, fresh ground is best

½ teaspoon almond extract (optional)

1 teaspoon sea salt

1 cup dried, chopped apricots (organic, unsulfured, sun-dried are best)

1 cup raisins, currants, or chopped dates

Preheat oven to 325°. Mix oats, nuts, and seeds into large bowl. Lightly heat other ingredients, except dried fruit, in a saucepan, and then pour over oat mixture, tossing thoroughly. Spread this mix onto cookie sheet or baking pan. Bake for about 20 minutes, stirring granola occasionally, until evenly toasted. Let cool and then toss in large bowl with dried fruit (if you like the chewy component in your granola). Store properly in closed containers. Use as a snack or a cereal.

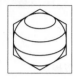
Cold Rice Salad Variation

—Serves 6

6 cups cooked brown rice

1 cup green and/or
  red pepper

4 green onions,
  chopped

4 radishes, sliced

½ cup fresh parsley
  chopped

½ cucumber, peeled
  and diced (optional)

½ cup roasted
  sunflower seeds

8–10 lettuce leaves

2 cups alfalfa sprouts

2 tomatoes, sliced

1 whole lemon, wedged

Mix rice with pepper, onions, radish, parsley, cucumber, and sunflower seeds. Place rice mixture in center of lettuce leaves, surround with alfalfa sprouts, and top with sliced tomatoes. If desired, sprinkle with salad herbs. Serve with lemon wedges. An olive oil vinaigrette or a nonfat yogurt vinaigrette would be ideal dressings.

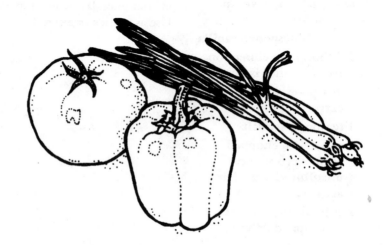

Rainbow Rice

—Serves 6–8

½ cup onion, chopped

½ cup red pepper,
chopped

½ cup carrot, chopped

½ cup yellow squash,
chopped

½ cup zucchini,
chopped

½ cup purple (red)
cabbage, chopped
(or beet or eggplant)

¼ cup green onions,
chopped

2 Tablespoons sunflower
or sesame oil (or
olive or canola)

2 teaspoons soy sauce
or to taste

½ cup water

6 cups cooked rice

1 cup parsley, chopped,
without stems

cayenne to taste (optional)

Cut vegetables lengthwise and then dice. Sauté the vegetables in oil in this order: onion, pepper, squashes, cabbage (eggplant or beet), and green onions, adding water and soy sauce, and stirring. Add cooked rice in clumps, stir into vegetables, and heat gently for 5 minutes. Leave covered and serve warm. Before serving, add parsley (and cayenne if desired). Good with a tofu or miso-tahini dressing (see seasonal recipes). This is a good cold salad as well.

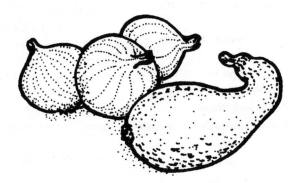

Chop Suey

—Serves 8–10

½ cup oil, i.e., soy,
canola, or sesame
(toasted optional)

1 cup green pepper, diced
(or celery, sliced)

1 cup onion, sliced
in crescents

2 cups button mushrooms,
sliced top to bottom

1 cup water chestnuts,
sliced

2 cups green cabbage,
shredded

1 cup Napa or Chinese
cabbage, shredded

1 cup bok choy

2 cups mung bean sprouts

3 cups water

½ cup arrowroot powder

½ cup soy sauce

cayenne pepper or chili
oil to taste (optional)

6–8 cups cooked rice

1 cup raw or toasted
almonds, slivered or
chopped (optional)

Use a heavy, large skillet or a wok for this chop suey dish. Heat wok or skillet first on medium heat. Add oil and then immediately add the vegetables, at 1–2 minute intervals, first adding pepper and onions, then the mushrooms and water chestnuts, then greens, and then bean sprouts, adding splashes of water up to 1 cup as needed. Have ready, mixed together in a bowl, the arrowroot (a thickener), soy sauce, cayenne or chili oil if desired, and 1–2 cups cool water until powder is dissolved. Stir liquid into vegetables, cover, and remove from heat. Serve over rice; it's nice.

If toasted almonds are desired, bake in oven on cookie sheet for 15–20 minutes at 300°, or buy already-roasted almonds at the store. For additional flavor, sprinkle some tamari soy sauce over almonds before roasting.

Additional foods to add or substitute for this Chinese meal are: tofu in cubes, bamboo shoots, snowpeas, green beans, celery, green onions, sliced carrots, broccoli florets, cauliflower, zucchini, and minced garlic or ginger, or just any "interesting" veggies on hand. Also, a sukiyaki dish can be made in a pot using about half the portions of above ingredients and about a cup or more water, leaving out the almonds, substituting carrots for the green pepper, and adding some clear rice noodles and chunks of tofu. Simmer about 10 minutes, and then add the greens, mung sprouts, and the arrowroot powder. For a little richer flavor, sauté the hard vegetables lightly in oil before adding to pot.

Sesame Salt (Gomasio)

A tasty seasoning for soup, salads, or grain and vegetable dishes. Roast sesame seeds in a dry skillet, stirring continuously, until a few begin to pop. Blend with sea salt, 1 part salt to 8–10 parts sesame seeds. Place in closed container and use as table seasoning.

○ WHEAT FREE

Wheat-free Pie Crust*   *—Makes 1 pie crust*

1 cup brown rice flour
1 cup oat flour
¼ teaspoon sea salt
2 Tablespoons sesame oil
⅔–¾ cup water

Lightly roast the flours in a skillet, stirring to toast but not brown. Combine all ingredients into a bowl and mix. Press mixture into oiled pie dish, spreading from center to edges to make a thin crust. Prebake for 10–15 minutes at 350°, remove and cool before adding pie filling. This recipe can also be used with whole wheat pastry flour and chopped walnuts.

The Universal Cracker Recipe**   *—Serves 6*

1 cup flour
½ teaspoon baking soda
  (optional)
¾ cup liquid (water,
  broth, or milk)
2 teaspoons oil
seasoning as you wish:
  garlic, herbs, seeds,
  nuts, or grated
  vegetables

Many health food stores offer specialty flours: corn, barley, millet, buckwheat, oat, lima bean, garbanzo bean, tapioca, potato flour, rice, and so on. You can also make your own using a hand mill or a small electric nut and seed grinder, available at health food stores. To make crackers, experiment with the following recipe until you get the consistency and taste you want. You'll be surprised how easy it is, and you avoid the problems of yeast, sugar, additives, preservatives, etc.

Combine flour and baking soda. Blend in liquid. Add oil and seasonings. Pour onto lightly oiled cookie sheet. Bake at 375° for 5–10 minutes. Flip and bake 3 more minutes.

---

* A variation from *The Self-Healing Cookbook* by Kristina Turner, published by Earthtones Press.
** from Dr. Braly's *Optimum Health Program* by James Braly, M.D.

○ MILK/EGG FREE

"Tofu Sour Cream" and "Tofu Mayonnaises," from the *The New Laurel's Kitchen*, are milk- and egg-free recipes for those with allergies and are also low in fat for individuals who like creamy sour cream or mayonnaise but are watching their waistlines or cholesterol levels.

Tofu Sour Cream

—Makes 1 ½ cups

¼ cup lemon juice

2 Tablespoons oil

1 Tablespoon light miso

¼ teaspoon mustard

(2 Tablespoons water)

1 Tablespoon shoyu
  (or other flavoring)

1 cup tofu (½ pound)

This makes a tasty substitute for plain sour cream. You won't need the water with soft tofu, but with firm tofu you probably will.

Blender: Place all ingredients except tofu in blender. Add tofu bit by bit, blending smooth with each addition. If the mixture stops moving, turn off blender and stir, then blend again. Add tofu and repeat until all is included.

Processor: Put it all in and process until creamy smooth.

Tofu Mayonnaises

Follow the directions for "Tofu Sour Cream," using the ingredients listed.

Russian

1 Tablespoon white miso

1 Tablespoon
  prepared mustard

2 Tablespoons oil

3 Tablespoons
  cider vinegar

dash pepper

pinch chili powder

½ teaspoon dill weed

⅛ teaspoon paprika

½ pound tofu

Oriental

1 Tablespoon shoyu
  or dark miso

3 Tablespoons rice
  vinegar

white part of 2 green
  onions, minced

2 teaspoons ginger,
  minced

2 Tablespoons oil

sliver fresh garlic, minced

½ pound tofu

French Onion

2 Tablespoons oil
  sautéed with:

½ small onion, minced

1 clove garlic

½ small carrot, grated

pinch chili powder

⅛ teaspoon paprika

2 Tablespoons cider
  vinegar

⅛ teaspoon black pepper

½ pound tofu

More Tofu: A couple of good tofu salads are "Eggless Egg Salad" in *The Enchanted Broccoli Forest* (page 76) by Mollie Katzen, published by Ten Speed Press, and "Marinated Tofu Salad" from *The Airola Diet and Cookbook* (page 112) by Paavo Airola, published by Health Plus Publishers.

○ BUTTER FREE SPREADS

Two tasty, low-fat, butter-free, spreadable vegetable butters by Kristina Turner from her book *The Self-Healing Cookbook* are "Sweet Carrot Butter" and "Sesame Squash Butter."

Sweet Carrot Butter —*Makes 1 small bowl*

4 cups carrots, sliced
½ cup water
pinch of sea salt
1 heaping Tablespoon kuzu, dissolved in 2 Tablespoons water
1–2 Tablespoons sesame tahini

Sweet, creamy, and super as a spread on whole wheat toast, rice cakes, or even waffles . . .

Slice carrots in 1-inch chunks and place in pressure cooker with water and salt. Bring to pressure, turn down, and simmer 10 minutes. (If you don't have a pressure cooker, steam 20 minutes). Puree carrots in blender, with ½ cup liquid from pressure-cooking or steaming. Dissolve kuzu in cool water, mix with carrot puree, and reheat. Stir until it bubbles (kuzu must be heated thoroughly to thicken). For buttery flavor, stir in sesame tahini.

Sesame Squash Butter —*Makes 1 small bowl*

1 cup mashed, cooked buttercup or butternut squash
3 Tablespoons sesame seeds*
1 teaspoon mellow white or chick-pea miso
dash of cinnamon
water

Carrot butter was my #1 favorite until I invented this!

Steam, bake, or pressure cook the squash, then mash. Roast sesame seeds by stirring in a skillet over medium heat until they smell toasty and crumble easily between thumb and forefinger. Grind into a butter in the blender or suribachi. Mix in squash, miso, and cinnamon and add just enough water to make a creamy spread.

---

* Fresh roasted and ground sesame seeds add a special taste and aroma. In a rush? Substitute tahini.

○ SEED CHEESE AND YOGURT (DAIRY-FREE AND RAW)

These recipes are a bit esoteric or eccentric, but for the highly vitalizing raw-food diet, seed cheeses and yogurt can provide very important nutrition. It does take some artful preparation, however, to make them right. Here are recipes from *The Hippocrates Diet and Health Program* (Avery Publishing Group) by Ann Wigmore. First make:

Rejuvelac

½ cup soft pastry
wheatberries (24-hour
   sprouted are best)
spring or filtered water

Grind wheatberries and put ¼ cup each in 2 large jars. Fill jars almost to top with water and cover with cheesecloth and an elastic band. Allow the mixture to sit for 3 days. On the fourth day, pour off Rejuvelac, straining out berries and sediment. Store unused Rejuvelac in the refrigerator. It will keep several days. Start a new batch twice a week.

Seed Cheese   —*Makes about 2½ cups*

1½ cups hulled, raw
   sunflower seeds
½ cup hulled, raw sesame
   seeds
1 cup Rejuvelac or spring
   or filtered water

Soak seeds 8 hours and sprout for 8 hours. After this time, pour Rejuvelac into a blender. Blend at high speed, slowly adding seeds until all are blended to a smooth paste (approximately 4 minutes). Pour the mixture into a glass jar, cover with a cloth or towel, and set aside for 4–8 hours. If Rejuvelac is not available, use water and let mixture sit 2 extra hours. Or, save ¼ cup from a previous cheese culture and mix it with the new batch. After the 4–8 hours have elapsed, pour off the whey by inserting a wooden spoon down one side of the jar to form a tunnel and spilling the liquid into the sink. Store it tightly covered in the refrigerator. Refrigerated, the cheese will last 5 days.

Seed Yogurt   —*Makes about 4 cups*

1½ cups hulled, raw
   sunflower seeds
½ cup sesame seeds
2 cups Rejuvelac or spring
   or filtered water

Follow the same procedure as for "Seed Cheese" (previous recipe), only set mixture aside for no more than 6 hours. Stir and refrigerate.

Bean Spreads (or Dip)

—Makes 2 cups

Basics:
2 cups cooked beans,*
mashed
1 Tablespoon oil
1 small lemon, juiced
1 clove garlic, pressed
½ onion, chopped
cumin to taste
salt to taste

Herbs and
Seasoning Choices:
green pepper or chili
pepper, chopped
parsley, chopped fine
green onions, chopped
½ teaspoon cumin
½–1 teaspoon
chili powder
1 teaspoon basil
½ teaspoon oregano
½ teaspoon coriander
¼ teaspoon thyme
1 teaspoon mustard
1–2 Tablespoons
red wine vinegar
1–2 Tablespoons
sesame tahini

You may use garbanzos, white beans, split peas, black-eyed peas, pinto, kidney, or black beans. Besides using one of these beans, this recipe can be made with a variety of tastes, using many different ingredients. To make a dip, add a little more water, lemon juice, and some oil.

Mash or blend beans with oil, lemon, garlic and onion, then add cumin and salt and 2–3 other herbs and seasonings selected from the list of choices. Add any other ingredients of choice. Can use as sandwich spread, or serve with crackers and vegetable sticks; celery and cucumber are good choices. As a sandwich with sliced tomato and sprouts or lettuce, it provides a nutritious meal.

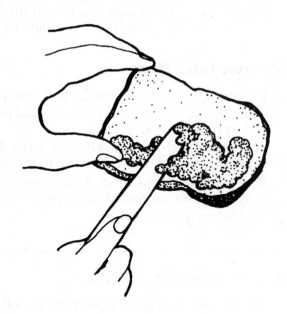

* See earlier discussion on cooking beans.

○ SPECIAL SNACKS FOR KIDS (AND THEIR FOLKS)

There are so many poor-quality treats available for kids that contain sugar, refined flour, preservatives, and dangerous artificial coloring, that I want to include a few treat recipes that children will like. Some of the recipes in this chapter may not be acceptable to many kids' usual tastes; however, there are probably more dishes that will. Some of the pastas, most breakfasts, burgers, and dips should go over fairly well. Basic grain dishes, the fruit kanten, sunshine bars, and the cookie recipes will likely be a hit. Any of the spicier recipes can also be toned down for family meals as well.

Other healthy snacks appreciated by children include: popcorn, granola, and dried fruits. However, minimize use of dried fruits, as they can be constipating. Soaking dried fruits overnight allows them to be hydrated and often more tasty.

Kids and most anyone will love "natural" french fries, or baked fries. Cut potatoes into strips. Place on pan and bake for 10–15 minutes at 350° until golden brown (bake with a little olive oil and salt or garlic salt and cayenne for more spicy baked "fries.") There are many fatty or sugary meals and snacks that we can make in healthier ways. Have fun in the kitchen and let your children play and create with you; they'll love it.

Frozen Juice Pops

Preferably, use bottled, nonsugared, naturally pressed juices. Choices of juices: orange, papaya, orange-papaya mix, tropical punch (a good one), apple or apple mix such as apple boysenberry, grape, etc.

Some juices, such as grape, will work better diluted with a little water; in general, for less sweet juice pops, add some water to the juice.

Pour juice into Popsicle containers and freeze. There are many new containers available in various shapes. Ice cube trays can also work, the shape is just harder to eat.

A great summer treat!

Dr. Elson's Nice Cream

Frozen desserts made of fresh fruit can only be made in certain types of juicers or food processors. I used to make "nice cream" in a Champion brand juicer, which was also good for nut butters. Use a hookup that pushes out everything that goes in. Freeze peeled bananas, then push whole bananas through the juicer; they will come out as creamy banana "nice cream," a real taste treat. Carob powder, carob chips, coconut pieces, or walnuts can also be run through with the bananas for a "nice cream" variation.

Fresh frozen peaches, strawberries (trimmed), or other berries can also be used straight or mixed with bananas. I have even thrown in some frozen kiwis, peeled first of course.

Yogurt Freezes

There are also many choices for these frozen yogurt treats. Many fruits will work well. Either mash the fruit and add the yogurt, or puree the fruit in the blender with a little honey or pure maple syrup, and add water or lemon juice for a tangy taste. Use plain regular, low-fat, or nonfat yogurt. Mix the yogurt in with the pureed fruit or blend all together. Can add chopped walnuts or almonds, coconut flakes, carob powder, or natural flavorings for variation. Pour mixture into freezable cups or scoop into Popsicle containers.

Some sample yogurt freezes include:

- **Banana Yogurt Freeze**—mash 2 ripe bananas with ½ teaspoon of honey or maple syrup and ½ teaspoon lemon juice; mix in 1 cup of yogurt, and freeze. For carob or cocoa banana, mix in 2 Tablespoons of carob powder or 1 Tablespoon pure cocoa.
- **Banana-Papaya**—mash 1 medium banana with ¼–½ fresh papaya and ½ teaspoon lemon juice—or blend to puree. Mix in 1 cup yogurt.
- **Apple**—puree 1 cup fresh apple without skin or use 1 cup applesauce, add 2 teaspoons honey, a pinch of cinnamon, and mix in 1 cup yogurt.
- **Strawberry**—puree 1½ cups strawberries with 1 Tablespoon honey and a splash of water. If using frozen, thawed berries, do not add water. Mix in yogurt and freeze.
- **Other berries** or fruits, such as peaches or nectarines, can also be used. Take 1–2 cups fresh or fresh frozen fruits, blend with 1 Tablespoon honey and a cup of plain yogurt. Freeze in cups or Popsicle containers.

Nut Milks

—Makes 1–2 cups

¼–½ cup nuts, preferably unsalted, raw whole nuts, or fresh coconut pieces (chopped or broken pieces of nuts or shredded coconut can also be used)

¾–1½ cups purified water

1–2 teaspoons pure maple syrup

1–2 pinches sea salt

Some milk-free, nutrient-rich beverage treats can be made in a blender with a variety of nuts, water, and a touch of maple syrup and sea salt. Almonds, Brazil nuts, cashews, or coconut can be used.

Put nuts in blender or food processor, mash to pulp, then cover with twice the level of water. Blend about 30 seconds, adding half of the maple syrup and salt. Pour nut milk through strainer into bowl and transfer to a storage jar. Place nuts back into blender and repeat blending with the remaining water, maple syrup, and salt. You may vary the proportions according to taste. Strain out the liquid "nut milk." Refrigerate and serve as a drink or on cereal. Lasts several days, refrigerated (use pure coconut milk within 24 hours). The leftover nut pulp can be used in cooking, such as in grain/vegetable dishes, or in baking.

Halvah

—*Makes 15–20 pieces*

1 cup ground sesame seeds
    or 1 cup raw tahini
    (sesame seed butter)

3–4 teaspoons honey
    (hardened, crystalline
    works best)

¼ cup raisins (optional)

2–3 Tablespoons shredded
    coconut (optional)

This is a rich, high-protein, high-oil, and high-nutrient treat.

Mash ingredients together in a small bowl and roll into balls or make into small bars. Roll on shredded coconut if desired. Can mix in 1–2 teaspoons of carob for carob halvah. Can also mash in banana for a tahini-banana mix that is very tasty.

Tahini Candy*

—*Serves 4*

¼ cup almonds

½ cup tahini

4 Tablespoons
    maple syrup

¼ teaspoon
    almond extract

1 Tablespoon
    carob flour

¼ cup grated coconut

Preheat oven to 425°. Spread the almonds on a baking sheet and roast in the oven for 5 minutes. In a small mixing bowl, blend the tahini, maple syrup, and almond extract, beating vigorously for 3 minutes until a stiff ball forms and the oil begins to separate; stir in the carob flour. As the mixture stiffens, press the dough against the sides of the bowl with a spoon to expel the oil, then pour off. Allow the dough to sit for 1–2 minutes. Remove the almonds from the oven. Press and drain the dough again and place in a napkin or paper towel; squeeze to absorb excess oil. Chop the almonds and add to the mixture. Place the mixture on a piece of wax paper (so it won't stick to the chopping board) and roll into a cylinder shape. Slice the roll into bite-sized pieces and cover with grated coconut.

Fruit Bars

—*Makes 10–12 bars*

½ cup honey

1 cup rolled oats

½ cup raisins

½ cup sunflower seeds

¼ cup of chopped dates
    or dried apricots

Heat honey in saucepan and stir in other ingredients. Pour into pan and let dry. Cut into bars and refrigerate or serve.

* This recipe is offered by Annemarie Colbin from *The Book of Whole Meals* (page 208), published by Ballantine Books.

Seasonal Menu Plans and Recipes

This section is divided into the four seasons and includes a specific four-day menu plan for each followed by recipes oriented to that season. There will also be some additional recipes for each season to provide some variety and adaptability for the vegetarian and omnivore alike. A nutritional analysis of these four diets will follow the winter recipes. The *italicized* food selections in the menu plans will have a specific recipe following the four-day menus. Enjoy!

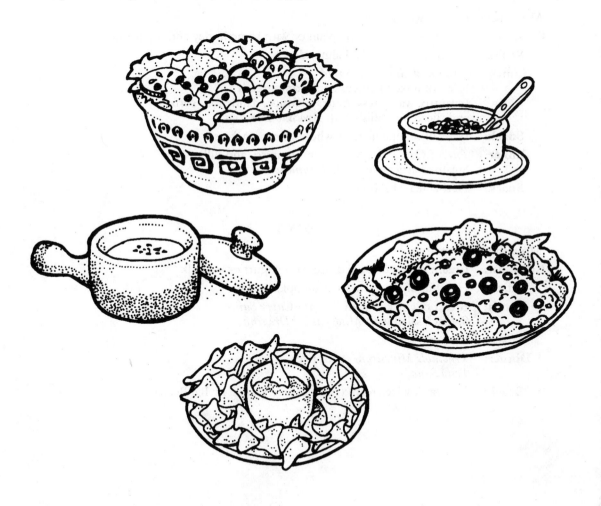

○ SPRING MENU PLAN

Spring is our purification season, with more fresh foods, especially greens, and more liquids. Start each day with two glasses of purified water, one with half a fresh lemon squeezed into it, and some stretching exercises.

DAY 1

Morning:	one or two oranges
Breakfast:	Cream of wheat or rye, plain or with some honey and oil or butter
Snack:	one handful of soaked almonds
Lunch:	*Pasta and Garbanzo Salad* Salad of mixed lettuces and spring greens (cilantro, watercress, miner's lettuce, dandelion, sorrel) and sliced red radish with *Avocado Dressing*
Snack:	Glass of orange juice or whole wheat crackers
Dinner:	*Pureed Carrot Soup* (with lemon, miso, and dill) Steamed artichokes with *Tofunaise*
Snack:	Herbal tea with honey

DAY 2

Morning:	Grapefruit
Breakfast:	Cream of rice or puffed rice with yogurt or soymilk
Snack:	Handful of raw or roasted pumpkin seeds
Lunch:	Breast of chicken with *Tomato-Caper Sauce* Spinach salad with *Miso-Tahini Dressing*
Snack:	Rice cakes
Dinner:	*Vegetable Minestrone* (with rice) *Pesto Sauce*
Snack:	Rice or Soy ice cream (such as Rice Dream or Ice Bean)

DAY 3

Morning:	one or two apples
Breakfast:	Oatmeal cooked with raisins
Snack:	one handful of sunflower seeds
Lunch:	Broiled fresh fish (halibut, sea bass, or swordfish) Oven roasted potatoes with rosemary Salad of mixed greens with vinaigrette of olive oil, balsamic vinegar, garlic, mustard, and sea salt
Snack:	Carrot and celery sticks, or granola
Dinner:	*Couscous Salad*
Snack:	Baked apple with raisins

DAY 4

Morning:	Strawberries
Breakfast:	Corn puffs or flakes with soymilk
Snack:	Handful of soaked filberts (hazelnuts)
Lunch:	*Polenta* with *Tomato-Lentil Sauce* Grated parmesan cheese (optional) Small green salad with vinaigrette
Snack:	Raw carrot and celery sticks
Dinner:	*Watercress Bisque* *Sweet and Sour Tempeh or Tofu*
Snack:	*Strawberry-Rhubarb Pudding*

Pasta and Garbanzo Salad

—*Serves 6*

1½ cups whole wheat
   spirals or bows

4 cups cooked or sprouted
   garbanzo beans

1 teaspoon thyme

1 teaspoon marjoram

1 clove garlic, minced

6 Tablespoons extra virgin
   olive oil or to taste

⅛ teaspoon cayenne pepper

tamari to taste

½ Tablespoon sea salt

Cook pasta in water and salt. Drain and combine with garbanzos, herbs, and garlic. Season with olive oil, cayenne, tamari and/or sea salt. Serve hot or cold. For a whole meal, you can also add some fresh veggies and a splash of rice vinegar.

Avocado Dressing

—*Serves 6*

2 medium avocados

1 lemon, juiced

1 teaspoon salt or
   tamari to taste

½ cup water

⅛ teaspoon cayenne pepper

1 clove garlic

Blend all ingredients well and toss with salad.

Pureed Carrot Soup

—*Serves 6*

7 cups water

12 carrots, cut
   into pieces

¼ lemon with peel

2 Tablespoons light
   miso or to taste

2 Tablespoons fresh dill

Bring water to a boil. Add carrots and lemon. Cover and simmer until carrots are tender, about 20 to 30 minutes. Remove lemon and discard. Puree in blender or food processor with miso and garnish with fresh dill. (A pureed carrot soup using carrots, onion, garlic, and celery with a squeeze of fresh ginger is a spicier autumn choice. Topped with some Sesame Salt (see page 574), this variation is very tasty.)

Tofunaise

—Serves 6

1 block tofu (6–8 ounces)
1 Tablespoon
  brown rice vinegar
½ teaspoon salt or to taste
½ teaspoon
  ground coriander
1 teaspoon Dijon
  mustard (optional)
1 Tablespoon olive oil

Blend all ingredients.

Tomato-Caper Sauce

—Serves 6

1 Tablespoon olive oil
1 clove garlic
1 chili pepper
1 28-ounce can peeled
  tomatoes, or 1 pound
  fresh, peeled tomatoes
¼ cup of chopped
  black olives
2 Tablespoons capers
sea salt to taste

Heat oil over medium flame and sauté garlic and chili pepper until slightly golden. Remove and add tomatoes. Simmer with lid ajar for about 20 minutes. Add olives and capers and simmer 5 more minutes. Salt to taste. Serve over baked breasts of chicken.

Miso-Tahini Dressing

—Serves 6

1 Tablespoon light miso
3 Tablespoons toasted
  sesame tahini
1 Tablespoon
  brown rice vinegar
¼ teaspoon rice malt
  or honey
3 Tablespoons water

Blend all ingredients well. If a thinner consistency is desired, add more water.

587

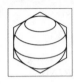

Vegetable Minestrone   *—Serves 6*

1½ quarts water
1 strip kombu sea
    vegetable (optional)
½ cup brown rice
1 Tablespoon fresh
    or ½ Tablespoon
    dried thyme
1 Tablespoon fresh
    or ½ Tablespoon
    dried marjoram
2 leeks, cut into
    ½-inch pieces
1 potato, cut into cubes
2 stalks celery, chopped
3 carrots, cut into pieces
1 cup broccoli florets
1 cup sweet peas
Sea salt to taste

Bring water, kombu, rice, and herbs (if using dried) to a boil, and simmer for 30 minutes. Add leeks, potato, celery, and carrots, and simmer 15 minutes longer. Then add broccoli florets, sweet peas, and herbs (if using fresh), and simmer another 10 minutes. Remove kombu, salt to taste, and serve.

If using leftover cooked rice, simmer vegetables in same order and add 1½ cups of rice at the end. Cooking time is approximately 25–30 minutes. Serve with "Pesto Sauce" (next recipe).

This soup is also very good served cold with a sprinkling of olive oil.

Pesto Sauce   *—Makes about 1 cup*

1 bunch fresh basil or
    spinach, clean and
    with stems removed
1 Tablespoon light miso
1 clove garlic
½ cup pine nuts
    and/or walnuts
4 Tablespoons olive oil
parsley (optional)

Puree all ingredients well in a blender or food processor. Some fresh parsley can be added to blender to enhance the green. If too thick, dilute with a little water. Pass at the table and add to "Vegetable Minestrone" (previous recipe). Of course, this dairyless pesto can be used for pastas or grain vegetable dishes if you so desire. A more traditional (and fattening) pesto sauce will use grated Romano cheese and olive oil.

Couscous Salad

—*Serves 6*

2 cups whole wheat
    couscous

3 cups boiling water

¼ cup chopped
    black olives

¼ cup capers

1 red bell pepper, cut
    into small pieces

1 stalk celery, cut
    into small pieces

2 green onions,
    sliced thinly

1 cup parsley, minced

¼ cup olive oil

2 teaspoons ume vinegar
    (or 1 Tablespoon lemon
    juice with ½ teaspoon
    sea salt), or to taste

¼ teaspoon
    cayenne pepper

lettuce leaves

cherry tomatoes

Place couscous in a bowl and pour boiling water over it. Cover and let sit for 10 minutes. Fluff with fork. Add olives, capers, vegetables, and parsley and toss with olive oil, ume vinegar, and cayenne. Serve over a bed of lettuce garnished with cherry tomatoes.

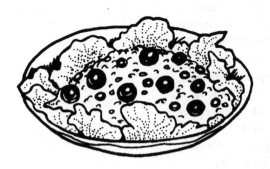

Polenta

—*Serves 6*

9 cups water

1 teaspoon sea salt

3 cups polenta
    (corn grits)

Polenta is excellent the day after. It can be baked, broiled, or grilled.

Bring water and salt to a boil. Slowly add polenta while stirring constantly with a whisk until well mixed. Lower flame to minimum, cover pot, and simmer until polenta has thickened, about 40 minutes. Stir occasionally to avoid burning the bottom. Transfer the polenta to a glass loaf pan, and let set for 5 minutes. Cut into squares and serve with "Tomato-Lentil sauce" (next recipe).

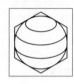

Tomato-Lentil Sauce   *—Serves 6*

½ onion, chopped finely

1 carrot, chopped finely

1 stalk celery,
  chopped finely

1 clove garlic, minced

2 Tablespoons olive oil

16 ounces fresh
  peeled tomatoes
  or 2 8-ounce cans

1 cup lentils

1 cup mushrooms,
  coarsely sliced

sea salt and pepper
  to taste

Parmesan cheese
  (optional)

Sauté onion, carrot, celery, and garlic in oil until onions are limp and transparent. Add tomatoes and lentils and simmer 30 to 40 minutes with lid ajar. Add mushrooms, cook 5 minutes longer, and season to taste with salt and pepper. Serve "Polenta" (previous recipe). Excellent also over pasta or whole grains. If desired, sprinkle Parmesan cheese over sauce.

Watercress Bisque   *—Serves 6*

1 onion, chopped finely

1 carrot, chopped finely

8 cups water

2 bunches watercress
  (about 8 cups),
  chopped coarsely,
  including stems

2 Tablespoons
  light miso or
  to taste

lemon wedges
  to garnish

Water-sauté onion and carrot until onion is limp and transparent. Add water and chopped watercress, cover and simmer for 20 minutes. Puree in blender or food processor with miso. Serve garnished with a lemon wedge.

Sweet and Sour Tempeh or Tofu —*Serves 6*

¼ cup water

¼ cup tamari

½ teaspoon ground
   coriander seed

1 clove garlic, minced

2 packages tempeh
   (1 pound) or 3 blocks
   tofu (about 1 pound),
   cut into 1-inch squares

¼ cup arrowroot flour

peanut or rice bran
   oil for deep frying

Mix water, tamari, coriander, and garlic together. Dip tempeh or tofu cubes in mix and coat with arrowroot flour. Heat oil in a wok or skillet, and deep fry tempeh or tofu until golden. Drain well on paper towel. For low-fat recipe, avoid frying by omitting arrowroot and oil; marinate tofu or tempeh and bake at 350° for 15–20 minutes. Serve with "Sweet and Sour Sauce" (next recipe).

Sweet and Sour Sauce —*Serves 6*

1½ cups water

1 cup rice syrup

4 teaspoons tamari

2 Tablespoons
   rice vinegar

1 Tablespoon tahini

½ teaspoon grated
   fresh ginger

1 Tablespoon kuzu,
   diluted in 1 Tablespoon
   cold water

2 green onions,
   chopped finely

Combine water, rice syrup, tamari, vinegar, tahini, and ginger and bring to a boil. Add diluted kuzu and stir until sauce thickens. Add green onions. One use for this sauce is to pour over "Sweet and Sour Tempeh or Tofu" (previous recipe).

Strawberry-Rhubarb Pudding

—Serves 6

5 cups strawberries, sliced

2 cups rhubarb, diced

3 Tablespoons maple syrup or to taste

1 teaspoon grated lemon rind

2 Tablespoons agar-agar flakes

1 Tablespoon kuzu, diluted in 2 Tablespoons cold water

Bring strawberries, rhubarb, maple syrup, and lemon rind to a boil and sprinkle in agar-agar flakes. Simmer until all flakes are dissolved (about 10 minutes). Add dissolved kuzu and stir until mixture thickens. Transfer to a bowl or individual cups and refrigerate until set. Garnish with strawberry slices and a sprig of mint.

Additional Spring Recipes

Complete information on the books used for these additional recipes will be noted in the *Recipe Book Bibliography* at the end of this chapter.

Lime Garlic Shrimp

—Serves 4–6

from *Tropic Cooking* by Joyce LeFray Young

2 pounds medium shrimp, cleaned, peeled, and deveined

¼ cup butter or margarine (canola oil is a better choice)

4 cloves garlic, minced

1 cup minced green onions

¼ cup freshly squeezed lime juice

coarsely ground black pepper

Tabasco or other hot sauce to taste

¼ cup freshly chopped parsley

Lime is a perfect fruit for the diet-conscious; it adds a nice zest to many dishes, without adding any calories to speak of. Be careful not to overcook the shellfish!

Prepare the shrimp and set aside.

In a large sauté pan, melt the butter or margarine. Add the garlic and green onions and sauté until the onions turn bright green. Add the shrimp and lime juice. Maintain the heat and cook just briefly, until shrimp turns pink. Stir in the black pepper, hot sauce, and parsley.

Serve over fluffy rice or on toasted, buttered rolls.

Green Jade Soup

—Serves 4

from *The Tao of Cooking* by Sally Pasley

3 dried Chinese
mushrooms

4 cups vegetable stock

⅓ cup carrots, peeled and
cut in 1-inch matchsticks

¼ cup thinly sliced
green onions

½ cup thinly sliced
mushrooms

about 10 spinach leaves

3 Tablespoons soy sauce

Soak dried mushrooms in 1 cup boiling water for 20 to 30 minutes, until soft. Drain and reserve stock. Slice in thin strips.

Bring reserved mushroom stock and vegetable stock to a boil in saucepan. Add carrots, green onions, and both kinds of mushrooms and simmer for 3 minutes. Add spinach leaves and soy sauce and cook for a few more minutes, until spinach is just wilted. Taste for seasoning.

Serve this simple, clear soup with nori rolls or tempura. You may also add thin Japanese noodles for a more filling soup.

Watercress Salad

—Serves 4

from *The Airola Diet and Cookbook* by Paavo Airola

1 bunch fresh watercress

¼ pound fresh mushrooms,
washed and sliced

1 cup mung bean sprouts

1 Tablespoon chopped
fresh parsley

1 green onion, chopped

3 Tablespoons
cold-pressed olive oil

1 Tablespoon
red wine vinegar

⅛ teaspoon sea salt

dash of cayenne pepper

Wash the watercress and tear into bite-sized pieces. Combine the watercress with the sliced mushrooms, bean sprouts, parsley, and green onion. Make a dressing with the olive oil, red wine vinegar, sea salt, and cayenne and pour over the salad, or use "Pollution Solution Dressing" (next recipe).

Pollution Solution Dressing

—Makes about 2 cups

from *The Airola Diet and Cookbook* by Paavo Airola

1 cup mayonnaise or
   Tofunaise (see recipe
   on page 587)

1 ripe tomato, chopped

1 small dill pickle,
   chopped

2 Tablespoons
   chopped onion

2 Tablespoons chopped
   green pepper

3 cloves of garlic, minced

2 teaspoons honey

1 Tablespoon plain yogurt

1 Tablespoon lemon juice

1 Tablespoon algin powder
   (sodium alginate)

1 Tablespoon
   brewer's yeast flakes

2 teaspoons
   lecithin granules

1 teaspoon kelp

½ teaspoon sea salt

dash of cayenne pepper

This salad dressing is specially formulated to minimize the damage from environmental pollution. It contains factors that have been shown to be effective in protecting the body from the toxic effects of heavy metal poisoning, such as from lead, mercury, and cadmium, as well as minimizing the damage from X-rays and other sources of harmful environmental radiation. Can use with any salad.

Combine all the ingredients and mix well. Store in the refrigerator.

Rice and Vegetable Salad

—Serves 4

from *The Book of Whole Meals* by Annemarie Colbin

1 carrot

½ bunch watercress

4 green onions

2 celery stalks

2 cups cooked
   brown rice

Shred carrot with a potato peeler. Remove the stems from the watercress; chop green onions and celery stalks. Now combine the vegetables in a salad bowl, stir in the rice, and toss with "Creamy Parsley Dressing" (next recipe).

Creamy Parsley Dressing

—*Serves 4*

from *The Book of Whole Meals* by Annemarie Colbin

2 ounces soft tofu
2 Tablespoons tahini
½ cup water
2 Tablespoons brown rice
   vinegar (or lemon juice)
½ teaspoon sea salt
   or to taste
1 handful washed parsley

Place all ingredients in a blender and puree until creamy. Pour approximately ¼ cup of the dressing on the "Rice and Vegetable Salad" (previous recipe). Toss well.

Zucchini Flowers with Tofu Filling

—*Serves 6*

by Eleonora Manzolini

12 zucchini flowers
½ cup whole wheat
   pastry flour
1 cup mineral water
1 cup tofu, crumbled
1 Tablespoon light miso
12 Kalamata olives,
   pitted, or 6 sun-dried
   tomatoes, soaked
peanut oil for
   deep frying
pinch of salt

Remove pistils from zucchini flowers and soak flowers in cold water for 20 minutes or longer. The longer they are soaked, the crisper they will be.

Place flour and mineral water in freezer for 15 minutes. In a bowl, mash together tofu and miso.

Remove zucchini flowers from water and place on a paper towel to dry. When dry, put 1 teaspoon of the tofu/miso mixture and then a pitted olive or half a sun-dried tomato into the top part of each flower. Roll up and place on a plate with a paper towel.

Heat oil in a skillet.

Quickly mix together flour, mineral water, and salt using a whisk. Dip each flower into the batter and deep fry until golden. Remove from oil with a slotted spoon and place on a plate with a paper towel.

Note: For lower fat and to avoid fried foods, the zucchini flowers can be baked at 450° for 10 minutes or until golden.

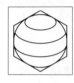

Pasta with Greens and Feta

—Serves 4 to 6

from *Still Life With Menu* by Mollie Katzen

6 Tablespoons olive oil

4 cups chopped onion

7–8 cups (packed) mixed bitter greens, washed, dried, and coarsely chopped (I used 1 medium-sized bunch each spinach and escarole)

salt to taste

¾–1 pound penne, fusilli, shells, or some comparable short, substantial pasta

½–¾ pound feta cheese, crumbled

freshly grated Parmesan cheese, to taste (optional)

freshly ground black pepper

Here is a painless way to slip some of those ultranutritious bitter greens into your diet. You can use any combination of kale, mustard, collard, dandelion, escarole, chard, or spinach. I especially like escarole and spinach together.

The instructions call for "short, substantial pasta," and I have suggested a few forms. This kind of sauce, with tender pieces of onion and bite-sized flecks of greens, studded with soft crumbs of feta cheese, adheres best to small, shapely units of pasta. Each mouthful of this dish packs in a beautiful integration of textures.

The sauce can be made a day or two ahead of time. Reheat it gently on the stove when you put up the pasta water to boil.

Heat the olive oil in a deep skillet or Dutch oven. Add the onions and cook for about 10 minutes over medium heat, stirring occasionally. Meanwhile, put the pasta water up to boil.

Add chopped greens to the skillet, salt lightly, and stir until the greens begin to wilt. Cover and cook 10–15 minutes over medium-low heat.

Cook the pasta until al dente. Just as it becomes ready, add the crumbled feta cheese to the sauce. (Keep the heat on low as you add the cheese.)

When the pasta is done, scoop it out with a strainer (in however many batches it takes), hold it over its cooking water momentarily to drain, then add it directly to the potful of sauce. Mix thoroughly.

Cook the completed dish just slightly over low heat for a few minutes. Add a small amount of Parmesan, if desired, and a generous amount of freshly ground black pepper. Then serve immediately, preferably on warmed plates.

Other nice spring choices include the "Spring Vegetable Salad" and "Cold Hunan Noodles with Sesame and Greens" from *Still Life With Menu* (pages 28 and 90) by Mollie Katzen, Ten Speed Press.

SPRING FOODS*

Fruits

Avocado
Date
Grapefruit
Jicama
Lemon
Lime
Loquat
Olive
Orange
Plum
Strawberry
Tangelo
Tangerine

Vegetables

Artichoke	Leeks
Asparagus	Lettuce
Beets	Butter
Beet greens	Greenleaf
Bok choy	Iceberg
Broccoli	Redleaf
Brussels sprouts	Romaine
Cabbage	Miner's lettuce
Cauliflower	Mint
Carrot	Mushroom
Celery	Mustard greens
Chard	Nettle
Chickweed	Parsley
Chicory	Radish
Chives	Rhubarb
Cilantro	Sorrel greens
Collard greens	Spinach
Comfrey	Sprouts
Dandelion greens	Sugar peas
Green garlic	Watercress
Green onion	
Green peas	
Kale	

Sprouts

Grains	Beans
Barley	Aduki
Buckwheat	Garbanzo
Corn	Lentil
Rice	Mung
Rye	
Wheat	**Seeds**
	Alfalfa
	Clover
	Radish
	Sunflower

Grains	Beans
Sprouted	Fava
	Sprouted

---

*These are the foods that are naturally available in the spring. This may vary slightly between locales. Some are the winter crops, such as cabbage or cauliflower, and others will not be available until later spring, after the early growing time.

Of course, foods that can be dried after their harvest or that are naturally contained in a protective coating for storage, are available throughout the year in most areas. These include the whole grains, beans, seaweeds, seeds and nuts. Although they are often used, they would not be classified as "Spring Foods."

For more complete information on the Seasonal Diets, see *The Seasonal Food Guide* poster from Celestial Arts, Berkeley, CA.

○ SUMMER MENU PLAN

In summer, we consume more liquids and raw, fresh fruits and vegetables, salads, and a lighter diet in general, and we are usually more active. This is a good season to experiment with special diets, such as fasting, or a raw food diet. The *italicized* food selections in the menu plans will have a specific recipe following the four-day menus.

DAY 1

Fruit: Fresh berries

Breakfast: *Breakfast Rice*, or puffed rice or rye flakes with yogurt

Snack: Soaked almonds

Lunch: Salad of mixed greens, raw spinach, chives, grated carrots, tomatoes, and tuna fish (or a mixture of bean sprouts or tofu salad for the vegetarian) with vinaigrette of avocado or olive oil, lemon juice, Dijon mustard, herb salt, and cayenne

Snack: Peaches

Dinner: *Stuffed Bell Peppers*, steamed Swiss chard sprinkled with roasted pumpkin seeds, minced garlic, olive oil, and soy sauce or tamari.

Snack: Rice cake with apple butter, or papaya

DAY 2

Fruit: Plums

Breakfast: Cream of wheat, *Crepes with Fruit*, or *Scrambled Tofu*

Snack: Wheat crackers or sprouted wheat toast with tahini

Lunch: Cold pasta salad with fava beans, fresh basil, lightly steamed asparagus tips, and baby (or sliced) carrots, and black olives with garlic oil, sea salt, and cayenne, served over a bed of lettuce

Snack: Cherries

Dinner: *Chicken "en Chemise"*; steamed artichoke with dilled tofu mayonnaise; watercress and baby lettuces with safflower oil, balsamic vinegar, and sea salt

Snack: *Fruit sorbet*

DAY 3

Fruit:	Oranges
Breakfast:	Granola with *Fruit Kanten*
Snack:	Walnuts
Lunch:	Broiled halibut basted with marinade of tamari, sesame oil, garlic, fresh thyme, and fresh marjoram; vegetable melange of lightly steamed sweet peas and carrots served with fresh arugula and a vinaigrette of olive oil, lemon or balsamic vinegar, and a pinch of sea salt
Snack:	Apricots
Dinner:	*Moussaka*, salad greens with vinaigrette
Snack:	Strawberries, blackberries, or fresh figs

DAY 4

Fruit:	Grapefruit
Breakfast:	Corn flakes with soymilk or Cornbread with *Peanut-Apple Butter*
Snack:	Sunflower seeds
Lunch:	Fresh corn on the cob with sweet, unpasteurized butter; *Mexican Salad Bowl*
Snack:	Banana
Dinner:	*Baked Dill Salmon*, green beans, *Salad of Belgian Endives*
Snack:	Fresh berries

Breakfast Rice

—*Serves 6*

1½ cups raisins

1 Tablespoon grated
    lemon rind

1 cinnamon stick or
    ½ teaspoon powder

1½ cups apple juice

5 cups leftover cooked rice

½ cup walnuts or almonds,
    coarsely chopped and
    lightly roasted

Simmer raisins, lemon rind, and cinnamon stick (or powder) in juice for a few minutes, until raisins are plump. Add rice, simmer a few more minutes, turn off heat, add walnuts or almonds, and let stand covered for 10 minutes or longer before serving.

Stuffed Bell Peppers

—*Serves 6*

6 bell peppers

3 Tablespoons
    sesame oil

1 clove garlic, minced

1 cup tempeh,
    crumbled, or
    1 cup cooked beans
    (white, navy, or aduki)

2 cups cooked
    leftover rice

2 green onions,
    chopped finely
    including green part

3 Tablespoons fresh
    cilantro, chopped
    or 1 teaspoon
    coriander powder

2 Tablespoons salsa
    (optional)

sea salt to taste

Preheat oven to 400°.

Cut tops off peppers and set aside. Scoop out seeds and white part and discard. Rinse peppers and turn over on wooden board to drain.

Heat oil (or water for lower fat) in skillet and sauté garlic and tempeh until golden brown. Add rice, green onions, cilantro, and salsa and mix well. Salt to taste and fill peppers with the mixture. Place peppers in Pyrex or other oven-proof dish, put tops back on them, and bake at 400° for 30 minutes.

A sauce can be made to cover peppers before baking. Either top simply with 3–4 ounces of grated Monterey Jack cheese, or blend 4 ounces of tofu with 1 Tablespoon tamari, 1 teaspoon of tahini, and 2–3 Tablespoons of water, depending on consistency desired.

Crepes with Fruit
—*Serves 6*

Batter:

2 cups whole wheat
   pastry flour

¼ teaspoon salt

2 Tablespoons
   corn oil (optional)

4 cups sparkling
   mineral water

Place flour and salt in a bowl, and if using oil, work it in with your fingers until it is evenly distributed. Add mineral water slowly stirring quickly with a whisk. Do not stir too much; the mixture should be bubbly. Use immediately.

Oil a crepe pan or a 9-inch cast-iron skillet, and heat over medium flame. Pour ¼ cup of crepe batter into the center of the hot pan and tilt the pan quickly in all directions, so that the batter covers the bottom of the pan evenly. Cook about 5 minutes or until the edges of the crepe begin to shrink. Lift crepe with a spatula and turn over. Cook another 2 minutes. Place crepes on individual plates, spread filling over each crepe, and roll up.

Note: This is a light and low-fat crepe; the bubbly water takes the place of egg to make the crepes fluffy.

Filling:

1 cup apple juice

3 cups seasonal fruit
   such as peaches,
   berries, apricots

pinch of salt

2 Tablespoons kuzu
   or arrowroot powder,
   diluted in 3 Tablespoons
   cold water or juice

Bring juice, fruit, and salt to a boil and simmer for a few minutes. Add dissolved kuzu and stir until mixture thickens.

Scrambled Tofu (lighter than eggs, and low-fat)   *—Serves 6*

3 8-ounce tofu cakes

1 Tablespoon light miso

1 Tablespoon sesame oil

1 cup mushrooms, sliced

¼ cup black olives, minced

2 medium tomatoes,
seeded and chopped

1 Tablespoon turmeric

¼ teaspoon cayenne,
or to taste

sea salt to taste;
soy sauce is also fine

¼ cup fresh parsley or
cilantro, minced

2 green onions,
sliced thinly

Place tofu in a bowl with miso and mash together thoroughly. Heat oil in skillet and sauté mushrooms for a few minutes. Add tofu mixture, olives, tomatoes, and turmeric. Stir together well, cover and simmer over low flame for 5 minutes. Season to taste with cayenne and sea salt or soy sauce, add parsley or cilantro and green onions, and serve. Add or substitute onion and garlic, carrot (diced or grated), and celery slices for variety. To vary flavor try nutritional yeast, thyme or rosemary, and dill. For spicy, egg-colored scrambled tofu, substitute ½ teaspoon curry powder for the turmeric.

Chicken "en Chemise"   *—Serves 6*

6 chicken breasts

6 pieces parchment paper

1 stalk celery, minced

1 onion, minced

1 teaspoon thyme

1 teaspoon marjoram

1 teaspoon herb salt

freshly ground
black pepper or
cayenne pepper

6 Tablespoons
lemon juice

6 Tablespoons dry
white wine (optional)

parsley to garnish

Preheat oven to 375°.

Season chicken breasts on both sides and place on paper squares. Place celery, onion and herbs on the chicken, add lemon juice, pepper, and wine, and fold ends of paper upward to form a little package. Bake for 30 minutes. Before serving garnish with fresh parsley.

Note: You can use a covered Pyrex baking dish for baked chicken breasts not "en chemise."

Fruit Sorbet   *—Serves 6*

4 cups fresh
   orange juice

3 Tablespoons
   maple syrup

2 Tablespoons grated
   orange rind

2 cups fresh or
   frozen strawberries,
   chopped, or local
   berries, whole

fresh mint sprigs
   for garnish

orange slices for garnish

Blend first four ingredients together in food processor or
blender. Transfer to a bowl and freeze for 2–3 hours, until
solid. Break into large chunks and blend again until creamy
and smooth. Return to the bowl and freeze again for about
30 minutes. Serve in individual parfait glasses with a sprig
of mint and a slice of orange.

Fruit Kanten   *—Serves 6*

7 cups apple juice

6 Tablespoons
   agar-agar flakes

1 teaspoon
   vanilla extract

1 cups fresh
   strawberries, or other
   seasonal fruit, sliced

3 cups granola

Bring juice and agar-agar flakes to a boil and simmer
covered until flakes have dissolved, about 10 minutes.
Add vanilla. Arrange fruit in the bottom of a rectangular
shallow glass pan and pour juice over it. Chill until set.
Cut into squares and serve this natural "jello" topped with
granola. This recipe can also be made in individual glass
cups or parfait glasses.

Moussaka
—*Serves 6*

2 large eggplants,
in ¼-inch slices

3 Tablespoons olive oil

1 large onion, sliced
into crescents

2 large tomatoes, peeled,
seeded, and chopped

½ cup white wine
(optional)

sea salt to taste

2 cups cooked chickpeas

1 Tablespoon
fresh oregano

3 Tablespoons fresh basil

1 cup feta cheese,
crumbled (optional)

Preheat oven to 300° and bake eggplant for about 10 minutes, or until tender enough to be pierced with a fork. Heat olive oil in a skillet, and sauté onion until limp and transparent. Add tomatoes, wine, and salt. Cook uncovered for 2–3 minutes. Add chickpeas and herbs and cook a few minutes longer. Place one layer of eggplant slices in the bottom of a casserole dish, cover with chickpea mixture, then sprinkle feta, add another layer of eggplant, and so on until all ingredients are used. Top with feta, cover, and bake 20 minutes at 350°. Remove cover and bake another 5 minutes.

Corn Bread
—*Makes 1 loaf*

1 cup whole wheat
pastry flour

1 cup cornmeal
or corn flour

1 Tablespoon baking
powder (aluminum-
free, if available)

⅛ teaspoon sea salt

¼ cup sunflower
seeds (optional)

¾ cup soymilk

¼ cup water

¼ cup corn oil

¼ cup pure maple syrup

⅛ teaspoon
vanilla extract

This is a healthy, milk-free, sweet breakfast corn bread. For a richer, spicier, milkier bread, see the "Rich Jalapeño Corn Bread" recipe from Fast Vegetarian Feasts *by Martha Rose Shulman in the Autumn recipes.*

Preheat oven to 350°.

Mix flour, cornmeal, baking powder, salt, and sunflower seeds in a bowl.

In a separate bowl, beat soymilk, water, corn oil, maple syrup, and vanilla together using a whisk.

Combine wet and dry ingredients. Stir a few times. Do not stir too much or the dough will become tough.

Pour into oiled loaf pan and bake at 350° for 45 minutes to 1 hour. Check with a toothpick; when it comes out clean, the bread is done.

Peanut-Apple Butter

—Makes 1 cup

¾ cup apple butter
    or apple sauce
¼ cup peanut butter

Blend together until smooth.

Mexican Salad Bowl

—Serves 6

3 Tablespoons fresh
    lemon juice

2 teaspoons mustard

1 Tablespoon ume
    vinegar (or apple cider
    and sea salt) or to taste

3 Tablespoons tahini

4 Tablespoons water

2 heads butter or other
    green lettuce, shredded

2 green onions,
    sliced finely

1 cucumber, grated

1 small bunch red
    radishes, grated

4 cups cooked
    black beans

2 Tablespoons
    minced cilantro or
    1 teaspoon ground
    coriander (optional)

Blend lemon juice, mustard, vinegar, tahini, and water together to make the dressing. (For a more Mexican dressing, use 3 Tablespoons salsa, 1 Tablespoon sesame oil, and ½ teaspoon salt or 1 teaspoon tamari.) Assemble all other ingredients in salad bowl and toss with dressing.

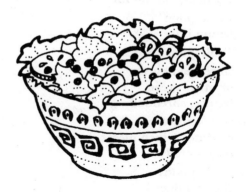

Baked Dill Salmon　　　　　　　　—*Makes 6*

2 Tablespoons soy sauce

2 Tablespoons
　lemon juice

6 salmon fillets

6 lemon slices

6 tomato slices

6 sprigs of fresh dill

Preheat oven to 375°.

　Mix together soy sauce and lemon juice, and dip salmon fillets in mixture to coat both sides. Place the fillets in a large baking dish; place a lemon slice, a tomato slice, and a sprig of dill on top and then cover with lid or foil. Bake about 20 minutes.

Salad of Belgian Endive　　　　　—*Makes 6*

1 Tablespoon light miso

1½ Tablespoon tahini

1 Tablespoon
　lemon juice

3 Tablespoons water

1 large head butter
　or other green
　lettuce, shredded

6 large endive,
　cut into ½-inch pieces,
　horizontally

4 Tablespoons
　chives, minced

Blend miso, tahini, lemon juice, and water together and toss with salad, or use Miso-Tahini Dressing (see recipe page 587).

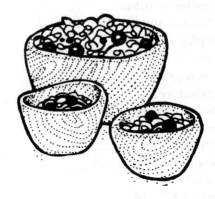

Additional Summer Recipes

Full information for the books used for these recipes will be at the end of this chapter in the *Recipe Book Bibliography*.

Fresh Corn and Tomato Soup —*Serves 4*

from *The New Laurel's Kitchen* by Laurel Robertson, Carol Flinders, and Brian Ruppenthal

½ onion, chopped
1 stalk celery, chopped
(dash cayenne pepper)
1 whole clove garlic
1 Tablespoon oil
5 ears corn
(4 cups off the cob)
4 good-sized tomatoes
½ cup water
½–1 teaspoon salt
(handful fresh coriander leaves, lightly chopped)

A thick, creamy, coral-colored soup with a truly superb flavor.

Sauté onion, celery, cayenne if desired, and garlic in oil in a heavy 2-quart pan until tender. (This amount of oil will be enough if you keep the heat low and stir frequently.)

Strip corn from cobs with a small, sharp knife. Remove stem end of tomatoes and cut up coarsely.

Add corn and tomatoes, water, and salt to sautéed vegetables. Bring to a boil; then reduce heat to low and simmer, covered, until corn is tender, about ½ hour.

The soup is pretty now, but even better if you take your courage in hand and proceed with the next step: purée it all. Return to pot, thinning with a little more water if you want, and correct the salt. Heat, stirring in coriander leaves just at serving time.

Russian Beet Salad

—*Serves 4*

from *The Enchanted Broccoli Forest* by Mollie Katzen

8 healthy (2½-inch diameter) beets

½ cup cider vinegar

1 medium clove of garlic, crushed

2 teaspoons honey

½ cup minced red onion

2 green onions, minced (whites and greens)

1 medium cucumber, seeded and finely chopped

2 hard-boiled eggs, chopped

2 Tablespoons fresh dill, minced or 1 teaspoon dried dill

2 cups mixed sour cream and yogurt

salt and black pepper, to taste

Boil the beets, whole, for about 20–25 minutes. Rinse under running water as you rub off their skins. Chop into ½-inch bits, and while they are still warm, marinate them in vinegar, garlic, and honey. Let stand 30 minutes.

Add all remaining ingredients. Mix well, and chill until very cold.

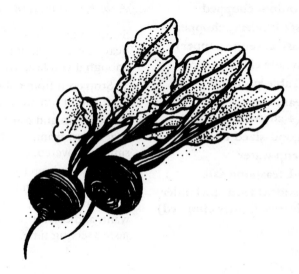

Israeli Salad

—Serves 4–6

from *The Enchanted Broccoli Forest* by Mollie Katzen

**2 young (6-inch)
cucumbers**

**2 medium-sized,
ripe tomatoes**

½ cup sliced radishes

**2 minced green onions,
including green part**

1 large, minced dill pickle

**1 medium-sized bell
pepper, minced**

**½ cup sliced,
pimiento-stuffed
green olives**

**½ cup minced Spanish
or red onion**

**½ cup (packed) finely
minced fresh parsley**

½ cup olive oil

juice from 1 large lemon

salt and pepper, to taste

Optional additions:
   **little cubes of
   cream cheese, yogurt,
   or sour cream on top**

Cut cucumbers and tomatoes into small cubes. Toss all ingredients together gently and chill. You can make this several hours ahead of serving time. It's nice to serve this in a glass bowl, because it's colorful.

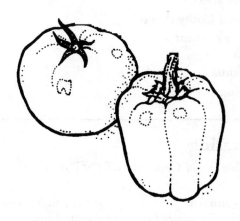

Tao Salad

—Serves 1

from *The Tao of Cooking* by Sally Pasley

3 cups lettuce, torn in
   bite-sized pieces
3 sliced raw mushrooms
3 tomato wedges
3 cucumber slices
½ cup grated Colby cheese
toasted whole wheat
   croutons
alfalfa sprouts
Tao dressing

Arrange lettuce on a large plate and top with remaining ingredients. Use plenty of croutons, sprouts, and Tao Dressing (next recipe).

Tao Dressing

—Makes 1 ⅓ cups

from *The Tao of Cooking* by Sally Pasley

⅓ cup mayonnaise
   (Tofunaise for lower fat)
⅓ cup yogurt
1½ Tablespoons
   cider vinegar
½ teaspoon salt
pinch black pepper
½ teaspoon finely
   chopped parsley
⅛ teaspoon basil
⅛ teaspoon dill weed
3–4 spinach leaves
⅔ cup salad oil
   (cold-pressed safflower,
   sunflower, or soy oil)

Combine all ingredients except salad oil in a blender and puree until smooth. Turn blender on low speed. While motor is still running, slowly pour in oil in a thin stream. When all the oil has been absorbed, turn blender on high speed and blend for a few more seconds to thicken.

Zucchini with Garlic and Tomatoes

—Serves 4

from *The Tao of Cooking* by Sally Pasley

2 Tablespoons olive oil

**1 teaspoon or more
finely chopped garlic**

**2 Tablespoons finely
chopped onion**

**1 tomato, peeled
and chopped**

**1½ pounds zucchini,
sliced in ¼-inch
thick rounds**

**2 Tablespoons finely
chopped parsley**

salt and pepper to taste

**2 Tablespoons
breadcrumbs**

**2–3 Tablespoons freshly
grated Parmesan cheese**

Heat oil in a skillet. Add garlic and onion and cook 3 minutes. Add chopped tomato and cook, stirring often, for 5 minutes.

Blanch zucchini 3 minutes in boiling, salted water. Drain well.

Add cooked zucchini to skillet with chopped parsley and season with salt and pepper. When heated through, transfer to a serving dish and sprinkle with breadcrumbs and grated cheese. Serve immediately.

Serve over rice or with a fish dish.

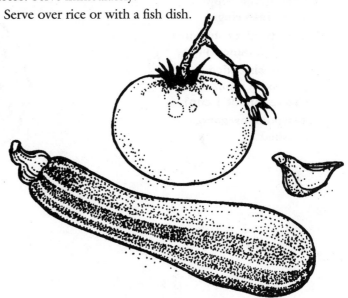

Rice Crust Pizza

—Serves 6

from *Eat Well, Be Well Cookbook* by Metropolitan Life Insurance Company

3 cups cooked
   brown rice

2 eggs beaten (or
   2 whites and 1 yolk)

1 15½-ounce jar
   pizza sauce (or
   homemade tomato
   sauce, see page 570)

1 small green pepper,
   sliced into rings

¾ cup sliced mushrooms
   (about 3 ounces)

4 ounces shredded
   part-skim mozzarella
   cheese (about 1 cup)

½ teaspoon oregano,
   crushed

Preheat oven to 400°F. Oil a 12-inch pizza pan. In a large bowl, combine rice and eggs. Spread onto pizza pan, making a ½-inch rim. Bake about 15 minutes. Reduce oven temperature to 375°F. Spread sauce over crust evenly. Top with pepper rings and mushrooms. Sprinkle with cheese and oregano. Bake about 10–15 minutes until cheese melts.

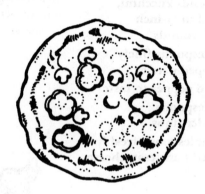

Couscous Casserole

—Serves 6-8

from *Stress, Diet, and Your Heart* by Dean Ornish, M.D.

2 cups broccoli florets

4 ripe tomatoes, peeled (see Note)

1 teaspoon safflower oil, plus additional for baking dish

1 onion, diced

1 clove garlic, minced or put through a press

1 teaspoon grated fresh ginger

½ pound (2 cakes) tofu, diced

1 teaspoon paprika

2 Tablespoons vinegar

1 Tablespoon mild-flavored honey

3 cups cooked couscous (1½ cups raw)

Steam the broccoli 5 minutes, drain, and refresh under cold water. Set aside.

Slice two of the tomatoes and set aside. Puree the rest in a blender or food processor.

Heat the 1 teaspoon oil in a heavy-bottomed skillet and add the onion and garlic. Sauté until the onion begins to soften. Add the ginger, tofu, tomato puree, paprika, vinegar, and honey. Simmer this mixture together over a medium flame, uncovered, for 10–15 minutes.

Preheat the oven to 325°.

Toss together the tomato-tofu mixture and the couscous. Fill a lightly oiled 2- or 3-quart baking dish with this mixture. Decorate the top with alternating rows of sliced tomatoes and broccoli. Cover with foil or a lid, and heat in the oven for 20–30 minutes.

Note: To peel tomatoes, drop into boiling water for 20 seconds, drain, and run under cold water.

Pasta with Marinated Vegetables —*Serves 4-6*

from *Still Life With Menu* by Mollie Katzen

3 red or yellow
  bell peppers

12 medium-sized fresh
  mushrooms, cleaned,
  stemmed, and sliced

2 6-ounce jars marinated
  artichoke hearts
  (including all
  their liquid)

15–20 cherry
  tomatoes, halved

12–15 large fresh basil
  leaves, minced (easiest
  to use scissors)

3–4 cloves garlic, minced

¾ teaspoon salt

6 Tablespoons olive oil

2 Tablespoons
  red wine vinegar

12–15 oil-cured olives,
  pitted and minced

1 pound fettucine or a
  tubular-shaped pasta
  like penne

½ cup grated
  Parmesan, Romano,
  or Asiago cheese

Be sure to give the vegetables time to marinate. Twenty-four hours of marinating time is optimal. You can get all the other vegetables ready while the peppers are roasting, and thus streamline the whole operation.

The hot pasta can be combined with room-temperature vegetables, but the dish tastes even better if all components are heated first. Warm the vegetables in a microwave or heat them gently in a large skillet over low heat. The drained pasta can be added directly to the skillet, along with the cheese. (Use a strainer or skimmer to transfer the pasta directly from its cooking water to the vegetables, saving yourself the trouble of traveling to the sink with a heavy hot kettle.)

Preheat oven to 350°. Place the peppers on a baking sheet and roast for 20–30 minutes, turning every 5–8 minutes or so, until the skin is fairly evenly blistered all over. Remove from the oven, and immediately place in a plastic or paper bag for about 5 minutes. Remove from the bag. When they are cool enough to handle, peel off the skin with a sharp paring knife (it should come off easily), and remove stems and seeds. Slice the peppers into strips, and place them in a large bowl.

Add all remaining ingredients except pasta and cheese, and mix well. Cover and let marinate a minimum of several hours.

Cook the pasta in plenty of boiling water until al dente. Drain, and combine with the marinade, adding the cheese as you mix it. Serve immediately.

Spicy Coleslaw
by Dr. Haas

—*Serves 4*

2 cups green cabbage,
    grated

1 cup red cabbage, grated

1 cup carrot, grated

½ cup black olives, diced

½ small onion, diced,
    and/or 2 cloves garlic,
    minced and pressed

½ cup almonds, slivered
    (optional for crunch)

2 Tablespoons mayonnaise
    or Tofunaise (page 587)

salt to taste

1 Tablespoon olive oil

1 teaspoon apple cider
    vinegar or juice of
    1 medium lemon

¼ teaspoon black pepper

¼ teaspoon red pepper
    (more for very spicy)

Grate cabbages and carrots, place in bowl, and mix in olives, onion, garlic, and almonds, if desired. Mix together mayonnaise, oil, vinegar or lemon juice, and spices, and stir into coleslaw. Refrigerate to cool before serving. I served this at my birthday party and it was a big hit!

Banana Yogurt Freeze
from *Fast Vegetarian Feasts* by Martha Rose Shulman

—*Serves 4*

4 large or 8 small,
    ripe bananas

1 cup plain,
    low-fat yogurt

2 teaspoons vanilla,
    or more, to taste

Freshly grated nutmeg
    to taste

Peel the bananas, cut in chunks, and freeze in plastic bags. They take 24 hours to freeze solid.

Place the yogurt and vanilla in a food processor and add the banana chunks. Using the pulse action of the food processor, process until almost smooth. Then process for several seconds until the mixture is completely smooth. Add nutmeg to taste, adjust the vanilla, and serve. Or hold in the freezer for up to 2 hours (it will become too hard if frozen any longer).

615

Sunshine Bars   *—Serves 2 dozen*

from *The New Laurel's Kitchen* by Laurel Robertson, Carol Flinders, and Brian Ruppenthal

1 cup orange juice

**1 cup dried apricots,
  loosely packed**

½ cup honey

½ cup oil

1½ cups rolled oats

1 cup whole wheat flour

½ cup wheat germ

1 teaspoon cinnamon

½ teaspoon salt

**1 cup raisins,
  partly cut up**

**⅔ cup toasted
  almond meal**

Preheat oven to 350°F.

Heat orange juice to a boil. Put dried apricots in pan, bring to a boil again, and turn off heat. Cover pan and let apricots absorb juice until tender enough to cut with a sharp knife, but not really soft.

Meanwhile, mix honey and oil. Stir oats, flour, wheat germ, cinnamon, and salt.

Drain apricots and add the juice to the honey-oil mixture.

Chop apricots coarsely and stir into dry ingredients along with raisins and almond meal. Combine wet and dry ingredients and press mixture into an oiled 9- x 13-inch baking dish. Bake about 30 minutes. Keep an eye on them! Cookies made with honey brown quickly.

Allow to cool completely before cutting.

Some other summer recipes for your reference include:

- Several for gazpacho, a classical cold summer soup, from *The Airola Diet and Cookbook* (page 157) by Paavo Airola, *The Moosewood Cookbook* (page 31) by Mollie Katzen, and "Avocado Gazpacho" from *The Tao of Cooking* (page 78) by Sally Pasley.
- "Chilled Cucumber Soup" and "Summer Vegetable Soup" from *The Moosewood Cookbook* (pages 30 and 15) by Mollie Katzen.
- "Spinach or Chard Soup" (also nice in spring) and "Lentil Tomato Mint Soup" from *The Tassajara Recipe Book* (pages 58 and 59) by Edward Espe Brown.
- A tabouli recipe from *Seasonal Salads from Around the World* (page 72) by David Scott and Paddy Byrne.
- "Indian Summer Casserole" from *Still Life With Menu* (page 128) by Mollie Katzen.
- "Pasta with Cottage Cheese or Ricotta and Tomato Sauce" from *Fast Vegetarian Feasts* (page 208) by Martha Rose Shulman.

SUMMER FOODS*

Fruits

Apricot	Nectarine
Avocado	Orange
Berries	Peach
Blackberry	Pear
Blueberry	Plum
Boysenberry	Prickly pear
Loganberry	Tangelo
Ollalieberry	Tangerine
Raspberry	Tropical fruits
Strawberry	Banana
Fig	Breadfruit
Grapefruit	Cherimoya
Lemon	Guava
Lime	Mango
Melons	Papaya
Cantaloupe	Passionfruit
Casaba	Pineapple
Crenshaw	Zapote
Honeydew	
Musk	
Persian	
Watermelon	

Vegetables

Artichoke	Sugar peas
Beet	Tomato
Bell pepper	Watercress
Cabbage	
Celery	
Chili pepper	**Beans**
Chive	Green beans
Corn, fresh	Sprouted beans
Cucumber	
Eggplant	**Nuts & Seeds**
Green beans	Sprouted
Green peas	
Lettuce	**Grains**
Okra	Sprouted
Parsley	
Radish	
Rhubarb	
Spinach	
Squash (soft)	
Crookneck	
Scallop	
Zucchini	

*These are the foods that are naturally available during the summer season in most areas. For more information regarding seasonal listings and food use, see *The Seasonal Food Guide* poster and booklet, published by Celestial Arts, Berkeley, CA.

○ AUTUMN MENU PLAN

Autumn gives us richer and denser foods that require more heat to prepare; these include whole grains, dried legumes, and hard squashes. Thus, there are more cooked foods, more calories, fats, and protein, less liquids, and often a few added pounds. Regular exercise, including stretching to maintain or improve flexibility, is also important during this more contractive time. The *italicized* food selections in the menu plans will have a specific recipe following the four-day menus.

DAY 1

Fruit:	Apple
Breakfast:	Oatmeal with yogurt, raisins, and maple syrup
Lunch:	*Fillet of Sole Florentine*; baked or steamed carrot and beet mélange served over steamed beet tops with a splash of olive oil, lemon juice, and sea salt
Snack:	Granola
Dinner:	*Lasagna*; salad greens with vinaigrette
Snack:	Baked apple

DAY 2

Fruit:	Grapes
Breakfast:	Twice-cooked rice with *Prune and Apricot Compote*
Snack:	Pumpkin seeds
Lunch:	Baked potato with *Avo-Miso-Tofu Topping*; grated carrots, red and green cabbage salad with vinaigrette sprinkled with toasted sunflower seeds or sliced hard-boiled egg
Snack:	Soaked prunes
Dinner:	Brown rice with aduki beans; steamed broccoli and cauliflower with *Walnut-Miso Sauce*
Snack:	*Carob-Tofu Mousse*

DAY 3

Fruit:	Cantaloupe or other melon
Breakfast:	Cornflakes, cooked millet, or *Millet Breakfast Cake with Orange Sauce*
Snack:	Filberts or pecans
Lunch:	*Turkey Breast*; *Wilted Spinach Salad*
Snack:	Blackberries
Dinner:	*Millet Croquettes*, *Brazilian Feijoada* (black beans); salad greens
Snack:	Popcorn

DAY 4

Fruit:	Pear
Breakfast:	Cream of wheat or whole wheat toast with peanut-apple butter
Snack:	Walnuts
Lunch:	*Grilled Swordfish with Pineapple Mustard*; *Warm Red Cabbage Salad*
Snack:	Apple
Dinner:	*Pasta alla Boscaiola*; salad greens with lemon and olive oil
Snack:	*Pears in Black Cherry Juice*

Fillet of Sole Florentine

—Serves 6

6 sole fillets

1 Tablespoon
fresh oregano

sea salt to taste

6 teaspoons lemon juice

6 Tablespoons dry
white wine (optional)

3 cups fresh
spinach, chopped

¼ teaspoon
grated nutmeg

lemon wedges

Preheat oven to 350°.

Place fillets in baking dish and sprinkle with oregano, salt, lemon juice, and wine. Bake for 5 minutes. Remove from oven and add spinach and grated nutmeg. Return to oven and bake an additional 3–4 minutes, or until spinach is wilted. Serve with wedge of lemon.

Lasagna

—Serves 6

2 Tablespoons olive oil

1 cup minced shallots

1 bunch spinach, chopped

1 teaspoon nutmeg

12 lasagna noodle
strips, cooked al dente
(slightly undercooked)
and drained

6 cups tomato sauce

2 cups leftover,
cooked beans

1 cup ricotta cheese, or
1 cup tofu mashed
together with
1 Tablespoon
light miso

sea salt to taste

freshly ground black
pepper to taste

Preheat oven to 350°.

Heat oil in skillet and sauté shallots until transparent. Combine with spinach and nutmeg.

In a large baking dish, layer lasagna strips, tomato sauce, beans, spinach mixture, and ricotta, until lasagna is used up. Season with salt and pepper. Finish with a layer of tomato sauce and top with ricotta cheese. Cover and bake at 350° for 20–30 minutes.

Prune and Apricot Compote —*Serves 6*

12 cups water
pinch of salt
3 cups prunes, pitted
3 cups dried,
  unsulfured apricots
1 Tablespoon grated
  lemon rind

Bring water and salt to a boil. Add prunes, apricots, and lemon rind, cover, and simmer for 1 hour adding more water if necessary. Serve fruits with their juice.

Avo-Miso-Tofu Topping —*Makes 2 cups*

1 large, ripe avocado,
  seeded and peeled
½ cup tofu, crumbled
1 Tablespoon light miso
2 Tablespoons
  lemon juice
1 teaspoon
  Worcestershire sauce
½ teaspoon Tabasco

Blend all ingredients together until smooth and creamy.

Walnut-Miso Sauce —*Makes 2 cups*

1 cup roasted (or raw)
  walnut pieces
1 Tablespoon
  light miso or to taste
1 Tablespoon rice vinegar
½ Tablespoon
  stoneground mustard
4 Tablespoons water
½ teaspoon
  maple syrup or honey

Blend all ingredients together until smooth.

621

Carob-Tofu Mousse
—Serves 6

2 blocks firm tofu
  (about one pound)
2 Tablespoons
  almond butter
3 Tablespoons maple syrup
1 Tablespoon vanilla
¼ cup water
3 Tablespoons grain coffee
  (Peru, Postum, Cafix)
6 Tablespoons toasted
  carob powder

Blend tofu with almond butter, maple syrup, and vanilla until creamy.

Bring water to a boil and dissolve grain coffee and carob powder in it. Mixture should have the consistency of a cream. Add to tofu mixture and blend again until very smooth. Serve in individual parfait glasses.

Millet Breakfast Cake with Orange Sauce
—Serves 6

1 Tablespoon corn oil
1 cup dry millet
3 cups apple juice
¼ teaspoon salt
¾ cup shredded coconut
1 Tablespoon vanilla
½ cup raisins

Preheat oven to 350°.

Oil a 2-quart casserole. Combine millet, juice, and salt in a saucepan and bring to a boil. Remove from heat and blend coconut with some of the millet and juice. Return to heat and add remaining ingredients. Simmer a few minutes, pour into casserole and bake for 45–60 minutes, or until firm. Allow to cool before cutting, or serve in Pyrex dish.

Serve with "Orange Sauce" (next recipe).

Orange Sauce
—Makes 2 cups

2 cups orange juice
½ teaspoon grated
  orange rind
½ teaspoon grated ginger
pinch of salt
¼ cup maple syrup
1½ Tablespoons
  kuzu dissolved in
  2 Tablespoons cold water

Bring orange juice, orange rind, ginger, salt, and maple syrup to a boil. Add dissolved kuzu and stir over low flame until thickened.

Turkey Breast   —*Serves 6*

3 Tablespoons olive oil

herb salt to taste

1 teaspoon thyme

1 teaspoon majoram

6 turkey breast fillets

1 medium onion,
    finely chopped

1 celery stalk,
    finely chopped

3 cups mushrooms, sliced

3 Tablespoons dry
    white wine (optional)

freshly ground pepper

Heat oven to 350°.

Combine olive oil, salt, and herbs. Place turkey breasts in a roasting pan and baste with oil/herb mixture. Bake at 350° for 10 minutes, basting when necessary. Remove turkey from oven, turn over and repeat procedure for another 10 minutes or until done, depending on thickness of fillets.

In a skillet, sauté onion and celery over medium heat until onion is limp and transparent. Add mushrooms, stir and sauté for a few minutes, add wine and cook for 5 minutes longer.

Top each turkey fillet with the mushroom mixture.

Wilted Spinach Salad   —*Serves 6*

3 bunches spinach
    (about 12 cups),
    coarsely chopped

1 red onion,
    sliced into rings

1 red bell pepper, chopped

6 Tablespoons olive oil

2 Tablespoons
    balsamic vinegar

sea salt to taste

1 cup feta cheese,
    crumbled (optional)

½ cup roasted walnut
    pieces (optional)

Place spinach in a pot or skillet over medium flame and stir until just limp; it should be bright green. Combine with onion rings and pepper, and toss with oil, vinegar, and salt to taste. Sprinkle feta and walnut pieces on top and serve warm.

Millet Croquettes

—Serves 6

3 cups cooked millet
2 Tablespoons soy sauce
1 small onion, grated
2 carrots, grated
½ cup parsley, minced
2 egg whites, beaten

Combine all ingredients and mash together well. Form into flat 2-inch patties and bake for 5 minutes. Remove from oven and using a spatula, turn patties over and bake for another 5 minutes or until golden.

Brazilian Feijoada

—Serves 6

1–2 Tablespoons
   olive or canola oil
1 large onion, chopped
2 cloves garlic, minced
2 stalks celery, chopped
2 carrots, chopped
4 cups black beans,
   cooked
1 large tomato,
   seeded and chopped
1 bay leaf
1 teaspoon
   ground coriander
1 cup red wine
   (optional)
1 cup soup stock
tamari to taste
¼ teaspoon cayenne

In a heavy-bottomed pot, heat oil and sauté onion, garlic, celery, and carrots over medium flame, stirring constantly until onion is transparent and limp.

Add beans, tomato, bay leaf, coriander, and wine. Cook uncovered for a few minutes. Add stock, cover and simmer for 15 minutes, or until liquid is almost absorbed. Remove 1 cup of beans, blend or mash, and return to pot. Season with tamari and cayenne.

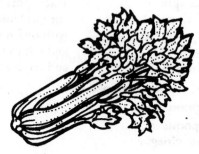

Grilled Swordfish with Pineapple Mustard —*Serves 6*

1 Tablespoon tamari
1 Tablespoon lemon juice
1 Tablespoon grated,
    fresh ginger
6 swordfish steaks
1 cup pineapple chunks
1 Tablespoon whole grain
    (stone-ground) mustard

Combine tamari and lemon juice in a bowl. Squeeze the juice from the grated fresh ginger through a cheesecloth or garlic press into the bowl. Dribble mixture over fish steaks and broil for 5 minutes. Turn fish over, dribble sauce over other side, and broil another 5 minutes or more depending on thickness of steaks.

In a blender or food processor puree the pineapple with the mustard. When fish is done, remove from the oven and spread a Tablespoon of the pineapple mixture on top of each steak.

Warm Red Cabbage Salad —*Serves 4–6*

1 head red cabbage
1 small onion, sliced
½ cup sweet peas
5 Tablespoons olive oil
3 Tablespoons
    rice vinegar
1 Tablespoon
    ume vinegar or
    sea salt to taste
½ cup roasted walnuts
    (optional)

Cut cabbage lengthwise into 4 pieces, then slice into ¼-inch strips. Steam until soft, about 3–5 minutes.

Sauté onion until limp and transparent and add to cabbage together with peas.

Combine olive oil, rice vinegar, and ume vinegar or sea salt and toss with cabbage. Sprinkle roasted walnuts on top and serve warm.

Pasta alla Boscaiola
—*Serves 6*

⅛ pound dried cepes or shiitake mushrooms

1 onion, chopped

2 cloves garlic, minced

½ pound mushrooms

1½ pounds tomatoes, peeled, seeded, and chopped

sea salt to taste

1½ pounds whole wheat pasta spirals

3 Tablespoons olive oil

3 Tablespoons parsley, chopped

Soak dried mushrooms in water for 30 minutes. Drain and chop. In a skillet sauté onion and garlic over medium flame, stirring constantly until onion is transparent. Add fresh mushrooms and cook for 5 minutes. Add soaked mushrooms and tomatoes. Season with salt and simmer, covered, for 20 minutes, or until cooking water has evaporated.

Cook pasta in water and salt. Strain, add mushroom sauce, olive oil, and parsley, and mix.

Pears in Black Cherry Juice
—*Serves 6*

6 firm pears

8 cups black cherry juice

¼ cup fresh ginger, peeled and cut into matchsticks or grate 1 Tablespoon ginger and press out into cherry juice

6 Tablespoons kuzu diluted in 6 Tablespoons cold water

6 sprigs mint

Place pears, juice, and ginger in heavy-bottomed pot and pour juice over them. The juice should half cover them. Cover and simmer until pears are soft but not mushy. Pierce with a toothpick to see if they are done. Remove pears from pot and place on a serving platter or on individual plates. Add dissolved kuzu to simmering juice and stir until thickened. Pour 1 cup of the sauce over each pear and garnish with a mint sprig.

Additional Autumn Recipes

Full information on books used for these additional autumn recipes are noted in *Recipe Book Bibliography* at the end of this chapter.

Garlic Soup —*Serves 6*
from *The Airola Diet and Cookbook* by Paavo Airola

1½ quarts water
4 potatoes
1 carrot
2 stalks celery
1 onion
2 large bulbs (heads)
    of garlic
½ teaspoon thyme
dash of oregano
dash of cayenne
sea salt to taste

Bring the water to a boil. Cut the potatoes, carrots, celery, and onion into ½-inch pieces, and place in the boiling water. Break the garlic bulbs and peel the individual cloves. Place them in the soup together with the spices. Cook the soup over medium heat for 20–30 minutes. When the soup is ready, it can be served in either of two ways:

Strain and serve as a clear broth with 1 raw egg dropped into each serving; or

Eliminate eggs and puree in the blender and serve as a "cream of garlic" soup.

Kasha Cream with Sunflower Seeds —*Serves 4*
from *The Book of Whole Meals* by Annemarie Colbin

1 cup kasha
    (buckwheat groats)
4 cups water
    (or more for
    thinner consistency)
½ teaspoon sea salt
½ cup sunflower seeds
shoyu (natural
    soy sauce) to taste

Grind the kasha in a blender, coffee mill, or handmill. In a 2-quart sauce pan, blend the kasha with 1 cup water until smooth, then add the remaining water and salt. Bring to a simmer, stirring constantly until it thickens. Cover and simmer for 15 minutes, stirring occasionally and adding water as needed. When the kasha has finished cooking, add the sunflower seeds and serve. Allow each person to season individual portions with shoyu to taste.

Thai Garlic Soup   —*Serves 6*

from *Still Life With Menu* by Mollie Katzen

**4–5 Tablespoons
  minced garlic**

**2 Tablespoons
  peanut oil**

**6 cups light stock
  or water**

4–5 teaspoons soy sauce

1 scant teaspoon salt

**3 cups coarsely
  shredded cabbage**

**2 medium-sized
  carrots, cut on
  the diagonal in
  1-inch lengths**

**1 stalk celery,
  chopped (optional)**

**a few mushrooms,
  sliced (optional)**

**crushed red pepper,
  to taste (if you go
  lightly on this it
  lends an intriguing
  and subtle touch)**

Don't be scared off by the amount of garlic here! It mellows amazingly as it cooks. The result is a light and gentle first course that can either precede a dramatic entree or be a soothing, small meal all by itself.

In a deep saucepan or Dutch oven sauté the garlic in oil over medium heat until it starts to turn brown. (This will take only a few minutes.)

Add remaining ingredients, and bring to a boil. Lower the heat and simmer, covered, about 10 minutes, or until all the vegetables are tender.

Taste and adjust seasonings. Serve immediately or store for reheating later. (Unlike many other soups, this one is not delicate, and reheats readily.)

Split Pea Soup

—Serves 6

by Dr. Haas

2 cups green split peas

8 cups water

1 onion, chopped

**1 large or 2 medium
carrots, sliced**

**2–3 cloves garlic,
minced or pressed**

**1 Tablespoon oil,
safflower or peanut
(optional)**

¼ teaspoon sea salt

**black or red pepper,
cumin, or curry
powder to taste
(optional)**

**1 Tablespoon miso
(optional)**

**2 Tablespoons parsley,
chopped**

Rinse peas. Place peas and water in pot and bring to boil. Optionally, lightly sauté onion, carrot, and one clove minced garlic in oil in soup pot, add water and peas, then bring to boil. Simmer on low heat for 30 minutes. Add remaining pressed garlic and seasonings. Simmer another 30 minutes or until carrots are soft. If adding miso, dissolve in small amount of water and stir into soup at end. Serve with parsley.

For a more complete meal, add 2 cups of cooked rice to pot at midway, or make croutons from whole grain bread by cubing several slices and baking them at 350° for 15–20 minutes. Serve with a large green salad.

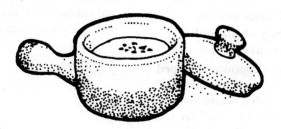

Veggie Burgers

—Serves 4

adapted by Dr. Haas from *The Self-Healing Cookbook* by Kristina Turner

1 carrot, grated

1 onion, diced

1 clove garlic, minced

2 teaspoons green onions, chopped fine

½ cup chopped parsley or spinach (optional)

2 cups cooked millet, tofu, or cooked soybeans

1–2 Tablespoons sesame oil

1 Tablespoon tamari

1–2 eggs, beaten,

½ cup whole grain bread crumbs

2 Tablespoons chopped almonds, peanuts, or roasted sesame seeds (avoid for low fat and easier digestion)

½ teaspoon thyme

½ teaspoon sea salt

Lightly sauté carrots, onions, garlic, green onions, and greens in sesame oil. Transfer to bowl and mix in millet or the mashed soybeans or tofu along with other ingredients. Mix with wooden spoon to a pasty burger consistency, adding water if necessary. Make into patties and sauté on skillet or, even better, bake in oven on cookie sheet at 350° about 40 minutes or until golden brown. Or, form into loaf and bake at 375° until brown. If desired, melt cheese on burgers and serve with choice of trimmings—buns or toast, sliced tomatoes, lettuce or alfalfa sprouts, catsup, mustard, relish, or Tofunaise (see page 587).

Combine with salad, steamed vegetables, corn on the cob, or for a classically American treat, some french fries– but do not fry your potatoes; cut into long strips, like fries, and bake at 350° until golden brown. Salt lightly and serve with homemade catsup. The kids will love 'em.

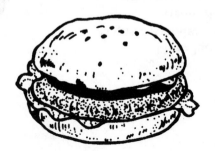

Confetti Quinoa

—Makes 3 cups

from *The New Laurel's Kitchen*, by Laurel Robertson, Carol Flinders, and Brian Ruppenthal

1 cup raw quinoa

2 cups water

¼ teaspoon salt

½ medium onion,
   finely chopped

¼ each, red and green
   bell pepper, seeded
   and finely chopped

1 teaspoon olive oil

2 Tablespoons chopped,
   toasted almonds or
   ¼ cup sliced water
   chestnuts

2 Tablespoons chopped
   fresh coriander leaves

Quinoa ("Keenwa"), sacred staple of the ancient Incas, still grows on the high slopes of the Andes—but also, nowadays, on the high slopes of the Colorado Rockies. Quinoa appeals to natural foods enthusiasts for its good nutrition (its balance of essential amino acids is close to ideal) and to gourmets for its unique texture and delicious flavor. Quinoa cooks in just fifteen minutes, and it's so delicate, so light and fluffy, that you can hardly believe it is a whole food. The flavor is appealing, and not quite like anything else, either. It bears some resemblance to couscous, and can be used in much the same way. It shines in dishes where you'd normally use bulghur wheat or millet.

Rinse quinoa thoroughly in a fine sieve. Bring two cups of water to a boil, then add salt and quinoa and bring to a boil again. Cover, reduce heat to a low simmer, and cook for 15 minutes.

Meanwhile, sauté onion and pepper in olive oil. Combine with grain. Just before serving, stir in almonds or water chestnuts and coriander leaves. Check salt.

Tempeh Cacciatore
—*Serves 4*

from *The New Laurel's Kitchen*, by Laurel Robertson, Carol Flinders, and Brian Ruppenthal

1 medium onion, slivered

½ cup chopped green bell pepper

2 Tablespoons olive oil

1 clove garlic, minced

1 cup sliced, fresh mushrooms

2½ cups tomatoes, peeled and chopped

⅓ cup red wine

1 bay leaf

½ teaspoon oregano

1 teaspoon basil

8 ounces tempeh, cubed

2 Tablespoons shoyu

Sauté onion and pepper in 1 Tablespoon olive oil over low heat until onion is translucent; then stir in garlic and mushrooms and cook another 5 minutes or so. Add tomatoes, wine, bay leaf, oregano, and basil and bring to a boil. Reduce heat and simmer for 10 minutes.

Meanwhile, in another small skillet or wok, sauté tempeh in remaining 1 Tablespoon oil, stirring frequently, until it browns slightly. Add to sauce along with shoyu, and simmer over low heat to marry the flavors (best if it can simmer at least half an hour). Serve on a bed of whole grain spaghetti or brown rice.

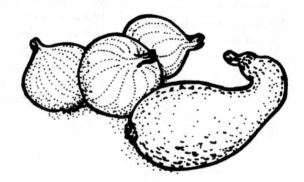

Rich Jalapeño Corn Bread
—Serves 12

from *Fast Vegetarian Feasts* by Martha Rose Shulman

1½ cups yellow cornmeal

½ cup whole wheat flour

¼ cup untoasted
wheat germ

½ teaspoon salt

½ teaspoon baking soda

2 teaspoons
baking powder

3 large eggs (or
1 yolk and 3 whites
for lower fat)

2 cups buttermilk or
1 cup plain low-fat
yogurt mixed with
1 cup milk

1 Tablespoon honey

2–4 jalapeño peppers,
seeds removed,
chopped

2 Tablespoons butter
(or corn oil)

For me nothing goes with a bowl of beans better than a thick piece of jalapeño corn bread. This one is almost like cake. You can, of course, omit the jalapeños, and have a delicious regular corn bread. (Also, there is a milk-free corn bread recipe in the Summer section.)

Preheat the oven to 375°F (190°C). Place a 9-by-9-inch (25 cm × 25 cm) baking pan or a 9-inch (25 cm) cast-iron skillet in the oven.

Sift together the cornmeal, whole wheat flour, wheat germ, salt, baking soda, and baking powder. In another bowl, beat together the eggs, buttermilk, and honey. Stir in the jalapeños.

Stir the wet ingredients into the dry. Mix together until blended, but do not beat.

Slide out the oven rack holding the hot baking dish or skillet, put in the butter, and return to the oven for a minute. When the butter begins to sizzle, remove the pan from the oven. Using a pastry brush, brush the pan with the butter and pour off any remaining butter into the batter. (Or avoid all butter and just grease the pan with corn oil.) Stir to combine, then pour the batter into the hot baking dish and set in the oven. Bake 30–40 minutes, until the top begins to brown. Cool in the pan, or cut into squares and serve hot.

633

Szechuan-Style Sweet and Sour Chinese Cabbage   —*Serves 4*

from *Fast Vegetarian Feasts* by Martha Rose Shulman

2 Tablespoons tamari

2 Tablespoons vinegar

1½ Tablespoons
mild honey

1 Tablespoon cornstarch

1 Tablespoon sesame oil

1 Tablespoon safflower oil

½–1 teaspoon hot red
pepper flakes, minced,
dried hot red pepper
(seeds removed)

1 Tablespoon miso
(optional)

2 pounds Chinese cabbage,
sliced crosswise into
2-inch pieces

2–3 cups hot, cooked
grains, such as millet,
couscous, or brown rice

This is a provocative dish for those who like spicy food. The miso gives it a satisfying, gutsy flavor.

Mix together the tamari, vinegar, and honey. Stir in the cornstarch. When it is dissolved, stir in the sesame oil. Set aside.

Heat the safflower oil (or canola) in a wok or large, heavy-bottomed skillet over moderate heat and add the red pepper and optional miso. Stir-fry for a few seconds and add the cabbage. Stir-fry for 2–3 minutes, until the cabbage begins to wilt, then add the tamari mixture. Cook for 1 minute, or until the cabbage is glazed. Serve immediately, with the hot, cooked grains.

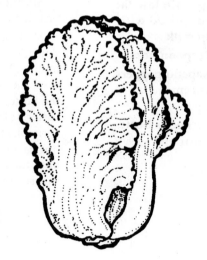

Carrot Bread
—4 large or 5 smaller loaves

from *Cosmic Cookery* (out of print) by Kathryn Hannaford

6 quarts carrot pulp
3 cups honey
1 cup oil
4 cups whole wheat flour
2 cups soy flour
2 Tablespoons cinnamon
1 Tablespoon nutmeg
4 cups sunflower seeds
4 cups currants or raisins

A good way to use the carrot pulp from making carrot juice.

Preheat oven to 325°.

Oil 1 large cookie sheet.

Mix thoroughly carrot pulp, honey, and oil. Sift the dry ingredients together, mix in the sunflower seeds and currants, and add to the carrot pulp mixture. Mix until all flour has been absorbed by carrot pulp. Mold by hand into loaves and bake on oiled cookie sheet at 325°.

Carrot Hash Browns
—Serves 3

from *Fit For Life* by Harvey and Marilyn Diamond

2 Tablespoons butter
1 teaspoon safflower oil
3 medium carrots, peeled and finely grated
3 medium all-purpose potatoes, peeled and finely grated
½ small white onion, finely grated
½ teaspoon sea salt (optional)

In large skillet, melt butter and oil. Add carrots, potatoes, and onions. Add seasoning. Sauté until browned on one side. Flip over and sauté on second side until browned. Break apart into small chunks, or serve in wedges cut from the round.

Shrimp Creole

—Serves 4

from *Eat Well, Be Well Cookbook* by Metropolitan Life Insurance Company

4 teaspoons vegetable oil

½ cup chopped green pepper (about ½ small)

½ cup chopped celery (about 1 rib)

½ cup chopped onion (about ½ medium)

1 garlic clove, minced

1 28-ounce can whole tomatoes, chopped, including liquid

¼ teaspoon crushed red pepper

1 bay leaf

½ teaspoon thyme, crushed

20 medium shrimp, shelled and deveined (about 10 ounces with shell; 8 ounces cleaned)

1 Tablespoon sherry

2 cups cooked rice

In medium saucepan heat oil over medium heat. Add green pepper, celery, onion, and garlic and cook about 5 minutes, until tender. Add tomatoes and liquid, red pepper, bay leaf and thyme; heat to boiling. Reduce heat to low; simmer uncovered about 30 minutes, stirring often, until reduced slightly. Add shrimp and sherry; cook about 4 minutes longer until shrimp turns pink. Remove bay leaf and discard. Serve over rice.

Other special autumn recipes that I have found include:

- "Kale and White Bean Soup" and "Chickpea and Spinach Soup" (also for summer), from *The Tassajara Recipe Book* (pages 60 and 61) by Edward Espe Brown.
- "Autumn Vegetable Soup," "Chinese Vegetable Soup," and "Pad Thai" to go with "Thai Garlic Soup" can be found in *Still Life With Menu* (pages 76, 89, and 209) by Mollie Katzen.
- "Baba Ganouj," a Syrian eggplant and tahini dip, from *The Tao of Cooking* (page 62) by Sally Pasley.
- "Spice Street Salad" and "Spicy Almond Dressing" from *Seasonal Salads from Around the World* (pages 81 and 137) by David Scott and Paddy Byrne.
- "Vegetable Stew" from *Moosewood Cookbook* (page 127) by Mollie Katzen.
- "Hot Tofu and Sesame Noodles" from *The Enchanted Broccoli Forest* (page 193) by Mollie Katzen.

AUTUMN FOODS*

Fruits

Apple
Berries
  Blackberry
  Cranberry
Dates
Fig
Grapes
Jicama
Mandarin orange
Melons
Pear
Persimmon
Plum
Pomegranate
Quince
Rosehips

Vegetables

Bell pepper
Broccoli
Burdock root
Cabbage
  red
  green
  Napa
Carrot
Cauliflower
Chayote
Corn, fresh
Cucumber
Daikon radish
Eggplant
Garlic (dried)
Gingerroot
Horseradish
Jerusalem
  artichoke
Leeks
Lettuces
Okra
Onions
Parsnips

Potatoes
Pumpkin
Rutabaga
Shallot
Spinach
Squash (hard)
  Acorn
  Banana
  Butterup
  Butternut
  Delicata
  Hubbard
  Spaghetti
Squash (soft)
Sweet potato
Tomato
Turnip
Yam

Grains (cooked)

Amaranth
Barley
Buckwheat
Corn
Millet
Oats
Quinoa
Rice
Rye
Wheat

Beans

Aduki
Black
Blackeye
Carob
Garbanzo
Great Northern
Kidney
Lentil
Lima
Navy
Peanut
Pink
Red
Soy
White

Nuts

Almond
Brazil
Cashew
Filbert
Macadamia
Pecan
Pignolia
Pistachio
Walnut

Seeds

Flax
Pumpkin
Sesame
Sunflower

*Many foods are available in the autumn harvest. For more information on seasonal eating see *The Seasonal Food Guide* poster and booklet, published by Celestial Arts, Berkeley, CA.

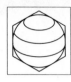

O **WINTER MENU PLAN**

The winter diet is often the richest, warmest, and heaviest of the seasonal diets. It includes more cooked foods, fewer fresh foods and cold drinks, and more teas and soups to keep the body warmer. And, of course, we may need more rest and dream time in the winter. The *italicized* food selections in the menu plans will have a specific recipe following the four-day menus.

DAY 1

Fruit:	Pear
Breakfast:	Sweet potatoes; cream of wheat; or *Cracked Wheat* with *Raisins and Walnuts*
Snack:	Sunflower seeds
Lunch:	*Cream of Broccoli Soup* (optional); *Roasted Turkey* with *Mushroom Sauce*, steamed greens, such as kale or chard
Snack:	Mandarin orange
Dinner:	*Stir-fried Vegetables with Tempeh or Tofu*; served over whole wheat pasta
Snack:	*Oatmeal Spice Cookies*

DAY 2

Fruit:	Orange
Breakfast:	Oatmeal or seven-grain cereal with stewed fruit
Snack:	Filberts or pistachios
Lunch:	*Curried Chicken Breast*, coleslaw
Snack:	Granola (see page 571 or buy some)
Dinner:	*Millet, Squash, and Aduki Bean Stew*; steamed kale with olive oil, garlic, and soy sauce
Snack:	*Apple-Raisin Compote*

DAY 3

Fruit:	Apples
Breakfast:	Baked acorn squash with sesame salt, or buckwheat cream (ground buckwheat, boiled) with raisins and sunflower seeds
Snack:	Soaked almonds
Lunch:	*Snapper Parmentière*; *Arame carrots, Scallions, and Corn*; steamed greens
Snack:	Popcorn
Dinner:	*Lentil Soup with Barley and Dulse*; salad greens and sprouts
Snack:	*Pumpkin Pie*

DAY 4

Fruit:	Kiwis
Breakfast:	Cream of rice with yogurt and honey
Snack:	Walnuts
Lunch:	*Butternut Bisque*; poached fish with steamed broccoli and cauliflower, or *Norimaki Sushi* as a vegetable substitute
Snack:	Dates or rice cakes with apple butter
Dinner:	*Rice-Lentil Loaf* with *Green Sauce*; steamed kale or chard with caraway seeds
Snack:	Baked apple

Cracked Wheat with Raisins and Walnuts   —*Serves 4–6*

1½ cups cracked wheat
1 cup raisins
½ cup walnuts
¼ teaspoon sea salt
½ teaspoon cinnamon

Combine all ingredients in a pot and bring to a boil. Reduce heat and simmer covered for 40 minutes.

Cream of Broccoli Soup   —*Serves 6*

1 cup water
¼ teaspoon salt
3 cups broccoli, chopped
1 cup low-fat milk
1 cup low-fat yogurt
1 small onion,
  finely chopped
1 Tablespoon light
  miso or to taste

Bring water and salt to a boil, add broccoli and cook for 20 minutes. Add milk and yogurt and cook a few more minutes. Puree in blender or food processor with miso.

In a small skillet sauté onion over medium flame, stirring constantly until golden. Add to soup.

For a dairyless version of the soup use a very loose oatmeal mixture (¾ cup rolled oats cooked in 3 cups water, then blended) instead of the milk and yogurt.

Roasted Turkey   —*Serves 4–6*

3 Tablespoons
  lemon juice
2 Tablespoons tamari
⅛ teaspoon cayenne
1 clove garlic, minced
6 turkey breast fillets
3 Tablespoons
  arrowroot flour

Combine lemon juice, tamari, cayenne, and garlic in a bowl. Dip turkey fillets in marinade and dust with arrow-root flour on both sides. Place in a baking dish and bake at 350° until done, about 15–20 minutes on each side depending on thickness of fillets, basting with marinade. Serve topped with "Mushroom Sauce" (next recipe).

Mushroom Sauce

—Makes 3 cups

½ cup onion, minced

2 Tablespoons light oil,
such as safflower or
canola

6 cups fresh
mushrooms, sliced

½ teaspoon sea salt
or to taste

½ cup dry white wine
(optional)

½ cup chicken or
vegetable stock

1 Tablespoon kuzu
diluted in
3 Tablespoons
cold water

½ cup parsley, minced

Sauté onion in oil for 5 minutes or until transparent.
Add mushrooms and salt, sauté one minute longer,
stirring well. Lower flame, cover, and simmer for
10–15 minutes. Uncover, add wine and allow alcohol
to evaporate over a high flame, for a few minutes. Add
stock, lower flame, and add kuzu stirring until thickened.
Adjust seasoning, stir in minced parsley, and serve over
"Roasted Turkey" (previous recipe).

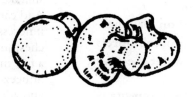

Stir-fried Vegetables with Tempeh or Tofu
—Serves 6

1 block (8 ounces) tofu
  or pack (6–8 ounces) of
  tempeh cut into cubes

1 large onion,
  cut into windowpanes

1 cup fresh (or
  reconstituted dried)
  shiitake mushrooms

1 cup vegetable stock

2 carrots,
  sliced on diagonal

1 cup broccoli florets

½ cup water chestnuts,
  sliced

1 cup bean sprouts

1 clove garlic, minced

2 Tablespoons grated
  fresh ginger

tamari or soy sauce
  to taste

3 Tablespoons
  toasted sesame oil

cayenne to taste

If using tempeh, bake or steam for 10 minutes before sautéeing. To cut onion into windowpanes, cut in half lengthwise, then cut each half into 3 or 4 sections lengthwise, depending on size of onion. Then slice each section crosswise into ¼-inch pieces. Remove stems from shiitake mushrooms and reserve to make stock. Slice mushrooms.

In a wok or large skillet, sauté onion over medium flame until it starts putting out its juice. Add ½ cup of stock and bring to a rapid boil over a high flame. Add shiitake mushrooms, cover and simmer for 5 minutes. Add carrots and sauté for a few minutes adding stock if necessary, then add tofu or tempeh, broccoli, water chestnuts, bean sprouts, and garlic in that order. Sauté a few more minutes or until broccoli is bright green. Squeeze fresh grated ginger through a cheesecloth and add to vegetables. Stir and cook a minute longer. Remove from heat, season with tamari, toasted sesame oil, and cayenne.

Oatmeal Spice Cookies

—2 dozen cookies

**2 cups whole wheat
 pastry flour**
1 cup rolled oats
pinch of salt
¼ teaspoon allspice
¼ teaspoon nutmeg
¼ teaspoon ginger powder
½ teaspoon cinnamon
½ cup water
½ cup corn oil
½ cup maple syrup
**½ cup carob chips
 (optional)**

Preheat oven to 375°. Combine flour, oats, salt, and spices in a bowl. Mix water, oil and maple syrup together well using a whisk. Add liquid ingredients to dry ingredients and mix together well to form dough.

Shape pieces of dough into cookies and bake for 10 minutes on each side. For variation, add a half cup of carob or cocoa chips to recipe.

Curried Chicken Breast

—Serves 6

1 onion, minced
**2 Tablespoons safflower
 oil (optional)**
6 chicken breasts
sea salt to taste
1 cup chicken stock
½ teaspoon cumin powder
**½ teaspoon
 coriander powder**
½ teaspoon ginger powder
**¼ teaspoon asafoetida
 (optional)**
**1 Tablespoon
 curry powder**
1 cup pineapple, diced
**1 Tablespoon kuzu,
 diluted in 1 Tablespoon
 cold water**

In heavy skillet, sauté onion in oil until translucent and limp, add chicken breasts, season with salt, sauté until golden, turn over and sauté other side until golden. Add ½ cup stock, cover and simmer until chicken is cooked. Pierce with a fork or paring knife to check; if no blood comes out, it is done. Remove chicken breasts and keep warm.

Add cumin, coriander, ginger, asafoetida, and curry to the skillet. Stir and cook until fragrant about 3–5 minutes, adding the rest of the stock a little at a time.

Puree pineapple and add to sauce. Simmer a few more minutes and add dissolved kuzu to simmering liquid stirring until thickened. Serve over chicken breasts.

Millet, Squash, and Aduki Bean Stew —*Serves 6*

1 cup aduki beans

1½ cups millet,
   dry-roasted in
   skillet first

4 cups water

1 piece kombu seaweed

1 small butternut
   or acorn squash,
   seeded and chopped

tamari to taste

Place beans, millet, water, and kombu in a pot and bring to a boil. Reduce heat and simmer covered for 30 minutes. Arrange squash chunks on top of the millet and beans. Simmer 30 minutes longer. Season with tamari.

Apple-Raisin Compote —*Serves 6*

4 apples, cored
   and chopped

1½ cups apple juice

1 cup raisins

1 cinnamon stick

3 cloves

1 teaspoon grated
   lemon rind

1 Tablespoon kuzu
   dissolved in
   2 Tablespoons
   cold water

1 teaspoon
   vanilla extract

Bring apples, juice, raisins, cinnamon, cloves, and lemon rind to a boil and simmer until soft, about 15 minutes. Add dissolved kuzu to simmering liquid and stir until thickened, then add vanilla.

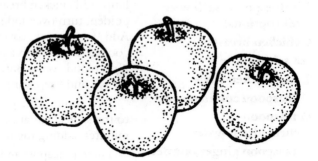

Snapper Parmentière
—*Serves 6*

1 medium butternut
   squash, sliced
1 Tablespoon olive oil
sea salt to taste
1 onion, sliced
6 fillets of snapper
   (or whole fish,
   3–4 pounds)
black pepper to taste
4 celery stalks, minced
1 onion, minced
1 clove garlic, minced
1 carrot, minced
1 bay leaf
parsley
1 Tablespoon dried thyme
1 Tablespoon dried
   oregano

In a glass baking pan make a layer of squash slices. Sprinkle with olive oil and salt and top with a layer of onion slices. Rub fish fillets with salt and pepper and place celery, minced onion and garlic, carrots, bay leaf, parsley, and part of the thyme and oregano on top. Roll fillets up and secure with a toothpick. Place them in the baking dish, sprinkle with the rest of the herbs, salt, and ground pepper. Cover and bake for about ½ hour. This dish can be done using a whole fish. In that case you would choose a snapper of about 4 pounds, stuff it with the herbs and vegetables, and place it belly down in a baking dish of the same size as the fish. Cover and bake for about 1 hour in preheated 350° oven.

Arame Carrots, Scallions, and Corn
—*Serves 6*

1 package arame seaweed
   (about 2 ounces)
1 cup carrots, sliced
   thinly on diagonal
2 Tablespoons toasted
   sesame oil
1 bunch scallions
   (green onions),
   sliced thinly
   including green part
1 cup corn kernels
tamari to taste

Soak arame in water for about 20 minutes.

In a heavy-bottomed pot sauté carrots in sesame oil over medium flame for about 5 minutes. Add arame and 1 cup soaking water. Cover and simmer for 20 minutes. Add green onions and corn and season with tamari, then turn off heat and let sit for 5 minutes before serving.

Lentil Soup with Barley and Dulse

—Serves 6

1 Tablespoon safflower
  oil (optional)

1 medium onion,
  chopped

1 stalk celery, sliced

2 carrots, sliced

1 cup barley

12 cups water

2 bay leaves

2 cups lentils

1 strip kombu seaweed

2 Tablespoons
  dark miso or
  to taste

Shredded dulse
  (optional, or to taste)

In a heavy-bottomed soup pot sauté in oil if using (can sauté without oil by using the vegetables' natural juices), onion, celery, and carrots, until onion is limp and transparent. Add barley, water, and bay leaves. Cover and simmer for 20 minutes. Then add lentils and kombu, and simmer for another 30 minutes. Discard kombu and bay leaves. Remove 1 cup of soup and blend with miso. Return to pot. Garnish with shredded dulse.

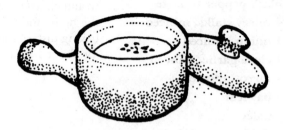

Pumpkin Pie

—Makes 1 pie

Crust:

⅔ cup rolled oats

½ teaspoon salt

⅓ cup ground almonds (in blender or food processor)

⅔ cup whole wheat pastry flour

3 Tablespoons maple syrup

½ teaspoon vanilla

2½ Tablespoons water

Mix dry ingredients in food processor. Mix wet ingredients in a bowl. Combine wet and dry ingredients and mix together well. Pat into oiled pie pan.

Filling:

2 cups pumpkin, pureed

1½ cups soymilk

⅓ cup maple syrup

1 teaspoon cinnamon

½ teaspoon ginger

½ teaspoon salt

½ teaspoon allspice

⅛ teaspoon clove powder

3 Tablespoons oat flour, toasted in dry pan

Preheat oven to 350°.

Mix all ingredients together well or blend in food processor. Put into pie crust and bake for 40 minutes.

647

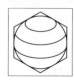

Butternut Bisque

—*Serves 6*

1 medium butternut
squash, washed
thoroughly

5 cups water

½ teaspoon salt

¼ teaspoon cumin

¼ teaspoon
coriander powder

¼ teaspoon ginger powder

¼ teaspoon garlic powder

6 Tablespoons yogurt

½ cup chopped, toasted
almonds for garnish

Cut butternut squash in half, scoop out seeds and cut into
1-inch cubes. Place in soup pot with water, salt, and spices.
Bring to a boil and simmer covered until you can pierce the
pieces easily with a fork, about 30 minutes.

Puree in blender or food processor, adjust seasoning,
and serve with a Tablespoon of yogurt in each cup and a
sprinkle of chopped toasted almonds.

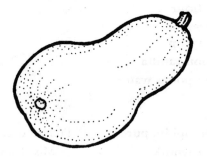

Norimaki Sushi

—Serves 4–6

4 green onions

1 medium carrot,
cut into 4 strips

4 sheets of nori seaweed

2 cups pressure cooked
brown rice, or 1 cup
rice overcooked with
3 cups water

2 dill pickles, cut into
strips

wasabi (Japanese
horseradish) to taste

shoyu (natural soy
sauce) to taste

Bring a little water to a boil in a small pot and quickly blanche green onion and carrot strip.

If you can, find toasted nori in your local health food store or Oriental market. If not, toast each sheet by holding over a flame or baking it in the oven or toaster oven for 2 minutes at 250°.

Place a nori sheet on a counter or sushi mat and spread about ⅓ cup of rice on it starting closest to you and leaving about ¼ of the nori at the bottom. Make sure the rice is spread out evenly and reaches the edges of the nori on both sides. Keep a bowl of cold water handy since you will need to moisten your hands frequently to handle the sticky rice.

Lay a green onion, a few carrot strips, and a few pickle strips across the center of the rice layer, making sure the vegetable strips reach the edges. Moisten your hands and lift the sushi mat. Your fingers should be on top of the rice and your thumbs beneath. Roll the mat forward pushing down with your fingers and up with your thumbs. Make sure not to roll the mat into the sushi. When you reach the end of the rice, lightly moisten the nori and seal. Squeeze gently and remove mat. Refrigerate first before slicing, or if serving immediately, carefully slice the roll with a very sharp knife.

Make a paste with the wasabi powder and water and place a dab of it on each roll. Be careful not to use too much since it is very strong. Serve with shoyu for dipping.

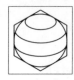

Rice-Lentil Loaf

—Serves 6

1 onion, minced

1 carrot, chopped
into small pieces

1 stalk celery, chopped
into small pieces

2 Tablespoons
sesame oil

1 Tablespoon rosemary

½ Tablespoon sage

2 cups leftover
cooked rice

2 cups cooked lentils or
leftover thick lentil soup

2 Tablespoons tamari

Preheat oven to 350°.

Sauté onion, carrot, and celery in oil until onion is limp and transparent, then add rosemary and sage and sauté a few minutes longer.

Add rice, lentils, and tamari and mix together well.

Place mixture into an oiled loaf pan and bake covered for 20 minutes. Remove cover and bake another 10 minutes. Let sit for a few minutes before slicing. Serve with "Green Sauce" (next recipe).

Green Sauce

—Makes 2 cups

2 cups water

1 Tablespoon toasted
sesame oil

¼ cup roasted walnut
pieces (optional)

4 Tablespoons tamari,
or to taste

¼ cup finely minced
parsley

1 Tablespoon kuzu
diluted in ¼ cup
cold water

Bring water and oil to a boil. Add walnut pieces and tamari. Stir in diluted kuzu and simmer until thickened. Add parsley. Serve over "Rice-Lentil Loaf" (previous recipe).

Additional Winter Recipes

Full information on the books used for these additional winter recipes is provided at the end of this chapter in *Recipe Book Bibliography.*

Russian Soup

—Serves 4

from *The Book of Whole Meals* by Annemarie Colbin

½ cup chick peas (garbanzos)

½ cup kidney beans

1 cup barley

8 cups water

1 onion

1 carrot

1 turnip

¼ small head cabbage, shredded

2 Tablespoons corn or sesame oil

1 teaspoon sea salt

2 Tablespoons shoyu (natural soy sauce) or to taste

1 handful parsley, chopped

Wash the beans and chickpeas separately, then soak each separately in 2 cups cold water for 8 hours; or bring to a boil, simmer for 2 minutes, and allow to soak in the warm water for 2 hours.

Drain beans; add fresh water to cover. Bring the beans and chick peas to boil; reduce heat, cover, and simmer for 30 minutes. Then combine the beans and chick peas with their cooking water in a 4- to 6-quart pot. Add the barley and remaining 4 cups of water; cover and bring to a simmer, cooking for 40 minutes.

Chop the onion, dice the carrot and turnip, and shred the cabbage. Heat the oil in a large skillet over medium heat; add the onion and sauté, then add the rest of the vegetables, stirring well after each addition. Continue to sauté for 10–15 minutes. Now stir the vegetable mixture into the beans and barley; add more water if needed, and simmer for 25 minutes. Season. Garnish the soup with chopped parsley and serve.

Note: For cabbage leaves to be tender, this recipe may need to be baked longer. However, the presteaming will usually be enough.

Russian Cabbage Borscht

—Serves 4–5

from *Moosewood Cookbook* by Mollie Katzen

1½ cups thinly sliced
  potato

1 cup thinly sliced beets

4 cups stock or water

1½ cups chopped onion

2 Tablespoons butter

1 scant teaspoon
  caraway seeds

2 teaspoons salt

1 stalk chopped celery

1 large, sliced carrot

3 cups chopped cabbage

black pepper

¼ teaspoon dill weed

1 Tablespoon +
  1 teaspoon cider vinegar

1 Tablespoon +
  1 teaspoon honey

1 cup tomato puree

Topping:

sour cream, dill weed,
  and chopped tomato

Place potatoes, beets, and water in a saucepan, and cook until everything is tender. (Save the water.)

Begin cooking the onions in the butter in a large kettle. Add caraway seeds and salt. Cook until onion is translucent, then add celery, carrots, and cabbage. Add water from beets and potatoes and cook, covered, until all the vegetables are tender. Add potatoes, beets, and all remaining ingredients.

Cover and simmer slowly for at least 30 minutes. Taste to correct seasonings.

Serve topped with sour cream, extra dill weed, chopped fresh tomatoes.

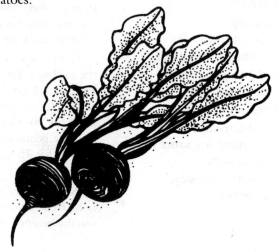

Hot and Sour Soup

—Serves 6

from *Fast Vegetarian Feasts* by Martha Rose Shulman

6 dried Chinese
    mushrooms
    (about 1 ounce)

8 cups water

4 vegetable bouillon cubes

6 green onions, sliced,
    white part and green
    part separated

2 cakes (½ pound)
    tofu, slivered

2 Tablespoons dry sherry
    or Chinese rice wine

¼ cup cider vinegar
    or Chinese rice wine
    vinegar, or more to taste

2 Tablespoons tamari,
    or more to taste

2 Tablespoons cornstarch
    or arrowroot

¼ cup cold water

2 eggs, beaten (optional)

¼ cup carrot, cut in
    2-inch matchsticks

¼ cup bok choy
    or celery cut in
    2-inch matchsticks

¼–½ teaspoon freshly
    ground black pepper,
    cayenne, or chili pepper
    to taste.

This soup is a favorite of mine, and one of the easiest and best I know of. It's light and warms you with its slightly piquant, vinegary broth. Even without the traditional pork (or chicken blood, which is often an ingredient in traditional recipes) it's a true Hot and Sour Soup.

Before you begin cutting the vegetables, place the mushrooms in a small bowl. Bring 2 cups of the water to a boil and pour over mushrooms. Cover and let stand 15 minutes. Meanwhile, prepare the other vegetables.

Place the remaining 6 cups water and the bouillon cubes in a large saucepan. Drain the mushrooms in a strainer over a bowl and add their liquid to the soup pot. Bring to a simmer. Cut the mushrooms in slivers and add them to the stock, along with the white part of the green onions. Simmer 5 minutes and add the tofu. Simmer 5 more minutes and stir in the sherry, vinegar, and tamari. Dissolve the cornstarch or arrowroot in the ¼ cup cold water. Stir into the soup and bring to a gentle boil, stirring.

Drizzle the beaten eggs into the boiling soup, stirring with a fork or chopstick so that the egg forms shreds. When the soup becomes clear and slightly thickened, remove from the heat. Stir in the pepper (be generous— this is the "hot" part of the soup) and adjust vinegar and tamari.

Distribute the carrots, bok choy or celery, and the green onion tops among the bowls and ladle in the soup. Serve at once, passing additional pepper and vinegar so people can adjust hot and sour to taste.

Hot and Sour Dressing

—Makes 1 ½ cups

from *Stress, Diet, and Your Heart* by Dean Ornish, M.D.

3 Tablespoons
   sesame tahini

4 Tablespoons cider or
   white wine vinegar

1 teaspoon hot red
   pepper powder or
   flaked red pepper

2 Tablespoons lemon juice

1 teaspoon
   mild-flavored honey

1 Tablespoon finely
   minced or grated
   fresh ginger

1–2 cloves garlic,
   finely minced

1 Tablespoon finely
   minced green onions

1 Tablespoon safflower oil

1 Tablespoon chopped
   fresh coriander
   (cilantro), optional

½ cup water

freshly ground pepper
   to taste

In a blender or food processor, blend all the ingredients together until smooth. Refrigerate until ready to use. Shake before tossing with the salad.

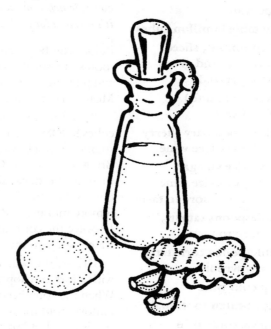

Kasha with Mushrooms, Water Chestnuts, and Celery

from *Fast Vegetarian Feasts* by Martha Rose Shulman

1½ cups buckwheat
  groats, washed

1 egg, beaten

3 cups boiling water

1 Tablespoon safflower oil

1 small onion, chopped

1 clove garlic, minced or
  put through a press

1 cake (½ pound) tofu,
  diced (optional; will
  complement the protein)

1 Tablespoon tamari
  (if using tofu)

2 stalks celery, sliced

½ small can water
  chestnuts, drained

salt and freshly ground
  pepper to taste

*This is the innards for the "Cabbage Leaves" (next recipe)
or this recipe can be used by itself as a hearty grain dish.*

Mix the buckwheat groats with the egg, and stir together to coat well. Heat a heavy, dry skillet and add the groats. Stir over medium heat until all the egg is absorbed and the groats are beginning to toast. Add the boiling water. When the mixture comes to a boil, reduce the heat, cover, and simmer 20 minutes, or until the liquid is absorbed. Meanwhile, prepare the vegetables.

When the kasha is cooked, heat the oil in a large, heavy-bottomed skillet and sauté the onion with the garlic until the onion is just beginning to get tender. Add the optional tofu and tamari, and sauté 3 minutes. Add the mushrooms and sauté, stirring, for a minute, then add the sherry and sauté 3 minutes. Stir in the kasha, and cook another 2–3 minutes. Season to taste with salt and freshly ground pepper. Serve hot.

Cabbage Leaves Stuffed with Kasha, with Creamy Tofu Sauce

—Serves 4

from *Fast Vegetarian Feasts* by Martha Rose Shulman

For the cabbage leaves:

2 cups Kasha with Mushrooms, Water Chestnuts, and Celery (preceding recipe)

12 large green cabbage leaves

For the Tofu Sauce (makes1 ½ cups):

2 cakes (½ pound) tofu

1 Tablespoon miso

1 Tablespoon sesame tahini

½ cup plain low-fat yogurt

1 Tablespoon lemon juice

pinch of freshly grated nutmeg

Just in case you're considering freezing this, don't. The cabbage leaves become like cardboard.

Preheat the oven to 350°. Oil a 2-quart baking dish. Steam the cabbage leaves for about 3 minutes, in a large, covered saucepan or wok, until tender and pliable.

Rinse under cold water and drain on paper towels.

In a blender or food processor, blend together the ingredients for the tofu sauce until smooth.

Place 2 heaping Tablespoons kasha mixture in the middle of each cabbage leaf. Spread a teaspoon of sauce over the kasha. Fold in the sides of the leaf and roll up, starting at the stem end. Place seam-side down in the baking dish.

Pour ½ cup (120 water in the dish and cover with foil or a lid. Bake for 20 minutes. Top with the remaining sauce and serve.

Note: For cabbage leaves to be tender, this dish may need to be baked longer. However, the presteaming step will usually be enough.

Vegetarian Chili

—Serves 6–8

from *Moosewood Cookbook* by Mollie Katzen

2½ cups raw kidney beans

1 cup raw bulghur

1 cup tomato juice

4 cloves crushed garlic

1½ cups chopped onion

olive oil for sauté
(about 3 Tablespoons)

1 cup each, chopped:
celery, carrots, and
green peppers

2 cups chopped,
fresh tomatoes

juice of ½ lemon

1 teaspoon ground cumin

1 teaspoon basil

1 teaspoon chili powder
(more, to taste)

salt and pepper

3 Tablespoons
tomato paste

3 Tablespoons dry
red wine

dash of cayenne
(more, to taste)

Put kidney beans in a saucepan and cover them with 6 cups of water. Soak 3–4 hours. Add extra water and 1 teaspoon salt. Cook until tender (about 1 hour). Watch the water level, and add more, if necessary.

Heat tomato juice to a boil. Pour over raw bulghur. Cover and let stand at least 15 minutes. (It will be crunchy, so it can absorb more later.)

Sauté onions and garlic in olive oil. Add carrots, celery, and spices. When vegetables are almost done, add peppers. Cook until tender.

Combine all ingredients and heat together gently— either in kettle over double boiler, or covered, in a moderate oven. Season to taste. Serve topped with cheese (or low-fat yogurt) and parsley.

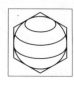

Spicy Nut Sauce

—Makes 1 cup

from *Dr. Braly's Optimum Health Program* by James Braly, M.D.

**2 Tablespoons chopped
green pepper**

1 small onion, minced

1 Tablespoon oil

1 cup chopped tomato

¼ teaspoon salt

**½ teaspoon chopped
jalapeño pepper or
¼ teaspoon cayenne
pepper**

**⅓ cup nut meal
(walnuts, pecans,
or sunflower seeds,
ground)**

¼ cup water

Sauté green pepper and onion in oil until tender. Add tomato and cook for 5 minutes or until soft. Stir in salt, pepper, and nut meal. Gradually add water, stirring to make a creamy sauce. Heat through and adjust spices to taste. May serve over grain and/or vegetable dish.

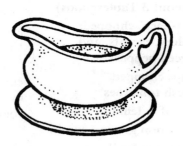

Basmati Rice 'n' Eggs
—Serves 4–6

by Bethany ArgIsle

3 cups basmati rice

5 cups water

6 eggs

6 green onions,
  chopped fine

1 small bunch cilantro,
  chopped fine

3 ripe tomatoes

¼ cup olive oil

3 Tablespoons
  low-salt soy sauce
  or mineral bouillon

¼ teaspoon
  cayenne pepper

2 Tablesoons toasted
  sesame oil

Basmati is known in the East as the "rice of kings."
It is light with a flowery fragrance.

Rinse rice thoroughly until water is clear. Add fresh water two finger breadths above rice and boil rapidly over moderate heat. Do not burn.

Soft boil eggs 3–4 minutes; then, run under cold water and peel. Wash and chop separately the green onions, cilantro, and tomatoes; place in individual bowls for personal serving garnish.

Add rice, eggs, oil and all seasonings to large bowl and mix lightly. Taste and balance seasonings as desired. Add garnish according to individual taste.

Leftovers are a lot of fun and can be planned the day before by making more of this dish than needed. Get out your wok or skillet and heat it over a hot flame. Then add first a half cup of purified water or a quarter cup of olive oil or rice bran oil. Immediately add rice and eggs with any lightly steamed vegetable such as green or red bell or chili peppers—or you can prebroil fresh, organic turkey sausage or soy sausage, chop, and add to dish. Add green onions a minute before dish is done. Cilantro and tomatoes can be used for garnish.

Soya Carob Nut Brownies

—Makes 30–35 brownies

from *Cosmic Cookery* (out of print) by Kathryn Hannaford

2 cups oil
2 cups honey
4 cups water
1 cup coconut
4 cups presifted whole
  wheat pastry flour
2 cups carob powder
1 cup soy milk powder
2 Tablespoons
  baking powder
1 Tablespoon sea salt
2 cups walnut pieces

Preheat oven to 350°.

Oil one 1-inch deep cookie sheet lined with waxed paper (9½ inches by 15 inches).

Combine the first 4 ingredients in a large bowl, mixing well. In another bowl, mix together the next 5 ingredients. Sift the dry ingredients gradually into the liquid ingredients, beating well after each addition. Beat until the batter is smooth, and then fold in the chopped nuts. Spoon the mixture into the oiled cookie sheet, filling it ½ full (½ inch). Bake at 350° until a toothpick inserted into the center of each pan comes out clean. Remove to cooling racks before frosting with "Carob Icing" (optional; recipe below).

Carob Icing

—Makes 6 cups

1 cup water
½ cup oil
1 cup honey
1 cup carob powder
1½ cups skim
  milk powder
½ cup soy
  milk powder

Mix the first 3 ingredients in a bowl. Sift the last 3 ingredients into the liquid, one at a time, beating well after each addition. The icing should be thick enough to harden on the cake. It should not be sticky, nor too hard. Add more skim milk powder if necessary.

Tofu Banana Cream Pie —*Serves 8*

from *Stress, Diet, and Your Heart* by Dean Ornish, M.D.

1 cup granola

2 teaspoons
   ground cinnamon

safflower oil for pie pan

1 pound (4 cakes) tofu

1 cup nonfat yogurt

¼ cup apple juice

3 Tablespoons
   mild-flavored honey

2 teaspoons vanilla
   extract (more to taste)

3 large ripe bananas

½ teaspoon nutmeg

juice of 1½ lemons
   (more to taste)

3 Tablespoons whole
   wheat flour

½ cup fresh strawberries

People often can't believe that they're eating tofu when they eat this low-fat dessert. It's creamy and rich, much like a cheesecake.

Preheat the oven to 350°.

Mix together the granola and 1 teaspoon cinnamon.

Brush a 9- or 10-inch pie pan or an 8-inch springform pan lightly with safflower oil and sprinkle the granola evenly over the bottom.

Blend together the tofu, yogurt, apple juice, honey, vanilla, 2 bananas, nutmeg, 1 teaspoon cinnamon, the juice of 1 lemon, and the whole wheat flour in a blender or food processor until completely smooth. Make sure there are no little chunks of tofu left unblended.

Pour into the prepared baking dish and bake in the preheated oven for 50 minutes, until the top is just beginning to brown. Remove from the oven and cool, then chill several hours.

Before serving, slice the remaining banana and toss with remaining lemon juice. Cut the strawberries in half, and decorate the top of the pie with the banana slices and strawberries.

Other winter recipe references:

- "Curried Squash and Mushroom Soup" from *Moosewood Cookbook* (page 12) by Mollie Katzen.
- "Russian Winter Salad" and "Spiced Beet and Walnut Salad" from *Seasonal Salads from Around the World* (pages 116 and 109) by David Scott and Paddy Byrne.
- "Hot and Spicy Stir-Fried Vegetables" from *The Tao of Cooking* (page 126) by Sally Pasley.
- "Potato Carrot Kugel" (noodle pudding) from *The New Laurel's Kitchen* (page 269) by Laurel Robertson, Carol Flinders, and Brian Ruppenthal.
- "Noodle Kugel" and "Tofu Noodle Kugel" from *Fast Vegetarian Feasts* (pages 318 and 319) by Martha Rose Shulman.

WINTER FOODS*

Fruits		*Vegetables*	
Apples	Pear	Bok Choy	Spinach (New Zealand)
Granny Smith	Anjou	Broccoli	Sprouts
Pippin	Watermelon	Brussels sprouts	Squash (hard)
Red Delicious	Persimmon	Burdock root	Acorn
Cranberry	Pomegranate	Cabbages	Butternut
Dates	Tangelo	Carrots	Delicata
Dried fruits	Tangerine	Cauliflower	Hubbard
Apple		Chard	Spaghetti
Apricot		Daikon radish	Sugar pumpkin
Coconut		Garlic	Sweet potato
Mango		Ginger	Turnip
Papaya		Jerusalem artichoke	Yam
Pear		Kale	
Peach		Leeks	*Nuts & Seeds*
Pineapple		Onions	same as *Autumn*
Prune		Parsnip	
Raisin		Potatoes	
Grapes		Rutabaga	*Beans & All Grains*
Jicama		Seaweeds	see *Autumn*
Kiwifruit		Agar, Kelp,	
Kumquat		Arame, Kombu,	
Mandarin orange		Dulse, Nori,	*Sprouts*
Navel orange		Hijiki, Wakame	Seeds, Grains, & Beans

*These are the foods that are naturally available to many areas during the winter. For the colder and snowy climates, most winter foods must have been dried and stored to provide our nourishment. *The Seasonal Food Guide* poster and booklet, also by Dr. Haas and published by Celestial Arts, gives further information on the seasonal diets.

NUTRITIONAL ANALYSIS OF THE SEASONAL DIETS

Constituents	RDA	Spring	Summer	Autumn	Winter
Calories	1300–2000	1500	1500	1650	1880
Carbohydrates (g.)	200	190	180	200	225
Cholesterol (mg.)	under 300	100	160	105	130
Fats (g.)	25–75	55	48	54	65
Protein (g.)	56	60	65	70	76
Fiber (g.)	NE(10)	10	10	12	15
Water (liter)	2.5	2.6	2.9	2.7	2.8
Vitamins					
Vitamin A/Beta-Carotene (IU)	5000	14000	14000	18000	22000
Thiamine (B_1) (mg.)	1.4	1.5	1.3	1.4	1.7
Riboflavin (B_2) (mg.)	1.6	1.6	1.4	1.6	1.8
Niacin (B_3) (mg.)	18	20	19	18	24
Pantothenic Acid (B_5) (mg.)	5	6	6	9	11
Pyrodoxine (B_6) (mg.)	2	3	3	2.6	3.4
Cobalamin (B_{12}) (mcg.)	3	0.6	1.0	0.6	1.3
Folic Acid (mcg.)	400	450	400	460	480
Vitamin C (mg.)	45	175	200	180	240
Vitamin E (I.U.)	15	14	10	12	15
Vitamin K (mcg.)	300	340	240	500	320
Minerals					
Calcium (Ca) (mg.)	800	500	640	490	800
Copper (Cu) (mg.)	2.0	3.1	7	3.4	38
Iron (Fe) (mg.)	10–18	16	18	16	18
Magnesium (Mg) (mg.)	350	340	340	360	440
Potassium (K) (g.)	2.5	3.2	3.1	3.5	4.4
Phosphorus (P) (mg.)	800	1150	1200	1100	1400
Sodium (Na) (g.)	2	1.4	1.5	1.4	2.4
Zinc (Zn) (mg.)	15	12	20	13	16

NE — Not established.

Note: Values, of course, will vary with the quality and amount of food consumed. The seasonal diets, mostly vegetarian and low fat, reveal slightly low values for certain nutrients in these analyses. Vitamins and minerals to watch include most of the B vitamins, especially B_{12}, calcium, zinc, and iron for women. These diets are very high in Vitamin A and potassium levels, and low in cholesterol and sodium. You can do an analysis of your diet using a book that includes food values or with a practitioner who uses a special nutritional service.

○ GLOSSARY

New and Unusual Foods

Agar-Agar—Flakes made from sea vegetables used to jelly desserts (aspics) and dressings. One Tablespoon agar flakes will jelly one cup of liquid.

Amazake—Creamy sweetener or beverage made from sweet brown rice; rich in flavor and easy to digest. Great over cereal instead of milk.

Arrowroot—Starch flour made from the root of the manioc plant. Used in sauces and desserts as a thickener.

Barley malt—Dark brown, complex carbohydrate sweetener made from sprouted barley. Similar to honey.

Bulghur—Whole wheat that has been cracked, partially boiled, and dried; used to make tabouleh.

Carob—The pod of the tamarind tree, or St. John's Bread; used as an alternative to chocolate.

Couscous—Cracked, partially cooked wheat. Different from bulghur in that it is cracked smaller and traditionally made from refined wheat. Whole wheat or even rice couscous are sometimes available.

Daikon—Long white radish with a sweet-pungent flavor. Cooked daikon helps dissolve fat and reduce mucus; fresh daikon helps in the digestion of oily foods.

Dulse—Mild-tasting purple sea vegetable, high in protein, natural iodine, iron, and other minerals. Must not be cooked.

Fig pep—Water extract of dried figs, high in iron and minerals; used as a sweetener much as molasses.

Gomasio—Dry-roasted sesame seeds and sea salt; used as a seasoning.

Job's tears—Also called Hato mugi, a Japanese type of barley, very sweet tasting and flavorful.

Kombu—Thick, wide, dark green sea vegetable used in making soup stock or cooked with beans to make them more digestible.

Kuzu—Rocklike starch made from the Kudzu plant. Used as a thickener for sauces or gravies. Also called the macrobiotic aspirin. A drink made from 1 cup of hot water, 1 Tablespoon of kuzu (dissolved first in 2 Tablespoons cold water), and 1 umeboshi plum will reduce flu or hangover symptoms.

Mirin—Sweet cooking wine made from whole sweet rice.

Miso—Protein-rich fermented bean and grain paste made from soybeans, brown rice or barley. Miso is used in soups, main dishes, sauces, and dressings. It aids digestion and circulation. It is best bought unpasteurized and should not be boiled.

Mochi—Sweet brown rice pounded into a cake. Placed into the oven it puffs up layered with vegetables in a casserole. It can also be added to soups in small pieces.

Nori—Crispy thin sheets of pressed sea vegetable. Nori contains several minerals and B vitamins. It is mostly used in making sushi.

Polenta—Coarse ground whole corn used in many Mediterranean dishes.

Ponzu—Sweet and pungent condiment made from soy sauce, citrus juices, and mirin. Great over grains and vegetables or for marinating fish or tofu.

Quinoa—The mother grain of the Incas; a complete protein grain similar to millet. Cooks in 20 minutes.

Rice syrup—Sweet, thick syrup made from brown rice. A complex carbohydrate sweetener similar to honey in consistency and color, but a little less sweet.

Seitan—A hearty, high-protein food made from whole wheat gluten. It has a meatlike, chewy texture and is commonly used in many oriental dishes. It is made without salt, is very low in fat, and has no cholesterol.

Shiitake—Flavorful mushroom used in traditional Japanese cuisine and folk medicine. Shiitake mushrooms are complete proteins and are a rich source of B vitamins.

Soy milk—Milklike liquid made from soybeans. Good for use in cereals, for cooking, or as a drink. Common packaged brands include Edensoy, YoSoy, and Vitasoy. Fresh soy milk should not be used in cooking.

Sweetleaf—Best of all sweeteners. It is made from the Stevia plant, is ten times sweeter than sugar, and has no calories. Good for diabetics and hypoglycemics alike, as well as people with Candida concerns.

Tahini—Smooth butter made from hulled and ground sesame seeds. Sold raw or roasted. Can be used as snack on bread or crackers, or for dips and dressings.

Tamari—Rich natural soy sauce, a by-product of making miso. Used as a salty seasoning for foods.

Tempeh—High-protein, whole-grain, cultured food made from organic soybeans and, often, brown rice or other grains. Easy to digest, very low in fat, and has no cholesterol. Apart from plain there are marinated tempehs on the market, such as tempeh "cutlets," tempeh "lemon broil," and tempeh "temptations," as well as tempeh burgers of various kinds.

Tofu—High-protein soybean curd, versatile and with no cholesterol.

Umeboshi plums—Zesty sour and salty pickled plums that stimulate digestion. They are used in some macrobiotic cooking. They are suggested to balance the blood, and may help in motion sickness, too.

Unrefined oil—Vegetable oil that has been mechanically cold pressed and has not been filtered. It retains its natural color, aroma, and nutrients. It has not been chemically bleached, deodorized, or deflavored and contains no preservatives, additives, anti-foaming agents, and anti-oxidants. Some excellent brands include Spectrum and Eden.

Wasabi—Light green Japanese horseradish powder that is mixed with water and made into a paste. It is a hot condiment traditionally eaten with sushi.

○ RECIPE BOOK BIBLIOGRAPHY

Airola Diet and Cookbook, Paavo Airola (Phoenix, AZ: Health Plus Publishers, 1981). Paavo Airola provides some very simple and vital recipes; a good overall program for lighter eating. This book can be ordered directly from the publisher by writing to Health Plus Publishers, P.O. Box 22001, Phoenix, AZ 85028.

Book of Whole Meals: A Seasonal Guide to Assembling Balanced Vegetarian Breakfasts, Lunches, and Dinners, Annemarie Colbin (New York: Ballantine Books, 1985). Annemarie Colbin has many fine yet simple recipes in this macrobiotic-oriented book. This book can be obtained directly from the publisher by calling (800)733-3000 (toll free). Her newest publication is *The Natural Gourmet.*

Cosmic Cookery, out of print, Kathryn Hannaford (Stockton, CA: Starmast Publications, 1974).

Dr. Braly's Optimum Health Program: For Permanent Weight Loss and a Longer Healthier Life, out of print, James Braly (New York: Time Books, 1985).

Eat Well, Be Well Cookbook, Metropolitan Life Insurance Co. (New York: Fireside, 1986). A lower-fat, "heart healthy" version of an American-type diet; not totally away from the use of sugar and chemicals, but has many interesting recipes.

Fast Vegetarian Feasts, rev. ed., Martha Rose Shulman (New York: Dolphin Books, 1986). One of the best ones I've seen: well-organized, good recipes from basic natural ingredients; low fat; and even a seasonal orientation. Love it!

Fit for Life, Harvey Diamond and Marilyn Diamond (New York: Warner Books, 1987). Although the focus is more on food philosophy, there are a number of simple, wholesome, and tasty recipes.

Hippocrates Diet and Health Program, Ann Wigmore (Garden City Park, NY: Avery Publishing Group, 1984). A unique book for the diet-conscious who enjoy sprouts and raw foods. Purifying, vital, and extremely healthy.

New Laurel's Kitchen, 2nd ed., Laurel Robertson, Carol Flinders, and Brian Ruppenthal (Berkeley, CA: Ten Speed Press, 1986). Very popular, well-rounded, and good for the basics. The original version was too heavy in milk products and sugar for optimum health; the new version published by Ten Speed Press is much improved.

Seasonal Salads from Around the World, David Scott and Paddy Byrne (Pownal, VT: Garden Way Publishing, 1986). A mixture of the exotic and simple; a lot of choices for international salad recipes.

Self-Healing Cookbook: A Macrobiotic Primer for Healing Body, Mind and Moods with Whole, Natural Foods, 2nd, rev. ed., Kristina Turner (Grass Valley, CA: Earthtones Press, 1988). A really healthful, practical, and easy-to-use recipe book.

Still Life With Menu Cookbook, Mollie Katzen (Berkeley, CA: Ten Speed Press, 1988). A beautiful and elegant book with some wonderful recipes. Mollie Katzen's new cookbook follows her popular *Moosewood Cookbook* and *Enchanted Broccoli Forest: And other Timeless Delicacies*, both of which are somewhat high in dairy fats.

Stress, Diet, and Your Heart, Dean Ornish (New York: New American Library, 1984). Dr. Dean Ornish has a winner here as far as the many healthful, creative recipes; a special book for heart patients. Look for his new book, Dr. Dean Ornish's Program for Reversing Heart Disease.

Tao of Cooking, Sally Pasley (Berkeley, CA: Ten Speed Press, 1982). A nicely balanced book with many simple, tasty recipes; it has been popular for many years.

Tassajara Recipe Book: Favorites of the Guest Season, Edward Espe Brown (Boston: Shambala Publications, 1985). One of the series of popular Tassajara books, this one has a multitude of nutritious vegetarian recipes. However, the recipes generally contain too much fat, milk products, and sugar.

Tropic Cooking, Joyce Lefray Young (Berkeley, CA: Ten Speed Press, 1987).

PART FOUR

NUTRITIONAL APPLICATION:
SPECIAL DIETS AND SUPPLEMENT PROGRAMS

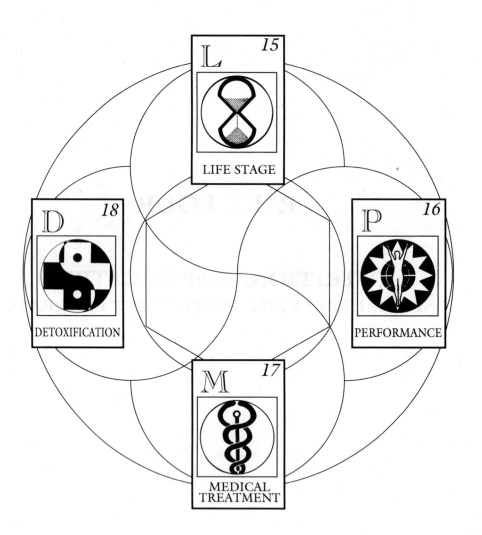

Introduction

Infancy to Immortality

This is a very important section for those interested in the life-supporting and therapeutic application of nutrition during the various states and stages of life, when afflicted with certain conditions, or to help change and enhance health. In the following 34 programs I offer some simple, basic guidelines regarding food and diet choices and special supplement suggestions to help heal a variety of problems, and support stress periods in our individual evolution. With all of the basic information I have provided up to this point, this part of the book gives you the Nutritional Application to take your health into your own hands.

The first goal of these programs is that of all nutrition scientists and practitioners—to avoid deficiencies of nutrients. The second is to help provide all the nutrients in the right amounts to maintain healthy function. This may be more than the RDAs in many cases. The third, which is especially important to the nutritionally aware physician and individual, is to use nutrition in a way that supports optimum health. This more orthomolecular approach is what we in my office call a Performance Enhancement Program, or PEP.* The idea here is to have sufficient levels of all of the necessary nutrients available in the blood and tissues so that these nutrient-rich fluids bathe the cells with all of the nutritional-biochemical metabolites required for an efficient and balanced metabolism. Also, higher amounts of some nutrients may provide some additional functions that lower levels do not; examples of this include the anti-inflammatory and antiviral effects of vitamin C or the cholesterol-lowering effect of niacin at levels of intake much higher than the RDA. Although we do not really know whether certain supplements are always necessary, many clinicians and scientists believe that such support adds an extra measure of safety to our health program, particularly to avoid deficiencies.

My overall goal is to help you to be your own doctor as much as possible. The Western medical system does not currently work this way. It is oriented to the diagnosis and treatment of disease using drugs and surgery primarily; it is not centered around evaluating people's lives in relation to their health, and educating them in living healthfully. If this were done, medical practices and hospitals would focus more on preventive and nutritional medicine, lifestyle and stress management, and supportive encouragement to eat well, exercise, curb excesses and abuses, normalize weight, stop smoking, as well as other ways to live that generate optimum individual and planetary health.

The more we can do to understand our needs, growth, and changes to support our health and correct any minor or recurrent malfunctions of our magnificent body, the easier our life will be. **The key to preventive medicine is education.** Nutritional Application is a key component of "self-help." Using vitamins, minerals, oils, herbs, as well as special foods and diets (including fasting and milder forms of detoxification), can all help in the process of healing and wellness. Part Four of *Staying Healthy With Nutrition* will help you apply this "nutritional know-how" to your life, and to share it with friends and family.

Preventive medicine and nutrition are now growing rapidly in popularity. They have moved, I believe, out of their infancy and toddler years into childhood and adolescence, when the acquisition of new knowledge is very exciting. This growth in knowledge and its practical application to health care and longevity is a result of the blending of science and nature. Combining new research in clinical biochemistry and nutrition with the resurgence of pesticide-free natural foods grown in healthy soils and with more natural remedies available for healing, we now have a chance to improve the field of nutritional medicine and therefore our health.

Still, I believe, much of medicine and a great percentage of doctors are very limited by a lack of basic and clinical nutritional knowledge. The practice of nutrition in mainstream medicine is carried out by dieticians who consult with doctors or work in

---

*The trademark on this name is held by Jeffrey H. Reinhardt, a nutritional biochemist and friend whom I have worked with for many years.

672

hospitals to prescribe diets for special problems. Here, nutrition is still in its infancy, with stunted or very slow growth; this frustrating situation exists because the minds of the people in control are hard to change. However, with the new information becoming available through research and clinical experience, the future of nutritional medicine looks exciting. We are realizing that there may be a big difference between treating and preventing deficiency, on the one hand, and providing optimum levels of dietary macronutrients and micronutrients, on the other.

Dietetics, the practice of diet therapy, has focused on five main areas: (1) weight loss and gain; (2) treatment of deficiencies, as with iodine for goiter and vitamin D for rickets; (3) support or rest for specific organs, such as a low-fat diet for gallbladder problems or avoiding spices for stomach ulcers; (4) special diets for metabolic problems, such as low-sugar for diabetes or low-salt for hypertension; and (5) elimination of harmful substances, such as caffeine and alcohol. Dietetics, like medicine, is mostly "disease-oriented" and often focuses on short-term therapeutic diets to be followed until we feel better, when we then return to our "normal" diet and lifestyle. I believe that this is a very limited approach. It overlooks the fact that some of the things we do or eat may play a part in creating our basic health problem in the first place. The concept that "when we are sick we need to totally reevaluate our life and create a new plan," which I believe is essential to good medicine and healing, has not been fully embraced by the general public, physicians, or insurance companies; however, more and more people are approaching their lifestyle and health in this way.

The Standard American Diet, as I have already shown, is not very healthy; in fact, it is quite SAD. We need to change the diet to one based on more wholesome, fresh foods, rather than go on a special temporary therapeutic plan. After many years of digestive abuse, these more natural foods may feel foreign and appear hard to digest and utilize. With a little time, however, this type of diet will feel much better.

Current dietetic policies and applications are responsible for school and hospital food, which is notoriously poor, even though it attempts to apply the established concepts of good nutrition and a balanced diet. These diets fall far short of supporting the optimal learning abilities of children or the healing process of ill people. All of us need good, vital nutrition to grow, heal, and be alive. The schools and hospitals are where we need the health-conscious master chefs. Surrounding these institutions should be beautiful gardens full of fresh foods to nourish both the professional staff and workers, as well as the students and patients. These changes will be a good beginning and give us a fairer chance to make it through life.

The current choices in a standard hospital menu include:

(1) a regular diet, which could run the spectrum from good to atrocious; (2) a soft diet, of overcooked and pureed foods; (3) a liquid diet, which is low in fiber and includes strained gruel, broth, juices, coffee, tea, and gelatin; and (4) a clear diet, only broth (from bouillon cubes), canned juices, and coffee or tea. There also might be modifications of the regular diet, such as a calorie and carbohydrate restriction for

diabetes, a low-salt diet for high blood pressure, or a low-fat or low-cholesterol diet for heart disease. These modifications are important, but they are really just a first step. If medicine is not aimed at helping people to change in order to treat or prevent future problems, it will only correct the immediate difficulty so that we can continue our health-threatening lifestyle with the least interruption necessary. This is both short-sighted and very costly.

This book, and especially Part Four, is oriented toward changing old habits and advocates thinking and living in new ways, with programs geared toward healthful goals. These often include long-range lifestyle habits or foods and nutritional supplements required to attain and maintain these health goals. Many of the suggestions are based on scientific research and population studies, others on my own or other practitioners' experiences, and more on common sense, logic, or intuition. Some of these programs even encompass my latest theories.

Overall, the programs that I suggest should be safe for most anyone; however, if there are specific medical concerns, consult your doctor or a practitioner who can be a judge of a nutritionally supportive program. Many of the diets or even supplement plans will not be oriented to the long term; I will note that where appropriate. Most of the nutrient suggestions are estimates of the best levels, based on both research and experience, but definitely in safe ranges with regard to potential nutrient toxicity. Most people handle these supplement levels very well. Occasionally, however, some people, such as those with allergies, food intolerances, chemical sensitivities, or certain digestive disorders, will experience symptoms, such as headache, diarrhea, nausea, or flushing, in response to a particular nutrient. These people will need to adjust their program. Discontinuing the supplements for a few days and then restarting, adding a new one daily, will help isolate the supplement that elicits the negative response.

The programs here offer a basic plan. Ideally, we want to work with a doctor or other experienced practitioner to have an evaluation and then to set up a carefully designed program to meet our individual needs. Often, specific tests, such as a biochemical profile, diet and digestive analyses, mineral or vitamin blood levels, an immune system analysis, or allergy tests, will be performed to help assess any of our special needs. Also, we should always remember that even with all the new and creative nutritional supplements available, nothing replaces a good diet.

Not everyone has to take the supplements as suggested. With normal levels of nutrients in the body, a good balanced diet of wholesome foods, low stress, and minimal pollution exposure, much supplementation may not be necessary all the time. Maybe a few times a year, such as at seasonal transitions or with certain problems, a specific supplement program can be used for a month or so. With many health problems, additional nutrients at higher levels may be helpful; these can often be tried as a first level of treatment before prescription drugs. Following some of the other guidelines or trying some of the herbs mentioned in the programs may be very helpful as well. Overall though, because of the problem that many people have in finding wholesome foods, with the soil depletion of minerals and the loss of nutrients in the storage and cooking of foods, I would suggest that some low-level supplementation is needed most of the time.

It is usually best to take vitamin and mineral supplements after meals, as they are naturally part of foods and are best tolerated and utilized in this way. Herbal remedies are often taken between meals to assist their medicinal activities; however, if they are not tolerated well, they can also be taken after meals. Vitamin C can be taken following meals if it is used only a couple of times per day, as it can help the absorption of many minerals, especially when taken as ascorbic acid. Usually some of the vitamin C we take should contain the bioflavonoids, which are also important nutrients. If vitamin C is taken many times daily, it can easily be taken between meals or at bedtime as well. Buffered vitamin C powders or tablets with alkaline minerals such as calcium or magnesium are usually taken alone at bedtime, between meals or one to two hours after meals so as not to weaken hydrochloric acid's digestive function. In general, I am more in favor of simple supplement tablets or powders than the big time-release tablets that may not be digested well, especially in people with weak digestion. Also, I prefer that supplements be taken two or three times over the course of a day; this gives the body a better chance to assimilate the nutrients and improve utilization. After breakfast and dinner are good times to take our general nutrients. For some people, however, lunch and evening will be more convenient. Most of us can adapt these general guidelines to fit into our lifestyle.

If we wish to initiate any of these programs, we should first look at what we are currently doing and what may need to be adjusted. We can then implement more of the suggestions as we feel comfortable with them or as the situation warrants. The recommendations also take into consideration the fact that people are different. That is why ranges of intake levels are sometimes given, or higher than RDA amounts listed, so that they will cover those who are weaker or need increased nutrient levels.

With some of the more serious medical conditions for which we might be under a doctor's care, it is best to consult with your doctor first and get his or her advice. Though we all seek open-minded physicians, some may be unreceptive to anything that differs from their viewpoint or "current medical thinking." If we are open to exploring nutrition and supplements for our condition or lifestyle and our physician is not, we might consider finding someone who will work with us toward the goals we want to pursue. By doing this, we will, I believe, positively influence our medical system by helping to inform physicians of new public interests and stimulate them to seek more knowledge of nutrition and natural medicine. That is how I initially became interested in this field—through patient requests and demands.

Medicine has always been changing, and there has always been a strong force of tradition trying to hold it back. This is also the situation in each of us who tries to change. There is usually an evolutionary part of us that is trying to stimulate and guide us toward our new self, lifestyle, or work, while another part of us is used to the old habits and tries to hold us back with fears or reasons not to change. These fears, which may also come from a spouse, a parent, or a friend as well as from ourselves, can take over and stop the process of natural evolution, or at least slow it temporarily. Eventually, it is to be hoped, we will realize that the old self does not really die; it gets incorporated into the new person that we become.

Any change in medicine, just like change in ourselves, is difficult. The more support we have, the better. This book and others, my medical practice and others like it, are intended to offer support and guidance for change. The following thirty-four programs offer some specific ways for us to incorporate nutritional medicine into our lives and health care. These diets and supplements will usually fit into what we are already doing. **They are not meant to take the place of a doctor's advice or prescribed medications.** But if, after a time, we feel better, we may then be able to let go of our medicines and then maybe even of our exterior doctor. Going from a state of health where we need a doctor's care to one where we can use a doctor to help us evaluate and support our health is a big step. Cooperative health care involves an evolutionary step which empowers us to become an important part of the decision-making regarding our health. Good luck!

PART FOUR—CONTENTS

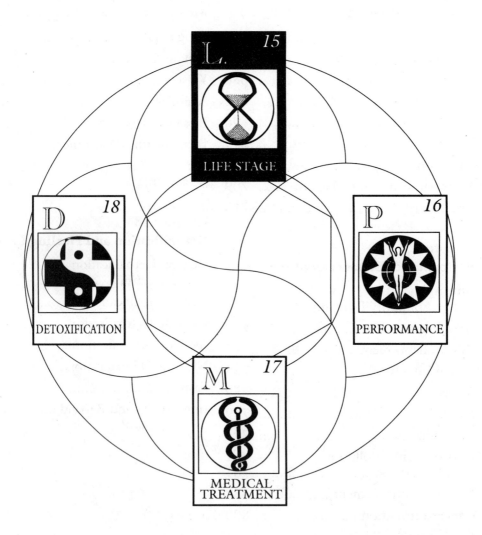

15 L. LIFE STAGE

16 P PERFORMANCE

17 M MEDICAL TREATMENT

18 D DETOXIFICATION

Chapter 15

Life Stage Programs

T his initial set of programs applies to the different stages of life with special sections on the hormonal changes that most women experience. I offer simple discussions of the various age groups to help you understand the changing nutritional needs during growth and development. The emphasis is to support a positive and healthy life-style with some reference to potential poor habits that could lead to health difficulties.

At the completion of each of these *Life Stage Programs,* suggested amounts of essential nutrients are listed. Many of these nutrients can be obtained from foods; often, however, additional supplementation may be desired to ensure that we acquire all the nutrients we need to support optimum health. Many common "vitamin" supplements contain at least the RDA levels, while other products will contain higher levels than are commonly accepted as "necessary" and possibly more adequate to the individual in need, such as during increased stress or illness. With a healthy diet in a healthy individual, these supplement programs may not be used all the time, but more during transition times or with any common symptoms such as fatigue. However, as I have discussed in other areas of this book, with the stresses under which we live and the potential deficiency of nutrients in even our natural, unrefined foods, it is wise for most of us to use some daily insurance supplementation.

This whole section is really about diet and health for the family, so I have kept it fairly simple, suggesting what to avoid in your diet and emphasizing healthful plans. The programs for infancy through adolescence are relatively short discussions of basic needs and concerns for those years rather than detailed examinations of all the potential problems. The same is true for the adult programs, which are followed by sections on women's health—pregnancy, lactation, birth control pills, premenstrual syndrome and menopause. The chapter ends with a thorough discussion of nutrition in relation to the aging process and the elderly.

Infancy

We might as well begin with the beginning of life. The time preceding birth, when the baby is still inside its mother, is an important period of growth and development, and at that time as well as after birth, the baby's health is very dependent on the mother's nourishment. Even the several months before a woman becomes pregnant are important. She must eat good amounts of wholesome foods to have enough energy and nutrients for her child and herself, both before and after birth. (See the programs for *Pregnancy* and *Lactation* later in this chapter.)

Nutrition is the key to growth and development. Baby's first food is mother's milk, which is uniquely formulated to meet his or her growth needs, provided mother eats an adequate diet. Initially, breast milk colostrum has the fluid and nutrient levels, such as zinc, that correlate with the baby's needs. As initial milk comes in, it is higher in fat and fatty acids, important to early developmental needs of the brain and the immune and nervous systems. Later, its fat content decreases and the protein and carbohydrate levels increase to meet the nutritional needs for general growth and development. With a good diet, mother's milk exclusively can support the baby for six months or more. Besides eating well, the mother should also avoid pharmaceutical drugs when possible and chemicals such as nicotine, alcohol, and caffeine. Occupational and even home chemical use should be avoided as well. Pesticides, such as DDT and more recently used chemicals, may contaminate food and get into breast milk, so whenever possible, organic or homegrown produce is ideal.

There are many reasons why breastfeeding is the best thing for both mother and baby. Initially, breastfeeding stimulates uterine contractions, reducing bleeding and bringing the uterus back to its normal size. It provides the intimate bonding of the mother and baby, so connected for the previous nine months, and it is convenient because mother always has baby's food with her; it is also less expensive, but above all breastfeeding is the healthiest choice for the child. Also, the output of calories to baby helps the mother to bring her weight back toward its pre-pregnancy level.

For baby, breast milk provides the right nourishment. It has more available iron, vitamins A and C, niacin, potassium, and the right amino acids for growth than any natural or formulated substitute. It not only has nutritional advantages but immunological ones as well, as the mother can pass her protective antibodies to her child. Recent studies show that breastfed babies are healthier than bottle-fed babies—they have fewer allergies, they are leaner, and thay have lower cholesterol levels—and this remains true in later years as well.

More than 95 percent of mothers can breastfeed if they wish. Many of those who have trouble can find help and reassurance from a breastfeeding support group such as

La Leche League or from a midwife friend, or a neighbor who has breastfed. Relaxation and increased fluid intake will also facilitate breastfeeding. Luckily, the number of mothers who breastfeed has been increasing over the last couple of decades, even among career-oriented women.

There are really not many good substitutes for mother's milk. It has been shown that 100 percent whey formula is probably the best choice. Goat's milk, slightly diluted, can also be used if the whey formula is not tolerated. A little soy milk can also be used after three or four months. Cow's milk is best avoided; it has a different amino acid balance than other substitutes, has more fats, and is more allergenic. The whey formula is very low allergenically, even less than goat's milk and soy milk. Formulas may be used in an emergency, but I generally do not recommend them because of their unnatural and synthetic makeup.

A common problem during the first six months is infant colic. It is more common in first children but may occur in any. Some psychological stresses may influence colic, but it may also be affected by the mother's diet. Cow's milk consumed by the mother may be a factor; excessive sugar or salt intake may also worsen colic. Often a decrease in the mother's milk product consumption will reduce the colic symptoms. Some extra B vitamins, calcium, magnesium, and potassium taken by the mother may help reduce colic in the baby as well as reduce mother's intestinal gas. Also, mother must constantly remember to eat well so that she does not become depleted during nursing.

Babies need more calories and protein per pound than any other age group. Goat's milk, and even cow's milk, with their protein, fat, and calorie content, are potentially valuable foods in moderation (if tolerated well) for rapidly growing babies (after eight to ten months) and children. The "dairy" problem comes in when adults continue to use milk and its products as a regular part of their diet. Lifelong use of milk is one of the biggest misconceptions and mistakes in nutrition. Consumption of dairy products should be greatly curtailed by the adult population, and by those children and teenagers sensitive to milk. If infants and children develop any recurrent congestive problems, such as excessive nasal mucus or ear infections, it is suggested they go off all cow's milk products for a time (several weeks) to see if their problems improve.

When and what to feed infants is a rather controversial issue as well. Some parents try to feed solid foods to their little babies at four months or sooner. This is a big mistake. Infants will do fine on milk alone. The trend is returning to later rather than earlier feeding. Premature feeding can lead to poor digestion, increased allergy, and obesity. There may appear to be increased growth, but it could be just increased fat. Skin-fold measurements are used now along with growth and development charts to show whether this is the case. Increased fat at this time can lead to increased numbers of fat cells, which will increase the likelihood of adult obesity. Premature feeding may also influence later eating habits. Five to six months is the earliest and six months probably the best time to begin feeding that little being any solid foods. Waiting until six months of age gives baby time to develop his or her digestive tract and immunological system to reduce the likelihood of allergy.

Initial foods should be simple, natural, and pureed to assist digestion. The true flavors of food are best; avoid the use of sweetened or salted foods, especially refined sugar and refined flour foods. First foods may be pureed or cooked fruits, cooked and pureed vegetables, and cooked cereal grains (formulated for baby). These foods along with mother's milk will provide the proper nourishment for this time of rapid growth. Egg yolks can also be added to the diet, but avoid egg whites as yet, as the albumin protein is more allergenic.

At seven to eight months, a few teeth may start to appear. Toast can be used for teething. Some meats can be added now; these should be baked or broiled and then finely chopped or pureed. Potatoes, baked or boiled and mashed, along with other vegetables, may also round out the menu.

From eight months to one year, babies may do some serious eating. They may be more independent, adventurous, and enthusiastic with food. They will try more new foods, and the diet can become more well-rounded. Whole eggs may be used as a good source of protein now. Milk consumption may be reduced, but it is still a regular source of nourishment. Infants may wean at this time, though many mother-baby teams will continue nursing for another year or more, especially with the aid of a breast pump for working mothers. Foods and meals should be simple. Make as much of your own foods as possible; jars and cans of foods should not be used exclusively.

After one year, the infant's diet may shift. Food needs for growth are less now as the rate of growth slows down. Many parents become concerned because it appears that the child isn't eating, but this is usually fine. Eating habits may change, food likes and dislikes develop. Try not to make eating a battle, and avoid games and rewards. Let the child eat; he or she will communicate his or her needs. Just offer nourishing foods and avoid sweet treats. Balance the diet over days, not at each meal, so that meals can be simple. Most healthy children eat only what their bodies need.

In regard to supplements to the diet in the first two years, most parents are more comfortable with a moderate insurance formula that at least covers the child's Recommended Daily Allowances (RDAs). Some parents and pediatricians feel that for healthy babies on breast milk and infants eating a good diet, additional supplements are not really needed.

When a vitamin formula is used, it is often a liquid supplement in the first year, and after that a flavorful chewable. For toddlers, the multiple should contain all of the B vitamins, vitamins C, E, and A. Basic minerals such as calcium and iron, as well as zinc, magnesium, manganese, and even a little chromium and selenium can also be included. I suggest more natural, chemical-free supplements, without sugar and artificial food colorings and flavors. The bigger companies with inexpensive vitamins may not believe that synthetic, treated chemical formulas are of concern, but many doctors and parents nowadays would certainly rather avoid those products.

The following chart shows the levels of vitamins and minerals suggested for this age group at the beginning of life. Some values are slightly higher than the RDAs to provide that extra margin of safety, particularly to cover those infants who may need more of some nutrients than others or for those who might be sick and need higher amounts of certain vitamins or minerals. Later sections suggest what nutrients might be needed in higher amounts in specific health situations; do not, however, use the levels suggested for adults. Talk to your doctor or refer to specific literature to find appropriate dosages for specific age groups.

Infants have been overdosed on some vitamins because of parents' misunderstanding of authors' suggestions. Vitamin A toxicity is probably most common. **Do not overuse vitamin A or D or cod liver oil,** which is high in both, or the minerals calcium, phosphorus, or iron. Breastfed babies can get a bit deficient in vitamin D unless they get a little sunlight exposure. Babies need a balanced diet and lifestyle, too.

Breast milk is usually low in fluoride, and though fluoride use is still debatable, it appears relatively safe to supplement, and thus many parents and doctors use fluoridated vitamins to protect against tooth decay. However, if mother drinks fluoridated water, it is now recommended NOT to give fluoridated vitamins to breastfed babies since it comes through the milk. Also, no fluoride supplements should be used at any age if the water is fluoridated.

DAILY NUTRIENT PROGRAM—INFANTS AND TODDLERS

	Birth–6 Months	*6 Months–1 Year*	*1–2 Years*
Calories	115/kg.	105–110/kg.	1,200–1,400
Protein (grams)	2.2 g./kg.	2.0 g./kg.	22–25 g.
Vitamin A	2,000 IUs	2,000 IUs	2,500 IUs
Vitamin D	400 IUs	400 IUs	400 IUs
Vitamin E	5 IUs	6 IUs	8 IUs
Vitamin K	15 mcg.	25 mcg.	30 mcg.
Thiamine (B$_1$)	0.4 mg.	0.6 mg.	0.8 mg.
Riboflavin (B$_2$)	0.5 mg.	0.7 mg.	0.9 mg.
Niacin (B$_3$)	6 mg.	8 mg.	10 mg.
Pantothenic acid (B$_5$)	3 mg.	3 mg.	4 mg.
Pyridoxine (B$_6$)	0.4 mg.	0.6 mg.	1.0 mg.
Cobalamin (B$_{12}$)	1.0 mcg.	2.0 mcg.	2.5 mcg.
Folic acid	40 mcg.	60 mcg.	100 mcg.
Biotin	50 mcg.	50 mcg.	50 mcg.
Vitamin C	40 mg.	60 mg.	100 mg.
Calcium	400 mg.	600 mg.	800 mg.
Chloride	0.6 g.	1.0 g.	1.2 g.
Chromium	50 mcg.	60 mcg.	80 mcg.
Copper	0.7 mg.	1.0 mg.	1.5 mg.
Fluoride	0.3 mg.	0.6 mg.	1.0 mg.
Iodine	50 mcg.	60 mcg.	80 mcg.
Iron	10 mg.	15 mg.	15 mg.
Magnesium	70 mg.	90 mg.	150 mg.
Manganese	0.7 mg.	1.0 mg.	1.5 mg.
Molybdenum	60 mcg.	80 mcg.	100 mcg.
Phosphorus	300 mg.	500 mg.	800 mg.
Potassium	0.7 mg.	1.0 mg.	1.5 mg.
Selenium	40 mcg.	60 mcg.	80 mcg.
Sodium	0.3 g.	0.6 g.	0.9 g.
Zinc	4 mg.	6 mg.	10 mg.

Childhood

For children ages two to twelve, it is very important to instill good eating habits and avoid overindulgence in refined sugars and flours and high-fat, fried fast foods. Children need a lot of nourishing foods to provide them with all of the important nutrients for growth; though physical growth is a little slower in this age period than it is in infancy or during adolescent years, mental growth is relatively rapid.

Creating healthy eating patterns begins with encouraging the consumption of good quality, wholesome foods, which is a lot easier when parents eat this type of diet. Children's tendencies are toward the sweets, treats, and salted snacks and away from vegetables, the important food group that probably offers the greatest nutritional challenge for parents. Try to be creative with veggies; most children prefer raw vegetables to cooked, so try more raw veggies. Basically, offer whatever vegetables the children like and maintain the fruits, grains, and protein foods.

Many children like to help and be part of their nutrition. Support this by reaching agreements and creatively inspiring their food choices and by teaching them to prepare food and feed themselves at an early age. Avoid soft drinks and excessive poor quality, "treat" foods, and offer more nourishing snacks, such as fruits, cheese or yogurt, nuts, crackers, or popcorn. Avoid nutritional adversity—battles and hassles around meal-time, and rewards of sweets such as ice cream, cake, or candy, or just dessert, for eating their vegetables. Bribery and rewards may emphasize the treats and lessen the value of the more healthful foods. Again, getting children involved in meal planning and preparation as they get older is often helpful. Having them assist in preparing their school lunch will give them more identity with it and pleasure in eating it. Good eating habits will generate good nutrition and thus a good mind and good actions.

For preschool kids, ages two to five, this is often a time of slower growth, and sometimes these children will decrease their food intake. Parents may be concerned, but usually these kids are fine. Offer them wholesome foods. Avoid bribing. Just keep offering them the foods they need, and be a good example yourself. Keep their diet low in refined foods, chemical foods, and sweet, salty, or fried foods. Children this age like to eat with their hands, especially finger snacks, so give them small pieces at meals when appropriate.

For school children, ages five to twelve, it may get a little tougher. Often likes and dislikes will limit their diets. Food games lose their charm, and rebellion may begin. On the other hand, many kids in this age group will become more cooperative and want to be helpful and accepted and thus may really attempt to eat well. A good breakfast is essential for these children going off to school. Eating hot, whole-grain cereals will provide a good source of morning energy (the sugary cereals may be more stimulating,

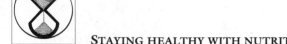

but the boost is short-lived and may be followed by a depressed period); some protein, such as eggs, will also provide sustaining energy. Given the current level of institutional (school) nutritional awareness, it is best to sack a good lunch for your child and to encourage them to eat it at lunchtime. However, there are always outside influences at their age, such as other children or television, that will attempt to undermine the healthful eating habits you have tried to develop in your children. Setting a good example (to not only do as we say, but also as we do) is the best influence parents have on the overall nutritional patterns of their young ones.

Many parents overestimate their children's needs and the amount of food required (which we do for ourselves as well). It is best to create simple meals and serve smaller portions more frequently throughout the day. Needs for calories and many of the basic nutrients will vary from ages two through ten. Obviously, with increased size and activity, the older children will need more food, which they naturally will eat. The more we can support them in avoiding empty calories, the better chance they will have of optimum growth. During the middle years, the average youngster will gain between five and eight pounds and grow about one-half inch per year, provided they have the nutrients they need. Support a healthy amount of physical activity in place of laziness or too much TV and telephone.

As insurance to prevent nutrient deficiencies, many parents want their children to take some supplements. Chewables are still a favorite, though as they grow, many kids can swallow pills and capsules. Powdered formulas can be added to foods. The nutrient levels shown in the table reflect the RDAs plus a little insurance for the special needs of children between the ages of two and eleven.

DAILY NUTRIENT PROGRAM—CHILDHOOD

	2–4 Years	*4–6 Years*	*6–11 Years*
Calories	1,300–1,600	1,600–2,100	2,100–2,800
Protein	23–28 g.	30–35 g.	35–45 g.
Vitamin A	2500 IUs	3000 IUs	4000 IUs
Vitamin D	400 IUs	400 IUs	400 IUs
Vitamin E	15 IUs	20 IUs	25 IUs
Vitamin K	30 mcg.	40 mcg.	60 mcg.
Thiamine (B_1)	0.8 mg.	1.0 mg.	1.5 mg.
Riboflavin (B_2)	1.0 mg.	1.2 mg.	1.6 mg.
Niacin (B_3)	10 mg.	12 mg.	17 mg.
Pantothenic acid (B_5)	4 mg.	4 mg.	5 mg.
Pyridoxine (B_6)	1.0 mg.	1.5 mg.	2.0 mg.
Cobalamin (B_{12})	3 mcg.	4 mcg.	5 mcg.
Folic acid	150 mcg.	250 mcg.	350 mcg.
Biotin	75 mcg.	100 mcg.	150 mcg.
Vitamin C	100 mg.	150 mg.	200 mg.
Calcium	800 mg.	800 mg.	850 mg.
Chloride	1.0 g.	1.5 g.	2.0 g.
Chromium	80 mcg.	120 mcg.	200 mcg.
Copper	1.5 mg.	2.0 mg.	2.5 mg.
Fluoride	1.5 mg.	2.0 mg.	2.5 mg.
Iodine	80 mcg.	100 mcg.	125 mcg.
Iron	15 mg.	12 mg.	12 mg.
Magnesium	200 mg.	250 mg.	300 mg.
Manganese	2.0 mg.	2.5 mg.	3.0 mg.
Molybdenum	125 mcg.	200 mcg.	300 mcg.
Phosphorus	800 mg.	800 mg.	800 mg.
Potassium	1.5 g.	2.0 g.	2.5 g.
Selenium	100 mcg.	150 mcg.	200 mcg.
Sodium	1.0 g.	1.3 g.	1.8 g.
Zinc	10 mg.	10 mg.	10 mg.

Adolescence

The teenage years are trying times in a lot of ways, especially in terms of nutrition. Adolescence is indeed a period of high nutritional risk, when the increased demands for nutrients are often met with poor choices of foods, unhealthy eating habits, and deficient intakes of calories and protein as well as many vitamins and minerals.

Adolescence usually begins at age 10–12 in girls and 12–14 in boys. There are not only new demands, but also many physiological changes because of the sexual hormones being released. Body composition also shifts, with girls increasing their percentage of fat and adding curves, while boys tend to increase protein and muscle development. During these years, young men may gain 15–20 pounds in weight and 4–5 inches in height per year, while girls may add 13–18 pounds and grow 3–4 inches yearly. The main years of growth are between ages 11–16 years for girls, 13–18 years for boys.

The nutritional problems of adolescence are probably related to the rebellious nature of these years. Teenagers eat what they want and when; they are hard to feed and harder to influence regarding dietary changes. Peer pressure is great. They often have limited food intake and poor nutrition, with a diet high in sweets and refined foods, fried foods, fast foods, and junk foods. The adolescent diet is often very high on the glycemic index, meaning more rapidly absorbing sugars. A diet higher in the complex carbohydrates such as whole grains and legumes will help to balance this. Luckily, though, for many teenagers the great demands for nutrients to support growth will increase their appetite for more concentrated protein foods and nutrient-rich foods. Some active adolescent males in particular may easily consume 4,000 calories daily.

Boys generally tend to eat enough food, but they may be deficient in nutrients because they often avoid vegetables, whole grains, and other whole foods. Teenagers who eat more refined foods without taking supplements commonly develop deficiencies. Teenage girls tend to eat less, as they are concerned about their weight, and the changes in fatty tissue increase this concern. Thus, they also may consume a diet deficient in nutrients. With the beginning of the menstrual cycle, there are greater demands for iron and other nutrients as well. Problems of bulimia and anorexia nervosa are more common in teenage girls, and will be discussed further in the *Weight Gain* program in Chapter 17. Teenage pregnancy can be a huge problem because of poor nutrition and deficiencies existing before pregnancy begins, let alone the challenge to a developing emotional system. Poor nutrition during pregnancy or prior to it greatly increases the risk of complications.

Obesity in adolescence usually results from poor food choices and laziness or lack of exercise. Other habits can also lead to weight gain. For example, more average daily time spent watching TV is associated with higher weights, also resulting from less activity and more snacks. With increased calorie intake during these growth years, there is an increase in the number and size of fat cells. This can lead to lifelong weight problems. Diet changes, sensible eating, and exercise are the best ways to counteract excessive weight gain, even in youngsters. Like eating habits, exercise habits are often created early in life, and once set, are harder to change. This is also true for attitudes toward health and life. These factors—eating and exercise patterns, and attitudes—are all important in generating long-term health.

Teenagers need to realize the importance of good nutrition, which can help a great deal in promoting nice-looking skin and general good looks. Dental caries are more common in adolescence, probably due to hormonal changes, a poor diet high in refined sugars, and mineral deficiencies. A more wholesome diet along with regular brushing and flossing will also promote healthy teeth.

We can help adolescent children best by being understanding and supportive. Our advice should be mild, with suggestions for modifications such as avoiding certain foods and trying others. Parents can be good influences by being good examples, eating well themselves, and not buying junk and refined snack foods for the home. Keeping nourishing snack foods such as fruits, nuts, and yogurt on hand and preparing wholesome meals will help youngsters make the best food choices.

A big concern in recent years is the wide availability of fast foods. These tend to contain high levels of salt, fat, and additives and low amounts of fiber and other vital nutrients. Protein is usually adequate; sugar may be excessive. If fast foods are not eaten too frequently (more than once weekly), they are not a big cause for concern. (And now, the fast food restaurants are offering healthier salads and nonfried foods.) However, a regular diet of soda pops, breads, cheese, sweets, and snack foods (which can be eaten at fast food places or at home and school) can be more of a problem. The protein content of such a diet may be low, and the B vitamins and vitamins C, A, and E are often deficient. Minerals may be the biggest problem. Calcium and iron are needed in high amounts in these growth years, and they are frequently not obtained in adequate amounts from diet alone. If soft drinks are substituted for milk, both calcium and vitamin D may be low. Zinc and manganese are also concerns, as are the trace minerals chromium and selenium. Those extra high nutrient foods such as brewer's yeast, molasses, wheat germ, and nuts can be added to fruit smoothies to increase the dietary nutrients. Teenagers may accept these kinds of suggestions.

The recommended overall diet plan is a balanced one containing vegetables, including some greens; nuts; whole grains; fruit; and higher-protein foods (dairy and meats) to provide the needed B vitamins, C, calcium, zinc, and iron. Vegetarian teenagers need to be even more conscious nutritionally, making sure they obtain many high-nutrient and wholesome foods. (See Chapter 16, *Vegetarianism* program.) To assure that growing teenagers obtain all the nutrients they need to support their heavy growth demands, a general multiple vitamin and mineral supplement is highly recommended. Girls especially need extra iron. Other needs may also be increased under certain circumstances; these are discussed in later programs.

FOUR ASPECTS OF LIFE AND NUTRITION

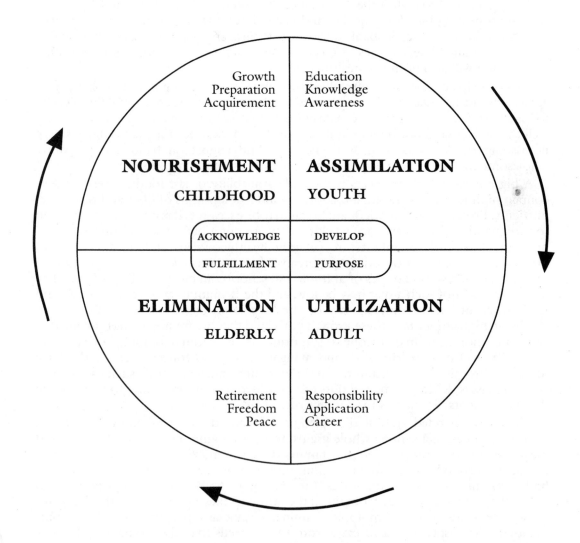

Growth
Preparation
Acquirement

Education
Knowledge
Awareness

NOURISHMENT

ASSIMILATION

CHILDHOOD

YOUTH

ACKNOWLEDGE

DEVELOP

FULFILLMENT

PURPOSE

ELIMINATION

UTILIZATION

ELDERLY

ADULT

Retirement
Freedom
Peace

Responsibility
Application
Career

The following nutrient levels suggest the RDAs (and slightly above) for two age groups of the adolescent years: 12–15 and 16–18. After that, the adult programs are used. There are, of course, nutritional supplements for young people that contain higher levels of vitamins and minerals that can also be used as additional support. Many teenagers will do well on these products as they ensure good levels of most nutrients.

DAILY NUTRIENT PROGRAM—ADOLESCENCE

	12–15 Years	*16–18 Years*
Calories	boys, 2,600–3,000	boys, 2,800–3,000
	girls, 2,000–2,300	girls, 2,000–2,200
Protein	boys, 45 g.	boys, 56 g.
	girls, 46 g.	girls, 46 g.
Vitamin A	5,000 IUs	5,000 IUs
Vitamin D	400 IUs	400 IUs
Vitamin E	30 IUs	30 IUs
Vitamin K	150 mcg.	150 mcg.
Thiamine (B_1)	1.5 mg.	1.5 mg.
Riboflavin (B_2)	2 mg.	2 mg.
Niacin (B_3)	18 mg.	18 mg.
Pantothenic acid (B_5)	10 mg.	10 mg.
Pyridoxine (B_6)	2.5 mg.	2.5 mg.
Cobalamin (B_{12})	5 mcg.	5 mcg.
Folic acid	400 mcg.	400 mcg.
Biotin	200 mcg.	200 mcg.
Vitamin C	300 mg.	300 mg.
Calcium	1,200 mg.	1,200 mg.
Chloride	3 g.	3 g.
Chromium	200 mcg.	200 mcg.
Copper	2–3 mg.	2–3 mg.
Fluoride	2.5 mg.	2.5 mg.
Iodine	150 mcg.	150 mcg.
Iron	18 mg.	18 mg.
Magnesium	350 mg.	400 mg.
Manganese	5 mg.	5 mg.
Molybdenum	500 mcg.	500 mcg.
Phosphorus	1,200 mg.	1,200 mg.
Potassium	4 g.	4 g.
Selenium	200 mcg.	200 mcg.
Sodium	2.5 g.	3.0 g.
Zinc	15 mg.	15 mg.

Adult Men

A dult males, like all other segments of our population, have their own special needs. Much of the information in this volume relates to both men and women; here we will look at the differences between the genders with regard to nutrition. In this program, we will review the requirements for a male's optimum physical, mental, and sexual functions, as well as his specific nutritional needs.

We want to think of life as long, healthy, and happy. How do we create that? Heredity and nutrition are probably the two most influential factors governing longevity. Other aspects of lifestyle, such as work, activity, exercise, stress levels, and chemical exposure, are also important. More subtle aspects, such as purpose, creativity, attitude, and often spiritual awareness, may also be core factors. I believe that the state of our nutrition, our general attitude toward life, and how we handle stress can influence our health and longevity more than anything else; they can maximize our potential or hasten our demise. Many specific nutrients protect us and enhance our energy and physiological potential as well.

Men (and humans) in this modern age, however, have departed from the basic aspects of supportive living. We have moved away from the land and manual labor to a frenetic lifestyle in cars and offices, eating on the run, working more with our minds than with our bodies. These increased stresses require greater nourishment than we have needed under low stress conditions. Unless we fill this vital nutrient gap, our energy, stamina, and productivity can be diminished. Obtaining quality foods and taking the relaxed, receptive time to eat them need to be more of a life priority. Most active, productive men need a good supplement program to protect them from illness and deficiency symptoms and increase their longevity by reducing chronic degenerative disease patterns.

Many parts of this book deal with nutrition's effect on our major diseases—cancer, cardiovascular disease, and diabetes. Even though the average life span in the United States has increased greatly (from 47 years for males born in 1900 to 72 years for those born in 1980), much of this is due to better prenatal and infant care, immunizations, and the use of antibiotics to treat acute infections. Now, many adult chronic, degenerative diseases result from regular overeating and from choosing the wrong foods, such as those high in fat and sugar, and too many refined foods. At the same time, too little of the wholesome, nutritious foods may contribute to suppressed immunity, increased infection rates, and susceptibility to cancer. It is important that men (and all people) find the right balance in diet and lifestyle. This includes all of the nutritional suggestions discussed previously—eating more fresh fruits and vegetables, whole grains, legumes, nuts, seeds, fresh fish, and, if desired, occasional lean poultry or animal meats, free of chemicals and antibiotics. Limiting the fatty, refined, and sugary foods, such as milk products, processed meats, fried foods, breads, candies, and pastries, while minimizing the use of caffeine, alcohol, and nicotine will help produce a healthier and longer life.

Most men with good energy levels can use regular detoxification periods (discussed in detail in later programs). Regular fasting or "cleansing," yearly (in springtime), seasonally, monthly, or even one day weekly, is a great preventive medicine tool; it may also help to reenergize the will and instincts. Difficulties may arise when we overwhelm our capacities to handle our foods, chemicals, emotions, thoughts, and so on. We may also begin to feel "backed up" when our abilities to digest, assimilate, and eliminate these many potential life stressors are reduced. Constipation, back pain, allergies, and sinus congestion, as well as certain cardiovascular diseases and gastrointestinal problems are the results of this type of lifestyle autointoxication. Many of these problems will respond well to a cleansing program. Refer to the *General Detoxification and Fasting* programs in Chapter 18. These cleansing periods offer us a good chance to reevaluate our life and make a new plan for health, work, or whatever else we may need to renew ourselves. Most men do not usually consider this practice, but those who do respond very well. In my experience, women are more likely to embrace these more evolutionary (or traditional) aspects of cultural medicine, hygienic practices, and healing; women are also usually more receptive to change and learning. Men, of course, need these renewing processes also; women, however, require fasting programs less frequently, because their problems more commonly result from nutritional deficiencies. Ultimately, we all need to find a balance, ever-changing, of course, that will keep us well and not require much detoxification.

Sexual energy and vitality are also important male issues, especially if we are going to get along well with our mate, lover, or friends. Safe sex is a big concern today, but if we do not have the energy for sex, we can forget these more adventurous subjects. Sexual function is supported by good diet and nutrient intake. The healthy diet should provide adequate protein and essential fatty acids as well as some cholesterol (eggs, dairy foods) or plant sterols, as are found in olive oil; these foods provide some of the precursors of certain sex hormones.

Several endocrine organs aid in normal sexual function. The thyroid gland, necessary for proper energy level and metabolism, is supported by iodine and B vitamins, particularly thiamine and pantothenic acid. Testicular function is vital to normal production of testosterone, the hormone most essential to male sex drive. Adrenal androgen hormones also support testicular activity and sexual development in men. Vitamin E and zinc may be the big two when it comes to sexual energy support. Vitamins A, C, and E and folic acid as well as essential fatty acids are all important to sperm production. The minerals calcium, magnesium, zinc, and sulfur, as well as vitamin B_{12}, inositol, and vitamin C are found in healthy sperm and so also may be necessary to fertility.

Adrenal function is important for sexual function, both physiologically and in terms of energy level. Many nutrients support healthy adrenal function—vitamins A, C, and

E, the B vitamins, especially pantothenic acid, and essential fatty acids. Factors such as stress, worry, excess mental activity, and regular sugar and caffeine use may contribute to weaker adrenal function.

If a man has a decreased sex drive, some extra zinc, magnesium, and vitamin B_6 may be helpful. With impotence, vitamins C and E, B complex, and calcium, plus some counseling to explore the psychological factors, will provide support. Herbs, such as ginseng root, which is a good tonic herb, can raise general and sexual energy levels. Also, reducing the use of sedative-type drugs, such as alcohol, and nicotine, which interferes with circulation, and generally reducing stress may all help. Much sexual dysfunction has to do with mental stresses and fears of intimacy. Massage and body therapy give an important balance to a busy lifestyle, as does regular exercise. All of these may be helpful in improving both energy levels and sexual vitality.

For men who experience premature ejaculation, there may be many factors involved. Among these are not enough practice or enough sex, poor circulation, and even allergies. Histamine, a chemical in our cells and blood, controls ejaculation. If this chemical is too high, as it often is with allergies, ejaculatory rate may be increased. Low histamine levels may slow this rate and in some men may even cause problems with ejaculating. Niacin and fatty acids tend to increase the release of stored histamine, while calcium and the amino acid methionine may lower it. So extra calcium and amino acids with higher methionine levels could help in certain cases of premature ejaculation. (For more on sex and nutrition, see the *Sexual Vitality* program in Chapter 16.)

Men, like women, have special nutrient needs to maintain their energy and sexuality. Men usually need at least the RDAs for all nutrients, with less iron and more magnesium and B vitamins than women. Otherwise, the requirements for a good nutritional foundation are really not very different. Men may need additional iron, particularly if there is any problem with bleeding, anemia, or if they are vegetarians. (Some recent research, however, suggests that excessive iron in men adds to their risk for cardiovascular disease due to iron's oxidative irritation of the blood vessels and the liver cells.) Men will also obviously need more calories and protein to support their generally larger size and often higher activity levels. The number of calories needed by men will vary with their desired weight and activity level. The male "couch potato" may need to reduce his caloric intake by eating fewer munchies, drinking less beer, and restricting his intake of foods high in fats and sugar.

The Nutrient Program shown in the table offers guidelines for men "on the go" between the ages of 19 and 65. The values listed range from minimum requirements to more optimum levels. (The basic RDAs are listed at the end of Chapter 13.) For certain nutrients, such as calories, fats, iron, and sodium, the lower numbers may be more appropriate. These values represent a combination of diet and additional supplements, and certain essential nutrients, such as sodium, chloride, fluoride, phosphorus, and vitamin K are not usually taken above dietary levels. If such nutrients as iron, calcium, copper, iodine, and potassium are sufficient in the diet, these are not usually added unless there are specific problems with digestion and/or assimilation. Important extra support for men may come from B vitamins, vitamins C and E, beta-carotene, magnesium, manganese, selenium, and zinc.

ADULT MEN'S NUTRIENT PROGRAM
RANGE (RDAS TO OPTIMUM SAFE LEVELS)

Calories	2,100–3,500
Fiber	8–20 g.
Protein	50–75 g.
Fats	50-75 g.

Vitamin A	5,000–10,000 IUs	**Calcium***	800–1,200 mg.
Beta-carotene	5,000–20,000 IUs	**Chloride***	2–5 g.
Vitamin D	200–600 IUs	**Chromium**	200–500 mcg.
Vitamin E	30–800 IUs	**Copper**	2–3 mg.
Vitamin K*	150–600 mcg.	**Fluoride***	1.5–4.0 mg.
Thiamine (B$_1$)	1.4–50.0 mg.	**Iodine***	150–300 mcg.
Riboflavin (B$_2$)	1.6–50.0 mg.	**Iron***	10–15 mg.
Niacin (B$_3$)*	20–200 mg.	**Magnesium**	400–800 mg.
Pantothenic acid (B$_5$)	7–250 mg.	**Manganese**	3.0–10.0 mg.
Pyridoxine (B$_6$)	2.5–100 mg.	**Molybdenum**	150–500 mcg.
Cobalamin (B$_{12}$)	3–200 mcg.	**Phosphorus***	800–1,200 mg.
Folic acid	400–800 mcg.	**Potassium***	2–6 g.
Biotin	150–500 mcg.	**Selenium**	200–400 mcg.
Choline	50–500 mg.	**Sodium***	1.0–3.5 g.
Inositol	50–500 mg.	**Zinc**	15–60 mg.
PABA	10–50 mg.		
Vitamin C	60–2000 mg.		
Bioflavonoids	100–500 mg.		

*These nutrients are noted because they are required for health; however, for men, they are usually adequate in the diet and do not require supplementation. Some calcium or iron may be taken occasionally in a multiple, or if the man is a strict vegetarian.

** Mixed niacin and niacinamide; 50 mg. or more of niacin may cause nausea, tingling, and flushing initially, but could help to lower the cholesterol levels. (See Niacin in Chapter 5).

Adult Women

Women also have special needs. On a very basic level, they need to love and be loved, to create, to express their feelings, and to express their being. (Men, of course, also have these basic needs.) Each woman is a special jewel that shines in her own way and she has her particular requirements for life.

Women also have special nutritional needs. During the menstruating years (between ages 13 and 50, varying individually), their need for iron to replace lost red blood cells is high. They also need adequate amounts of other nutrients, such as the B vitamins, iodine, calcium, and magnesium—more, I think, than the RDAs suggest.

One of the main concerns with women is that their food intake may not be adequate. Physical activity levels may be low, and often there is low calorie intake related to dieting to stay thin. This may result in inadequate nutrient intake to meet nutritional requirements. Very active women may also eat lightly to keep their weight down, and without adequate supplements, this can lead to deficiencies.

On the other hand, some women put on weight very easily and have a difficult time losing it. Even low-calorie diets may not do the trick. Increased activity levels with a moderately caloric, balanced, high-vegetable, lean-protein diet may help them to reduce. Checking the thyroid hormone levels, assessing the caloric intake/utilization relationship to weight and energy maintenance and activity levels, and integrating and optimizing these will be helpful. (This is, of course, a wide concept.) Also, basic multivitamin plus additional supplements, particularly extra B vitamins, such as B_6 and B_{12}, plus potassium, calcium, and magnesium, will also be helpful. (For more on this, see the *Weight Loss* program in Chapter 17.)

Sexual vitality is also very important to women. A number of nutrients are important in supporting the sexual organs, sexual functions, and a normal menstrual cycle. Adrenal support and function are very important for women as well as for men. The adrenal glands help us deal with stress and give us sexual energy. Stress, allergies, and high amounts of sugar intake can weaken these important glands, and this may be exacerbated by nutritional deficiency. The adrenals need adequate levels of vitamins A, C, and E, essential fatty acids, and B vitamins, particularly pantothenic acid. Chromium and adequate levels of amino acids will also help reduce sugar cravings and thus help support the adrenals.

The female ovaries secrete estrogen and progesterone, which control the menstrual cycle. These hormones are influenced by the pituitary gland in the brain; the pituitary is influenced by higher brain centers, which are in turn affected by emotions, moon cycles, weather, and the seasons. This female hormonal balance is, therefore, a delicate one that needs a lot of support. It requires sufficient levels of B vitamins, especially folic acid and niacin, plus zinc and vitamin E. Certain fats and cholesterol are important precursors of female hormones, mediated through the liver's biochemical processes. Drug and alcohol use, which can stress the liver, may weaken this sensitive hormonal function. Also, some women's cholesterol levels are too low, especially those who are strict vegetarians, and this may be related to low hormonal levels and early menopause.

During the actual menstrual cycle, women tend to lose iron in the red blood cells; there are also tendencies to lose calcium and zinc. Copper levels usually increase, as they do with the use of birth control pills, which contain estrogen. During and after menstruation, women can take a little extra iron, magnesium, calcium (vitamins D and C will help absorption), zinc, and vitamin B_6. Copper should be avoided above dietary levels or above the usual 1–2 mg. in a general supplement. A good protein diet with extra B complex and vitamin C is recommended also. Extra calcium and magnesium, ideally in the citrate or aspartate forms, may be helpful for menstrual cramps. Niacin (50–100 mg.) might also be beneficial. Though it may not be easy, women should try to avoid too many sweets during the pre- and postmenstruation times.

When women become pregnant or breastfeed, they have greatly increased requirements for calories, protein, and many vitamins and minerals, especially calcium, magnesium, and iron. If birth control pills are taken (not recommended), many nutrients are needed in greater amounts. More zinc and less copper and iron, more vitamin B_6, a basic B vitamin formula, and vitamins E and C should be taken.

Menopause can be a very stressful time, filled with changes, stresses, and various symptoms—fatigue, irritability, hot flashes, headaches, cramps, and depression are a few. Continuing to take estrogen hormones helps reduce these symptoms, but there are also many possible aids to be found in diet, lifestyle, nutritional supplements, and herbs. Vitamin E, A, calcium, magnesium, zinc, and B vitamins may help. Female herbs such as dong quai (angelica root) have been shown to reduce symptoms too. After menopause, calcium needs and bone health are the greatest concern unless extra hormones are taken. (See the following programs for *Pregnancy, Lactation, Birth Control Pills,* and *Menopause* for further discussions of these subjects.)

In my experience, most women do best on a low- to moderate-calorie diet that includes a good amount of protein and vegetables, some whole grains, and fairly few fruits and sweet foods. Milk products are tolerated by some, but they can be weight-increasing foods, especially with lots of cheese. Some low- or nonfat milk and plain yogurt seem to be the best utilized.

Women also need to exercise and stay fit, especially if they are thinking of having babies, working at a high-stress job, or working at all regularly out in the world. A good exercise program maintains energy, vitality, and figure better than TV and munchies.

Women have different nutrient needs than those of men. They may need fewer calories but only slightly less protein and the same amount or more of many of the essential nutrients. That is why they need a more compact (good nutrient/calorie ratio), nourishing diet of high-quality foods. The requirements for most minerals are the same, but women need more iron, almost double men's level. Vegetarian women must focus more intently than others to get adequate iron in their diet, since the foods containing the most available iron are meats and liver. But it can be obtained from many other foods, supplements, or cooking in cast-iron cookware. Women need a little less magnesium than men, but I find that many women actually require even more calcium-magnesium, especially when they exercise. The following table lists the nutrients needed by the average active, healthy woman as insurance to maintain her health. The amounts shown range from the RDAs to optimum levels, and include a combination of dietary intake and additional supplements. Nutrients such as protein, fats, vitamin K, chloride, fluoride, phosphorus, potassium, and sodium are not usually taken above dietary levels. Most others will be part of basic supplements.

ADULT WOMEN'S NUTRIENT PROGRAM RANGE
(RDAS TO OPTIMUM SAFE LEVELS)

Calories	1,500–2,500		
Fiber	8–15 g.		
Protein	45–65 g.		
Fats*	40–70 g.		
Vitamin A	4,000–10,000 IUs	**Calcium**	850–1,200 mg.
Beta-carotene	5,000–20,000 IUs	**Chloride****	2–4 g.
Vitamin D	200–400 IUs	**Chromium**	100–400 mcg.
Vitamin E	30–800 IUs	**Copper**	2–3 mg.
Vitamin K**	100–300 mcg.	**Fluoride****	1.5–3.5 mg.
Thiamine (B_1)	1.0–30.0 mg.	**Iodine****	150–300 mcg.
Riboflavin (B_2)	1.2–30.0 mg.	**Iron**	18–30 mg.
Niacin or		**Magnesium**	350–700 mg.
Niacinamide (B_3)	15–100 mg.	**Manganese**	2.5–15 mg.
Pantothenic acid (B_5)	7–250 mg.	**Molybdenum**	150–500 mcg.
Pyridoxine (B_6)	2–50 mg.	**Phosphorus****	800–1200 mg.
Cobalamin (B_{12})	3–200 mcg.	**Potassium****	2–5 g.
Folic acid	400–800 mcg.	**Selenium**	150–300 mcg.
PABA	5–50 mg.	**Sodium****	1.5–4.0 g.
Biotin	150–500 mcg.	**Zinc**	15–30 mg.
Choline	50–500 mg.		
Inositol	50–500 mg.		
Vitamin C	60–1,000 mg.		
Bioflavonoids	125–500 mg.		

*Total fats include olive oil and fish/salmon oil with EPA and DHA, but a low amount of saturated fats.

**These nutrients are listed because they are required in the diet (they have RDAs), although they are not usually added to formulae or taken as extra supplements.

Pregnancy

Nutrition during pregnancy is probably the most important aspect of this magical creation of life. Good nutrition before and during pregnancy can make the difference between health and sickness and support the general constitution of your child for life. The key word for pregnancy is EAT—and that means to eat well, not overeat or eat junky, high-calorie, empty nutrient, or high-fat or salty foods, but highly nourishing foods. The woman's body needs more of everything—calories, protein, calcium, iron, zinc, B vitamins, and most other vitamins and minerals.

A very important factor in a healthy pregnancy is the woman's pre-pregnancy condition. The risk of nutrient depletions is greatly enhanced during pregnancy and lactation. To enter this demanding period with illness, bad habits, or any nutritional deficiency, such as anemia, may mean a troublesome pregnancy and years of recovery. So if you are thinking about having children, even vaguely considering the possibility, begin early to care for yourself. This applies to men as well. Nutritionally healthy men will provide healthier, more functional sperm and probably healthier children. My advice to people planning a pregnancy is to prepare themselves by having a complete evaluation—physical, general biochemistry, diet and nutrient analyses—and then get on a good diet and supplement program. Changing health-damaging habits such as smoking, regular alcohol or caffeine use, and other drug use is definitely a wise move.

In *Nutrition in Health and Disease*, Myron Winick, M.D., calculates that it takes an estimated 75,000 calories to make a baby, or about 300–400 extra calories per day. The average woman will need 2,400–2,600 calories per day during pregnancy, and even more in the last trimester. This means about 15–20 percent more calories than usual. An extra few hundred calories can be consumed pretty easily, but if they come from sweets or other empty-calorie foods, they will not provide the extra nourishment needed. Wholesome foods are a necessity, and concentrated or nutrient-dense foods are crucial if a mother-to-be wants to get much of her requirements from food. Women need a higher nutrient/calorie ratio in pregnancy.

Protein. Besides more food and more calories, pregnant women need nearly twice as much protein as the 45 grams usually required; 75–85 (even up to 100) grams of protein are needed daily during pregnancy. Some preliminary research, however, points out that too much protein intake during pregnancy can lead to some problems, such as larger babies and thus, more difficult birthings, and postmature babies. This area needs further study. During pregnancy, women need adequate good quality protein within a balanced diet. This protein supports the tissue growth of both the fetus and the new tissues made by the mother. Common protein foods are meat, fish and poultry, eggs, and dairy foods. Nuts, seeds, grains, and legumes are also important. The lacto-ovo-vegetarian will need sufficient grains, legumes, seeds, nuts, eggs, and dairy foods. I do not suggest strict veganism during pregnancy. Although it can be done, it does not have the same degree of safety as eating a wider range of protein foods, let alone the added calcium and iron needed. Even though vitamin B_{12} may be absorbed better by vegetarians than by meat-eaters because of their needs, it is not found in many vegetable foods. Traces may be found in foods such as peanuts, sunflower seeds, sprouts, kelp and other seaweeds, and soybean products, particularly tempeh, miso, and soy sauce. Seafood, however, has much higher levels of vitamin B_{12}.

Calcium is also very important. Calcium needs in general are more than 50 percent greater during pregnancy, particularly the second half. If the mother is not obtaining sufficient calcium, her body will pull it from her bones to nourish the growing fetus. At least 1,200 mg. of calcium are needed daily, and this is difficult to obtain from the diet alone unless more dairy products and fish are eaten. Calcium helps form the baby's bones and teeth and aids muscle and heart function, blood clotting, and nerve transmission. Besides fish and milk products, calcium foods include whole grains, nuts and seeds, leafy greens, sea vegetables, and other vegetables. Meats contain some calcium, but their high phosphorus level may interfere with calcium utilization.

Iron is another crucial nutrient, needed to help build blood cells in the mother and fetus. Iron also aids in disease resistance and elimination. The iron needs more than double, to at least 30–60 mg. per day and likely more. Estimates suggest that women need somewhere between 15–20 mg. absorbed, and absorption is only about 10–20 percent of that ingested (see *Iron* discussion in Chapter 6), thus pregnant women need an intake likely over 100 mg. daily (and if anemic, probably more). It is difficult to get that high an iron intake from the diet alone unless we live on liver, molasses, wheat germ, and eggs, and most of us would not enjoy that much. If the mother-to-be does not obtain enough iron from her diet, she will deplete her iron stores. With these reduced, her demands to make more blood cells will not be met, and anemia will occur, usually accompanied by fatigue and poor endurance. Thus, almost all pregnant women take an iron supplement with their vitamin program. Since iron is not absorbed efficiently, more is needed to increase its availability; taking it two or three times daily also improves the chances of obtaining enough. Some women have trouble handling iron supplements; certain formulas may be handled more easily than others (again, see the *Iron* discussion in Chapter 6, on *Minerals*). Good animal sources of iron include beef liver, red meats (beef, lamb, and pork), eggs, chicken, and salmon. Vegetable sources are: seaweed, brewer's yeast, molasses, millet, prunes, raisins, mushrooms, chard, spinach, and most nuts, seeds, and legumes.

Zinc is another important mineral that can be deficient in pregnancy and is needed to aid normal development of the immune system in the fetus. Zinc is found in the same foods in which iron is found, with additional amounts in shellfish, especially oysters.

Folic acid is another crucial nutrient during pregnancy. It is needed to help form red blood cells, to aid the growth and reproduction of other cells, and to support the development of the nervous system in the fetus. Folic acid also helps stimulate the mother's appetite. Needs are doubled during pregnancy, to 800 mcg. daily. Folic acid is found in leafy green vegetables, whole grains, yeast, fish, dairy foods, and organ meats.

Other nutrients are also needed at increased levels. The needs for vitamins A, C, E, and B_6 all go up. I do not suggest megadoses of vitamin C during pregnancy because the effects of this have not been clearly determined. However, regular intake of 50–100 mg. several times daily will help utilize iron, calcium and magnesium, folic acid, zinc, and vitamin A. Other minerals, such as iodine, magnesium, and sodium, are also needed in increased amounts. For years, obstetricians were advising pregnant women to avoid sodium, but now they are suggesting that they use it as usual. For most women, some added salt is fine, and they can eat foods that naturally contain sodium, such as celery, beets, red meats, cheese, eggs, and scallops. The craving that some women have for pickles, olives, or sauerkraut may be related to a need for sodium. While more salt is needed to build the blood volume, there are limits, and very salty foods, such as potato chips and pretzels, should be avoided. Excessive salt intake can lead to problems of water retention, elevated blood pressure, and further risks to the mother and baby.

Another change that has been suggested in the field of obstetrics involves the healthy level of weight gain during pregnancy. Even 20 years ago, doctors suggested that women limit their weight gain to 20 pounds, and even a limit of 10–15 pounds might be suggested. Now the goal is more like 20–25 pounds, or about 20 percent of ideal weight, and it has recently been shown that women who gain even 30–40 pounds, especially from good food, deliver larger and very healthy babies. The average weight gain is around 25 pounds, but 25–35 is fine. Most of the weight (10–13 pounds) is gained in the last trimester, about 8–12 pounds during the mid trimester, and only 3–4 pounds during the first three months.

As emphasized, the mother needs more of everything during pregnancy because she has to make a new being. And Mother Nature has provided the inner baby with the mechanisms to get what it needs from the mother whether she has extra or not. As I have stated, the baby can pull minerals, vitamins, and protein from the mother's bones, organs, tissues, and other storage areas. This can leave the mother depleted, which can take a long time, even years, to correct. Besides making a new baby, these nutrients are needed to form the placenta, to increase the size of the uterus and breast tissue, and to create amniotic fluid. Mother's blood volume increases by 25–50 percent, and more fluids, iron, B_{12}, folic acid, zinc and copper, calcium, magnesium, and proteins are needed to support this new blood. Storage levels of most nutrients must be obtained from the diet as well.

So what is the best diet for our mother-to-be? First, she should eat a well-balanced diet containing all the food nutrients, with an increased amount of calories, usually about 300–400 more per day than usual. Weight-reduction programs during pregnancy are definitely taboo except for the obese and under careful supervision. (Weight Watcher's actually has a program for pregnant and nursing women.) There is much less worry about weight gain and sodium use now than there was years ago, as both these factors may contribute to a healthy pregnancy and child. It is really the quality of the weight gain that is important—that is, the building of the necessary tissues rather than just adding fat.

A wholesome diet is crucial to avoid wasted calories from junk foods and sugary snacks and to provide plenty of nutrient-rich foods to satisfy the increased needs for most of the vitamins, minerals, and protein. More dairy products, animal meats, whole grains, and vegetables will help a lot. Nutrient-rich foods for pregnancy that will help guard against dietary deficiencies include eggs, fish, poultry, organ meats, milk products, red meats, whole grains, wheat germ, nuts and seeds, yeast, molasses, seaweeds, and leafy green vegetables. Some of these should be eaten daily. For a more specific food plan for pregnancy, see page 707.

NUTRIENT-RICH FOODS THAT WILL HELP GUARD AGAINST DIETARY DEFICIENCIES DURING PREGNANCY

eggs	whole grains
fish	wheat germ
poultry	yeast
organ meats*	molasses
milk products	seaweeds
red meats	leafy green vegetables
nuts and seeds	

*only from organically raised animals; these foods are really more like medicines

---

A high-fiber diet with whole grains, fruits, and vegetables is also important for good bowel function to avoid constipation, a common problem of pregnancy. At least six to eight glasses of good drinking water should be consumed daily besides some milk and herb teas. The top herbal choice is raspberry leaf tea, which is thought to tone up the uterus. Herbal folklore claims that a cup of raspberry leaf tea drunk daily during pregnancy will assure a healthy labor.

Exercise is also very important during pregnancy, as always. Keeping the body limber, loose, and toned is necessary to a healthy pregnancy. Do exercise; don't get lazy. It is important for good circulation, and can help prevent constipation, varicose veins, and a flabby tummy. Regular stretching, movement classes, and even aerobic-type activities, such as indoor and outdoor bicycling, swimming, and hiking, will help maintain vitality. If you have not been exercising much prior to becoming pregnant, begin slowly with stretching and light activities. Also, avoid impact aerobics, jumping rope, and horseback riding—but keep moving. Regular, quiet internal "exercises," such as meditation and visualizations, are important to prepare for all the body changes, emotional shifts, and a smooth labor and healthy baby.

It is particularly important during pregnancy to avoid drugs of all kinds. Caffeine and alcohol should be minimized to occasional use only and are better avoided completely. Nicotine use is best eliminated, as it is associated with many problems in the pregnancy, birth, and health of the infant as well as the mother. It is also wise to avoid chemicals of all kinds—in foods, at work, and in the home. Many chemicals will pass through the placenta to the baby. Though the placenta protects the baby from many harmful substances, there are very few that it blocks completely. Pesticides or metals can be concentrated in the fetus. Sugar substitutes such as saccharin, artificial flavors, food dyes, and nitrites should be eliminated from the diet. Nitrosamines formed from nitrates and nitrites (found in hot dogs, bacon, and other lunch meats) have been shown in animal studies to produce cancer in the offspring. Good levels of vitamin C in the body can block nitrosamine formation.

Any pharmaceutical drug use should be carefully monitored by the doctor or midwife. All drugs would be best avoided if possible. Many drugs may interact with body nutrients and increase the risk of deficiency. Pregnant women need to be very careful to avoid drug and chemical exposure, because it is very hard to do any detoxification during pregnancy. The body is in a building up, gathering state and will utilize most everything that comes into it or store it away for later use.

Nutritional changes and support may help remedy some of the common problems of pregnancy. Morning sickness with nausea and vomiting is especially common during the first few months. This problem is likely a result of biliary or liver activity. During the night, the liver works to eliminate toxins, which are thus in the system on awakening. A good diet and avoidance of fatty foods, alcohol, and other liver-irritating drugs before pregnancy is helpful in minimizing morning sickness. Vitamin B_6 aids liver metabolism. The active metabolic form is the pyridoxine precursor, pyridoxal-5-phosphate (P5P), because it enters directly into the functioning metabolic cycle. Usually, supplementing 25–50 mg. of B_6 three times daily will help reduce the symptoms of morning sickness. Occasionally, higher amounts are needed. If these higher levels are used, it is wise to continue smaller amounts for a while to prevent pyridoxine withdrawal in mother or baby; higher dosages, however, are usually not required all the way up to delivery time, because intestinal symptoms decrease after the first few months. Other supplements helpful in morning sickness include vitamins B_{12}, C, and E and extra magnesium and potassium. Herbs are often helpful as well. Raspberry leaf, peppermint, or ginger root teas have been effective for some women.

Dietary changes are the best way to handle morning sickness. A reduction of fatty food intake and an increase in carbohydrates may be helpful. A higher fiber intake keeps intestines moving, which helps elimination and detoxification. Acidic foods, such as citrus fruits or juice, and iron supplements or milk may increase nausea and vomiting. Small, frequent meals and snacks of carbohydrate or protein can be best tolerated. Munching on a few soda crackers or dry toast upon awakening may help alleviate early morning nausea. Don't worry, this too shall pass; and breathing and relaxing also help.

Pregnant women and their husbands and families need to be understanding and adaptable, especially in regard to diet. Food cravings can be wild, food consumption goes up, and sometimes a woman's whole life becomes centered around food. And these can be obstacles. The digestive tract is more sensitive, and as the pregnancy progresses, the size of the stomach shrinks due to the growing womb. Often food intolerances or many new likes and dislikes develop. To adapt, the diet may shift to frequent small and simple, but nourishing meals. Nutritious liquid meals are a good choice. From protein powders to fruit or vegetable smoothies, these drinks can be packed with nutrients. One possibility for building and nourishing mother and baby is the "Baby Shake," an adaptation of the "Pregnancy Cocktail" described by Fred Rohe in *The Complete Book of Natural Foods.*

THE BABY SHAKE

Blend Together:

½–1 cup apple juice	1–2 teaspoons blackstrap molasses
1 banana	1–2 teaspoons nutritional yeast
½–1 cup yogurt	1 Tablespoon wheat germ
1 raw egg	1-2 Tablespoons honey or pure maple syrup
½–1 cup low-fat milk	⅓ teaspoon kelp

This can be adapted to your special desires and the flavors you can tolerate. If something in the drink doesn't appeal to you, avoid it and try something else. Other fruits or juices can be used, or no juice and just milk, a banana, or another fruit as a base. Adding water will make it more dilute, which some women will tolerate better. Flavorings such as vanilla or almond or a handful of raw almonds, coconut, or sunflower seeds can be added and blended. In regard to food-combining, when different foods are blended together as a drink, they seem to be better tolerated. However, if you do not handle this mixture well, simplify the drink and just use a banana, yogurt, and milk or water, along with some yeast or wheat germ and a little sweetener. Overall, your Baby Shake can be very tasty and nourishing.

Later in pregnancy, when labor is just beginning, take some extra calcium-magnesium to help reduce the pain of contractions and muscle aches and spasm. About 1,500–2,000 mg. of each has been helpful to some women. This can be repeated later if labor is extended. If a caesarean section is going to be done, it is wise to take extra tissue-healing nutrients (vitamins A and C, and zinc) prior to and after the procedure, for several days to several weeks if possible. (See the *Surgery* program in Chapter 17.)

As for regular supplements during pregnancy, usually a high-potency multiple or special prenatal formula with plenty of iron should be taken. If nausea occurs with the supplement, try to take it later in the day with meals. The nutrient plan shown in the table gives the ranges from the MDR (minimum daily requirement) for pregnancy to what I feel is the optimum insurance level.

For special problems, such as anemia, more iron may be needed. Consult your doctor or midwife. Of course, not all of these nutrients will be used as supplements. Many of them, such as sodium, chloride, fluoride, and potassium are obtained from the diet. However, depending on the dietary intake of various nutrients, such as calcium, zinc, or B vitamins, or individual blood measurements, any specific nutrient can be further increased by supplement use to give the necessary intake.

(Also note: in the next program, *Lactation,* more specifics of the pregnancy diet are discussed.)

NUTRIENT PROGRAM FOR PREGNANCY
(RANGE—RDA TO OPTIMUM)

Calories*	2,300–3,200		
Fiber	10–15 g.		
Protein*	75–90 g.		

Vitamin A*	6,000–10,000 IUs	**Calcium***	1,200–1,600 mg.
Beta-carotene	10,000–15,000 IUs	**Chloride+**	2–4 g.
Vitamin D	400–600 IUs	**Chromium**	200–400 mcg.
Vitamin E*	50–400 IUs	**Copper**	2–3 mg.
Vitamin K	100–400 mcg.	**Fluoride+**	1.5–3.5 mg.
Thiamine (B$_1$)	1.5–50 mg.	**Iodine*+**	175–350 mcg.
Riboflavin (B$_2$)	1.5–30 mg.	**Iron*#**	40–80 mg.
Niacin (B$_3$)	16–100 mg.	**Magnesium***	450–1,000 mg.
Pantothenic acid (B$_5$)	7–250 mg.	**Manganese**	2.5–15 mg.
Pyridoxine (B$_6$)	2.6–100 mg.	**Molybdenum**	150–500 mcg.
Cobalamin (B$_{12}$)	4–200 mcg.	**Phosphorus*+**	1,200–1,600 mg.
Folic acid*	800–1,200 mcg.	**Potassium+**	2–5 g.
Biotin	200–500 mcg.	**Selenium**	150–300 mcg.
Choline	50–250 mg.	**Sodium*+**	2.5–4.0 g.
Inositol	50–250 mg.	**Zinc***	20–40 mg.
PABA	10–50 mg.	**Essential fatty acids****	2–3 teaspoons
Vitamin C*+++	80–1,000 mg.		
Bioflavonoids	100–250 mg.		

*Requirements for these nutrients are increased during pregnancy.

+These nutrients are required for health, yet are not usually taken as additional supplements.

#Iron intakes include diet plus additional supplementation of 30–60 mg. daily.

++More vitamin C can be used for short periods for colds, flu, and so on.

**Fatty acids come from olive oil, flaxseed oil, or other nutritious cold-pressed vegetable oils.

Lactation

Breastfeeding is an important part of the pregnancy and birth process and the best way to nourish the new infant. It is also helpful for the mother to balance her pregnancy. Nursing not only is a calorie and fluid outlet, helping mother reattain her pre-pregnancy weight, it is often vital to her emotional and psychological well-being and to the bonding with the new baby. In addition, the hormone released during breastfeeding, oxytocin, helps contract the uterus back to normal size and health.

Nutritional requirements are much the same as during pregnancy, with even higher requirements for many nutrients and reduced needs for a few. After all, we are feeding a growing baby. An infant requires about 2–3 ounces of milk per pound of weight, so a newborn of seven pounds needs about 18 ounces of milk daily; as he or she grows, more milk is required. Each ounce of milk has about 20 calories, so mother is giving out 300–400 calories a day initially, and more as the baby grows. She needs 200–500 more calories per day than even during pregnancy and 500–1,000 more than before it, depending on her weight. Some mothers will consume fewer calories after birth in order to lose weight, but this is not wise. Too great a reduction in calories can diminish milk production (as can resuming cigarette smoking). Mother should naturally lose weight during breastfeeding, and as she reduces her level of nursing, she may also lessen her calorie intake.

Water is the main ingredient of mother's milk, so adequate fluid intake is essential. At least three quarts of liquid are recommended daily, including water, juices, and milk. Mother's diet should also be high in nutrients, mainly from eating those good, wholesome foods. High protein levels are still required, though a little less is needed than during pregnancy; calcium, magnesium, and iron requirements are also similar. Vitamins C and A, zinc, and iodine are needed in higher levels. Folic acid requirements decrease by 25 percent as the mother's blood volume decreases. Extra B vitamins may be helpful (for stress and fatigue related to sleep deprivation), as breast milk is fairly low in them, but high-dosage B vitamin pills are best avoided during lactation. Specifically, high amounts of vitamin B_6 can reduce milk production.

Good nourishment is essential to prevent depletion of mother and to provide the right nutrients for baby. Remember, the food that mother eats provides the nutrients in her milk and thus the infant's nutrition. Many of the nutrient-rich foods suggested for pregnancy should be consumed—dairy products, eggs, fish, other animal foods, whole grains, vegetables, especially leafy greens, and vitamin C fruits. Standard food-group orientation suggests more portions of most everything. The summary of food group needs for nonpregnant, pregnant, and nursing women shown here is adapted from *Mowry's Basic Nutrition and Diet Therapy* by Sue Rodwell Williams.

GENERAL PREGNANCY NUTRITIONAL PLAN

	Servings per Day		
	Nonpregnant	*Pregnant*	*Nursing*
Milk foods—low-fat milk (avoid skim), cheese, yogurt, butter (1 serving = 1 cup milk or yogurt, or 3–4 oz. cheese)	2	3–4	5–6
Cereal grains (1 serving = about 1 cup grain or 1 slice of bread)	3	4–5	5
Vegetables—raw yellow or dark green (1 serving = 1 cup)	1	2	2
Other vegetables (1 cup)	1	2	2
Vitamin C foods—citrus, berries, peppers, tomato (1 serving = 1 cup)	1	2	2
Eggs (1 serving = 1 egg)	1	1–2	1–2
Meats—fish, poultry, or lean red (1 serving = 3–4 oz.)	1	1–2	2–3
Legumes (1 serving = 6 oz.)	1	1–2	1–2

For vegetarian women, it is wise to eat the recommended amount of the dairy products and eggs to meet protein and calcium needs, as well as to eat more whole grains and legumes. If milk consumption is minimized, more tofu, legumes, nuts and seeds, and leafy greens and some calcium supplement are recommended. More care in balancing the diet is usually necessary whenever the diet limits specific food groups. Additional protein powder or supplemental amino acids (free form), as powder or capsules (750–1,500 mg. daily) may be useful if the protein intake is not sufficient.

For healthy breastfeeding, mother's comfort is important. To maintain good milk production, use both breasts regularly and relax before and after nursing. Remember, good fluid and nutrient intake is essential for successful nursing and thus to the growth and development of the baby. Many women tell me that using olive or coconut oil on their nipples keeps their skin healthier and aids nursing. (See earlier *Infancy* program for further discussion of nursing.)

The nutrient program shown in the table gives the range of values from the minimum requirements to the optimum amounts for the needs of lactation. Refer to the table in the previous section on *Pregnancy* for comparison with the nutrient needs listed here. The following program refers to the combined intake of diet and nutritional supplements. Chloride, fluoride, phosphorus, potassium, and sodium are not usually supplemented unless shown by testing to be needed.

NUTRIENT PROGRAM FOR LACTATION
(RANGE—RDAS TO OPTIMUM)

Calories*	2,600–3,500		
Fiber	15–30 g.		
Protein*	65–90 g.		

Vitamin A*	7,000–10,000 IUs	Calcium*	1,200–1,600 mg.
Beta-carotene	5,000–15,000 IUs	Chloride+	2–4 g.
Vitamin D	400–600 IUs	Chromium	200–400 mcg.
Vitamin E*	60–400 IUs	Copper	2–3 mg.
Vitamin K	100–400 mcg.	Fluoride+	1.5–3.5 mg.
Thiamine (B₁)	1.6–25.0 mg.	Iodine*	200–400 mcg.
Riboflavin (B₂)	1.7–25.0 mg.	Iron*	50–100 mg.
Niacin (B₃)	18–100 mg.	Magnesium*	450–1,000 mg.
Pantothenic acid (B₅)	7–250 mg.	Manganese	2.5–15 mg.
Pyridoxine (B₆)	2.5–100 mg.	Molybdenum	150–500 mcg.
Cobalamin (B₁₂)	4–200 mcg.	Phosphorus*+	1,200–1,600 mg.
Folic acid*	600–1,000 mcg.	Potassium+	2–5 g.
Biotin	200–500 mcg.	Selenium	150–300 mcg.
Choline	100–250 mg.	Sodium+	2.5–4.0 g.
Inositol	100–250 mg.	Zinc*	25–40 mg.
PABA	25–100 mg.		
Vitamin C*	100–2,000 mg.		
Bioflavonoids	125–250 mg.		

*These nutrients are needed in higher than usual amounts during lactation.
+These nutrients are required in the diet, although they are not usually supplemented.

Menopause and Bone Health

Menopause represents a major transition period in the lives of most women. That is why it is called the "change of life." Women experience a decreased production of sex hormones by the ovaries, and many times there are symptoms representative of estrogen deficiency and withdrawal. Men may also experience some "change of life," but usually this is fairly mild compared to what women experience.

Most women enter menopause between the ages of 45 and 50, but it may occur anywhere between 40 and 55. Those whose ovaries are surgically removed before they have entered menopause will almost immediately experience menopausal symptoms and often are placed on estrogen alone or hormone replacement therapy (HRT), using estrogen and progesterone to simulate their natural cycle. While estrogen therapy or HRT is helpful to most women, there are potential risks and side effects, so many women eventually want to shift to a more natural program and go off synthetic hormones. The discussion here is therefore oriented toward a natural program of diet, nutritional supplements and herbs to minimize menopausal symptoms and enhance vitality.

The symptoms of menopause include a change in the frequency or volume of blood flow of the periods (or actual cessation of menstrual periods), irritability, hot flashes and night sweats, emotional swings, headaches, depression, insomnia, loss of sex drive, and weight changes. More internal metabolic shifts, such as the bone loss of calcium, may also occur.

There are many factors that influence the intensity of symptoms and probably even the time they appear. A poor diet, emotional stress, and lack of exercise may lead to an increase in symptoms, particularly when these lifestyle habits have been going on for years. Women who become aware of these relationships prior to menopause and change their habits to help build themselves up with diet and supplements, and deal with their stressful issues will most assuredly have an easier time. Not all women have a difficult menopause; some may not even experience symptoms at all.

A good diet along with supportive nutritional supplements and stress management may help to delay the onset of menopause and reduce symptoms when it does occur. Of other positive lifestyle habits, regular exercise is the most important. It strengthens the bones and improves calcium metabolism. It may also help mobilize some stored estrogen from the fatty tissues, which may make for an easier transition. Outdoor exercise, such as walking, bicycling, swimming, golf, or tennis, will add sunlight and thus aid the body's vitamin D production, and so improve calcium utilization.

During menopause, it is wise for women to get adequate sleep and even take naps if they feel tired. Menopause can often be a time of lowered energy. Stress reduction and dealing with the concerns and worries about aging are important. Embracing maturity and wisdom adds a positive attitude and supports this process. Drinking plenty of water helps keep the body vital and young, with the internal processes functioning best.

A diet that contains vital and wholesome foods will support a stronger life force and the ability to better handle changes. As I have emphasized throughout this book, a vital diet is one that includes fresh fruits and vegetables, whole grains, nuts, seeds, and legumes; with fish, poultry, eggs, milk products, and cold-pressed oils used in moderation; and sugar, refined flour products, other refined processed foods, cured meats, fried foods, and chemicals avoided.

A diet with good quantity and quality of protein and one high in B complex foods may help delay the onset of menopause by supporting the pituitary gland, which regulates the ovaries and the female cycle. (It appears that strict vegetarian women and those with low cholesterol levels have an earlier menopause than more omnivorous women; further research in this area may help us to understand more about diet, cholesterol, and menopause.) Some of the protein foods suggested are fish, milk products such as yogurt and cottage cheese, eggs, whole grains and legumes, nuts, and seeds; foods high in B vitamins are green vegetables, whole grains, wheat germ, and yeast. Good levels of pantothenic acid, choline, and inositol also aid the adrenal and pituitary functions. Special foods that offer high amounts of vitamins, minerals, and energy include brewer's yeast, molasses, lecithin, and kelp (or other seaweeds). These can be used with milk or juice to make a high-nutrient drink.

Osteoporosis is a loss of bone minerals, density, and bone strength, particularly of the spine and long bones of the arms and legs; it is a common problem of menopausal women. Osteoporosis is a difficult problem to diagnose. Regular x-rays are not that sensitive, and they reveal bone loss only after it is fairly significant. The new technique available to measure bone density, photon absorbtiometry, is more sensitive at assessing early osteoporosis. Generally, though, women should be aware of early warning signs, such as periodontal disease, changes in the curvature of the spinal column, such as a "dowager's hump," or pain in the middle or lower back. The most important factor is preventing the loss of bone calcium; this is much easier than correcting bone loss after it occurs.

To prevent osteoporosis, it is wise to eat a good diet and maintain an adequate calcium intake through foods and supplements in the years before menopause. Many people eat a diet that is much higher in phosphorus than in calcium. This can lead to improper bone metabolism and loss of bone calcium. Meats, nuts, seeds, poultry, boneless seafood, and even whole grains have a much higher phosphorus than calcium content. Soda pops have added phosphates, increasing their phosphorus level. One advantage of using milk products is that they have a very good calcium-to-phosphorus ratio, with actually slightly more calcium. Eggs and many vegetables, especially the green leafy veggies, also have lower phosphorus content.

Premenopausal women should regularly consume 1,000–1,200 mg. of calcium per day. Supplementing some calcium without phosphorus will usually balance out these nutrients. Adding about 500–1,000 IUs of extra vitamin D and 500–800 mg. of magnesium per day will help the calcium be best utilized and protect against osteoporosis. Adequate boron, a trace mineral, in the diet and supplements to include 2–3 mg. is also shown to aid calcium utilization. A diet containing good amounts of fish, leafy greens, whole grains, and dairy foods will support healthy bones. Phosphorus, zinc, copper, and manganese are also important to building strong bones. If osteoporosis is present, research suggests that estrogen therapy may help slow its progress and even improve the bone health, though it also poses risks. Fluoride, 2–4 mg. per day in foods or even taken as a supplement, has been shown to strengthen bones, but it, likewise, may have other concerns.

When estrogen is used during or after menopause, it is wise to follow a program similar to that suggested for users of birth control pills (if the woman still has a uterus, a progestin agent should also be used to simulate the natural cycle and to protect the uterus from cancer development). Extra vitamins C, E, and B_6, extra zinc, and minimum copper intake are the main suggestions. It is clear that estrogen or hormone replacement therapy does prevent osteoporosis, possibly better than any other program, especially with a good diet, adequate calcium intake, and plenty of exercise. Regular exercise has clearly been shown to minimize bone loss, especially postmenopausally. Weight-bearing exercises, such as walking, tennis, or golf, help to strengthen the bones, probably more than swimming. When taking estrogen, usually less calcium is needed than when no hormones are used. Still, a natural program such as the one described here will help prevent osteoporosis and ease the symptoms and transition of menopause. (For more on osteoporosis, see the *Calcium* discussion in Chapter 6.)

Younger women also can develop osteoporosis, usually due to a poor diet, low calcium intake, and excessive vigorous exercise. Dancers, gymnasts, and long-distance runners have this problem most commonly, and it is exaggerated with anorexia and weight loss. These young women often have associated low body fat, low estrogen levels, and irregular or nonexistent menstrual periods. A more nourishing diet, reduced activity, and calcium-vitamin-mineral supplements can help to correct this problem and prevent future ones.

For menopausal hot flashes, irritability, and/or night sweats, supplemental calcium and vitamins D and E will often help. Dong quai herb has also benefited many women with those symptoms. Two capsules taken two or three times daily is the standard usage in this regard. Ginseng has also been helpful, especially when there is associated fatigue. Other herbs that work are some of the female tonics, such as the cohosh herbs, unicorn root, and licorice root. The FE-G and female formulas described in the section on *Premenstrual Syndrome* in Chapter 17 may also be helpful in menopause, as they seem to support estrogen production by stimulating the female organs. Sarsaparilla root has been used as a female herb, and valerian root can be used for insomnia and irritability. Calcium-magnesium is helpful for muscle and back pains or cramps. Kelp tablets have been used to support thyroid function, which helps women through the changes of menopause. Iron is still needed in premenopausal amounts until there is no more bleeding; then the iron requirements decrease from 18–10 mg. per day.

The nutrient program presented here includes dietary plus supplemental needs. Nutrients such as chloride, phosphorus, fluoride, sodium, and potassium are usually not supplemented, but obtained from diet. The ranges allow for individual comfort in using the higher amounts, which may be best for this program. (See the following program for the *Elderly* for further information. The programs on *Anti-Aging* and *Anti-Stress* in Chapter 16 may also provide assistance to the menopausal woman.)

MENOPAUSE NUTRIENT PROGRAM

Protein	45–80 g.		
Vitamin A	5,000–10,000 IUs	Copper	1–2 mg.
Beta-carotene	15,000–20,000 IUs	Fluoride*	2–4 mg.
Vitamin D	400–1000 IUs	Iodine*	150–300 mcg.
Vitamin E	800–1,000 IUs	Iron	10–18 mg.
Vitamin K*	150–400 mcg.	Magnesium+	600–1,000 mg.
Thiamine (B$_1$)	50–100 mg.	Manganese	2.5–15 mg.
Riboflavin (B$_2$)	25–50 mg.	Molybdenum	150–500 mcg.
Niacinamide (B$_3$)	50–100 mg.	Phosphorus*	800–1,000 mg.
Pantothenic acid (B$_5$)	100–750 mg.	Potassium	3–5 g.
Pyridoxine (B$_6$)	50–250 mg.	Selenium	100–300 mcg.
Cobalamin (B$_{12}$)	30–100 mcg.	Zinc	15–30 mg.
Folic acid	400–800 mcg.		
Biotin	50–500 mcg.	*Optional:*	
Choline	500–1000 mg.	Lecithin	500–1,000 mg.
Inositol	500–1000 mg.	Primrose oil or	1,000–2,000 mg.
PABA	200–400 mg.	other	1,000–2,000 mg.
Vitamin C	1–3 g.	GLA-containing oil	or 4–6 capsules
Bioflavonoids	250–500 mg.	Hydrochloric acid (with meals)	1 or 2 tablets
Boron	2–3 mg.		
Calcium+	1,200–1,500 mg.	Digestive enzymes (after meals)	1 or 2 tablets
Chromium	150–400 mcg.		

*These will not usually be supplemented in the diet, or for fluoride, it may be in the water.
+The dietary levels of calcium and magnesium should also be considered in these totals.

The Elderly

This program is designed primarily for people over age 65, an age group that continues to increase in numbers in our society. An important point I would like to state early is that we need to care for ourselves in our younger years so that we can stay healthy in our older ones. Also, our society needs to learn to better care for our elders and to incorporate them into a meaningful life to keep them feeling useful and youthful.

Being old or aging is as much a state of mind involving how we live and our attitude toward life as it is a physical condition. Of course, our genetics are also important. Some people become old in their 50s and 60s, while others only really start to age (or degenerate) a year or two before they die in their 80s or 90s. Psychologically, even some young people are old. They are limited and resist change and lose the positive energy and love of life. Youth, like age, is really a state of mind.

With regard to nutritional status, elderly people are sometimes even more difficult to nourish than teenagers. Many are resentful or rebellious and eat an unbalanced diet consisting of a limited number of foods. Malnutrition is fairly common in the elderly, with low calorie and protein intakes, as well as many deficiencies of important vitamins and minerals. Many elders eat less because of such reasons as apathy, diminished sense of taste and smell, poor teeth, low income, or inability to obtain or prepare foods, and they further have reduced digestion and absorption, which makes their intake needs even higher than usual. The government RDAs become relatively meaningless for the elderly; they simply need more nutrients!

Many old-age problems, such as insomnia, anorexia, fatigue, depression, diminishing eyesight and hearing, fragile bones, and fractures, are a result of poor diets and nutritional deficiencies. This can also lead to a weakened immune system and more infections. The thymus gland, which produces the important T lymphocytes that mediate the cellular immune system and help to regulate antibody formation, tends to diminish in activity with aging—especially with a low vitality diet, living under stress, and possible emotional factors, such as loss of friends and relatives, anxieties of aging and loneliness, and depression—thus leading to problems of weakened resistance, infections, and sometimes cancer. Tissue weakness due to lack of cellular support can lead to decreased skin protection and increased aging of the skin. Free-radical formation and a reduction of neurotransmitter chemicals, such as acetylcholine, gamma-aminobutyric acid (GABA), glycine, L-glutamine, norepinephrine, and serotonin, caused by deficiencies of amino acids and the B vitamins including inositol and choline—all may contribute to aging, internally and externally, mentally and physically. (This is discussed further in the *Anti-Aging* Program in Chapter 16.)

Most elderly people have reduced production of gastric hydrochloric acid, which minimizes the breakdown of complex carbohydrates, fats, and proteins. The general function of the other digestive organs, such as the pancreas, which produces digestive enzymes, is also reduced. Often the digestive lining does not function as it once did, and absorption of nutrients, particularly minerals, decreases.

COMMON DEFICIENCIES IN THE ELDERLY

Calories	Potassium	Vitamin B_1
Protein	Zinc	Vitamin B_2
Fiber	Chromium	Vitamin B_6
Fluids	Iron	Vitamin B_{12}
Calcium	Copper	Folic acid
Magnesium	Vitamin A	Vitamin C

Many elderly people simply do not obtain enough calories. Calorie count can be easily increased with more food, but it is important that it be more nutrient-rich food, so that the important vitamins and minerals are also provided. Less protein may be needed for tissue production, but because of poorer assimilation, as much protein as usual is needed. Amino acid intake is necessary to build cells, for energy, and for tissue repair.

Fiber, in foods and as a supplement, is very important to colon health and function. It reduces the incidence of colon cancer and possibly other types of cancer, as well as pulling some chemical toxins from the body. Eating more fresh fiber foods, such as vegetables and whole grains, offers many other benefits as well. Extra bran (insoluble fiber) or psyllium (soluble fiber) will help bowel function when natural-fiber foods are not eaten in sufficient quantities. Constipation, a common problem in the elderly, can be reduced and eliminated with adequate fiber and water.

Fluid intake by older people may also be low. Drinking enough clean water is crucial to good internal organ function for clearing impurities and for waste elimination. It also keeps the skin healthier and prevents dehydration, which may lead to all kinds of problems.

A number of common vitamin and mineral deficiencies occur in the elderly, mainly from not consuming enough fresh, nutrient-rich foods. Vitamin A is commonly low, and this can lead to poor vision, dry skin, and weakened immunity. Thiamine and riboflavin (B_1 and B_2) may not be adequate in the diet because of low intake of whole grains, and this may affect the skin and energy level. Pyridoxine (B_6) is often low, especially with avoidance of whole foods and with eating refined flour products. Folic acid may be deficient because of avoidance of leafy greens, and vitamin B_{12} may be inadequate because of both low intake and poor absorption. Folic acid and vitamin B_{12}

are important for building blood cells and for energy. Supplemental B_{12}, even through injections, is often helpful for enhancing energy levels in the elderly. Vitamin C intake may also be inadequate, because of avoidance of citrus fruits and fresh, raw vegetables; this deficiency may lead to poor tissue health, healing abilities, and disease resistance.

The diets of the elderly population are often deficient in many minerals. In fact, deficiencies of minerals and hydrochloric acid (HCl)—needed for adequate absorption of most minerals, such as iron, calcium, and zinc—are very common. This inadequacy of digestion by limited production of HCl (and digestive enzymes) may well in fact be one of the most common health factors affecting the elderly, though it may be less obvious than some more externalized problems. Vitamin B_{12} absorption may also be low because of weak intrinsic factor, which is produced by the same parietal cells that produce hydrochloric acid. Calcium intake is one of the biggest concerns. Calcium deficiency is more common in women than in men. Low-calcium foods, lack of exercise, low hydrochloric acid, and poor digestion lessen calcium availability. Antacids, especially those containing aluminum, are best avoided because of their interference with calcium absorption and the possibility of aluminum toxicity, which has been implicated in Alzheimer's disease and other types of senility. Avoiding both aluminum cookware and the storage or heating of foods in aluminum foil are also good ideas. Imbalances among calcium, phosphorus, and magnesium and possibly low levels of vitamin D also affect calcium bone metabolism. Magnesium in the diet (whole grains, nuts, seeds) may also be low, while phosphorus intake is often normal or elevated, and excess phosphorus may allow even more bone loss when calcium is deficient. Occasionally, older people with arthritis avoid calcium with the support of their doctors. However, there is no reason for that. With arthritis, calcium is being lost from the bones and may precipitate in the joints, but this is a result of the mineral imbalance. Calcium is needed in balance with phosphorus, magnesium, boron, and vitamin D.

Decreased absorption and limitations in the diet may affect the levels of most of the minerals as well. Iron may be low, but fortunately there is less need for it in the elderly. If anemia is present, check for iron levels as well as B_{12}, folic acid, copper, and protein. Iron-rich foods such as meat, even liver, may be used occasionally for their good protein and other nutrient contents. Copper, important to many energy and enzyme systems, can be obtained from whole grains, nuts, seeds, and many vegetables, and is very high in oysters. Zinc, which is necessary for immune function, acid-base balance, tissue healing, and the prevention of aging, is also often inadequate in the diet. Low immune function due to zinc deficiency is frequently a factor in infections, cancer, and cardio-vascular problems. Zinc is present in many of the same foods as copper.

One of the most commonly deficient minerals is chromium, which is sparse in the soil and foods, and often poorly absorbed. Chromium is important to the proper use of blood sugar, functioning in glucose tolerance factor (GTF) to support the function of insulin. Supplemental chromium is often helpful, and brewer's yeast, if tolerated, is one of the better foods for supplying this mineral.

715

Potassium may also be deficient, because of low intake of vegetables and higher intake of salt. Sodium, chloride, and potassium are the body electrolytes that help balance acid-base chemistry and fluid movement. With weakened kidney function, which is not uncommon in the elderly, electrolyte imbalances occur. Adding potassium in food and supplements and diminishing salt intake will help restore the balance.

Many medicines may interfere with mineral absorption and function. Antacids may bind calcium, as mentioned earlier, as well as other minerals, such as zinc or magnesium. Many diuretic drugs stimulate the kidneys to clear more potassium, lessening body stores. When these drugs are prescribed by a physician, this is often carefully watched, and potassium may then be supplemented. But the diuretics, which are commonly used by the elderly, also increase clearance of zinc, magnesium, and other minerals, and these are not always replaced, so that deficiencies of these minerals can result. Antibiotics can reduce colon flora, a source for the production of B vitamins and vitamin K. This can limit many intestinal functions in any age group. Laxatives can also cause loss of nutrients, and mineral oil, used more frequently years ago, can bind the fat-soluble vitamins A, D, E, and K.

Dietary factors that should be monitored include excessive consumption of simple sugars and total fats. Intake of sugar, refined foods, and other nonnutrient calories should be minimized. High intakes of sugar will increase blood fats, which will speed up aging and atherosclerosis. Dietary fat is also best kept at a minimum. Lower levels of stomach acid and reduced production of digestive enzymes make fat harder to process. There are more nutritious foods than the fatty foods, though some dairy products, if tolerated, may be helpful. Low-fat or nonfat milk is probably better than whole, unless we are trying to gain weight.

Prevention of aging is very important. There are many aspects to this; the psychological ones are the most significant. The time to prevent growing old is between the ages of 40 and 60, when a good, well-balanced diet high in vitamins, minerals, and other basic nutrients, and low in fats and refined foods is crucial. Of course, this type of supportive nutrition does not become less important in the senior years. How we lived yesterday affects us today, and what we do today will influence our future. Our whole attitude toward life and how we live our days is really what we are looking at here. The way we feed ourselves is an outcome of our self-image, knowledge, conditioning, education, self-love, and desire to live and be healthy.

The diet of the elderly should contain a variety of foods. This is often a challenge because of past experience, eccentric likes and dislikes, economics, and the state of health of the teeth and oral cavity. Good teeth or dentures are very important to a healthy diet. Sometimes, whole food groups may be omitted because of inability to chew them. If chewing is a problem, more fresh vegetable juices should be drunk; pureed foods, particularly vegetables, and cooled whole-grain cereals will add a lot of nutrition. Even balanced protein-nutrient drinks may be better than not eating. All of these foods add water content to the diet as well.

Sufficient fluids and fiber are crucial to any elder's diet. Fluids are important to prevent constipation and dry skin. Keeping everything moving in the tissues, circulatory system, and intestinal tract is a vital part of feeling good. Stagnation due to poor flow and dehydration can shut us down physiologically and psychologically. Good flow on all levels is essential to regaining health and staying well. Fluid intake should be enough to produce three to four pints of urine a day. More water, herbal teas, juices, and soups, as well as fresh fruits and vegetables (all water-content foods) will help.

The older body usually uses fewer calories, while the percentage of body fat may rise. Problems of both underweight and overweight occur commonly in the elderly and are often harder to correct at this time of life. At this age, a little (5–10 pounds) excess weight is probably healthier than being underweight. Being too heavy, though, is hard on the bones; in addition, obesity increases the risk of cardiovascular disease and cancer. The three health monitors we do not wish to let rise too much as we age are blood pressure, cholesterol levels, and weight. To maintain weight, it is wise to eat a diet containing the calories required for our ideal weight at ages 25–30. A nutritionist, dietician, or doctor should be able to help with calculation of these caloric needs.

Remember, though, those calories need to contain nutrients. Some meats and dairy products may be used to obtain appropriate amounts of protein and vitamin B_{12}. Supplemental amino acids with good levels of methionine and lysine are helpful for protein building when protein food intake or energy is low, since they may be more easily utilized as they do not need to go through digestion. It is important to include plenty of fresh fruits and vegetables (raw and steamed, and even vegetable juices and soups), and the whole-grain cereals and legumes. These high-nutrient foods contain some calcium and other nutrients that are helpful to bone health.

Older people who are not currently on a wholesome diet can make a slow transition over one or two months to more natural foods. This means a reduction of refined foods, canned and packaged foods, and devitalized foods. It may be helpful to make these changes gradually, so as to allay the threat of upheaval. Though it is more difficult to change our ways as we age, these positive changes are still possible and very helpful. Remember, if we eat vital foods, we will be vital!

Think of a few people in their 60s, 70s, or 80s. What do you think has led to their degeneration or to their health and vitality? What are you planning for your anti–aging program? Have you already begun?

Avoiding overeating and underactivity is important, because this nondynamic duo can be disastrous. Likewise, a poor appetite can result from lack of exercise with poor utilization and circulation of previously obtained nutrients. Exercise is necessary at all stages of life, and it is no different for the elderly. Not only will it improve the appetite and the desire for better foods, it may significantly improve our attitude toward life. Exercise is a key to bone health, helping prevent osteoporosis. It will also improve other functions—digestion, assimilation, and circulation, as well as muscle tone. Walking, swimming, and dancing are probably the best all-around exercises for older folks, though any may be suitable depending on past history and present condition. If you are not exercising regularly, it is wise to build up endurance slowly to a good active program. It will help in all walks of life.

Often there may not be as much enthusiasm for good nutrition, exercise, and life in general in the elderly. When the body is not working as well, it is not as much fun to take it out for a spin. That is why it is so important to care for ourselves well in earlier years so that we can maintain our vitality and spirit. Creating more support programs for the elderly, plus training programs for those who care for the elderly, will help our society and each of us in our later years.

Loneliness and isolation from family and other loved ones are common for the elderly. Death of a spouse may leave the remaining partner without the enthusiasm or capability to care for him or herself. Encouraging and supporting these folks to attend group or community meals and find new friends can make a big difference. Sharing meals and visiting with relatives may have a special meaning and be a primary encouragement to living. Extended family and local community meetings and meals, especially if they have good food, can be very supportive to many elderly people. Engaging one another in exercise activities, such as walking, hikes, or classes, will help in socializing with peers and boosting morale. Interactive, nurturing therapies, such as counseling or massage, can be very helpful at reducing resistances and enhancing physical energy and flexibility. Our society also needs to learn better how to incorporate this growing age group (in years and in numbers of people) into the functioning community. Connecting our elderly people with the support or care of young children, I believe, is an ideal approach. Young children and elderly people often seem to have a special magic together.

For single people who cook mainly for themselves, here are some suggestions to economize, be practical, and still eat well. Sharing cooking and meals with a friend or two will allow easier preparation, easier shopping, and reduced costs, especially if the friends take turns shopping and cooking. The more people that food is prepared for, the lower the cost per person. If you are cooking just for yourself, buy smaller quantities of food and prepare simpler meals. With many foods, it is wiser to make extra portions, enough for a day or two. Soups, grains, and casseroles will refrigerate well and can be used over two or three days. Meat dishes and other foods can be packaged in individual meal sizes and frozen for later use. If the appetite is not too good, it is still wise to eat regularly, with smaller, nutritious meals. Many quick-fix foods should be on hand; eggs, yogurt, and instant whole-grain cereals are some examples. Nutritional yeast and molasses can be used in blender fruit drinks, with or without milk, a raw egg, and a piece or two of fruit such as banana or pear (if this is supported by the digestion; it's not perfect food combining).

Prune juice and bran are common laxative foods to help keep the elimination regular and avoid the problem of constipation. A morning or evening drink made with 4–6 ounces of prune juice, 2–4 ounces of water, a quarter or half lemon, and 2 tablespoons of wheat or oat bran should do the trick.

Overall, good nutrition is a vital part of any senior's health plan—one of the best buys in the health insurance market. Maintaining regular activity and exercise is equally important. Drinking plenty of pure water, avoiding processed and chemical foods, and eating lots of fiber foods, such as the fruits, vegetables, and whole grains, are basic nutritional guidelines for staying healthy. Avoiding or minimizing the use of unnecessary pharmaceutical medications and other drugs, such as nicotine, caffeine, and alcohol, is also important. Most of the above suggestions will help to prevent or slow the aging process. Additional antioxidant nutrients are also a good idea. Many of these free-radical scavengers are included in this program (they are further discussed in the *Anti-Aging* program in Chapter 16).

**IMPORTANT FACTORS TO
GOOD HEALTH FOR THE ELDERLY**

Regular meals
Low-fat, high-fiber diet
Exercise
Nutritional supplements

There are many herbs that may be helpful to aging people, including ginseng root, Gingko biloba, and gotu kola leaf. Ginseng has long been used in the Orient to relieve fatigue and strengthen people. Known as the "longevity" herb, it is used regularly by elderly Chinese men and women to slow the aging process. Ginseng tea bags, powder, or concentrate can be used in hot water to make tea and a couple of cups drunk daily. One or two capsules of powdered ginseng root can be taken twice daily to give a feeling of greater strength. Raw pieces of the hard root can be sucked or chewed, but this is not as potent as the tea. Be aware that excessive use of ginseng root can elevate the blood pressure (as can licorice root) and possibly irritate the gastrointestinal mucosa. The trace mineral germanium has been found to be in high concentration in ginseng. Gingko biloba, another popular oriental herb from the leaves of an ancient tree, has been more recently used in this country to help with circulatory problems, senility, and hearing disorders (see further discussion of these herbs in Chapter 7).

Gotu kola herb is more popular in India, where it also has an ancient tradition. It acts as a brain stimulant, strengthening the memory and other mental powers. Gotu kola can be taken as a tea or in capsules, by itself or with other herbs. In Western medicine, a drug that has been fairly popular among the elderly population (as well as with young men who want to appear alert and quick-witted) is hydergine. It is a cerebral stimulant that improves memory and mental clarity, with very few side effects. It is now used very commonly in people with senility and poor memory.

Among elderly men, prostate enlargement affecting urine flow and possibly leading to prostate surgery is very common. A swelling of the fibromuscular prostate gland can result from such factors as a high-protein, high-fat diet and insufficient activity, both physical and sexual. A diet that is low in chemicals, fried foods, and fats in general and high in fresh foods with good liquid and nutrient content will help things to move better and keep the prostate healthy. Regular exercise and stretching, especially yoga-type inverted positions, and maintaining some sexual activity also offer preventive benefits. Nutrients such as vitamins A, C, and E and other antioxidants, especially zinc, may be helpful in reducing or preventing prostate problems. Herbs such as saw palmetto berries, corn silk tea, parsley, ginger root, marshmallow root, juniper berries, and uva ursi have also been helpful to many men with prostate problems. An encapsulated formula with some of these herbs taken three times daily or a tea drunk two or three times daily could be tried for a month or two. Refer to an herbal text for further information on these and other herbs related to the prostate or the aging process.

Most people in their later years would be helped by an easy-to-digest, well-balanced vitamin and mineral formula for nutritional insurance. There are very few people over 60 who do not have some symptoms of early chronic illness—the body degenerates slowly, blood vessels get clogged, senses may diminish, and digestion and assimilation may weaken. So it is wise to use a nutritional supplement to ensure the best chance for the body to get plenty of what it needs for proper functioning. Many of the nutrients offer some protection against inflammation, regulate blood clotting, improve immune function, and improve fat metabolism by helping the body to handle cholesterol and triglycerides. Several high-quality powdered and encapsulated general formulas, which are easier to digest and assimilate, are available from companies such as Nutricology in San Leandro, California; DeBuren International in Mill Valley, California; Karuna Corporation in Novato, California; and TwinLab, in Ronkonkoma, New York. There are many others; check your local health food store or pharmacy.

As with the other programs, the nutrient ranges in the table here are from minimum needs, which may be obtained through diet and/or a basic daily supplement, to optimum insurance levels, which may require higher-dose formulas or even vitamin injections. For the elderly, because of poor digestive function, a powdered general formula taken a few times daily will improve the chances of absorbing sufficient amounts of many important, though hard-to-assimilate nutrients. Many seniors are also helped by digestive aids such as extra hydrochloric acid prior to meals and pancreatic enzymes in between meals to improve the breakdown of food. Some of the formulas I mentioned above, such as DeBuren's Optimum I and II, also contain these digestive aids to help the nutients be better utilized.

When high amounts of supplemental fiber, such as wheat bran, are used (I recommend eating more high-fiber foods), more vitamins and particularly more minerals may be needed to make up for those pulled out through the colon by the fiber. Extra B vitamins are often needed to support function. Usually, double levels of most of the B vitamins are suggested. I think doubling the intake of most of the hard-to-absorb minerals, such as chromium and zinc, can help as well.

Remember, common deficiencies in the elderly include vitamins A, B_1, B_2, B_6, B_{12}, and C, folic acid, and the minerals calcium, magnesium, zinc, iron, chromium, and other trace minerals. Calcium, magnesium, and vitamin D are important to support a continued healthy skeleton. Plenty of water and good quality vegetable oils (cold-pressed) are also important to keep the skin and tissues healthy. The following table offers some guidelines for setting up a good supplement program.

DIETARY NUTRIENT PROGRAM FOR THE ELDERLY*
(RANGE—RDA TO OPTIMUM)

Calories	Men —1,900–2,600
	Women —1,600–2,200
Protein	60–80 g.

Vitamin A	5,000–10,000 IUs	**Chromium**	200–500 mcg.
Beta-carotene	10,000–20,000 IUs	**Copper**	2–3 mg.
Vitamin D	200–600 IUs	**Fluoride***	1.5–4.0 mg.
Vitamin E**	60–1,000 IUs	**Iodine***	150–300 mcg.
Vitamin K	100–300 mcg.	**Iron**	10–20 mg.
Thiamine (B_1)	1.5–50.0 mg.	**Magnesium**	400–800 mg.
Riboflavin (B_2)	1.5–50.0 mg.	**Manganese**	3–15 mg.
Niacin (B_3)	16–100 mg.	**Molybdenum**	150–500 mcg.
Niacinamide (B_3)	50–100 mg.	**Phosphorus***	800–1,200 mg.
Pantothenic Acid (B_5)	7–500 mg.	**Potassium***	2–5 g.
Pyridoxine (B_6)	2.5–50.0 mg.	**Selenium**	150–300 mcg.
Pyridoxal-5-phosphate	20–50 mg.	**Silicon**	50–100 mg.
Cobalamin (B_{12})**	10–500 mcg.	**Sodium***	1.5–3.0 g.
Folic acid	400–800 mcg.	**Zinc**	15–60 mg.
Biotin	150–400 mcg.		
Choline	250–1,000 mg.	**Hydrochloric acid**	5–10 g.,
Inositol	250–1,000 mg.	**(as betaine or**	or
PABA	25–100 mg.	**glutamic acid)**	1–2 tablets
Vitamin C	60–3,000 mg.	**(prior to or**	
Bioflavonoids	125–500 mg.	**with meals)**	
Boron	1–2 mg.	**Digestive enzymes**	1–2 tablets
Calcium	800–1,500 mg.	**(pancreatic enzymes)**	
Chloride*	2.0–4.0 g.	**(after meals)**	
		Flaxseed or cod liver oil	1 Tablespoon

*As with other life stage support programs, nutrients easily available, such as sodium, chloride, phosphorus, sulfur, and potassium, are not usually supplemented unless there is a deficiency. Of these, potassium may be more commonly supplemented due to poor nutrition or medication.

**Can go up to 1600–2400 IUs for intermittent claudication.

***Vitamin B_{12} is commonly used as an injection in the elderly, at least several times a year, to help build up tissue stores.

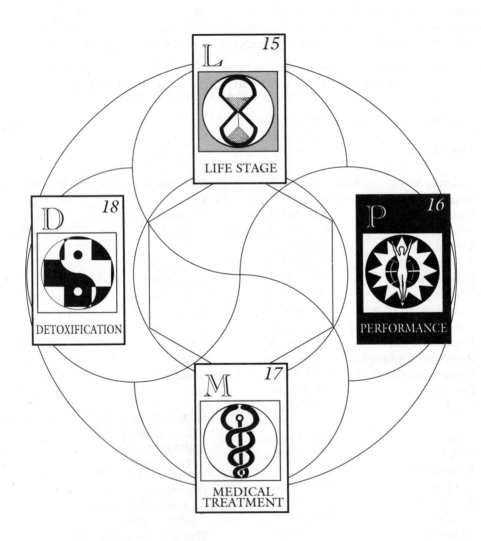

L **15**
LIFE STAGE

D **18**
DETOXIFICATION

P **16**
PERFORMANCE

M **17**
MEDICAL
TREATMENT

Chapter 16

Performance Enhancement Programs

Yep! This is the chapter for PEP! These special Performance Enhancement Programs focus upon optimizing certain body areas such as our skin or immune function; preventing problems in special situations, such as when eating a vegetarian diet, traveling, or doing extensive exercise; protecting us from certain chronic conditions, such as the negative effects of pollution, or from developing cancer or cardiovascular disease; supporting our life processes, such as our sexuality, minimizing the aging process, or reducing stress.

So much of our health is up to us. We can only realize with time and experience that the more energy, work, and commitment we put into our health and well-being on all levels, the better body and function, i.e., performance, we will manifest.

These PEPs are designed to give you the information and know-how to take the best care of yourself, have your body perform optimally and help you be your own best diagnostician should certain problems occur. The next chapter, *Medical Treatment Programs*, is more geared to fixing health problems; for those programs, you will need to learn more medicine (which will be discussed) to understand better how your beautiful body-machine works so you know what is going on when it is not running right.

Some of medicine is mechanical, but much is not. An intuitive art can never be replaced by technology. Your own self-awareness in regard to your spectrum of health is part of your goal. Learning to listen to what is out of sync and adapt your lifestyle, by changing your diet, taking certain supplements, reducing or increasing activity level, or changing life direction in some way, are your basic tools for healing—and believe me, they can aid your body to repair many existing and potential problems. Just being able to listen to and attune your inner self and make the necessary shifts based on whatever messages you receive is the beginning and the foundation of true healing and being your own doctor.

Anti-Aging: The Longevity Program

In this section, the basic process of physical and mental aging as it relates to many of the chronic degenerative, and sometimes fatal, diseases will be explored. This program can be used in conjunction with other programs, such as *Immune Enhancement*, *Anti-Stress*, *Cancer Prevention*, *Sexual Vitality*, *Cardiovascular Disease Prevention*, and *Skin Enhancement*. For example, since this *Anti-Aging* plan may help to prevent both cellular and DNA changes, reduce the level of mutagenic cells and decrease the impact of environmental chemicals, it may help us prevent the twentieth-century plague of cancer.

This program can also take us beyond just learning to be healthy; it can lead to an enhancement of vitality in our elderly years so that we can experience the fruits of our years of labor and embrace more the wisdom and joys of life. Aging is not inevitable. To live 100–110 years in a healthy state is not out of the question if we just take care of ourselves in regard to diet, exercise, and the many other factors discussed here. Though it may be difficult in our younger years, we will look back and know the worth of our efforts as we enjoy feeling good and staying youthful. The goals of this program are twofold: first, to increase longevity by preventing and decreasing the potential for and progression of degenerative disease and, second, to improve the vitality and tissue health of the body through proper nutrient support.

There is, of course, a wide individual variation in the aging process. Genetics and constitutional factors will make some people more predisposed to problems in such areas as the cardiovascular system and circulation, skin, or memory. But with better care and by following some of the guidelines of this program, those less fortunately endowed can increase their potential and lengthen their years on Earth, while those genetically well-endowed people will further increase their health and longevity.

The aging process does not have to reach a level that interferes with function. The Baltimore Longitudinal Study of Aging, almost 30 years old itself with no gray hair, has shown that many healthy older people can have cardiovascular systems and memories as functional as those of much younger people. It is true that to keep the body fit, we need to exercise it, and to keep the mind sharp, we must also give it a regular workout. Unless there are specific health problems, particularly with the circulation, our memory should not really diminish until a late stage of life. Similarly, sexual hormones, particularly in men, are present and active in the later years, most assuredly in those who have been sexually active and who have maintained their activity into their 60s, 70s, and 80s. Sex is not just young people's activity.

The program presented here can be employed by anyone over 40 years of age, especially those who wish to begin the protective, antiaging process early, though it can also be utilized in later years. This *Anti-Aging* program can also be useful to those under stress or with demanding jobs, as well as people who push themselves in work or have trouble dealing with day-to-day demands. People who live in cities and those whose work or life exposes them to chemicals may benefit from many of the suggestions here. Those on diets of processed foods, red meats and cured meats, and other chemical foods would do well to change these habits and follow the *Anti-Aging* plan for at least six months to experience the benefits. Smokers, alcohol drinkers, and those who have used other drugs that contribute to body breakdown are also candidates for this program, which can reverse some of the damaging effects. There are other programs for most of the above-mentioned concerns in Part Four.

Problems of the Aging Process

The most common problems of aging affect the cardiovascular and nervous systems, as in atherosclerosis and senility. Others include arthritis, cancer, diabetes, certain immunological diseases, gastrointestinal problems, such as diverticulosis, and skin diseases. People with these problems or those who want to prevent them can utilize either this program or one more specific to their condition. Here we explore some of the common physiological effects of aging that generate many of these diseases. Most of these lifestyle-related diseases, of course, come about when we do not take the best care of ourselves. Many subtle and gross changes in the cardiovascular and respiratory systems lead to poor delivery of oxygen and nutrients to the tissues. In conjunction with an insufficiency of the necessary nutrients coming into the body, this is the most important underlying factor in most problems of aging. Many other changes occur in the heart and circulation prior to the diminished nutrient supply. A reduction in heart pumping action with decreased lung capacity reduces oxygen delivery and increases carbon dioxide buildup. An increase in blood vessel stiffness and blood pressure with age also diminishes circulation. Many aspects of living, such as smoking, a high-fat diet, and lack of exercise, affect these changes. Other diseases, such as diabetes and hypertension, contribute to further problems of atherosclerosis, abnormal heart function, and reduced circulation.

The nervous system can also be affected, with a slowing of nerve conduction, loss of brain weight, reduced reflexes, and a decrease in memory and learning capacity. Dementia or senility may result from the diminishing nervous system function along with the cardiovascular effects of reduced circulation. Brain neurotransmitters are vital to nerve conductivity and brain function. Acetylcholine, norepinephrine, and serotonin, the three main neurotransmitters, are all produced and affected by dietary nutrients, such as choline, pantothenic acid, and the amino acids tyrosine, phenylalanine, and tryptophan. Acetylcholine supports brain function, memory, and sexual activity; norepinephrine also affects sexual and general energy levels, memory, and learning; and serotonin aids relaxation and sleep.

Alzheimer's disease, a common form of senile dementia (loss of mental capacity), has received a lot of attention recently. It often begins earlier (in the 50s) than other types of senility. Theories as to its cause range from aluminum toxicity or sensitivity to an autoimmune process to a virus infection affecting the brain. Cigarette smoking clearly increases the risk of Alzheimer's. Microscopic brain cell and brain tissue changes described as "neurofibrillary tangles" are classic in Alzheimer's disease; the diagnosis is most often accomplished by excluding other possibilities. The main effect seems to be on the "cholinergic" system, which is governed by the neurotransmitter acetylcholine, but other neurotransmitters are probably affected as well. Many treatments have been tried, without much success. Clearing excess aluminum and reducing aluminum intake may be helpful. Lecithin or choline supplements have been helpful in some people.

Other body systems affected by aging include the musculoskeletal system and the gastrointestinal, genitourinary, and endocrine organs. There is often a loss of muscular strength and coordination with aging. There is often some thinning of spinal discs and bones in general, degeneration of cartilage and ligaments, and the loss of tissue elasticity and flexibility. With aging there is a loss of height and an increase in bone fractures. Arthritis becomes more common with the years and leads to greater joint wear and tear. The hips are a common site for both joint pains and arthritis in the elderly.

Good digestive function is important to proper assimilation of nutrients. This begins with good teeth. Teeth are made up of minerals, nutrients that are not well absorbed when there is low stomach acid and pancreatic digestive enzyme function. Good colon function and elimination are also important to prevent constipation and diverticular disease, common problems with aging. Kidney function may also diminish with aging, inhibiting clearance of excess nutrients, chemicals, and toxins. The prostate and sexual organs also need good blood and energy supply to keep them functioning properly.

Many hormonal changes also occur with aging. The basal metabolic rate and thyroid hormone function may diminish, thus decreasing the energy level. Weakened glucose tolerance can lead to more problems with diabetes. Body fat percentages usually increase with age, even with the same dietary intake. Immune functions may also be reduced with the "scavenger" white blood cells becoming less effective, allowing an increase in infections. Cell repair and elimination of defective cells may lessen, leading to an increased incidence of cancer. Autoimmune problems from a misguided immune system may also occur.

Many habits and activities affect these common changes of aging. Factors that increase aging and degeneration include smoking, excess alcohol, fats and chemicals in food, poor or deficient diet, overeating, stress, pollution, and laziness. Psychological factors influencing aging include extreme emotions, negativity, resisting positive suggestions and support, getting trapped in ruts, and hanging onto depression, loneliness, anger, and grief. A positive attitude and psychological health will greatly increase longevity and delay "getting old."

Theories of Aging

My own combined theory of aging is that **stagnation** is the key—stagnation of bioenergy circulation and stagnation of the digestive tract and bowels. Good colon function to prevent toxin buildup, regular exercise to stimulate energy production and circulation of the blood and lymph, dealing properly with extreme emotions and stresses, and maintaining a positive attitude all help to support vitality and circulation on all levels. Chemical irritants and nutritional deficiencies accelerate the aging process. We need to maintain proper food acquisition, digestion, assimilation, and elimination to have long-term health and minimize the aging process. We also need to have all the nutrient building blocks available to the cells and tissues when they need them. This requires eating wholesome, nutritious food, as well as proper digestion and assimilation.

AGING THEORIES

Stagnation and toxicity
Aging clock and hormones
Cross-linking of proteins
Free radicals
Errors in DNA
Changes in brain
Autoimmunity
Stress

The aging clock theory regards the aging process as programmed by an inherent, preset number of possible cellular divisions. Our individual set of cell divisions and the time between them determines our life span. Different cells have different division rates. Lifestyle factors such as stress and nutrition, degenerative changes, and immunological and hormonal health can affect our inherent cell division potential or the length of time between cell divisions. Our genes are most closely influenced by nucleic acids, RNA and DNA. When RNA is affected, it may influence cell activity, protein building, and tissue repair and healing. Basic wear and tear and random insults to our genes can speed up our aging process. Chemicals, microorganisms, random toxins, and nutritional or functional deficiencies (such as reduced digestive enzyme production) all affect this important cellular process.

As far as we know, at present there is no hormone or code that causes death or self-destruction. But there are many subconscious, self-destructive tendencies such as not taking care of ourselves in the best ways possible. As we age, we must attend to minimizing internal aging to maintain vitality and tissue health. This is accomplished in part by eating light and staying light, but eating well. It is the synergy of nutrient and emotional deficits and depletions that contributes to both aging and the subsequent dying process.

The cross-linking theory suggests that molecular changes occur in the protein molecules of body tissues that cause microfibers to be laid down against the normal direction of other tissue fibers. This creates aging through loss of elasticity, stiffness, and degeneration. This may always be going on as the underlying mechanism for tissue change, inflammation, and degeneration, but it is more likely a result of the biochemical process of free-radical formation.

The free-radical theory, currently the most accepted aging hypothesis, offers an explanation of the basis of degenerative disease. It suggests that free radicals—unstable, reactive molecules with a free electron—seek to latch onto whatever they can find. When they are not countered by antioxidant nutrients, they may attack cell membranes, fat molecules, or tissue linings. Free radicals are generated by the metabolism of oxygen and other chemicals. Singlet oxygens, hydroxyl ions, peroxides, and superoxide molecules are some of the products of oxidation. Unsaturated fats, certain reactive chemicals, both inhaled and consumed in food or water, microbes, and smoking cigarettes all generate free radicals.

The antioxidants, also termed "free-radical scavengers," protect us by binding the free radicals. When we get sufficient levels of these antioxidants, such as vitamins E and C, selenium, and beta-carotene (vitamin A precursor) in our diet or as supplements, we can neutralize the free radicals and prevent cellular and tissue damage. Our body produces *superoxide dismutase* (SOD) and *glutathione peroxidase* (GP), enzymes that also counteract free radicals. These enzymes, however, are themselves unstable and are not specifically helpful as supplements because they are metabolized very rapidly and are not readily absorbed. By keeping our liver and its cells functioning well, we can support the production and function of these important antioxidant enzymes.

Other aging theories include **errors in DNA** (which could be generated by free radicals), chemical exposure, general toxicity, and basic genetic tendencies. **Changes in brain** function and the regulation of balance in the hormonal and nervous systems may also be at the core of the aging process. **Autoimmunity** and a general breakdown of immune function is another theory of degeneration; **stress**, which likely increases free-radical formation, may itself be at the heart of the aging process, as well as diminishing other vital physiological processes. The general process of aging probably involves combinations of all of the above theories working together in varying ways within each individual.

Diet and Supplements

The diet and supplement plan that will best provide us with the basic and special nourishment we need to maintain health and prevent aging includes the following guidelines:

- **Regularly undereat**. Avoid obesity; eat more low-calorie foods, such as vegetables, especially those high in beta-carotene.
- **Minimize fat intake**. The diet should be low in saturated and animal fats, with only moderate intake of vegetable-oil foods and cold-pressed vegetable oils and very low intake of fried fats or oils. Overall, not more than 25 percent of the calories in the diet should come from fat.
- **Focus the diet on complex-carbohydrate-containing foods** to acquire more fiber and sustained energy without overconsumption and congestion. Complex carbohydrates such as whole grains (specifically, brown rice, millet, oats, barley, buckwheat, and whole wheat), legumes, potatoes, and other starch vegetables and squashes are the key to any diet for longevity.
- **Protein intake should be moderate**—no more than 50–70 grams daily—with an increase in vegetable proteins such as nuts, seeds, and whole grain/legume combinations to about 75 percent of the dietary protein intake.
- **Eat a chemical-free diet** as much as possible. Most chemicals have some toxic properties, and many generate free-radical production. Some, such as certain pesticides and the nitrates and nitrites in cured meats, can even be carcinogenic in the body.
- **Moderate salt, sugar, alcohol, nicotine, and caffeine**. Each of these has specific irritating properties; however, regular nicotine use is the worst in regard to aging.
- **Drink plenty of good drinking water**, free of toxic pesticides and other chemicals. Proper hydration is important to skin health, digestive function, proper elimination, and all bodily functions.
- **Follow the *Anti-Aging* program** for micronutrients and antioxidants presented in the table below.
- **Use periods of detoxification**, or cleansing, to balance and rest the body's systems. Fasting or cleansing, I feel, is the missing link in Western nutrition. It is very important to regenerate optimum function and to enhance elimination. It helps improve many body functions, including the important digestion-assimilation-elimination cycle (see the programs on *Fasting* and *General Detoxification* in the last chapter for more information).

Supplements are important to the *Anti-Aging* program. First, a general and complete multivitamin-mineral formula is recommended. There are now more high-quality multivitamins that contain additional antioxidants; because these extra nutrients counteract so many disease processes as well as stress, likely the underlying cause of many problems. In addition to a general formula, the following nutrients are specific to the *Anti-Aging* program (the first seven are antioxidants):

- **Vitamin E** is an important antioxidant nutrient when taken in doses well above the RDA, usually at least 400–1,000 IUs daily. Vitamin E protects cell membranes and in particular prevents lipid irritation and breakdown. It also counteracts some of the negative effects of air pollution chemicals and metals.

- **Selenium** is an antioxidant mineral that works synergistically with vitamin E; that is, together they have a better effect than each separately. The selenium-containing enzyme, *glutathione peroxidase*, protects cellular membranes and irritation from metals. Selenium deficiency is associated with an increased risk of cancer, and adequate selenium intake is correlated with a reduced incidence of malignancy, particularly of the breasts, colon, and lungs, common sites of cancer.

- **Beta-carotene** is another cancer-preventing antioxidant nutrient. As an anti-aging nutrient, this form of vitamin A is better than retinol (from animal sources). Beta-carotene is a dual vitamin A molecule that can be split easily in the small intestine or liver. Vitamin A deficiencies are associated with an increased risk of cancer, particularly cervical and lung cancer. Beta-carotene specifically protects smokers from lung cancer (it reduces but does not eliminate the risk) in amounts of 25,000–40,000 IUs daily taken in one or two doses.

- **Vitamin C** is a crucial antioxidant nutrient. It is also an anticancer nutrient, as it has been shown to reduce cervical dysplasia, an early stage of cancer, and to prevent the conversion of nitrites to the carcinogenic nitrosamines. Ascorbic acid specifically protects cell membranes from viruses and may prevent chemical irritations. It also helps to lower blood fats, thus decreasing cardiovascular disease risk, and reduces irritation from cigarette smoke and air pollution.

  Bioflavonoids, found in many vitamin C foods, may also have antioxidant properties. Adequate amounts of bioflavonoids in the diet can help strengthen and protect blood vessels, improve enzyme activity, and may even help reduce the incidence of cataracts. Vitamin C supplements should contain some bioflavonoids.

- **L-Cysteine** is a sulfur-containing amino acid that acts as a free-radical scavenger, binding and neutralizing those irritating molecules. It aids detoxification, in part by supporting the liver in producing and storing glutathione, a tripeptide (protein) that is part of an important antioxidant enzyme system. L-cysteine gives cellular and tissue protection from chemicals as well. This amino acid is usually taken with vitamin C to protect the kidney from forming stones made of cystine (a by-product of cysteine metabolism). The recommended dose is 250 mg. of L-cysteine with 1 gram of vitamin C twice daily. If this amino acid is taken regularly, it is wise to also take a general formula containing the other required amino acids.

- **Zinc** also has mild antioxidant effects through its function in the enzyme *superoxide dismutase*, a free-radical scavenger. Zinc also contributes to immune support. A daily dose of 30–60 mg., including diet, is part of the *Anti-Aging* plan.

- **Manganese and copper** act as mild antioxidants, mainly as support, along with zinc, of the *superoxide dismutase* (SOD) enzymes, which metabolize the superoxide free radicals.

- **Fiber** is necessary as part of the diet and as a supplement. It helps colon elimination and may reduce the likelihood of cancer, especially in the breast and colon. Low-fiber, high-fat diets have been associated with an increased incidence of colon cancer.

- **Water** is a vital part of the "fountain of youth" program. It helps all the body functions, nourishes the skin, and is necessary for good elimination.

- **Calcium** protects against carcinogenic changes of the cells in the colon lining. It is also important to energy (ATP) production, heart and nerve function, good teeth, and bone health, protecting against osteoporosis.

- **Magnesium** protects the cardiovascular system by supporting heart function and preventing vascular spasms. It also aids in relaxation by reducing nervous tensions, an important part of staying healthy. Magnesium is also necessary for amino acid metabolism and energy (ATP) production.

- **Chromium** supports glucose tolerance, often reducing sugar cravings and possibly the incidence of diabetes, and also helps to lower blood cholesterol, thereby helping to prevent the main degenerative disease, atherosclerosis.

- **Molybdenum** is another trace mineral that may play a role in inhibiting cancer.

- **Niacin** is the active circulatory stimulant form of vitamin B_3. This nutrient helps improve circulation and also lowers cholesterol, two factors that reduce the risk of cardiovascular disease.

- **Vitamin B_{12}** helps keep energy up and protects nerve coverings. B_{12} is needed in the production of red blood cells and in the synthesis of DNA and RNA, important rebuilding processes in the body.

- **Folic acid** also helps in RNA and DNA (and red blood cells) production, but only in dosages higher than the 400 mcg. RDA. A dose of 1–2 mg. twice daily is commonly prescribed in Canada for this supportive function.

- **RNA**, as is found in foods such as the blue-green algae, chlorella, spirulina, and wheatgrass, all high in chlorophyll as well, help slow the aging process. RNA supplements have not been shown, however, to be very effective in actually increasing RNA in the tissues.

- **Choline**, as is found in lecithin, supports production of cell membranes and the important neurotransmitter acetylcholine.

- **Omega-3 fatty acids**, such as EPA and DHA, help reduce cholesterol and cardiovascular disease risk. Flaxseed oil contains both these omega-3 and omega-6 essential fatty acids.

- **L-carnitine** is a nonessential amino acid that helps to balance fat metabolism (utilization) and support energy production within the cell and in the muscles. L-carnitine may also reduce body fat and weight, which is important to longevity.

- **Coenzyme Q₁₀**, also called ubiquinone, improves the function of the cardiac muscle, our body's most important pump for longevity. It also may enhance specific immune functions.

- *Lactobacillus acidophilus* and other intestinal bacteria are also important at times to support the normal colon ecology and for the breakdown of food and production of colon vitamins. Reimplanting healthy bacteria may also help reduce other organisms, yeasts, or parasites.

- **Organic germanium** (trace mineral complex, germanium sesquioxide) is an oxygenating nutrient that I am sure future research will demonstrate to possess antiaging properties.

- **Mucopolysaccharides**, or chondroitin sulfates, may have a role in reducing inflammation, which can be a culprit in aging, and in reducing the risk of cardiovascular disease and arthritis. These substances, found in mussels and oysters, also help keep the collagen tissues and cells strong. Though the research so far has not substantiated the usefulness of mucopolysaccharides, the clinical responses have been favorable.

- **Hydrochloric acid** and digestive enzyme support may be helpful, particularly if these substances are deficient in our bodies. Proper breakdown and utilization of food nutrients are essential to staying healthy. Poor digestion can lead to many problems, including increased incidence of allergy; furthermore, improper assimilation of undigested foods can ultimately lead to increased nutrient deficiencies as well as free-radical formation from food reactions.

Herbs

Herbs have long been known for their benefits in cleansing the body and blood, protecting us from irritants and cancer cells, and supporting longevity. Those that I think are best for these purposes are garlic, ginseng root, capsicum, also known as red or cayenne pepper, and gotu kola.

- **Garlic** has some antiviral, antifungal, and antibacterial properties. It also probably has some anticancer function. Garlic helps to stimulate liver and colon detoxification and aids in reducing both blood pressure and cholesterol levels, which reduces the risk of cardiovascular disease.

- **Ginseng root**, known as the "longevity herb," has been used for centuries in the Orient to improve energy, especially in the elderly. Ginseng seems to support the adrenal glands and the immune function, though further tests are needed to confirm this. There are many kinds of ginseng; the red may lead to a mild increase in blood pressure, while the white varieties may help reduce it. Ginseng should not be used regularly in an antiaging program unless there is fatigue. It may be used three or four times a year, with a few capsules taken daily for a week or two or a tea prepared from the root, drunk over several days.

- **Capsicum** is a very interesting herb. A spicy bush-berry, cayenne helps to stimulate both the circulation and elimination. It also acts as a mild diuretic, increasing kidney cleansing. Cayenne is a natural energy stimulant that, unlike coffee, helps to reduce the blood pressure as well as the cholesterol level.
- **Gotu kola** has long been used by the East Indians for a variety of conditions. It is used in an antiaging program as a memory and brain stimulant and has been known as a longevity herb, likely for its effect on mental and physical vitality. Gotu kola has a diuretic effect and has been used as a glandular tonic in both men and women.

In the future, more and more specific nutrients and herbs will be used to slow down the aging process and enhance health, mainly by reducing stress and supporting immune function. Immune enhancement and a greater understanding of the relationship between immunology and health will probably be the basis of our future medicine.

Unless we get involved in serious cloning of cells and tissues or in cryobiology, the freezing of cells, tissues, and whole bodies to prolong or regenerate life, it is going to be up to each of us to live according to the health-sustaining laws of nature and the universe. A total revamping of the diet, with nutrient-rich, wholesome foods and a focus on regular undereating, will support us best. Reducing chemical exposure by cleaning up the environment will also be necessary for greatest longevity. Learning to reduce and manage stress in our daily lives and generate an attitude of enthusiasm and love for life is crucial to our future health and happiness.

The specific nutrient program I recommend for antiaging is shown in the following table. The values given are averages for men and women of different sizes and shapes. Ranges are shown for most values to allow for some flexibility in individual application. Unless otherwise noted, these amounts are to be taken daily, usually divided into two or three portions over the course of the day. Amounts consumed in the diet can be taken into consideration for nutrients such as folic acid, calcium, or iron; excess iron should not be taken unless you are being treated for iron deficiency or are monitored by a nutritional specialist. This supplementation program may be used for one month several times yearly for healthy people in their 40s and 50s, and then more regularly in the later years or with particular aging concerns. For specific medical conditions, using more specific programs discussed later may be more relevant.

ANTI-AGING NUTRIENT PROGRAM

Calories	1,600–3,000	Calcium	800–1,200 mg.
Protein	50–75 g.	Chromium	200–500 mcg.
Fats	40–70 g.	Copper	2–3 mg.
Carbohydrate	250–400 g.	Iodine	150–200 mcg.
Fiber	10–20 g.	Iron	
Water	1.5–3.0 qt.	men and post-menopausal women	10–15 mg.
		menstruating women	18–30 mg.
Vitamin A	10,000 IUs	Magnesium	600–800 mg.
Beta-carotene	25,000–50,000 IUs	Manganese	5–15 mg.
Vitamin D	400 IUs	Molybdenum	100–500 mcg.
Vitamin E	400–800 IUs	Selenium, preferably as selenomethionine	200–300 mcg.
Vitamin K	300 mcg.		
Thiamine (B_1)	10–50 mg.		
Riboflavin (B_2)	10–50 mg.	Silicon	100–200 mg.
Niacin (B_3)	50–100 mg.	Zinc	
Niacinamide (B_3)	50–100 mg.	men	30–60 mg.
Pantothenic acid (B_5)	250–500 mg.	women	25–50 mg.
Pyridoxine (B_6)	25–200 mg.	L-amino acids complex	1,000 mg.
Pyridoxal-5-phosphate	25–50 mg.	L-cysteine	500 mg.
Cobalamin (B_{12})	50–250 mcg.	L-carnitine	250–500 mg.
Folic acid	1,000–2,000 mcg. (1–2 mg.)	Coenzyme Q_{10}	30–60 mg.
		Flaxseed oil	1–2 t.
Biotin	500 mcg.	Organic germanium	75–300 mg.
Choline	250–1,000 mg.		
Inositol	500–1,000 mg.	*Others:*	
Vitamin C	2–6 g.	Hydrochloric acid (with protein meals)	5–10 grains (1–2 tablets)
Bioflavonoids	250–500 mg.		
		Digestive enzymes (including bromelain) (after meals)	2–3 tablets
		Wheat germ oil	4 capsules
		Mucopolysaccharides	100–500 mg.

Anti-Stress

In the future, stress may come to be seen as the primary contributing cause of most disease. Research continues to link stress to more and more symptoms and diseases, both acute and chronic. Stress is inevitable in today's world and, of course, we need a certain amount to function. The key is to be able to manage our level of stress.

What is stress? It is our reaction to our external environment as well as our inner thoughts and feelings. Stress in essence is our body's natural response to dangers, the "fight or flight" mechanisms—the body's preparedness to do battle or flee from danger. This response involves a complex biochemical-hormonal process, which we will discuss shortly.

Stress in today's world is mainly a result of continuous high demands that are imposed on us by work, family, and lifestyle, or that we impose upon ourselves through our desire to accomplish. Mild stress acts as a useful motivation for activity and productivity. But when the stresses in our life are too extreme or too many, this may result in all kinds of problems. Some people consistently overreact to their day-to-day life. However, most of us might be overwhelmed only when we have an increased intensity or number of stresses, such as excessive demands all at once leading to a continuous feeling of not having enough time or energy to do what we feel we must do. Others respond stressfully to intense emotional experiences, personal changes, extreme weather, or overexposure to electronic stimuli, all of which can weaken us.

Stress can generate many symptoms and diseases, mediated by changes in immune function, hormonal response, and biochemical reactions, which then influence body functions in our digestive tract and our cardiovascular, neurological, or musculoskeletal systems. A wide variety of problems such as headache, backache, and infection, even heart disease or cancer in the long-term, may result.

Our brain and pituitary gland respond to stress by releasing adrenocorticotropic hormone (ACTH). This stimulates our adrenals to increase production of the hormones epinephrine, norepinephrine, and cortisol. Other hormones that affect metabolism and water balance may also be released. Epinephrine and norepinephrine, known as the adrenalines or catecholamines, are the main stimuli to the stress response. They stimulate the heart, increase blood pressure and heart rate, and constrict certain blood vessels to increase blood flow to the muscles and brain and to decrease it to the digestive tract and internal organs, preparing us for the "battle" with the "danger," wherever it is. Adrenaline also raises blood sugar, as it stimulates the liver to produce and release more glucose (and cholesterol) into the blood so our cells will have the energy we need. All of this results in an increased rate of metabolism. Stress experienced around the time of eating thus diverts the energy needed for efficient digestion.

During times of increased stress and greater demand, our body's nutrients are used more rapidly to meet the increased biochemical needs of metabolism, so we require increased amounts of many of these nutrients. The diet and nutrient plan presented here is specifically designed to reduce these negative biochemical effects of stress. There are also many other important aspects of handling this modern-day problem, primarily psychological and lifestyle approaches to stress management. Soon, there will be a medical specialty designed to deal solely with stress-induced diseases. In fact, most specialties now have some set of symptoms or a diagnosis in their field of expertise related to these psycho-emotional/stress-induced diseases. The problem is that most doctors are not trained to do more than diagnose them, and often these diagnoses, such as "irritable bowel" or "spastic colon," tension headaches, or neurogenic bladder disease, are made primarily by excluding the "real diseases." Often, only tranquilizers, psychotherapy, or biofeedback are available in most circles of medicine, and this approach may be limited. There is a lot more that each of us can do to better manage our stress.

Who will benefit from this *Anti-Stress* program? It is mainly for those who are routinely subjected to high demands, particularly mental demands, and who suffer from "intellectual performance anxiety." People in this group are mostly office workers, people who must sit and be productive for eight to ten hours a day with little physical outlet, such as the executive or office worker, although they also might be salespeople, flight attendants, mechanics, nurses, or journalists. The *Anti-Stress* program is also suitable for people undergoing short-term periods of increased stress because of personal changes or other events that increase energy demands, such as divorce or marriage, death of a loved one, relocation, job change, or travel.

Many of the conditions discussed in this chapter are related in some way to stress—for example, athletes experience extra physical stress and executives experience more mental stress; stress is also a factor in the aging process. Stress can occur at all levels of our being. There are physical, emotional, mental, and spiritual stress factors involved in almost all diseases. Particular medical conditions that have a high stress component include asthma and allergies, cardiovascular and gastrointestinal diseases, arthritis, and cancer. Surgery, viral conditions, and environmental chemical exposure may be short-term problems with high stress components. Thus, aspects of this program may apply to many of the other programs. Check other discussions as they may tie into your particular concerns.

TYPES OF STRESS

- **Physical stress**—exercise, hard labor, birth
- **Chemical stress**—environmental pollution such as exposure to pesticides and cleaning solvents, and the personal use of chemicals, such as drugs, alcohol, caffeine, and nicotine
- **Mental stress**—high responsibility, long hours, perfectionism, anxiety, and worry
- **Emotional stress**—anger, fear, frustration, sadness, betrayal, bereavement
- **Nutritional stress**—vitamin and mineral deficiencies, protein or fat excesses or deficiencies, food allergies
- **Traumatic stress**—infection, injury, burns, surgery, extreme temperatures
- **Psycho-spiritual stress**—relationship, financial or career pressures; issues of life goals, spiritual alignment, and general state of happiness

COMMON STRESS FACTORS

- **Attitude toward self**
- **Personal financial state**
- **Moving**
- **Traffic tickets**
- **Tests in school**
- **Meeting someone new**
- **Raising children**
- **Demands at the office**
- **Job and career challenges**
- **Promotion, job loss**
- **Emotional challenges**—personal relationships, fear, anger, loneliness
- **Family changes**—marriage, divorce, separation, a new baby
- **Physical challenges**—weather changes, extreme climates, athletic events
- **Health challenges**—illness, injury, surgery, chemical exposures
- **Life changes**—adolescence, aging, pregnancy, menopause

Please realize, though, that stress is not the situations or incidents themselves; rather, real stress comes from the way we react to them. For stress to arise and negatively influence our health, we must experience something as a danger. When we do, anxiety is generated, which we often experience as fear or a feeling of threat to our survival. If we view stress positively, we see it as simply a survival response. But if we cannot handle the stress, we may experience the symptoms and diseases of stress. Learning to adapt our attitude and find suitable outlets for our stress is a very important long-range plan.

As stated earlier, the normal biochemical response to a sense of danger is stimulation of the adrenal glands to release increased levels of hormones, particularly the catecholamines—epinephrine (adrenaline) and norepinephrine. The catecholamines are cardiovascular stimulants that increase heart rate, constrict blood vessels, stimulate the brain, and affect every other body system to prepare it for "fight" or "flight"— that is, handle the danger or hit the road. The problem comes in when there is really no physical danger but our body reacts as if there were. Then, if greater physical demands and activity do not provide an outlet for the increased adrenal activity, it may be turned inward and play havoc with our physiology and organs, as well as with our emotions and our mind.

Though all parts of our body are affected by stress, certain areas seem to be more sensitive than others. In my estimation, the digestive tract is the most easily influenced, followed by the neurological and circulatory systems and the muscles which accumulate some of the tensions as well as toxins from metabolism. The psychological outlook and welfare of the individual are also strongly affected by acute and chronic stress.

How the damage comes about involves the mechanisms of constant adrenal stimulation along with free-radical production (see *Anti-Aging* program for a full discussion) and immune suppression. Stress produces irritating molecules that generate immunological changes, damage cells, and inflame organ and blood vessel linings. Stress responses also "eat up" more important nutrients which can lead to deficiencies and allow the other stress response changes to damage the tissues even more. Stress has been shown to decrease protective antibodies and reduce the important T lymphocytes that function in the cellular immune system. Chronic stress is clearly a culprit in the generation of aging and degenerative diseases.

In addition to the increased demands on the adrenal cortex, certain mechanisms affect the stomach and pancreas and thus our digestion. Stress initially increases stomach hydrochloric acid production, leading to indigestion, heartburn, gastritis, and ulcer problems. With increased acid levels, however, the pancreas is stimulated to release alkaline enzymes to help balance the acidity. With chronic stress, this can lead to hypochlorhydria (low stomach acid) and reduced function of the pancreas. This may result in poor digestion and assimilation of nutrients and thus vitamin and mineral deficiencies as well as the development of food allergies due to improper breakdown of the bulk foodstuffs and the subsequent absorption of larger molecules, which may be immunogenic.

There is also a weakening of the adrenal response with chronic stress, whether the stress is from regular sugar intake (adrenaline helps rebalance blood sugar) or from other physical or emotional demands. When the adrenals do not respond, we may have a more difficult time coping with the stress, and when this inability to cope sets in deeply, we may feel like giving up. We might experience depression, hopelessness, or even death, which can result from the serious diseases that arise with a severely weakened immune system. That is why it is so important to avoid the vicious cycle of trying to meet high demands by pushing ourselves with poor nourishment, poor sleep, and lack of fun. A whole field of medicine, called *psychoneuroimmunology*, is arising to deal with our new knowledge about the relationship among stress, immunity and brain functions, and disease, examining such problems as AIDS, cancer, and chronic viral conditions. Though we have learned a lot about stress and its influence on disease in recent years, there is still a great deal more to learn regarding the physical mechanisms involved in immune interaction. This, I believe, is going to be the dominant medical field of the future.

STRESS-RELATED SYMPTOMS AND DISEASES

Fatigue	Indigestion	Infections
Irritability	Diarrhea	Eczema
Headaches	Constipation	Psoriasis
Muscle tension	Peptic ulcer	Allergies
Neck and back pains	Irritable bowel	Asthma
Atherosclerosis	Loss of appetite	Nutritional deficiencies
High blood pressure	Anorexia nervosa	Premenstrual symptoms
Diabetes	Weight changes	Sexual problems
Arthritis	Insomnia	Psychological problems
Cancer	Depression	

For people with elevated stress levels, I suggest a variety of stress-reducing activities to minimize the dangers of this underlying cause of disease.

VARIOUS THERAPIES FOR STRESS

- **Have more fun.** Do things that you enjoy and that help you to relax.
- **Express your feelings.** Emotions need regular venting, and unexpressed emotions are the building blocks of stress, pain, and illness.
- **Get good sleep.** Poor sleep or sleep habits do not let your body really rest, discharge tensions, and recharge.
- **Learn relaxation exercises.** These can help a great deal in reducing stress through letting go of mental stresses and experiencing moments of inner peace. This quiet, "nothing happening" space is where, I believe, the healing process begins.
- **Exercise.** Regular physical exercise is one of the best ways to clear your tensions and feel good, with more energy and a better attitude toward life.
- **Develop good relationships.** It is important to have friends in whom you can confide and find support. Those who love and accept you and will advise but not judge you are your true friends. It is also very meaningful to be a true friend to another.

- **Experience love and satisfying sex.** A primary relationship that is loving, sensual, and sexual can also be a major stress reducer. Having an understanding, accepting, and warm being (most often human) to receive your hardworking body and mind can be the best therapy available. However, if you do not have this in your life, there are many other therapies that are helpful. Often, an intense relationship can also be a stressor. It is important to find a balance in all you do, in each endeavor and in your life as a whole.

- **Change perceptions and attitudes.** When ideas or views are not serving you, it is wise to examine and adapt them. It is important to learn to respond to life's situations and not react. This is a true response-ability! Hanging onto frustrations, holding grudges, and accepting the victim-blame game are not in your best health interests. It serves you to look at the big picture and step out of the little struggles. Ask why you might need to experience these challenges and try to view them as opportunities for growth and learning. Applying more spiritual principles to life is very useful and often helps solve many of the conflicts involved in finding greater peace of mind and heart. Find and experience self-love, self-respect, and self-worth.

There are many positive things to do with regard to diet and nutrition, as well as many things to avoid. This program is designed to counteract and reduce the negative biochemical and physiological effects of stress and to minimize the specific stressing agents, such as the wide variety of drugs, both street and prescription. Caffeine, nicotine, and alcohol are all irritating drugs. Many over-the-counter and prescription drugs may also cause physiological problems and irritate us physically or mentally.

A **diet** of high-nutrient foods is essential for people under stress, because stress increases cellular activity which leads to increased nutrient usage. The resulting depletions may aggravate the damaging effects of stress. Also, less food may be consumed during times of stress, as the digestive tract may be a little upset; and the higher nutrient foods make up for lower consumption. However, some people who are stressed tend to push themselves and not take good care of themselves, avoiding meals, especially wholesome ones, and snacking on quick-energy or fast foods. They may be martyrs who feel that they must serve the cause and there is no time for such things as eating properly, or they may just be too busy and forget to eat. These people are usually not overweight; on the contrary, they need to be reminded to eat. This unrelenting push without feeding the stomach (and every cell) can lead to acid irritation of the digestive organs and ulcers. Then the cycle of antacids starts and further poor digestion and assimilation is the final outcome.

Probably the best type of diet for the fast-track people with intellectual performance anxiety is three to five small but wholesome meals a day, like the *Warrior's Diet* discussed in Chapter 9, *Diets*. Lots of water is important to keep us well hydrated and to help counteract stress by circulating nutrients. Avoiding stress around meals is very important. Try to rest and relax before and after eating, even if just for a minute or two of placing your body in a receptive state for the nourishment coming in—rather like clearing the computer of its active program so that it can receive new information. If there is time to take 10–15 minutes before and after meals, that is even better, especially after large meals. Listening to relaxing music also helps.

A detoxification-type diet may be useful at times of intense stress, and it is often a natural response to these increased demands. Drinking lots of liquids, such as water and juices, and reducing heavier meals that may not be handled well can help us lighten up when life gets "too heavy." A response of overeating and food abuse can only make matters worse. Juices, soups, and salads, for example, can nourish us well without creating great demands on our body and digestion, which may not be working well at the time. Our energy level and productivity may rise with lighter eating as well. A lighter, cleansing diet may help us through times of short-term stress. Some food intake may enable our body to assimilate the supplements that can also be of value. A good supplement plan is imperative to our *Anti-Stress* program. Stress depletes so many of our body's nutrients that it is difficult to obtain the levels we need from food alone unless we spend eight hours a day shopping, preparing food, and feeding ourselves—and that is not too realistic.

Nutrients that are commonly depleted by stress include the antioxidant vitamins A, E, and C, the B vitamins, and the minerals zinc, selenium, calcium, magnesium, iron, potassium, sulfur, and molybdenum. Because of increased metabolism and use of energy, our stressed body utilizes more carbohydrates, proteins, and fats, especially the fatty acids. Unrelenting stress, however, is not the basis for a healthy weight-loss program.

The B vitamins and vitamin C are the main constituents of many antistress formulas. They are all significantly depleted by stress and the stress-related problems may be compounded by deficiencies resulting from poor nutrition prior to the time of increased stress. All of the B vitamins are important here. Pantothenic acid, or vitamin B_5, may well be the most important antistress nutrient of the B complex. Along with folic acid and vitamin C, it is necessary for proper function of the adrenal glands. Niacin, enough to generate the niacin flush, may be useful in counteracting some of the biochemical effects of stress. Vitamins B_1, B_2, B_6, biotin, and PABA are also helpful. I recommend taking higher than the RDA of all of the B vitamins, spread out in two or three portions, all taken before dark, since they can be stimulating; it is wise to let the mind and body relax as it gets toward bedtime. I suggest more minerals in the evening, as they tend to help in relaxation. However, if evening work is important or there are evening meetings, a good B complex supplement can be taken after dinner. The B vitamins may even have a relaxing effect on some people, and they could be used by them in the evenings to calm the nerves. A regular B vitamin, with 25–50 mg. each of most of the Bs, for example, will be used and eliminated by the body within a few hours. Such tablets or capsules can be taken several times daily. Time-release B vitamins, which do not have to be taken so often, are also commonly used. Many people do better with hypoallergenic or yeast- and wheat-free B vitamins. Although our body will utilize some of the B vitamins taken at any time, most vitamin and mineral supplements are best assimilated after a meal.

Vitamin C supplementation is also very important for stress. Vitamin C, or ascorbic acid, may indeed be the single most essential antistress nutrient. It offers cellular protection, immune support, and adrenal support to produce more cortisone and epinephrine. Vitamin C is also an important antioxidant that helps protect against fat peroxidation, including restoring vitamin E after it is oxidized. Vitamin C is very rapidly utilized and minimally stored in the body. Therefore, regular usage, even four to six times daily, is ideal. A dosage of 1–2 grams per day is recommended, although as much as 8–10 grams may be used for severe problems related to stress. One or two of the vitamin C dosages taken each day should contain the bioflavonoid C complex, including rutin and hesperidin.

In addition to extra B vitamins and C, I suggest an antioxidant program such as described for the *Anti-Aging* program. Vitamin A and beta-carotene, vitamin E and selenium, and the amino acid L-cysteine are all part of this. As with vitamin C, these antioxidants sacrifice themselves (through oxidation) to balance out the free radicals.

Minerals are also important, with potassium, calcium, and magnesium heading the antistress list. Potassium is essential for most crucial physiologic activities. Calcium is vital to nerve transmission and regular heartbeat as well as immune function. It aids both relaxation and muscle tone. Magnesium is a tranquilizing mineral that helps balance the nervous system and supports heart function. An Epsom salt (magnesium sulfate) bath (with 1 cup) can be very relaxing. In general, a dosage of 600–1,000 mg. of calcium and 400–800 mg. of magnesium daily, in addition to diet, is recommended, with most of it being taken in the evening before bed.

Calcium and magnesium can also be used to balance the stomach acid. For acute or early stress with hyperacidity, these alkaline minerals taken before meals can be a helpful antacid. With chronic stress, when stomach acid is more often low, taking them before bed is better. Pancreatic function is often low as well with chronic stress, and additional pancreatic enzymes after meals may be helpful.

Minerals that are helpful for their immune and enzyme support, such as *superoxide dismutase*, include zinc, copper, manganese, and selenium. Chromium may be useful in allaying sugar cravings, while potassium is important to prevent heart irregularities and muscle cramps and to balance the hypertensive effects of sodium when salt is used in excess. Like vitamin C and the Bs, minerals are best taken in several portions for optimum absorption and utilization. Taking the important ones such as calcium, magnesium, iron, or zinc by themselves will reduce competitive absorption between them and produce higher levels of each in the blood.

Supplemental amino acids may allow better protein utilization and energy balance, especially when digestion is poor. The powdered, L- form amino acids are easily utilized by the body, much more easily than steak, though the meat has other nutrition (and possibly other toxins). The antioxidant amino acid, L-cysteine, promotes liver function and detoxification. L-glutamine is helpful for proper brain function, especially with stress. Methionine may also be protective against stress through its support of fatty acid metabolism and other functions. L-tyrosine and L-phenylalanine may help reduce stress-induced high blood pressure, while L-tryptophan can be used for relaxation and sleep.

SLEEP-AID NUTRIENT COCKTAIL

Vitamin C,* 500–1000 mg. (helps mineral absorption)
Calcium, 500–750 mg.
Magnesium, 350–500 mg.
Potassium, 300–500 mg.
L-Tryptophan, 500–2,000 mg. (if available)
Relaxing herbs, such as valerian, chamomile, vervain,
  catnip, hops, or linden flowers

Begin with just the C, calcium, and magnesium. If that doesn't work, add 500 mg. of L-tryptophan, increasing the dosage if necessary by 500 mg. every three days, up to 2,000 mg. If you still have no relief, try an herbal sleep-inducing formula, beginning with one or two capsules and building up if needed. Celestial Seasonings' Sleepytime tea has helped many people. Drinking a warm cup of it or another nighttime relaxant tea is a helpful addition to a calming-down routine. Some people also enjoy a warm cup of whole milk before bed for its tranquilizing effect, if the digestion will handle it.

*A mineralized ascorbic acid powder with calcium, magnesium, and potassium can be used in a drink.

Herbs may be useful in the *Anti-Stress* program as well. Licorice root, and its active extract DGL, have a soothing and anti-inflammatory effect, and may be useful for stress. Valerian root, by itself or in combination with other herbs, has a tranquilizing effect and can be used before sleep or as a muscle relaxant, either as a tea or in a capsule. Catnip leaf can tame that wild or ferocious feeling and is a safe herb to improve the recharging quality of our catnaps. Ginseng root, as a tea or in capsules, is often thought of as a stimulant but is commonly used as an antistress herb. It strengthens deeper energies and the ability to handle life, and it is definitely better in the long run than coffee. White ginsengs, such as northern or white Siberian, tend to be safer for the blood pressure (too much red ginseng can elevate it). Gotu kola leaf is a good herb for mental stress. Like ginseng, it is very popular in the Eastern cultures. Two formulas that I have used for patients are made by Professional Botanicals: RLX ("relax"), which contains skullcap, passion flower, celery seed, musk root, lupulin, and hops, and RST ("rest") or Sleepeaze, which contains passion flower, valerian root, black cohosh root, German chamomile flowers, lupulin, and lemon balm.

Some practitioners use adrenal glandular tablets to support the extra adrenal demands during stress. Many people respond well to this treatment if they feel comfortable taking beef adrenals. I personally do not. Adrenal cortical extract (ACE) has been

743

a popular injection for a number of years for stimulating energy and treating a variety of problems, such as allergies, hypoglycemia, and fatigue. This appears to be less commonly used and harder to obtain, likely because of medical politics. It was not particularly unsafe; its effectiveness and safety were not well enough established to satisfy the FDA.

Some of the freeze-dried, blue-green algae products have also been useful because of their mild detoxifying and energizing effects. They also seem to reduce some mental stress. I personally like how I feel when I take chlorella or spirulina. They also provide protein and all the essential amino acids.

The following table shows my recommended Anti-Stress Nutrient Program. The amounts listed are the total day's intake (in addition to the diet), which I recommend splitting into three portions. Where ranges are shown, these are to accommodate individual needs and ability to handle higher amounts of these nutrients.

ANTI-STRESS NUTRIENT PROGRAM

Water	2–3 qt.	Calcium	600–1,000 mg.
		Chromium	200–400 mcg.
		Copper	2–3 mg.
Vitamin A	7,500–15,000 IUs	Iodine	150–200 mcg.
Beta-carotene	10,000–25,000 IUs	Iron	10–20 mg.
Vitamin D	400 IUs	Magnesium	350–600 mg.
Vitamin E	400–1,000 IUs	Manganese	5–10 mg.
Vitamin K	200–400 mcg.	Molybdenum	300–800 mg.
Thiamine (B$_1$)	75–150 mg.	Potassium	300–500 mg.
Riboflavin (B$_2$)	50–100 mg.	Selenium	200–400 mcg.
Niacin (B$_3$)	50–150 mg.	Zinc	30–60 mg.
Niacinamide (B$_3$)	25–100 mg.	L-amino acids	1,000–1,500 mg.
Pantothenic acid (B$_5$)	500–1,000 mg.	L-cysteine	250–500 mg. with vitamin C
Pyridoxine (B$_6$)	50–100 mg.		
Pyridoxal-5-phosphate	25–75 mg.	*Optional:*	
Cobalamin (B$_{12}$)	50–250 mcg.		
Folic acid	500–1,000 mcg.	Hydrochloric acid with meals for chronic stress	5–10 grains
Biotin	150–500 mcg.		
PABA	50–100 mg.		
Choline	500–1,000 mg.	Pancreatic enzymes (after meals)	1–2 tablets
Inositol	500–1,000 mg.		
Vitamin C	4–8 g.	Adrenal glandular	50–100 mg.
Bioflavonoids	250–500 mg.	Chlorella	1–2 packets or 6–12 tablets daily
		Licorice root	2–4 capsules

Skin Enhancement

In this section I discuss what it takes to keep our skin looking young and healthy—what we can do for it, what to avoid, and some dietary guidelines and supplement suggestions. Many aspects of lifestyle, including stress, cigarette smoking, and sun-bathing or ultraviolet (UV) tanning may lead to premature aging of the skin. I also review some of the many acute and chronic skin disorders that occur at various ages or throughout life. Fortunately, most of these problems eventually heal on their own. I will briefly examine these with a focus on nutritional influences and treatment, trying to be a bit more helpful than the lighthearted maxim of the Dermatologist: "If it's dry, wet it; if it's wet, dry it out. If that doesn't work, use cortisone."

The skin is our largest organ. It functions as a protective covering, a key sensing organ, an oil producer, and an important organ of elimination. Through regular evaporation and perspiration, the skin can clear all kinds of toxins to help maintain internal balance. The skin must be well nourished to stay healthy. It needs good circulation through its millions of tiny capillaries, good nerve function, and a ready supply of nutrients to aid its rapid growth.

Our skin surface is the intermediary between the external and internal environments and reflects the health of the underlying organs and our internal body function. By looking at the skin, tongue surface, eye tissue, and hair quality, I can get a good idea of an individual's general health, vitality, and internal balance. In Chinese medicine, the skin coloration or hue around and under the eyes reflects the subtle balance among the Chinese five elements. For example, a greenish hue may suggest a liver/gallbladder imbalance. In this system, the colors are related to different organs as shown in the following chart.

Color	Organ	Element
Green	Liver, gallbladder	Wood
Red	Heart, small intestine	Fire
Yellow	Spleen, stomach	Earth
White	Lungs, large intestine	Metal
Blue	Kidneys, bladder	Water

The condition of the skin and tissue around the eyes can suggest certain other problems. Signs of fatigue and increased aging lines or dark circles under the eyes may indicate stress; the Chinese would diagnose weak adrenal-kidney energy. Water or kidney imbalance may show up as puffiness, while colon congestion or imbalance might be represented by wrinkled bags under the eyes or a white coloration. Allergies may be revealed by slightly puffy or pitted dark circles, even looking like black and blue "shiners" under the eyes when severe. As the skin is an eliminating organ, the general skin health may tie into functions of the lungs, colon, kidneys, and liver. In Chinese medicine, many skin problems are treated by strengthening the function of these organs.

To keep our skin healthy, it is most important to take good overall care of ourselves, as the skin's well-being is dependent on the health of the rest of our body. Drinking adequate amounts of water may be the single most important factor in healthy skin and good eliminative functions. Two quarts of quality drinking water per day is the suggested average, but this may vary for different individuals, according to a number of factors. More water is needed with a rich, fatty diet than with a lot of fruits and vegetables; with a high activity level than with a sedentary lifestyle; with hot, dry weather than with cold and damp; in summer than in winter; and with constipation than with normal bowel function. We must each find our own balance of fluid intake. It is wise to drink regularly upon awakening, between meals up to about a half hour before eating (it keeps the appetite down, too), and whenever thirsty. Water is the best liquid for us, followed by herb teas, fruit juices, and mineral waters; we should avoid caffeinated beverages, sugary drinks, and soda pops.

Increased Water Needs	*Decreased Water Needs*
Rich, fatty diet	Diet high in fruits and vegetables
Activity and exercise	Sedentary
Hot, dry climate	Cold, damp climate
Summer	Winter
Constipation	Normal or loose bowels

NO SMOKING! for healthy skin. The smoke and chemical irritation, besides causing a variety of serious medical conditions, causes rapid aging of the skin, especially around the mouth and eyes. Smokers notoriously have many more age lines around those areas than nonsmokers of the same age. The effect of tobacco smoke on the aging process is due mainly to an increase in free radicals, which are damaging to the skin cells in the dermis as well as to the cells in our inner organs and tissue linings. Smoking has a drying effect and also exposes smokers and others to many toxic chemicals (such as carbon monoxide) and metals (such as cadmium), which may cause more chronic irritation internally. For similar reasons, avoiding or protecting ourselves from other chemicals, at home, at work, and especially in foods and pharmaceuticals is also important to healthy skin.

Ultraviolet (sun) light is known to be damaging to the skin and results in more rapid aging and dryness of the skin, as can be seen in many a farmer, construction worker, or sun worshiper. The changes in the ozone layer make sun exposure more dangerous than ever. Care must be taken with sunbathing or using sun lamps, because excessive ultraviolet light exposure can eventually reduce skin elasticity and tone. Along with dehydration or nutrient deficiencies, this may lead to rapid skin aging.

Skin care with moisturizing and beauty products requires a fine balance between nurturance and chemical exposure. I recommend natural products whenever possible. A number of companies now produce natural skin care products that can help rehydrate dried skin, relubricate skin with oils, and protect the skin from heat, cold, chemicals, and the sun. Sunscreens are very popular now with the current knowledge of the sun's chronic damaging effects on the skin. Beauty creams with aloe vera, clay packs, herbal wraps, honey or egg white facials, and dry-brush massaging are some ways to clean, detoxify, and nurture our epidermis. Saunas and sweats are also helpful in clearing impurities through the skin.

Diet and Supplements

The diet that supports healthy skin includes high-nutrient, high-water-content foods such as fresh fruits and vegetables. These important foods should be consumed daily, as fresh fruits eaten alone in the morning and vegetable salads at lunch or dinner. Cooked vegetables with proteins or starches are also recommended. The essential fatty acids found in the vegetable oils, seeds, and nuts are also necessary to nourish our skin and keep the texture and vitality strong. Cold-pressed olive oil and flaxseed oil are, I think, the best sources of essential fats. Olive oil is stable to heat; however, flaxseed (linseed) should only be used uncooked. Some of the cold-pressed polyunsaturated oils, such as safflower, soy, and sunflower, can also be used in moderation but should not be used for frying or cooking; sesame oil can be used in cooking, sparingly. Some cholesterol-containing foods, such as eggs, poultry, and occasionally even meat, may be used. Fresh fish is one of the better, slightly lower-fat animal foods.

Water is very important to help carry nutrients throughout the body and to flush out toxins. Adequate protein intake, along with good protein digestion and assimilation, is essential to make available the amino acids vital to tissue building and rapid cellular turnover in skin. Two amino acids, L-cysteine and L-proline, are especially important here. A high-fiber diet consisting of whole grains, legumes, and vegetables is helpful to detoxify the colon regularly and prevent accumulation of colon toxins going through the body causing tissue toxicity, which can lead to problems in the skin. Vitamin A and beta-carotene foods are helpful to skin health, as are zinc- and silica-rich foods.

Supplements for healthy skin include a multivitamin and mineral, antioxidant nutrients to counteract free-radical damage, and the essential fatty acids. Water intake, as stated, is essential to healthy skin tissue. Fiber, such as bran or psyllium seed husks, helps prevent colon stagnation and general body toxicity which easily affects the skin. Vitamin A and beta-carotene are important to fat-soluble vitamins that play a role in preventing acne, blemishes, and dry skin and may help to prevent skin cancer. Vitamin A deficiency can lead to all kinds of skin problems. The antioxidant function of beta-carotene is useful as well. Ascorbic acid (vitamin C) provides more antioxidant free-radical protection in the blood and body fluids, and helps to reduce some of the aging effects of smoke or chemicals. Vitamin E and selenium also perform this function, especially with regard to fats. Selenium may also reduce the risks of skin and other cancers. Zinc is needed in cell repair, for DNA, RNA, and enzyme production, and to keep the immune function strong. Silica is thought to strengthen the skin, hair, and nails; after all, it is highly concentrated in the coverings (skins) of most fruits, vegetables, and grains. The B vitamins are essential to healthy skin. Niacin, pyridoxine, riboflavin, and thiamine deficiencies are all associated with skin disorders. Biotin supports skin health as it helps our body synthesize fats and proteins, and utilize carbohydrates. Vitamin B_6, or pyridoxine, is needed for cell division and protein synthesis, both important skin functions. Essential fatty acids (EFAs) are vital to skin tissue health; these are found in many oils, such as olive and linseed oils. Cod liver oil is high in vitamins A and D and other nutrients, but it also may concentrate impurities. Eicosapentaenoic acid (EPA), the main omega-3 fish oil, also has some nourishing qualities for the skin, besides protecting against cardiovascular disease. Gamma-linolenic acid (GLA), as found in evening primrose oil, does the same and has also been used successfully for some cases of eczema and as a mild anti-inflammatory. The amino acids are essential to protein building, cell division, and tissue health and repair and are certainly important to functioning skin. The sulfur-containing amino acids, such as L-cysteine and methionine, are especially important skin amino acids. Tyrosine (and copper) help in skin and hair pigmentation.

SKIN-SUPPORTING NUTRIENTS

Water	Calcium	Essential fatty acids
Fiber	Selenium	Olive oil
Vitamin A	Zinc	Cod liver oil
Beta-carotene	Silica	Linseed oil
Vitamin C	B vitamins	Omega-3 fatty acids (EPA)
Vitamin E	Vitamin B_6	Gamma-linolenic acid (GLA)
	Biotin	All amino acids
		L-cysteine
		L-proline

Common Skin Conditions

Skin problems include dry skin, dandruff, acne, poison oak or ivy and other types of contact dermatitis, and psoriasis. There are, of course, a variety of bug bites or infections that generate self-limited skin eruptions. Some, like staphylococcus infections, which commonly cause painful boils, may require the use of antibiotics or a more long-range detoxification/blood purifying program in addition to topical care of the problem.

Dry skin is a fairly common problem that can give rise to painful cracks and fissures, or at least a look of low vitality. Dry skin may result from poor nourishment, dehydration, or soap and chemical exposure. Certain hormonal problems, such as low thyroid function, could also lead to xeroderma (dry skin); any problem like this would need to be found and corrected. With dry skin, more water is usually indicated, as are the essential oils. Supplemental olive oil internally and externally will usually be helpful. A supplement formula with vitamin A and beta-carotene, the B vitamins, and zinc is also useful.

Dandruff is a form of dry skin of the scalp. Often this results from an improper diet high in certain fats, such as hydrogenated fats and fried fats, and deficient in important essential fatty acids, which are found in the vegetable oils and fresh nuts and seeds. Lots of mental activity and poor water intake usually underlie a dandruff condition. Food allergies or deficiencies of the B vitamins, beta-carotene, and minerals, such as zinc, are also possible causes. Seborrheic dermititis is a specific oil-based irregularity of the skin and scalp. Selenium sulfide (Selsun) shampoos are often helpful in the treatment of dandruff. An overnight olive oil wrap may remoisturize the skin and clear the snowstorm. To apply such a wrap, shampoo and let hair almost dry, or just dampen it slightly. Apply cold-pressed olive oil and massage it into the scalp. Wrap with a towel and sleep, then shampoo in the morning. Additional amounts of nutrients such as vitamins A, B_6, C, and E, zinc, selenium, and essential fatty acids may help correct the dandruff problem from the inside out.

Acne, a common problem in teenagers, results from a combination of hormone stimulation, production of irritating fatty acids by certain bacteria, stress, and poor diet. Acne vulgaris (the medical name) is tied to an overproduction of the oil in the sebaceous glands of the skin. More water intake, eliminating fried foods and hydrogenated fats from the diet, and taking extra vitamin A and zinc will often reduce acne outbreaks. Food allergies and intestinal yeast overgrowth also seem to increase acne problems. Extra essential fatty acids, such as one or two tablespoons of cold-pressed flaxseed oil daily, plus the B vitamins, extra pantothenic acid, calcium, and sulfur, may help. Aloe vera gel applied to the skin, and goldenseal powder and comfrey compresses may protect and help heal the acne sores. Oral antibiotics such as tetracycline (the most commonly used), a topical erythromycin gel, or a dangerous pharmaceutical, Accutane, can be effective in more serious, nonresponsive cases of acne.

Insect bites or contact (allergic) dermatitis from plants, chemicals, or metals may respond to local application of various poultices, such as baking soda or comfrey root or goldenseal powder, applied to the skin and covered with a bandage. This is often beneficial for poison oak sores, for example. Increased levels of vitamin C, often with additional A and zinc, may be helpful for insect bites. Higher levels of thiamine, or vitamin B_1, such as 50–100 mg. two or three times daily, may repel insects such as mosquitoes or fleas as they dislike the thiamine odor that is eliminated through the skin. The other B vitamins should be taken along with the B_1 to prevent imbalances.

Psoriasis is a more complex problem, associated with well-demarcated raised red patches on the skin with a silvery scale. It most commonly occurs around the elbows and knees, that is, at the hard or stressed surfaces. It may also appear around the scalp and, in fact, can occur anywhere. Its exact etiology is not known, though psoriatic skin does show a very rapid cell division—it is skin that is growing too fast. Whether this is an immunological, genetic, or stress problem, or all three, is not known for certain, though stress definitely seems to aggravate psoriasis. A recommended treatment plan for this condition includes relatively low fat and protein content in the diet; more high-water content, high-nutrient foods; extra vitamin A and/or beta-carotene, zinc, vitamin C, bioflavonoids, and liquid lecithin; in addition, a sulfur-based ointment used regularly on the lesions with alternate applications of aloe vera gel. Following some of the guidelines in the *Anti-Stress* program may be helpful as well.

Herbs

Herbs useful in maintaining healthy skin or treating some conditions include comfrey leaf and root, topical aloe vera gel, yellow dock, horsetail (springtime), licorice root, parsley, cayenne pepper, and garlic. Comfrey's healing properties help strengthen tissues of the skin, tendons, ligaments, and bone. This herb can be used both internally and externally. Yellow dock and cayenne work mainly to help detoxify the liver and blood. Parsley acts as a diuretic and may help clear toxins as well. Licorice helps the digestive and adrenal functions. The cortisonelike activity from the adrenal glands helps the skin tissue maintain its tone and elasticity. Excess cortisone, usually from medicines, may cause very bad stretch marks (striae) and many other side effects. Garlic is also a purifier, and it is known to reduce skin cancer potential.

In his fascinating book, *The Scientific Validation of Herbal Medicine*, Daniel B. Mowrey recommends an herbal skin formula for general cleansing or itching and dry skin of many disorders, such as acne, eczema, and psoriasis. It includes chapparal, to cleanse and decrease mutagenic cells; dandelion root for liver and blood detoxification; burdock root and yellow dock root for blood purification (these are often helpful for eczema); echinacea for immunological support (it also reduces boils and skin ulcers, helps cleanse lymph, and stimulates white blood cell production); licorice root; kelp; and cayenne. This is a powdered formula taken in capsules, from several a day for maintenance or purification up to 10–12 a day to treat particular skin conditions. A steam facial using flowers such as rose petals is very cleansing and relaxing. Boil a pot of water, drop some rose, calendula, or marigold flowers in it, and sit over the steam with a towel over your head for 10–15 minutes. Follow with a little lotion or your preference of skin care products.

The general program for skin enhancement shown in the following table is intended for people with dull or lackluster skin, dry skin, or a chronic skin condition. Aspects of other programs, such as the *Anti-Stress* program, *Anti-Aging* program, or the *Detoxification* programs, may be combined with this program. Smokers should follow the *Nicotine Detoxification* program as well. Remember, too, that worry and extreme emotion tend to increase our aging process and wrinkle our skin. "Don't make those faces; your face may freeze that way"—not really; we should express ourselves, but to take good care of our skin, we should take care of our whole body. Focus on this program for a few months. Evaluate your skin and general health before and after, and work to incorporate healthy habits as well, such as drinking water, exercising, and eating well.

SKIN ENHANCEMENT PROGRAM

Water	2–3 qt.
Protein*	50–75 g.
Fats*	40–65 g.
Fiber	10–15 g.

Vitamin A	10,000–20,000 IUs	Iodine	150 mcg.
Beta-carotene	15,000–25,000 IUs	Iron	10–18 mg.
Vitamin D	400 IUs	Magnesium	300–500 mg.
Vitamin E	400–600 IUs	Manganese	10 mg.
Vitamin K	150–300 mcg.	Molybdenum	500 mcg.
Thiamine (B$_1$)	25–50 mg.	Selenium, as selenomethionine	200–300 mcg.
Riboflavin (B$_2$)	25 mg.	Silicon	200 mg.
Niacin (B$_3$)	50 mg.	Sulfur	400–800 mg.
Niacinamide (B$_3$)	100 mg.	Vanadium	200 mcg.
Pantothenic acid (B$_5$)	250 mg.	Zinc	45 mg.
Pyridoxine (B$_6$)	50 mg.		
Pyridoxal-5-phosphate	50 mg.	L-amino acids	1,000 mg.
Cobalamin (B$_{12}$)	100 mcg.	Essential fatty acids from olive oil and	1–2 Tbsp. on food
Folic acid	800 mcg.		
Biotin	500 mcg.	Flaxseed oil, or	2 tsp. as supplement
PABA	100 mg.		
Inositol	500 mg.	Primrose oil	4–6 capsules
Choline	500 mg.	Lactobacillus acidophilus	1 billion or more organisms per dosage
Vitamin C	2–4 g.		
Bioflavonoids	250 mg.		
Calcium	600–800 mg.		
Chromium	200 mcg.		
Copper	2 mg.		

*With increased caloric needs, and for bigger and more active people, these numbers may be higher to maintain 30 fat (9 cal./g.) and 12–15 protein (4 cal./g.).

Sexual Vitality

While most species of Earth use the sexual act for procreation, humankind may be the only one for which sex is a pleasure, sport, and obsession. Along with money, hunger, and desire for power, sex is a primary motivating force. It is a basic instinctual urge that all humans experience at some time, and the sexual/sensual component of a relationship is often necessary to keep it strong and healthy.

Many changes have occurred in our sexual focus in the last quarter century. It is no longer oriented just to erections, marathon sex, and multiple partners, though that might be the interest for some. We now have more responsibilities for our own and each other's health. Safe sex—not transmitting diseases or creating unprepared-for pregnancies—is definitely both sensible and in vogue. Condoms are back, birth control is important, and knowing your partner is crucial to health. There have always been some built-in dangers with sexual activity, from syphilis to gonorrhea to herpes and now AIDS. As the dangers grow, often so do the mystique and adventure of sexuality.

Nowadays, people are more monogamous, attempting to focus on loving and supporting one another, looking more for growth and learning and less for control and dependency. Relationship vitality is important and often secondary to sexual vitality; love that binds us must reach many levels, emotional and spiritual as well as physical. Few relationships last over the long term that are based on good sex alone, just as few endure without a decent sexual relationship. Ultimately, love is the overriding principle, and with love, physical sharing and enjoyment are manifest.

Stress and nutrition are important factors in sexual vitality. Stress, particularly mental stress in the form of worry, overwork, and financial concerns, can interfere with sexual energy and expression. On the other hand, sexual problems themselves can be a source of anxiety and unhappiness. Resolving relationship problems often requires some psychological assistance. Guilt can be a big psychological block to adequate sexual energy. In many situations, there has not been a clear emotional separation from a parent or a previous loved one, and subconscious feelings of incest or adultery may be undermining the experience. Fears of certain fantasies becoming reality may also create anxiety interference. There are all kinds of potential sexual problems. In this section, however, we concentrate more on supporting a healthy sexual function rather than the wide range of sexual dysfunctions and infertility.

For normal function, we need both healthy organs and a balanced, working endocrine system, producing the necessary hormones. Low pituitary function may lead to decreased development of the sexual organs, early menopause in women, and impotence in men. Weak adrenals may reduce the desire and strength for sex and increase sensitivity to stress. Low thyroid may cause a lack of desire or capacity for sex. In men, low testicular function decreases sex drive and sperm production. In women, low estrogen slows sexual maturity, decreases breast size, and retards egg maturation. Estrogen-progesterone imbalance can create many menstrual cycle variations and symptoms.

For a fulfilling sexual relationship, women particularly need to feel love and to have energy without fatigue, a hormonal balance that allows peaceful emotions, and some level of relaxation with a good sex drive. Men need good circulation to create a penile erection, physical vitality, and good hormone function. Lust often encourages more passionate sex. This is most common early in a relationship, when fantasy and sensuality arouse the sexual desires of both sexes. But for a longer run and repeat performances, some other qualities must be present in the relationship.

A big obstacle to a longer-range satisfying sexual relationship is boredom or complacency. Becoming used to each other, along with the little day-to-day irritations or conflicts, can easily interfere with the sexual energy of either or both partners, and soon, sex may be a rare occurrence, decreasing in frequency from daily or weekly to monthly or even less often. Bringing a feeling of freshness, fantasy, romance, and new energy into the relationship and bedroom will often revive the sex life. Creativity in a relationship is important.

There is no reason why sexual activity has to decrease in later years, though for most people, it usually does become less frequent. The changes that come with age still allow sexual function; realistically, however, it is not the same as it is in a young person. Women have lower hormone levels later in life unless they go on hormone replacement, but they can still maintain sexual vitality and drive, with or without hormones. Men usually have less decrease or a less distinct cutoff in hormone levels, which are more necessary for their sexual function. As long as there is good circulation and cardiovascular health, both sexes can maintain a good sex life. Obesity, poor diet, mental and emotional stress, and cardiovascular disease are some common conditions that can interfere with sexual vitality.

The Chinese have a concept about the frequency of ejaculation and orgasm for men and women that is described in the fascinating book *The Tao of Sex and Loving* by Jolan Chang. According to this theory, men are meant to have frequent erections, lots of sex, and only rare orgasms. Regular ejaculations drain the kidney/adrenal chi (energy) and possibly lead to fatigue, decreased vitality, or lower back weakness in men. When the adrenals are weakened, there is also lower ability to handle stress. Men can learn to have more complete orgasms without ejaculation with special techniques described in the book. Women are meant to have as many orgasms as they wish, which are energizing to them. And if the man is not releasing all the time, he will have more sexual vitality to satisfy his partner. Sound intriguing?

Many other factors seem to affect sexual desire and performance. Alcohol, nicotine, coffee, marijuana, and sugar are some of the pleasure drugs that may reduce sexual vitality, as can many pharmaceuticals, such as tranquilizers, antihypertensives, particularly beta-blockers, and birth control pills or hormones. Other factors that may influence sexuality include genetics, childhood upbringing, personal attitudes, and basic hormone levels. For example, men with higher testosterone levels and better adrenal function usually will have more sex drive.

As mentioned earlier, stress levels also can interfere directly with sexual function and drive. Often, underlying worries about money, job, and so on take our minds off sex. A recent study revealed that men who received raises or promotions at work increased their sexual frequency; the reverse happened to those who were demoted or whose pay was decreased. (For more understanding of stress aspects, see the *Anti-Stress* program. Further discussion of sexuality is found in the programs for *Adult Men, Adult Women,* and *The Elderly.*)

Nutrition can also have a lot to do with sexual vitality, which clearly decreases with malnourishment. The focus of the diet is on antiaging and a healthy cardiovascular system. A wholesome diet low in fat and high in fiber and complex carbohydrates is a good place to begin. Any diet (and lifestyle) that maintains good circulation and normal weight and contains high-vitality fresh foods will lead to better sexual function. A good protein intake is important, but excessive protein may interfere with sexuality. Likewise, adequate dietary fats and fatty acids are required for normal hormonal function. Cholesterol is a precursor of several sexual hormones, and if it is too low, this may lead to impaired sexual function and vitality.

Regular exercise is also very important to reduce stress and anxiety and support a healthy heart. However, excessive exercise, especially in women, can reduce fertility, hormone levels, menstrual periods, and sex drive, so balance is important here as well.

Many of the foods traditionally believed to improve sexual function are from the ocean. Fish are thought to be good for brain and sexual function, especially the shellfish, such as oysters and clams. This may be because of their high levels of zinc. High-zinc foods have been thought to support male prostate function; pumpkin seeds, an old prostate helper, are high in zinc. Also from the ocean come the very-high-mineral seaweeds, which seem to support sexual function. Celery, especially celery root, is thought to be a mild aphrodisiac. Milk products such as cheeses and ice cream may have a sedative effect on sexual energy.

There are many specific supplements that influence sexual vitality, particularly vitamin E and zinc. Vitamin C, niacin, and the amino acid arginine also seem to support sexual function. Many glandular formulas are available, and some men and women may experience improvement with them. The idea that if we eat the organs or organ extracts from other animals to offer some essential help to our own corresponding organs is not a new concept and does make some sense, but there is no good research to substantiate the effectiveness of doing this.

As for many other programs related to age and stress, a general multivitamin and antioxidant formula is a good idea. Extra vitamin E may be helpful for sexual vitality and fertility, but this is still hard to prove in humans. The essential fatty acids are important to tissue strength and membrane integrity and fluidity. Niacin, the flushing

NUTRIENTS FOR SPECIFIC SEXUAL ORGANS

Brain	*Pituitary*	*Adrenal*	*Thyroid*
B vitamins	B vitamins	Vitamin A	Iodine
Choline	Pantothenic acid	B vitamins	B vitamins
Calcium	Niacin	Pantothenic acid	Thiamine
Magnesium	Vitamin E	Niacin	Vitamin E
Potassium	Zinc	Thiamine	Tyrosine
L-amino acids		Vitamin C	
Tryptophan		Vitamin E	
		Essential fatty acids	

Testes and Sperm*	*Ovaries*
Vitamin E	B vitamins
Zinc	Niacin
Vitamin A	Folic acid
Vitamin C	Vitamin E
Folic acid	Zinc

*Sperm contains calcium, magnesium, zinc, sulfur, vitamin B_{12}, vitamin C, and inositol, so these are likely important also. ATP (energy) is an absolute requirement for sperm motility, so nucleic acids, especially inosine, are important for fertility.

form of vitamin B_3, acts as a vasodilator, increasing blood flow to the skin and many other parts of the body. Some people also experience sexual stimulation from this niacin flush. Zinc seems to be especially related to male fertility and sex drive. Low zinc levels may lead to impotence, a low sperm count, and a loss of sexual interest. However, taking more than 100 mg. daily is not recommended as this can reduce immune function and absorption of other minerals, such as copper and manganese. Prostate health and testosterone hormone production may also be influenced by zinc. Vitamin C is associated with sperm motility, and male infertility has been related in part to vitamin C deficiency. Besides vitamin C, the bioflavonoids, along with vitamins A and E, and the mineral zinc, are important to healthy mucous membrane tissue and function. L-arginine, an amino acid, is also somehow tied to sperm production. In a study cited by Dr. Sheldon Hendler in *The Complete Guide to Anti-Aging Nutrients*, 4 grams per day of arginine increased low sperm counts in 80 percent of the men tested. Many of them were then able to naturally father children. Selenium may mildly stimulate sexual energy; manganese may also be related to sex drive; and molybdenum may have an as-yet-undetermined influence on sexual function. Pantothenic acid provides pituitary and adrenal support and, thus, indirectly improves testosterone production in men. Folic acid is a B vitamin helpful for both ovarian function and sperm production, and it, along with beta-carotene, vitamin E, and selenium, may reduce the production of abnormal cells. Iodine supports the thyroid gland function, which improves both the desire and capacity for sexual activity.

A number of herbs seem to influence sexual function and enhance sexual vitality, in addition to the many botanicals that have been used for treating various sexual maladies. Ginseng root is the classic example of a sexual strengthening herb. It is used more for men than for women, though when the lack of sexual energy is a result of fatigue, ginseng may help in both sexes. The aphrodisiac and sexual power capacities of ginseng, however, are only anecdotal and not supported by research; its main benefit may be its effects in supporting general vitality. Dong quai and Fo-ti tieng are two other herbal roots used in traditional Chinese medicine. Dong quai is a female herb that acts as a blood purifier, antispasmodic for cramps, and as a hormonal tonic. Fo-ti tieng, or *Polygonium multiflore*, is used more in males as a kidney tonic and diuretic, and to enhance fertility. It is also used for blood sugar programs. Both herbs can be taken in capsules or boiled to make tea. Damiana leaf has an historical reputation as an aphrodisiac and a stimulant of sexual activity. Good-quality (fresh, dried) damiana has helped many people stimulate their sexual appetites. Saw palmetto herb is best known for its treatment of male prostate problems. It and damiana have been used together to enhance sexual health. Both are also employed for respiratory difficulties. Licorice root seems to possess some estrogenic properties and has been used in many female tonifying formulas. It may be useful for reproductive health and for treating infertility. Sarsaparilla root contains "building block" chemicals that stimulate the synthesis of steroid sex hormones.

The following table lists the supplement suggestions for maintaining or strengthening sexual energy. Following this, along with a good diet, a low anxiety level, a little romance, and a springtime picnic with the one you love, will keep all your body parts alive from the top down and from your toes up. Keep loving yourself and others to feel young and lively.

SEXUAL VITALITY NUTRIENT PROGRAM

Water	2 qt.
Protein	50–70 g.
Fats	50–75 g.
Fiber	15–20 g.

Vitamin A	10,000 IUs	Copper	women—2 mg.
Beta-carotene	20,000 IUs		men—3 mg.
Vitamin D	400 IUs	Iodine	225 mcg.
Vitamin E	800 IUs	Iron	women—18 mg.
Vitamin K	300 mcg.		men—10 mg.
Thiamine (B$_1$)	50 mg.	Magnesium	350 mg.
Riboflavin (B$_2$)	50 mg.	Manganese	10 mg.
Niacin (B$_3$)	50 mg.	Molybdenum	500 mcg.
Niacinamide (B$_3$)	50 mg.	Selenium	200 mcg.
Pantothenic acid (B$_5$)	500 mg.	Silicon	100 mg.
Pyridoxine (B$_6$)	50 mg.	Zinc	women—30 mg.
Pyridoxal-5-phosphate	50 mg.		men—60 mg.
Cobalamin (B$_{12}$)	100 mcg.	Flaxseed oil	1–2 t.
Folic acid	800 mcg.	L-amino acids	1,000 mg.
Biotin	500 mcg.	Inosine	150–300 mg.
Inositol	500 mg.	Herbs	
Choline	500 mg.	see previous discussion	
Vitamin C	2–3 g.	in this program	
Bioflavonoids	250 mg.		
Calcium	650 mg.		
Chromium	200 mcg.		

Athletes

This is a program that I am really excited about, partly because I like to think that I am an athlete. I believe that this program can really make a significant difference in the fine-tuning and longevity of the competitive athlete. The nutritional misconceptions among sports people are great, and the diets, protein concoctions, and vitamins they are taking may even be dangerous.

Although there may be some differences between the body builder and the marathon runner, they are both required to push their bodies to the limit. Increased activity levels, sweating, and tissue wear and tear mean a need for special support. Any intelligent athlete also should know how important it is to balance workouts with proper stretching exercises to maintain flexibility, and with toning exercises as well as some aerobic activity for cardiovascular health. Aerobic exercise—continuous, repetitive movement of large muscle groups (legs or whole body) for more than 10–15 minutes—uses oxygen more efficiently, plus it burns fat. Our maximum aerobic exercise heart rate (calculated simply) is 220 minus our age. Depending upon our physical state, we will usually exercise at a range from 70–85 percent of our maximum.

A concern I see in my practice is the "ex-athlete," such as the college jock who was in training for years on a special high-protein, high-fat diet. Such people usually handle this type of diet well enough in their early years because of the high amount of exercise they did. However, when they entered the work world instead of professional sports and changed their lifestyle but not their diet, they gained weight and clogged their arteries. This is also true for retired sports professionals. Changes in activity levels require changes in diet, both total calories and types of food eaten. Such people need to keep exercising as well as change their diets to reduce the chances of early death from cardiovascular disease. No one should ever really become an ex-athlete anyway; exercise is for life. It represents a commitment to health.

One of the big problems with athletes is that regular training and vigorous workouts allow them to get along with the worst kind of diet. The body uses up everything and needs more. Exercise is as important as or more important than a good diet, but implementing both together is the optimum; this duo is the best plan for weight reduction and maintenance. Regular exercise improves metabolism and calorie/ nutrient use, reduces cardiovascular disease risk, osteoporosis and diabetic risks, while it improves oxygenation and psychological attitude. Competitive or professional athletes also require a balanced exercise program supported by proper nutrition.

Athletics is affected by a lot of nutritional controversies, and it may be hard for athletes to know what is good for them. High-protein diets, lots of meat, protein powders, salt tablets, special vitamin pills, and now carbohydrate loading to prepare for

759

endurance and competitive efforts—these are just a few of the topics. I do not support high-protein diets or protein powders, although in some cases these may be helpful. People in active training do have some increased protein needs, but too much animal protein and powders can stress the kidneys and contribute to toxic metabolic products in the colon and body.

Salt tablets are almost always unnecessary—water and high-nutrient foods and occasional salted snacks will replace what is needed. Potassium and magnesium are needed as much as or more than sodium chloride. High-fat diets are also contraindicated. Muscles need glycogen (a carbohydrate) for their fuel, and carbohydrates give us the sustained energy we need for athletic activity. Thus, a basic complex-carbohydrate diet is the healthiest focus, with some added special dimensions for training.

Regular vigorous exercise obviously increases our demands for most everything, particularly calories and nutrients. Exercise improves our elimination and our metabolism, which means we need to nourish ourselves regularly. Physical exercise is also a stressor that may increase free-radical formation, so that additional antioxidant nutrients may be required. The physical stresses of vigorous exercise may also cause tissue irritation and breakdown, which we can counteract with natural anti-inflammatories, such as vitamins E and C and *bromelain* enzyme, and with amino acids to build up the tissues again. Regular sweating also causes the loss of many nutrients, particularly water, Vitamin B_1, and some minerals—sodium, potassium, chloride, and magnesium are probably the most significant.

If all of these processes and nutrients are not balanced, nutritional deficiencies may result. Then, injuries can occur more easily, bone or muscle loss or breakdown may result, and this can all interfere with athletic performance. We prevent injuries with proper care in nutrition, adequate stretching and warm-ups, proper cool-downs, and adequate liquid intake. In the competitive world, the slightest changes may make a great difference—sometimes the difference between losing and winning. For professional athletes, of course, this could affect their livelihood.

Diet for the athlete in training and/or for performance is centered on the complex carbohydrates—whole grains and their products, such as pasta, legumes, potatoes and other starchy vegetables—along with some good-quality vegetable and/or animal protein, fruits, and a low-to-moderate fat intake. Athletes, like everyone else, need a well-balanced diet with a high nutrient intake. The increased activity generates the need for a higher amount of calories, protein, and other nutrients than the less active person requires. For weight control or maintenance, we need to vary our calorie intake with our activity level. When the season is over or we take time off or just stop exercising for some reason, we need to change our diet and consume less calories, fats, and proteins.

A high-fat diet is definitely out for athletes. It slows them down and can increase the body fat percentage, something that is taboo for the active athlete. For many of us, the fatty flavor of foods is the more addictive aspect of the diet, and with any lessening of physical activity, the higher-fat foods will clog the blood vessels and increase cholesterol and heart disease risk. Athletes should definitely avoid fried foods, high-fat meals, lunch meats, bacon, ham, and any foods cooked in animal fats. The higher-protein, lower-fat foods such as fish and poultry are better than the red meats. Some nuts and seeds, high in essential oils and protein, can be used as well.

Protein is very important for athletes, but the subject of how much and which proteins are best needs a lot of clarification. Protein intake in general should be less of a focus in the diet. Excess protein intake can produce certain minor problems, including clogging of the colon and stress on the kidneys. More protein than is needed for tissue building and its other functions merely gets used for energy or must be eliminated. The complex carbohydrates, though, are used much more efficiently for energy needs or for storage for later use. So, for best efficiency and performance, I believe that a diet based on complex carbohydrates with adequate, but not excess, protein is ideal.

Athletes (and regular exercisers), however, do need some extra protein with increased activity, but it should be increased in proportion to calories. People who are trying to gain weight, those wanting to build muscle, or those in heavy training do need additional protein, sometimes up to 150–200 grams daily, to stay in positive protein balance, especially when the calorie intake goes up near 3,000 a day. Some protein powders and amino acid formulas can be used to augment the protein balance. Aerobic-type exercises may slightly increase protein needs but not as much as body-building activities. Some extra protein intake, still along with a high-complex-carbohydrate, low-fat diet, will support muscle bulk while maintaining body fat levels. Young athletes need even more good protein foods than adults but should still focus on the complex carbohydrates for proper development. Again, avoid high-protein diets that exclude other important foods, particularly the complex carbohydrates, fruits, and vegetables. For building muscle, it may be better in many cases (especially when extra calories are not needed) to use good-quality supplemental amino acids or protein hydrolysates containing peptides to provide the cells and tissues with what they need to build and repair, rather than eating an excess of heavier flesh food proteins.

Complex carbohydrates provide the sustaining long-term energy, proteins the tissue building, and fats the lubrication and tissue support. This type of diet is also high in fiber, which allows good elimination. It is wise for serious athletes and health-conscious people to avoid excessive use of alcohol, regular cigarette smoking, and stimulants such as caffeine in coffee, tea, and cola beverages. Some iron-rich foods are especially important for female athletes or active runners, as their red blood cells may be broken down more rapidly. High-iron foods include red meats and liver (organic only), shellfish such as oysters, leafy greens, prunes, and mushrooms. With anemia, higher doses of supplemental iron may be needed.

Carbohydrate loading is a fairly new concept in the athletic world. It is based on the fact that complex carbohydrates such as grains, pastas, pancakes, and whole grain breads increase available energy, improving the stamina and ability to work. Here is how carbohydrate loading works. Four or five days before an endurance-type event, we increase our exercise and reduce our complex carbohydrate intake to about 40–50 percent of our diet, and eat more protein, fats such as dairy products and eggs, and fruit. This depletes the glycogen in our muscles and liver. Then, two to three days before the event, we increase complex carbohydrates to 70–75 percent of our diet, eating at least three big meals of carbohydrates, plus some proteins and fats. This increases the stored glycogen in the liver and muscles. Glycogen, the storage form of glucose, is easily converted to the simple sugar that is used by all cells and tissues for energy. Glycogen is then burned first for energy; if more energy is needed, fat will be utilized, and that works well too. If there is very low body fat, proteins in tissues may also be converted to energy. All of these macronutrients will need to be replaced. Some athletes report that carbohydrate loading increases sexual energy too. For any athletes with fatigue, carbohydrates will often help. Adding more grains, pasta, cereals, breads, vegetables, and fruit may also add strength and endurance.

GENERAL BALANCED DIET FOR ATHLETES

Carbohydrates—50–60 percent of total calories
    10–20 percent simple—fruits, most vegetables, and any special "treats"
    40–50 percent complex—whole grains, legumes, starchy vegetables

Proteins—15–20 percent (maximum 25 percent)
    animal—fish, poultry, meats, eggs, dairy
    vegetable—nuts, seeds, legumes

Fats—25–30 percent
    saturated—meats, eggs, dairy products
    unsaturated (more than half)—nuts, seeds, vegetable oils, avocado

---

One of the biggest nutrient concerns in athletes is water depletion. With heavy training, be it strenuous or extensive activity, large water losses can occur, and drinking water is the only way to remedy this. Long endurance events also increase the need for fluids. Any activity where sweating occurs sets up an even higher requirement for water than the usual one and a half or two quarts per day. Water, which should be our main liquid, has many essential functions. It supports the whole process of sweating and elimination of toxins, it nourishes the skin and other tissues, and it is the medium in which our blood cells circulate and everything in our body lives. Dehydration from low fluid intake leads to weakened tissue perfusion (circulation of blood with oxygen and nutrients), fatigue, and poor performance.

In addition to water, extra minerals must be replaced. These can be added to the water or replaced with food consumed following exercise. Prepared fluid-replacement drinks are good in concept, but many contain chemicals and are overly sweet. For fluid replacement, it is best to avoid sugary drinks or even lots of fruit juices. Diluted fruit juices with minerals would be helpful. I use a vitamin C powder with calcium, magnesium, and potassium designed by Allergy Research Company/Nutricology, sometimes adding some powdered amino acids.

For long events, a little sweet liquid, such as fruit juice, can be added to the water to provide some calories and energy. Water should be drunk in the couple of hours before an event to rehydrate the tissues and then, if there is extended competition or workout, sipped throughout the activity. No colas, caffeine, or alcohol should be consumed prior to or during a race or any exercise. Salt tablets are also best avoided.

Nutritional supplements are often helpful in improving athletic performance. A good-quality, high level multivitamin/mineral is crucial, one whose total daily dosage is contained in 3–6 capsules or tablets; this is best taken several times daily to ensure regular availability. Many B vitamins, such as thiamine, riboflavin, niacin, and pantothenic acid, are lost more rapidly with exercise and need more replacement.

Minerals are of major importance, as many are eliminated and need replacement to prevent muscle cramping, reduced cellular support, and other weakened physiological functions. Potassium chloride is lost during exercise through sweat. It is an important electrolyte for nerve conduction and muscle and heart function and is often useful in preventing spasms. Extra potassium, about 100–200 mg., is helpful after periods of exercise, along with potassium-rich foods eaten throughout the day. Calcium and magnesium are also important, a bit more so for women than for men. The calcium-magnesium cellular exchange supports muscle contraction and relaxation, nerve conductivity, cellular and bone strength, and delivery of oxygen to the muscles. From 600–1,000 mg. of calcium and 400-600 mg. of magnesium daily (above the diet) in two portions is suggested. Taking these supplements after exercise and before bed is the minimum. Iron is especially needed by women to maintain the red blood cells' hemoglobin to carry oxygen; iron is also part of the muscle protein myoglobin. Without enough iron, energy and endurance are usually poor, which is not promising for athletic performance. Chromium is also lost in higher amounts during exercise; at least 200 mcg. are needed daily to help prevent or reduce any risk of sugar metabolism problems.

The antioxidant nutrients are important to reduce tissue irritations, inflammations, and loss of energy caused by free radicals. Vitamin A and beta-carotene, vitamin E, selenium, and vitamin C are all part of the athlete's PEP. Loss of vitamin C, essential to connective tissue strength, is also increased with exercise. Joggers need extra C to prevent bone and ligament injuries, and ascorbic acid may be helpful in reducing all kinds of musculoskeletal irritation and injury. The vitamin C-mineral formula I mentioned previously is not only useful for assimilating the vitamin C, but is also an easily absorbable formula that replaces several important minerals. A complete mineral tablet can also be taken with it. Silicon or silica, usually derived from the horsetail herb *Equisetum arvense*, is important for maintaining elasticity and flexibility in the tissues.

Nutrients and Exercise

- **Water**—essential to cell respiration and circulation
- **Antioxidants (vitamins A, C, and E; selenium, L-cysteine)**—protect against tissue, joint, and cell irritation by reducing free radicals and oxidation of fats
- **Bioflavonoids**—improve vitamin C effectiveness; serve as anti-inflammatory agents

B Vitamins

- **B_1**—generates energy
- **B_2**—improves cell oxidation
- **B_3**—energy metabolism
- **B_5**—adrenal support; boosts energy
- **B_6**—enhances performance by metabolism of amino acids and proteins
- **Folic acid and B_{12}**—red blood cell formation; adequate oxygen delivery
- **Biotin**—carbohydrate metabolism; generates energy
- **Choline**—supports brain and nervous system

Minerals

- **Calcium**—bone metabolism; muscle and nerve function
- **Iodine**—thyroid support
- **Iron**—blood cells and oxygen
- **Magnesium**—muscle and nerve function; with potassium, improves endurance
- **Manganese**—tissue strength and cellular function
- **Potassium**—muscle and nerve function; improves endurance
- **Zinc**—improves performance; growth and tissue repair

Amino Acids (all L- forms)

- **Leucine, isoleucine, valine**—muscle energy
- **Carnitine**—fat utilization, energy generating
- **Arginine**—growth hormone; muscle building
- **Lysine, ornithine**—work with arginine
- **Tyrosine**—thyroid hormone and neurotransmitters
- **Tryptophan**—good sleep
- **Phenylalanine**—improves mental performance; may reduce pain of exercise
- **Aspartic acid**—brain support
- **Proline**—tissue support

Others

- **Enzymes (*trypsin, bromelin, papain, pancreas, superoxide dismutase*)**—reduce inflammation
- **Coenzyme Q$_{10}$**—supports heart function
- **Octacosanol**—increases stamina, long-term effect
- **Liver**—boosts energy
- **Adrenal, heart, thyroid extract**—individual organ support
- **Dimethylglycine**—improves oxygen utilization
- **Gamma-linolenic acid**—anti-inflammatory
- **Inosine**—energizing through ATP formation
- **Germanium sesquioxide**—energizing through facilitating electron transport

For adequate amino acids, a general formula of the L- forms (not D or DL) is best. Usually, two or three portions are taken daily, after exercise and/or after meals. An L-amino formula higher in L-tyrosine and L-phenylalanine may be more stimulating and physically energizing. L-proline will support the syntheses of collagen for membranes, ligaments, and tendons. Some extra magnesium and pyridoxal-5-phosphate, the active form of vitamin B$_6$, may improve the metabolism of the amino acids in the liver and could be used as well after a workout.

Other amino acids useful for athletes could be used only in addition to the general formula. L-carnitine is an important one. It is peculiar in that it is not used in the formation of body tissues but can be made in the liver and kidneys from other amino acids, methionine and lysine, along with niacin, vitamins B$_6$ and C, and iron. It is found in few foods other than animal meats. Carnitine is thought to be helpful in preventing cardiovascular disease, aiding weight loss, and improving athletic performance. It aids in fat metabolism and energy production in the cells' mitochondria by improving utilization of fats. It is a good amino acid supplement for people who exercise.

The combination of L-arginine and L-lysine has also been shown to improve exercise endurance and strength, according to Rita Aero and Stephanie Rick in *Vitamin Power* (Harmony Books, New York, 1987). Two to three grams of arginine and one gram of lysine taken together stimulate growth hormone and protein building. (Other authors, such as Pearson and Shaw of *Life Extension*, have suggested an arginine-ornithine combination.) These combinations help put the body into a positive nitrogen balance, meaning that more protein is being made in the tissues than is being broken down and eliminated. These can be taken together in an amount of about 1,000 mg. each at night after days of heavy workouts, up to four or five times a week, when the other amino acids are taken as well during the day.

The branched-chain amino acids (BCAAs) are leucine, isoleucine, and valine, all of which are essential. In our bodies, these comprise about one-third of our muscle tissue. For people working on muscle building, supplementing the BCAAs can be helpful to this process. Having enough of these amino acids can prevent tissue wasting (protein loss) with exercise. Taking 1–3 grams of each of these amino acids has an anabolic (building) effect on muscle tissue similar to that experienced with steroid treatment, but without the risks and side effects (although they are also not as potent anabolically). When the BCAAs are used it is necessary to take them together, about half an hour to an hour before a workout. Taking 50 mg. of vitamin B_6 or pyridoxal-5-phosphate, its active metabolite—will aid the utilization of the BCAAs. It is also wise to take additional amino acids, including extra L-tryptophan and L-tyrosine, because the BCAAs are so rapidly used that they can interfere with the absorption of these other amino acids.

A number of other supplements have been associated with increased athletic strength and endurance. None has been clearly shown to be effective by the little research done, but many an athlete has described feeling better when using these products. I will leave it up to you to try these "bioenergetic boosters" and see what they do for you.

Octacosanol is said to increase endurance, possibly by improving energy metabolism in the muscles. It is obtained mainly from wheat germ oil, where it is found in high concentration. Bee pollen and other bee products, such as royal jelly, definitely provide some simple carbohydrate energy, and many people feel uplifted and supercharged when using them. They also provide various minerals plus possibly some yet-to-be-discovered power agents. Pangamic acid (see *Vitamin B_{15}* in Chapter 5) is no longer available in the United States, but it is highly touted in Russia for its healing powers and endurance enhancement. Dimethylglycine, or DMG, is the form that people take now to get some of the pangamic acid precursors. Though it is not really clear how this product works, many people describe benefits from its use. Another precursor nutrient that I really like is inosine; used at a dosage of 300–500 mg. daily, inosine helps to release oxygen from hemoglobin. It is the precursor of adenosine, which is the building block for production of ATP, the energy molecule for cellular metabolism.

A formula that I use regularly and before exercise is Oxynutrients by Nutricology in San Leandro, California. It contains 150 mg. of inosine per capsule, plus dimethylglycine, L-carnitine, organo-germanium, coenzyme Q_{10}, and more nutritional energizers. One capsule two or three times daily or two capsules 30 minutes before exercise really makes a difference. I also use it in patients with fatigue or viral problems, and have been receiving excellent reports.

Various body therapies, such as massage, acupressure, and chiropractic skeletal alignment, have helped many athletes perform better. Sexual activity also may add that extra charge for better performance, but this is controversial. Many athletes avoid sexual relations prior to competition. It may, however, be a very relaxing and energizing practice.

Herbs have been used in many ways for the various problems encountered by athletes as well as for increasing performance. Ginseng root has been known to increase stamina. It is a general tonic and also has some antistress properties. Cayenne pepper is a natural stimulant that may raise the metabolism and increase energy levels. Comfrey is a common herb for musculoskeletal injuries. It has some mild anti-inflammatory effects, and I have seen comfrey leaf work "magically" for healing sprains. To use it for this purpose, wrap lightly steamed leaves (or chew them and make a poultice) over the wound and then cover with a cloth. Leave on, if possible, for a few hours. Also, drinking an herbal tea containing comfrey root and the silica-containing spring horsetail will support the healing process. White willow bark contains natural salicylates and thus possesses anti-inflammatory properties. It is available in tablets or capsules and can be used like aspirin for sore joints or muscle aches. *Bromelain* is an enzyme from pineapple and is available as a supplement; it too has mild anti-inflammatory effects, and aids digestion of vegetable protein in the gastrointestinal tract.

Vigorous workouts cause muscle and tissue irritation and inflammation, which can lead to soreness after exercise. This is commonly due to lactic acid buildup and free-radical formation. Antioxidant nutrients, more water, and some anti-inflammatory nutrients and herbs may help reduce some of that soreness when it is bothersome. Also, warm baths, massage, and a long, slow walk will help restore the feeling of being loose and ready for more vigorous exercise.

The program shown in the following table is designed for the serious athlete as well as anyone who is seriously working out to achieve top physical condition by improving strength, flexibility, and endurance. When we work out this way, it affects every other aspect of our life. The amounts listed for each nutrient are the day's total suggested intake, usually taken in several portions throughout the day. Good luck and keep exercising. It's worth it!

ATHLETES' NUTRIENT PROGRAM

Calories*	2,000–3,500
Water*	2–3½ qt.
Protein*	75–150 g.
Fats*	60–100 g.

Vitamin A	5,000–10,000 IUs	**Molybdenum**	500 mcg.
Beta-carotene	15,000–25,000 IUs	**Potassium**	2–3 g.
Vitamin D	400 IUs	**Selenium**	250–400 mcg.
Vitamin E	400–1,000 IUs	**Silicon**	100–200 mg.
Vitamin K	300 mcg.	**Zinc**	women—15–30 mg.
Thiamine (B$_1$)	75 mg.		men—30–60 mg.
Riboflavin (B$_2$)	25–75 mg.		
Niacin (B$_3$)	50 mg.	*Optional:*	
Niacinamide (B$_3$)	100 mg.	**L-amino acids**	1,500 mg.
Pantothenic acid (B$_5$)	1,000 mg.	**L-carnitine**	500–1,000 mg.
Pyridoxine (B$_6$)	50 mg.	**L-arginine**	1,000–1,500 mg.
Pyridoxal-5-phosphate	100 mg.	**L-lysine**	1,000–1,500 mg.
Cobalamin (B$_{12}$)	100 mcg.	**L-proline**	500 mg.
Folic acid	800 mcg.	**Branched-chain**	1,000 mg. each
Biotin	500 mcg.	**amino acids**	(before workouts
Choline	500 mg.	**(leucine, isoleucine,**	with 50 mg.
Inositol	500 mg.	**valine)**	vitamin B$_6$)
Vitamin C	2–5 g.	**Bromelain**	100–200 mg.
Bioflavonoids	250–500 mg.		(2,000 mcu/g.)
		Pancreatic enzymes	200–400 mg.
Calcium	600–1,000 mg.	**(after meals)**	(1–2) tablets
Chromium	250–400 mcg.	**Lactobacillus**	1–2 billion organisms
Copper	2–3 mg.	**Dimethylglycine**	25–50 mg.
Iodine	150–250 mcg.	**(before exercise)**	
Iron	women—20–25 mg.	**Coenzyme Q$_{10}$**	30–60 mg.
	men—10–15 mg.	**Flaxseed oil**	2–3 t.
Magnesium	400–650 mg.	**Gamma-linolenic**	
Manganese	5–15 mg.	**acid (GLA)**	160–400 mg.
		Octacosanol	2–4 capsules
			(250–500 mg.)

---

*Varies from women to men and with the extent of exercise.

Executives and Travel

This program is specifically for business people with persistently high-stress lifestyles. I call it a program for "executives" because most of us associate executives with a very busy life with lots of responsibilities and tight travel schedules; however, any of us may fit into this category. We are all the "executives" of our own lives.

While similar to the *Anti-Stress* program, this one focuses on a particular kind of stress—the high mental and physical demands placed on the "work athlete." These demands often include regular and/or varied chemical exposures, such as inhaling carbon monoxide and other chemicals when driving on freeways, working in smoke-filled offices, or flying in airplanes sprayed with chemicals. Such a lifestyle also may mean frequent eating at restaurants, creating a need for special nutrient protection (and enhancement), and regular travel by car or airplanes, especially across time zones where jet lag may be a problem. This program is really for anyone whose demanding lifestyle means having peak energy and a clear head for longer hours than nine to five.

Many of the habitual stimulants add to already existing stresses. Coffee and doughnuts, let alone cigarettes, play havoc with all the body systems and deplete our energies. Driving in traffic, exposure to smog or chemicals at work, quick snacks on the run, fast foods, sugary treats, big meals at meetings, a little extra alcohol—all are added stressors. With poor diet, being too busy to exercise regularly, and the many stresses of work, we may soon be lying in bed trying to recover our energy and see where we fell off of our healthy life path. We all need to be aware of how the many factors of our lifestyles affect us, and then recover our balance through change. Anyone who smokes or drinks too much coffee or alcohol can refer to the programs for those particular problems in Chapter 18 and create a plan to stop, or at least reduce the excessive use. This program, however, will also help counteract some of the deleterious effects of those drugs and habits.

Most of us find ways to handle our lifestyle stresses from day to day or week to week. We may take little vacations every month or so. If we are strong and healthy to start with and take decent care of ourselves, we should be able to sustain a hardworking schedule almost indefinitely; from a spiritual perspective, though, we all need that special time, even a few weeks, every so often to reevaluate and reprogram our lives. For most of us, this occurs only every few years, for some it takes place yearly, others may always be in this process. Part of staying healthy is learning to listen to our inner voice and timing and keep nourishing our essential being so that we do not need to break down or get sick to reattune.

The general executive nutritional plan includes food low in fat and high in nutrients and water content, with substantial amounts of fresh fruits and vegetables, whole

HEALTHY CHOICES FOR DINING OUT

	Choose	*Avoid*
Breakfast	fresh fruit juice	fried and scrambled eggs
	fruit and yogurt	omelettes
	oatmeal	bacon
	other whole grains	sausage
	granola	baked goods
	soft-boiled eggs	sugar products
Lunch	fish	hamburgers
	pasta	hot dogs
	salad	fried foods
	fruit	lunchmeat sandwiches
	cottage cheese	alcohol
Dinner	big salads	steak
	whole grains	ham and pork chops
	pasta	heavy sauces
	vegetables	alcohol
	fish or poultry	rich desserts
Snacks	mineral water	soft drinks
	fresh fruit	candy bars
	vegetable sticks	coffee
	almonds	

grains, some animal or vegetable proteins, and adequate good drinking water. It is wise to maintain our real energy sources instead of relying on fake caffeine-nicotine stimulation, excess alcohol, and sugary treats and sweets such as candy or doughnuts. Occasional use is okay, but when any of these become a regular habit or a crutch, there is potential for trouble. It is also smart to avoid high-fat and fried foods such as burgers, hot dogs and other cured meats, and nonnutrient, chemical foods such as soft drinks and refined baked goods. Basically, we need our new, healthy American diet, more like the Ideal Diet discussed in Chapter 13—a balanced diet of wholesome meals, with plenty of the fresh foods, especially in the spring, summer, and early autumn. Eating out at restaurants, where lots of hidden chemicals or potentially dangerous nutrients such as excess fats, salt, or additives may be used, can be a real challenge. When traveling, I usually carry some of my regular foods with me on the plane and use them for salads over the first day or two away, which is my "danger zone" for getting off my basic diet plan. Drinking lots of water (which I also carry with me, as I do not drink airline or tap water) while traveling and the first couple of days after traveling helps me prevent getting out of tune in bowel function and sleep patterns. If I will be eating in restaurants I will limit myself to one main meal daily and eat light snacks during the day.

It is also wise for the busy executive to take a moment to relax before and after meals to let go of tensions or worries that may affect digestion. Gastrointestinal problems are not at all uncommon with the busy executive types. Since you may not have much time to go to the doctor, aren't you better off taking care of yourself?

Regular exercise is, of course, essential for any hardworking executive. It reduces stress, helps clear toxins through sweating, and keeps us fit to continue our endeavors. And we would best adapt our attitude to view exercise as fun, convenient, and lifelong, rather than a chore or hassle. There are a multitude of excuses that can interfere with the lifesaving and life-generating benefits of regular exercise. Qualities that we develop internally also help us in our external life. Flexibility developed through stretching and yoga is essential to handling life's stresses. Strength gained from weight lifting, Nautilus machines, or calisthenics and endurance from aerobic activities, such as dancing, running, bicycling, or swimming, will help get us through some of those tougher days. Swimming is especially nice because the water also has a tranquilizing effect.

All executives need a relaxation plan. Wisdom suggests an occasional weekend or at least one day "away from it all" to recharge, play, let go, and get our minds off business. Whatever helps us relax is worthwhile, whether it be reading, a walk in the woods, healthy exercise, going to museums, or hot baths. Plan it ahead, and keep the schedule! Good sleep is essential to staying on top of a demanding lifestyle. If sleep is a problem, check the *Anti-Stress* program for advice. With extensive travel, a bath or hot shower, a steam or occasional massage can all be very useful for staying fit. Massage can clear tensions and bring relaxation; I think it is an absolute necessity for a busy lifestyle.

If we feel stuck and want to change any area of our life, be it job, relationship, or location, counseling often facilitates the process of looking inward. It can help us get a clearer picture of our needs and desires and set up a new plan; therapists can also help us learn relaxation and stress management skills. It may be that we need a change in our attitude so that we do not feel so trapped, or we may really need to change our life externally to create improved health and happiness.

The stress of a busy lifestyle increases our demands for many nutrients, so a multi-vitamin supplement is recommended. Extra B vitamins are essential for anyone under stress. Whereas the exercising athlete needs more minerals and amino acids, the "worker athlete" needs more B vitamins to meet the different kind of mental stress demands. The Bs are best taken two or three times daily, mainly after breakfast and lunch.

Vitamin C is also important—stress eats up C as well as the Bs. Ascorbic acid, or buffered vitamin C if there are acid stomach symptoms, is best taken regularly three, four, or more times daily, one gram after each meal and before bed, along with extra calcium and magnesium at bedtime to help relax the nerves and calm the sleep. Calcium and magnesium are alkaline minerals, they can "buffer" the mildly acidic ascorbic acid.

With stress, there is also increased need for pantothenic acid as well as vitamin C to support the adrenal glands. Digestive enzymes may also be helpful to aid digestion and assimilation of nutrients. With long-term stress, adrenal glandulars may help support our counterstress functions. With exposure to chemicals and the general stress-induced, free-radical toxin production, the antioxidant nutrients are also needed daily. Vitamin A, beta-carotene, vitamin E, selenium, and zinc are all helpful for their protective functions.

Amino acids may be very helpful for busy executives on the go. A formula with a higher amount of tryptophan and less tyrosine and phenylalanine will be more relaxing, which may be particularly helpful when there is a lot of air travel. L-cysteine aids the body's detoxification processes, and can be added, more with travel.

A nutrient program for travel is very important for busy people who fly regularly, including airline pilots and flight attendants. We must counteract the effects of many potential hazards, such as ozone and radiation exposure at high altitudes, cigarette smoke (less so now), lower oxygen levels, air pollution, alcohol, food chemicals, pesticide sprays, airport stress, and time zone changes. Water intake to avoid dehydration is really most important. The air inside a plane is very dry and dehydrates us rapidly. Alcohol consumption adds to the problem, and coffee and nicotine are mild dehydrating agents as well. Thus, constipation, headaches, and fatigue can result from the dehydration as well as from the stress effects of flying. Increasing fluids and vitamin C before, during, and after plane flights will definitely help. I usually take an herbal laxative such as aloe vera capsules, Laci-Lebeau tea, or a mixture of herbs called Lower Bowel Tonic when I fly. My whole life seems to back up when my bowels slow down. I often get a colonic irrigation before I leave for long trips. That usually makes the trip smoother, plus I feel lighter and more positive. I also take extra B vitamins for travel stresses, and additional antioxidants to balance out chemical and radiation exposures.

Flying across time zones, particularly from west to east against the sun, affects our body's natural biorhythms—nature's time clock. It changes our usual light cycle and thus affects our pineal and pituitary glands, which influence most of our hormonal and energy systems. Extra L-amino acids along with and vitamin C will help counter jet lag. A high-complex-carbohydrate meal and additional tryptophan along with extra water intake will provide relaxation and good sleep. It is best to reattune our bodies to our new time zone, including eating, sleeping, and activity cycles, rather than live in the old. An L-amino acid formula with a high proportion of tryptophan is more relaxing, especially to the brain, than a formula with more tyrosine and phenylalanine, which compete with tryptophan in the brain and is more likely to be stimulating. But many people find that the tyrosine-phenylalanine combination, 1,000 mg. of each, works better for them for jet lag. In *The Immune Power Diet*, Stuart Berger, M.D., notes that this amino combination, along with 1,000 mg. vitamin C and 100 mg. vitamin B_6, taken before sleep, is what works best for him, especially after flying from west to east. Extra L-tryptophan taken at night along with vitamin C and calcium and magnesium will help us to relax and get a good night's sleep. Carrying a tape deck with some relaxing music is also useful during the flight and for sleep. Also, doing some exercise and stretching after landing, followed by a warm bath or sauna, a massage, and a light meal, is a great way to recharge in a new city, and does wonders for jet lag. These approaches are integral parts of a jet-set lifestyle. Try them!

Some herbs may also help provide a calming effect with travel and with a highly stressed, busy lifestyle in general. There are two phases to this program—energizing and relaxing. To strengthen the active part of this cycle, herbs such as ginseng, a general tonic, or gotu kola leaf, a mental energizer, can be used. I might also suggest various coffee- or caffeine-substitutes rather than using and abusing coffee. Yerba mate is a mildly caffeinated herb that may be part of some herbal stimulating formulas, such as Celestial Seasonings' Morning Thunder. Various mixtures of roasted roots, such as barley or chicory, are mildly stimulating but have no caffeine; Cafix and Pero are very flavorful examples.

The more calming herbs that may be helpful for the busy executive include valerian root and chamomile. These can be made into a tea or taken in capsules. A cup of warm chamomile tea or a mixture such as Sleepytime (even two bags per cup) drunk before bed often makes for a pleasant sleep. Catnip leaf tea is sometimes tranquilizing, as are linden flowers and hops. Calms homeopathic tablets also work very well for aiding sleep; use as directed on the bottle. There are many possible nighttime relaxing teas or encapsulated formulas available. These are often a lot more helpful and healthful than using alcohol or sleeping pills, and they produce no hangover!

The following program can be used either on a regular basis or during periods of high stress. The total amounts can be spread throughout the day in two or three portions.

EXECUTIVES' AND TRAVELERS' NUTRIENT PROGRAM

Water	2–3 qt.
Fats	under 70 g.

Vitamin A	5,000–10,000 IUs		**Copper**	2 mg.
Beta-carotene	15,000–30,000 IUs		**Iodine**	150 mcg.
Vitamin D	400 IUs		**Iron**	10–18 mg.
Vitamin E	400–800 IUs		**Magnesium**	350–500 mg.
Vitamin K	300 mcg.		**Manganese**	10 mg.
Thiamine (B$_1$)	75–150 mg.		**Molybdenum**	500 mcg.
Riboflavin (B$_2$)	25–75 mg.		**Selenium**	200 mcg.
Niacin (B$_3$)	50–100 mg.		**Zinc**	30 mg.
Niacinamide (B$_3$)	50–100 mg.			
Pantothenic acid (B$_5$)	500–1,000 mg.		**L-amino acids**	1500 mg.
Pyridoxine (B$_6$)	100 mg.		**L-tryptophan**	500–1500 mg.
Pyridoxal-5-phosphate	50 mg.		(before bed, if available)	
Cobalamin (B$_{12}$)	100–200 mcg.			
Folic acid	800 mcg.			
Biotin	300 mcg.		*Optional:*	
Inositol	500 mg.		**Adrenal glandular**	100–200 mg.
Vitamin C	4–6 g.		or	
Bioflavonoids	250–500 mg.		**Ginseng root powder**	2–4 capsules
			Herbal relaxing	2 capsules
Calcium	600–800 mg.		formula	or as directed
Chromium	200 mcg.			

Vegetarianism

S ome aspects of vegetarianism have been discussed in Chapter 3, *Protein*, and this type of diet was more fully described in Chapter 9. Here I explore the particular nutrient needs of those following a vegetarian diet, as well as reviewing briefly the many advantages and a few disadvantages of this most humane diet.

Vegetarianism has a long history, and a primarily vegetarian diet is still the most common type on the planet. Even in America, most people's diets were mainly vegetarian until the turn of the twentieth century, when beef consumption began to increase; it continued to increase steadily until only recently.

A change to a vegetarian diet automatically reduces intake of both protein and saturated fats unless there is a marked increase in consumption of dairy foods and eggs. One of the biggest problems with the contemporary American diet, which I have discussed earlier, is the focus on (or obsession with) protein as the staple of the diet. This is probably responsible for the increase in cardiovascular diseases and cancer because it also naturally increases the intake of saturated fats. We need to return to a focus on whole grains, legumes, and vegetables to give us the high-complex-carbohydrate, high-fiber, high-nutrient, and low-fat diet that is so essential to good health and longevity.

Vegetarianism is indeed becoming more popular again. It has support from the American Heart Association and the American Cancer Society, who in their subtle way are finally acknowledging that diet is an important component of health and disease. Many more diet books and cookbooks are focusing on the vegetarian diet, and more athletes, business people, and others are adopting this diet and lifestyle plan.

It is clear to me that vegetarianism makes a statement about both health and planetary consciousness. In a provocative new book, *Diet for a New America*, John Robbins discusses the inhumane treatment of animals and the waste of resources (water and land) by the cattle and poultry industries. Our diet says a lot more about us than just our personal tastes, as Mr. Robbins tells us on the book cover: "How your food choices affect your health, happiness, and the future of life on earth." We all need to be more vegetarian even if we are not "exclusively" vegetarian. Supporting the current carnivorous planetary program is a factor that creates pollution, economic imbalance, and relative starvation, and this is what, I believe, we are trying to change for the health and peace of our future generations—our children.

In my experience, vegetarians often adopt many other positive health habits in addition to eating more naturally. Those who are vegetarians more for health than for religious reasons tend to eat wholesome foods, avoiding the refined flour and sugar foods and other empty-calorie treats, which are also vegetarian "foods." I believe that even the Seventh-Day Adventists, the most celebrated group of vegetarians, at least in the medical literature, could have a much healthier diet and better statistics if they would adopt these principles. Still, as a group, they have lower triglyceride and cholesterol levels and a lower incidence of cancer, heart disease, and obesity than the meat-eating population. A decrease in chronic diseases and an increase in longevity go hand in hand with vegetarianism.

Among the potential disadvantages of vegetarianism are that a no flesh food product diet often makes it more difficult to balance our intake all of the necessary nutrients, particularly protein, vitamin B_{12}, iron, and zinc. Calcium deficiency, in general a big concern, seems not to be as common in vegetarians as had been thought. Adequate protein can easily be obtained, as discussed later in this section. Vitamin B_{12}, or cobalamin, is consistently a problem for vegetarians, especially for the pure vegetarian, or vegan, who eats no animal foods at all—not even milk products or eggs. Vitamin B_{12} is most plentiful in red meats, and some is found in other animal foods, but most plant proteins are fairly low in this "red" vitamin. Brewer's yeast, tempeh (fermented soybeans), and some sprouts have small amounts of B_{12}. Vitamin B_{12} deficiency leads to poor metabolism of protein, fats, and carbohydrate; problems in building the coverings of nerves; and a low red blood cell count, called pernicious anemia. Fortunately, though, B_{12} is stored in the tissues at levels high enough to last for several years of low intake. I believe that a vegetarian's body, or the body of anyone who has a particularly low intake of a nutrient, will naturally develop better absorption of that nutrient. Very few long-term vegetarians whom I have evaluated have had low blood levels of vitamin B_{12}. Extra B_{12} as a supplement (the sublingual tablets are currently the best source of oral B_{12}) will usually prevent any deficiency unless there are problems with the stomach making "intrinsic factor" or with the liver's ability to store this vitamin (see the discussion of *Vitamin B_{12}* in Chapter 5).

A vegetarian diet can also be an important part of a good therapeutic plan for many problems. It is more cleansing or detoxifying than the usual higher-fat and higher-protein diets, because it usually contains a greater percentage of dietary fiber and the watery fruits and vegetables. In terms of the body's nutritional cycles of cleansing, building, and balancing, the vegetarian regime is very effective in cleansing, beneficial in balancing if it is well-planned and implemented, and generally less effective in its building powers. (For that reason, I do not recommend a vegan diet for children or teenagers or during pregnancy or lactation, where I feel more building and strengthening are needed. The lacto-ovo type of vegetarianism, though, should work fine.) It might be wise for all of us to eat a vegetarian diet every so often, such as a day or two a week, one week a month, or even more often during spring and summer. Variations of the vegetarian diet can be used for detoxification as discussed later in Chapter 18. A fast or cleansing diet may be a useful remedy for many types of congestive problems. With sickness, though, I usually suggest more complex carbohydrates in the diet, with higher intake of water and water-containing foods; this helps avoid dehydration and usually improves vitality.

Some choose vegetarianism for spiritual reasons, feeling that it elevates us to our higher vibrational levels and enhances sensitivity. Meats and animal foods pull us down into our earthly realms of sexual instincts, aggression, and desire for power. Often, someone eating a completely vegetarian diet will want to move away from the busy, active life of most cities where the hustle and bustle requires a more aggressive energy. When I lived for years in the country as a vegetarian, we used to describe going into San Francisco on business as a "meat loaf" day.

The vegetarian diet composed of "organically grown" foods comes the closest to following the general nutritional guidelines recommended throughout this book. A high-fiber, high-complex-carbohydrate, nutrient-rich diet composed mainly of whole grains, legumes, vegetables, fruits, nuts, and seeds will provide all the nutrients we need. Whether vegetarian or not, this should be the basic foundation of all health-oriented diets. It is also more alkaline and higher in most vitamins and minerals than any other type of diet. Only small amounts of milk products, eggs, or various animal fleshes might be added to the vegetarian diet to make it easier to obtain the necessary calcium, iron, and B_{12}.

Protein is always the big topic of discussion when it comes to vegetarianism. Eating complementary proteins, such as grains or seeds with legumes, or eggs or dairy foods with any of the vegetable proteins, is the usual suggestion for obtaining adequate protein. This is because each specific vegetable protein is low in one or two of the essential amino acids so that when eaten alone it does not provide equivalent levels of all the essential amino acids required to build our tissue proteins. When we eat some legumes, which are high in lysine and isoleucine and low in tryptophan and methionine, with grains, which have the opposite strengths and weaknesses, we obtain all of our essential amino acids in more equal levels. If the digestion of proteins and the assimilation of amino acids and peptides is normal, then a minimum daily requirement of protein should be in the range of 40–50 grams (about 1½–2 ounces).

Several noted authors have recently suggested that we do not need to be as concerned about complementary proteins as was previously thought. Frances Lappé, who proposed the idea of complementing proteins in *Diet for a Small Planet*, now suggests that our body can find the needed amino acids when any plant protein food has been eaten over the day. Though I have felt that this might be true, I have not seen any conclusive research, which might be hard to conduct, about this issue. On the other hand, it would seem that when there is any malnutrition and subsequent deficiency or low body stores of certain nutrients, in this case amino acids, it would be more difficult to manufacture necessary body proteins from consistent meals containing incomplete proteins eaten over several days. In that situation, or when food intake analyses or blood tests suggest inadequate protein intake or assimilation, we then must focus more on protein consumption and, possibly, digestion. Otherwise, a balanced vegetarian diet should pose no concerns about adequacy of protein intake.

Given the current knowledge and an attitude of "better safe than sorry," I still suggest combining vegetable proteins at meals or at least in the same day to create a complete profile of essential amino acids. Protein deficiency, though much rarer than most people fear, can cause some problems. With a more stressful lifestyle or a high level of athletic activity, protein needs may be increased, and thus, more high-protein foods are required. Fatigue is a common problem in vegetarians with low-protein diets. Weight loss and low body weights are also more likely with this type of diet. Another concern I have is that amino acids and proteins are very important to the immune system. I commonly see lower white (and red) blood cell counts in vegetarians, likely due to not having all the cell-building nutients available, particularly protein. If the immune system is weakened by a low nutrient availability, especially in combination with high stresses, infectious disease is much more likely. In the digestive analyses of my patients I also see a higher amount of parasites and intestinal yeast overgrowth present in the vegetarians. This may be due to the lower protein and higher sweet diet which appears more common with inadequate protein intake—more vegetable-based foods are higher in carbohydrates and sweet flavors, plus many vegetarians crave sweet foods. It may also result from a more alkaline system, which supports growth of parasites and yeasts, or low immunity. In most of these cases, I recommend a higher-protein, wholesome food diet. I may even suggest the additional L-amino acids to ensure that all are present for immune functions, though most amino acid formulas are not "vegetarian derived."

There is also some concern that a high-fiber vegetarian diet does not provide enough of the important minerals such as zinc, manganese, copper, iron, and calcium, or that the phytic acid in grains combines with these minerals in the intestinal tract and reduces their absorption. Recent research described in Dr. Stuart Berger's *How to Be Your Own Nutritionist* suggests that after a few weeks of high-fiber vegetarianism, our body improves its absorption of zinc, iron, calcium, and copper. In any event, I recommend a good mineral supplement program to ensure that we ingest enough of these nutrients. The mineral intake should be in balance, because a high amount of one mineral may interfere with the absorption of the others; this is especially true for zinc and copper or calcium and magnesium.

As part of the supplement program, I suggest a general multiple-nutrient formula, vegetarian-derived, of course. Additional calcium-magnesium is suggested if there is low intake of dairy products. Extra vitamin D will enhance calcium absorption, and this is particularly important during the less sunny months and for those who avoid the sunshine. I encourage taking extra zinc (and copper and manganese to balance with zinc) because it is so important and dietary deficiencies are common, even in vegetarians. I often suggest additional iron, especially if the red blood cell count is low; menstruating women frequently need higher amounts of iron. It is wise for vegetarians to have blood counts done occasionally (every year or two) to make sure that anemia is not developing.

In regard to supplemental vitamin B$_{12}$, I suggest it for all strict vegetarians. It is contained in almost all multiple formulas, though even higher amounts are often wise, at least several times yearly for a month or so. Vitamin B_{12} may often help with problems of fatigue. If there is any problem with absorption (this can be checked by monitoring blood levels), vitamin B_{12} injections would be indicated. An amino acid formula or protein powder may also be useful if there is any fatigue, excessive weight loss, or concern about inadequate protein ingestion, digestion, or assimilation.

The following table offers a basic supplement plan as insurance for those on a vegetarian diet. Some naturalists do not like to take "vitamins," as they are not whole foods, but extracts of foods or synthetic preparations, but in many instances I feel that they are indicated. They are suggested here as a means for prevention of depletions and deficiency diseases. If we eat very well, balance our foods, maintain low stress levels, stay attuned to our body functions, and occasionally test body nutrient states and biochemical functions, then we might be able to avoid supplementation. However, I recommend at least short-term periods, several times yearly, of more intense nutrient intake to ensure proper availability of all the micronutrients.

VEGETARIANISM NUTRIENT PROGRAM

Calories	1,800–3,000*
Protein	50–70 g.

Vitamin A	5,000–10,000 IUs	**Calcium**	500–800 mg.
Beta-carotene	10,000 IUs	**Chromium**	200 mcg.
Thiamine (B$_1$)	25 mg.	**Copper**	2 mg.
Riboflavin (B$_2$)	25 mg.	**Iodine**	150 mcg.
Niacin (B$_3$) or	50 mg.	**Iron**	men—15 mg.
Niacinamide (B$_3$)	50 mg.		women—25 mg.
Pantothenic acid (B$_5$)	100 mg.	**Magnesium**	350–500 mg.
Pyridoxine (B$_6$) or	50 mg.	**Manganese**	5–10 mg.
Pyridoxal-5-phosphate	50 mg.	**Molybdenum**	300 mcg.
Cobalamin (B$_{12}$)	100–250 mcg.	**Selenium**	200 mcg.
Folic acid	400 mcg.	**Silicon**	100 mg.
Biotin	500 mcg.	**Zinc**	30 mg.
Choline	250–500 mg.		
Inositol	250–500 mg.		
Vitamin C	2 g.	**Lactobacillus**	2 billion organisms
Bioflavonoids	250 mg.		
Vitamin D	400 IUs	*Optional:*	
Vitamin E	400 IUs	**L-amino acids**	1,000 mg.
Vitamin K	150–300 mcg.		

*Depends on the size, age, and the activity level of the individual.

Environmental Pollution and Radiation

There are many reasons for concerns about environmental pollution and radiation exposure in this day and age. This is more true around big cities, but even in the rural sections of this nation, air and water contamination is spreading, and pesticides are a danger everywhere. Unless we want to go live in the wilderness, we need to be aware of many environmental toxins and learn how to protect ourselves from them; however, the wilderness is likely to be contaminated these days as well. Also, the air and waterways transport industrial and agricultural pollutants, and radioactive fallout may affect living things anywhere.

Environmental pollution has become a major political and health issue for all of us. The issue of short-term profit versus the health of our planet and ourselves is what we are really addressing. Many of the specific issues and individual environmental toxins, as well as the politics involved, are discussed in detail in Chapter 11. This section also examines some of the specific toxins but is primarily designed to offer a general program on how to minimize, handle, and protect ourselves from the many environmental pollutants and their effects upon us.

Exposure to environmental pollution is inevitable. A healthy human can adapt to mild and periodic exposure to pollutants in our air, water, and food. Some chemicals are easier to avoid than others. We have more control over what we take into our body than what goes into our air and water. Healthy food choices, such as "organic" produce and purified water, and avoiding food additives, cigarettes, and home chemicals will certainly diminish our risks.

Our immune defenses, gastrointestinal and liver functions, and other systems of elimination all play an important role in handling and clearing body toxins. With increased or prolonged exposure or with a diminished ability to handle chemical contamination for a variety of reasons, such as a weakened immune system or a liver overworked with excessive demands from processing certain drugs or consuming too much fat in the diet, our interaction with these toxins can have many damaging effects. The damage may range from mild tissue irritation or immune suppression to an increase in the formation of carcinogenic cells. If these processes continue unchecked, cancer could develop. (See Chapter 11 for a discussion of chemical carcinogenesis.)

Understanding the hazards and where and how we are exposed to these environmental dangers is an important beginning. Our greatest insurance is maintaining a healthy, functioning body and immune system through positive lifestyle habits, such as eating a wholesome diet, exercising regularly, minimizing stress and maintaining positive attitudes. In addition, many nutrients in our diet and extra nutritional supplements can both support needed functions and protect against possible dangers.

This program is designed for people subject to regular (daily) environmental exposure, such as those living in a smoggy industrial city, as well as for people who are chronically or acutely exposed to particular chemical agents. These include artists, chemical workers, metal workers, electronics workers, people who use pesticides, printers, those exposed to x-rays, either as technicians or as patients, and those who work around or at nuclear or other power plants.

The basic guidelines for staying healthy in an increasingly polluted environment involve avoiding certain subtle dangers, protecting ourselves against others, and taking positive personal and political actions.

It is wise to live, if possible, where the air is relatively clean, or, if we cannot, to invest in a home air purifier and to take protective supplements. Stopping smoking and avoiding others' cigarette smoke are also important steps. Making sure our water is clean wherever we live means testing it and possibly investing in a good quality, solid-carbon-block filter or reverse osmosis water purifier to ensure that water, our most important "nutrient," does not add to our contamination (see Chapter 1, *Water*). Buying and eating "organic" foods as much as possible will also help to minimize further exposure to pesticides and other chemicals used to treat food. Growing our own garden is an even better idea and will orient us toward eating more fresh and wholesome food. Avoiding overuse of chemicals at home is also a good idea, as is reducing exposure at work whenever possible. Commonly used steroid drugs can suppress our immune function and reduce our natural defenses' ability to protect us from toxins and microorganisms as well as lead to slower healing. These steroid drugs with their complex and suppressive effects should be avoided, and if possible, natural healing should be supported and encouraged.

Avoiding excessive sun exposure, especially of the face and particularly in fair-skinned individuals, is very important. There has been a marked increase in skin cancer in recent decades, thought to be a result of the thinning of the ozone layer caused by air pollution with chlorofluorocarbons. This means that the sun's ultraviolet rays are less filtered and more dangerous now than they were 25 years ago. A sunscreen, 10–15 SPF, is suggested whenever sun exposure will last longer than an hour. Many natural sunscreens contain PABA, a B vitamin. (For more ideas on healthy survival, see the *88 Survival Suggestions* at the end of Chapter 11.)

Our nutritional plan to counteract exposure to environmental pollutants and radiation begins with a diet that will keep us healthy and not compromise our immune functions with irritating or allergenic foods. That means a diet that provides adequate, balanced protein, is high in complex carbohydrates and low in fat and sugar, and includes plenty of fresh fruits and vegetables. A minimum of four to six glasses of purified water, as well, helps keep everything moving and favors elimination of toxins. Remember, "dilution is the solution to pollution." Taking "medicinal" baths can also be used for detoxification of certain pollutants and radiation exposure.

HEALING BATHS

Metal or chemical exposure—use the *Clorox bath*, which helps remove pollutants through skin. Add 1 cup Clorox bleach to hot bath; soak for 15–20 minutes.

Radiation exposure—try this *salt-soda bath*—a good suggestion following airline flights or long hours at a computer. Add 1 pound each of sea salt and baking soda to hot bath; soak until bath is cool.

Energizing detoxification bath—add 2 cups apple cider vinegar to hot bath; soak 15–30 minutes. Can be used for radiation exposure in place of salt-soda.

Bath Therapy Salts—available in stores to add to bath water for relaxation and relief of muscle aches.

Because chemical bombardment can lead to a weakened immune system, an increase in allergies, and more symptoms and disease, avoiding foods high in chemicals is definitely part of the plan. Some people become hypersensitive to the chemicals in the environment as a result of chemical exposures, and foods can be a major factor. The most important food additives to avoid are the food colors found in so many artificial foods and the nitrates and nitrites used in cured meats, such as bacon, ham, bologna, and salami. Artificial flavors and other food additives, such as sulfites and MSG, should also be avoided.

Chlorophyll-containing foods, such as the greens—lettuces, spinach, chard, and kale—are good choices, as are the cruciferous vegetables, such as cabbage, cauliflower, broccoli, and brussels sprouts, which are thought to be anticancer foods (these should all be "organic," as these skinless vegetables may concentrate chemicals). All of these foods, as well as most sprouts, are good sources of vitamin K; these cruciferous vegetables are also known to protect us from cancer development. Foods rich in beta-carotene, such as these same cruciferous vegetables, as well as carrots and sweet potatoes, will add more of this antioxidant nutrient. Some freshly made vegetable juices daily, with carrots, greens, and others, adds a vitalizing and purifying drink. Miso, a fermented soybean paste used for soup broth, is known to protect against pollution and radiation. Seaweeds, high in natural metal-chelating algins, are likewise useful antipollution foods. They are also high in minerals. Some authorities believe that yogurt and other fermented milk products help protect against pollution. Extra kelp (seaweed powder), brewer's yeast, or liquid lecithin may also give additional support.

ANTI-RADIATION SOUP —*Serves 2*
by Bethany ArgIsle

4 ounces tofu, cut in small squares

1 ounce kombu or nori, cut in strips

3 cups purified water

1 Tablespoon miso paste (or to taste)

1 lemon

1½ cups cooked brown rice

1 Tablespoon toasted sesame oil (optional)

green onions, chopped (optional)

cilantro, chopped (optional)

For "Anti-Radiation Soup," add the tofu and seaweed (nori or kombu) to boiling water and simmer for a few minutes. Stir in some miso paste for flavor (do not boil the miso), add juice of lemon and the optional ingredients if desired, cover, and let sit for 15–20 minutes. Serve with brown rice—eaten separately or stirred into the soup. This macrobiotic dish was shown to reduce radiation sickness after the Hiroshima bombing and will probably protect us from some of the hazardous effects of x-rays and metal exposures.

_____

Many vitamins, minerals, and other nutrients can counteract some of the actions of environmental toxins. A good-quality "multiple" will provide many of them. The antioxidant nutrients will decrease the potential of free-radical toxicity. Vitamin A provides immune support and tissue protection. Beta-carotene specifically reduces the carcinogenicity of many chemicals, especially airborne ones and the chemicals in cigarette smoke; it also helps decrease the negative effects of ionizing radiation. Vitamin C protects the cells and tissues against the effects of water-soluble chemicals such as carbon monoxide, metals such as cadmium, and metabolic by-products such as carcinogenic nitrosamines made from nitrites. At least several grams of ascorbic acid daily are needed for this protection. Vitamin E, about 400–800 IUs, and selenium, 200–300 mcg., work together to protect the cells from pollutants including ozone, nitrogen dioxide, nitrites, and metals, such as lead, mercury, silver, and cadmium. For environmental protection, the sodium selenite form of selenium may not be as effective as the more direct-acting selenomethionine form, especially in regard to its detoxifying function.

Many minerals are useful in this program. Zinc is probably most important as an immune strengthener and tissue healer that is needed for the functioning of many detoxifying enzymes, thus helping to protect the cells from pollutant toxins. As an example, zinc, as well as copper and manganese, function in the *superoxide dismutase* system to detoxify oxygen free radicals which might be generated from ozone and photochemical smog. Calcium and magnesium help to neutralize some colon toxins and decrease heavy metal absorption from the gastrointestinal tract.

The B vitamins are also important. A B complex formula with sufficient thiamine, pantothenic acid, and niacinamide is usually helpful. Niacin, the B_3 "flushing" form, has an interesting role in the purification process, especially with many chemicals and pesticides. A combination of high amounts of niacin and other vitamins and minerals, long saunas, fluids, and exercise offers a very purifying process. There have even been claims of improvement of symptoms from Agent Orange (2,4,5T) toxicity with the use of this kind of detoxification program. This type of program is usually carried out over periods of about two or three weeks. It can even be done on occasion after recent exposure or excessive drug intake (see *General Detoxification* in Chapter 18).

Lipoic acid, a cofactor in the metabolism of pyruvate, is another interesting relative of the B vitamins. It is not essential in humans, but it does have some medicinal effects and is safe. It helps protect the liver and aids in detoxification, particularly for the effects of radiation. This vitamin can be taken at levels of about 100 mg. daily for these effects.

The sulfur-containing amino acids have a protective and detoxifying effect. L-cysteine, the primary one, may help neutralize many heavy metal toxins and toxic by-products (aldehydes) of smoking, smog, alcohol, and fats through its precursor role in the formation of glutathione, a tripeptide essential to the action of several important enzymes, particularly *glutathione peroxidase*. Since glutathione itself is not very stable or thought to be well utilized as an oral supplement, L-cysteine appears best utilized for this protective purpose. Methionine, another sulfur-containing amino acid, also has mild detoxification and protective functions.

Fiber, both the insoluble type, such as wheat bran, and the more soluble psyllium husks, encourage natural detoxification in the colon, binding toxins and reducing absorption of metals. Another chelating fiber is the algin molecule, sodium alginate, that comes from seaweeds. It can be utilized as a supplement to decrease absorption of minerals, especially the heavy metals and radioactive metals used in nuclear power plants and medical testing. The chlorophyll-containing algae, such as chlorella and spirulina also provide this chelating effect, though more mildly than the alginate extracts. Several studies have shown a decreased absorption of radioactive strontium (Sr_{90}) as well as barium, silver, mercury, cadmium, zinc, and manganese with the use of oral alginates. Two other nutrients that are popular in antioxidant and antistress energizing formulas are the enzyme *superoxide dismutase* (SOD) and dimethylglycine (DMG). Although there has been little supporting research on the oral use of these nutrients, many people who take them describe improved energy and mental clarity.

Regarding radiation exposure, the first suggestion is to avoid it whenever possible. Minimize irradiating medical tests. Particularly avoid medical body scans, which may require injection of radioactive metals such as cobalt 60, iodine 131, or technitium 90. With x-rays, shield the thymus gland, an important immunological organ in the upper chest. When dental x-rays are taken, ask the dental technician for a thyroid (neck) screen. The dentist should have a lead "thyroid collar" available. Do not live near a nuclear power plant or an industry that employs radioactive wastes or toxic chemicals. Also, do not eat fish caught from waters containing effluents from these factories. Frequent high-altitude airline flights increase radiation exposure. Avoid irradiated foods that may be treated with nuclear waste containing cobalt 60 or cesium 137. We do not "officially" know the effects of consuming treated food, but I am not overly optimistic. (See Chapter 11, sections on *Food Irradiation* and *88 Survival Suggestions.*)

With any radioactive iodine tests or exposure to iodine fallout, take kelp or iodine for several weeks before and after the test to occupy the iodine-binding sites (unless, of course, this will interfere with the test) so that the least amount of the radioactive element will stay in the body.

Strontium 90 competes with calcium and also lowers vitamin D. Taking extra vitamin D, calcium, and magnesium plus kelp and algin, pectin and lecithin, and L-cysteine may reduce absorption and speed elimination to prevent strontium 90 from getting stored in the bones.

Radiation causes many undesirable internal reactions, especially in the most prolific tissues, such as the gastrointestinal tract and skin. Radiation therapy may affect the appetite, tastes, and the ability to eat. Radiation is cumulative, and many things may add to it, from color TV and microwaves to x-rays and fallout exposure. We need a good protective program! When living in areas with high background radiation, it is wise to take higher amounts of antioxidants regularly.

Several writers have offered guidelines for protection against the effects of radiation. Paavo Airola, in *How to Get Well*, suggests a plan of high amounts of vitamin C with rutin, extra pantothenic acid, brewer's yeast, yogurt, vitamin F or essential fatty acids, inositol and lecithin, and lemon juice or lemon peel. Stuart Berger's guidelines in *The Immune Power Diet* include extra potassium, 1200 mg. of calcium, and 800 mg. of magnesium in addition to his usual environmental protection plan of 4–6 grams of vitamin C, 600 IUs of vitamin E, 100 mg. of zinc, and 20,000 IUs of beta-carotene. In *The Complete Guide to Anti-Aging Nutrients*, Sheldon Hendler recommends vitamins C and E, niacin, and copper to protect against the effects of x-rays and environmental toxins.

In addition to radiation, this program will also help against environmental pollut-ants, including a number of toxic chemicals, such as carbon monoxide, ozone, sulfur dioxide, and nitrogen dioxide from the air, various pesticides and volatile hydrocar-bons, food additives such as nitrites and sulfites, and toxic heavy metals such as lead, cadmium, and mercury. Cigarette smoke is a big problem, mainly for those who choose to smoke or cannot quit. (A *Nicotine Detoxification* program is offered in Chapter 18.)

A number of herbs and food extracts can be used to help detoxification and decrease the risks from environmental pollution. The algins, mentioned earlier, help clear metal and radiation toxins. Fibers such as wheat (or oat) bran and psyllium seed husks help to increase toxin elimination. Alfalfa, rich in chlorophylls and vitamin K, may help reduce tissue damage with radiation exposure. Apple pectin also helps bind and clear intestinal metal and chemical toxins. In *The Scientific Validation of Herbal Medicine*, Daniel Mowrey recommends a formula for environmental pollution including alfalfa, algin (from seaweed or algae), wheat bran, apple pectin, and kelp. These help to decrease the toxicity of chemical and metal pollutants; in addition, this high-fiber formula helps to reduce cholesterol levels and is often useful in treating colds and flus, where bowel elimination is so important. Extra vitamin E and fish oils containing DHA and EPA as well as an antioxidant formula with additional vitamin C may make this formula work even better. Of course, we as a culture must pay heed. Even our potential healing sources (water, food, oils, etc.) can become toxic if we do not care for Earth's environment.

The table on the following page concentrates on the nutrients that protect against damage by toxins and free radicals. These nutrients offer protection by providing immune support, antioxidant and anticancer effects, and detoxification. The amounts listed are daily totals, usually taken in several portions over the course of the day.

ENVIRONMENTAL POLLUTION AND
RADIATION PROGRAM

Water	2–3 qt.			
Fiber*	12–18 g.			

Vitamin A	10,000–15,000 IUs		**Iodine**	150–300 mcg.
Beta-carotene	15,000–30,000 IUs		**Iron**	15–20 mg.
Vitamin D	400 IUs		**Magnesium**	350–650 mg.
Vitamin E	800–1,000 IUs		**Manganese**	15 mg.
Vitamin K	500 mcg.		**Molybdenum**	600 mcg.
Thiamine (B$_1$)	25–75 mg.		**Selenium,**	
Riboflavin (B$_2$)	25–75 mg.		**as selenomethionine**	300 mcg.
Niacin (B$_3$)	150 mg.		**Silicon**	100 mg.
Pantothenic acid (B$_5$)	1,000 mg.		**Zinc**	60 mg.
Pyridoxine (B$_6$)	50–100 mg.			
Pyridoxal-5-phosphate	25–50 mg.		**L-amino acids**	500 mg.
Cobalamin (B$_{12}$)	100–200 mcg.		**L-cysteine⁺**	500 mg.
Folic acid	800 mcg.		**L-methionine⁺**	250 mg.
Biotin	500 mcg.		**Lipoic acid**	100 mg.
PABA	100 mg.		**Chlorophyll**	6 tablets or 2 tsp.
Choline	1,000 mg.		**Sodium alginate**	300–600 mg.
Inositol	1,000 mg.			
Vitamin C	6,000 mg.			
Bioflavonoids	500 mg.			
Calcium	600–1,000 mg.			
Chromium	400 mcg.			
Copper	3 mg.			

*A high-fiber diet and/or 6 g. each of wheat bran and psyllium husks.
⁺Take with three times the amount of vitamin C.

Related programs
  Anti-Stress, Immune Enhancement, Cancer Prevention, and *General Detoxification*

Immune Enhancement

Our immune system is the most dynamic body component in determining our state of health or disease. It will be the basis, I believe, of future breakthroughs in medicine. There is a great deal of evidence from current and past research demonstrating life's effects on human immune function and our immune system's influences upon our health. These investigations provide a continuous flood of knowledge about the sensitive balance and many levels involved in our wellness. *Psychoneuroimmunology*, which provides a bridge between psychology and the nervous and immune systems, now plays an essential role in medicine.

Our immune system constantly interacts with our internal environment, protects us from our external environment, and provides the inherent knowledge to sense the difference between friend and foe. For many reasons, including genetics and individuality, some of us may be overactive or too underactive in our defenses, and this can create a great variety of health problems, such as allergies, infections, and cancer.

There are many components to our immune system—organs, bone marrow, cells, antibodies, chemicals, and the nutrients that help nourish and generate them. Most of these cells and tissue constituents are part of what is called in medicine the reticuloendothelial system, which plays a "defensive role in inflammation and immunity" (*Dorland's Medical Dictionary*) and in the formation and destruction of blood cells. Our immune system protects us from viruses, bacteria, yeasts and fungi, foreign proteins, and cancer cells. It provides two kinds of protection: Innate (inborn) nonspecific immunity and specific learned or acquired immunity. Specific immunity depends on "humoral" (antibodies and chemicals carried in the blood) and cellular (white blood cells) responses, which can be immediate or delayed.

The thymus-derived lymphocytes (T lymphocytes or, simply, T cells) run the cellular defense and the delayed immune reactions. T cells, specifically T-helper lymphocytes, guide the B cells to produce antibodies (each cell produces only one specific antibody), a process that takes a three-to-five or more days induction period, often the time of infection by new viruses. Reexposure to the same virus will create a more rapid antibody response. This is our important immune memory and there are "memory B cells" that circulate in the blood to respond to subsequent infections. The T-helper cells stimulate immune activity, especially B cell activity, whereas the T-suppressor cells slow down certain functions such as antibody formation, usually after a problem has been handled. Another important cell which is neither a T or B cell or a phagocyte is the NK (natural killer) cell. The T lymphocytes also send messages to (and receive messages from) the macrophages and other phagocytes to "attack" virus-infected cells and foreign organisms, either by engulfing or marking them. Other T cells can also be cytotoxic to virus-infected cells. All of these important T lymphocytes originate in the bone marrow and mature in the thymus gland, the "king" of the immune system. B lymphocytes also originate in the bone marrow and may mature there, in the spleen, lymph nodes, and elsewhere; they are programmed to become the antibody factories or the plasma cells, which are formed from B cells and also produce the specific antibodies.

IMMUNE ANATOMY

Organ Tissues	Non-specific* Defenses	Antigen-specific+ Defenses
skin	skin	macrophages
thymus gland	mucous membranes	T cells
bone marrow	mucus secretions	T-helper cells
spleen	cilia	T-suppressor cells
lymph nodes	neutrophils	natural killer cells
tonsils	lysosomes	B cells
adenoids	iron-binding proteins	plasma cells
Peyer's patches	other chemical mediators	antibodies—IgA, IgE,
(small intestine)	stomach acid	IgG, IgM, IgD
appendix	lysozymes in tears, saliva	complement system
liver		interferon

---

*Not mediated by antigen stimuli.
+Mediated through antigen proteins

To explain the entire immune anatomy and interrelationships would take a book or two, but I feel that few other relevant and explanatory notes are important here. The skin and mucous membranes, including the cilia (tiny hairs) lining these membranes and the mucus itself, are all first lines of nonspecific, physical defense by providing a physical barrier against invasion. The lymphatic system is really the secondary circulatory system that removes foreign cells and proteins, which it eventually dumps into the blood to be broken down and eliminated. The lymphatic system itself has no pump, and thus relies on muscle activity and exercise for the lymph to circulate. That is one reason why I believe that physical stagnation increases the chance of infections, and conversely, exercise improves resistance. Lymph nodes are storage sites for cells along the lymphatic system. There are hundreds of these nodes throughout the body. When infection is present, these nodes can commonly be felt in the area closest to the infection. Predominant lymph nodes are in the neck, groin, or axillary regions. The tonsils, adenoids, the appendix, and Peyer's patches along the small intestine are other important lymphoid tissues. The thymus, bone marrow, and spleen are all sites for immune cell maturation. The liver is also important to immune function, because it helps to detoxify many substances in the body that could be taxing to the immune system.

The phagocytic white blood cells are important in immune surveillance first as the frontline defense patrolling the body. They engulf foreign substances and microorganisms and then can kill or dissolve them by their chemicals. The neutrophils and macrophages work through oxidative destruction. The NK cells kill by secreting a *phospholipase* enzyme, which dissolves the lipid protection of cells containing viruses or other germs. The NK cells may also release a series of chemicals called interleukins, such as interleukin 2 (IL_2), which act as mediators in T lymphocyte functions and proliferation as well as other possible functions. Zinc may help in the production and function of NK cells as well as T and B cells. Besides the basic T and B cells, and the helper and suppressor T cells, and helper-suppressor ratio, special IL_2 receptor positive cells and Ta_1 positive cells, which are actively dividing T cells, can be measured by specialized T cell or immune system blood studies to reveal the status of current immune functions. Leukotrienes and prostaglandins (E_2 series) are other chemicals that are implicated in inflammatory and allergic reactions. More of these are produced when the diet is high in arachidonic acid, found mainly in saturated animal fats.

The complement system releases chemicals in the serum that can lyse, or break apart, antibody-coated cells and microorganisms. Lysozymes and enzymes in tears and saliva can also lyse certain microorganisms. Interferon is an antiviral substance produced by T lymphocytes and macrophages. Iron-binding protein in phagocytic cells also plays a role in protecting against certain infections.

As with other body systems, immune balance is the key. A number of important factors in life influence immune health; unfortunately, there are many more factors that suppress it than enhance it. The basic aging process usually reduces our immune competence. Allergies and infections may do this also, though initially these may stimulate immune activity. Surgery, radiation and chemotherapy, all standard Western cancer treatments, as well as some antibiotic therapy, can weaken immune function, which is not ideal for healing or prevention of cancer in the future. Stress responses, such as that caused by business activity or travel, can lower immunity, as can all varieties of intense emotional and psychological experience. Low self-esteem, emotional extremes, or loss of a loved one may reduce lymphocyte and NK cell numbers and function. Many drugs and chemicals, from steroids (and possibly steroidlike agents, such as excess vitamin D or progesterone) and other anti-inflammatory agents to sugar, alcohol, and marijuana, can be immune suppressors. The external environment can also be detrimental to the normal functioning of the immune system. Photochemical smog, industrial chemicals, pesticides, and certain antibiotic residues in meats as well as a high-fat diet may tax the immune system further. Even excess intake of the polyunsaturated fatty acids (PUFAs) from vegetable oils may increase free-radical formation and affect immunity. Nutritionally, low protein intake and vitamin A and zinc deficiencies are most relevant to immune suppression; a deficiency of essential fatty acids and other essential nutrients, such as pyrodoxine, pantothenic acid, and selenium, may also contribute.

IMMUNE SYSTEM SUPPRESSORS

aging
allergies:
  pollens
  dust
  food
infections:
  viruses
  bacteria
  yeasts and fungi
  parasites
surgery
radiation
chemotherapy
drugs:
  cortisone and other steroids
  anti-inflammatories
  adrenalin
  insulin
lack of sleep
airplane travel
stress:
  social
  work
  financial

emotional extremes
  depression
  loneliness
overeating
high-fat diet
  (including excess PUFAs)
sugar
excess iron
malnutrition (especially in
  infants and the elderly)
nutrient deficiencies:
  vitamins A, C, and E
  B vitamins, especially B_5,
    folic acid, B_6, and B_{12}
  zinc and selenium
  essential fatty acids
  protein
chemicals in diet and environment:
  phenol and formaldehyde
  hydrocarbons
  air/water pollution
drugs, recreational:
  marijuana, nicotine
  cocaine, amphetamines
  alcohol

A major concern is that immune suppression or weakness can predispose us to infections as well as cancer; these diseases may generally deplete our energy level and vitality. Overwork, multiple stresses, and lack of rest, exercise, and sleep tend to deplete our energies, our strength, and our ability to defend ourselves. This leaves us more vulnerable to outside influences. I believe that these imbalances of lifestyle, along with emotional and other psychological factors, are the basis of immune weakness.

Besides immune compromise, problems of hyperimmunity seem also to be more common nowadays. Allergies are the main example of immune overactivity; however, the autoimmune diseases appear more prevalent as well. In these diseases, such as thyroiditis (Hashimoto's), rheumatoid arthritis, and lupus erythematosus, our immune system aberrantly makes antibodies to our own body tissues, which then leads to

IMMUNE SYSTEM SUPPORTERS

self-love	zinc	rotating diet
interpersonal love	selenium	low-fat, low-sugar diet
positive attitudes	iron*	wholesome foods
laughter	copper	dietary protein
affirmations	vitamin C	chemical-free diet
breathing	bioflavonoids	chemical-free home and work
relaxing	vitamin A	filtered, purified water
meditation	beta-carotene	fasting
exercise, yoga	vitamin E	essential fatty acids
herbs:	pyridoxine	adequate digestive function
garlic	pantothenic acid	digestive enzymes, such as
licorice	folic acid	*bromelain, papain,* or
echinacea	vitamin B$_{12}$	*trypsin*
goldenseal	amino acids:	thymus glandular**
ginseng	arginine	allergies, infections, and
dimethylglycine	ornithine	fever***
coenzyme Q$_{10}$	carnitine	
organo-germanium	cysteine and glutathione	
staphage lysate	possibly lysine and taurine	

* Excess iron can increase oxidation and weaken immunity.

** Possibly also spleen, thyroid, and adrenal glandulars as long as these are free of pesticides and viruses that could cause disease.

*** May initially stimulate immune activity and then be suppressive.

inflammation, pain, or malfunction of those organs or tissues, as the case may be. We have a great deal more to learn about these autoimmune diseases (and allergies for that matter) in the coming years.

On the positive side, a balanced and optimistic attitude, healthy lifestyle habits in regard to diet, and basic care of the human body will support the optimal function of not only our immune system but our entire body. As I have said, there are not many specific agents that increase immunity. Our immune function is optimum when we supply our body with the necessary nutrients, take time to relax and recreate, and do not block and weaken our natural vital energy circulation through the other factors that are listed as immune suppressors. Adopt more of these lifestyle-related immune supporters!

For whom is this immune enhancement program best suited? It can be employed by those people with chronic fatigue, particularly secondary to viral infections, or by anyone with repeated illnesses or infections who needs a stronger immune defense system. People under stress, both physical and psychological, need to strengthen their immune systems. Really, anyone subject to several of the factors listed in the "immune suppressors" chart might benefit from this *Immune Enhancement* program, which is not really dissimilar from the programs for *Anti-Aging* and *Cancer Prevention*. People who have cancer or have had cancer will want to make sure they include many of the recommendations in this program as well.

Our immune functions can be evaluated in a variety of ways. If we are healthy and full of energy and do not get many infectious diseases, it is not likely that we need any blood tests for our immune system; it is probably normal. But if we are easily fatigued or get recurrent colds, flus, or other infections by viruses, bacteria, yeast, or parasites, our immune system may be out of balance or deficient in one or more functions.

The most common blood test that indicates immunological activity is a simple, inexpensive complete blood count, or CBC. Particularly important is the white blood cell count (WBC). The differential count gives us the percentages of the basic WBCs— polymorphonucleocytes (PMN-phagocytes), bands (PMN-percursors), lymphocytes (the immune directors, including T and B lymphocytes although they are not specifically noted), and the other less common monocytes (scavengers), eosinophils (allergy cells), and basophils.

Through another blood test, the specialized T and B cell study provides a sensitive index of the immune system. A complete test provides absolute levels and relative percentages of T cells and B cells, T-helper (T_H) cells, T-suppressor (T_S) cells, Natural Killer (NK) cells and the helper/suppressor (T_H:T_S) ratio. This T_H:T_S ratio is currently the most generally utilized monitor of immune function. It may be elevated in problems such as infections or allergies, or decreased in other infections or in acquired immune deficiency syndrome (AIDS). The T_H:T_S ratio can be monitored over the course of certain illnesses to determine the effectiveness of treatment. In healthy people, it is also thought to be one of the better objective monitors of more subtle immune status. More finite measurements of immune status may be available soon, such as the level of interleukin 2. Other tests that may also be relevant in an immunological evaluation include antibody (Ig-immunoglobulin) levels, complement, interferon, routine blood and liver function tests, and allergy tests for both environmental and food allergens.

Reducing any active allergic response through avoidance, desensitization, and detoxification may help to reduce the immunosuppressant effects of existing allergies. More generally, avoiding chemicals and other factors from the immune suppressor list may also minimize any immune function weaknesses. Further measures for immune support include the ideas presented in other programs, *Executives and Travel* or *Anti-Stress*. Intense, as well as chronic, unrelenting stress and emotions are real concerns in weakening immunity. Preventive care in lifestyle, diet, and supplements is ultimately most important.

The immune-supporting diet plan includes the common sense suggestions discussed in Chapter 13, *Your Ideal Diet*, as well as suggestions from the programs for *Allergies, Anti-Stress,* and *Cancer Prevention.* A low-chemical, low-sugar, and low-fat diet is mandatory! A rotating diet, without regular use of milk or its products, eggs, wheat, corn, sugar, and yeast or other specific foods to which one may be allergic, is suggested.

Wholesome foods free of chemicals and pesticides are the best. Care must be taken to prevent food exposure to microorganisms, including parasites, as they may have a deleterious influence on our immune health. Low chemical intake is important. This means avoiding both chemicals in foods and chemical consumptive habits, such as alcohol, caffeine, cocaine, marijuana, and nicotine—as is always the case for optimal health. A water purification system which removes chemicals is also a good investment for our health (See Chapter 1).

Care must be taken to obtain sufficient dietary proteins and L- amino acids that help form the immune tissues and antibodies. For proper protein production, adequate amounts of pyridoxine, pantothenic acid, folic acid, magnesium, and zinc are very important. The essential fatty acids are also required for cell and tissue health. On the other hand, excess protein and saturated fats are "clogging" to the vascular and lymphatic systems and may suppress immunity. Fasting and detoxification diets can strengthen immune functions and reduce immune overload and reactions, as can be seen in allergies and infections or autoimmune problems such as rheumatoid arthritis. The reduced intake of allergenic substances and the cleansing of potentially allergenic materials from the body can reduce many symptoms and allow the T lymphocytes to restore balance and reduce their hyperreactivity.

With regard to specific supplements, it is most important to prevent deficiencies of many vital nutrients, such as vitamins A and C and zinc, by following the previous suggestions and eating foods high in these nutrients. Additional supplements, if not excessive, are insurance, possibly in the face of poor digestion and assimilation, to provide adequate nutrients to the cells and tissues.

Useful supplements for immune enhancement begin with a basic multiple that includes the essential vitamins and minerals plus the important antioxidant nutrients. If the multiple does not provide adequate amounts of the antioxidants such as vitamin C, vitamin E, beta-carotene, zinc, and selenium, then an antioxidant formula or additional specific nutrients are needed to reach the optimum levels. Of course, this program is designed for those with some immune suppression or those who want to enhance a sluggish immune system. The positive side of those many important nutrients whose deficiency leads to weakened functions is that adequate levels support or stimulate those actions.

Vitamin C is probably the most important of the antioxidant nutrients. A higher level of intake than usual, about 4–10 grams if tolerated, can help in antibody response and in some white blood cell functions. Vitamin C has also been shown to increase production of interferon, a substance with antiviral and, possibly, anticancer effects. Vitamin C levels have been found to be commonly decreased in the presence of such situations as surgery, stress, and progressive disease, as well as colds and other infections, especially those of viral origin. In these situations, it is needed in increased amounts. The vitamin C-complex nutrients, such as rutin and other bioflavonoids, may also have mild antioxidant, synergistic effects. Bioflavonoids appear to act with vitamin C to potentiate its anti-inflammatory properties and improve cellular defense against various microbes. Quercetin, a type of bioflavonoid, has also recently been found to function as an immune supporter and antihistamine.

Nutrient Deficiency*	Immunologic Problems Related to Deficiency
Vitamin A	Reduced cellular immunity, slow tissue healing, increased infection rate, lowered IgA levels (which affect defense at the mucous membranes).
Vitamin C	Decreased phagocyte function, reduced cellular protection, and slow wound healing.
Vitamin E	Decreased antibody production and response; with selenium deficiency, lowered cell-membrane integrity.
Vitamin B_5	Lowered humoral immunity, increased irritation of stress.
Vitamin B_6	Lessened cellular immunity, slow energy metabolism.
Vitamin B_{12}	Decreased lymphocyte proliferation and PMN bacteriocidal activity.
Folic acid	Reduced blood cell production, perhaps increased cervical cancer.
Zinc	Decreased T and B cell function and thymic hormones; increased infection rates, and slow healing.
Iron	Decreased cellular immunity and neutrophil activity. (Excess iron can also impair bacteriocidal activity.)
Selenium	With vitamin E deficiency, antibody response is lowered; increased cellular carcinogenosis.
Copper	Lowered resistance to infection.

*Adequate levels of these nutrients will support or enhance these immunological functions.

Two nutrient pairs—Vitamin A and zinc, and Vitamin E and selenium—are also essential. Selenium, as sodium selenite or selenomethionine, and vitamin E stimulate antibody production and strengthen cellular immunity. Zinc and vitamin A are also needed for cellular immunity, increasing T cell activity and the function of the phagocytic white blood cells. Both are important to tissue healing. Beta-carotene is useful as a vitamin A precursor, also aiding in wound healing and protecting against carcinogenesis.

Some B vitamins are particularly helpful. Vitamin B_6 aids immunity and antibody formation and is probably the most important of the B vitamins. Vitamin B_{12} may help stimulate immune function, more readily when injected as oral absorption is slow. Pantothenic acid is helpful in combating stress, and B_1, B_2, and B_3 may provide subtle immune help by providing a balanced complement of the B vitamins. This helps the overall antibody production. Folic acid is also needed for normal cellular function.

In addition to zinc and selenium, the most important minerals are iodine, iron, copper, and magnesium, though basic levels of manganese, molybdenum and chromium are also important. Iodine is required in the neutrophil killing of microbial invaders. Iron improves resistance against infection by increasing cellular metabolic efficiency and immune activity; it supports the lymphocytes and neutrophils (phagocytes) and can improve bacterial killing. Excessive iron intake, however, can also be immunosuppressive (it increases oxidation), enhance microbial growth, and reduce phagocytic cellular activity. Copper also improves resistance to infection and should be increased to balance out zinc intake. Like iron, too much copper can have deleterious effects, so careful monitoring is important.

Water, fiber, adequate protein, and essential fatty acids (EFAs) are all crucial to a healthy body and immune system. Water helps to flush out impurities and, with fiber, helps to clear colon toxins. EFAs found in nuts, seeds, and vegetable oils, as well as gamma-linolenic acid (GLA) help increase the anti-inflammatory prostaglandin E_1 (PGE_1), while eicosapentaenoic acid (EPA) may slightly reduce immunity. However, EPA also decreases the level of PGE_2 prostaglandins, which can be inflammatory and irritating and may produce a false or unnecessary immune response that is part of many illnesses. A mixed-oil formula with a high proportion of EFA and GLA is probably best used here.

The antioxidants and other nutrients help counteract the free-radical irritants. These unstable, free-radical molecules include superoxides, peroxides, hydroxyls, singlet oxygens, and hypochlorites. Vitamins C and E are helpful modulators of free radicals in general; along with zinc, copper, and manganese, they help reduce superoxides through *superoxide dismutase* enzymes. Selenium supports the production of the enzyme *glutathione peroxidase*, which counteracts peroxides, stimulates immune response, and protects against many toxins. Riboflavin subtly assists at maintaining electron balance.

The sulfur-containing amino acids, L-cysteine and methionine, are also "free-radical trappers" and part of a general antioxidant program. Other amino acids that are useful for immune enhancement include L-arginine and L-carnitine. L-arginine stimulates thymus activity and the number and activity of the T lymphocytes. L-carnitine, which can be synthesized from lysine with the help of vitamin C, also helps enhance immunity possibly by stimulating the utilization of fats, and thus increasing energy (ATP) production while preventing oxidation and free-radical formation.

For either immune suppression or protection from colds and flus, vitamins A and C and zinc are recommended. Together these nutrients activate the thymus gland and increase production of thymosin, one of the thymus hormones, which in turn improves T cell and natural killer lymphocyte numbers and activity. Thymosin injections can also be used to stimulate the cellular immune response. If stress is the key element that weakens immunity, then additional adrenal or thyroid glandular support may help. Other possible immune supporters we may wish to use include organogermanium (Ge-Oxy 132), dimethylglycine (DMG), and coenzyme Q_{10}. A formula that includes all these plus other energy enhancing nutrients is Oxynutrients formulated by Dr. Stephen Levine of Nutriology in San Leandro, California.

If we are sick with an infection or we feel like we are getting sick, I suggest increasing the supplemented levels of vitamin A to 25,000–50,000 IUs, vitamin C to 4–8 grams, and zinc to 50–100 mg. I would also add garlic, which is a natural antibiotic, and goldenseal, which is thought to improve immunity, to help clear wastes through liver tonification, and to have antimicrobial properties. After we are feeling better and ready for recovery, we can add ginseng root to help rebuild our energies. Licorice root is another herb that can be used for stress-related immune problems. It seems to support energy and adrenal balance, and has been shown to improve interferon production.

It is a good idea not to reduce fevers unless they are very high (over 103°F). Fevers have a purpose, in both children and adults. They help in detoxification, immune stimulation, and increasing metabolism and, in some cases, killing the microorganism. Intake of fluids and minerals needs to be increased with fevers to counteract the body losses.

Exercise is also very important to immune function. Regular activity increases the circulation of nutrients and the cellular immune components. And remember, muscle activity is necessary to circulate our lymph fluid. Squeezing our brain with thousands of thoughts does not make the lymph flow. Circulation of blood, lymph, energy, thoughts, and feelings is important to the vitality and health of our body, mind, heart, and spirit, and to our immune system. Don't worry, be healthy!

IMMUNE ENHANCEMENT NUTRIENT PROGRAM

Water	2½–3 qt.		Calcium	600–1,000 mg.
Calories	1,500–2,500		Chromium	200 mcg.
Protein	60–80 g.		Copper	3 mg.
Fats	50–75 g.		Iodine	150 mcg.
(20–30 percent of caloric intake)			Iron	10–20 mg.
			Magnesium	300–600 mg.
Fiber	10–20 g.		Manganese	5–10 mg.
			Molybdenum	300 mcg.
Vitamin A	10,000 IUs		Selenium, as selenomethionine	300–400 mcg.
Beta-carotene	15,000–30,000 IUs		Zinc	45–60 mg.
Vitamin D	400 IUs			
Vitamin E	600–800 IUs		L-amino acids	1,000 mg.
Vitamin K	150–300 mcg.		L-cysteine	250 mg.
Thiamine (B₁)	50 mg.		L-arginine	500 mg.
Riboflavin (B₂)	25–50 mg.		L-carnitine	500 mg.
Riboflavin-5-phosphate	25–50 mg.		Thymus gland	100 mg.
Niacinamide (B₃)	50 mg.		Essential fatty acids* or Flaxseed oil	3–6 capsules
Niacin (B₃)	50 mg.			
Pantothenic acid (B₅)	500 mg.		GLA (evening Primrose or Borage seed oil)**	3–6 capsules or 200–400 mg.
Pyridoxine (B₆)	50 mg.			
Pyridoxal-5-phosphate	50 mg.		EPA (fish oil)***	2–4 capsules or 200–400 mg.
Cobalamin (B₁₂)	200 mcg.			
Folic acid	800 mcg.			
Biotin	500 mcg.		Organo-germanium	100–250 mg
Vitamin C	4–10 g.		Dimethylglycine	50–100 mg.
Bioflavonoids	250–500 mg.		Coenzyme Q₁₀	30–60 mg.

*Not necessary if two or more teaspoons of fresh (uncooked) cold-pressed vegetable oils are consumed daily.
**Use with allergies or inflammatory problems.
***Use if blood fats are relatively high.

Cancer Prevention

$\mathbb{S}$ ince cancer has become the plague and one of the greatest fears of the modern technological, chemical age and, overall, cancer treatment, other than for certain malignancies, has not to date been very successful, prevention of cancer is the only sensible approach. The relationship of diet to cancer came of age in the 1980s. With our new knowledge, we can clearly now do something about the threats of cancer and our future. Caring for ourselves and others as if we really love life and have a desire to live will win over all possible disease!

Chapter 11, *Environmental Aspects of Nutrition*, contains a fairly detailed discussion of cancer—its genesis, potential offending agents, dietary concepts, prevention ideas, and so on. Here I want to focus more on general nutrition and supplements and their importance in preventing cancer.

Two decades ago, it was difficult to find any major institutions, doctors, or groups like the medical associations or the American Cancer Society, that would admit that there were any ties between cancer and nutrition. Now the nutritional and environmental influences on the genesis of cancer, the second biggest killer of the American adult population, have been fairly well accepted as key components in this disease. A big breakthrough came with the 1977 *Senate Select Committee's Dietary Goals for the United States*, listing cancer as one of the major degenerative diseases (cardiovascular disease and diabetes are others) that are linked to improper diet. The committee's suggestions of lower fat, higher fiber, and more natural foods are definitely a part of the cancer-prevention diet. An important report called *Diet, Nutrition and Cancer*, compiled by the National Academy of Sciences and released in 1982, gave further credence to the relationship between diet and cancer and offered more specific dietary suggestions. And in 1988, the U.S. Department of Health and Human Services published a major manuscript by C. Everett Koop, M.D., entitled *The Surgeon General's Report on Nutrition and Health*. It discusses the relationships between nutrition and our common degenerative diseases, including cancer.

But cancer is a multifactorial, multidimensional disease. While nutritional and environmental influences are definite components, physiological, social, emotional, psychological, and spiritual factors are also important. Therefore, the prevention and treatment of cancer must deal with all of these aspects of life.

The aging process itself increases cancer risk, but particularly if we do not take good care of ourselves. Poor nutrition can lead to many functional problems, such as lowered immunity and slower cell repair. The increased exposure to carcinogens is no help either. (See more on this in the *Anti-Aging* Program). To much of the medical profession, cancer prevention means primarily early detection—more exams, x-rays, mammograms, and biopsies—so that the necessary surgery, drugs, and radiation can be applied sooner to prevent an untimely death. However, prevention of cancer is much more than early detection—it means not creating the disease. A good diet and stress management are important cancer preventives. A strong, healthy immune (defense) system is also an essential part of this plan (see the preceding program on *Immune Enhancement*). With a strong immune system, even the few cancer cells that might be regularly generated would be easily removed from the body. Put simply (according to current thinking), it takes both the disease of the cells and the failure of the immune system together to create cancer—in other words, the effect of potential carcinogens on an already unstable body.

Michio Kushi, author of the in-depth text *The Cancer Prevention Diet*, believes that cancer is caused not so much by carcinogens per se as by the imbalance in the body caused by improprieties of diet that allows the agents to create problems. He advocates the "unified theory of disease," which sees the internal imbalance between yin and yang as the primary cause of cancer and most diseases. It is the "duality," or seeing of body parts or diseases as separate from our entire being, that allows us to treat even the mildest of symptoms as an enemy and not as an ally trying to guide us in a new direction. As we continue to approach our health in this way, we create further diversions from unity and manifest more-difficult-to-treat acute and chronic problems. Cancer itself, as is true of most disease, can be seen as a lack of harmony with our environment and a diversion from our inner truth.

This program is suitable for most everyone, especially those in a high-cancer-risk group. That includes men and women over 40 or 50 years old and people with a family history of cancer, especially women with a family history of breast cancer. Smokers, people with a dietary history that includes cancer risks, and those who have been exposed to known carcinogens will also benefit.

What really causes cancer? Is it a virus or genetic code, the effect of carcinogens on cellular growth, or a weakened immune system? Is it a poor, "cancer-promoting" diet? Or does it have to do with the psychological factors influenced by stress, poor attitude, or low self-esteem? We do not really know; cancer seems to be linked to all of these factors. Family history is definitely a factor, and if someone in our families has had cancer, that should increase our watchfulness for this disease as well as encourage us to use early detection procedures.

Discussion of cancer risks and promoting factors could easily fill a book. I want to keep it simple. Below I list the eleven main cancer risks, followed by a more extensive discussion of various factors that may add to our chances of developing cancer sometime in our lives. One of the difficult tasks in researching many cancer risks is that cancer can often take 30–40 years from the time of exposure to a carcinogen for it to manifest as a physical tumor. But the following list clearly shows that the promotion of cancer involves almost exclusively diet, environment, and lifestyle. Problems that result from pharmaceutical medicines or viral conditions that weaken immunity and allow

CANCER: KEY RISK FACTORS

1. **Smoking**
2. **Dietary excesses**—fats (mainly saturated, fried polyunsaturated oils, and cholesterol); protein; obesity (calories)
3. **Undernutrition**—deficient fiber and nutrients such as vitamins C and E, beta-carotene, selenium
4. **Occupational chemicals**
5. **Food chemicals**—pesticides, additives, hormones
6. **Air and water pollution**
7. **Excess sunlight and radiation**
8. **Certain pharmaceutical drugs**—estrogen, metronidazole (Flagyl), lindane (Kwell), or griseofulvin
9. **Alcohol**
10. **Viruses**
11. **Psychological influences**—such as personal changes, loss of loved one, grief, divorce

---

cancer to develop more easily are probably rarer, and usually even the factors that predispose us to these conditions are areas over which we have some control.

Smoking, mainly of cigarettes, is a primary cancer risk and is correlated with nearly all lung cancer. It is also a factor in cancers of the mouth, throat, and larynx and possibly others. Pipe and cigar smoking produces higher incidences of mouth cancer but less of lung. Cigarette smoke acts synergistically with alcohol, asbestos, and other carcinogens in air, water, and food to further increase cancer risk and rates. It is likely that naturally grown tobacco rolled in untreated paper poses less cancer risk; the chemical production and treatment processes involved in manufacturing a pack of cigarettes are definitely an added cause for concern. Regular marijuana smoking may also be a factor in cancer, though more research on this is needed. Cigarette smoking is clearly the largest and most preventable cancer risk.

Excess fats in the diet definitely increase the incidence of breast, colon, and prostate cancer and possibly others, such as uterine or ovarian cancer. The fats of most concern include saturated animal fats, as found in meats and dairy products; fried or rancid oils; hydrogenated and refined oils, and cooked polyunsaturated fatty acids (PUFAs). Rancid oils and foods cooked in oils cause more free-radical irritation (as do high amounts of PUFAs), mainly from lipid peroxides, and these act as mutagens and carcinogens. Excess protein in some studies correlates with cancer rates, but most of the higher protein foods also contribute to higher fat levels and this type of diet will often lead to more general body congestive and degenerative processes.

Obesity is definitely correlated with higher cancer rates. Colon, rectum, and prostate cancer rates are higher in obese men, while obese women have increased risks of cancer of the breast, cervix, uterus, ovary and gallbladder. It is not totally clear whether the risk is posed by the obesity itself, higher caloric intake, or by the many associated factors, both nutritional and psychological (overweight people tend to hold things in).

Deficiencies of many nutrients are implicated in some cancers. Low fiber in the diet is probably the biggest culprit, mainly in the increasing problem of colon cancer. Slow transit time through the intestinal tract, allowing more contact to carcinogens, may be the main factor here. Many specific nutrient deficiencies have been correlated with various cancers. Vitamin A and beta-carotene deficits increase the incidence of lung and mouth cancer, especially among cigarette smokers, and are also implicated in cancers of the skin, throat, prostate, bladder, cervix, colon, esophagus, and stomach. Also of concern is selenium deficiency, which we now know may increase the risk of many cancers, mainly of the breast, lungs, colon, rectum, and prostate, as well as skin, pancreas, and intestinal cancer and leukemia. Vitamin C may reduce the carcinogenicity of nitrosamines and other chemicals; vitamin C deficits may increase cervical, bladder, stomach and esophageal cancers, as well as the general carcinogenic process. Vitamin E deficiency definitely weakens the body's ability to balance rancid oils and free radicals, and this increases cancer risk. Other mineral deficiencies implicated in cancer include molybdenum deficiency in esophageal and stomach cancer; zinc deficiency in cancer of the prostate, colon, esophagus, and bronchi and general immune system weakening; and possibly iodine and iron deficiencies.

Occupational chemicals are a topic of great concern. Many workers at home or in jobs are exposed to a wide range of chemicals with varying carcinogenicity. Possible agents include nuclear radiation and fallout, chemicals used in dry cleaning and other cleaning supplies, benzene, coal tar and its derivatives, asbestos, arsenic, PVC, gasoline and petroleum products and other hydrocarbons, pesticides, cosmetic chemicals, and many others. A more detailed discussion is included in Chapter 11, *Environmental Aspects of Nutrition*. Cigarette smoking also increases the risks from these occupational hazards.

Food chemicals are another big topic. There are many possible carcinogens, most of minimum risk but often cumulative, and we have much to learn about possible interactions of multiple carcinogens. Chemicals may be added to food during growth, manufacture, or preparation, and some are even made by the foods themselves or in combination with other microorganisms.

POSSIBLE FOOD CARCINOGENS

Additives—food colors, flavors, nitrates, and nitrites.

Saccharin—implicated (still unclearly) in bladder cancer.

Hormones—in meat, possibly even DES, which was recently banned.

Pesticides—sprayed on foods before and after harvesting.

Aflatoxin—produced by molds on peanuts, other legumes, and possibly other foods; may cause liver cancer.

Coffee—questionably implicated in bladder cancer. Decaffeinated coffee may be treated with carcinogens such as trichloroethylene or methyl chloride.

Sugar—may weaken immunity and increase cancer risk.

Nitrates and nitrites—common in preserved and smoked meats, such as ham, bologna, salami, corned beef, hot dogs and bacon; may convert to carcinogenic nitrosamines.

Pickled or salt-cured foods—may influence stomach and digestive lining.

Barbecuing—creates protein changes and production of benzopyrene, a mild carcinogen. Charbroiled meats and burnt toast may also be concerns.

Mushrooms—may contain toxic hydrazines.

Potatoes—when bruised or green.

Other foods—cottonseed oil, cocoa, mustard, black pepper, horseradish, fava beans, parsley, celery, alfalfa sprouts, parsnips, and figs all may contain mild carcinogenic substances. (Some of the agents produced by these plants may act as natural pesticides.)

Water pollution may involve a great many chemicals; metals, pesticides, PCBs, vinyl chloride, carbon tetrachloride, and gasoline are a few examples. Contamination of underground water tables may spread rapidly. Air pollution may also contain many carcinogenic substances from the nitrous and sulfur gases to hydrocarbons, carbon monoxide, and so on.

Excessive sunlight is implicated in skin cancer and excess radiation for cancer in general. Light-colored skin, cosmetic chemicals, and nutrient deficiencies, as well as the changes in Earth's ozone layer due to pollution, may also be factors in skin cancer. X-rays can produce leukemia and other cancers; this probably involves other precipitating factors, such as exposure to other carcinogens and/or low levels of necessary antioxidant nutrients.

Pharmaceutical drugs have a cancer-producing potential that has been well studied, at least in animals. Estrogen hormones, for postmenopausal use or as birth control pills, are factors of concern in women, though the latest research suggests less correlation with both breast and uterine cancers than was previously thought. Metronidazole (Flagyl), a commonly used antibiotic for bacteria and parasites, poses cancer risks, as does lindane (Kwell), a pesticide used on the skin for mites and lice. Griseofulvin, an antifungal agent, also poses mild cancer risks. In my opinion, steroid drugs, commonly used for suppressing all kinds of natural and unnatural body responses, have definite potential through immune suppression for increasing cancer risk. I believe there should be more research done regarding the implication of steroid use in the incidence of postinfections and cancer.

Alcohol has also been implicated in some cancers, such as cancers of the mouth, larynx, esophagus, and pancreas. These risks are increased when alcohol use is combined with cigarette smoking. Alcohol abuse is also often associated with poor diet and many nutritional deficiencies.

Viral diseases have been implicated in a variety of cancers. For years, genital herpes infections were thought to increase cervical cancer rates. It is now shown that the human papilloma virus responsible for the common venereal warts are more closely tied to cervical cancer than are herpes viruses. Vitamin A, folic acid, and selenium deficiencies may also be involved in cervical cancer. Cytomegalic and Epstein-Barr viruses have been considered as factors in cancer, possibly through mutagenic cellular effects, and may contribute to certain lymphomas or leukemias.

Psychological factors and the role they play in cancer is a fascinating topic; an increasing amount of research is being done in this area. It is clear that in some cases, a significant loss or perception of loss of a loved one occurred between one and two years prior to the diagnosis of cancer. This gives us another insight into the idea that it may take years, even 30–40, for a cancer to develop; cancer can also be a rapidly occurring and progressive disease.

There may indeed even be a cancer-type personality. The cancer disease process may be more prevalent in individuals who do not easily form close bonds or love relationships and do not easily express their feelings such as anger or frustration or who internalize most of their feelings, not necessarily aware that they even have any. These people might also show passive, compliant, or overly nice behavior and have low self-esteem. When such people experience unresolved loss of a loved one through death or divorce, a sense of helplessness or hopelessness may set in and weaken the immune system. Research seems to indicate that the feisty, tough scrappers who do not easily accept others' opinions or condemnation of themselves and can readily express their own feelings do much better with cancer, recovering more rapidly and more commonly than the more passive, accepting types. Bernie S. Siegel, M.D., discussed this area of personality and cancer extensively in his wonderful book *Love, Medicine and Miracles*. He reported that children who developed cancer also had shown some of the aforementioned traits, with a definite correlation with loss or perceived loss of a loved one—usually a parent but possibly a sibling or even a dog—in their early years. Excessive stress and psychological traumas all influence our immunity and increase our cancer risk. It is possible that the relationship between cancer and psychology can be summarized by the statement that cancer or any stress-related illness can result from a deep or chronic challenge or threat to our personal identity, roles, or relationships.

It is clear that cancer is not a simple disease to understand, diagnose, or treat. There are many types of cancer, each with its own set of predisposing factors, growth rates, treatment options, and so on. What is common to all, though, is the uncontrolled growth of aberrant cells which endangers healthy tissues, function, and life. Still, each person with cancer is an individual, and I believe that in most situations, many factors are involved in the genesis of the cancer. Our focus in this program, however, is to minimize our risks and prevent cancer, which now afflicts more than one in every four people at some time in their life and eventually touches nearly every family in the Western world. It is obvious that we should avoid smoking and the smoke of others, minimize the use of carcinogenic chemicals at home and at work, and do our best to breathe clean air and drink good water. We should also minimize our exposure to radiation. Reducing time in front of the television and computer screens will lower our exposure. Not living near nuclear power plants is important; limiting airline flights may help. Exposure to medical, dental, and chiropractic x-rays can be decreased. Many practitioners in each of these professions overuse regular radiation to follow patients. Routine chest x-rays for hospital admissions, for detecting tuberculosis or other lung or heart disease, or for employment are often unnecessary. Routine dental x-rays can be taken every five years instead of at the usual two-year intervals. Chiropractors often x-ray the entire spine; this can be very helpful, but it should not be done more than once or twice in a decade. Care can be taken to use the best equipment with the least radiation exposure and leakage. Whenever possible, x-ray films should be shared among practitioners, rather than each one taking new films.

Fear of the future in a world overwhelmed by individual unconsciousness is a cancer generator. If we are a contributor to our planetary demise, then cancer or other diseases may be the interest on our investment.

—*Bethany ArgIsle*

Positive Action

In addition to all of these things to avoid, there are also many positive things to emphasize to reduce our cancer risks. Diet (low fat, high fiber) and nutrients (extra vitamins A, C, and E, and selenium) can be very helpful. These are discussed in more detail below.

Positive steps toward early detection of cancer are also important. Although healing from cancer may be difficult, it is clear that the earlier it is found, the better the chances for survival (though this viewpoint is not universal). The current consensus is still that regular breast self-exam, Pap smears, prostate exam and sigmoidoscopy, colonoscopy (looking in the colon), and possibly routine mammography, may be to our advantage in early detection. Of course, it is advantageous only to those who have cancer; the high percentage of people with normal results have gone through the expense of time and money and often some pain.

It is important to keep ourselves physically and psychologically fit through exercise and working on our attitude. Regular exercise definitely improves our attitude and energy for life, as well as being a good immune supporter. When we are distressed or confronting important issues, dilemmas, or crises, it is wise to seek help to process our feelings if we are not able to handle them fully ourselves. A good friend and confidant can help, or a trained therapist may be beneficial. We all need to break the association of seeing a psychologist or therapist with being "crazy" and, instead, look at therapy as an important part of preventive medicine. Being able to deal with life's stresses as a challenge rather than with despair, helplessness, hopelessness, or other internalized feelings that make us feel that there is no escape is essential, not only in preventing cancer but for general health as well. Most of us still play out childhood patterns and our individualized attitudes of trust and self-image affect our adult relationships and everyday life, and this does not serve our best or most-evolved interests. Astute, interactive therapy and/or hypnotherapy can help point out these old patterns and replace them with new, more helpful ones to improve our potential for experiencing love and success in most areas of our lives.

Stress management techniques, relaxation and visualization exercises, and meditation are all useful self-help processes that may be learned. Developing a spiritual or universal perspective about our world and our involvement with life is also important for interpreting and coping with challenging experiences such as cancer. Michio Kushi suggests that a complaining, arrogant, rigid, and competitive character makes one more susceptible to degenerative disease, while a healthier approach may be peaceful, grateful, flexible, and cooperative.

The Cancer Prevention Diet usually involves a moderate to major change in the average person's dietary habits. Even the most traditional nutrition books now suggest the following as the main components of the *Cancer Prevention Diet*:

- **Lower fat intake** to about 20 percent of total calories (25–30 percent is more realistic; the average has been 42 percent). A maximum of 65 grams of fat per day is suggested; 50 grams is better. That represents 450 calories (9 cal./g., 9x50=450) of fat daily, or 20 percent of a 2,250-calorie diet. More of the fats should be the mono- and polyunsaturated types with a reduction of saturated fat intake, and little or no consumption of refined and heated oils.

- **Increase dietary fiber** to improve colon function mainly by increasing complex carbohydrates in the form of whole grains and lots of vegetables, along with some fruits, all of which contain high amounts of many of the important nutrients.
- **Increase fresh fruits, vegetables and whole grains.**
- **Maintain ideal weight and avoid obesity.**
- **Avoid smoking.**
- **Avoid smoked, salted, pickled and barbecued foods.**

The seven dietary suggestions of the American Cancer Society (ACS) are very similar:

1. **Avoid obesity.**
2. **Cut down on total fat intake.**
3. **Eat more high-fiber foods**, including whole grains, fruits, and vegetables.
4. **Include cruciferous vegetables**, such as cauliflower, broccoli, and cabbage.
5. **Include foods rich in vitamins A and C.**
6. **Lower alcohol consumption.**
7. **Lower intake of salt-cured, smoked, or nitrite-containing foods.**

So we begin with a high-nutrient, low-fat, high-fiber diet. More specifically, protein intake should be about 15 percent of the diet—from 12–18 percent, and not more than 20 percent, or 100 grams (400 calories) per day. Complex carbohydrates could make up about 60 percent of the diet, which would greatly increase the fiber intake. Up to 40 grams daily of fiber is not unrealistic. Foods high in fiber and water content to promote good bowel function and a diet and lifestyle supportive of healthy adrenal glands (minimize stress and sugar), liver (minimize chemicals and alcohol), thyroid (less stress and radiation exposure), and thymus/immune system (see *Immune Enhancement* program to review immune suppressors and supporters) are all important in keeping cancer risks low. In addition to vitamins A and C, we want to increase dietary intake of the B vitamins, especially folic acid, vitamin E, selenium, beta-carotene, and zinc. The diet should be low in alcohol, salt, coffee, and, obviously, chemicals and preservatives in foods.

Our low-fat, cancer-prevention diet focuses on starches, such as whole grains, legumes, potatoes, pastas, and squashes, along with fruits and vegetables and some other protein foods, such as small amounts of meats, preferably fish and poultry, nuts and seeds, and occasional eggs or milk products if tolerated. The overall best foods for cancer prevention include organic white meats of poultry and fish, whole grains, vegetables, especially organically grown cruciferous ones, and fruits, such as citrus fruits. The worst are high-fat, chemical foods and smoked, barbecued, or pickled foods.

CANCER PREVENTION: DIETARY SUGGESTIONS

Emphasize: (organic if possible)	*Avoid:*
cruciferous vegetables	high-fat foods
other vegetables	hydrogenated fats
whole grains	synthetic or high-chemical foods
fruits	smoked foods
poultry	pickled foods
fish (untreated)	barbecued foods
legumes	excess polyunsaturated oils
some nuts and seeds	alcohol
seaweeds/sea vegetables	high-calorie diets
	high-cholesterol diet
	low-fiber diet
	environmental chemicals
	excessive proteins

A primarily or exclusively vegetarian diet is generally helpful in preventing cancer. All studies of people on vegetarian diets showed reduced incidences of a variety of cancers, including the common ones of the colon, breast, and prostate. The macrobiotic (primarily cooked grains and vegetables) and vegan diets (avoiding eggs and milk) probably pose even a lower risk than the classically researched Seventh-Day Adventist diet; although both these diets contain wholesome foods, they must be watched for deficiency problems. A macrobiotic diet has become popular among people who are suffering from cancer or concerned about preventing it. Such a diet focuses on whole grains (50–60 percent); vegetables (25–30 percent), mainly cooked; soups (5–10 percent); and beans and sea vegetables (5–10 percent). Michio Kushi discusses the macrobiotic diet and its application to cancer in great detail in his book, *The Cancer Prevention Diet.* Also refer to Chapter 9, *Diets,* in this book.

Certain vegetables from the cruciferous family have recently been recognized as having anticancer properties. These include broccoli, brussels sprouts, cabbage, kale, bok choy, and cauliflower. They increase the levels of the enzyme *aryl hydroxylase* in the liver, lung, and intestines; this enzyme detoxifies many carcinogens and blocks their action. It may be the indoles and isothiocyanates in these foods that activate the enzymes. Other foods that may increase the action of *aryl hydroxylase* include spinach, lettuce, mustard greens, kohlrabi, turnips, and parsnips. Chlorophyllic greens and wheatgrass also may have a positive anticancer effect through their purification and detoxification functions.

Since I consider the genesis of cancer largely a result of autointoxication, chemical exposure, stagnation, and congestion (physical, mental, and emotional), I believe that periodic detoxification diets and fasting are appropriate for most people as a preventive to degenerative disease and to generally improve clarity and vitality. Juice fasting or a fruit and vegetable detoxification diet also helps us reflect on and reevaluate our diets, attitudes, life priorities, and personal path. This enhances our evolutionary process which I feel is essential to "staying healthy." For more information on *Fasting* and *Detoxification*, see Chapter 18.

The Ideal Diet, as discussed in Part Three, is basically a good anticancer diet as well. It is a moderately low-fat, low-calorie, high-fiber diet that includes many of the nutrient-rich foods, such as fruits, vegetables, whole grains, legumes, seeds, nuts, and the low-fat animal proteins if desired. It is adapted to the seasons, which allows better availability of organically grown local produce, extremely important in minimizing intake of potentially dangerous chemical carcinogens.

I was very impressed with a recent publication by the American Institute for Cancer Research entitled *An Ounce of Prevention*. It is a four-volume series, one volume for each season, presenting a low-fat, high-fiber, chemically light, healthy-looking diet with a focus on practical recipes. It was very pleasing to my heart to see each volume devoted to a particular season, with colors and all, containing recipes rich in the naturally grown foods. This is the concept that I have been advocating for over a decade. The new seasonal back-to-nature diet approach is catching on again and leading the way back to greater nutritional health and vitality.

Let us now explore some of the anticancer nutrients. There are three main avenues for defense against cancer, and each has specific nutrients that will support that function:

1. **Strengthening the immune system**—vitamins C and E, vitamin A and beta-carotene, zinc and copper, and the B vitamins folic acid, riboflavin, pyridoxine, and pantothenic acid.
2. **Avoiding or neutralizing carcinogens**—vitamins C and A, selenomethionine, and the amino acid L-cysteine.
3. **Preventing DNA and cellular damage**—vitamin A, vitamins C and E, beta-carotene, and the minerals selenium, zinc, and manganese.

The diet I have suggested will provide adequate levels of most of these nutrients if the foods are digested and assimilated. High amounts of fruits and vegetables will provide lots of vitamins C and A, beta-carotene, and some of the B vitamins. Whole grains will give us more B vitamins, some vitamin E and most minerals. Good-quality proteins will provide amino acids and cysteine. With a more vegetarian and low-fat diet there can be slight deficiencies, such as vitamin E, and, depending in some cases on the soil content, zinc and selenium, both of which may require supplementation.

Vitamin A and beta-carotene are also important anticancer nutrients that support normal cellular differentiation of the tissues and internal linings. Vitamin A may prevent cancer cell formation by inhibiting the binding of carcinogens to the cell wall; similarly, beta-carotene may protect the DNA in the nucleus of the cell by decreasing

810

the bonding of chemicals to the membrane around the nucleus, which contains the DNA, our basic life material. Both of these nutrients are antioxidants that scavenge free radicals, particularly singlet oxygen molecules. Decreased levels of vitamin A are associated with increased rates of cancer of the lungs especially, and also of the mouth, esophagus, bladder, cervix, and stomach. Beta-carotene has been shown to be deficient in a large proportion of smokers who develop lung cancer, as it seems to specifically protect cells of the mucous membranes. It has also been shown to be low in people who develop cancers of the throat, skin, prostate, and colon and is probably protective against those cancers as well. Due to its stronger antioxidant functions, beta-carotene is likely the better anticancer nutrient than the retinol form of vitamin A. Zinc, which is needed to form the retinol-binding protein (for vitamin A), may also be low in people who develop cancer. Vitamin A and especially beta-carotene are found mainly in fruits and vegetables, such as carrots, sweet potatoes, squashes, greens such as spinach and broccoli, seaweed and blue-green algae, bell peppers, apricots, and cantaloupe. Vitamin A in the retinol, or animal, form is found in fish, eggs and liver.

Vitamin C is involved in all three of the cancer defense functions and is obviously an important nutrient. It is one of the main antioxidant nutrients, protecting cell and mucous membranes and vascular linings from free radicals generated by carcinogens and other molecules. Even though the use of ascorbic acid in cancer treatment is controversial, it is important to use for cancer prevention. This vitamin is abundant in foods such as citrus fruits, cruciferous vegetables, and peppers. With the current stresses and chemical exposures in our society, and the inability to acquire high levels of vitamin C from our diet, I usually suggest some regular supplementation, at least 2–3 grams daily, though even 500–1000 mg. (0.5–1.0 gram) is probably sufficient for most of its protective functions. Rutin, one of the vitamin C-complex nutrients, or bioflavonoids, found in various foods and herbs, may also have some anticancer properties.

Anti-Cancer Aspects of Vitamin C

1. Is an antioxidant.
2. Stimulates T lymphocytes to produce interferon, which decreases virus reproduction.
3. Supports thymus function, specifically in strengthening the cytotoxic and killer T lymphocytes, and supports antibody responsiveness.
4. Reduces the production of nitrosamines (a strong carcinogen) from dietary nitrates and nitrites from the soil and those added to smoked or processed meats, and those we produce through our own digestion and metabolism.
5. Reduces stomach, esophageal, and bladder cancers by means of its multiple protective effects on mucous membranes (this needs more research).
6. Has been shown, along with folic acid, to minimize cervical dysplasia and cancer, where these nutrients have been measured at reduced levels.

Vitamin E functions best with adequate levels of selenium as selenomethionine, and vice versa, as antioxidants and cell membrane protectors. Vitamin E is found naturally in vegetable oils and nuts and seeds, with a little in the germ of whole grains such as wheat and rice. It reduces carcinogen production and strengthens immune cells and cell membranes against the penetration of viruses and toxic chemicals.

Selenium helps regulate the *glutathione peroxidase* enzyme, a strong antioxidant enzyme. Low selenium levels in the soil and in our body are clearly associated with increased rates of leukemia and cancers of the breast, lungs, colon, rectum, prostate, ovary, skin, and pancreas. If soils are low in this mineral, the foods grown in them will not contain much selenium. It is wise to increase selenium-rich foods, such as the whole grains and legumes or brewer's yeast, if tolerated, as well as to take a supplemental 100 mcg. per day to be safe. High copper levels can reduce selenium absorption and utilization as well.

Zinc is another important mineral. It is an immune supporter and is important to the formation and function of many enzymes that work on detoxifying chemicals. Low levels of zinc in the body have been associated with higher rates of prostate, bronchial, esophageal, and colon cancers. Low levels of molybdenum in the soil have also been shown to be associated with increased levels of esophageal cancer. Calcium protects against colon cancer by protecting and correcting irregular cells in the colon. Other minerals that may have anticancer qualities include iron and iodine.

Fiber is another important anticancer substance and is a part of many foods which can also be taken as a supplement, such as psyllium seed husks or the bran of wheat or oats. Adequate dietary fiber improves intestinal transit time and binds carcinogens, thus reducing exposure to them. A high-fiber diet clearly reduces the incidence of colon cancer and diverticular disease (and may lower blood cholesterol), whereas a high-fat, low-fiber diet increases the risk of colon, breast, and other cancers.

Lactobacillus acidophilus is, I believe, a useful anticancer agent, mainly to prevent colon cancer. Lactobacilli cultures in the colon decrease other bacteria that can change bile salts into irritating carcinogens, as well as reduce yeast overgrowth and inflammation that result from these organisms, which also contribute to allergies and immune suppression.

A few other immune-supporting nutrients include gamma-linolenic acid (GLA), extracted from evening primrose oil or other sources; GLA helps increase certain prostaglandins that support lymphocyte immune activity, and there is some indication that it has an anticancer effect. More research is also needed on the anti- or procancer effects of L-arginine, a semiessential amino acid. L-carnitine may also be helpful for improving fat utilization, as poor fat metabolism and free-radical fat molecules can cause cellular and tissue irritation. Organic germanium may also be effective in cancer prevention, although it is more clearly useful in cancer treatment.

BHA and BHT are antioxidant food chemicals (preservatives) that some researchers feel have potential to lower chemically induced cancers; other authorities believe these chemicals are too toxic to use as supplements. I prefer the natural antioxidant nutrients that are commonly found in foods.

Garlic and echinacea are thought to help support immune function, and thus may play a role in preventing cancer. Aside from garlic, no herbs have been studied well enough to determine their possible cancer preventive effects. (There may be some herbs, both Western and Eastern, that have anticancer effects; these will be discussed more in *Staying Healthy with Modern Medicine*, my next book, which will include cancer therapy. Among those that may have properties effective in preventing cancer development are intestinal detoxicants, such as the algins and kelps; herbal blood cleansers (alteratives) such as chapparal, cayenne pepper, burdock and yellow dock roots, and blue flag root; colon cleansers such as rhubarb root and black walnut; diuretics and kidney cleansers such as cleavers, uva ursi and dandelion; lymph cleansers such as echinacea; and nutritives, such as alfalfa.

The following program is particularly geared to protect those with added cancer risks, although it may also be used periodically, for a month or two several times yearly, for the average individual. With aging, or during times of stress or emotional traumas, this program may also be helpful. The following values can include nutrients in the diet and/or additional supplements.

CANCER PREVENTION NUTRIENT PROGRAM

Water	2 qt.
Calories	1,500–2,500
Protein	50–75 g.
Fats	40–65 g.
Fiber	15–30 g.

Vitamin A	5,000–10,000 IUs		Iodine	150–200 mcg.
Beta-carotene	15,000–30,000 IUs		Iron	10–20 mg.
Vitamin D	400 IUs		Magnesium	300–600 mg.
Vitamin E	400–800 IUs		Manganese	5–10 mg.
Vitamin K	150–300 mcg.		Molybdenum	250–500 mcg.
Thiamine (B$_1$)	50–100 mg.		Potassium	300–600 mg.
Riboflavin (B$_2$)	25–75 mg.		Selenium, preferably	200–300 mcg.
Riboflavin-5-phosphate	25–50 mg.		as selenomethionine	
Niacinamide (B$_3$)	50–100 mg.		Silicon	100–200 mg.
Niacin (B$_3$)	50 mg.		Vanadium	150–300 mcg.
Pantothenic acid (B$_5$)	250–500 mg.		Zinc	30–60 mg.
Pyridoxine (B$_6$)	50–100 mg.			
Pyridoxal-5-phosphate	25–50 mg.		Lactobacillus	1–2 billion organisms
Cobalamin (B$_{12}$)	100 mcg.		Garlic oil or powder	2–3 capsules
Folic acid	800 mcg.		Essential fatty acids,	2–4 capsules
Biotin	500 mcg.		or Flaxseed oil	1–2 teaspoons
Vitamin C	3–6 g.		Gamma-linolenic acid	4 capsules
Bioflavonoids	250–500 mg.			or 200–300 mg.
			L-amino acids	1,000 mg.
Calcium	850–1,200 mg.		L-cysteine	250 mg.
Chromium	200–400 mcg.		L-carnitine	500 mg.
Copper	2–3 mg.			

Cardiovascular Disease Prevention

Well, this is the biggie! With a little effort on each of our parts and a willingness to change, we can make a big difference in the incidence of this nation's number one killer, cardiovascular disease (CVD). Heart and blood vessel disease are not inevitable; in fact, they are preventable in most cases. It is very clear from every major study in the last decade that diets high in saturated fats and cholesterol, which would consist of regular intake of red meats, dairy foods, and eggs, are directly correlated to the incidence of CVD and its complications, whereas a low saturated fat, low cholesterol diet greatly lowers the risk of these diseases.

The main disease process at the base of the cardiovascular diseases is atherosclerosis, or hardening and clogging of the arteries. (Arteriosclerosis is the generic term referring to hardening of the arteries. Atherosclerosis refers to the disease process of artery plaqueing and is the term I will use in this text.) Atherosclerosis involves the thickening and narrowing of our blood vessels that occurs somewhat in most people, but with certain risk factors it can progress very rapidly and lead to early demise, even in their 40s or 50s. Atherosclerosis commonly affects the coronary arteries, which deliver blood to the heart muscle itself. This biggest cardiovascular concern causes a great deal of limitation and chest pain, or angina pectoris. When advanced, this coronary artery disease can result in a myocardial infarction (MI, heart attack, or "coronary"). Heart attacks are clearly the most common cause of death in the United States and the Western world. Other areas of the body may also be affected with atherosclerosis. Disease of the carotid arteries of the neck affects our mental faculties; atherosclerosis of the leg arteries decreases our ability to walk without pain; and clogging of the pelvic arteries affects our sexual performance.

Hypertension, or high blood pressure, is often a hidden multifactorial problem and the most common CVD; the main pathologic process involved in hypertension is atherosclerosis. The narrowing and hardening of the arteries increase their resistance and pressure and makes the heart work harder, which can then wear down this vital muscle. Untreated hypertension may lead to further heart disease including heart attacks and congestive heart failure, as well as to cerebrovascular accidents (stroke).

For nearly half a century, cardiovascular disease has been the number one cause of mortality and morbidity in the United States and in most of the Western world. At the turn of the century, it was not even in the top ten. In underdeveloped countries where people live on a more natural, "native" diet, there is a low incidence of CVD. In the United States, the many CVDs account for over 50 percent of all deaths. Of course, people live longer now, which allows for the development of more degenerative disease, but there is also more middle-age weight gain in a more sedentary population

815

that eats more fats and refined foods than in the past. These last three factors are fairly easy to change (if change is ever easy) and form the basis of preventing these now common diseases.

Cardiovascular Diseases	Results
Atherosclerosis	Angina pectoris (chest pain)
Hypertension	Limitation of movement
Coronary artery disease	Memory loss
Carotid artery disease	Cerebrovascular accident (stroke)
Peripheral artery disease	Cardiac arrhythmias
Heart disease	Myocardial infarction
	Congestive heart failure
	Valvular heart disease*

*Especially mitral and aortic disease from high blood pressure.

Hypertension and heart disease are not inevitable results of aging. In countries where populations eat a diet low in fats, cholesterol, and salt there is very little or no hypertension in comparison to countries whose people eat those richer foods. The 90-year-olds in Hunza society appear to be free of CVD and have normal blood pressure. To keep the blood pressure low with age and minimize the atherosclerotic process we need to do the following:

- Eat a diet low in saturated fats, cholesterol, salt, and processed, refined foods (both fats and sugars).
- Eat high-fiber foods.
- Eat plenty of whole grains, fruits, and vegetables.
- Exercise or have a regular, active lifestyle, especially including walking.
- Keep body fat low.

There has already been some progress; in the last twenty years, the previous rapidly rising death rate from CVDs began leveling off and decreasing, likely due to better coronary care, CPR education, public education, and drug control of high blood pressure. Since 1968, there has also been greater dietary awareness, an interest in exercise, and an effort to diminish cigarette smoking. It is clear that a good (lower fat, more vegetarian) diet, regular exercise, weight reduction, and stress modification can reduce the symptoms of atherosclerosis, hypertension, and angina pectoris as well as decrease the risk and incidence of CVD in general. So why is it still so prevalent? Often, people must be hit over the head before they will acknowledge new information and change long-term patterns. On both an economical and educational level, the big

816

industries fight changes that might affect their status and income. The meat, dairy, and egg megabusinesses still try to deny the relationship between their foods and high cholesterol levels and cardiovascular disease—advertising their products as being good for everybody and providing literature to young children to encourage the regular use of their foods. Now other businesses, such as fast food chains, are getting into the educational act claiming that a hamburger, fries, and a milkshake are a balanced meal. Kids are already influenced by advertising for sugary and refined food products.

Even with the improvement of the last 20 years, there are still well over a half million deaths per year from heart attacks and strokes (down from the previous 1 million yearly). About a third of the 1.5 million people who have "coronaries" each year die from those attacks. Nearly 50 million Americans have some CVD, mostly high blood pressure (over 35 million) and coronary artery disease (CAD, about 5 million), with many more people who are undiagnosed. Our cholesterol level, a key contributing factor in CVDs, can only be determined with a blood chemistry analysis, while hypertension often does not reveal itself prior to its being found on a physical exam. When either elevated cholesterol levels or high blood pressure are found, cardiovascular damage may already have begun. Because it is difficult for people to know if they have high blood pressure, it has been labeled the "silent killer." Here, we will first look at the many risk factors for CVD, and then examine the underlying disease process, atherosclerosis.

The cardiovascular risk factors are commonly classified into the primary factors—of which there are three: **cigarette smoking, high cholesterol,** and **high blood pressure**—and the secondary of which there are many. Some of these significant factors in the genesis of CVD include obesity and being overweight, genetics, stress, a sedentary lifestyle, diabetes, and alcohol abuse. Many authorities feel that, even more than the moderate or high fat and cholesterol intake, it is the many nutritional deficiencies that arise from our present-day nutrition and that affect our cholesterol metabolism which lead to increased atherosclerosis. Deficiencies of vitamins C, E, and B_6 and selenium are the main concerns. Other relevant nutrients are magnesium, chromium, niacin, essential fatty acids, and fiber. The types of fats consumed in the diet and the deficiency of the essential fatty acids, linoleic and linolenic, are felt by some authorities to be the source of the CVD problem. Udo Erasmus describes this in his book, *Fats and Oils,* in which he also suggests that the heated and hydrogenated "modern" oils used for cooking and frying are a big concern. Thus, margarines are a concern in regard to the atherosclerotic process. The increased consumption of homogenized milk fat in the standard milk appears to be linked with cardiovascular problems. An article by Wayne Martin in the November 1989 *Townsend Newsletter for Doctors* provides a great deal of support for the theory that cholesterol itself is not the culprit it is thought to be in the atherosclerotic process, but it is the hydrogenated and homogenized fats used and consumed in so many foods that are the disease-causing factors.

Regarding minerals, the calcium-magnesium interchange and the sodium-potassium relationship affect hardening of the arteries and blood pressure. Even copper

CARDIOVASCULAR DISEASE RISKS

Primary	Secondary	Others
High cholesterol*	family history of hyperlipidemia	caffeine
Hypertension	maleness	soft water
	obesity	hypothyroidism
Smoking	stress (type A)	cadmium toxicity
	lack of activity (heart exercise)	
	diabetes	
	aging (with other risks)	
	nutritional deficiencies:	nutritional deficiencies:
	vitamin C	chromium
	vitamin E	niacin (B_3)
	selenium	fatty acids
	vitamin B_6	fiber
	magnesium	zinc
	potassium	copper

Another way of categorizing these risk factors is:

Personal Factors	Disease Relationships	Behavior Patterns
family history	diabetes	smoking
gender	high blood pressure	diet (high or low-fat)
age	hyperlipidemia (types II and IV)	overweight
stress level	high cholesterol	stress, overwork
personality (type A)	elevated lipoproteins (high LDL-HDL ratio)	exercise (low to high)
overwork, time pressure, etc.	high triglycerides	nutrient deficiencies
overweight	hypothyroidism	water choices
		substance abuse: sugar, alcohol, caffeine, and other drugs
		regular use of: homogenized milk, margarines, and hydrogenated fats

_____

*Due to heredity and/or a diet high in fats and cholesterol.

and zinc deficiencies and imbalance may be related. It is clear however, that the saturated fats and cholesterol in the diet are linked to CVD in all animals studied, including the human species. Carnivorous animals, such as dogs and cats, seem relatively immune to high-fat diets. Possibly understanding their protection will give us further insight into CVD prevention.

The relationship of cholesterol has been and continues to be the biggest controversy in this area. Current thinking is that high blood cholesterol, especially with higher LDL cholesterol (the "bad" kind) and lower HDL cholesterol (the "good" kind, because it picks up used cholesterol and carries it back to the liver), is a significant factor correlated with atherosclerosis, coronary artery disease, and early death. The very large Framingham study showed that people with a blood cholesterol level of 260 mg. had three times the incidence of myocardial infarctions that those with levels of 195. Lowering cholesterol levels by whatever means—diet, weight loss, exercise, and even drugs—decreased the risk of heart attacks. Yet there may be other variables; this cholesterol picture may just be the surface factor.

Some authors, such as Richard Kunin, M.D. and Michael Lesser, M.D., feel that the metabolism of cholesterol, which uses many vital nutrients, is the real problem. With adequate nutrient levels, reasonable amounts of dietary cholesterol will not cause the problems we are seeing. Our liver makes cholesterol, which we need for many functions such as the production of hormones (estrogen and testosterone), vitamin D, and bile. A natural feedback mechanism should reduce our production when we consume cholesterol-containing foods. There may be certain factors, yet unknown but possibly genetic and nutritional, that interfere with this feedback mechanism. B vitamins, vitamins C and E, magnesium, manganese, and zinc are all needed for cholesterol metabolism, and if these are low, this waxy fat cannot as easily get into the cells to function and sludges around in the blood, clogging up our vessels. This is rather like the process in adult diabetes, where the sugar cannot get into the cells and stays in the blood, causing problems.

In *Mega Nutrition*, Dr. Kunin suggests that the rapid rise in CVD was associated with three important dietary changes besides an increase in fat intake that were as significant as or even more significant than cholesterol. First was the refining and milling of flour which removed many of the nutrients that are important to cholesterol metabolism. Second was the use of chlorinated water which was popularized and spread throughout the country. Chlorine tends to bind and reduce levels of vitamin E which acts as an important protector of the vascular lining. Third, homogenized milk also hit in the 1940s. Homogenization changes the fat composition of milk so that it is not as easily metabolized and passes more readily through the liver. This, I believe, is a big factor in the increase in CVD.

These theories have some backing, but are not generally accepted. More research is needed to verify that we can still eat a reasonable amount of high-fat and high-cholesterol foods such as eggs, meats, milk, and butter, and still not develop CVD, as long as our diet is nutrient-rich and meets all of our needs. Until then, I believe that there is more than enough research evidence to prove that eating a diet low in fat, especially saturated fat, and cholesterol, along with the other changes that I suggest, is still the best thing to do. We still need fats in our diet, but mainly the natural essential fatty acids found in nuts and seeds, fish, and grains and beans. These oils are necessary for many vital functions and also help release bile products from the liver and gallbladder. Bile is made from cholesterol and thus is one of the ways to eliminate cholesterol from the body.

Cholesterol is part of many of the foods that omnivores eat. It is contained only in animal foods, such as meats, eggs, and milk products. The average daily intake in the United States is 500 mg. for men and about 350 mg. for women. Women are somewhat protected from CVD during their child-bearing years by their female hormones. The new suggested maximum for cholesterol intake is 300 mg., not much more than contained in one egg yolk (275 mg.). It is probably ideal, especially for those at risk for CVD, to consume less than 150 mg. of cholesterol daily. That is the reason for the big push to a more vegetarian diet. (A strict vegetarian diet, meaning no eggs or milk products, can sharply reduce an elevated cholesterol level in one month, possibly as much as 100 mg./dl. (deciliter), or 100 mg. percent.)

Cholesterol is easy to absorb and hard to eliminate. It appears that the higher our blood cholesterol level, the greater our risk of CVD. Below 180 mg. percent poses a low risk; 180–200 mg. percent is a good range; over 200 mg. percent clearly increases our CVD risk, while over 250 mg. percent gives us a high risk. (LDL and HDL levels are also important within the total cholesterol value; see discussion below.) The average adult has a blood cholesterol level between 200 and 220 mg. percent. So there is work to be done. There is no known deficiency disease with cholesterol; many people apparently do well with little or no cholesterol intake. The body still makes it, though with certain chronic illnesses or liver impairments, blood cholesterol levels may fall to very low and probably functionally deficient levels. Cholesterol helps in tissue repair and other important functions mentioned previously.

Many doctors feel comfortable working with the total cholesterol value alone. Reducing it through smoking cessation, control of diabetes, hypertension, or obesity, dietary changes, or exercise programs can offer some security in disease prevention. It is now known that even a small increase in cholesterol can lead to a marked increase in coronary disease and heart attacks; the main research studies suggest that every 1 percent we lower a high cholesterol, we reduce our heart disease risk by 2 percent. So even mild decreases in cholesterol are helpful.

In recent years, more practitioners are using the cholesterol subfractions—HDL and LDL (VLDL may also be significant). These represent lipoproteins, or fat-protein molecules, that carry the nonimmersible fats through the blood. The high-density lipoprotein (HDL) carries cholesterol back to the liver from the bloodstream and is thought to be protective by taking the extra cholesterol out of the blood. Low-density

820

lipoproteins (LDLs) transport cholesterol through the blood to the cells and usually comprise most of the blood cholesterol. Very low density lipoproteins (VLDLs) also keep cholesterol in circulation and may contribute to atherosclerosis. The total cholesterol/HDL ratio and/or the LDL/HDL ratio can be observed as a relative measurement of CVD risks.

Smoking, being sedentary, and consuming saturated fats in the diet lower protective HDLs. Exercise, a high-fiber diet, and alcohol increase HDL, though alcohol also produces irritating effects on the liver and vascular system, and may increase total cholesterol. Increased LDL levels can be caused by increased consumption of saturated fats and sugar, deficient levels of vitamin C or chromium, and high copper or iron levels. The various fats have different effects on cholesterol. Saturated fats lead to more LDL and VLDL. The monounsaturated fats tend to have a neutral influence on cholesterol levels, while the polyunsaturated fats tend to lower total cholesterol but may also likewise lower the good HDLs.

DIETARY FATS

Cholesterol-Rich Foods	Saturated Fats	Monounsaturated Fats	Polyunsaturated Fats
egg yolks	butter	olive oil	vegetable oils:
liver	cheese	olives	sesame
other organs	milk	almonds	safflower
pâtés	red meats	pecans	sunflower
milk fat	poultry	peanuts	corn
fatty meats	coconut oil	cashews	soybean
	palm oil	avocados	walnut
	margarine	fish	

Other fats contained in foods that have beneficial effects on cholesterol are the omega-3 fatty acids, EPA and DHA, found in coldwater fish such as salmon, mackerel, and sardines. This fairly recent important discovery, as well as other essential nutrients, especially magnesium and pyridoxine, are discussed in more detail below.

Smoking is another crucial factor and an instigator of not only our number one killer, cardiovascular disease, but also our number two life destroyer, cancer. Day-to-day smoking sensitizes our vascular system and heart. Nicotine damages the vascular lining, increases heart rate, and decreases oxygen delivery, with further carbon monoxide intoxication. Smoking also increases LDL cholesterol levels and possibly poses an additional risk of increased levels of beta-VLDL (currently under research). Cadmium, which is a blood pressure elevator, and other toxic minerals are also found in cigarette smoke. Nicotine also increases arterial constriction, which further limits oxygen and nutrient delivery to the cells and tissues. And chronic cigarette smoking clearly increases our chances of having atherosclerosis and hypertension with all of their complications. Thus, cigarette smoking by itself includes all three primary risk factors for CVD.

Hypertension is not only another major risk factor, but also occurs as a result of atherosclerosis itself. High blood pressure is defined as one over 140/90 mm Hg (millimeters of mercury, a pressure reading). Normal blood pressure (BP) should range from 100/70 to 120/80. The higher number represents the systolic BP, the BP while the heart pumps; while the lower number represents the diastolic BP during the rest between beats. The blood pressure itself is basically the pressure that the blood exerts on the arterial walls. An elevated diastolic pressure has a worse affect on the genesis of atherosclerosis than does a high systolic pressure. Even a diastolic pressure between 80 and 90 is associated with an increased risk. High blood pressure puts strain on the blood vessels, the heart, and the kidneys (especially important in controlling the BP).

Many doctors consider a BP in the range from 140/90 to 160/95 to be only mildly elevated, though it definitely increases risk. This is the area of "borderline" hypertension that we can do most about. Hypertension, like CVD in general, is affected by a number of risk factors. Weight, diet, family history, gender, race, stress, smoking, and lack of exercise are some of the main ones; there are many more. Suffice it to say here that it is a major disease, limiting and shortening the lives of nearly 50 million people in the United States and many more times that in the entire world. And it is a disease we can do something to prevent. The CVD prevention program applies to high blood pressure as well, and clearly, lowering elevated blood pressure by whatever means possible reduces the risk of heart disease, heart attacks, and strokes.

Obesity is another major risk factor in CVD, contributing to both atherosclerosis and hypertension. Being overweight raises blood pressure, increases blood fats, reduces HDL, and usually minimizes exercise, as well as increasing diabetes incidence. This all speeds up the atherosclerotic process and the occurrence of coronary artery disease. By decreasing obesity, we can decrease many of the above-mentioned CVD risk factors at one time.

Stress factors also contribute to CVD. The type A personality has an increased risk, more indirectly, through poor diet, caffeine use, and increased adrenaline output, which raises blood pressure. The hard-driven, ambitious type A person is constantly creating his or her life under the pressure of time, with the attitude that there is never enough time to do all there is to do, or that it should be done faster. Some authorities further attribute to this personality a low awareness of spiritual or philosophical values, or a low religious orientation, with a perspective basically geared toward work and running around the world. These type A people could benefit from stress reduction to help them in relaxation, and from exercise, especially with a sense of fun, to aid in letting go of the ever-riding tensions.

Lack of exercise is also a problem in CVD. The heart and circulation need regular, even vigorous exercise to keep them strong. Remember, the heart is a muscle that needs to work out. We will look more at exercise as a positive preventive to cardiovascular disease in the discussion below.

Drinking "soft" water is definitely a risk. It replaces the minerals calcium and magnesium in normally CVD-protective water with sodium mainly, which has a tendency to increase blood pressure and worsen atherosclerosis. Areas where people drink "soft" water have higher incidences of CVD and heart attacks. It is best to drink spring or well water for its beneficial minerals as well as to prevent chemical exposure. And water is definitely better for us than caffeine and alcohol. Caffeine increases heart rate and blood pressure and adds the risk of cardiac arrythmia. Alcohol is a suppressant but also an irritant and is a minor risk factor itself in CVD.

Family history is not something we can do much about, but our knowledge of it can motivate us to take extra special care of ourselves and more diligently apply the program outlined here. Certain genetic traits may influence cholesterol metabolism and levels of production of cholesterol and other fats. It appears that some people actually make more cholesterol (or perhaps clear less or use less) than others. This increases their risk of vascular problems. Specific genetic (familial) problems of fat levels are described in medicine. These are termed "hyperlipidemias," the lipid disorders, and include five types. Types II and IV, the most common, cause high cholesterol and high triglyceride levels, respectively. Type IV is the most common and is thought to result more from familial eating patterns than from genetics. It also can proceed to problems in sugar metabolism. These disorders can be revealed by a blood test.

A history of hyperlipidemia disorder or a family history of coronary heart disease, high blood pressure, diabetes, or obesity put us at increased risk for developing some type of CVD. This means we need to enhance our prevention efforts, which may require many changes, depending on our current lifestyle. Cardiovascular disease really needs to be prevented in childhood. Atherosclerosis often starts in children, as can hypertension. Avoiding the typical high-fat, high-sugar, and high-salt foods and snacks and fried oils can make a big difference. Keeping the weight normal and getting plenty of exercise is the way to go. In some manner, television is a cardiovascular disease risk as it encourages a sedentary life and poor food choices are highly advertised. Dietary suggestions for children with CVD risk and obesity will be discussed later in this section.

It is important to remember that effects of risk factors are cumulative. Just being overweight is not a big problem if our cholesterol and diet are okay or if we do not smoke, but if we are an overweight, sedentary smoker with high blood pressure and a poor diet, we will not be living on that path very long.

I would like to discuss the process of atherosclerosis so that we have a clearer picture of this basic degenerative disease affecting the lives of millions. Atherosclerosis is the hardening of the inner arterial walls with lipids (mainly cholesterol), smooth muscle cells from the blood vessel walls themselves, and calcium. This process, which is stimulated and added to by platelets and white blood cells, forms the plaque, or atheromas. Atherosclerosis can begin early with these fatty streaks in the blood vessel walls. Many teenagers with high-fat diets have plaque in their arteries. The fries, shakes, burgers, and hot dogs that are so prevalent in our culture's diet, along with the deficiencies that arise from high intake of sugar and refined foods (there often is not much room left for many nutrient-rich foods), predispose our youth to this early hardening of the arteries.

The basic process of atherosclerosis is thought to begin with minor microinjuries to the vascular linings. These tiny wounds stimulate the overgrowth of muscle cells and attract and attach the fat/cholesterol and platelet aggregation along with calcium precipitation to eventually form a small fibrous scar that begins to narrow the opening of the artery. (Cholesterol is a waxy fat/sterol that is attempting to heal the irritated or injured tissues; it's really trying to help!) This arterial plaque reduces the blood flow and also decreases the strength and elasticity of the vessel wall. This can predispose us to increased blood pressure and aneurysms (ballooning of the artery), which can then lead to bleeding, strokes, or other, milder consequences.

These tiny injuries to the blood vessels involve many contributors, but the mechanism by which they occur is via free-radical pathology, not dissimilar to most inflammatory and cellular changes. We discussed the formation of these irritating molecules in the *Anti-Aging* and *Anti-Stress* programs, and the development of diseases such as arthritis and cancer.

Free-radical formation and the process of atherosclerosis involve many factors, most of which we have discussed. Saturated and hydrogenated fats in diet, elevated fats and cholesterol in the blood, hypertension, smoking, carbon monoxide, and deficiencies of nutrients such as vitamins C and E, chromium and selenium, are some of the main ones. Other contributing factors include infection, allergy, particularly from antigen-antibody complexes formed from food proteins, and abnormal platelet activity. Platelet function is important; it helps our blood to clot when this is needed. However, an increased adhesiveness can be a big problem, especially in those with already thicker, fatty blood or with irritated tissue linings (saturated fats thicken the blood). Platelets produce a substance called thromboxane A_2, which increases platelet stickiness and stimulates clot formation. It also stimulates increased productivity of the smooth muscle cells in the blood vessel walls. Contributors to increased platelet adhesiveness are smoke, excess fats, especially LDL cholesterol, diabetes (high blood sugar), and many nutritional deficiencies, such as vitamins A, C, E, B_3, and B_6 and the minerals calcium, magnesium, zinc, and manganese. This overfunction of platelets is thought to increase the progress of certain diseases, mainly cardiovascular in nature, and especially atherosclerosis, but also arthritis, diabetes, and cancer.

Atherosclerosis can be a slow process. The disease may not cause problems for many years and then the symptoms can begin and progress rapidly, as a blood vessel usually must be more than half (more like 70–80 percent closed before it creates difficulty. A full clot—that is, a thrombosis—will lead to blocked circulation and often death of the tissues to which the blood vessel leads, unless there is existing collateral

824

circulation to that area. This is how a heart attack develops, with atherosclerosis in the significant coronary arteries. In coronary artery disease, 70–80 percent closure will more likely lead to chest pain, the symptom of angina pectoris. If an atheroma or clot breaks off from its blood vessel attachment, it will move through the blood until it reaches a vessel that it is too large to pass through and then clog up that vessel, which can be disastrous. Clots in the blood vessels also can stimulate arterial spasm, which often worsens symptoms.

Atherosclerosis affects the vascular, mainly the arterial, system and commonly leads to problems in the heart, kidneys, brain, ears, and sexual organs. The heart, or coronary, blood vessels are the biggest area of concern. The effect on the kidney (renal) circulation can lead to hypertension. Carotid artery disease directly influences brain circulation, which can lead to memory problems, hearing loss, perhaps dizziness or vertigo, senility, and strokes. Transient ischemic attacks (TIAs) affect the state of consciousness with intermittent loss of blood flow. Poor circulation is the biggest cause of decreased sexual function and impotence in middle-aged or older men.

The best way to evaluate the presence or state of CVD is by a thorough workup. A history will describe any possible symptoms tied to circulatory compromise or block-age, the result of atherosclerosis. A physical exam will not usually tell much unless there is some heart abnormality, poor circulation, or elevated blood pressure. The blood pressure (BP) should ideally be under 120/80 in adults and 110/70 in children. Any elevation puts a patient at higher risk, and calls for closer follow-up. The BP can go up just from the nervousness of being in a doctor's office, so it needs to be checked under more normal circumstances if it is abnormal. However, if it goes up under the stress of visiting a doctor, it likely goes up with other stress also.

An electrocardiogram, or EKG, is a measurement of the heart rhythm and electrical activity. This is positive only after problems already exist. Neither an EKG nor a chest x-ray is preventive; they simply show the presence of disease after it occurs and offer very few cues that would point out potential future problems, as can the blood pressure or blood level of cholesterol, HDL, and LDL. Many doctors are encouraging patients to treat cholesterol levels over 200 mg./dl. with diet, exercise, and even drug therapy. Increased blood levels of triglycerides, sugar, and uric acid are also of concern. A more extensive test for the heart is an echocardiogram using ultrasound, which can pick up more subtle changes in the heart muscle and its internal valves. Angiography, the injection of dye into the blood to study the circulation through the heart or any area of the body, is done more commonly these days to measure the circulatory status. It is performed before cardiac bypass surgery and is itself very risky, expensive, and possibly painful.

The best approach to cardiovascular disease is, of course, prevention. To prevent CVD, our overall plan includes not smoking; preventing and/or controlling obesity, high blood pressure, and diabetes; exercising and staying fit; eating a low-fat, more vegetarian diet; and monitoring and keeping our levels of cholesterol low, both in our diet and in our blood. For high-risk people, the program needs to be more vigorous. They need clear dietary guidelines and good follow-up care if they are to have a good chance of reducing development of CVD potential and its associated morbidity and mortality of later years. Not smoking, more aggressive control of obesity, hypertension, or diabetes, and a more strict low-fat diet are really mandatory.

GOALS FOR DECREASING CVD RISKS

Quit or minimize smoking
Lower and control blood pressure
Lower total cholesterol
Lower LDL cholesterol
Increase HDL cholesterol
Lower weight if overweight
Increase aerobic exercise

To Lower Cholesterol and LDL

Decrease total fats in diet
Decrease saturated fats in diet
Decrease cholesterol in diet
Increase essential fatty acid
  (polyunsaturates) foods in diet
Use more monounsaturated oils,
  such as olive or canola
Increase fiber
Use psyllium husks
Add oat bran
Increase complex carbohydrates
Decrease caffeine and nicotine
Supplement nutrients:
  Vitamins B_6, B_3, C;
  chromium; EPA; garlic

To Increase HDL Cholesterol

Get regular aerobic exercise
Do not smoke
Decrease weight
Supplement nutrients:
  essential fatty acids; niacin;
  EPA; fiber; garlic; L-carnitine

Much research is being conducted to investigate whether atherosclerosis is reversible. There is no question that its progress can be slowed through diet and exercise. However, whether it is possible to actually reverse it and clear the vessels of plaque is still questionable, although many authors, including myself, feel that it is possible and recent studies suggest this. Some studies show that a low-fat, low-cholesterol diet can result in increased cardiac output and a reduction of blood fats, which it is thought will decrease fatty plaques over time. A comprehensive research experiment conducted by, among others, Dean Ornish, M.D. and discussed in *Stress, Diet and Your Heart* suggests that exercise, stress reduction, and better diet result in marked improvement in almost all patients with CVD, in terms of both symptom reduction and enhanced performance ability. This is now proven in his new book, *Dr. Ornish's Program for Reversing Heart Disease.*

Many of the significant risk factors contributing to CVD can be lessened through dietary influences. These risks include high blood pressure, high cholesterol, (especially high LDL levels), high triglyceride levels, and obesity, as well as many cases of diabetes. High fat consumption, low fiber intake, and excess salt and sodium intake are influential nutritional risks. Proper diet alone can decrease cholesterol levels by 30 percent or more, although this usually requires some radical dietary shifts. Smoking and lack of exercise, the main nondietary habits (cardiovascular risk factors) involved, often require similar changes of willpower as does diet; and furthermore, we need a feeling of positive self-worth to even gather the force to make these successful changes.

The primary dietary focus of the **cardiovascular disease prevention diet** is fat intake. The diet should be low in fat in general and particularly low in saturated fats (animal fat plus coconut and palm oils) and the hydrogenated fats (all margarines) and oils such as used for frying foods. These are mainly poor-quality vegetable oils used so commonly in commercial food preparation and restaurant cooking. Avoiding these oils is highly recommended. It is clear that a diet high in saturated fats and cholesterol leads to increased blood cholesterol levels and increased atherosclerosis. In my clinical experience, homogenized, pasteurized milk and dairy fats seem to drive cholesterol to high levels. A quart or more of whole milk daily or regular intake of ice cream can lead to cholesterol levels over 300 mg./dl.; and thus, going off these foods can dramatically lower the cholesterol.

To prevent atheroschlerosis, a low-fat, low-cholesterol, and high-fiber diet is recommended. Fiber reduces CVD risk in many ways. It binds cholesterol and fats and lessens their absorption. It subsequently decreases blood cholesterol and LDL and increases protective HDL cholesterol. Increased fiber levels—and we are talking about 20–30 grams daily, which often requires supplemented fiber—will also help reduce blood pressure levels in those with elevations.

Fat intake should be reduced from the average 40–45 percent to a maximum of 25–30 percent of total calories; even lower levels, 15–20 percent, are suggested. With supplemental fatty acids or the use of good-quality cold-pressed vegetable oils to obtain our necessary linolenic acid, even lower fat intake can be consumed safely. This, however, is very difficult unless we eliminate a wide variety of common foods, including all fried foods, meats, milk products, butter, cheese, eggs, nuts, and seeds, which also clearly reduces protein intake.

Currently, the average American fat intake ranges from about 100–150 grams per day. Of course, men usually consume more than women, and many people with some food awareness consume less. In diet analyses, however, I commonly see this range, even up to and over 200 grams daily. At 9 calories per gram, 125 grams means 1,125 calories per day of fat. If that represents the average of about 40 percent of total calories, it would mean a diet of about 2,800 calories a day, which would add weight to most folks other than athletic men. If we eat 100 grams (900 calories) of fat daily, and that is one-third of our total calories, that means a total of 2,700 calories a day; if fats are a more healthful 25 percent of the diet, that means a total of 3,600 calories, more than most people consume. Realistically, fat intake levels must be no higher than 50–75 grams a day to create a calorie range of 1,800–2,700 with a diet containing 25 percent fat.

The types of fat consumed are also important. More unsaturated (poly- and monounsaturated) than saturated fats are suggested; that means a higher intake of vegetable oils and polyunsaturated-fat-containing foods. Beef, for example, has a ratio of saturated to polyunsaturated fat (S:P) of around 15:1, whereas the ratios in poultry and fish are closer to even. Vegetable fats found in nuts or seeds have an even lower S:P ratio. The polyunsaturates tend to be more beneficial to our levels of fat and cholesterol than the saturated fats found in milk, eggs, and meat. However, the polyunsaturated fats are unstable and not only lower total cholesterol but may also reduce the important HDL; the monounsaturated fats are probably better. Be careful of the hydrogenated polyunsaturates (many margarines and cooking oils); they have increased saturated fats and unusable, trans-fatty acids (mirror image molecules of the natural cis-fatty acids), and are even less desirable than the fats from butter, milk, or meat. Excess polyunsaturates also have added cancer and heart disease risks, possibly because of oxidation and the potential formation of free radicals. Overall, a minimum of fats is suggested, with avoidance of many of the less healthful unsaturated fats, such as refined cooking oils, margarines, mayonnaise, and artificial dressings and creamers, which also contain questionable chemicals. It is fairly clear that the total fat intake has an important influence on blood cholesterol as does the proportion of saturated fats or cholesterol-containing foods, so this needs to be an important area of focus.

Particularly helpful oils are contained in the coldwater fish such as salmon, mackerel, sardines, and herring. These contain EPA (eicosapentaenoic acid) and DHA (dicosahexaenoic acid), which have a positive effect on lowering cholesterol and triglycerides. It is now considered that these are CVD-prevention nutrients and that consuming these oil-containing fish two or three times a week will be to our cardiovascular benefit. EPA can also be used as a supplement to the diet.

In addition to a low-fat and high-fiber intake, a low-salt and low-sugar diet is also suggested. Avoiding salted and pickled or cured foods, especially meats, is suggested for health. Excess sugar, because it increases calories, weight, and blood fats, is an indirect risk factor in CVD; it is not healthy for many other reasons. More complex carbohydrates, including mostly whole grain and vegetable foods, are definitely in our favor for CVD prevention. The starch-centered diet, along with exercise, is the basis of the Pritikin program to reduce and prevent CVD. Nathan Pritikin was one of the more vigorous proponents of this excessively low-fat diet.

DIETARY SUGGESTIONS TO REDUCE CVD RISK

- **Eat more fruits and vegetables.**
- **Eat more whole grains.**
- **Use low-fat snacks.**
- **Reduce fat intake to 25–30 percent of the diet.**
- **Reduce cholesterol intake to less than 300 mg. per day.**
- **Reduce consumption of egg yolks to three to five per week.**
- **Minimize use of whole milk and its products; use low-fat or nonfat milk products.**
- **Avoid red meats; eliminate all cured meats and lunchmeats.**
- **Limit the use of nuts and seeds, not more than a handful daily.**
- **Avoid excess intake of avocados, olives, crab, and shrimp.**
- **Eat more coldwater fish, such as sardines and salmon.**
- **Use fresh, monounsaturated, mechanically pressed oils, such as olive or flaxseed oils, to provide the essential fatty acids.**

Children and Cardiovascular Disease

CVD prevention may need to start in young people, even preteens and adolescents, particularly if there is early obesity or a family history of heart disease. Weight, blood pressure, and cholesterol levels can be followed in these higher risk children. Diet modifications may be begun early with a lower-fat diet, primarily by reducing the animal fat and fried food consumption; this is accomplished by minimizing the intake of such foods as burgers, hot dogs, french fries, chips and excessive cheese, ice cream, and even milk products overall. Low-fat or nonfat dairy products can be used with these young people, yet still be a diet which contains adequate levels of protein, essential oil-containing foods, calcium foods, and even eggs, though these should not be consumed excessively. Encouraging more fruits, vegetables, whole grains, nuts and seeds, and some low-fat dairy foods will provide an adequate fiber, lower-fat diet with adequate calcium and calories. Some fish and poultry and occasional meat will support the protein needs very well, yet there are now many more vegetarian-oriented teenagers and young adults in our society who do very well.

With children who eat a lot of fast foods, ice cream, pizza, cookies, sodas, and other exciting modern day treats, the challenge is to get them to eat more wholesomely. Parents should provide these "treat" foods to their children only after they eat their more nutritious foods, and then only occasionally. Wholesome suggestions include replacing some soda and cookie snacks with low-fat milk, yogurt, and crackers; adding oat bran to cereals, meat loaf, or casseroles; using whole grain cereals in place of sugary ones as well as using cooked whole grains at meals; substituting Popsicles and fruit juice bars for fattier ice cream; using some low-fat cheeses such as cottage cheese or mozzarella (pizza with cheese and vegetables, not with fatty meats, is acceptable, even once or twice weekly); encouraging vegetables and fruits, with skins, even green salads when possible; and buying cookies and treats with low saturated fats and low sugar, such as fig bars, animal or graham crackers, ginger snaps, or the newer fruit-juice-sweetened cookies. We as parents also need to set a good example ourselves by our good food choices and by not overeating. Also, not snacking while watching television is suggested.

There is some controversy among authorities about the diet of the young in regard to CVD risk. Some believe that all children should be on a low-fat diet, at least lower than our current 40 percent national average. Most definitely, many of the poor-quality, refined foods should be avoided. Clearly, children who are obese or who have cholesterol levels over 200 mg./dl. should work to correct these states, and those who have families with CVD should be watched more closely. But overall, the higher-protein, higher-fat diet so consistent throughout the Western world does lead to increased growth and size of children and adults. Many cholesterol-rich foods, such as milk, cheese, meats, and eggs support the growth spurts. Yet, consumption of these foods are also associated with reduced longevity secondary to degenerative disease. My inclination has been to feed children this richer diet with more protein-fat foods, though it would still need to be a wholesome one, avoiding the junk, sweets, and fried oils. Then, as they move into their later teens and early adulthood, prepare them to shift their diet focus to a more natural, lower-fat, more vegetarian plan, with regular exercise supported along the way.

Herbs and Supplements

In addition to the oily coldwater fish, specific CVD-prevention foods include garlic, which has a fairly strong cholesterol- and blood-pressure-lowering effect, and onions and cayenne pepper, which have milder effects. These three foods are also herbs that are used in blood cleansing and thinning; garlic specifically lowers blood clotting potential. Soybeans and soy products such as tofu and tempeh may have a positive effect on cholesterol and atherosclerosis; besides all are low in fat and high in protein. Paavo Airola suggests other good foods for reducing CVD risk. These include the grains millet and buckwheat, sunflower seeds, okra, potatoes, asparagus, apples, and bananas, as well as yeast, lecithin, and linseed oil. Linseed (flax) oil has a high amount of the omega-3 fatty acids, such as EPA and DHA, and is a less expensive supplement to help reduce cholesterol levels. Linseed oil also contains the essential fatty acids (EFAs), linoleic and linolenic, which may help reduce blood fat levels and fatty deposits. Cold-pressed flaxseed oil is also readily used by our bodies in the important EFA functions, but it is a very fragile oil and must be fresh and then protected from light, heat, and oxidation.

FAT REVIEW

Agent	Cholesterol Effect	Effect on LDL-HDL Ratio*
Saturated fat	↑	↑(↑LDL)
Monounsaturated fat	↓ or =	= HDL
Polyunsaturated fat	↓	= or ↑(↓HDL)
EPA	↓	↓(↓LDL)
Lecithin	↓(possibly)	=
Smoking	↑	↑(↓HDL)

*The lower ratio has a lower risk of CVD.

FATTY ACID CHART

Oils	Omega-3 %	Omega-6 %
Linseed (Flax)	50–60	15–20
Walnut	5–10	20–30
Soy	5–10	40
Safflower	0.5	70
Sunflower	0.5	65
Corn	0.5	60
Cottonseed	0.5	50
Olive	0.5	10

Most of the common vegetable oils are high in the omega-6 fatty acids, as are borage seed and evening primrose oil, though they contain mainly gamma-linoleic acid (GLA). Soybean oil and walnut oil are higher in the omega-3s, and linseed oil is highest. All of the EFAs, both omega-3 and omega-6, help in cell membrane support and prostaglandin synthesis. They also help in the transfer of oxygen in the lungs and are essential to growth in the young.

Fruits are also recommended. They have some nutrients, and are high-water-content cleansing foods that make the diet more alkaline. A diet of only fruit and vegetables for a week or two is a good way to realkalinize our body and blood, which aids detoxification and lowers blood fats. A more acidic, richer diet creates more mucus, and thicker, more viscous blood, and lymphatic congestion.

I think of atherosclerosis as being much like the crud that builds up in water pipes because of various chemical or mineral imbalances that allow particle precipitation. I then think of fasting on juice or water as a means of cleaning that sludge from the blood vessels and organs. Fasting definitely reduces blood fats and blood viscosity so that blood flows better. It also reduces weight and blood pressure, and I believe fasting is very useful in the prevention and treatment of CVDs. Of course, fasting is not a diet but a supervised therapy. See more on this in the *Fasting* program in Chapter 18.

Cholesterol-Lowering Nutrients	Other Nutrients That Reduce CVD Risk and Complications
Fiber	Vitamin B_2
Garlic	Vitamin E
EPA	Selenium
Niacin	Beta-carotene
Vitamin B_6	Zinc
L-carnitine	Magnesium
Vitamin C	Calcium
Chromium	Potassium
	Inositol
	Choline
	Coenzyme Q_{10}
	Gamma-linolenic acid

There are a number of important nutrients, both in the diet and as supplements, that help prevent cardiovascular disease. Three of these important aids to reducing cholesterol and CVD risk are fiber, garlic, and the fish oils, EPA and DHA.

Fiber, both in the diet and as a supplement, has been shown to have several positive effects. It reduces blood pressure, cholesterol, and LDL and raises HDL. Apple pectin, oat fiber, psyllium husks, and locust bean gum have all been shown to reduce cholesterol and LDL. By reducing LDL while maintaining or raising the HDL cholesterol, this reduces the LDL/HDL ratio and therefore lowers the CVD risk. Alfalfa seed meal is high in saponin, an agent that is thought to be lipotropic, that is, it improves the utilization of fats.

Garlic, as a supplemental powder or oil, or used freely in the diet, has a positive effect on reducing triglycerides, cholesterol, and LDL, while raising HDL. Studies have shown that higher amounts of garlic, such as 10–15 grams daily, produce these effects without toxicity and that garlic reduces platelet stickiness and clotting. The sulfur-containing amino acids and other sulfur components of garlic may be what helps reduce these fats by their effect on cholesterol synthesis.

Omega-3 fatty acids—marine lipids, fish oils, EPA and DHA, or whatever other names we give them, and alpha-linolenic acid, found in some vegetable oils—have a number of positive effects for both CVD prevention and treatment. EPA (eicosapentaenoic acid), the main oil in fish (and flax/linseed oil), helps reduce lipid blood levels and plaque formation, thereby lessening atherosclerosis. It thins the blood and reduces platelet aggregation, a process that is relevant in atheroma progression and thrombosis. Specifically, fish oils reduce cholesterol but not the important HDL, whereas most vegetable oils lower both. EPA probably works by reducing platelet thromboxane secretion and increasing the prostaglandin E_3 series, which are anti-inflammatory agents. It also has been shown to have an effect on decreasing the activity of monocytes, which are phagocytic white blood cells involved in atheromas through adherence to the blood vessel wall. Aspirin, commonly used in medicine in low dosages to reduce clotting risks, decreases platelet stickiness as well as stimulating prostaglandin synthesis, but it also reduces platelet function and can have various side effects. Animal fats, in contrast to fish oils, increase platelet stickiness, which tends to clog the blood, reducing circulation and oxygenation. In addition to a low-fat diet and exercise, EPA is a good agent to help in reducing cardiovascular risk through its just-described effects. However, its ability, in my experience, to lower cholesterol and LDL is not dramatic, though, in occasional people it may be the best agent. Also, the higher amounts of EPA oil needed to lower lipid levels can be caloric, cause intestinal upset, and may adversely affect carbohydrate metabolism. Clearly, a low-fat diet can offer the most dramatic effect on cholesterol levels initially.

A number of other nutrients help reduce cholesterol. Chromium supplementation has been shown to lower LDL and raise HDL, reducing CVD risk. Pyridoxine (B_6) deficiency may increase plaque formation, as may vitamin C deficiency. Vitamin C treatment improves cholesterol metabolism and can also reduce total cholesterol and LDL levels, as well as the incidence of postsurgical clots. Niacin in dosages over 100 mg. clearly has a cholesterol-lowering effect and has also been shown to reduce risk of recurrence of heart attacks and to improve the circulation in general. Supplementing niacin, vitamin B_3, has become a popular therapy for reducing cholesterol. Increasing amounts up to 2–3 grams daily definitely helps to lower blood fats; however, many people do not tolerate well the "niacin flush" and other symptoms often associated with niacin supplementation. L-carnitine helps in fatty acid metabolism. One study suggests that it increases prostacyclin, a prostaglandin that dilates coronary arteries, possibly as a result of decreased platelet thromboxane levels. A dosage of 250–500 mg. of L-carnitine twice daily is suggested as a CVD preventive. Coenzyme Q_{10} is another favorable nutrient for cardiac and lipid function. This can be taken in dosages of 20–30 mg. twice daily.

Antioxidant nutrients are also important to protect tissue and vascular linings from free-radical irritants. Vitamin E is a strong antioxidant, especially for preventing the oxidation of fats. Low vitamin E levels have been associated with increased platelet stickiness. Studies to determine its cholesterol-lowering and cardiovascular-protection effects have been inconclusive, but I feel that it should definitely be a part of a CVD prevention program for its protection against free radicals. An amount of 600–800 IUs can be taken in a dosage of 600–800 IUs daily. Selenium, vitamin E's functional partner, helps protect the cells and tissue linings, as well as decreasing cadmium's blood-pressure-raising effect. Low selenium levels have been associated with an increased incidence of heart disease and strokes as well as of cancer. Beta-carotene is also protective of tissue linings and may improve oxygen utilization and reduce platelet clumping, thus decreasing clotting potential. Zinc may also be protective against CVD, as it aids tissue healing and immune function, but high amounts, over 100 mg. per day, may raise cholesterol levels.

Other nutrients that may play a role in CVD prevention are vitamins B_5 and B_2 and several minerals. Pantothenic acid (B_5) and riboflavin (B_2) help in lipid metabolism. Calcium is needed for normal heart function and nerve transmission. Low calcium, especially in combination with increased sodium, as is found in soft water, increases blood pressure. Thus, excess sodium in the diet should be avoided. Like calcium and magnesium, potassium is a very important nutrient for normal heart function; it helps to balance out some of the detrimental effects of elevated sodium. Depletion of copper may also increase the risk of CVD, so it is needed in sufficient, though not excessive, amounts. Inositol and choline may help reduce blood pressure and atherosclerosis, though the results of research on this are controversial. There has also been some suggestion that gamma-linolenic acid (GLA) from evening primrose oil or other sources helps reduce blood clotting potential. Lecithin is another nutrient often recommended for CVD prevention. High amounts of it have been shown to decrease cholesterol levels, but in these amounts, this oil is highly caloric and contains high levels of phosphorus, which can affect calcium metabolism. Lecithin can be obtained naturally from whole grains, soy products, nuts, seeds, and vegetable oils.

Magnesium may be the single most important nutrient in CVD protection, especially when it is deficient. We want to make sure we get sufficient magnesium, which is found readily in the whole grains, nuts, and seeds and many vegetables. Magnesium is important to heart function and tissue health. It can actually dilate coronary arteries (and thus reduce angina) and increase the collateral circulation. Low heart tissue levels of magnesium have been found in heart attack victims and may contribute to coronary artery spasm, which reduces or closes off blood flow. Magnesium also helps normalize the heartbeat (a deficiency increases sensitivity to arrythmias), the blood pressure, and the heart's sensitivity to toxins and to the effect of norepinephrine. I am certain that sustained, adequate magnesium levels will reduce the incidence of fatal heart attacks. Another important function of magnesium is that it helps keep calcium in circulation so that it does not precipitate in tissues, a big factor in atherosclerosis, as well as in kidney stone formation and other problems of abnormal calcification. Along with calcium, magnesium helps maintain the electrical stability of cells, especially in the heart muscle. Alcohol causes a loss of magnesium through the kidney, as do diuretic drugs. Magnesium in foods and as supplements is a good tranquilizer and also aids in blood pressure control.

A few herbs can be helpful in cardiovascular disease prevention. As mentioned previously, these include garlic and cayenne pepper. Ginger root helps with the circulation, while hawthorn berries are the safest effective heart tonic. Many herbs can be used in CVD as heart tonics, as diuretics in hypertension, and for improving general circulation.

Lifestyle factors helpful in reducing CVD, besides reducing smoking, especially, and avoiding excessive caffeine and alcohol, are exercise and stress management. Before the technological age, exercise was part of everyday life; now it must be a special activity. The reality is that, to be healthy, we must trade all the time we save in faster travel, mechanical devices, and easier cooking and cleaning and put that time into exercise.

EXERCISE BENEFITS IN
CARDIOVASCULAR DISEASE PREVENTION

Strengthen heart muscle
Improve oxygen delivery
Lower pulse rate
Lower blood pressure
Lower blood fats, cholesterol, and triglyceride
Raise protective HDL cholesterol
Reduce stress
Improve attitude toward life

In a healthy person, the resting heart rate may range from 50–65 beats per minute for men and 55–70 for women. An unfit person may have a rate in the 80s or 90s. A good exercise program will strengthen the heart muscle and help to reduce the resting heart rate as well as to lower blood pressure and blood fats, while raising HDL cholesterol, thus lessening atherosclerosis risk. It is clear that regular aerobic exercise is crucial to maintenance of a healthy circulatory system with a strong heart, which will then be able to deliver more blood and more oxygen to the tissues.

When starting an exercise program, we should walk more and monitor our pulse and even our blood pressure. It is important to find an exercise program that is enjoyable, as stress reduction is another advantage of exercise. It is a good idea to vary our activity and to do proper warm-ups and cool-downs. We should also avoid big meals before exercising and stop if any pain develops during the activity to attempt to assess any problem. If the pain persists, check it out with a doctor. If it has been months or years since we exercised, if we are overweight or out of shape, or if we have any health problems, we definitely should have a thorough checkup before beginning any serious exercise program. An exercise-treadmill test will tell us whether the heart and blood pressure respond normally to vigorous activity.

Managing stress is an important key to cardiovascular health. We all experience stress, and it has its uses; however, we must counteract its negative effects, which include increased blood pressure and heart rate and free-radical generation. We may also need to develop or maintain a generally positive attitude toward life, whether that takes counseling, taking more vacations, learning relaxation techniques, or religious/ spiritual seeking. We need to spend time with our family and with ourselves. For many people, exercise is an important aid to stress reduction.

When we are stressed, we often tend to eat a poorer diet with less nutritious food choices. We speed through meals and may consume more caffeine to get going and more alcohol to slow down at the end of the day. These habits need to be changed, which will often help reduce stress. Busy people need to give themselves time for rest and relaxation to keep their own sanity and health, especially for their cardiovascular system. (Also, see the *Anti-Stress* program earlier in this chapter.)

835

If all of these suggestions do not help reduce risk factors and cholesterol, there are some pharmaceutical drugs that may be used to at least reduce cholesterol. These are suitable mainly for people with high blood fat levels or those who will not change their diet. The most commonly used one, cholestyramine, or Questran, blocks cholesterol absorption. It is effective but does have side effects, such as indigestion, bloating, and constipation. Mevacor, or lovastatin, is a relatively new drug that has become popular very quickly. It is quite effective with only mild side effects, if any. There are also many drugs to control hypertension, which is very important to reduce CVD risk. If lifestyle changes cannot reduce blood pressure, these may be needed.

Some doctors offer "chelation" therapy treatments, which is controversial, to reduce atherosclerosis. This is a series of moderately expensive intravenous infusions of EDTA, a mineral-chelating molecule, which binds calcium from the blood and possibly from arterial plaque and removes it through the kidneys. Some patients experience dramatic benefits, but research to date has not been very promising. I personally would definitely try it before "the knife" if I were experiencing cardiovascular disease symptoms, but I am not enthusiastic enough about it to use it in my practice.

If we cannot prevent or get control of our CVD, we can always take moderately toxic drugs to control our blood pressure or have a triple or quadruple bypass operation that requires sawing our chest in half—neither of which sounds very appealing. It is much wiser to work diligently in our earlier years to do all we can to reduce our CVD risk. Though not everyone can prevent atherosclerosis and degenerative cardiovascular disease, many can. It is worth a try.

CARDIOVASCULAR DISEASE PREVENTION
NUTRIENT PROGRAM

Calories	1,500–2,500*
Fats	40–70 g.
Fiber	15–25 g.

Vitamin A	5,000–10,000 IUs	**Iodine**	150–225 mcg.
Beta-carotene	15,000–25,000 IUs	**Iron**	10–20 mg.
Vitamin D	200 IUs	**Magnesium**	400–750 mg.
Vitamin E	600–800 IUs	**Manganese**	5–10 mg.
Vitamin K	150–300 mcg.	**Molybdenum**	300–500 mcg.
Thiamine (B$_1$)	50–75 mg.	**Potassium**	300–500 mg.
Riboflavin (B$_2$)	25–75 mg.	**Selenium**	200–300 mcg.
Niacinamide (B$_3$)	100 mg.	**Silicon**	100 mg.
Niacin (B$_3$)	50–1,000 mg.**	**Vanadium**	200 mcg.
Pantothenic acid (B$_5$)	250–500 mg.	**Zinc**	30–60 mg.
Pyridoxine (B$_6$)	50 mg.		
Cobalamin (B$_{12}$)	100 mcg.	**Flaxseed oil**	1–2 tsps. or 2-4 capsules
Folic acid	600 mcg.		
Biotin	300 mcg.	**EPA (fish oil)**	2–4 capsules (200–600 mg.**)
Choline	500 mg.		
Inositol	500 mg.	**Coenzyme Q$_{10}$**	40–60 mg.
Vitamin C	3–6 g.	**L-carnitine**	500–1,000 mg.
Bioflavonoids	250–500 mg.	**Garlic**	4 capsules
Calcium	650–1,000 mg.		
Chromium	300–500 mcg.		
Copper	2–3 mg.		

*Depends on size and activity level
**Dosage can be increased slowly, and depends on cholesterol level, taking more niacin or EPA for higher levels.

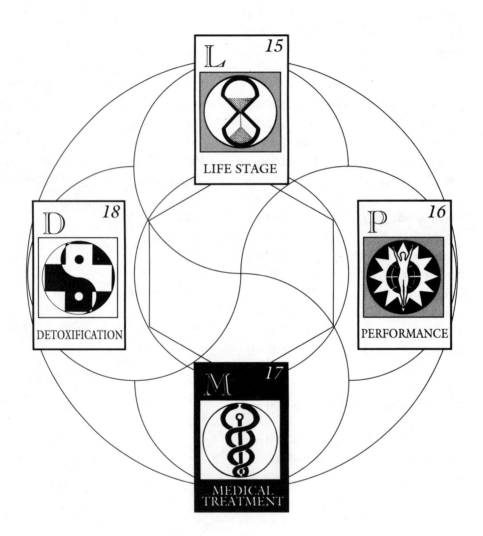

Chapter 17

Medical Treatment Programs

Medical doctors are trained mostly in the diagnosis and treatment of disease and there is really so much to learn about this highly technical science that it takes many years to learn to practice well. However, it may take even more years of experience (and personal growth), seeing what does and doesn't work, to progress into *the art of medicine*. Only recently, though, has medical education returned to its roots and begun to show interest in nutrition, environmental medicine, natural remedies, healing arts, basic communication skills, and interest in how people's lives and attitudes both cause and influence their diseases and healing. As this occurs, it requires more personal experience and growth during medical training to help develop the true art of healing. It is my belief that doctors with special interest and insight in these above-mentioned areas of training have more to offer their patients. Yet, even with an increasing number of doctors interested in more humanitarian and natural medicine, it is still difficult to find practitioners who are willing to go beyond symptom/ disease treatment into correcting the causes of problems and healing lifestyles and lives.

Giving patients more responsibility and involving, and even encouraging, them in self-healing care is, I believe, another dimension of medical practice. Doctors who only diagnose and treat with drugs and surgery are ignoring an entire field of preventive medicine and patient education, in the same way as medical reactionaries who refuse to accept the potential benefits and proven necessity, especially in acute cases, of Western medicine are also ignoring an entire field. As more and more doctors (and individuals) begin experiencing the effects that dietary changes, natural therapies, herbal and nutritional supplements, and inner techniques have in stimulating healing, it can only help our health care delivery and markedly reduce the costs involved.

There are many philosophies and dietary approaches, and much of this nutritional practice is outside the current "standard medical" field. I am working to bring nutritional and medical practice together into nutritional medicine through more scientific assessment and individual treatment programs. This may require an in-depth evaluation of one's diet and nutritional status, specifically for vitamin and mineral levels, immune function, and any food allergies. (See *Appendix* for specific tests.) Then with this information and the understanding, guidance, and support needed to carry it through, we can design a most effective and appropriate program for a given unique individual.

Clearly, our lifestyle affects our health—nutrition is important, as are our attitude and behavior, and exercise and stress levels. By addressing these areas we can more easily prevent many problems. Clearly, it is easier to prevent disease than to heal it after it occurs, when much more energy, time and money are needed to return to health.

I often tell patients that what they experience as symptoms and disease are not the real problems, they are a result of their lives—what they eat, do, and feel, and their deeper issues, attitudes, beliefs, and emotions. I really believe that doctors and all healers need to work with people and their lives, and not just their diseases. As Bernie Siegel, M.D., points out in his recent book, *Peace, Love, and Healing,* doctors need to learn how to treat people's whole lives; if we do that, their diseases heal more easily. I have long considered myself a philosopher-physician in the school of the ancient Chinese practice, guiding people in how to live in harmony with their environment, seasons, emotions, and lives. This is a forever job, but at least it is a J-O-B that is also a J-O-Y, as Bethany ArgIsle advises.

This chapter brings together specific discussions of various medical concerns, and the factors that contribute to these problems with some philosophy and ways of understanding them in relationship to our lives. I also offer a complete nutritional approach, using diet and natural remedies, nutritional supplements, and herbs, to work on the biochemical healing process for these conditions.

Of course, there are many other potential medical problems that exist; however, I have discussed only a few common nutritional medicine concerns in this text. *Staying Healthy with Nutrition* focuses on disease prevention; it stresses healthy nutrition and personal-planetary lifestyle. Currently, I am conducting more extensive research and writing on other medical nutrition areas, such as fatigue, viral conditions, arthritis, asthma, gastrointestinal problems including parasites, diabetes and hypoglycemia, cardiovascular disease, cancer treatments, and the nutritional factors of mental health. These will be included in the third of the *Staying Healthy* trilogy, *Staying Healthy with Modern Medicine,* which will also include paradigms of future health care delivery systems.

Use this information to support your standard medical care or as your main therapeutic regimen, as the case may be. The following and final chapter, *Detoxification and Healing Programs,* will provide more specific ways to help clear disease from our bodies and to eliminate some of the abusive, irritating substances that provide the basis for degenerative disease. I plan to give you my formula and foundation for health and longevity.

840

Weight Loss

This is a very common and complex health topic. Most Americans are heavier than their optimum weight, so in that sense they are overweight, but most are not obese, which I would define as as being overweight to a degree that clearly increases our health risks. Being overweight could also be defined in terms of what we think and feel about ourselves, as the psychological attitude toward our weight is so very important. Some people, mostly young women, may think that they are overweight and eat sparingly, when they are actually malnourished and underweight.

Most "overweight" people are very fickle about their weight-control regimens. They will try any and many programs, mostly short-term crash diets that focus on calorie restriction or a single food group, such as the high protein diet. The up-and-down weight syndrome may lead us to the path of lifelong obesity.

Quick weight loss is not the aim of this program. That is relatively easy to do time and again. The only healthy and effective long-range weight reduction plan is to have a balanced and healthy lifestyle such as described throughout this book, and to find the diet and eating habits that allow us to reach and maintain our "right" weight.

Working to change our dietary habits and following the many guidelines and diet suggestions discussed here can really make a difference. With moderate to active regular exercise, we can all be close to our optimum weight. We must realize, though, that this optimum weight may not be quite as low as that of the body we idolize or even as low as that listed in the ideal weight charts. Heredity, conditioning, and metabolism, as well as percentage of body fat, will influence what is ideal, or healthy, for each of us.

Significant excess weight—more than 30 pounds—and more extreme obesity are some of the bigger health concerns of the Western world. The over-intake and under-utilization of food and the storage of excess fuel in our body as fat and waste create a serious nutritional disease. This problem contributes to many more serious diseases, such as cardiovascular disease, cancer, and diabetes—the three most life-threatening, chronic degenerative conditions in our society. Obesity is an important risk factor in all of them; in addition it causes a general decrease in longevity.

MEDICAL PROBLEMS RELATED TO OBESITY

Diabetes	Arthritis
High cholesterol levels	Gout
Atherosclerosis	Varicose veins
Hypertension	Gallbladder disease
Heart disease	Liver disease
Kidney disease	Menstrual problems
Cancer	Infertility
Strokes	

3M Keys to Weight Loss: Mother—Motivation—Metabolism

Mother. Weight problems begin early; the majority of overweight adults had some problem with their weight as children or adolescents. Genetics clearly plays a part, but our ability to distinguish its effects from those of conditioning and environmental stimuli is very limited. We can say that children of overweight parents have a greater tendency to be overweight. Our mother is usually the first one to feed us, and early on we develop patterns of eating and relating that often influence us for life. And for many this pattern with mother continues, with moms trying to nourish us on many levels throughout life. Counseling concerning the relationship with mother helps many overweight people clarify the issues and desires related to food and may allow new motivations to come forth.

Motivation. Most overweight people know that ups and downs in weight do not work. Fad diets may be fun, but they are usually frivolous, because 80–90 percent of people who lose weight with them then regain the weight lost or sometimes even more, and this is less healthy than just staying the weight we are. We need a lifetime plan, and this is where motivation comes in. Gathering our deeper strength by focusing on the long-range vision as well as the quick benefits, and continually telling ourselves that we can do it, is what will help to overcome our weight problem. It has been conditioned very deeply. Most people think more about the immediate benefits of the slimmer body or better appearance, often believing it will please another, than the lifelong health risks of being overweight. Emphasizing both may help improve motivation.

Overeating and poor habits are hard to change but easy to develop. I know from experience. It is easy to simply say change the diet, but without the motivation and the ability to break through our psychological barriers, it is very difficult to make major changes. I found it very successful to first change the types of foods I ate to a more natural-food diet. Sugars, fats, and refined foods can easily be replaced with more wholesome choices. These refined and rich foods may increase our hunger as well as add low-nutrient calories. (Complex carbohydrate foods fill us with fewer calories and reduce our appetite.) Thus, reducing their intake usually makes a difference in calorie and nutrient intake, and often in our metabolism and general health, which will influence our weight. Then we can move on to deal with our more difficult habits. Isolating and eliminating allergenic/addictive foods is difficult only for a few days. Then, eating a variety of foods will minimize other possible allergens in the diet. Really, we need to create a new, stable lifestyle approach to give us the right body weight and energy, and the effective level of metabolism to maintain them.

Metabolism. There are several theories regarding the effects of our metabolism on our weight, and I am convinced that they each describe important factors. Our basal metabolic rate (BMR) is the rate at which our body burns calories to maintain its functions at rest. It is affected by our gender, age, diet, activity level, thyroid function, amount of sleep, amount of body fat, body temperature, weight, and likely, by our genetics. We need a certain number of calories to maintain our weight with a regular exercise level. We can calculate our acceptable calorie intake by figuring the number of calories required to meet our basic needs (BMR) and adding to it the extra calories used in exercise and mental activity. Formulas for doing this are provided in many nutrition books, such *Jane Brody's Nutrition Book.*

OVERWEIGHT—THEORIES AND CAUSES

General	Specific
Metabolic rate	Excess calories and/or fats
Set point	Excess sugar refined foods
Fat cell type and number	Overeating
	Slow liver metabolism
Family Influences	Nutrient deficiencies
Heredity	Low thyroid function
Eating patterns	Lack of exercise
Food choices	Food allergies
Family relationship	Yeast infections
Food as security substitute	Parasites
Psychological attitudes	Insulin insensitivity
Self-image within family	Emotional factors
	Fat body self-image

"Set point" theory is a newer way of describing this complex metabolic process. This theory applies to what our body "thinks" is normal and the set point is actually the amount of body fat our body tries to maintain. Obese people have a higher set point than trimmer ones. This may be related to the number of fat cells, which may in turn be tied to genetics and early eating patterns.

The set point theory suggests that our body works like a thermostat. When we diet and consume fewer calories, our body reacts as if a starvation crisis is upon us, with compensatory responses, such as lowering the BMR, the rate at which we burn calories, in an attempt to conserve calories and weight. The end result is that we can maintain the same weight on fewer calories. This theory makes sense, considering our long-term experiences with weight reduction.

Regular dieting, especially the low-calorie starvation diet, is met with ever greater difficulty in maintaining weight loss and often results in faster rebounds. As our weight goes up and down, our metabolism seems to slow, as it does with age, and it becomes harder and harder to lose weight. Once established, our personal set point and level of body fat are not easily influenced. Our set point, and thus our weight, might even go up. Our body really needs regular exercise and a long-term, steady, lower-calorie diet plan to adapt to a lower weight and better energy efficiency, or "turning our thermostat down."

The "fat cell" theory also applies here, and seems to correlate with the "set point" philosophy. It has been shown that we each develop a specific number of fat cells in our body. This mainly occurs at certain times of life—before birth, during infancy, and during the adolescent growth phase. This may be genetically determined, but it also appears that if we are overfed or overeat during these times, we may create more fat cells. At other times, as in our adult life, we increase only the size of our cells. When we take in more calories than we use, our cells and fat stores get bigger. So a trim person may have a lower number of cells, or the same number of smaller cells than a heavier person, but when we lose weight and become thinner, our fat cells become smaller.

This process involves primarily "white" fat found mainly in the fat cells that lie under our skin. This is our energy, or calorie storage fat. The "brown" fat, or the "good" fat, actually burns calories for body heat. This fat is deeper and surrounds and protects our organs. Normal fatty acid metabolism supports and nourishes the brown fat. The storage, or white, fat is where our body puts the extra calories from dietary sources that we do not utilize. When we diet regularly or our weight goes up and down, our internal weight control system fears starvation and will store more fat as energy for the future. With repeated weight loss and weight gain, the same number of calories in our diet may keep us at a higher weight because we have a higher set point.

When we have developed more fat cells during our growth periods (infancy and adolescence), we will tend to have more fat, a slower metabolism, and a higher set point, and we will be more likely to have a higher weight. Once this pattern develops, such as by being overweight early in life, it is very hard to change. It takes work and a new self-image! Regular exercise and increasing exercise capacity are the main physical ways to improve the set point and lose weight and then to be able to maintain our weight with a reasonable number of calories. This is a far healthier approach than taking thyroid pills or one of the many possible diet stimulants.

Other ideas about individual wieght suggest two opposing views. One school says that people are thin because they do not overeat as much as fat people, since they are guided more by internal signals of hunger and the types of food that their bodies want. Overweight people on the other hand respond more to external signals, such as the presence of food or other people and social situations, or they may react more emotionally to the normal internal messages.

Others believe that obese people do not really eat a great deal more than thin people; they just have a different set point and a slower metabolic rate. Heredity and early conditioning play a major role here. Heavier people's food choices may not be as wholesome as those of thin people, with higher-fat and higher-calorie foods predominating. Malnutrition from nutrient deficiencies and food allergies can also be influential. Obesity is really a combination of these many factors. Of course, most of us know overweight people who eat a lot of food. Then again, we may know overweight people who eat lightly, as well as trim people who can really put it away. Most overweight people, I believe, have overeaten at some point to develop their capacity for obesity, unless there is some hormonal imbalance, which is not very common.

We need to start as early as possible to achieve dietary control. Children need both wholesome, nutritious foods and loving guidance! Only about 10 percent of elementary school children are overweight, yet between 20 and 30 percent of high schoolers are at least moderately obese. To lose weight and maintain it, behavior must change. Behavior modification is a form of therapy that can be effective in helping us change from an overweight person to a trimmer one. This can be practiced by ourselves or with the help of a close friend, spouse, or diet "buddy," but a behavioral or other counselor can often assist with it.

An important beginning is to try to get in touch with our level of hunger. Most "fat" people do not eat from hunger; in fact, many rarely experience this natural guide to eating. Using an eating diary to evaluate what, when, and where we eat, how much, our level of hunger, and what else we are doing at the time can be very revealing. An example of this form is found in *Taking Charge of Your Weight and Well-Being* by Joyce Nash and Linda Ormiston (Bull Publishing Co., Palo Alto, CA., 1978). Keeping such a diary for several weeks can help us to see more clearly our relationship to eating. We can then make a plan incorporating our new, positive habits and use new rules to change our behavior in weak areas. For example, if we snack while we make dinner or pick at the leftovers in the kitchen, we can make a commitment to eat food only at the dining room table and allow no eating in the kitchen or when standing. It may be difficult at first; constant awareness is needed. Behaviorists claim that it takes three weeks to change a habit and create a new one, so keep at it. Part of our eating behavior is affected by psychological aspects, such as our self-image, relationships to family or partner, sexuality, and general stress. Often, counseling is important to help change behavior to meet our dietary challenge.

Successfully achieving a new weight means changing our diet, not "going on a diet." When we return to our old, "normal" diet, we will create the same body we had before, and likely add another pound or three. First we change our diet by substituting wholesome foods for the more high-calorie and chemical foods in the diet. Next, we work to create good habits. The following list offers some suggestions for behavior patterns, food choices, and activities to help reach and maintain our optimum weight.

Before beginning a new diet plan, a health evaluation may be important, especially for those with recent weight gain or symptoms of medical problems. Before embarking on any low-calorie diets, we should have a complete exam, general biochemistry panel, and, if over 45, an electrocardiogram. A complete thyroid hormone panel is often useful to rule out low thyroid function, which could be a cause of weight gain or difficulty in losing weight. Blood fats, protein, potassium, and calcium levels are also important monitors in the process of weight loss. A positive side effect of diet change and weight loss is reduction of blood cholesterol and triglycerides and high blood pressure, yet also watching for mineral depletions, particularly of potassium, is a good idea.

A food allergy evaluation may be a valuable step on the path to a trim and healthier body. Many people have internal reactions to foods, with increased immune response, cellular irritation, and many possible symptoms. These can cause inflammatory activity and water retention, as well as poor utilization of other foods. Currently, the best way to isolate problem foods is a blood test that measures levels of IgG antibodies to specific food antigens (the protein stimuli of the food). This reveals delayed or "hidden" food allergy or hypersensitivity. Measuring IgE levels can determine foods causing more immediate reactions, such as hives, asthma, or eczema, though these reactions are relatively uncommon, which is why skin tests, which measure the IgE reactions, are not very helpful. Cytotoxic testing, looking at cellular reactions, is no longer used because interpretations of its results were too subjective. Antibody measurement is more reproducible.

Testing food reactions ourselves by trying different foods in the diet and observing how we feel can be very useful for the astute person, but the reactions may involve other variables besides the foods. TV doctor Dean Edell feels that the best method is double-blind testing—giving patients encapsulated dried foods as well as placebos, without the patient or tester knowing which is which, or even what food is being tested. This is a good method, but it is time consuming, and it assumes that food reactions occur so dramatically and immediately that people can be aware of them. Some reactions do happen at once, but many are more subtle and occur 12–24 hours later. Avoiding the causes of these quieter internal reactions contributes to the body's fine-tuning and makes weight loss easier. Food allergy testing followed by a rotation diet avoiding the reactive foods plays an essential part in reaching and maintaining optimum weight and health (see more in the *Allergy* program in this chapter).

Several possible diets can be used as long-term plans for people who have problems maintaining their optimum weight. These are all generally healthier diets than those of the general population. There are literally thousands of quick-weight-loss, low-calorie, nutrient-deficient diets available to consumers. That is not what we are looking for to achieve our goals. I do not usually recommend fasting for weight loss, but if someone wants to lose a quick five to ten pounds in a short period of time, I will work with them,

BEHAVIOR PATTERNS FOR OPTIMUM WEIGHT

- Focus on decreasing caloric intake and increasing calories out (exercise).
- Eat most foods early in the day for best utilization of calories.
- Drink eight to ten glasses of water daily, but not with meals.
- Drink two glasses of water 30 minutes before meals to reduce appetite.
- Eat slowly and chew food well.
- Limit treats and refined foods; avoid sodas and chemical foods.
- Eat lots of fruits and vegetables—as snacks, too.
- Walk a lot and exercise regularly.
- Avoid fats in the diet—they are more caloric.
- Use only low-fat or nonfat milk products.
- Minimize salad dressings, cream soups, and meats.
- Lessen or avoid alcohol and caffeine; minimize salt intake.
- Rotate foods—eat a variety; isolate allergenic foods and avoid them.
- Practice food combining.
- See a nutritionist to help with the eating plan or for food-habit counseling.
- Use smaller plates and portions.
- Fill up first on lower calorie foods, such as soups or vegetable salads.
- Avoid high-calorie snacks and desserts.
- Wait 10–15 minutes before taking seconds—hunger will decrease.
- At restaurants, avoid overeating and take any extra food home.
- Take at least 20–30 minutes to eat a meal, even snacks.
- Eat at only one or two places in the home.
- Sit and relax before eating.
- Avoid eating while watching TV, driving, or doing other things.
- Shop for food only after eating, not when hungry.
- Practice eating only when hungry.
- Create a schedule for eating.
- Plan meals and food choices ahead, snacks included.
- Carry food with you to work or when going out so that you have the right choices.
- Put snacks and sweet foods away at home.
- Stay out of the kitchen, cupboards, and refrigerator unless preparing food.
- Plan activities to occupy your free time when you might snack.
- Tell family and friends to support you and not push food.
- If you blow it, go right back to your plan, and do not make it an excuse to indulge.
- Weigh yourself only once every week or two.
- Learn about food, fats, calories, and so on, so you know what you are doing.
- Keep a good self-image and positive attitude toward life.
- Allow yourself to indulge (within reason) once weekly without guilt or self-judgment.
- Realize that it is ultimately up to you.

after an evaluation, with the overall intention of using that period to create a new eating plan to be used when the fast is over. Fasting is very valuable at increasing food awareness and sensitivity to both bad and good foods and eliminating addictive food and eating patterns, so that people can come back to eating with new enthusiasm and attention. A one-day-a-week fast on water or juices can be a valuable tool for many people who want to lose or maintain weight as it reemphasizes the importance of food choices and food awareness.

The essential aspects of a healthy weight-loss diet are lean protein (for example, fish and poultry), low fat, and lots of vegetables. High-fiber foods, with some complex carbohydrates, are also helpful, especially with an orientation to vegetables and vegetable-protein combinations such as grains and legumes. Eating a variety of foods and rotating those foods every few days is important. Cold-pressed vegetable oils are the main fats, with some low-fat dairy products if tolerated. Saturated and hydrogenated fats are minimized. Refined sugar and flour foods, including baked goods, candy, sodas, and other sweets, are avoided. Alcohol is out, and caffeine is minimized. We need to drink lots of water instead to support normal weight and healthy skin and internal functions.

Meals are restructured to include a a moderate breakfast, great lunch, and light dinner. Snacks are low-calorie foods, such as fruits, vegetables, popcorn, or crackers. Overeating is prohibited. We must take breaks during big meals to let the body balance and let us know whether it needs more food. It usually does not; we really require a lot less food than our overweight mind tells us. Our satiation meter needs to be turned down, and that will take a golden key, which is not always easy to find. It may require going through our past, our emotional and psychological barriers, to find our creative spark and drive to be our best self and not let food interfere with this path of power. It really takes responsibility and a commitment to our new body-to-be, and a knowledge and belief that we can do it. We need to think more about eating to survive and feeding our body with the best possible fuel. Taking the time to eat, chewing each bite thoroughly, is essential to short-term digestion and absorption and the long-term health of the whole digestive tract. Being aware of the process of eating and of what food is eaten is a must.

Specific diets for weight loss and/or weight maintenance

- The fish-fowl-vegetable diet
- The allergy-rotation diet
- The high fiber-starch diet
- The Haas plan—the Ideal Diet

The fish–fowl–green vegetable diet is a fairly healthy weight-loss diet that should be used for one or two months at the most. Several pounds a week can be lost fairly easily with this diet even with only moderate activity. It includes fresh ocean fish, tuna, shrimp, and trout, organic poultry, and green vegetables, both raw and cooked—all to be eaten in the quantity desired (within reason, of course). One piece of fresh fruit and one cooked egg daily are also suggested. This provides good balance, though it is fairly low in fiber. Some bran and/or psyllium can be used to support bowel function. Salad dressing should be limited to one or two tablespoons daily of vegetable oil, such as olive, with some fresh lemon juice or vinegar. If no oils are used, an essential fatty acid supplement should be added. Herbal teas and/or spring or distilled water are the main fluids. Some clear soup broths are acceptable. Daily fluid intake should be eight to ten glasses (8 ounces), with two glasses being drunk first thing in the morning and 30–60 minutes before each meal. A general multivitamin or the program given at the end of this section should also be used daily for health insurance.

The high fiber-starch diet is another weight loss/maintenance alternative. This is not exclusively starches—it includes some fruit, green vegetables, and protein foods—but the main foods are the whole grains, legumes, pasta, potatoes, and starchy vegetables, such as carrots and squashes. These high-fiber complex carbohydrates when eaten at the beginning of a meal will provide bulk and thus decrease the appetite and give a feeling of fullness. They are also relatively low-calorie foods because they are low in fat, but only if they do not have sauces, gravies, butter, or oil added to them. The complex carbohydrates also provide a consistent energy production and can stabilize the imbalance that some people experience. Vegetables can be consumed as desired, at least several cups daily. They are also low in calories. A couple of pieces of fruit daily are suggested. Dairy foods, red meats, and any fried, fatty, or refined foods are avoided, as are sweets. One meal, early in the day, can include a concentrated protein, such as fish, poultry, eggs, or, for strict vegetarians, some tofu, nuts, seeds, or beans. This diet can be a good weight-loss plan for overweight vegetarians, especially if they avoid excessive grains and sweets. Soups and salads are helpful. Water intake is eight to ten glasses daily for this diet also. A multivitamin product can be used, along with some extra B_{12}. Care should be taken that iron and calcium intake are adequate; these and other minerals might be supplemented, though most should be found in sufficient amounts in this diet.

The allergy-rotation diet is becoming more popular for weight loss as well as for general health, especially when there are food allergies present. The Ideal Diet described in Chapter 13 is a modified rotation diet; also see the upcoming *Allergy* program. When food allergies are suspected, we should be tested or guided by a doctor or nutritionist, and any foods shown to be a possible problem should come out of the diet for one to two months, depending on the degree of sensitivity. After that time, individual foods can be tested again (this is called a "challenge"), but only one per day. If we seem to be addicted to any foods, that is, we crave them and eat them every day, sometimes even at every meal—those foods should be completely removed from the diet for at least several weeks before testing them, although avoiding them even for only four days will allow our body to be sensitive to their true effects. If we can be aware enough of our diet to know which foods are doing what, then we can know which foods to eliminate. This rotation diet can be very well balanced since it includes a wide variety of foods.

To desensitize to other possible food allergies, a rotating diet means setting up a four-day rotation plan—any food eaten on one day must be excluded from the diet for the next three days. For example, if apples, corn, or peas are eaten on Monday, we would not eat them again until Friday. This diet is not very easy to initiate, but once started is not too difficult. It does, however, require limiting restaurant eating and preparing most of our own foods. Just planning foods and meals and preparing food ahead of time creates better eating habits. Eliminating allergenic foods also reduces water retention through reduced immune reactions and secondary inflammation and may allow us to feel much better while we trim.

The Ideal Diet discussed in Part Three is very good for weight reduction and maintenance for most people provided we limit the quantities of food consumed. It is a well-balanced diet that incorporates aspects of all the previous diets. It is a rotation diet, good for food allergies; it has a high fiber content from the whole grains and vegetables; it is low in fat; and it contains good-quality protein. To reduce calories further, the morning nut snack can be replaced with another fruit.

BASICS OF THE IDEAL DIET

Early morning	one or two pieces of fruit
Breakfast	starch, such as a cereal grain or potatoes
Midmorning snack	fruit
Lunch	protein and green and other vegetables
Midafternoon snack	vegetable or fruit
Dinner	starch or protein with vegetable
Evening snack	vegetable or fruit, if needed

Water should be consumed as usual—eight to ten glasses per day, mainly drunk about one hour before meals—and a basic multivitamin/mineral supplement could be used, including essential fatty acids or some fresh vegetable oil, one or two teaspoons daily. (Refer to the *Seasonal Menu Plans* and *Recipes* in Chapter 14 for more ideas.) More water and fiber and more filling low-calorie foods will help in decreasing the appetite. Water and fiber are the two most useful and inexpensive nutrients for weight reduction and maintenance. They will also support good colon function, which is helpful to detoxification and reducing food cravings. Lowering fat intake and absorption (fiber also does that) and increasing foods high in vitamins and minerals as well as supplemental nutrients will also support optimum metabolism and aid in weight loss.

Exercise is also crucial. Few weight-loss programs are effective without increasing physical activity. To lose weight or mass, we need to reduce intake and increase output. Reducing fat stores and adding muscle improves energy utilization by using more calories for active metabolic tissues. Exercise also improves general metabolism and vitality and lowers that important "set point," allowing us to maintain lower weight and body fat with the same food intake. At a good level of exercise, the body will burn more calories than usual, even 12 hours afterward. Regular exercise is clearly needed to keep fat off.

Daily exercise is essential. If we are just starting out, we should first begin slowly and build to a regular daily program. If we make it a habit, we will really see the benefit. Then, at most we might skip it for one day a week, but only if we must, and then we should stretch and walk anyway. Some aerobics activity is ideal, even 20–30 minutes a day, five or six days a week. Our body stores energy, not as calories, but mainly as fat. Aerobic-type exercises will burn and reduce fat stores, without reducing muscle tissue (weight-loss programs without exercise can cause muscle loss). One to two hours daily of activity is fine; we must make the time to do it. We can add brisk walks to the more strenuous activity as we get into shape. A 30-minute walk about a half hour after meals is just the thing to further help digestion and assimilation. With more exercise, our vitality, endurance, and ability to handle stress and life all improve. Try it!

I want to say more about those two previously mentioned factors that are very important to healthy and easy weight loss—water and fiber. Water works in a variety of ways to promote both weight reduction and general well-being. In his article "Water: How 8 Glasses a Day Keeps Fat Away," taken from *The Snowbird Diet,* Donald S. Robertson, M.D. (coauthored by Carol Robertson) states that "incredible as it may seem, water is quite possibly the single most important catalyst in losing weight and keeping it off. Although most of us take it for granted, water may be the only true 'magic potion for permanent weight loss.'" Dr. Robertson also suggests that "water suppresses the appetite and helps the body metabolize stored fat, helps maintain proper muscle tone, clears wastes and may help relieve constipation." More water is needed by overweight people; for those who tend to retain fluid, drinking plenty of water will help rebalance the improperly distributed body fluids. During weight loss, Dr. Robertson suggests about three quarts a day, each drunk over a 30-minute period—one quart in the morning, another at noon, and a third between 5 and 6 P.M. or thereabouts, depending on dinnertime. The water should be consumed about 30 minutes before meals to help hydrate us and reduce the appetite. The water should be cool to cold, because extra calories will then be burned to warm it. This can become a lifetime habit.

Sufficient fiber in the diet supports good colon function and helps to eliminate wastes that are released during weight loss. Especially if the diet is low in fiber foods, we may add supplemental fiber as psyllium seed husks and bran. Psyllium is a soluble fiber that will increase bulk and reduce the appetite. It has also been shown to reduce fat absorption by coating the intestinal tract. When olive oil is also used, it will help mobilize some of the toxins in the intestines and carry them out, while the psyllium will reduce the oil absorption and thus calorie intake. Insoluble wheat or oat bran fiber can also help in detoxification as well as in stimulating the colon function.

Other digestive supporters include liquid chlorophyll. A teaspoon or so added to water twice daily will help nourish the intestinal lining and improve digestion. With better assimilation, our tissues and cells are more nourished and there may be fewer cravings and less desire for food. Ginger-lemon water can help with circulation and diuresis, as well as support liver and gallbladder function. Even just lemon water—half a small lemon squeezed into water—drunk 15–30 minutes before meals will help digestion and utilization of fats. The new flavored mineral waters (no calories) can be used as a beverage, up to two or three cups daily. These drinks, because of the carbonation, are somewhat filling. Common flavors include lemon, lime, orange, cola, root beer, cherry, and cherry-chocolate.

Many other supplements can be helpful during and after weight loss. A general vitamin/mineral supplement is very important, especially when we are on special diets that may not be perfectly balanced (very few are) or if we take in fewer than 1,500 calories daily. Extra minerals are essential to prevent deficiency, especially with high fiber intake, which may reduce mineral absorption. Amounts over the RDAs are needed for iron, zinc, copper, manganese, and molybdenum. Calcium is especially important to prevent bone loss, as less calcium is also absorbed with the fiber. Magnesium is also cleared in the gut as well as through the kidneys, and so a good intake is needed. Vitamin B_6 will help provide a diuretic effect during weight release.

Since weight loss involves a mild process of detoxification, with the body burning fat and other tissues (without proper exercise, the body loses muscle as well), some antioxidant nutrients are suggested to handle the extra toxin load. Vitamin C, 1–3 grams daily in two or three portions, and vitamin E and selenium, usually taken together in the morning, are suggested. L-cysteine can also be used; this amino acid helps liver and intestinal detoxification processes.

Other amino acids have been recommended by some authorities. A general L-amino acid formula can be used; Dr. Stuart Berger suggests taking it about 30–60 minutes before meals, as certain amino acids, such as phenylalanine, may help reduce the appetite. In *Vitamin Power,* Stephanie Rick and Rita Aero cite research that suggests that a combination of arginine and lysine, 1,500 mg. each, taken before bed can help weight loss by increasing growth hormone production and improving fatty acid metabolism and general energy. I have been more impressed with L-carnitine's help in weight loss, as it supports the efficient use of fats in the body. The usual plan is 500 mg. taken twice daily, with the morning and evening meals.

Various fatty acids may also be taken to stimulate weight loss by improving fatty acid metabolism. An essential fatty acid formula can be used. Most obese people need more good polyunsaturated fats to balance their lipid metabolism. Gamma-linolenic acid from evening primrose oil and eicosapentaenoic acid (EPA) from fish oil are both precursors to different prostaglandins and may also be helpful. Some chronically obese people will respond to supplementation with essential fatty acids and evening primrose oil. Cold-pressed linseed (flax) oil is high in both omega-3 (EPA and alpha-linolenic) the omega-6 (linoleic and others) fatty acids and is a less expensive way to obtain these oils. Usually, three or four teaspoons a day are sufficient if fats are avoided in the diet. When taking additional fatty acids, it is wise to supplement the many cofactors that help in fatty acid metabolism. These are zinc, magnesium, beta-carotene, and vitamins A, C, niacin, pyridoxine, and biotin. Vitamin E also aids our metabolism as well as prevents oxidation of the other oils.

WEIGHT LOSS SUPPORT PLAN*

- **Improving digestive effectiveness.** Poor breakdown of foods allows poor cell nutrition, which can lead to cravings and overeating. Hydrochloric acid, digestive enzymes, and pancreas may help.
- **Improving metabolism** (utilization efficiency) of carbohydrates, fats, and proteins, particularly the burning of fats for fuel. Their suggested supplements include carnitine, vitamin B_{12}, vitamin B_6, folic acid, choline, inositol, methionine, taurine, liver and thyroid glandulars, vitamin A, dimethylglycine (DMG), and gamma-linolenic acid (GLA).
- **Stimulating energy levels** with vitamin C, pantothenic acid, adrenal glandular, potassium, magnesium, manganese, chromium, octocosanol, and the branched-chain amino acids—leucine, isoleucine, and valine.
- **Reducing cravings,** especially for sweets, by using the amino acid glutamine, chromium, and by avoiding allergenic foods.
- **Suppressing the appetite** with the amino acids phenylalanine and tryptophan.

*Adapted from the book *Super Fitness Beyond Vitamins,* Michael Rosenbaum, M.D., and Dominick Bosco.

There are many herbs that can also be helpful during weight loss. Juniper berry is a good diuretic herb and helps in detoxification. Parsley leaf is also a diuretic, and peppermint leaf tea helps reduce the appetite for many people, as it is said to relax the stomach nerves. Chickweed herb, a spring green, has historically been known for reducing appetite and helping in weight loss. Bladderwrack is a type of sea vegetable; when taken with kelp, it will support thyroid function, and the high mineral levels of this herb aid general energy utilization. Garlic has also been used in weight-loss programs to help lower blood lipids and for detoxification.

In *The Scientific Validation of Herbal Medicine,* Dr. Mowrey notes that he never suggests chickweed because of the lack of backup research on it. Plantain (Plantago ovata) is a green with much more scientific support. The plantain fiber aids in weight loss by reducing cholesterol and triglyceride levels, by lessening fat absorption, and by its "appetite-satiating" effect. Dr. Mowrey's herbal formula for weight loss includes plantain, fennel seed, burdock root, hawthorn berry (to support heart function), kelp, and bladderwrack.

Losing weight effectively and healthfully and maintaining a proper weight is a complex and multifaceted process. Finding a diet that works for us is important, and creating

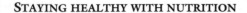

a good exercise program is essential for long-term weight control. Implementing our healthy diet almost always requires changes in various habits and relationships that affected our weight previously. Behavior patterns need to be altered in order to achieve a new relationship to food. Both behavior and motivation can be learned, but it takes work—repeated and sustained effort. Beginning to believe in ourselves and our success is also catalyst and a source of support in becoming who we want to be, with the body and energy we desire. We have to know we can do it, believe it, see it in our mind's eye, and feel it in our hearts to have the body, health, and life that we want—and then do the work it takes to maintain them.

The following supplement plan can be used during a weight-reduction plan when daily calorie intake is limited. The amounts for each nutrient are a daily total, which can be divided into three portions.

WEIGHT LOSS NUTRIENT PROGRAM

Water	3 qt.	Calcium	800–1,200 mg.
Calories	1,000–1,800	Chromium	400 mcg.
Fiber (includes diet	20 g.	Copper	2–3 mg.
plus bran & psyllium		Iodine	150–225 mcg.
supplements)		Iron	15–20 mg.
Psyllium	6–8 g. daily	Magnesium	500–800 mg.
(before meals)		Manganese	10 mg.
Bran	8–10 g. daily	Molybdenum	500 mcg.
(after meals		Potassium	1–2 g.
and at bedtime)		Selenium	200 mcg.
		Silicon	100 mg.
Vitamin A	10,000 IUs	Zinc	30–60 mg.
Beta-carotene	10,000–30,000 IUs		
Vitamin D	400 IUs	*Others:*	
Vitamin E	400–800 IUs		
Vitamin K	300 mcg.	Digestive enzymes	2–3 tablets
Thiamine (B$_1$)	75–150 mg.	(after meals)	
Riboflavin (B$_2$)	50–100 mg.	Adrenal glandular	50–100 mg.
Niacinamide (B$_3$)	75–150 mg.	L-amino acids	1,500 mg.
Pantothenic acid (B$_5$)	250–500 mg.	L-carnitine	1,000 mg.
Pyridoxine (B$_6$)	50–100 mg.	Phenylalanine	500 mg.
Pyridoxal-5-phosphate	50–100 mg.	(before meals)	
Cobalamin (B$_{12}$)	100–200 mcg.	Flaxseed oil	1 Tablespoon
Folic acid	600–800 mcg.	Olive oil	2 teaspoons
Biotin	500 mcg.	(with psyllium)	
Choline	500–1,000 mg.	(before meals)	
Inositol	500 mg.	Evening	
Vitamin C	3 g.	primrose oil	4–6 capsules
Bioflavonoids	250–500 mg.	Coenzyme Q$_{10}$	20–30 mg.
		Dimethylglycine	50–100 mg.
		Organic germanium	100–200 mg.

I'M TOO FAT TO EAT

Have you ever been too fat to touch your toes?
to blow your nose?
to get in or out of your clothes?
to smell a rose? to feel the wind blow?
to know, grow, show…

Now it is time for front row…

Too fat to eat,
Too fat to eat those sweets
Too fat to reach your feet
to reach your defeat.
O, O, deplete my fat—
Skinny rewards in the sun
skinny, skinny on the run
NOW, station N.O.W.
relaxation…concentration
regeneration…duplication
illumination…relation
that silent conversation—
can you hear it?
less material
more ethereal
Some people are skinny
& very much material
but that's immaterial

— *Lynn Segerblom & Bethany ArgIsle, written during a fast*

Weight Gain

This program is basically the opposite of Weight Loss with similar emphasis on avoiding junk foods, excessive fats, and other poor nutritional choices. People who want to gain weight need to eat more calories and more food. To most of the overweight population, this would be a dream come true, but for underweight people who have trouble gaining weight, it can be a real problem.

Like obesity, being underweight involves many factors. Undernourishment during infancy and adolescence or nutrient deficiencies of the mother during pregnancy can lead to a lower number of fat cells and thus the potential for lower amounts of fatty tissue. Genetics and conditioning are also factors. Thinness, of course, runs in families, as does obesity. Poor eating habits and low food intake are other causes of underweight. Illness can cause weight loss. Flus or debilitating diseases such as cancer can lead to loss of weight, which can be hard to regain, especially when those with these problems are not used to higher-calorie diets. Stress and anxiety are often found with low body weight. High-strung people and worriers can have trouble putting on weight. During times of extreme emotional upset, it may be difficult to eat, and that can be a problem. People who use stimulants such as caffeine and cigarettes are more commonly underweight than those who do not abuse these stimulants. The caffeine-cigarette combination generates a lot of nervous energy and frenetic mental activity. It may be productive for office work, but not for health.

Several medical problems can be associated with weight loss or the inability to gain weight. Thyroid problems, mainly hyperthyroidism, are the most common of these, and are associated with many other symptoms, such as a rapid heart rate, sweaty palms, and insomnia. Some psychologically related medical problems are also associated with underweight. Bulimia and anorexia nervosa are the two serious food-oriented maladies; they are, in fact, often symptoms of much deeper emotional, attitudinal problems. Treatment of bulimia, or voluntary vomiting, may require a combination of medical and psychological care. The cycle of regular overeating and vomiting is hard on the body, as it can irritate the upper gastrointestinal tract with hydrochloric acid and cause a loss of potassium and other nutrients. Bulimia may or may not be a part of anorexia nervosa, which is becoming a more common eating disorder.

Anorexia nervosa, loss of appetite due to nervous or psychological factors, mainly afflicts young women from ages 13–25. It commonly entails a delusion about weight and body image and a fear of eating food because of possible weight gain. Anorexics are often malnourished, deficient in both calories and nutrients. They may also be involved in regular vigorous exercise, such as aerobics or ballet, and may use laxatives, both of which may lead to further loss of body nutrients. And they may become socially separated because of a fear of group pressure toward eating.

Anorexia nervosa is a serious problem! People with this syndrome should receive immediate treatment with education, emotional support, understanding, and food. This problem is more common in the teen years, which is even more a concern because nutrient needs are very high and poor nutrition is more common in this age group. Fortunately, though, this eating avoidance (not really loss of appetite) usually passes in time.

There should also be care not to overdiagnose or overtreat young people who may watch their weight and eat sparingly. Just try to encourage eating of good-quality, lower-calorie foods and suggest a supplement program such as the one at the end of this section.

For people with problems of being underweight, a medical evaluation is usually needed, especially if the problem is recent. A general physical exam and blood chemistry test may rule out medical problems such as anemia, abnormal thyroid function, or even cancer. Mineral tests and a diet profile may assist in isolating nutritional deficiencies. Usually, though, if both parents were trim and the individual has been thin most of his or her life, no medical problems will be revealed. A faster metabolism and lower potential for fat storage are usually the explanation.

People with low weight who have difficulty gaining weight often need a combined program. Working with a psychologist, stress counselor, or hypnotherapist to deal with some of the psychological, attitudinal, and emotional factors may be helpful. Stress reduction such as through relaxation exercises, music, or meditation, can be important, especially for nervous or high-strung individuals. Learning to slow down internally and externally can improve metabolism and the assimilation of nutrients. Stopping smoking or the overuse of caffeine is very helpful at adding a few pounds, as it will often slow the metabolism, at least initially.

The other, primary focus for gaining weight is good nutrition—diet and supplements. In this area, the suggestions are the opposite of those for weight loss. Bigger portions, many meals along with extra snacks, and more healthy, easily digested, high-calorie foods are the foundation of the plan. Increasing calories is the key; an extra 500 calories per day over and above body requirements can lead to a pound a week weight gain. More yogurt and cheeses, nuts, avocados, rice, potatoes, and bread with some butter may be helpful and healthful for getting extra calories. This will also increase dietary fats somewhat; fats are more caloric than the complex carbohydrates or sweeter foods. If there is a low cardiovascular risk, with a moderate cholesterol level (175–210) and good blood pressure, even more fats, especially monounsaturated fats such as olive oil, can be consumed. Smokers are at a slightly greater risk of developing cardiovascular diseases with this higher-fat diet, though generally additional oils, seeds, butter and other milk products, and even meats, if those are tolerated, may be used to add weight. It is still wise to avoid fried foods and hydrogenated oils; an increase in vegetable fats, especially cold-pressed oils is wiser than adding more animal fats.

Often, underweight people experience symptoms of fatigue and coldness in the body. Fat helps to keep us warm, and low body fat with poor circulation will reduce vitality and warmth. Fatigue may also be related to nutritional deficiencies secondary to limited caloric diets and low intake. Vegetarians and people who eat macrobiotic diets tend to have lower weights, but these may be healthier weights if these people consume reasonable amounts of calories, protein, and vegetable oils—and mostly nutrient-rich foods. Still, these diets can more easily lead to deficient calorie intake, because they are lower in fats, and most of the foods consumed are low-calorie foods (better for weight loss). In these cases, more animal proteins can be therapeutic. Deep-water fish and organic poultry are best; but even "organic" red meat and liver may be helpful for deficient, tired, cold-type people. Low thyroid function and anemia can produce fatigue and coldness; however, hypothyroidism usually causes some weight gain also. Most often, low weight with fatigue results from inadequate nutrition. In the Chinese traditional energy system the imbalance that is associated with "weak Fire element" may lead to fatigue, low endurance, and coldness, although this symptom complex may be associated with either low or increased weight. These symptoms may also accompany anemia, a part of "weak Fire" or weak blood, and in this case more iron, as is found in the animal meats, poultry and fish, or as supplements, is the appropriate medicine. Folic acid, vitamin B_{12}, copper, and adequate protein intake, as well as regular exercise also help to build up the blood and improve the energy, endurance, and weight.

Another dietary suggestion for weight gain is to increase the size and number of meals. Three main meals and three or four snacks will help keep calorie intake up. A decrease in the bulky low-calorie foods and a focus on the higher-calorie ones will also help. It is good to eat the main course first (the opposite of the plan for losing weight). Follow the richer foods then with vegetables and salads, with lots of good dressing if there is room. Of the vegetables, eat mainly starchier ones, such as potatoes, carrots, beets, and squashes. Also, eat the starchy grains, such as rice, oats, and pastas. Sweets and desserts are really not very helpful; they tend to fill people with short-term energy without nutritional value and may actually lead to increased energy expenditure. Fluid intake just before or during meals is not recommended, as it reduces the appetite, and you will want to eat more to gain weight. Some alcohol, maybe one drink of a good wine, before a meal occasionally is helpful as it promotes relaxation and improves the appetite. Even bedtime snacks are appropriate when it comes to gaining weight, as long as it does not interfere with sleep.

Adequate rest and deep sleep are important to help the body slow down and relax the nervous tension that can eat up calories. Warm milk before bed with a little treat such as toast or a cookie can be useful to improve sleep and add calories. Avoiding stimulants that increase nervous energy, especially in the evening, is a very good idea. And again, stopping smoking is important to this program and life itself.

A regular exercise program should be followed, but it should be oriented more to toning and conditioning exercise, such as working with weights, to build up the body muscle, tissue density, and thus, increase weight. Vigorous aerobic activity, however, burns off more calories and may keep weight down (though some is useful to maintain endurance). Walks in the fresh air and nature may help us to stay fit and relaxed enough to be more receptive to food.

Some supplements are helpful in improving the potential for weight increase. A general multiple is, of course, suggested to provide all of the essential nutrients. Additional B vitamins taken several times daily may also help; most of the B vitamins aid the metabolism and assimilation of food and proper generation of energy (ATP). Essential fatty acids, as a supplement or as additional vegetable oil in the diet, are helpful from both a caloric perspective and a metabolic one. Amino acids are also effective when taken before meals. They stimulate the appetite and provide good protein synthesis capacity, thus helping to build the body. Overall, a moderate supplement (not high amounts) program is indicated, just to cover the basic needs for nutrients; we are not trying to increase the metabolism in general. People with significant weight loss or people who generally have low weight, say 10–15 percent below their ideal, need to focus more on "living to eat" rather than their usual "eating to live" plan, at least for a while, to bring up their weight.

WEIGHT GAIN NUTRIENT PROGRAM

Calories	2,500–3,500	Calcium	600–850 mg.
Protein	65–125 g.	Chromium	200 mcg.
Fat	60–110 g.	Copper	2 mg.
		Iodine	150 mcg.
Vitamin A	5,000–10,000 IUs	Iron	10–18 mg.
Beta-carotene	20,000 IUs	Magnesium	300–500 mg.
Vitamin D	400 IUs	Manganese	5–10 mg.
Vitamin E	400 IUs	Molybdenum	200 mcg.
Vitamin K	300 mcg.	Selenium	200 mcg.
Thiamine (B_1)	50–75 mg.	Silicon	50 mg.
Riboflavin (B_2)	25–75 mg.	Zinc	30 mg.
Niacinamide (B_3)	100 mg.	L-amino acids	1,500 mg.
Pantothenic acid (B_5)	100 mg.	(500 mg. before each meal)	
Pyridoxine (B_6)	50 mg.		
Pyridoxal-5-phosphate	25–50 mg.	Essential fatty acids	6 capsules
Cobalamin (B_{12})	50 mcg.	or Flaxseed oil	2 Tablespoons
Folic acid	600 mcg.	*Optional (if needed for better digestion):*	
Biotin	250 mcg.	Hydrochloric acid	5–10 grains
Vitamin C	1,500 mg.	(with protein meals)	
Bioflavonoids	250 mg.	Digestive enzymes (after meals)	1–2 tablets

Yeast Syndrome

The "yeast" problem with *Candida albicans* is one of the new medical concerns of the 1980s that will continue into the next century. It has been described by many prominent physicians, including C. Orian Truss in *The Missing Diagnosis,* William Crook in *The Yeast Connection,* and Keith Sehnert in *The Candidiasis Syndrome.* It is a very common problem, one of the most frequent I see, and is to me a medical adventure, because I learn a great deal while working with people with this problem. Often the therapy for yeast, or candidiasis as it is commonly known, will positively and dramatically change lives. The somewhat complex, multilevel treatment program has been effective in a high percentage of the people I have treated, and I have worked with hundreds with this problem to date.

FACTORS COMMON TO PATIENTS WITH YEAST SYNDROME

- Frequent or long-term use of antibiotics, such as tetracycline for acne
- Frequent use of broad-spectrum antibiotics for recurrent infections, such as in the ears, bladder, vagina, or throat
- Birth control pill use in women
- Premenstrual symptoms
- Recurrent vaginal yeast infections in women or prostate problems in men
- Regular use of cortisone-type drugs
- Cravings for sweets, breads, or alcohol
- Sensitivity to molds, dampness, and smells
- Mental symptoms such as depression, mood swings, or confusion
- Chronic fatigue, indigestion, or food reactions
- Recurrent skin fungus infections, such as ringworm, athlete's foot, "jock itch," or nail problems

---

The yeast syndrome is a controversial topic. Most traditional doctors do not want to hear about this condition and call it a "fad" disease, but those who will explore the possibility and look for it in their patients will be hard-pressed not to accept this problem as "real." One of the reasons, I believe, for medicine not really accepting the "yeast syndrome" is because the problem arises predominantly as a side effect from the use of commonly prescribed drugs—antibiotics, birth control pills, and corticosteroids.

The problem originates when a common yeast, *Candida albicans,* begins to over-grow in the intestinal or genito-urinary tract. It may be contracted initially through sexual contact. When other normal body microflora are killed off by antibiotics, the yeasts will then proliferate and coexist with the useful germs. Mild mucocutaneous infections (of the skin, vagina, throat, or bladder, for example) may develop in the yeast phase of this dimorphic organism. This common yeast is usually noninvasive (that is, it remains localized) except in the severely debilitated patient. However, with long-term infestation or with the weakened immune state that can result from a reduction of normal colon bacteria, the yeast can shift into its fungal form, wherein it develops rhizoids, or roots, that can be implanted in the intestinal wall or other mucosal linings. This allows absorption into the body of by-products (toxins) of fermentation and other antigenic material generated by the fungus. The body will then make antibodies to the *Candida albicans* organisms. This can lead to an immunological or hypersensitivity reaction that is manifested as the polysystemic disease for which this syndrome is now known.

The yeast problem thus occurs at two levels—the localized infections, of which skin rashes and vaginitis are the most common (intestinal overgrowth is also common), and the secondary and more serious systemic reactions. This problem can then produce such symptoms as recurrent skin fungus infections, examples being ringworm, athlete's foot, "jock itch," or nail problems; headaches; fatigue; cystitis or prostatitis; mental symptoms such as mood swings, poor memory or concentration, depression, or confusion; premenstrual symptoms; recurrent herpes infection; joint pains; cravings for sweets, bread, or alcohol; indigestion or food reactions; and sensitivity to molds, dampness, environmental pollution, cigarettes, and various smells.

This yeast syndrome is much more common in women than in men and seems to affect the hormonal balance, initially causing mild premenstrual symptoms of irritability, depression, fatigue, and swelling, and leading to actually abnormal and/or painful menstrual periods. I would estimate that a significant number of women with PMS have a problem with *Candida albicans,* and probably more than half the women with candidiasis have some uncomfortable premenstrual symptoms.

Diagnosing polysystemic candidiasis may involve several tests. Most doctors who work with this problem use a questionnaire such as the one provided by Dr. Crook in his book, *The Yeast Connection.* The scores indicate the likelihood of a yeast problem, and while not exact, this is a pretty accurate tool. Many doctors suggest a trial treatment program merely on the basis of an interview, exam, and questionnaire score, as the response to therapy is often a good indication of the presence of the problem. However, I like to have more objective monitors, so I perform two main tests, both reasonably inexpensive. One is a culture of a stool specimen to quantify the amount of *Candida albicans* (or other yeast) organisms present. This can then be repeated to measure the effectiveness of the program. Also, a sensitivity test that finds what substances will actually kill the yeast (in the lab, at least) can be done after the organism is isolated. The other test measures the blood levels of three antibodies (IgA, IgM, IgG) to the *Candida albicans* organism, performed by Immunodiagnostic Lab in San Leandro, California. If these antibodies are elevated, this suggests that some systemic reaction is occurring in the body (the stool reveals only an intestinal overgrowth), which may be correlated with more widespread symptoms. This test also gives us the opportunity to monitor the body's status over time to measure treatment response. Reducing yeast organisms in the body and replacing friendly bacteria will usually reduce elevated antibody levels.

Other tests may be helpful in determining coexisting medical problems. A study of the stool for ova and parasites may show these to be more commonly present in yeast carriers than in the average population, as often the same predisposing factors, poor digestion and low stomach acid, are present. Treatment may also be needed to eliminate these parasites. Creating proper colon ecology is a crucial factor in health, disease resistance, and many important body functions. When normal colon bacteria are present in sufficient quantities (which they may not be when other invaders are taking their place), they will actually produce many vitamins using the nutrient fuel provided them. Vitamin K and most of the B complex vitamins—niacin, B_{12}, pantothenic acid, B_6, biotin, and folic acid—are among these. Intestinal bacteria also aid final digestion of food, such as proteins and milk. With low colon bacteria counts, poor digestion, and an unhealthy intestinal lining, more food allergies may develop. A blood test measuring specific antibodies to many commonly allergenic foods may be indicated in some people with candidiasis, especially when there is a real problem with food intolerance. Frequently found reactions, indicated by greatly elevated IgG antibody levels, include reactions to both baker's and brewer's yeasts, wheat, milk, cheeses, mushrooms, and eggs. Many others are possible, but those are the ones I have found to be most common and most strong.

Three-Faceted Approach to Treatment of the Yeast Syndrome

1. Do not feed the yeasts foods upon which they thrive.
2. Reduce yeast growth through natural and pharmaceutical agents.
3. Reestablish normal intestinal ecology.

The overall approach to treating the yeast problem is threefold. The **first facet** is to refrain from feeding those "yeastie beasties" what they like to eat so they can thrive and divide. They live on mostly simple sugars and yeast and fermented foods. These include fruits, fruit juices, and dried fruits, sugary foods, refined flour products, alcoholic beverages, cheese, vinegar, breads, and other yeasted fermented food products, such as soy sauce. All these foods are avoided on the yeast diet.

What to eat? There are many recommended foods—fish, poultry, meat, lots of vegetables, some whole grains, nuts, seeds, and occasional eggs. (The antiyeast diet is more difficult for vegetarians, but definitely possible.) Some yogurt, especially acidophilus culture, is all right if milk is tolerated. Oils are obtained from some butter and more cold-pressed vegetable oils, such as olive, flaxseed, sesame, and sunflower. Legumes are often limited because they add to intestinal gas.

Basic meals include proteins and vegetables or, occasionally, starch and vegetables. For the first few weeks, the carbohydrates, including pastas and especially breads, are limited, with only some whole grain cereals being used. This lowers fiber intake, but usually other aspects of the treatment help colon function. The Ideal Diet discussed in Part Three, with certain modifications, will make a good Candida diet. The rotation is a good way to reduce food reactions. Initially, the diet includes no fruit, or only one piece a day, and none of the sweeter fruits, such as grapes, bananas, and melons. The starches are limited to one portion a day, and the meals are oriented toward proteins and vegetables.

This is a **special therapeutic diet,** and not necessarily a lifelong one, though many people like the way they feel on it. Intestinal symptoms decrease, energy improves, and itchy or irritated skin may start to heal with a decrease in sugar and yeasty foods. Also, some weight can be shed easily on this diet. This may be a problem for the already trim person, and lighter people need to emphasize regular eating to prevent weight loss.

After a few weeks, we can test ourselves with fruit, bread, other grain products, or cheese—of course, one food at a time, and only one daily—to see how we handle them. If they seem to cause no problems, we can then bring these foods into our diet on a rotating basis. Eventually, adding more whole grains and fiber will provide what I believe is a healthier diet. Different degrees of strictness with the diet may be necessary, depending on the severity of the problem. A more stringent diet might exclude all fruits; whole grains, particularly the glutinous ones—wheat, barley, and oats; herb teas and spices, which may contain molds; and many nuts, which can also carry molds.

ANTI-YEAST DIET PLAN

Emphasize		*Avoid*	
Vegetables—all	Beans	Sugar—all forms	Baked goods
Meats*	Nuts & Seeds	Alcoholic beverages	Vinegars
Poultry*	Butter	Fruit juices	Pickled vegetables
Eggs	Cold-pressed oils	Dried fruits	Cheese
Fish*	Lemon	Refined flours	Mushrooms
Whole grains	Fruit, fresh**	Breads	

*Vegetarians will need to use more whole grains, beans, and nuts and seeds but this higher carbohydrate diet does not really curb yeast as well. Furthermore, vegetarians seem to be more prone to yeast overgrowth because their diet is more alkaline and sweet, which supports the yeast.

**Limited to two pieces daily.

The **second facet** of the treatment is to diminish the amount of yeast present. This is what Western medicine is so good at accomplishing. Nystatin powder is the most commonly used pharmaceutical for initial treatment of intestinal yeast. Nystatin itself is made from a culture of certain bacteria and it will actually kill yeast. It is not readily absorbed through the intestinal mucosa, so basically it just handles the gastrointestinal yeast. Since it is most often given as pure powder dissolved in water, it will also kill some of the yeast in the oral cavity when it is gargled. A solution can be used to wash the sinuses as well by dissolving nystatin in saline solution and using a dropper or inhaling the solution. For men with candidiasis and recurrent prostatitis or genital or skin symptoms of yeast, or for women with recurrent cystitis or other systemic symptoms, I may prescribe a stronger antifungal agent called ketoconizole, brand name Nizoral. This is effective for most yeast problems, but it can be irritating to the liver, so its use must be watched closely. For people who do not respond well to Nystatin or other natural remedies, Nizoral may be indicated. The usual dosage is one 200 mg. tablet daily for three to six weeks if it is well tolerated. A new Nizoral-related drug, fluconazole, or Diflucan, is now available and, though expensive, may be a slight improvement over Nizoral. Other "azole" drugs are available from many European countries and Canada. These include clotrimazole, miconazole, tinadazole, and econazole. They have similar systemic antifungal action (most are also mild amoebicides), are less expensive, and are also less toxic on the liver.

During yeast treatment, symptoms may arise secondary to killing the yeast. This occurs most with Nystatin, at times with the natural therapies, and only occasionally with the systemic medicines. The symptoms might include headache, fatigue, a mild flulike syndrome, or an exacerbation of already existing symptoms. It may be helpful during "die-off" periods to clear the colon every two or three days with a water enema or have a colonic irrigation every week or two for several treatments. Adding some Nystatin to the water to introduce it directly into the colon may help clear some more yeast.

Natural remedies that help to reduce yeast by killing it or by interfering with its growth include caprylic acid, fresh garlic and garlic extract, and the herb, pau d'arco, or taheebo. Caprylic acid is a natural fatty acid extracted from coconut oil. It interferes with the growing and duplicating process of the *Candida albicans* does not actually kill yeast, but it is effective in reducing intestinal yeast levels. It must be used for a fairly long period. I often prescribe the caprylates to follow a two to three month course of Nystatin and use a caprylic acid product such as Caprystatin or Capricin for a few months also. The length of treatment for yeast depends on the degree of the problem, the response to the treatment, and the results of tests.

Garlic has been shown to kill some yeast in sensitivity tests in the lab. It can be added to the treatment regimen and often helps. Two capsules several times daily is the usual dosage, though good garlic may have a blood-pressure-lowering effect at that amount, which may detrimentally affect some people. Goldenseal root also has some antifungal properties. Pau d'arco, a Brazilian tree bark, has become a very popular herb in the treatment of yeast, allergies, and other immune problems. It can be taken in capsules, or tea made from the bark can be drunk several times daily. It seems to tonify or strengthen the gastrointestinal tract and may help reduce yeast.

The **third facet** of the yeast treatment involves restoring the colon to its natural state, mainly by reimplanting lactobacillus bacteriae. Acidophilus primary products used. There are a couple of other bacteria that are also helpful in the gut and used in some formulae. *Lactobacillus bifidus,* a cousin to provide some colon support in the adult. *Streptococcus faecium,* a friendly form of strep bacteria, also adds a helpful function by replacing the once-present yeast.

A formula that contains all three of these bacteria is produced and marketed by Klaire Laboratories in Southern California. This high-quality, milk-free product called Vital-Plex can be taken as a supplement during the yeast treatment. Another product that has been well researched is DDS-1, produced by UAS Laboratories. It is available in powder, capsules, and tablets. Studies at the University of Nebraska and Michigan State University have shown acidophilus DDS-1 to have many positive effects, as described by Keith Sehnert, M.D., in "The Candidiasis Syndrome, Old Problem, New Mystery." This acidophilus in the colon can produce acidophilin, which has an antibiotic effect on a number of potentially pathogenic colon bacteria. It also has been shown to inhibit growth of *Candida albicans* yeast. This product, as do most effective acidophilus cultures, helps restore bacteria that produce many B vitamins, including B_2, B_3, B_6, B_{12}, folic acid, biotin, and pantothenic acid. DDS-1 has also been shown to produce enzymes that help in digestion of proteins and milk sugar (lactose), and through its effect on fat metabolism, it has a mild cholesterol-lowering potential. Other research has revealed that DDS-1 and other lactobacilli may have antiviral effects with some viruses (herpes is one example) and anticancer effects, especially in the colon. I have seen lactobacillus treatment reduce the severity and recurrence of cold sores, genital herpes outbreaks, and canker sores, which may be a result of its correcting chemical or acid-base imbalance. By replacing putrefying bacteria in the mouth, throat, and upper intestinal tract, it has been seen to resolve bad breath as well as many symptoms of gastrointestinal upset, helping people's guts "feel more settled."

DDS-1 *Lactobacillus acidophilus* is discussed at such length here because it has been studied more extensively than others. However, there are other lactobacillus products that likely have similar effects, and these are being researched as well. Potency of the product is likely important. Many cultures now contain billions of live bacteria per dosage, rather than the few million that were once common. This should make them more effective, since the higher counts will allow a greater number of bacteria to actually reach the colon. Replacing the diminishing yeast with these physiologically active bacteria will help restore the colon's normal functions. Yeasts in the colon use up nutrients, rather than making additional ones, and they ferment foods, often leading to gas, bloating, abdominal discomfort, and flatulence. Reimplanting the colon with friendly bacteria helps to reduce many of the intestinal and digestive symptoms of candidiasis.

There are a number of other supplements that can help in treating the yeast syndrome. Supplemental hydrochloric acid with meals followed by digestive enzymes after eating can often help us to better break down and utilize our protein, fats, and food in general to make available the amino acids, essential fatty acids, and mineral micronutrients we need for healing. And they help to relieve digestive symptoms and make it easier for us to obtain the energy from the food. Healing the intestinal wall is an important part of clearing the candidiasis symptoms and reducing food reactions. Flaxseed or evening primrose oil and certain herbs can help with this.

For nutrient supplementation, a general multiple is used as a base, with some additional antioxidants to help handle certain toxic by-products, avoid immune suppression, and improve immune function. Organic germanium may be used to aid in this immune support and to improve the gut mucosa. Vitamin A, beta-carotene, and vitamin C are useful in the regulation of the yeast and support of the immune function. Extra magnesium is also a part of the program. Less zinc is suggested than in other programs, at least initially, as it possibly stimulates the Candida growth. Extra B vitamins, including biotin, provide support by replacing some of those lost because of the diminished colon bacteria that produce them. Coenzyme Q_{10} has been shown to have positive effects in yeast treatment as well.

Some of the nutrient oils may be used in the treatment of the yeast problem. In addition to garlic oil and the caprylic acid formulas, essential fatty acids (EFA), fish oil (EPA), and evening primrose oil (EPO) may be helpful, along with vitamin E. A product I have used that incorporates all of these oils is *Samolinic,* made and distributed by the Key Company. I might suggest a product such as this or separate portions of some of these oils if there seem to be many inflammatory or allergic symptoms.

The type of herbal treatment suggested for the yeast condition depends mostly on the other, coexisting problems. If there are premenstrual symptoms, diuretic herbs or female tonifying herbs may help (see the *Premenstrual Syndrome* program later in this chapter). With intestinal symptoms or upset, soothing digestive herbs may be helpful. Peppermint or chamomile teas are beneficial; capsules containing slippery elm bark and comfrey root powder can help heal the intestinal lining. Goldenseal root powder in short courses (one or two weeks) strengthens the mucous membranes, but it also stimulates liver detoxification, which can cause an increase in symptoms. Pau d'arco is a tonic herb that is often used in yeast treatment. Thyme oil has also been claimed to reduce yeast growth, but I have no experience with that.

Evaluating and treating the yeast syndrome is a real challenge for both doctors and patients. It takes patience and can often require a very long therapy as the body uses its very sensitive biofeedback process to let us know what is working. Often, Nystatin or other antifungal products must be taken for years, but usually will produce, within a few months, a marked change in the symptoms and a reduction in colon yeast colonization and blood antibodies to the yeast. Many people experience a profound and positive change in their health with proper diagnosis and treatment of this condition. However, we must also be careful not to overtreat and turn this medical concern into nothing more than the latest "fad" of the 1980s, as the medical profession would like. Yeast awareness is here to stay, and doctors and patients must be even more careful in their use of antibiotics, birth control pills, and the immune-suppressive corticosteroids.

YEAST SYNDROME NUTRIENT PROGRAM

Yeast-free diet	*see text*		
Vitamin A	10,000 IUs	Magnesium	400–800 mg.
Beta-carotene	15,000 IUs	Manganese	5–10 mg.
Vitamin D	400 IUs	Molybdenum	500 mcg.
Vitamin E	800 IUs	Selenium	300 mcg.
Vitamin K	300 mcg.	Zinc	15 mg.
Thiamine (B$_1$)	50 mg.		
Riboflavin (B$_2$)	25–50 mg.	Lactobacilli and other helpful microorganisms	4–10 billion organisms
Niacinamide (B$_3$)	100 mg.	Caprylic acid	300–600 mg.
Pantothenic acid (B$_5$)	500 mg.	Organic germanium	100 mg.
Pyridoxine (B$_6$)	50 mg.	Coenzyme Q$_{10}$	20–40 mg.
Pyridoxal-5-phosphate	50 mg.	Essential fatty acids*	4 capsules
Cobalamin (B$_{12}$)	50 mcg.	Gamma-linolenic acid* such as evening primrose oil	4 capsules
Folic acid	800 mcg.		
Biotin	1,000 mcg.	Hydrochloric acid (with meals)	1–2 tablets
Vitamin C	3,000 mg.		
Bioflavonoids	250 mg.	Digestive enzymes (after meals)	2–3 tablets
Calcium	600–1,000 mg.		
Chromium	500 mcg.	*Herbal Options:*	
Copper	2 mg.	Goldenseal root powder	2–3 capsules (2–3 weeks)
Iodine	150–225 mcg.	Pau d'arco	2–4 capsules or 2 cups tea
Iron	10–18 mg.		
		Garlic oil or garlic extract	4–6 capsules
		Echinacea freeze dried	2–4 capsules

*Flaxseed oil, 2–4 teaspoons daily, can replace these two products.

Allergies

The theories, problems, and treatments of allergies and hypersensitivities represent an enormous topic that could easily fill an entire book—in fact, many such books have been written by noted medical authors. This section discusses some of the basic concepts in the field of allergy, with an emphasis on new work related to this growing twentieth-century dilemma, particularly regarding the use of diet and supplements in treating both food and environmental allergies.

Allergies are a result of our physiological and biochemical interaction with the world around us and within us—with the foods, chemicals, and natural substances in our immediate environment that we ingest, inhale, or physically contact, and with various internal microbes and body tissues. Our body's immune system is designed to correctly identify and differentiate between self and nonself—that is, between what our body needs and what is foreign to it—and when it encounters foreign substances, it reacts by making antibodies or releasing certain chemicals, such as histamines. Of course, it is appropriate for us to make protective antibodies against infectious organisms, chemicals, and other foreign substances; pollens, molds, animal hairs, dust, and foods all contain protein antigens that stimulate some antibody response. The problem arises when we have an inappropriate response, or "hyperresponse." Then the antibodies attach to the antigens, causing a variety of internal reactions. Histamine and other chemicals are released into the system, causing an inflammatory reaction. These antigen-antibody (Ag-Ab) reactions affect the tissues and organs, mainly the skin, mucous membranes, lungs, and gastrointestinal tract. Symptoms commonly produced include itchy and watery eyes, runny and congested nose and sinuses, skin reactions, and rapid heart rate. Less obvious but still common allergic symptoms include fatigue, headache, intestinal gas or pain, abdominal bloating, and mood changes.

These allergic manifestations often are the result of multiple stressors and biochemical reactions. I often describe this to patients as the "cup runneth over" theory. Certain people may be reactive to specific environmental and food products, as I myself am. However, if our diet is relatively clean, our stress level is low, and our normal eliminative functions are working well, we will exhibit minimal, if any, symptoms. On the other hand, if we have too many stressors going into our cup—a high-demand schedule; a few dinners out with more bread, cheese and wine; a few extra worries; less exercise; and a little constipation—our cup may "runneth over" and we may experience sinus or upper respiratory symptoms, a skin rash, or other "allergic" problems. From a naturopathic viewpoint, allergic symptoms represent detoxification of any overly congested body; the traditional Chinese viewpoint suggests an imbalance of energies and organs. Western medicine has its own theories, which I also present.

Related to allergies are hypersensitivities, allergylike reactions that result from the repeated sensitizing of our body by certain substances, usually a protein antigen of foods or specific chemicals. Hypersensitivities are distinguished from immediate allergies by the fact that hypersensitivity reactions are usually delayed, with symptoms appearing several hours or longer after exposure, even up to one or two days later. They are mediated through T lymphocytes of the cellular immune system and delayed-type IgG antibodies rather than the IgE/mast cell/histamine system of rapid allergic responses. In regard to other allergic-type reactions, the term "hypersusceptibility" should be used to describe the rapid symptoms associated with environmental illness or exposure to environmental chemicals. This is likely a neuro-endocrine interaction rather than a true allergy.

Primary External Factors Causing Allergies and Hypersensitivity Reactions

- **Natural environmental substances**—mold spores, pollens from trees and grasses, dust (actually dust mites), animal hairs, and insects. These commonly produce upper respiratory symptoms in sensitive individuals. Itching, redness, and fluid (water and mucus) may affect the eyes, nose, sinuses, throat, bronchial tubes, and lungs.
- **Foods**—any food may be allergenic. Common ones include wheat, milk, eggs, corn, yeast, coffee, and chocolate. Even herbs and teas may lead to allergic symptoms. Food allergies may affect most body systems, with the gastrointestinal, nervous, respiratory, and skin areas affected the most.
- **Chemicals**—both environmental chemicals and food additives may create sensitivity. There are literally thousands of possibilities, including sprays, resins, hydrocarbons, pesticides, and so on. Some may weaken our immunity and allow further allergies to develop. Tobacco is a common allergen-containing substance to which many people are both addicted and allergic, a common duo according to our new understanding of allergies.

Pathways of Allergens into the Body*

- **Nose**—inhalation of environmental allergens.
- **Mouth**—ingestion of food and chemicals found in foods, water, and medicines.
- **Skin**—contact with various agents and injections of drugs and other substances.

We may also have internal "allergies," where our immune system reacts to our body's tissues as protein antigens, and actually forms specific antibodies to them. These antibodies then latch onto the antigen-coded organ tissues, where they may interfere with proper function and produce a wide variety of inflammatory symptoms and

---

*Depending on a variety of factors, some individuals are more sensitive to allergens that enter through a particular area.

diseases. More common areas affected include the thyroid gland, blood vessels, and joints, causing problems such as Hashimoto's thyroiditis, polyarteritis nodosa, and rheumatoid arthritis. These abnormal responses to normal tissues are termed auto-immune diseases. They are increasing in frequency and becoming one of the greater mysteries of modern medicine.

Common allergic problems include hay fever, eczema, contact dermatitis, and bronchial asthma. **Hay fever,** or **allergic rhinitis,** is characterized by sneezing, runny nose, itchy eyes, and postnasal drip. It is caused by reactions to pollens such as ragweed, trees, dust, grasses, molds, animals, and foods. It can be diagnosed by skin testing or blood antibody levels. Treatment may include avoidance of, or desensitization to, the allergens, or drugs such as antihistamines, decongestants, cortisone sprays or tablets, and cromolyn sodium nasal spray. Hay fever tends to run in families and is usually seasonal.

Hives, or urticaria, is characterized by red, itchy, and possibly painful wheals (bumps) on the skin. This condition may be caused by reactions to insect bites, chemicals (such as sulfites or food colors), drugs (such as aspirin or penicillin), or foods. Common foods causing hives are shellfish, nuts, citrus fruits, tomatoes, strawberries, chocolate, beef, pork, and mangoes. Avoidance is the key to treatment; antihistamines may relieve symptoms. When reactions are caused by drugs, more acute treatment may be needed. Genetics may play a role in this type of allergy, and prior sensitization to the specific agent is necessary for the reaction, as for most allergies.

Eczema (dermatitis) is characterized by dry, itchy skin, especially on the arms and legs. It is often hereditary, and it may be worsened by stress, sweating, or food allergies. Treatment involves lowering stress, avoiding soaps and detergents, use of cortisone creams and drugs, an elimination diet with avoidance of allergenic foods. Desensitization is usually not very helpful for this problem.

Contact dermatitis is characterized by an itchy, red, raised rash that may blister. It can occur anywhere on the body where contact to the allergen has been made. Common allergenic agents are poison oak or ivy, chemicals such as nail polish or soaps, plastics, metals, and fabrics. Medical treatment involves avoidance of known allergens and the use of antihistamine and cortisone drugs to reduce symptoms.

Asthma is characterized by difficulty in breathing, wheezing, coughing, and production of bronchial mucus. It is caused by a combination of genetic, allergic, and stress factors. It is commonly treated with drugs, avoidance and desensitization, and stress management. (This complex illness will be discussed in my next book, *Staying Healthy with Modern Medicine.*)

Headaches, alcoholism, and cigarette smoking may also involve allergy factors. Pain in the head, neckaches, and painful sensitivity to light, while they may be a result of stress or muscle tension, may also be caused by reactions to chemicals and foods. In such cases, the treatment would include rest, relaxation, pain relievers, and clearing of allergenic agents. Alcoholism often involves an allergic component with an addiction to grains and/or yeast (intestinal or vaginal yeast, skin fungus, or internal parasites or worms may also act as allergens as well as tissue irritants); it may also be a psychological disease with possible genetic predisposition, and may be related to a deficiency of trace mineral chromium (see Chapter 6), which is a key component of glucose tolerance factor. Treatment involves avoidance and therapy, possibly with the use of drugs or counseling. Cigarette smoking often involves an allergic addiction to either tobacco or the chemicals added to cigarettes. Treatment of nicotine addiction incorporates the elimination of the addiction, which may require counseling, will power, detoxification, and a change of lifestyle. (See programs on alcohol and smoking in Chapter 18.)

While there are a great many types of allergic reactions, almost all result from elevated levels of two different antibodies—immunoglobulin E (IgE) and immunoglobulin G (IgG), which occurs more with foods. IgE stimulates the release of histamine, causing immediate physiological activities. The common histamine response includes swelling, redness, itching, and possibly pain. The IgG antibody causes more delayed and long-term reactions. Some of the problems caused by the IgE reaction are hay fever, or pollen reactions, insect sting reactions, urticaria (hives) from ingested substances, such as foods or drugs, and atopic (hereditary allergy-mediated IgE) dermatitis or eczema. Many of these are fairly easy to observe and diagnose; however, reactions such as a change in energy level, decreased mental clarity, or digestive symptoms may be more difficult to acknowledge and to understand as allergic responses. IgG-mediated delayed types of reactions include many drug side effects; problems from exposure to chemicals, including tobacco; and most food allergies (that is why skin testing is not very useful for such allergies—it measures only IgE responses). Most allergy problems are a mixture of these different immunoglobulin-medicated reactions.

The main focus of traditional allergy practice is the diseases involving the IgE-histamine response—hay fever, eczema, and asthma. These are termed "atopies" (hereditary allergies); sensitive individuals have a genetic or at least familial propensity for experiencing these diseases sometime in their lives. These problems are more common in children and tend to regress with age. When such problems start later in life, they may be less genetically dominated and more related to other factors. Each of these conditions involves increased sensitivity to certain allergens. For example, an asthmatic or eczema sufferer may be allergic to eggs, wheat, or milk; hay fever sufferers are usually sensitive to pollen and environmental agents. Isolating the specific reactions and avoiding the agents that cause them, and/or using injection desensitization, may relieve the symptomatology. However, in all these cases, even with an elimination of symptoms, there is still the potential for the problem because of genetic or familial predisposition. Schools of natural healing or Chinese medicine may view these allergy problems in terms of body biochemical or energy imbalances and attempt to offer relief by correcting these difficulties. Nutritional medicine may have a lot to offer the allergic person by providing the optimum tissue and cellular nutrient levels that allow improved function and reduced allergic symptoms.

A deeper realm of allergy and immunology has fascinated many physicians in the last two decades. This is now incorporated into the field of clinical ecology. It involves our interaction with the environment and its effect on human health and disease. Clinical ecologists are physicians who evaluate and treat chronic illness on the basis of allergy, immune response (and immune weakness), and nutrition. Therapy may involve isolation from allergens, dietary changes, and an "orthomolecular" approach to nutritional supplements—that is, using higher amounts of various nutrients to support the body's functions and to alter abnormal physiology and correct functional or metabolic nutritional imbalances. Problems such as chronic fatigue, rapid aging, recurrent infections, arthritis, headaches, asthma, and mental illness have been treated successfully with this approach. The theories of "cerebral allergy" and "allergy-addiction" have been set forth by these pioneering physicians.

Herbert Rinkel, M.D., was probably the first to notice the problem of "cumulative allergic reactions," which led to his initial work on the "rotary-diversified" diet. This diet, and variations of it, have been used for over 50 years and each year more physicians employ the diet in their practices. The basic theory of many practicing physicians is that inappropriate immune responses produce antibodies to basically harmless and even usable macromolecules; these reactions may affect the normal body functions. Many of these reactions may be "hidden" or masked in the process of "allergy-addiction." In this case, foods may be acting on the body much like agents such as coffee, alcohol beverages, or tobacco—which are also common allergens. To avoid the withdrawal symptoms, we must regularly take in the specific substance. This type of reaction most commonly causes what are now called "cerebral allergies"— altered neurotransmitter reactions that affect the energy, emotions, and psyche. The theory is that certain allergenic antigens or antigen-antibody complexes cross the blood-brain barrier and cause these unusual reactions. Common cerebral symptoms include headache, dullness, lightheadedness, dizziness, anxiety, irritability, confusion, uncoordination, and depression. Lethargy, aggression, crying spells, insomnia, and even psychotic symptoms may also be experienced. Drs. Rinkel, William Philpott, and Marsha Mandell all have shown a fairly high percentage of food allergies in schizophrenic patients and those with other psychological disorders. Wheat, milk, and tobacco were most commonly found to be involved; "cerebral allergies" in particular can be most significant with the cereal grains. Food allergies may occur as a "fixed" reaction (stable over time), or "cumulative," increasing with repeated use and lessening with avoidance.

FOODS COMMONLY ASSOCIATED WITH SPECIFIC ALLERGIES

Headaches	Hay Fever	Childhood Allergies
wheat	milk	milk
chocolate	wheat	wheat
Migraine Headaches	nuts	eggs
alcoholic beverages	chocolate	artificial colors/flavors
cheese	colas	salicylates
chocolate	sulfites	peanuts
nuts	**Hives**	*less common:*
wheat	strawberries	rye
citrus fruits	tomatoes	beef
tomatoes	chocolate	fish
MSG	eggs	**Asthma**
nitrates	shellfish	wheat
eggs	mangoes	eggs
milk	pork	**Cerebral Symptoms**
Eczema	nuts	corn, wheat
eggs		milk
citrus fruits		soybeans
tomatoes		

The allergy-addiction syndrome related to foods is very common. These easily become "hidden" allergies, which may be involved in binge eating, overeating, weight gain, and general ups and downs that come from eating food. Cravings, even very subtle ones, often are part of this syndrome, but people who experience this might think that they just like a particular food and so eat it regularly. And when they eat it, they may feel a lift. This is thought to be a result of stimulation of beta-endorphins in the brain, which give us an "up" or euphoric feeling, as occurs with prolonged exercise.

Most addictions, especially to foods (and some street drugs), involve some allergy, but the allergic reactions may be masked, with repeated exposures producing no symptoms. A positive identification of the allergenic food cannot be made until it has been eliminated for four or more days; at times even avoidance for 24 hours might be enough to reveal the allergy. After a few days, trying the food by itself may produce a marked, abnormal response, and then we can see more clearly what has been happening. Much like an alcoholic with allergies to yeast and grains, people with such food addictions may tend to binge on the allergenic foods, especially when they are under psychological stress.

A wide variety of symptoms are possible with food allergy-addictions. Randolph and Moss's *An Alternative Approach to Allergies* offers a very advanced and somewhat complex analysis of the many theories and symptoms of food allergies, noting that the addiction occurs in two phases, stimulatory and withdrawal. During the stimulatory cycle, when we eat the food, we experience a decrease in symptoms; when we avoid it, we experience a "hangover" and an increase in symptoms. In the withdrawal phase, we experience initially a worsening of symptoms and then improvement. When we re-expose ourselves to the food, we often get a marked increase in symptoms and a clearer picture of the problem.

Children experience food reactions quite commonly. Cerebral symptoms may occur, leading to hyperactivity, poor attention, and difficulty in learning, as well as many other physical symptoms. Often, isolating the allergens, which may be foods and/or chemicals in foods, and eliminating them from the diet can make a huge difference in the life of the affected child, and consequently, in the lives of his or her parents and siblings.

What foods are most commonly connected to these allergies? Dr. Rinkel's research led him to conclude that "the constant, monotonous intake of any food promotes the development of a food allergy in a susceptible person." The foods he found most frequently to cause reactions were wheat, eggs, milk, coffee, corn, yeast, beef, and pork.

Although different practitioners report different lists of foods that they find to be commonly allergenic—for example, some include corn, soy products, cane sugar, or nuts, while others do not—all agree that wheat, milk, and eggs are the top three; yeast is another common allergen. All of these foods not only are consumed daily by most people but also are found as components of many other foods, giving us repeated exposures daily. In general, infrequently eaten foods less likely lead to allergies.

Causes of Allergies

The causes of allergies are, I believe, multiple. There is, of course, the genetic predisposition, which is clearly established in the atopic diseases of hay fever, asthma, and eczema but may also predispose us to many others. Eating habits during the first year of life may influence our potential for allergy more than anything else, even heredity. Feeding babies solid foods too early and not breastfeeding them is a primary way to cause allergies and, thus, produce many problems in infants. Cow's milk and baby formulas provide large molecules that are difficult for the infant's immature gastrointestinal tract and immune system to handle. Gluten allergy from early feeding of grains such as wheat, corn, and oats is also common. The best way to prevent allergies, particularly childhood ones, is to breastfeed a child exclusively for six months before introducing solid foods. (See *Infancy* program.) Even in adults, poor digestion, with low levels of hydrochloric acid or pancreatic enzymes, is an underlying cause of many food reactions.

The digestive process is tied to allergies, particularly to foods, as Dr. Michael Rosenbaum and Dominic Bosco clearly concur with in their book, *Super Fitness Beyond Vitamins*. The problem starts with incomplete digestion that results from improper chewing of food and poor action of hydrochloric acid, pancreatic enzymes, and bile. These are influenced by stress and by excessive fluid intake around meals. The incomplete digestion along with the "leaky gut" that comes from inflammation in the gastrointestinal mucosa—resulting from stress, the intake of fried and fatty foods, as well as chemicals, and the presence of parasites or *Candida albicans*—allow absorption of larger molecules that then generate an immune reaction. (Also, please note: Low-level infectious microorganisms may also create allergic propensity; I believe this is common with worms, other parasites, yeasts, and certain bacteria.) Chronic stress affects pancreatic and adrenal function which are tied to digestion, energy level, and food cravings.

The key here is to minimize food allergies by enhancing digestion—chewing well, eating good foods, lowering stress, and supporting digestive juices. Decreasing inflammation and healing the gut, treating any abnormally present microorganisms, supporting immune and glandular functions, and stimulating proper detoxification will all help minimize food reactions, and allergies in general. Many nutrients, which will be discussed shortly, can support all of these functions as well.

Toxicity in the environment is another probable cause for the increasing numbers of allergic people. Exposure to many more irritating and allergenic substances also may adversely affect our immune function. Today, many people are reacting to new synthetic products and pollutants in the air. Formaldehyde, hydrocarbons, and carbon monoxide in the air as well as many industrial or food chemicals found in food, such as the antibiotics, certain food colors, sulfites, MSG, and sodium benzoate, may all stimulate allergic responses as well as lower our immunity. There are many other chemicals that are not easy to diagnose or avoid. Living as natural a life as possible, avoiding polluted areas and chemicals, is the best we can do.

Stress also plays a major role in allergies by dysregulating immune functions and by weakening adrenal response. Stress can also directly influence our digestive function, which I believe can be a core factor in allergies. Chronic stress may lead to a reduction of hydrochloric acid output (initially it may raise HCl secretions) and digestive enzyme function, so that we do not break down our food properly. Absorption of larger food molecules into the blood may lead to increased antibody responses and subsequent allergies. Furthermore, the effects of stress on our immune system can lead to an increase in infections, which contribute to both environmental and food allergies. For example, parasitic intestinal infections may act as direct allergens and also increase other allergic responses. In addition, other aspects of stress, including emotional and mental stress, anxiety, and fatigue, all increase susceptibility to allergies. Menstrual stress (hormonal changes) also seems to increase allergic reactions.

Abuse of chemicals and refined foods is another factor that can cause or exacerbate allergies. This can also enhance stress levels and weaken immunity, and may lead to nutritional deficiencies—another problem that increases allergic sensitivity. Low nutrient levels of vitamin C, most B vitamins, vitamin A, and many minerals influence body function sufficiently to weaken allergic resistance.

Excess or repeated contact with particular foods and substances in the environment causes allergies. It usually takes a few days for our immune system, mainly our T lymphocytes, to be sensitized to an antigen and guide the formation of antibodies by B lymphocytes. After that, reactions to exposures are immediate and usually produce mild immune-inflammatory responses. Initially, histamine released by other cells causes some redness, swelling, and fluid release and also stimulates the T cell antibody activity. Later exposures create repeated antigen-antibody responses, which can have a variety of effects on the tissues and bodily functions.

Temperature extremes also influence many people's allergic problems and generally increase susceptibility to allergies. Quick changes of temperature, particularly going from heat to air conditioning, may themselves produce symptoms such as sinus congestion, skin rash, hives, or even asthmatic attacks.

The causes of allergies are indeed a complex issue. Everything from our genes to our spiritual awareness is a factor, with diet and stress levels being especially important. The traditional Chinese medical viewpoint suggests that allergies reflect internal balance or imbalance, mainly of the wood (liver) and metal (lungs and colon) elements, as well as being a result of general energy congestion. If that is the case, then rebalancing these organs within the entire energy system will help improve allergic symptoms. I have seen improvement with acupuncture treatments along with some liver and colon detoxification through diet and herbs.

Just as there are many causes, there are also many symptoms related to allergies, both gross and subtle, visible and invisible. Often acute symptoms such as fatigue, itching, or a runny nose can progress to a chronic problem with repeated exposure, especially to food allergens; such difficulties as headache, depression, or arthritis may follow. Really, any of the inflammatory "itis" diseases, such as colitis, arthritis, dermatitis, and bronchitis, can come from allergies.

Allergy Evaluation

Evaluating allergies is another complex and controversial issue. There are a number of tests available to evaluate environmental and food allergies. Skin testing is probably the best way to isolate specific environmental allergens, because these are harder to detect ourselves, especially for substances such as pollens. Molds may be a bit easier to isolate, as by noticing our reactions upon going into a damp house. Allergies to animals are often fairly simple to identify, though many of us deny our chronic reaction to our beloved cat or dog. There are many techniques for skin testing. I prefer the Rinkel method because it individualizes the analysis and treatment plan. Some doctors use group antigen testing, mixing a variety of pollens or animal danders together. This is simpler and usually less costly and time consuming, though not always as effective, especially in patients with more complex problems.

When it comes to foods, the source of most allergies, skin testing is not as useful. Only a small percentage of reactions may be found through this method. That is why traditional allergists believe that all the brouhaha over food allergies is unwarranted. But many allergy-oriented family doctors know that food allergies are indeed important, and the basis of many problems. (One of these is Dr. Theron Randolph, who set up an inpatient clinical ecology unit at a Chicago hospital, where he isolates people from most allergens and then tests them with one allergen at a time.)

POSSIBLE ALLERGY SYMPTOMS AND PROBLEMS

Fatigue	Runny nose	Weight gain
Headaches	Postnasal drip	Obesity
Learning disabilities	Sinus congestion	Weight swings
Hyperactivity	Canker sores	Binge eating
Emotional outbursts	Earaches	Overeating
Mood swings	Tinnitis	Frequent hunger
Irritability	Ear congestion	Joint pain
Depression	Recurrent ear infections	Swelling of hands or feet
Muscle aches	Cough	Arthritis, juvenile
Muscle weakness	Sore throat	Arthritis, rheumatoid
Anxiety	Hoarseness	Alcoholism
Disorientation	Chest congestion	Drug addiction
Poor thinking	Itching	Cigarette smoking
"Brain fag"	Hives	Asthma
Stomachache	Eczema	Hay fever
Diarrhea	Nonspecific rash	Regional ileitis
Constipation	Palpitations	Ulcerative colitis
Nausea	Tachycardia	Seizures
Vomiting	Edema	Bloating
Dark circles under eyes	Heartburn	Vaginal itching
Recurrent vaginitis	Loss of sex drive	

Some tests are fairly good for measuring food allergies; techniques have improved in recent years. The RAST (Radio Allergo Sorbent Test), which measures IgG or IgE antibodies to specific food antigens, is probably the best. It is costly, but it can give us the most accurate results for a large number of foods all at once. Cytotoxic testing, which measures the cellular response (mainly of white blood cells) to food antigens, has fallen into disuse because of lack of accuracy of many labs due to the subjective nature of the test. A newer, computerized technique, ALCAT, which measures white blood cell reactions to food antigens, may be a more useful test.

There are tests that completely evaluate and correlate allergic reactions to food with actual patient experiences. Self-testing or a clinical form of self-testing is really the best. These include a variety of techniques using a general method called provocative testing, where the patient receives sublingual drops of foods, ingests capsules containing powdered foods, or eats whole foods. Ideally, the patient does not know what food is being tested and has not eaten it for several days, for then reactions will be most clear. However, in a clinical setting, a patient may know what food is being tested, may have eaten it within the last 12–24 hours, and may have only 30 minutes to observe a reaction. All these factors make this type of test less accurate. It may take longer than the time allotted to react to a food, and our psyche often influences our reactions when we know what food is being tested. In addition, when several foods are tested on the same day, overlapping reactions may occur.

The best practical testing involves following an elimination diet and then consuming various suspect foods and watching for reactions over 24 hours. This means that only one food a day can be tested if the results are to be accurate. The absolute best test, of course, is a double-blind test, where neither the patient nor the clinician knows what food extract is in those funny little capsules and the specific reactions are quantified over a period of at least three or four hours, and even up to one or two days. This, however, is not very practical.

Food elimination testing is not really easy, because it requires self-discipline, but it is fairly simple in technique. It can be helpful for isolating not only what foods are involved but also what kinds of reactions occur from each food. As mentioned earlier, many food allergies (as well as "intolerances" and "sensitivities") and symptoms are masked by addictive behavior, so a food elimination plan is needed to uncover them.

The advantage of food elimination or avoidance and retesting is that it helps the body release these addictions, so that retesting the food will reveal the actual allergy. It is also inexpensive and offers us a valuable direct experience of our food reactions. Its disadvantages are that it is time consuming and sometimes difficult to fit into our everyday life and that the results are based on our subjective experience, so that accuracy is dependent on a significant short-term reaction (many food reactions are not immediate) and high awareness of our body's functioning. Yet, overall, food elimination testing can be very valuable. And if it does not reveal clear findings and we still suspect food allergies, then a blood antibody (RAST) test can be done.

The elimination diet involves avoiding any foods that are commonly reactive, that we suspect are causing reactions, or that we eat regularly. This is best done for from four to seven days before testing is begun. If symptoms persist, the avoidance period may need to be several weeks long. If after this time there is no improvement, either allergenic foods are still being eaten or, more likely, food allergy is not the problem.

Another testing method involves doing a short fast on water or juices, which will clear addictive foods and resensitize the body. In my first book, I describe a lengthy food elimination program whereby individual food groups are eliminated one by one until we get down to a few days of only juice and water before individual foods are tested. A simpler technique would be to eat a diet that contains only foods that are unlikely to be allergenic. These include all fruits except citrus; all vegetables except corn; white or brown rice (but no other grains; other starches could include hard squashes and sweet potatoes); turkey (and chicken if it is not regularly consumed); deep-sea whitefish—halibut, swordfish, sole (no shellfish or salmon); walnuts, almonds, and sunflower seeds (in moderation). However, if any of these foods have been eaten regularly or craved, they should be avoided. If symptoms develop during the avoidance (or testing) period, 1–2 grams of vitamin C should be taken every couple of hours. The buffered ascorbates with minerals or bicarbonate are usually helpful. Withdrawal symptoms are not at all common during the avoidance phase, but they may occur.

What to Eat for an Allergy Elimination Diet

- All fruits, except citrus
- All vegetables, except corn, tomatoes
- Brown or white rice
- Turkey
- White fish—halibut, sole, or swordfish
- Almonds, walnuts, or sunflower seeds

The best thing about food elimination is that it is usually an important part of the treatment as well as of the evaluation. After testing, the new diet becomes our individualized therapeutic diet. To test foods, though, only one food should be consumed at a time. This is termed a "challenge." Testing foods singly is the only way to really follow what our reaction, if any, will be. Since it is possible to react to chemicals, preservatives, and pesticides on foods, it is wise to use whole organic foods whenever possible.

There are two approaches to this testing method. The first is to eat "mono meals," consisting of a moderate to large portion of an individual food, and then to monitor any reactions to that food over the next three or four hours. In this way, several foods can be tested in a day. I generally suggest this method following a short fast because the body is in a cleaner state and able to respond more clearly to food challenges. For basic food testing, it may be more appropriate and simpler just to create a diet of foods found to be safe through the elimination phase and then build on that, trying new ones. Again, only one new food should be added at a time; adding only one per day is ideal rather than three of four, which could confuse our responses. Use the less potentially allergenic foods first, before attempting a wheat, egg, or milk challenge. Some people will want to try their most suspected foods first, and this can be all right, though it may interfere with further testing if there is a positive reaction.

If we do react positively to a food, then we eliminate it again for three to six weeks before retesting. This will help to reduce the allergy and reduce antibody levels, so that we may not react as much or even at all. Certain food reactions are fairly fixed, and we may need to completely avoid the foods that cause them. However, we will be able to tolerate most foods if we eat them infrequently or work them into a new "rotary-diversified" diet, where most foods are rotated on a four-day basis—part of our food allergy diet therapy.

It is important to keep a journal during food testing and record any reactions—how we feel before, immediately after, and in the several hours (even up to 12–24) after consuming a food. If we leave it all to memory, we may miss subtle reactions or forget what happened. This also increases our food awareness. Most of us have not been trained to observe how we feel after we eat a meal.

Monitoring our pulse rate is another aid to evaluating food reactions. If we take our pulse often enough to know our basic resting pulse and become efficient in the technique, we can record our pulse before and after consuming a food or meal. If it increases by more than 12–14 beats per minute after eating, one of the foods may be an allergen. We should check our pulse about five minutes after eating and at fifteen-minute intervals for the next hour. The "pulse test" devised by Arthur Coca, M.D., can be used as a more subtle physiological evaluation as well as to monitor alongside actual symptoms.

Allergy Treatment

Treatment of allergies is also rather diversified and somewhat complex. The standard medical approach is to use antihistamine or immunosuppressive steroid drugs to reduce symptoms; a more corrective approach involves the isolation of specific allergens through skin testing and then to do desensitization through shots, as well as avoid allergen exposure where possible. This is the usual procedure for environmental allergies and common problems such as hay fever and asthma; however as previously mentioned, this process is not very useful for discovering or treating most food reactions. For hay fever or asthma, cromolyn sodium works well but must be taken regularly for several weeks to be effective. There are obviously hundreds of drugs available for allergic conditions, but our focus here is to try to be drug-free. With drug or food reactions, the approach is usually avoidance of the allergenic agents, if they can be determined.

Most medical treatment for allergies is not curative but is aimed at reducing symptoms. Ideally, we want to correct and heal the body so that we become less congested and less allergic. Before even thinking about medical investigation and treatment, it is wise to do what we can ourselves first. Reducing stress, eating a good diet, and taking nutritional supplements will often work very rapidly to reduce allergic symptoms. The elimination diet or even a short fast can help us identify and handle food allergies. I personally would begin a detoxification program, use herbs and supplements, and probably have acupuncture treatments; I believe that this would give me the best chance for rapid recovery. If necessary, I will offer skin testing and desensitization to my patients, and this is also helpful; it is just more time-consuming and expensive. To help in allergy treatment, it is also important to pay attention to our gastrointestinal tract. If yeast infections or parasites are present, treating for these problems is often helpful. Many allergic people have weak digestion and are low in hydrochloric acid and digestive enzyme production, and supplementing these is often beneficial.

I believe that changing our diet itself can aid in preventing and treating all kinds of allergies, especially those to foods, which are very common. Often, just eliminating "reactive" foods from our diet can reduce symptoms of other allergies.

The most common diet for allergies is the standard four-day rotation plan (one of the basics of the Ideal Diet discussed in Part Three), emphasizing fresh, wholesome, unprocessed foods. For the very sensitive person, or for those with difficult digestion, prepare foods in easily digestible forms, such as soups or fresh juices. It takes four days for our body to clear the food we have eaten. By rotating this way, we prevent the

ALLERGY DIET

Eat whole, unadulterated foods
Diversify the diet
Rotate foods
Rotate food families
Eat only nonallergenic foods at first

chronic buildup of antibodies and reduce possible allergic reactions. After antibody levels decrease and these "reactive" foods again become tolerated, they should not be consumed regularly since they may generate reactions as before. Other foods should also be rotated to prevent becoming "sensitive" to them as well.

The high-water-content nutritious foods in the Ideal Diet will support the body's detoxification and healing processes. Eliminating reactive foods reduces cravings and allows satiety to be reached sooner; smaller amounts of better-quality foods are usually easier to digest. This diet usually produces steady weight loss in people who are overweight; normal-weight or underweight people will usually have less or no weight loss on the Ideal Diet, but may need to increase food intake for maintenance.

Fasting and detoxification programs are often very beneficial for allergic conditions. A body that is less "congested" is less allergic. In working with hundreds of allergic patients through the years, I have found short fasts to be helpful for a vast majority of people. With allergies, the focus of the "cleansing" fast is the liver and colon. Lemon water or the "lemonade fast" (see the *Fasting* program in Chapter 18) helps the liver, while general juice fasting with a cleansing of the colon through enemas or colonic irrigations can make an incredible difference.

For seasonal allergies that are fairly predictable, it is often helpful to do a fast a week or two before the usual onset of symptoms. This is most commonly in the spring, which is naturally the season for cleansing. The beginning of the spring is the best time to clear out bad habits and past addictions, and to create our new diet and lifestyle plan. Of course, after the fast, it is important to introduce foods slowly and to be aware of any reactions.

There are many nutrients and supplements that may be helpful in reducing allergic symptoms. I have often seen improvement with a simple program of a multiple vitamin-mineral supplement with an extra 2–3 grams of vitamin C and 500 mg. of pantothenic acid (B_5). The vitamins C and B_5 help to ameliorate the impacts of stress by supporting the weakened adrenals; the adrenal corticosteroids released can then minimize the allergic-inflammatory response. Vitamin C can also be used for any withdrawal symptoms or for reactions secondary to food intake, and higher levels have an antihistaminic effect.

Along with Vitamin C, its supportive bioflavonoids could be added. Many have anti-inflammatory and antiallergy affects. Quercetin is a particular one that has been shown in research to reduce histamine levels and allergy symptoms. My experience with myself and many patients is very favorable. An amount of 250–600 mg. daily in several doses is needed for the effect. Quercezyme Plus, a product by Enzymatic Therapy, is one I particularly like.

In addition to these above-mentioned nutrients, other B vitamins are also helpful. Folic acid, B_6, and B_{12} all support antibody formation. The pyridoxal-5-phosphate form of vitamin B_6 may be particularly helpful in the allergic patient. It has an apparent anti-inflammatory effect, and as the active metabolite of pyridoxine, it works more directly. It is possible that allergy patients do not phosphorylate pyridoxine very easily. Repeated, small doses of niacin (10–50 mg.) will cause release of histamine and may contribute to increased allergy symptoms initially. Regular niacin flushes, though, will within days reduce stores of histamine, which may then help lessen allergic symptoms; then, continued niacin use will maintain those lower levels of histamine and allergy symptoms.

Vitamin A, about 20,000 IUs per day, and zinc, 50–100 mg., are both helpful in alleviating allergy symptoms and in preventing infections. They also help to heal the gastrointestinal mucosa, along with vitamin C, and they improve or normalize the antibody response to antigens, which is often "out of whack" in people with allergies. Other minerals besides zinc, particularly manganese, may also be useful. Magnesium, selenium and chromium are also frequently beneficial.

The fat-soluble nutrients are also needed. Vitamin E, about 800 IUs per day, is a helpful protectant of membranes. Gamma-linolenic acid (GLA) from evening primrose oil, borage, or black currant seeds, is being found to be an effective nutrient in the reduction of allergic symptoms. This is probably due to the anti-inflammatory effects of the Series 1 and 3 prostaglandins that are formed from GLA. Six to eight capsules daily (200–400 mg. total GLA), divided into several portions, are usually effective. Other anti-inflammatory nutrients include EPA, vitamins A, B_5, B_6, and C, bioflavonoids, zinc, and the enzyme bromelain. The antioxidants, including beta-carotene, vitamin E, selenium, zinc, vitamin C, and dimethylglycine, may also help with inflammation and immune support.

L-amino acids can also be helpful by stabilizing energy levels and supporting immune components and functions. As mentioned earlier, people with allergies often have poor digestion, particularly for proteins; L-amino acids are a simple, quick way to obtain these building blocks. Digestive support is also very useful in allergic patients. Better breakdown, assimilation, and metabolism of foods reduces allergic components and irritations in the gastrointestinal tract and has often been seen to reduce symptoms as well. Taking hydrochloric acid tablets with meals, followed by digestive enzymes after eating, is a good beginning plan; of course, for anyone with hyperacidity, ulcer symptoms or other abdominal pains, this is not recommended. Many formulas, such as Zypan, made by Standard Process Labs, combine both digestive enzymes and hydrochloric acid in one tablet. When such formulas are used, usually two or three tablets (depending on meal size) can be taken just after meals (especially after meals that contain high amounts of proteins and fats).

Additional fiber can provide mild colon detoxification. Supplemental psyllium and bran can be added to a good high-fiber diet. Garlic in the diet can also help with detoxification, as can the supplement sodium alginate, which lessens possible heavy metal toxicity. Betonite clay (montmorillonite) is a strong absorbent that binds chemicals, metals and other impurities in the gut. It also, as do most of the fiber molecules, has the potential to bind minerals such as calcium and zinc.

A recently formulated physiological sulfur, methylsulfonylmethane (MSM), has been shown to have anti-inflammatory effects on the mucous membranes. Thus, it may be helpful for both food allergies (by helping to heal the gut) and for inhalant allergies. It also may be a useful nutrient for those with arthritis. MSM is a naturally occurring sulfur metabolite in human tissues and is present in high amounts in breast milk. A beginning amount is one 500 mg. capsule daily, going up to three or four capsules daily.

Other possibly helpful supplements, especially in the acutely allergic patient, include organic germanium (Ge-132) and possibly Coenzyme Q_{10} (CoQ_{10}) and superoxide dismutase (SOD), as per the experience of many practitioners, including Lester Rose, M.D., of San Jose, California. Dr. Rose has recommended for allergies, as well as for chronic candidiasis and chronic Epstein-Barr syndrome, a combination of Ge-132 (600 mg. daily tapering to 150 mg. over three weeks), CoQ_{10} (60 mg. twice daily), SOD (3 tablets upon arising), and a multiple without iron.

Many people also try a glandular supplement approach in treating allergies. Adrenal is often the first choice to support the body's ability to handle stress and allergies. Thymus gland tablets may help strengthen cell-mediated immunity, though this is not well proven. Liver extracts are also used sometimes. Another approach is to conduct a general evaluation of organ strengths and weaknesses and then to use particular glandulars to create the proper balance. If glands or extracts of glands are chosen, they should be free of pesticides, herbicides, and other agricultural chemicals as well as free of viruses.

Many herbs are commonly used in the treatment of allergies, to strengthen the immune system and lungs, to promote detoxification, and to reduce inflammation and histamine-mediated allergy symptoms. A good herbal allergy formula consists of ephedra, echinacea, wild cherry bark, white willow bark, mullein leaves, cayenne pepper, and garlic. Ephedra (ma huang) and echinacea are often used together. Ephedra causes vasoconstriction, echinacea improves the white blood cell response, and both have been shown to lower IgE levels. Wild cherry bark, coltsfoot leaf, and mullein leaves are lung-strengthening herbs; white willow bark is an anti-inflammatory; cayenne supports circulation; and garlic assists in detoxification.

Some other lung-strengthening herbs include pleurisy root, horehound, and licorice root. Licorice also supports the adrenals and soothes the digestive tract. Other soothing herbs include slippery elm bark and marshmallow root. Comfrey root, which contains the tissue-supporting nutrient allantoin, is useful for helping to heal the intestinal lining.

Some people have reported experiencing a reduction of local hay fever and pollen-allergy symptoms by the use of small amounts of bee pollen. Eating one to three grains at first and increasing the number of grains slowly over a period of a few weeks seems to have benefited some pollen allergy sufferers. I do not recommend this, however, because the types of pollens present may vary, and some may cause a temporary worsening of symptoms.

HERBAL ALLERGY FORMULA

Ephedra	Echinacea
Wild cherry bark	White willow bark
Mullein leaves	Cayenne pepper
Garlic	

Mix equal amounts into "00" capsules or a tea.
Take two capsules three times daily.

The following table presents suggested daily amounts, taken in several portions, of the essential nutrients and other supplements for reducing allergic potential and minimizing allergy symptoms.

ALLERGY NUTRIENT PROGRAM

Water	2–3 qt.
Fiber	10–15 g.

Vitamin A	20,000 IUs*	**Magnesium**	300–600 mg.
Beta-carotene	20,000 IUs	**Manganese**	10 mg.
Vitamin D	400 IUs	**Molybdenum**	500 mcg.
Vitamin E	800 IUs	**Selenium**	200 mcg.
Vitamin K	300 mcg.	**Sulfur (as methyl-**	
Thiamine (B$_1$)	50 mg.	** sulfonylmethane)**	500–1,500 mg.
Riboflavin (B$_2$)	50 mg.	**Silicon**	100 mg.
Niacin (B$_3$)	100 mg.	**Zinc**	60 mg.
Niacinamide (B$_3$)	50–100 mg.		
Pantothenic acid (B$_5$)	1,500 mg.	*Others:*	
Pyridoxine (B$_6$)	50–100 mg.	**L-amino acids**	1,500 mg.
Pyridoxal-5-phosphate	50–100 mg.	**L-cysteine**	250–500 mg.
Cobalamin (B$_{12}$)	100 mcg.	**Gamma-linolenic acid**	6 capsules
Folic acid	800 mcg.		or 240–480 mg.
Biotin	1,000 mcg.	**Lactobacillus**	1–2 billion organisms
PABA	150 mg.	**Coenzyme Q$_{10}$**	30–60 mg.
Vitamin C	4–8 g.	**Organo-germanium**	75–300 mg.
Bioflavonoids	250–750 mg.	**Dimethylglycine**	50–100 mg.
Quercetin	250–600 mg.	**Hydrochloric acid**	10–15 g.
		** (betaine)**	
Calcium	600–1,000 mg.	** (with meals)**	
Chromium	200 mcg.	**Digestive enzymes**	2–3 tablets
Copper	2–3 mg.	** (after meals)**	
Iodine	150 mcg.	**Bromelain**	100 mg.
Iron	18 mg.	** (between meals)**	
		Adrenal	100 mg.
		Thymus	100 mg.
		Liver	100 mg.
		Sodium alginate	300–450 mg.

_____

*Limit this amount to 6 weeks, then cut back to 5,000–10,000 IUs daily

Birth Control Pills

Birth control pills (BCPs) are both the most effective and the most hazardous form of contraception. Preventing pregnancy in this way is done by taking an oral dose of a combination of the hormones estrogen and progestin (synthetic progesterone) in amounts higher than the body's natural levels. This prevents the pituitary hormones that stimulate ovulation and fertilization of the egg from being released, and thus prevents pregnancy.

Though taking oral contraceptives regularly is 99 percent effective in birth control, there are many possible side effects. Weight gain, emotional swings, circulatory and vascular symptoms, and gastrointestinal upset are not uncommon. Blood clots, liver problems, and cancer are also possible, though relatively rare; these were more common in the 1960s with the higher-dose pills. Many women have difficulty with oral contraceptives, though many others seem to tolerate them well. The use of birth control pills is more common in young women and teenagers, which adds another dimension of uncertainty regarding the nutritional effects of these drugs.

Oral contraceptives may create certain nutrient deficiencies and excesses as well as increase the nutritional needs of the user. Most of the B vitamins, particularly pyridoxine (B_6) and folic acid, are needed in higher amounts when birth control pills are taken. The copper level usually rises, and zinc levels often fall. Thus, more zinc is needed as well. An increased need for vitamins C, E, and K may also result from the use of birth control pills.

In *Nutrition and Vitamin Therapy,* Michael Lesser, M.D., points out that birth control pills cause an alkaline imbalance in the vagina that may lead to increased susceptibility to infection. Extra ascorbic acid, 1–2 grams per day, may help balance the acid environment and prevent this problem. He and other authors also suggest that the increased blood levels of copper generated by oral contraceptive use may contribute to depression and emotional symptoms; additional manganese and zinc may reverse these symptoms. Sharon DeBuren, nurse practitioner and nutritionist, adds that the depression from BCPs is also neurochemical reaction to artificial steroids (female hormones), and from a lack of a women's own superior hormones—estradiol and natural progesterone secreted with ovulation. Iron levels may also rise, and less iron may be required because the pills often reduce the amount of menstrual blood loss, as well.

Because BCPs are metabolized by the liver before being eliminated, a diet low in other liver irritants is suggested. Alcohol, cocaine, and other drugs, pesticides and preservative chemicals in food, as well as fried foods should be avoided. Cutting down on refined foods and sugary treats is also suggested; these foods are "empty" calories and may cause further nutrient depletion. Avoiding nicotine and fried foods is also a good idea to prevent further vascular irritation. Teenage girls on "the pill" must also be particularly careful to avoid nutritional deficiencies, and all would be well advised to take a supportive nutritional supplement. Adequate intake of the antioxidant nutrients, such as vitamins C and E, selenium, and beta-carotene, can help reduce potential toxicity of oral contraceptives. The herb, milk thistle, contains silymarin and may be especially helpful.

A high-nutrient diet is the best prevention for problems. Low-fat protein levels and nutritious foods such as whole grains, vegetables, nuts, and seeds are also important. Eating lots of vegetables is the best way to prevent many mineral deficits and also maintain weight. And several teaspoons of cold-pressed vegetable oil, particularly olive oil, should also be used daily to ensure the intake of the essential fatty acids. All of the above-mentioned foods, along with protein intake from such foods as eggs, fish, poultry, dairy foods, and legumes, is a sensible approach. In addition to the usual female adult or teenage levels, if taking oral contraceptives it is recommended that intake of the following nutrients be increased to the levels listed:

Nutrient	Daily Amounts (in 1 or 2 doses)
Vitamin B_6	50–100 mg.
Vitamin B_{12}	50–200 mcg.
Folic acid	600–800 mcg.
Vitamin E	400–600 IUs
Vitamin C	1–3 g.
Zinc	20–40 mg.

Other B vitamins can also be increased to higher levels, such as an additional 25 mg. of each, to balance out the B complex. More antioxidants can also help reduce the deleterious effects of the drugs. These include beta-carotene, selenium, and possibly amino acid L-cysteine to complement the additional vitamins C and E.

Copper intake in supplements should be limited to 1 mg., though the increased zinc intake will help lower copper levels. Whole grains, nuts, seeds, and vegetables will ensure that copper requirements are met. Iron supplements may be decreased somewhat with use of birth control pills unless the menstrual periods are heavy or there is anemia. Iron needs are probably reduced from the usual 18 mg. to around 12–15 mg per day. All of these values can be checked occasionally by blood biochemistry profiles or evaluation of mineral levels to ensure proper individualized care.

NUTRIENT PROGRAM FOR ORAL CONTRACEPTIVES

Water	1½–2 qt.

Vitamin A	5,000–10,000 IUs	Calcium*	600–1,000 mg.
Beta-carotene	10,000–20,000 IUs	Chromium	200–400 mcg.
Vitamin D	200–400 IUs	Copper	1–2 mg.
Vitamin E	400–600 IUs	Iron	15–20 mg.
Thiamine (B_1)	25–50 mg.	Magnesium*	400–600 mg.
Riboflavin (B_2)	25–50 mg.	Manganese	5–10 mg.
Niacin or niacinamide (B_3)	25–50 mg.	Molybdenum	150–300 mcg.
Pantothenic acid (B_5)	50–250 mg.	Phosphorus	600–800 mg.
Pyridoxine (B_6)	25–50 mg.	Potassium	1–2 g.
Cobalamin (B_{12})	50–200 mcg.	Selenium	150–300 mcg.
Folic acid	600–800 mcg.	Zinc	30–60 mg.
Biotin	200–400 mcg.		
PABA	25–50 mg.	Fatty acids, olive, or Flaxseed oils	1–2 teaspoons
Vitamin C	1–3 g.		
Bioflavonoids	250–500 mg.		

*Calcium and magnesium are best supplemented as citrates or aspartates.

Premenstrual Syndrome

Premenstrual syndrome (PMS) is a recently described problem. Although the history of symptoms that occur around the menstrual cycle is ancient, it is likely that modern-day women, with increased demands and stresses, changes in nutrition, and new careers that take them away from their natural cycle and their connection to the home, garden, and nature, are particularly susceptible to such symptoms. Women might think about these symptoms as a call of the womb and the moon to be more attuned to their female cycle. It may not be easy, but I believe it is possible for women to stay connected to their female cycles and still be active and productive in the outer world. This may require more care in regard to nutrition and a supplement program that counteracts stress while supporting the female organs and hormone functions. Stress (and being out of touch with emotions or not following their true emotions) is definitely a big factor in women's premenstrual symptoms.

The current medical theories about PMS or, as it is sometimes termed, premenstrual tension (PMT), relate it to an estrogen-progesterone imbalance, particularly reactions to the increased estradiol levels. During the second half of the cycle, after ovulation, progesterone levels normally rise, while estrogen levels also rise slightly. These changes can influence water retention, causing some fullness of the uterus and other body tissues; this seems to be exaggerated premenstrually with the relatively deficient level of progesterone. Many of the symptoms, such as bloating, breast swelling and tenderness, fatigue, headaches, emotional irritability, depression, back pain, and pelvic pain, are probably a result of the water retention and subsequent emotional tension. Other hormonal and physiological factors, or effects on the immune system, may contribute to the problem as well. Less common symptoms include dizziness, fainting, cystitis, hives, acne, sore throat, joint pains and swelling, and constipation.

Low progesterone levels seem to be the main factor in PMS symptoms. Why progesterone levels may be low has not yet been determined, but many women seem to respond to treatment with progesterone in the second half of their cycle, from just after ovulation to the usual time of menstruation. A common treatment is to use vaginal or rectal suppositories containing progesterone (or even topical progesterone) once or twice daily. The newer treatment is oral, micronized progesterone that is not destroyed by the gastrointestinal tract or broken down by the liver. Usually, however, progesterone therapy is not needed, because most women will respond to a nutritional and herbal approach to treating PMS. Many nutrients are needed, but probably the two most important ones are vitamin B_6 (pyridoxine) and magnesium. B_6 helps to clear water through a diuretic effect on the kidneys. Usually 50–100 mg. once or twice daily will be effective. A complete B vitamin supplement is also necessary to prevent these higher amounts of B_6 from causing imbalances of other B vitamins. It has been theorized and shown in some studies that magnesium deficiency within the cells is also correlated with some of the PMS symptoms. Supplementing magnesium at amounts equal to up to one and a half times the calcium level, that is, about 800–1,200 mg., is helpful in reducing some PMS symptoms. Zinc is also an important mineral here.

Other possible menstrual irregularities, as discussed by Susan Lark, M.D., in the *PMS Self Help Book* (Celestial Arts, Berkeley, CA, 1984), have symptoms that may be related to low estrogen levels. Women with this problem often experience more of their symptoms after their period than before it. This low-estrogen state is far less common than the progesterone deficiency. Occasionally, tests to measure hormonal levels can be done at specific times of the month. However, these are expensive and not always easy to interpret (the range of normal is wide) unless done repeatedly. Generally though, as long as there are relatively regular menstrual periods, these ovarian and pituitary hormone levels will be within normal values. Other tests that may be abnormal include thyroid hormone levels, thyroid antibodies, or antiovarian antibodies, which may represent some autoimmune problems.

Another common symptom, not only of PMS but of most women's premenstrual time, is a craving for sweets. This desire is often enhanced in those with PMS, which brings up another important point. Women with PMS often have other correlating conditions that may contribute to symptoms. These include hypoglycemia (low blood sugar), candidiasis (an overgrowth of and hypersensitivity to the common yeast *Candida albicans*), food and/or environmental allergies, moderate to severe stress, and vitamin and mineral deficiencies. Whether these problems contribute to or are a result of the premenstrual and hormonal problems is not clear, but it is important to evaluate women for these conditions when they either have significant PMS symptoms or do not respond well to treatment. PMS is definitely aggravated by low blood sugar generated by stress and an intake of refined flour and sugar products.

From a dietary point of view, it is important to avoid the food stressors, irritants, and stimulants that, if they do not contribute to the PMS problem in the first place, definitely make it worse. These include sugars and refined foods, caffeine, alcohol, and chemicals. A diet that helps in reducing symptoms is a balanced, wholesome, and high-nutrient one, with lots of whole grains, leafy greens and other vegetables, good protein foods, and some fruits, but a minimum of fruit juice. A hypoglycemic diet of regular meals and protein-oriented snacks is often helpful. If there are yeast or allergy problems, a diet to help with those conditions (see previous programs) would be beneficial. If these problems are not present, extra brewer's yeast, with its high levels of B vitamins and minerals, can be a supportive food. Eating a variety of foods and a modified rotation diet (as is discussed in the *Allergy* program in this chapter) are also helpful in getting the wide range of important nutrients and maximizing food sensitivities. Some women also experience a reduction of symptoms through colon detoxification and a cleansing-type diet high in juices, soups, and salads. Intake of fiber as psyllium or bran started a week before symptoms usually begin will improve colon elimination, and an enema or colonic irrigation at the time symptoms begin might be helpful.

Premenstrual syndrome is more common in women in their 30s and 40s than in those in their 20s and teenage years. Dr. Lark points out a number of other factors associated with an increased likelihood of PMS problems—these include women who are or have been married, do not exercise, have had children, experience side effects from birth control pills, have had a pregnancy complicated by toxemia, have a significant amount of emotional stress in their lives, or those whose nutritional habits lead to certain deficiencies or excesses. Dietary factors that worsen PMS include foods high in refined sugars and fats, processed or chemical foods, caffeine drinks (coffee, tea, colas), alcohol (especially wine and beer with the higher carbohydrate level), chocolate products, eggs, cheese, red meats, and high-salt foods. A natural food diet, of course, will help alleviate the symptoms of PMS.

British physician Katherine Dalton, M.D., was one of the first to describe PMS and offer some therapeutic help. Guy Abraham, an obstetrician-gynecologist, has further classified PMS problems, a system that Dr. Lark also discusses in her book. The four main types are:

1. **Type A ("anxiety")**—a mixture of emotional symptoms: anxiety, irritability, and mood swings.
2. **Type C ("carbohydrates" and "cravings")**—sugar cravings, fatigue, and headaches.
3. **Type H ("hyperhydration"),** also known as Type W ("water retention")—bloating, weight gain, and breast swelling and tenderness.
4. **Type D ("depression")**—depression, confusion, and memory loss.

Other groups of symptoms include acne—oily skin and hair and acne—and dysmenorrhea (painful periods)—cramps, low back pain, nausea, and vomiting; recently classified as Type P for pain.

Dr. Susan Lark's *PMS Self Help Book* provides specific treatment plans for the different types of symptoms. The recommendations for the different types, including diet and suggestions, are all very similar. In her programs, all include some form of stress reduction, exercise, supplementation, herbal therapy, acupressure massage, and yoga postures.

For acne problems with PMS, extra vitamin A (20,000–40,000 IUs, mainly as beta-carotene) and zinc (20–40 mg.) are usually helpful. Choline and inositol, nutrients found in lecithin, may help nourish the skin; 500 mg. of each daily are recommended.

Dysmenorrhea and other pain problems respond well to higher amounts of magnesium, about 500 mg. more than calcium, as this has a nerve tranquilizing and muscle relaxing effect. Vitamin E (400–800 IUs) and vitamin B_6 (100–300 mg. daily) may also be helpful in reducing pain. Extra B vitamins and a general vitamin and mineral program are usually also necessary.

Anxiety symptoms, such as mood swings and irritability, often respond to extra B vitamins, particularly thiamine (B_1), 150–250 mg. per day, and pyridoxine (B_6), 200–300 mg. per day, with about 50 mg. each of the rest of the B vitamins. Using inositol and extra magnesium, such as magnesium citrate (which causes fewer bowel symptoms, especially diarrhea, than other magnesium salts), about 400–600 mg. daily, will help. Progesterone therapy may be most helpful for Type A, or anxiety, problems. A doctor must be consulted for this therapy. Also, phenylethanolamine (PEA), a substance found in certain foods, such as bananas, chocolate, and hard cheeses, may increase symptoms of anxiety. These foods should be avoided in this type of PMS.

For depression, added tryptophan (if available), 1,000 mg. before bed, may be helpful. If this does not help, or if it causes side effects, such as headache, Stuart Berger, in his *Immune Power Diet*, recommends trying another amino-acid, L-phenylalanine, in the same dosage. Zinc, vitamin B_6, and calcium/magnesium may also be beneficial in reducing premenstrual depression.

For women with the Type C, or sugar cravings, pattern, often associated with stress, fatigue, and headaches, confusion, or dizziness, a program that should help reduce these symptoms supplements the basic vitamin and mineral plan with additional B vitamins, particularly B_6, 200–300 mg. per day, and B_1, 150–250 mg. per day; chromium, 200–400 mcg.; vitamin E, 800 IUs; and vitamin C, around 6–8 grams per day. Eating frequent, small meals and avoiding sugar will also be helpful in reducing cravings.

For Type H with water or bloating problems, which can be the most troublesome, causing weight gain, breast tenderness, and general emotional upset, the basic B vitamins, including high amounts of B_6 and supplemental B_1, magnesium, potassium, vitamin E, and evening primrose oil (with GLA, gamma-linolenic acid, as the active ingredient), 1–2 capsules taken three times daily, may be very helpful. (I have seen evening primrose oil be helpful for many women with various PMS symptoms.) Also, with water retention problems, food allergy, particularly to wheat, may be a contributing factor. A trial of a couple of months of avoiding wheat products can aid in providing relief of symptoms. Sometimes the response can be dramatic. Regular exercise is also important in reducing this type of PMS.

Many herbs are helpful in treating PMS. Angelica, or dong quai, is a commonly used herb that acts as an energizer and female tonic when it is taken regularly as capsules (2 capsules twice a day) or as a tea. Ginger root acts as a circulation aid and mild stimulant and is helpful in getting some of that retained water moving. Other diuretic herbs include parsley and juniper berry. Licorice root is a good balancer and seems to provide an "up" feeling when drunk with some ginger as a tea. Their flavors tend to combine well. Valerian root or catnip tea will provide some relaxation when there is general anxiety or irritability. Sarsaparilla is a tonifying (strengthening) herb that supports the hormonal functions and may actually contain some hormones itself. There are also many herbal formulas for treating PMS and for strengthening the female functions. One that I have found helpful to my patients is FE-G (Female General Tonic), made by Professional Botanicals. It contains black haw, licorice, false unicorn root (estrogen-containing plant), ginseng root, ginger, and life root. I recommend 2 capsules two or three times daily, usually for three to six months if it appears helpful. In the first month

PREMENSTRUAL TENSION (PMT)

Type	Main Symptoms	Key Treatment Plans
PMT-A	Anxiety	Magnesium 400–600 mg. per day. Progesterone therapy. Low PEA diet–avoid chocolate, bananas, and hard cheeses.
PMT-D	Depression	Zinc 30–60 mg. per day. Vitamin B_6 100–300 mg. per day. Magnesium 400–600 mg. per day. Tryptophan 1,000–1,500 mg. before bed or 500 mg. two or three times daily.
PMT-H or W	Water retention	Avoid food allergens, particularly wheat. Potassium 1–2 grams per day, plus potassium foods. B complex vitamins with extra B_6, 50–200 mg. per day. Regular exercise.
PMT-P	Pain	Vitamin E 400–800 IUs per day. Magnesium 400–600 mg. per day. Vitamin B_6 100–300 mg. per day.
PMT-C	Cravings	Low-sugar diet. Frequent small meals. Chromium 200–400 mcg. per day.

or two herbs tend to work more slowly and must be taken over a longer period of time than stronger pharmaceuticals. There are many similar formulas available now for PMS and other female problems.

Some doctors also use glandular supplements in treating PMS. In *Super Fitness Beyond Vitamins* (New American Library, New York, 1987), Michael Rosenbaum, M.D., describes his success with the use of pituitary, particularly anterior pituitary, extract in treating stubborn PMS symptoms. Brain and pancreas glandular supplements may also be helpful, Dr. Rosenbaum points out.

There are also many nutritional supplement formulas available for premenstrual syndrome. The table below presents an all-encompassing nutrient program (most of these nutrients are best taken in two or three portions over the course of the day). This may be tailored for specific symptoms by application of the suggestions given earlier. Of course, many of the nutrients listed are consumed in the diet. Supplementation of sodium, potassium, chloride, fluoride, iodine, and phosphorus is usually not necessary, though additional potassium, about 1 to 2 grams, may be helpful in some cases. Even extra vitamins D and K may not be needed. The precursor of B_6 (pyridoxine), pyridoxal-5-phosphate, may actually be more effective than B_6 itself, because some people may not be able to easily convert the pyridoxine to its usable form. Both forms of vitamin B_3 are used; niacin offers some circulatory stimulation and flushing while niacinamide supports the general neuromuscular relaxation of B_3.

I have seen a high rate of success in the improvement and elimination of symptoms in women who change their diets and implement a regular supplement program. I have also heard other gynecologists, family doctors, and nurse practitioners claim that they see nearly an 80 percent success rate with a good program. Of course, learning to deal better with life stresses, relationships, and sexual issues will further increase the likelihood of success.

PREMENSTRUAL SYNDROME NUTRIENT PROGRAM**

Vitamin A	5,000–10,000 IUs	**Calcium**	800–1,000 mg.
Beta-carotene	10,000–20,000 IUs	**Chromium**	200–400 mcg.
Vitamin D	200–600 IUs	**Copper**	1–2 mg.
Vitamin E	400–1,000 IUs	**Iodine***	150–300 mcg.
Vitamin K*	150–300 mcg.	**Iron**	15–20 mg.
Thiamine (B$_1$)	50–250 mg.	**Magnesium**	750–1,500 mg.
Riboflavin (B$_2$)	50–100 mg.	**Manganese**	2.5–15 mg.
Niacin (B$_3$)	25–100 mg.	**Molybdenum**	150–500 mcg.
Niacinamide (B$_3$)	50–100 mg.	**Phosphorus***	800–1,000 mg.
Pantothenic acid (B$_5$)	50–500 mg.	**Potassium***	2.5–5.0 g.
Pyridoxine (B$_6$)	50–200 mg.	**Selenium**	150–300 mcg.
Pyridoxal-5-phosphate	50–150 mg.	**Zinc**	15–30 mg.
Cobalamin (B$_{12}$)	50–200 mcg.		
Folic acid	400–800 mcg.	**Gamma-linolenic acid**	3–6 capsules
Biotin	50–400 mcg.	**Eicosapentaenoic acid (EPA plus DHA)**	1–2 capsules
Choline	500–1,000 mg.	**L-amino acid formula**	1,000 mg.
Inositol	500–1,000 mg.	**L-tryptophan+ (before bed)**	250–500 mg.
PABA	50–100 mg.		
Vitamin C	1–3 g.	**L-phenylalanine (in 2 doses during the day)**	500–1,000 mg.
Bioflavonoids	250–500 mg.		

*These nutrients will not usually be supplemented.

+Only, of course, if L-tryptophan is available.

**Digestive enzymes, herbs, and glandulars may also be helpful in reducing PMS problems.

Pre- and Postsurgery (and Injuries)

This program, although it is simple, can really make a difference—a few changes and supplements can lessen stress, improve healing, and prevent infections after surgery. I have done my own independent research through the years, suggesting a program similar to this for my patients who have had elective surgery, and they have routinely told me that "the doctors and nurses couldn't believe how fast I healed and was up and about"—and invariably there were no complications. In addition, many medical studies reviewing postsurgical healing time and morbidity, particularly from infections, have shown that with a few basic nutritional supplements, namely vitamin A, vitamin C, and zinc, healing time speeds up; in addition, there are fewer complications, and people are out of bed and out of the hospital sooner.

Many doctors, particularly surgeons, resist these findings. I do not know whether this is due to economics or because they just do not want to believe that taking nutrients in higher dosages than "normal" is necessary. I would bet that having patients follow a few basic nutritional suggestions would improve both doctor and patient success. A good nourishing diet and additional vitamin C, vitamin A, and zinc with adequate fluid intake will usually do it. More recently, I have had patients scheduled for elective surgery tell me that their surgeons suggested they take additional supplements starting two weeks prior to their operations, so there may be some progress in regard to nutrition in the general medical profession.

I suggest that anyone having elective surgery should follow this program for three to four weeks prior to and four to six weeks after surgery. With emergency or urgent surgery, it is wise to begin taking the extra supplements as soon as possible and to eat the most nutritious diet available. This program will also work to support tissue healing following an injury, burn, or other traumas or with an infection or sickness that causes tissue damage. My surgical program is designed to increase the reuniting of collagen fibers, facilitate protein metabolism, and strengthen the immune system.

General measures important to healing include proper rest and sleep, fluid intake, and, of course, a nutritious and balanced diet high in fiber and low in fats and junk foods. High-quality protein foods (fish, poultry, eggs, nuts and seeds) are essential because tissue healing requires protein synthesis, so our body needs all of the important amino acids. A "healthy" intestinal flora is also important to health and healing. Additional *Lactobacillus acidophilus* culture may help replenish the colon. The diet should also contain adequate amounts of high-fiber foods (whole grains, vegetables, and legumes), calcium foods (greens, grains, nuts, and small amounts of dairy products), and foods containing essential fatty acids (some nuts, seeds, or vegetable oils). Congestive foods (excess dairy products, sweets, and baked goods) and fatty foods (fried foods, heavy meats, and ham and other cured meats) should be avoided.

Minimizing and handling stress is also essential to keeping the immune system strong, which is in turn important for preventing infections and supporting healing. It is wise to stay away from steroid drugs, both topical and systemic, as they suppress our immune system. Doctors tend to overprescribe and patients to overuse these steroid medicines. Smoking should be stopped or minimized if possible before surgery. Avoiding stimulating drugs, such as coffee and cocaine, and sedating drugs, such as alcohol and marijuana, prior to elective surgery, is also a wise idea.

I usually do not recommend that people fast or make any major diet revisions prior to surgery; rather, they should maintain a nutritious diet with some shifts toward the healthier practices mentioned above. If possible, people should be close to, or just above, their ideal weight for surgery. Obesity increases surgical risks (infection, poor healing), while underweight people often do not have sufficient energy reserves to heal rapidly.

Of course, I recommend a wonderful diet all of the time, but it is a good idea to begin increasing protein intake and adding the healing nutrients a few weeks before surgery to build up both the strength and the tissues. Usually, the diet can be a little lighter a few days prior to surgery, emphasizing more fruits, vegetables, and liquids along with the nutritional supplements. This will help lessen digestive organ stress.

Recovery from surgery takes time. The diet should be a little lighter initially, and low in fats. With any abdominal surgery, often a liquid or soft diet is necessary for a while. This is where protein and/or nutrient powders are useful. There are also more healthful suggestions than the bouillon, jello, coffee, and colas that might be served. Some examples are vegetable and meat broths, fresh juices, light soups, pureed carrots, squash, mashed potatoes, bananas, applesauce, or other fruits or vegetables, progressing to oatmeal, cream of rice cereal, and richer soups.

After surgery, it is sensible to eat foods as tolerated and as suggested by the doctor or the nutritionist, gradually resuming the nourishing, presurgery diet. Then after two or three months, when most tissue healing is complete and the body is stronger, a mild cleansing and detoxification may be initiated, especially if general anesthesia was used during the surgery or other potentially toxic drugs were used afterward.

This fine art of administering potentially lethal drugs to reduce pain, induce unconsciousness, and yet maintain life has progressed significantly in the past century. Many procedures are possible now that were only fantasies generations ago. Yet, many people realize that the anesthesia is often more difficult to recover from postsurgically than the actual cutting of tissues. Thus, I suggest using the least amount of drugs and the simplest anesthetic procedure possible; clearly the toxicity of anesthesia can be worse with suboptimal nutrition. Local anesthesia is clearly a big advance in medicine of recent years. Before general anesthesia, it is wise for people to nourish themselves well first with a high-nutrient diet containing good quality protein foods, and by taking supportive supplements to strengthen tissues and create nutrient reserves. The antioxidant nutrients (vitamins C and A, selenium, zinc, and L-cysteine) are suggested.

Vitamin E can be taken, but in lower doses (100–200 IUs) so that it does not affect blood clotting or tissue healing.

Most books on medical dietetics include many specific diets for various types of surgery. The program suggested here is more general and, I assure you, more healthful. The current hospital diet might make more economic sense, and it is probably the way that the bureaucrats who create these diets eat anyway, but it is not in the best interest of the patients. Our hospitals need to provide more nutrient-rich, healing diets, with more wholesome foods and liquids to help revitalize and nourish (and heal) the patients so that they can return to their normal lives as quickly as possible. Hospitals should also provide a hypoallergenic (low in wheat, yeast, corn, eggs, or milk) and low-chemical (no additives, binders, artificial colors) diet. If, as dieticians believe, "we do not need supplements if we eat a balanced diet," they should then clearly provide a chemical-free, hypoallergenic and wholesome diet. However, the RDAs do not apply to hospitalized and surgical patients; these people need more of most nutrients due to the stress and possible inadequate digestion and assimilation. In addition, the RDAs do not include many important nutrients, such as manganese, selenium, chromium, boron, and vanadium. Hospital diets should also be providing supplemental electrolyte powders to provide additional magnesium, and protein powders to support patients' healing and to prevent muscle wasting. I suggest, as Dr. Robert Haas does in his book *Eat to Succeed* (New American Library, New York, 1986) that people take their own nutritional supplements to the hospital; bring (or have family and friends bring them) good food, drinking water, and fresh juices; and encourage hospitals to provide more natural foods prepared with little or no saturated fats, salts, and chemicals or preservatives.

Another reminder for improved healing from surgery is to become active and involved in the healing process as soon as possible. Most surgeons and nurses are supportive of this practice and will provide encouragement. "Think/Feel healing"— know, believe, and see (through internal visual imagery) that complete recovery is taking place.

Several specific nutrients are particularly important in this program. Vitamin A in the retinol form helps in tissue healing and immune support. The beta-carotene form, provitamin A, adds further vitamin A and has an antioxidant effect. Vitamin C also improves collagen tissue healing and is needed in regular frequent amounts to replenish the increased amounts of vitamin C used during the stress of surgery and sickness. The bioflavonoids support the beneficial vitamin C effects and aid in tissue healing as well. Zinc is important to tissue healing and immune support through its function in a variety of enzymes. Magnesium also activates many enzymes useful in healing.

The B vitamins are needed, particularly extra riboflavin (B_2), which seems to help tissue repair, and pantothenic acid (B_5) to deal with the extra stress of surgery. Adequate vitamin K in our diet supports normal blood clotting, so important during surgery. Various other vitamins, such as B_1, B_3, B_6, and B_{12}, and other minerals, such as selenium, copper, iron, calcium, potassium, manganese, molybdenum, and cobalt, are also important to healing. Of course, with surgical blood loss, more iron may be needed in the recovery stage to build blood cells. Silica is useful to skin and tissues. *Bromelain,* the pineapple enzyme, has a mild anti-inflammatory effect and may be useful after surgery to aid in food digestion as well as to reduce micro blood clots (thrombi). Moderate levels of supplemental L- amino acids can be helpful, and some recent research suggests that additional amounts of L-arginine and L-lysine in particular aid tissue healing as well. The essential fatty acids (omega-3 and omega-6) are also very important to wound healing.

Healthy immune function is, of course, essential to healing and preventing infections. The antioxidant nutrients are useful in supporting the immune system, but for this program, a lower than usual amount of vitamin E is suggested, usually about 200 IUs and definitely not more than 400 IUs. Vitamin E has been shown in some studies to slow wound healing time, in contradiction of the popular belief that oral vitamin E and topical E are good for healing tissues; many vitamin E caps have been popped and the oil applied to the skin to help in healing. It would make sense to use vitamin A oil for this purpose, as it is a nutrient known for its tissue healing properties.

Herbs can also be used to support wound healing. Horsetail is very high in silica, a mineral that helps strengthen tissues, especially skin, hair, and nails. Goldenseal root is a tonic herb when taken internally and also has mild anti-infection properties. Used locally, it works as an antiseptic. It has been used effectively in helping heal wounds internally and externally, in strengthening mucous membranes, and in ulcer treatment. Comfrey leaf has always been believed to have healing properties when taken internally, though there is not much specific research data to support this observation. It is more often used externally for sprains and bone, muscle, and ligament injuries or internally for broken bones than for healing surgical wounds.

The following table lists the basic nutrients to be taken before and after surgery when possible. Usually, following this program for two to three weeks prior to surgery and four to six weeks afterward is sufficient. This program may also be used when recovering from wounds, injuries, burns, or infections. My experience has led me to believe that it will reduce healing time, reduce morbidity secondary to surgery, and lessen the duration of hospital stays.

PRE- AND POSTSURGERY NUTRIENT PROGRAM
(AND FOR HEALING INJURIES)

Water	2–3 qt.
Fiber	10–15 g.
Protein	70–100 g.
Fat	50–75 g.

Vitamin A	20,000 IUs*	**Copper**	2–3 mg.**
Beta-carotene	15,000 IUs	**Iodine**	100–200 mcg.
Vitamin D	400 IUs	**Iron**	20 mg.
Vitamin E	200 IUs	**Magnesium**	500–800 mg.
Vitamin K	300 mcg.	**Manganese**	10 mg.
Thiamine (B$_1$)	50 mg.	**Molybdenum**	800 mcg.
Riboflavin (B$_2$)	25–100 mg.	**Potassium**	2–3 g.
Niacin (B$_3$)	25 mg.	**Selenium, as**	
Niacinamide (B$_3$)	50 mg.	selenomethione	200 mcg.
Pantothenic acid (B$_5$)	1,000 mg.	**Silicon**	100–200 mg.
Pyridoxine (B$_6$)	50 mg.	**Sulfur**	400–800 mg.
Pyridoxal-5-phosphate	25 mg.	**Vanadium**	150–300 mcg.
Cobalamin (B$_{12}$)	200 mcg.	**Zinc**	60–100 mg.**
Folic acid	800 mcg.		
Biotin	300 mcg.	**L-amino acids**	1,000 mg.
Inositol	1,000 mg.	**L-arginine**	500–1,000 mg.
Vitamin C	4–6 g.	**L-lysine**	500–1,000 mg.
Bioflavonoids	500 mg.	**Lactobacillus**	2 billion organisms
		Bromelain	200–400 mg.
Boron	2–3 mg.		
Calcium	800–1,200 mg.		
Chromium	200 mcg.		

*20,000 IU vitamin A should only be used for four to six weeks, beginning a week or two prior to surgery and two to three weeks afterward. At other times, the amount should be limited to 5,000–10,000 IUs daily.

**Amount should be higher if more zinc is taken—about a 20:1 ratio of zinc to copper.

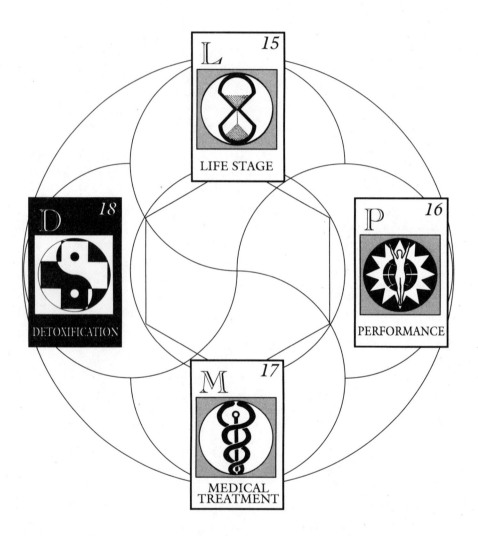

Chapter 18

Detoxification and Healing Programs

S o many problems in our Western society come from excessive use of foods and drugs. Abuses and addictions touch almost every person's life. This chapter deals with many of the dietary and substance abuses and ways to heal them.

To begin with, we must ask ourselves—as I suggest to people in their initial medical visit to my clinic—is there anything that we do everyday that we would be aware of missing if we would not do it? If so, this activity is a habit or addiction. Of course, there are positive habits. Yet there are many others that may negatively interact with life and health, and can lead to a variety of problems—physically, mentally, and emotionally.

Common addictions in our culture include sugar, various drugs, both pharmaceutical and recreational, caffeine, alcohol, and nicotine. Most adults have problems with one or more of these "drugs," and may even be aware of their habit/addictions and would like to change them, but they don't, can't, or won't for various reasons. In this day and age, we also must be aware of techno-traps, including TV, phone, computers, VCR, FAX, microwaves, and transportation.

I believe that fasting (and detoxification) is the missing link in the American (and Western) diet.

The seven programs contained in this chapter involve various aspects of these fasting and detoxification processes. I really believe that much disease, especially degenerative disease, comes from congestion and stagnation in the body (in the organs, tissues, circulation, lymph, and the cells), and that this congestion/stagnation disease can be cleared from our body. I have personally experienced it and seen it in hundreds of patients. This chapter's title, *Detoxification and Healing Programs*, suggests that I believe these processes, detoxification and healing, can be synonymous in many instances; of course, this is when applied to the right medical circumstances. The other side of disease, in very simplistic terms conceptually, originates from depletion and deficiency, and for these, fasting or cleansing dietary processes are not the answer; in fact, they may make matters worse. These and many other general concepts of detoxification are discussed in the first program, *General Detoxification and Cleansing*.

In the subsequent programs, I will discuss the problems with drugs (over-the-counter, prescription, and recreational) and ways to go about changing our lives to enable us to free ourselves from the shackles of highs and lows, prosperity and poverty, and abuses and addiction. From there, I have written specific programs for dealing with caffeine, alcohol, and nicotine; these three common addictions, particularly the latter two, can be very devastating to health and life. In each program, I will discuss the physiology of the specific drug, its hazards and ill effects, and special ideas and actions to help you handle and clear these addictive habits. This information can guide you in your changes, which—along with the psychological and life support that you may also need in order to love yourself enough to change your habits to live in more positive, life-generating ways—will then help you be successful in whatever changes you attempt.

The last two programs may take some growth and evolution to embrace; however, many people, as I am often surprised, are more than ready for this optimistic health information on the art of fasting and concepts of immortal living. Juice fasting is a powerful, healing tool, one of the greatest! It is a vehicle to freedom from addiction of all kinds. It helps us open to our true guidance, growth, potentials, and life. Fasting opens us spiritually and emotionally, and supports us in becoming more real in our lives, in doing what we believe and know in our hearts and spirits. With that openness and clarity, we can then embrace some of the more spiritual philosophy discussed in *Immortality and Beyond*.

General Detoxification and Cleansing

Now that I have devoted so many pages to nutrients, foods, diets, and special eating plans to support health and to treat a variety of disease states, it is important to emphasize a number of programs in the category of elimination—both the basic process of detoxification and programs that will help us cleanse specific common toxins and habits from our lives.

It is somewhat difficult to separate the concepts and practices of detoxification from those of fasting. Fasting, or the avoidance of solid food, as I use the term here, is one method of detoxification, probably the most effective, yet extreme, form. There are many other ways to detoxify.

Toxicity is of much greater concern in the twentieth century than ever before. There are many new and stronger chemicals, air and water pollution, radiation and nuclear power. We ingest new chemicals, use more drugs of all kinds, eat more sugar and refined foods, and daily abuse ourselves with various stimulants and sedatives. The incidence of many toxicity diseases has increased as well. Cancer and cardiovascular disease are two of the main ones. Arthritis, allergies, obesity, and many skin problems are others. In addition, a wide range of symptoms, such as headaches, fatigue, pains, coughs, gastrointestinal problems, and problems from immune weakness, can all be related to toxicity.

Toxicity occurs on two basic levels—external and internal. We can acquire toxins from our environment by breathing them, by ingesting them, or through physical contact with them. Chapter 11, *Environmental Aspects of Nutrition*, deals with chemical aspects of food and how they influence our lives and health. We all are exposed to toxins daily. We eat and drink them and impose them upon ourselves repeatedly and regularly. Most drugs, food additives, and allergens can create toxic elements in the body. In fact, any substance can have toxicity—water, sodium, and almost all nutrients can be a problem in certain circumstances.

On the internal level, our body produces toxins through its normal everyday functions. Biochemical, cellular, and bodily activities generate substances that need to be eliminated. The free radicals that have been discussed throughout this book are biochemical toxins. When these substances/molecules/toxins are not eliminated, they can cause irritation or inflammation of the cells and tissues, blocking normal functions on a cellular, organ, and whole-body level. Microbes of all kinds—intestinal bacteria, foreign bacteria, yeasts, and parasites—produce metabolic waste products that we must handle. Our thoughts and emotions and stress itself generate increased biochemical toxicity. The proper level of elimination of these toxins is essential to health. Clearly, a normal functioning body was created to handle certain levels of toxins; the concern is with excess intake or production of toxins or a reduction in the processes of elimination.

A toxin is basically any substance that creates irritating and/or harmful effects in the body, undermining our health or stressing our biochemical or organ functions. This may result from drugs which have side effects, or from patterns of physiology that are different from our usual functioning. Recreational drugs also usually have some harmful effects. The free radicals irritate, inflame, age, and cause degeneration of body tissues. Negative "ethers," psychic and spiritual influences, thought patterns, and negative emotions all can be toxins as well—both as stressors and by changing the normal physiology of the body and possibly producing specific symptoms.

Toxicity occurs in our body when we take in more than we can utilize and eliminate. Homeostasis means that our body functions are in balance. This balance is disturbed when we feed ourselves more than we can utilize or partake of specific substances that are toxic. Toxicity may depend on the dosage, frequency, or potency of the toxin. A toxin may produce an immediate or rapid onset of symptoms, as many pesticides and some drugs do; possibly, even more commonly, it may cause some long-term negative effect, such as asbestos exposure leading to lung cancer.

Of course, if our body is working well, with good immune and eliminative functions, we can handle our basic everyday exposure to toxins. The purpose of this section is to discuss ways to support the elimination of toxins, excessive mucus, congestion, and disease and to prevent, on a day-to-day basis, the buildup of toxicity. Through detoxification, we clear and filter toxins and wastes and allow our body to work on enhancing its basic functions.

OUR GENERAL DETOXIFICATION SYSTEMS

Respiratory—lungs, bronchial tubes, throat, sinuses, and nose
Gastrointestinal—liver, gallbladder, colon, and whole GI tract
Urinary—kidneys, bladder, and urethra
Skin and dermal—sweat and sebaceous glands and tears
Lymphatic—lymph channels and lymph nodes

Our body handles toxins by either neutralizing, transforming, or eliminating them. As examples, many of the antioxidant nutrients we have discussed so much may neutralize free-radical molecules. The liver helps transform many toxic substances into harmless agents, while the blood carries wastes to the kidneys; the liver also dumps wastes through the bile into the intestines, where much waste is eliminated. We also clear toxins through sweating, from exercise or heat. Our sinuses and skin may also be accessory elimination organs whereby excess mucus or toxins can be released, as with sinus congestion or skin rashes, respectively.

Detoxification occurs on many other levels as well. Physically, this process can help clear congestions, illnesses, and disease potential. It can improve energy. I believe that many "detox" processes can help rejuvenate us and prevent degeneration. Mental detoxification is also important. Cleansing our minds of negative thought patterns is essential to health; the physical detoxification also helps this mental process. Emotionally, detoxification helps us uncover and express feelings, especially hidden frustrations, anger, resentments, or fear, and replace them with forgiveness, love, joy, and hope. On a spiritual level, many people experience new clarity and/or an enhancement of their purpose of life during cleansing processes. A light detox over a couple of days can help us feel better, while a longer process and deeper commitment to a new way of life, such as eliminating certain abusive habits and eating a better diet, will help us really change our whole life.

Detoxification is part of a transformational medicine that instills change on many levels. Change and evolution are keys to healing. Enhancing elimination helps us deal with and clear problems from our past, from childhood and parental patterns to recent job or relationship stress. When our body has eliminated much of its toxic buildup, we feel lighter and are able to really experience the moment and be open for the future.

Detoxification is a relative term. Anything that supports our elimination can be said to help us detoxify. Doing nothing more than drinking an extra quart of water a day will usually help us eliminate more toxins. Eating more fruits and vegetables—the high-water-content, cleansing foods—and less meat and milk products will create less congestion and more elimination. There are many levels of the progressive detoxication diets, from these simple changes to complete fasting. I want to express some concerns about overelimination or overdetoxification, which I see occasionally. Some people go to extremes with fasting, laxatives, enemas, colonics, diuretics, and even exercise and begin to lose essential nutrients from their body. A negative balance can be created in this manner, such as protein or vitamin-mineral deficiencies though congestion from overintake and underelimination is a more common problem in this culture. I believe that the best and simplest way to look at symptoms and disease is in terms of excess (congestion) and deficiency; this is the basis of the traditional Oriental philosophy.

Elimination equals illumination.

Reduce excesses, but not excessively.

—ArgIsle-izms

Who Is Best Suited for Detoxification?

Almost everyone needs to detox, cleanse themselves, and rest their body functions at times. Cleansing or detoxification is one part of the trilogy of nutritional action, the others being building, or toning, and balance, or maintenance. With a regular, balanced diet, devoid of excesses, we will need less intensive detoxification. Our body has a daily elimination cycle, mostly carried out at night and in the early morning, up until breakfast. However, when we eat a congesting diet higher in fats, meats, dairy products, refined foods, and chemicals, detoxification becomes more necessary. Who needs to detoxify and when is based in part on individual lifestyle and needs.

More common toxicity symptoms include headache, fatigue, mucus problems, aches and pains, digestive problems, "allergy" symptoms, and sensitivity to environmental agents such as chemicals, perfumes, and synthetics. People who experience these and others on the list may benefit from diet changes or avoidance of the drug or agent that may be influencing the symptom. It may be important to differentiate allergic symptoms from those of toxicity to determine the appropriate medical care. The diet and detox program here is fairly similar to the *Allergy* plan discussed earlier and is often helpful in reducing allergic symptoms. Fasting can be extremely beneficial for people with allergies. Of course, there may be subtle characteristics of toxicity that differentiate it from other health concerns.

SIGNS AND SYMPTOMS OF TOXICITY

Headaches	Backaches	Runny nose	Fatigue
Joint pains	Itchy nose	Nervousness	Skin rashes
Cough	Frequent colds	Sleepiness	Hives
Wheezing	Irritated eyes	Insomnia	Nausea
Sore throat	Immune weakness	Dizziness	Indigestion
Tight or stiff neck	Environmental sensitivity	Mood changes	Anorexia
Angina pectoris	Sinus congestion	Anxiety	Bad breath
Circulatory deficits	Fever	Depression	Constipation
High blood fats			

Many common acute and chronic illnesses may be alleviated by a program of detoxification/cleansing, as they are basically created by short- and long-term congestive patterns. People with addictions to any substance may benefit from a detox program, even if it is only the temporary avoidance of the addictive agent or agents. Withdrawal symptoms that commonly occur with many drugs, including sugar, caffeine, and over-the-counter medications, are precipitated by detoxification. Many of the poisons (toxins) that we ingest or make are stored in the fatty tissues. Obesity is almost always associated with toxicity. When we lose weight, we reduce our fat and thereby our toxic load. However, during weight loss we release more toxins, and thus need protection through greater intake of water, fiber, and the antioxidant nutrients, such as vitamins C, E, and beta-carotene, selenium, and zinc. With exercise we can also turn fat into muscle (not literally) and help further detoxification.

PROBLEMS RELATED TO CONGESTION/STAGNATION/TOXICITY

Acne	Obesity	Prostate disease
Abscesses	Infections by:	Menstrual problems
Boils	Bacteria	Vaginitis
Eczema	Virus	Varicose veins
Allergies	Fungus	Diabetes
Arthritis	Parasites	Peptic ulcers
Asthma	Worms	Gastritis
Constipation	Uterine fibroid tumors	Pancreatitis
Colitis	Cancer	Mental illness
Hemorrhoids	Cataracts	Multiple sclerosis
Diverticulitis	Colds	Alzheimer's disease
Cirrhosis	Bronchitis	Senility
Hepatitis	Pneumonia	Parkinson's disease
Fibrocystic breast disease	Sinusitis	Drug addiction
Atherosclerosis	Emphysema	Tension headaches
Heart disease	Kidney stones	Migraine headaches
Hypertension	Kidney disease	Gallstones
Thrombophlebitis	Stroke	
Gout		

Of course, not all of these problems are solely problems of toxicity or completely cured by detoxification. Most of these diseases, and the majority of those factors, have to do with abuses, especially on a nutritional level. Often, these problems, many of which are discussed in other sections of this book, are alleviated by eliminating the related toxins and following this detox program.

What Is Detoxification?

Detoxification is the process of clearing toxins from the body or neutralizing or transforming them, and clearing excess mucus and congestion. Many of these toxins come from our diet, drug use, and environmental exposure, both acute and chronic. Internally, fats, especially oxidized fats and cholesterol, free radicals, and other irritating molecules act as toxins. Functionally, poor digestion, colon sluggishness and dysfunction, reduced liver function, and poor elimination through the kidneys, respiratory tract, and skin all add to increased toxicity.

Detoxification involves dietary and lifestyle changes that reduce intake of toxins and improve elimination. Avoidance of chemicals, from food or other sources, refined food, sugar, caffeine, alcohol, tobacco, and many drugs helps minimize the toxin load. Drinking extra water (purified) and increasing fiber by including more fruits and vegetables in the diet are steps in the detoxification process. Moving from a more to a less congesting diet, as shown in the accompanying table, will help us to move along the detox road.

Most Congesting ◄———					———► *Least Congesting*	
drugs	fats	sweets	nuts	rice	roots	fruits
allergenic	fried foods	milk	seeds	millet	squashes	greens
foods	refined	eggs	beans	buckwheat	other	herbs
organ meats	flours	baked	oats	pasta	vegetables	water
hydrogenated	meats	goods	wheat	potatoes		
fats						
More Potentially Toxic ◄———					———► *More Detoxifying*	

Detoxification therapy, as fasting, is the oldest treatment known to humans and is a completely natural process; and in many cases, as we listen to our inner guidance as animals do, we may apply this process to many illnesses and states of health and life. Many authorities claim the detox process helps clear wastes and old or dead cells and revitalizes the body's natural functions and healing capacities. Of the thousands of people that I know who have used cleansing programs, the vast majority have experienced positive and incredible results. As I said, I believe that fasting/cleansing/detoxification is the missing link in Western nutrition, and if we used this process more in our daily lives and our medical system, we could heal and prevent a great deal of disease. *Now is the time* for all of us in the world to listen—and to clean and clear our bodies, homes, offices, our relationships, towns, cities, countries and the entire planet, lest we perish from toxicity.

When Is the Best Time to Cleanse/Detoxify?

We need to incorporate nature's cycles with our own cycles. We may notice regular periods of congestion, and we may reduce or prevent these by following a more detoxifying program. Whenever we feel congested, our first step is to follow detox procedures, many of which we can fine-tune in time with our experience of what works for us. I have found personally that if I start to feel congestion or a cold coming on, then I can exercise and sweat, sauna or steam, drink loads of fluids, take vitamins C and A, and get a good night's sleep without eating much—and almost every time I will wake up healed! If I feel my bowels are backed up, I will usually take some herbs to stimulate them.

Each of us has a natural cleansing time when our body wants a lighter diet, more liquids, and greater elimination than intake. This occurs daily, usually in the night until midmorning; it may occur weekly but more commonly for a few days a month. Women, in particular, are aware of this natural cleansing time with their female cycle. In fact, many women do much better premenstrually and during their periods if they follow a cleansing program—more juices, greens, lighter foods, herbs, and so on—in the week before their menstruation.

The seasonal cycle is really the most important in regard to natural detoxification periods. If we can harmonize with these, we can do much to stay healthy. I discussed the relationship of the seasons to diet in other parts of this book, and in greater detail in my first book, *Staying Healthy with the Seasons*, and explore this further in the program on *Fasting*.

To summarize here, the seasonal changes are the key stress times in nature and the times where we most need to lighten up our outer demands and consumptions and turn more within to listen to our inner world that mirrors the natural cycles. Spring is the key time for detoxification; autumn is also important. At least a one- to two-week program is suggested at these times. In spring, we may eat more citrus fruits, fresh greens, and juices or try the Master Cleanser lemonade diet, while in autumn we may dine on other harvests, such as apples or grapes, and the many vegetables. Lots of fresh fruits and vegetables are appropriate when we are going into summer; and brown rice, vegetables, and soups may be best to simplify our diet when going into winter.

The sample yearly program provided here is designed for a basically healthy person who eats well. It would not be appropriate for those with deficiency problems such as extreme fatigue, underweight people, those who experience coldness, or those with heart weakness. There are even more contraindications for fasting, which releases more toxins than this program does. Releasing too much toxicity can make many sick people sicker; if that happens, they will need to increase fluids and eat again until they feel better. People with cancer need to be very careful about how they detoxify. Prior to or just after surgery is not a good time to detoxify, but after healing, say about four to six weeks later. Pregnant or lactating women should not do any heavy detoxification, though they can usually handle mild programs.

SAMPLE YEAR-LONG DETOX PROGRAM

Spring

For 7–21 days between March 10 and April 15, use one or more of the following plans:
- Master Cleanser (lemonade diet).
- Fruits, vegetables, greens.
- Juices of fruits, vegetables, and greens.
- Herbs with any of the above.
- These plans can be alternated and even include a 3–5 day supervised water fast.
- Remember to take time (about half as long as the fast) for the transition back to the regular diet.
- Elimination and food testing can also be done at this time.

Mid-Spring

3-day cleanse at new moon time in May as a reminder and enhancer of food awareness.

Summer

One week of fruits and vegetables and/or fresh juices to usher in the warm weather sometime between June 10 and July 4.

Late Summer

3-day cleanse of fruit and vegetable juices around the new moon time in August.

Autumn

7–10 day cleanse between September 11 and October 5, such as:
- Grape fast—whole and juiced—grapes, all fresh.
- Apple and lemon juice together, diluted.
- Fresh fruits and vegetables, raw and cooked.
- Fruit and vegetable juices—fruit in the morning, vegetables in the afternoon.
- Juices plus spirulina, algae, or other green chlorophyll powders.
- Whole grains, cooked squashes and other vegetables (a lighter detox).
- Mixture of the above plans.
- Basic low-toxicity diet with herbal program.
- Colon detox with fiber (psyllium, pectin, and so on) along with enemas or colonics.
- Preparing and planning new autumn diet, enhancing positive dietary habits.

Mid-Autumn

3-day cleanse on juices or in-season produce around new moon in late October/early November.

Winter

A lighter diet in preparation for the holidays (can be done between December 10 and January 5):
- Avoidance of toxins and treats, with a very basic wholesome diet.
- One week of brown rice, cooked vegetables, miso broth, and seaweed. Ginger and cayenne pepper can be used in soups.
- Saunas or steams and massage—you deserve it!
- Hang on until spring!

Where Can We Detoxify?

During basic, simple detox plans, most of us can maintain our normal life functions. In fact, energy, performance, and health often improve. For some though, detox may produce symptoms such as headaches, fatigue, irritability, mucous congestions, or aches and pains; any of the symptoms of toxicity may appear, though usually not. According to naturopathic theory, any symptoms that have previously been experienced may also be experienced transiently during detox/healing, and I have seen this occur. However, sometimes it is hard to know what is actually happening. Should we treat the problems that come up or simply watch them? Since my basic approach in medicine is to allow the body to heal itself and support the natural healing process whenever possible, that is what I try to do unless the person is very uncomfortable.

For many of us, especially the new or inexperienced, it is wise to begin any special programs, diet, or lifestyle changes with a few days at home. In time, experience will show what is best for us. Most of us can maintain a regular work schedule during a cleanse or detox program (we may likely be more productive), but it may be easier to begin a program on a Friday, as the first few days are usually the hardest. This is because some people may be more sensitive during cleansing to their work environment or to chemical exposures, for example. Also, certain individuals may be faced with temptations or the influence of other workers or family members challenging their decisions, and for this, knowing and trusting what they are doing and having the support of a professional or group will add to their comfort and willpower.

At the end of the first day, at around dinnertime, symptoms may begin to appear, with headache and fatigue the most common, and it is good to be able to rest and spend time in familiar surroundings without a lot of outer demands. By the third day, we usually feel pretty stable and ready for work life. However, many people like to start new programs on Monday and just know that they will do fine, using willpower and visualization to see it through. People often feel better than ever and are able to accomplish tasks and meet challenges more easily than usual. In fact, experienced fasters may fast during busy work periods to improve their productivity. Preparation and projection, clearing doubts and fears, and keeping a daily journal are all useful during this vital process and are crucial to any successful undertaking.

Why Detoxify?

We detoxify/cleanse for many reasons, mainly to do with health, vitality, and rejuvenation—to clear symptoms, treat disease, and prevent further problems. A cleansing program is ideal for helping us to reevaluate our lives, to make changes, or to clear abuses or addictions. It takes us through our withdrawal and reduces cravings fairly rapidly, and if we are ready, we can begin a new life without the addictive habits or drugs.

I cleanse because it makes me feel more productive, creative, and open to subtle and spiritual energies. Many people detox/cleanse—or, more commonly, fast on water or juices—for spiritual renewal and to feel more alive, awake, and aware. Christ, Paramahansa Yogananda, and many other religious figures and teachers have advocated fasting for health and for spiritual attunement. It really does help move our energies from our lower centers of digestion and elimination up into our heart, mind, and consciousness centers. Fasting will be discussed more in a later program.

Detoxification can be helpful for weight loss, though it is not a primary reduction plan; I think it is more important as a transition. However, anyone eating 4,000 calories a day of a fatty, sweet, and poorly balanced diet who begins to eat 2,000–2,500 calories of more wholesome foods will definitely experience detoxification, weight loss, and improved health.

We also cleanse/detoxify to rest our overloaded organs of digestion and our liver, gallbladder, and kidneys and allow them to catch up on past work. Most often our energy is increased and more steady. There are many reasons why we may want to cleanse.

REASONS FOR CLEANSING

Prevent disease	To be more:
Reduce symptoms	Organized
Treat disease	Creative
Cleanse body	Motivated
Rest organs	Productive
Purification	Relaxed
Rejuvenation	Energetic
Weight loss	Clear
Clear skin	Conscious
Slow aging	Inwardly attuned
Improve flexibility	Spiritual
Improve fertility	Environmentally attuned
Enhance the senses	Relationship focused

How Do We Detoxify / Cleanse?

I have touched on ways to detoxify throughout this section; the remainder is a discussion of general and specific diet plans, other activities, and supplements, including vitamins, minerals, amino acids, and herbs, to aid us in this healing process.

There are many levels to this part of the program. The first is to eat a nontoxic diet. If we do this regularly, we have less need for cleansing. If we have not been eating this way, we should detoxify first and then make permanent changes.

THE NONTOXIC DIET

- Eat organic foods whenever possible.
- Drink filtered water.
- Rotate foods, especially common allergens, such as milk products, eggs, wheat, and yeast foods.
- Practice food combining.
- Eat a natural, seasonal cuisine.
- Include fruits, vegetables, whole grains, legumes, nuts and seeds, and, for omnivarians, some low-fat dairy products, and fresh fish (not shellfish) and organic poultry.
- Cook in iron, stainless steel, glass, or porcelain.
- Avoid or minimize red meats, cured meats, organ meats, refined foods, canned foods, sugar, salt, saturated fats, coffee, alcohol, and nicotine.

Another aspect of the nontoxic diet is avoiding drugs—over-the-counter, prescription, and recreational types—and substituting natural remedies, such as nutrients, herbs, and homeopathic medicines, all of which have fewer side effects. Other natural therapies, such as acupuncture, massage, and chiropractic may help in treating some problems so that we will not need drugs for them. Avoiding or minimizing exposure to chemicals at home and work is also important. This lessens our total toxic load. Substituting natural cleansers, cosmetics, and clothes is helpful. There are many suggestions for these areas of life in Chapter 11.

The effects of the detoxification diet may vary. Even mild changes from our current plan may produce some responses, while more dramatic dietary shifts will produce a profound cleansing. Shifting from the most congesting foods to the least—eating more fruits, vegetables, grains, nuts and legumes and less baked goods, sweets, refined foods, fried foods and fatty foods—will help most of us detoxify somewhat and bring us into better balance, with more vitalized cells, organs, and body.

Maintaining the same diet but adding certain supplements can also stimulate detoxification. Fiber, vitamin C, other antioxidants, chlorophyll, and glutathione, mainly as amino acid L-cysteine, will all help (see the end program following this

915

discussion). Herbs such as garlic, red clover, echinacea, or cayenne may also induce some detoxification. Saunas, sweats, and niacin therapy have been used to cleanse the body. Simply increasing liquids and decreasing fats will shift the balance strongly toward improved elimination and less toxin buildup. Increased consumption of filtered water, herb teas, fruits, and vegetables and reducing fats, especially most fried food, red meats, and milk products will also help detoxification. This is a more structured, basic diet, but for most average Westerners, it will be a major shift to a cleaner diet. A vegetarian diet would also be a healthful step toward detoxification for those with some congestive problems. In general, moving from an acid-generating diet to a more alkaline one, as discussed in earlier sections in Chapters 10 and 12, will aid the process of detoxification. Acid-forming foods, such as meats, milk products, breads and baked goods, and especially the refined sugar and carbohydrate products, will increase body acidity and lead to more mucus production and congestion to attempt to balance the body chemistry, whereas the more alkaline, wholesome vegetarian foods enhance cleansing and clarity in the body. The right balance of acid and alkaline foods for each of us is, of course, the key.

A deeper level of the detox diet is one made up exclusively of fresh fruits, fresh vegetables, either raw and cooked, and whole grains, both cooked and sprouted; however, no breads or baked goods, animal foods and dairy products, alcohol, or nuts are used. This diet keeps fiber and water intake up and helps colon detoxification. Most people can handle this well and make the shift from their regular diet with a few days transition. Some people do well on a brown rice fast (a more macrobiotic plan), usually for a week or two, eating three to four bowls of rice daily along with liquids such as teas.

The next level of detoxification involves a diet consisting solely of fruits and vegetables, all cleansing foods. The green vegetables, especially the chlorophyllic and high-nutrient leafy greens, are very cleansing and supportive for purification of the gastrointestinal tract and the whole body. Ann Wigmore and her staff at the Hippocrates, or Optimum, Health Institute guides people in a wheatgrass and sprout cleansing program that is a wonderfully rejuvenating experience for many.

A raw foods diet is fulfilling for many people, very high in energy and nutrition. It contains lots of sprouted greens from seeds and grains such as wheat, buckwheat, sunflower, alfalfa, and clover; sprouted beans; soaked or sprouted raw nuts; and fresh fruits and vegetables. Cooking food is not allowed with this diet; eating foods raw maintains the highest concentrations of vitamins, minerals and important enzymes, and allows them to find their way into our body and cells. Many people feel that this is the best of diets; it can be health supportive over quite some time if it is balanced properly. Special seed cheeses and yogurt can be found in the recipe section of Chapter 14.

Other specialized detox diets include macrobiotics and diets that treat certain problems, such as a yeast overgrowth or allergies. Treating these problems properly, as discussed in the *Allergies* and *Yeast Syndrome* programs in Chapter 17, allows the body to reduce its irritating reactions and to heal.

Beyond the fruit-and-vegetable diet are the liquid cleanses or fasts. Juices, vegetable broths, and teas can be used to purify our body and life. Miso, a paste of fermented soybean, can be used during fasting. It provides many nutrients and supports colon function and the intestinal bacteria, which help detoxification. Spirulina, an algae powder, can also be helpful to many fasters when added to juices. It provides protein to meet body needs and may aid those who experience some fatigue with fasting. Consuming fresh, diluted juices from various fruits and vegetables is safe and helpful for many conditions described in this section. Fasting experts believe that it actually works better than a straight water fast, as it helps to eliminate wastes and old or dead cells while restoring and building new tissue with the easily accessible nutrients from the juices. Water fasting is more intense, often resulting in more sickness and less energy, than fasting with juices. Paavo Airola, one of the pioneers of fasting in America, states in *How to Get Well* and other books that "systematic undereating and periodic fasting are the two most important health and longevity factors." Dr. Airola lists fruit and vegetable juices that cleanse and help in the healing of specific organs (see more in the *Fasting* program).

A key to proper treatment at the proper time is to work with detoxification individually. It does take a sensitive person or a sensitive practitioner to find the right path. Detoxification experiences can range from subtle to intense. We have to look at a person's general health, physiological balance, energy level, and current life activities in order to set up the right program. There are a lot of possibilities. If unsure, start with your basic diet and move along the changes toward juice fasting and see how you feel. Take a couple of days for each step, and, if you feel fine, move to the next level, as described.

LEVELS OF DIETARY DETOXIFICATION

- Basic diet
- Eliminate toxins daily from more congesting to less (see chart on page 910); for example, drugs, sugar, fried foods, meats, dairy, etc. Take one to seven days.
- Fruits, vegetables, whole grains, nuts, seeds and legumes
- Raw foods
- Fruits and vegetables
- Fruit and vegetable juices
- Specific juices, Master Cleanser, apple, carrot-greens, etc. (See *Fasting* program)
- Water

When I set up a detox/cleansing program, I evaluate each individual with a history, physical exam, biochemistry tests, dietary analysis, mineral levels, and any other specific tests indicated to determine their status. Looking at the patient's current state of health, symptoms, and disease as an outcome of their diet, lifestyle, and inherent/

familial patterns, and then considering their health goals, we create the plan together. As is true with any healing process, the plan must be followed, reevaluated, and fine-tuned to make it work to its best potential.

If people are deficient in nutrients and/or energy, they may need a higher-nutrient, higher-protein building diet to improve their health rather than a cleanse. Fatigue, mineral deficiencies, and low organ functions may call for this more supportive diet. However, even in these circumstances, short cleanses, such as three days, can help eliminate old debris and prepare the body to build with healthier blocks.

Our individual detox programs can change, as our needs often vary with time. My own personal program has changed over the decades. Initially, fasts were very powerful for me, transformative and healing. Now I usually notice very little effect, as I feel much cleaner most of the time. If I do get congested with different foods, with travel, or when under other stresses, a few days of juices or just light eating will make a big difference. I ate a low-protein, high-complex-carbohydrate, vegetarian diet for a number of years. Now a mild detox for me consists of more strengthening protein-vegetable meals. Fresh fish with lots of vegetables satisfies and energizes me more now than in the past. The higher-starch meals led me to overeat more to feel nourished. This new diet has let me reduce calories and weight and feel stronger and healthier. And this too, I am sure, will change in time. Yes, detoxification is an individual affair, and many personal aspects are involved in devising a complete plan.

Colon cleansing is one of the most important parts of detoxification. Much toxicity comes out of the large intestine, and sluggish functioning of this organ can rapidly produce general toxicity. During a detox program, most people will work on some level with their colon. There are entire programs for colon detoxification available, such as Dr. Robert Gray's *Colon Cleansing* program, which includes a book and special supplements, found mainly in health food stores. A series of colonic water irrigations, best performed by a trained professional can be the focal point of a detox program, usually along with some cleansing diet and fiber supplements for toning and cleaning the colon. During a basic dietary detox program, other, more subtle colon stimuli are usually used to enhance colon action. These may include herbal or pharmaceutical laxatives, fiber and colon detox supplements, such as psyllium seed husks alone or mixed with other agents, for example, aloe vera powder, betonite clay, and acidophilus culture. Enemas using water, herbs, or even diluted coffee (stimulates liver cleansing) may also be used.

To improve elimination through the skin, regular exercise is important to stimulate sweating. Exercise also improves our general metabolism and helps overall with detoxification. Regular aerobic exercise is a key to maintaining a nontoxic body, especially when we are a little abusive of various substances. On the other hand, exercise increases the production of toxins in the body, so it must be accompanied by adequate fluids, antioxidants, vitamin and mineral replenishment, and other detoxifying principles already discussed. (Also, see the earlier *Athletes* program in Chapter 16.)

Regular bathing is essential to cleanse the skin of the toxins it has released and to open the pores to eliminate more. Saunas and sweats are commonly used to help purify the body through enhanced skin elimination. Dry brushing the skin with an appropriate skin brush before bathing is usually suggested, especially during detox programs, to cleanse the skin of old cells and invigorate it. Massage therapy, especially lymphatic and even deeper massage, is very useful in supporting our detox program. It stimulates elimination and body functions and promotes relaxation. Clearing tensions, worries, and other mental messes also makes for a more complete detoxification.

Resting, relaxation, and recharging are important to this rejuvenation process. During detox, we may need more rest, quiet time, and sleep, although more commonly we have more energy and function better on less sleep. Relaxation exercises help our body rebalance as our mind and attitudes stop interfering with our natural homeostasis. Practicing yoga combines quiet, yet powerful exercises with breathing awareness and regulation, allowing increased flexibility and relaxation. It may be appropriate for many to help balance more active and/or more contractive exercise programs, especially during detox and transition times.

Certain supplements may be used during most of these detoxification programs. However, general supplementation is less important in this detoxification program than in many of the other programs presented in this book or in the specific detox plans for drugs, alcohol, caffeine, and nicotine, when higher amounts of nutrients can ease the withdrawal transitions. For straight juice cleansing or water fasts, I usually do not recommend any supplements; however, I may suggest a couple of nutrients or herbs to stimulate the detox process. Potassium, extra fiber with olive oil to clear toxins from the colon, sodium alginate from seaweeds to bind heavy metals, and apple cider vinegar in water (1 tablespoon of vinegar in 8 ounces hot water) to help reduce mucus are among these. For people beginning to detoxify with transition diets, I often suggest a specialized nutrient program to help neutralize toxins and support elimination. With weight loss, toxins stored in the fat will need to be mobilized and cleared. More water, fiber, and antioxidants can help handle this.

The supplement program used for general detoxification is outlined in the table at the end of this section. It includes a low-dosage multiple vitamin/mineral to fulfill the basic requirements during the transitional diet. The B vitamins, particularly niacin, are important, as are minerals such as zinc, calcium, magnesium, and potassium. The antioxidant nutrients are also important. These include basic levels of beta-carotene, vitamin A and zinc, and vitamin E and selenium, with special focus on vitamin C, probably our main detox vitamin. Some authorities believe that higher amounts of vitamin A (50,000 IUs), vitamin C (8–12 grams), and vitamin E (1,000–1,200 IUs) are helpful in detoxification.

The liver is our most important detox organ because of its many metabolic fuctions. Certain authorities suggest liver-supportive nutrients and even a liver glandular during general detoxification. The liver needs water and glycogen (glucose storage) as glucuronic acid for many of its detoxification functions. A higher starch or carbohydrate diet with lower levels of protein and fats is helpful. This plan correlates with most of the previous detox diets I have suggested, from juices to brown rice and vegetables. The B vitamins, especially B_3 and B_6, vitamins A and C, zinc, calcium, vitamin E and selenium, and L-cysteine are all also needed to support liver detoxification.

Several amino acids are helpful in detoxification, particularly the sulfur-containing ones, cysteine and methionine. L-cysteine supplies sulfhydryl groups which help to prevent oxidation and to bind heavy metals, especially mercury (vitamin C and selenium also help with this). Cysteine is the precursor of glutathione, our most important detoxifier, and thus helps to counter many chemicals and carcinogens. Glutathione is part of detoxification enzymes, specifically *glutathione peroxidase* and *reductase*, which work to prevent peroxidation of lipids and to decrease many toxins, such as smoke, radiation, auto exhaust, chemicals and drugs, and many other carcinogens.

Glycine is a secondary helper. An amino acid that supports glutathione synthesis, it also decreases the toxicity of substances such as phenols or benzoic acid, the latter used as a food preservative. Other amino acids that may have mild detoxifying effects include methionine, tyrosine, and taurine. For more information on amino acid metabolism and uses, I suggest a book by Eric R. Braverman and the late Dr. Carl C. Pfeiffer entitled *The Healing Nutrients Within: Facts, Findings and New Research on Amino Acids.*

As mentioned earlier, another detoxification supporter is fiber, as psyllium seed husks, often combined with other detox nutrients, such as pectin, aloe vera, alginates, and/or colon herbs. This helps cleanse mucus along the small intestine, create bulk in the colon, and pull toxins from the gastrointestinal tract. When fiber is combined with one or two tablespoons of olive oil, it helps bind toxins and reduce absorption of fats as well as some basic minerals. Psyllium husks also reduce absorption of the olive oil, which is important, since it is caloric and it may have picked up fat-soluble chemicals that were released. In *Vitamin Power*, Stephanie Rick and Rita Aero suggest taking 2 grams each of psyllium and bran several times daily (with meals and at bedtime) along with one teaspoon of olive oil to help detoxify. Acidophilus bacteria in the colon help neutralize some toxins, reduce the metabolism of other microbes, and lessen colon toxicity. Supplemental acidophilus is often added to a detox program.

Remember, water should always be used during any type of detox program to help dilute and eliminate toxin accumulations. It is likely the most important detoxifier. It helps clean us through our skin and kidneys, and it improves our sweating with exercise. Eight to ten glasses a day (depending on our size and activity level) of clean, filtered water are suggested. Some authorities suggest distilled water for use during detox programs, since, because of its lack of minerals, it will draw other particles (nutrients and toxins) to it; however, I think it throws off our bichemical/electrical balance, and I prefer regular, purified water (see Chapter 1). Two or three glasses of water should be drunk 30–60 minutes before each meal and even at night to help flush toxins during our body's natural elimination time.

A special elimination process has been developed and used in some clinics to help in the detoxification of chemicals, especially pesticides and even pharmaceutical drugs. This program usually involves several weeks at a center with a therapy including a high-fluid and juice diet, exercise, and large amounts of niacin (vitamin B_3) with sauna therapies. The saunas are extended and may last for several hours daily, with breaks to drink fluids. The idea is to cleanse the hidden chemicals from the fat through juice cleansing, weight loss, niacin therapy, exercise, and sweats. Niacin is a vasostimulator and vasodilator, aiding circulation.

This "niacin-sauna" program is interesting and definitely has possibilities as an intense, medically supervised detoxification process. However, it is still experimental and does entail risks. Preliminary results are good, especially for people with symptoms caused by exposure to pesticides, such as Agent Orange, yet there are some drawbacks. Besides the cost and time required, the extreme detox can cause losses of nutrients, especially minerals, creating depletions from which it could take months to recover. Special attention must be given to ensuring proper nutrient restoration during and after this therapy. I think that this program, even short versions of it, can be used to help detoxify from most drugs, especially the recreational types, and daily abuses of alcohol and nicotine. Many of us can do a modified version on our own with the use of a sauna, a few days' juice fast, regular exercise, and supplemental niacin, beginning at 100–200 mg. and moving up to 2–3 grams daily. Be sure to replenish fluids and minerals. If there are medical problems, weakness, or fatigue, I would not suggest doing this without the advice and supervision of a physician.

Many herbs can support or even create detoxification. In fact, this area is really the strength, I believe, of herbal medicine. There are hundreds of possible herbs to be used for blood cleansing and cleaning the tissues or strengthening the function of specific organs. The old term for blood cleansers is "alteratives," which is the term used in many standard herbal texts. The following are some of the more important ones.

CLEANSING HERBS

Garlic—blood cleanser, lowers blood fats, natural antibiotic

Red clover blossoms—blood cleanser, good during convalescence and healing

Echinacea—lymph cleanser, improves lymphocyte and phagocyte actions

Dandelion root—liver and blood cleanser, diuretic, filters toxins, a tonic

Chaparral—strong blood cleanser, with possibilities for use in cancer therapy

Cayenne pepper—blood purifier, increases fluid elimination and sweat

Ginger root—stimulates circulation and sweating

Licorice root—"great detoxifier," biochemical balancer, mild laxative

Yellow dock root—skin, blood, and liver cleanser, contains vitamin C and iron

Burdock root—skin and blood cleanser, diuretic and diaphoretic, improves liver function, antibacterial and antifungal properties

Sarsaparilla root—blood and lymph cleanser, contains saponins, which reduce microbes and toxins

Prickly ash bark—good for nerves and joints, anti-infectious

Oregon grape root—skin and colon cleanser, blood purifier, liver stimulant

Parsley leaf—diuretic, flushes kidneys

Goldenseal root—blood, liver, kidney, and skin cleanser, stimulates detoxification

A GENERAL CLASSIFICATION OF HERBS USEFUL IN DETOXIFICATION*

Blood Cleansers	Laxatives	Diuretics	Skin Cleansers Diaphoretics
Echinacea	Cascara sagrada	Parsley	Burdock
Red clover	Buckthorn	Yarrow	Oregon grape
Dandelion	Dandelion	Cleavers	Yellow dock
Burdock	Yellow dock	Horsetail	Goldenseal
Yellow dock	Rhubarb root	Corn silk	Boneset
Oregon grape	Senna leaf	Uva ursi	Elder flowers
root	Licorice	Juniper berries	Peppermint
			Cayenne pepper
			Ginger root

Antibiotics		Anticatarrhals**	
Garlic	Echinacea	Echinacea	Hyssop
Myrrh	Propolis	Boneset	Garlic
Prickly ash	Clove	Goldenseal	Yarrow
Wormwood	Eucalyptus	Sage	

*Not usually for fasting or juice cleansing, but mainly for dietary detoxification—using herbs alone may be the most productive in some detoxification programs. Consult a naturopathically oriented doctor.

**anticatarrhals help eliminate mucus

SAMPLE DETOX FORMULA

Echinacea   *Garlic*
Goldenseal root   *Parsley leaf*
Yellow dock root   *Licorice root*
Cayenne pepper

Obtain powders (or ground herb), equal amounts of all of these herbs except half the cayenne, and put this mixture into 00 capsules. Take two capsules two or three times daily between meals.

General Detoxification Nutrient Program

The following list of supplements ties together many aspects of the detoxification process. The specific supplements to be used should take into account individual circumstances. The program can be carried out for varying lengths of time, from one week to one or two months. Further programs for special detox situations are described in the following sections. Remember to work on all the levels of detoxification and listen within for your true healing information.

GENERAL DETOXIFICATION NUTRIENT PROGRAM

Water	2½–3 qt.		
Fiber	20–40 g.		

Vitamin A	5,000 IUs	**Iron**	10–18 mg.
Beta-carotene	15,000 IUs	**Magnesium**	300–500 mg.
Vitamin D	200 IUs	**Manganese**	5–10 mg.
Vitamin E	400–800 IUs	**Molybdenum**	300 mcg.
Vitamin K	200 mcg.	**Potassium**	300–500 mg.
Thiamine (B$_1$)	10–25 mg.	**Selenium**	300 mcg.
Riboflavin (B$_2$)	10–25 mg.	**Silicon**	100 mg.
Niacinamide (B$_3$)	50 mg.	**Vanadium**	300 mcg.
Niacin (B$_3$)	50–2,000 mg.*	**Zinc**	30 mg.
Pantothenic acid (B$_5$)	250 mg.		
Pyridoxine (B$_6$)	10–25 mg.	*Optional:*	
Cobalamin (B$_{12}$)	50–100 mcg.	**L-amino acids**	500–1,000 mg.
Folic acid	400–800 mcg.	**L-cysteine**	250–500 mg.
Biotin	200 mcg.	**DL-methionine**	250–500 mg.
Vitamin C	1–4 g.	**L-glycine**	250–500 mg.
Bioflavonoids	250–500 mg.	**Psyllium seed**	4–8 g.
		Flaxseed oil	1–2 teaspoons
Calcium	600–850 mg.	**Olive oil**	3–6 teaspoons
Chromium	200 mcg.	**Liquid chlorophyll**	2–4 teaspoons
Copper	2 mg.	**Apple cider vinegar**	1–2 Tablespoons
Iodine	150 mcg.	**Acidophilus culture**	1–2 billion organisms
		Detox formula herbs:	4–6 capsules
		echinacea, yellow dock, goldenseal, garlic, parsley, licorice, cayenne pepper	

*May be used for special detox programs; see previous discussion.

Drug Detoxification

This program is important because it concerns problems common to a large number of people in our culture. Not just drug addicts but most people are habituated or addicted to one or more substances. Drug detoxification involves two main processes—changing our abusive habits and releasing the drugs from our lives.

Drug use is a huge problem; we are a drug culture, and literally thousands of substances are used extensively. Western medicine is likewise a drug-oriented system. We consume billions of pills yearly and spend many billions of dollars on them. These figures do not even include the everyday use of caffeine, alcohol, and nicotine.

Some preliminary concepts can help us prepare for drug detoxification. Most important is the relationship between states of being, symptoms, and our use of drugs. If we are slow or hyper, we may stimulate or sedate ourselves chemically. If we view a symptom as a problem, we may want to correct it with a drug. Although for immediate relief this may seem very practical, it is theoretically ludicrous and shows a complete misunderstanding of the design of the human body. Drug use and drug therapy rarely fix anything. Our symptoms are a warning sign of something wrong for which we must work to determine the cause. Symptoms are not the real problem, but results of deeper processes and causes. They are not an error on the part of our body; our body rarely errs. It responds to how we treat it. We must correct our internal imbalance by listening to our body and avoiding dietary and lifestyle abuses, which means limiting drug use.

It is very important not to devitalize our body if we can possibly avoid it. The first step for many people is to learn again to care for and love themselves and reinforce their desire to live. Much of drug use, at least the habitual type, is part of a syndrome of self-destruction. Pharmaceutical prescriptions and most over-the-counter (OTC) drugs are designed to help us feel better, yet often they are used for problems resulting from abusive or misguided habits.

Addiction is a tremendous personal, social, and economic problem in our culture. It both supports and drains our total economy. Our society and advertising world promote addiction. It begins with sugar, caffeine, nicotine, alcohol, and many foods, such as milk products. Our behavior regarding foods, particularly sweet ones, is conditioned very early and is very difficult to change.

Later, the coffee break becomes a reward, a refueling and rest stop in the intense workday. The caffeine and sugar stimulants are the prime mind/nerve provocateurs to continue to work more. Nervousness and hyperactivity are often associated with productivity, though they are really not comparable to steady, healthful energy; trying to perpetuate that artificially stimulated productivity eventually leads to reduced capacity, time lost from work, wasted money, and increased illness.

All drugs have some toxicity. Most have both physiological and psychological actions and addictive potential, with accumulated toxicity and some withdrawal symptoms when we try to give them up. Before going through any drug or chemical detoxification, it is wise to prepare and plan for it before we proceed. This is important both physically and psychologically. It is definitely helpful to have the aid of a physician, therapist, family member, or good friend for support. The withdrawal phase can be the most difficult time, and this can vary from a day or two to a week or more. It is often hard to differentiate the physical sensations from the underlying psychological involvement. The withdrawal phase is tied fairly closely to the drug addiction—the worse the withdrawal, the more likely we are to continue to use the chemical to prevent withdrawal. A psychological dependency easily develops.

After initial withdrawal, which is often tied to detoxification—that is, the natural release of the stored chemicals from the body—we need willpower and commitment to our original plan for eliminating the particular substance from our life. We also need to work on new behavior patterns, avoiding exposure, such as the people and places associated with our previous problem substances, at least for a while, until we develop more deep-seated new habits so that we have the strength to say no when we are exposed again. Behavior modification therapy can be very helpful.

Drug problems are common, and there are really no stereotypical drug addicts; they can be the affluent businessman, the housewife, the down-and-out "street" person, or anyone under pressure or with unmet psychological needs. Drug and substance abuse are an individual, family, and worldwide problem that can affect young and old, men and women.

The general approach in dealing with drug detoxification begins with admitting that there is a problem. Then we must gather our desire and willpower to accomplish what we set forth to do in our mind and heart. We really have to want to change. Sadly, this incentive often arises from illness or crisis rather than a true desire to be healthy, but many of us may enter through that door and still follow a healthy path.

In addition to a decisive plan and the necessary psychological support, a wholesome, well-balanced diet and nutritional supplements can be very helpful. During the transition, fasting or at least a cleansing diet is helpful to enhance purification and lessen the severity and length of the withdrawal period. I have seen people make incredible lifestyle changes with a week-long cleanse. It is very empowering and allows them to clarify their plan and goals while strengthening their willpower.

The key to dietary detox support is in increasing alkalinity and reducing acidity. Cravings and withdrawal are more intense with an acid state generated from an intake of acid-forming foods such as meats, milk products, and refined flours and sugars. All the fruits and vegetables are alkaline-forming in the body. A fruit and vegetable diet, juices and soups, or even water can be used temporarily. See the previous *General Detoxification* program for more complete instructions.

I do not suggest doing withdrawal and drug detox during illness or pre- or postsurgery, although sometimes it is unavoidable. Pregnancy is another concern, where it is so important to clear all unnecessary drugs, even over-the-counter (OTC) drugs, alcohol, nicotine, and caffeine. We must be careful, and a physician's help may be needed, but usually the basic daily abuses can be tapered off and eliminated over a few days.

Some supportive nutrients can be very helpful during drug elimination. Water is most essential to help clear our cells, tissues, organs, and body. "Dilution is the solution to pollution" is still one of my favorite cleansing statements, along with "Elimination equals Illumination," by Bethany ArgIsle. Extra fiber can also aid colon function and pull more toxins from the body.

A general increase in nutritional supplements is usually helpful in detoxification from drugs, with or without a change in diet, though better with, of course. Vitamin C and the other antioxidants—A and zinc, E and selenium, L-cysteine and other amino acids—are all useful, in addition to the basic vitamins and minerals. Glutathione, which is formed from L-cysteine in the body, helps to decrease the toxicity of most drugs and chemicals through its function in detoxification enzymes.

An orthomolecular approach to drug detoxification includes the B vitamins, minerals, a high amount of vitamin C, antioxidants, and L- amino acids. These work better with a food diet than with fasting, so the alkaline, fruit- and vegetable-based diet is best used with a high nutrient intake. With a more liquid diet, minimizing supplements is suggested, maybe using just vitamin C, some minerals, and an antioxidant formula, along with some herbs and chlorophyll.

Many people find the use of herbs beneficial in drug detoxification. Goldenseal root powder is probably the most important here. Its alkaloids help clear toxicity, and it stimulates the liver to better perform its detox function. One large or two small capsules three times daily before meals for one or two weeks can be helpful. Herbs that work as laxatives, diuretics, and blood or lymph cleansers can also be used in specific formulas. Valerian root and other tranquilizing herbs may also be very useful during excitatory withdrawal symptoms, such as anxiety or insomnia. Chlorophyll, taken as tablets or liquid, has a mild purifying and rejuvenating quality.

Pharmaceutical—Prescription and OTC Drugs

Any of the thousands of prescription and over-the-counter (OTC) drugs currently available and in common use can be toxic, especially when too much is used or when they are used for too long. Aspirin and other anti-inflammatory and pain-relieving drugs, tranquilizers, and antidepressants are all in very common use.

A key to preventing the need to detoxify from drugs is to not use them in the first place. Many people are turning to more natural therapies and remedies as better preparations and experience improve the efficacy of these modalities. Nutritional supplements, herbal remedies, and homeopathic medicines are commonplace substitutes for drugs; when used correctly, they support our body's natural healing powers and correct the internal organ/function/energy imbalances. Acupuncture is also helpful in this regard, as is chiropractic therapy. Massage and other body mechanics can be supportive both by allowing the body to heal naturally and by stimulating elimination during detoxification periods.

OTC products, more easily abused than pharmaceuticals because they can be readily obtained, are usually less toxic. Some symptoms commonly treated with the use of OTC drugs and the drugs commonly used are as follows.

Symptoms	*Drugs*
headache	aspirin, acetaminophen, ibuprofen
fatigue	caffeine, nicotine, No-Doz
insomnia	tranquilizers, antihistamines
colds, flus	antihistamines, decongestants
allergies	antihistamines, decongestants
constipation	laxatives, lubricants
diarrhea	Kaopectate, fibers
indigestion	antacids, Pepto-Bismol, Alka-Seltzer
excess weight	stimulants

Many of these drugs can create physical dependency, especially when there is a chronic problem or when there are withdrawal or rebound symptoms, as there are in allergy conditions, sinus congestion, and constipation. If problems persist we should consult our doctor or healer to help us determine the underlying cause and to correct that. If stress and worry are the cause of insomnia or if our poor food choices lead to our gastrointestinal symptoms, we need to handle these problems. Herbs or homeopathics often can be a more gentle remedy for some of these symptoms.

Aspirin and caffeine are two big OTC drug problems. Caffeine will be discussed thoroughly in the next program. Aspirin, a valuable drug, has been in common use for many decades, though its use is now decreasing because of its association with stomach irritation, allergies, Reye's syndrome, its effect on blood clotting, and the availability of acetaminophen and other anti-inflammatory drugs. Still, acetylsalicylic acid (aspirin), derived from coal tar, has over 50 million regular users in this country, and the average annual intake of aspirin products is more than 100 per person per year—over 20 to 25 billion tablets of this one agent alone used every year. Many aspirin products also contain other analgesics (pain relievers) and caffeine. Aspirin is also an anti-inflammatory agent and can reduce fevers (which is not always good, since fevers can be a natural healer), and it does this better than its counterpart acetaminophen (Tylenol, Datril). Both drugs are now commonly used as people experience more pain and degenerative, inflammatory disease, including cardiovascular disease where aspirin is used in regular low dosages to reduce blood clotting effects. Anti-inflammatory drugs in general are fairly easy to eliminate if we can eliminate the pain for which they are taken.

Stronger pain drugs include the new anti-inflammatories, such as ibuprofen (Medipren, Motrin), which has many possible side effects. Its use also can be avoided with correction of the problems that cause the symptoms. Even stronger prescription narcotics, such as codeine (found in many formulas; aspirin or acetaminophen with codeine is very commonly used); hydrocodone (Percodan); propoxyphene (Darvon); or even Demerol or morphine may be prescribed. All of these narcotic drugs are much more addictive, and thus more difficult to stop using.

Other Drugs—Street and Recreational

Street or "recreational" narcotics are also a big problem. These include opium, methadone, and especially heroin, and more recently "ice," "crack," "crunch," and "cripple." Over a half million heroin users are addicted to and possessed by this intravenous drug, which mixes euphoria with depression. This drug also reduces the appetite and libido, so food and sex, love and nurturing often lose importance, and users live just for the drugs. Specialized care is needed for narcotics withdrawal, and this section's suggestions may offer support during this process.

Using sleeping pills, tranquilizers, and antidepressants is another way to deal with life's frustrations and challenges. Valium has been a very popular drug, the most popular for a few years, but new drugs keep entering the race, and Ativan, Xanax, Halcion, and others are now also very popular. Barbiturates are less common now; they used to be the main sedatives but now are probably more frequently used on the street. All these drugs that slow us down, mainly by depressing our nervous system, act like alcohol, so review the *Alcohol Detoxification* program along with this one if these drugs are an interest or problem.

Stimulants, such as the amphetamines and cocaine, are on the opposite end of the spectrum from sedatives. They are very stimulating but also cause dramatic fluctuations in energy. They excite the nervous system and cause euphoria or irritability with resultant loss of appetite, hypersensitivity, and insomnia, usually followed by fatigue and depression. The amphetamines, such as Dexedrine, Benzedrine, methamphetamine, and Desoxyn, are somewhat less of a problem than they were in prior years (probably because there are better ways of getting high or losing weight), yet for anyone with an addiction to "uppers," they have a very dangerous and difficult problem. As with the narcotics, amphetamine withdrawal and detoxification often require professional assistance, although some people manage to do it on their own. The stimulant drugs in general are more deadly than most others, including narcotics, so it is very important to eliminate them if we want to live long and healthy lives.

A general detox program for a pharmaceutical or OTC drug involves first familiarizing ourself with its effects, side effects, addiction potential, and withdrawal symptoms (preferably, we do this before we use it). If we are using a drug, we must be able to acknowledge when we are addicted. We can tell this by some of the following characteristics:

Addiction

We need the drug to function.

We need it in ever higher doses.

We need it more frequently.

If we miss a dose, we begin to feel sick.

We have a history of abuse or addiction.

Some drugs are dangerous to stop. Going "cold turkey" from sedatives, stimulants, and narcotics can have serious consequences, including seizures. Tranquilizers may be needed to get us through the withdrawal phase. Overall, a plan should be made with the help of a professional, such as consulting a medical doctor or psychologist to help in withdrawal.

If we are slowing down or want to evaluate our drug use, we can record the dosage, time of use, and any reactions we may have and how long after taking the drug they occur. When we do stop, we should get busy to take our mind off the drug. There are now many more doctors and facilities, including hospital detox centers, that can help us deal with drug problems. Other therapies, such as counseling, biofeedback, behavior modification, and acupuncture, may help us in our plan to clean up our life and lessen our drug uses.

A few commonly used drugs will be discussed now—cocaine, marijuana, and the most common addiction, sugar. The other important drug habits, namely caffeine, alcohol, and nicotine abuse and addictions will be discussed thoroughly in subsequent programs.

Cocaine

Cocaine came into popular use in the United States with the introduction of Coca-Cola, when that drink had a lot of zip and addictive qualities. Since coca leaf extract was removed from Coca-Cola in 1903, the high sugar and caffeine content has been able to maintain the stimulating and addicting qualities, along with its depleting nature.

Cocaine is a central nervous system stimulant that produces an excited state shortly after it is inhaled ("snorted," "tooted") and a mild euphoria that lasts for 10–20 minutes, associated with an all-powerful "I can take on the world" kind of deluded feeling. It also increases the heart rate and blood pressure and reduces the appetite and financial reserve.

Cocaine is extremely addicting, both psychologically and physically (over time of course, not with one try; however, its withdrawal can be seen after any usage) and is very costly, often causing financial ruin to the addicted and his or her family. It can cause nasal, sinus, and mucous membrane damage when used intranasally, as it commonly is. It causes a cycle of excitability and depression that is often balanced with sedatives and then more stimulants. Speedballs (cocaine and heroin) and free basing (smoking it) are both extremely dangerous.

Cocaine withdrawal can be very difficult, particularly psychologically (the opiates, for example, seem to be more physically addicting).

COCAINE WITHDRAWAL SYMPTOMS

craving	runny nose	depression
anxiety	nasal irritation	apathy
sleepiness	fatigue	delirium
sleeplessness	muscle aches	seizures
irritability	weight gain	

With a good program, these symptoms can be minimized. An alkaline diet with lots of liquids, fruits, and vegetables and small amounts of whole grains and protein is helpful. Multivitamin/minerals with additional vitamin C and some antioxidants can smooth the withdrawal and support the healing transition.

For cocaine detoxification, as with healing from any drug, first we must acknowledge that we have a problem and decide to do something about it. We should get rid of all the drugs and paraphernalia and drop friends and associates that are tied to our drug problem. We can seek (and accept) the support of our spouse, friends, or relatives if we are comfortable with that. For actual withdrawal, we should prepare for symptoms with the aforementioned nutrients and the support of a professional. Tranquilizer drugs may be needed for a few days or longer, but these must be handled sensitively, as one addiction can easily replace another. Psychological counseling and/or a support group can help prevent any new addictions. Often it is helpful to become "addicted" to health for a while until we can work with our addictive personality, which can require longer therapy. During any transition or drug withdrawal, we should stay busy and exercise as much as possible, and stay away from parties where the problem drug may be used. Those who have a problem with cocaine or are tempted to use it again should talk to someone or check into a cocaine detox center. They can also call 800-COCAINE, a national line to help with this problem.

Dare I?
Dare I bend my brain on that Night Queen Cocaine
notice me . . .
I'm what you used to be
before you covered the door to your heart
with that lie, but now all you do is count
up how much you can buy
Composted Brains
Night Queen Cocaine
She'll suck you dry,
she'll pass you by
that Night Queen Cocaine.

—*Bethany ArgIsle*

Marijuana

Cannabis sativa (and *indica*), or marijuana, is the most commonly used illegal drug in the Western world. In the United States, it has become a megabusiness. For many years, it was thought to be fairly innocuous, but now most medical authorities believe that marijuana is not a harmless drug at all and that with regular use it can lead to many problems, both acute and chronic.

Of course, most things in moderation tend not to create any major problems, but cannabis is commonly abused and can be habit forming and psychologically addicting, with some mild physical withdrawal potential. The biggest concern is with children or teenagers—it tends to generate a nice relaxed feeling, but this "laid back" sensation may create an apathetic and irresponsible attitude toward life.

Marijuana "herb" probably has some positive medical potential. It is a good tranquilizer with fewer side effects than most. It has been shown to aid in general pain relief, and in glaucoma, it lowers the eye pressure; marijuana generally increases sensory awareness to our body and environment. However, it is not readily available for medical use.

Another side effect with regular marijuana smoking is that it can cause lung irritation and bronchitis, with an associated higher incidence of respiratory infections than in nonsmokers. Some preliminary studies suggest that it may even cause cancer (such as testicular cancer in men), but that would probably require excessive and/or long-term use. Further research is needed to evaluate this relationship and to differentiate the drug effect from that of possible pesticide exposure. Marijuana also has an effect on fertility. In men, it causes reduced testosterone levels, which may be associated with lack of aggressiveness, and can also reduce sperm count. In women, it lowers levels of prolactin, related to uterine function and breastfeeding, and is associated with irregular menstrual cycles.

Marijuana can also be an adrenal drain, lessening our ability to handle stress, and many regular cannabis smokers have associated hypoglycemic problems. The initial effect of smoking marijuana is an increased blood sugar. The "munchies" that are associated with "getting stoned" may be related to low blood sugar and reduced liver glycogen storage, setting up a craving for food, especially sweets. There is also some suggestion that marijuana sedates some of our immune functions, and I have classified it as an immune suppressant.

There can be emotional changes with both the smoking of and withdrawal from marijuana. Apathy or lack of motivation is common, though many people feel energized when stoned. Irritability and hostility are also common. Other personality changes are possible. Besides a craving to smoke, withdrawal symptoms include anxiety, hyperactivity, insomnia, anorexia, and depression.

For marijuana detoxification, as with other drugs, we must first decide that it is a problem and plan to stop, seeking support from companions. Avoid "pothead" friends and get rid of the "stuff" and associated paraphernalia. The tetrahydrocannabinol (THC), marijuana's active ingredient, gets stored in the body fat and liver, so as we detox, some of the withdrawal symptoms or flashbacks may surface, but usually they are pretty mild. With exercise, sweats, or weight loss, the fat will release toxins, but this is also helpful for a faster clearing. It is wise with marijuana withdrawal to avoid other drugs, tranquilizers, and cigarette smoke and to know and believe that we can stop it. As with alcohol and other only mildly toxic drugs, people seem to be able to use it occasionally for social or relaxation reasons, but when it becomes a regular habit, it is wise to avoid it completely.

Sugar

I wanted to include sugar in this program because I think it is easily the most commonly addictive food/drug worldwide. The traditional Chinese health system views the desire for sugar, or the sweet flavor, as a craving for the mother energy, a craving representing a need for comfort or security, whereas a desire for spicy or salty flavored foods might represent looking for the father energy or yang strength.

Although sugar addiction is common, for many people the craving is cyclical and usually mild (withdrawal also is usually mild physically), yet periodic strong cravings are possible. For those who are more sensitive to refined sugar, or any sweeteners, or for those who consume it in large amounts many times daily, many symptoms of abuse and withdrawal may occur.

Many nutritional authorities feel that the high use of sugar in our diet is a major nutritional culprit in disease. This includes sugar in all forms—from pure white beet or cane sugar, soda pops, and candies to honey and fruit juices. Sugar often replaces other, more nutritious foods, and it weakens our tissue health and body resistance. Microorganisms and insects love sweet, simple sugar foods, and a sweet diet allows greater

SUGAR ABUSE AND WITHDRAWAL SYMPTOMS

headaches	sugar cravings
visual disturbance	weakness
blurry vision	inability to concentrate
anxiety	depression
tachycardia	delirium
rage	

infestation with bacteria, fungi, and parasites, and then will support their growth, which may weaken our immunity. Reducing our entire dietary sugar load is important.

If we have a problem with sugar abuse, we can decide to change this and cut down on or eliminate this substance by avoiding many of the sweet foods. Many people who abuse sugar do not eat a wholesome diet and have nutritional deficiencies, hypoglycemia, and other problems, both physical and psychological. Let us also not forget the more severe problem of "sugar diabetes."

There are many other more nutritious nibbles to replace sugary foods. These include popcorn, rice cakes, vegetable sticks, fruits, nuts, seeds, and unsweetened granola. We should clear our house of unhealthy sweetened foods. Once sugar has been removed from the diet, it is still possible to use it again, but only as occasional treats, as it is not as readdicting as many stronger drugs. Many people who have kicked the sugar habit find that they no longer tolerate sugar very well.

AVOID SUGAR FOODS

candy	white sugar	cake
soda pop	fructose	cookies
ice cream	maple syrup	doughnuts
artificial juices	honey	liqueurs
fruit juices	chewing gum	wine

Nutrients that can help reduce the sugar craving and help in sugar withdrawal are the B vitamins, vitamin C, zinc, the trace mineral chromium, and amino acid L-glutamine. Chromium is the central molecule of glucose tolerance factor, which helps insulin work more efficiently at removing sugar from the blood and nourishing the cells. The amino acid L-glutamine, which can be used directly by the brain, has also been helpful in reducing sugar (and alcohol) cravings. A diet that is rich in whole grains and other complex carbohydrates, vegetables, and protein foods can also help stabilize the blood sugar and minimize the desire for sugar.

There are many other addictions to be aware of. We all find something to latch onto in order to feel connected. It is important to stay aware of these patterns so that we can step out of our dependency and gain perspective on our habits. Besides addictions to people, such as mother, father, spouse, or friends, many of us are addicted to our kids or animals. Some have addictions to work or money. Others are addicted to running around or talking and go through withdrawal when they stop and try to sit still and quietly. Still others are the opposite and are attached to inactivity. The telephone, television, and computer are even more common addictions in our technological age.

I would say that the addictive aspect of drugs and diet is emotional in nature. Dietary flavors, certain foods, and certain feelings we get from them and the drugs that we try are usually conditioned. Often, an ability to stop and see things clearly or to talk about them with a counselor will allow us to make the necessary transition from addiction to safe and balanced use of substances in all aspects of our life.

The following program is a general one for drug detoxification and for suppport during drug use. The ranges of many nutrients allow varying amounts to be used depending upon needs. During withdrawal, the higher levels may be used, with mid-range levels used during the three to six weeks of detox after the initial withdrawal. Lower ranges may provide basic support during general drug usage.

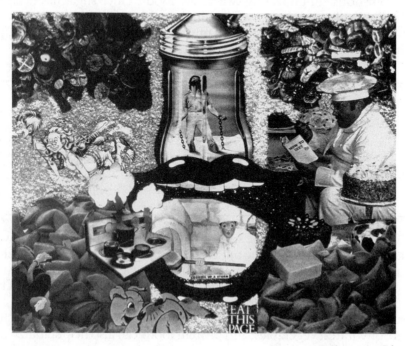

Bethany ArgIsle

DRUG DETOXIFICATION NUTRIENT PROGRAM

Water	2–3½ qt.		
Fiber	20–40 g.		

Vitamin A	10,000 IUs	**Iron**	10–20 mg.
Beta-carotene	20,000–40,000 IUs	**Magnesium**	400–800 mg.+
Vitamin D	200–400 IUs	**Manganese**	5–10 mg.
Vitamin E	200–800 IUs	**Molybdenum**	150–300 mcg.
Vitamin K	300 mcg.	**Potassium**	100–500 mg.
Thiamine (B₁)	25–100 mg.	**Selenium**	200–300 mcg.
Riboflavin (B₂)	25–100 mg.	**Silicon**	50–150 mg.
Niacinamide (B₃)	50–100 mg.	**Vanadium**	200–400 mcg.
Niacin (B₃)	50–1,000 mg.*	**Zinc**	30–60 mg.
Pantothenic acid (B₅)	250–1,000 mg.		
Pyridoxine (B₆)	25–100 mg.		
Pyridoxal-5-phosphate	25–50 mg.	**L-amino acids**	1,500 mg.
Cobalamin (B₁₂)	100–250 mcg.	**L-cysteine**	250–500 mg.
Folic acid	800 mcg.	**L-glutamine**	250–1,000 mg.
Biotin	300 mcg.	**Essential fatty acids,**	2–4 capsules
Choline	500–1,000 mg.	** or Flaxseed oil**	2–4 teaspoons
Inositol	500–1,000 mg.	**Goldenseal root**	3–6 capsules
Vitamin C	2–10 g.		
Bioflavonoids	250–500 mg		
Calcium	650–1,200 mg.+		
Chromium	200–500 mcg.		
Copper	2–3 mg.		
Iodine	150 mcg.		

*Increase dosage slowly.

+Higher amounts are needed for hyperactive withdrawal states, aches, or cravings.

Caffeine Detoxification

Caffeine has become a ubiquitous drug. Used originally in most cultures for ceremony or some daily stimulation, it has become a regular, overused energy stimulant in the Western world, with the United States leading in coffee and caffeine use.

Coffee, brewed from the ground-up coffee bean (*Coffea arabica*), is the major vehicle for caffeine consumption. In this country, more than a half billion cups are drunk daily, with most consumers drinking two or more cups, and more than ten pounds of coffee per person are consumed yearly. This food/drug mixture, often along with sugar and/or milk, is one of the most freely marketed substances in the world.

There are several basic areas of concern about this substance. I believe that a major one, possibly even more important than the caffeine itself, is the toxic chemicals used in the many stages of growing and marketing coffee. The easily rancified oils and the irritating acids contained in the beans offer further hazards. People trying to cut down by drinking "decaf" could even be exposed to dangerous chemicals unless they are drinking coffee prepared by the "water process" or Swiss process, which uses steam distillation to remove the caffeine. Otherwise, agents such as TCE (trichlorethylene) or methylene chloride used in the chemical processing may be contained as residues in the decaf coffee. More coffee-drinking concerns have arisen over the last decades as pesticide use and chemical processing have generally increased, though fortunately our coffee consumption has lessened over the last 40 years. In 1946, at the peak of use, yearly consumption was 20 pounds per person; since most children and some adults were not consuming any, many people were consuming a lot more than the 1,000-cup-a-year average. In 1979, estimated consumption was down to around 9 pounds per year, or about two cups per day per person. It has gone up slightly since then, here and in many other countries of the world, where it is also consumed in large quantities.

Another problem is caffeine's widespread use in so many products, such as soft drinks and many over-the-counter (OTC) drugs. All products containing caffeine should carry a warning saying something like, "Caffeine can be hazardous to your health. Regular use may be addicting and injurious." The problem here is less with the drug itself and more with the amounts consumed and the constant stimulation on which people depend many times daily. One big area of concern here is with children and teenagers, who may consume large amounts of caffeine in soft drinks. Cola naturally contains caffeine, yet many soft drinks have even more added. The caffeine creates an addiction to the drink.

Another concern is that caffeine addiction often occurs along with other substance abuses, nicotine and sugar most commonly. Caffeine, like sugar, overstimulates the adrenals and then weakens them with persistent or chronic use. First, sugar stimulates and weakens the adrenals, which creates fatigue. Then we use caffeine to keep us aware and awake, further depleting our adrenals, to which many respond by drinking more caffeine with sugar. In addition, people who overuse caffeine tend to need more tranquilizers and sleeping pills to help them relax or sleep.

Caffeine can be a lifetime drug for many. We begin with hot chocolate or chocolate bars, which contain some caffeine, move into colas or other soft drinks with caffeine, and then add coffee and tea. Many adults use caffeine daily, but this is slowly changing with education and experience revealing the long-range problems resulting from caffeine abuse.

Caffeine, one of the class of methylxanthine chemicals/drugs, is present in coffee and many other drinks and products. Another of the xanthines, theophylline, is found in black teas; it is also commonly used in medicine to aid in breathing. Theobromine, the third xanthine derivative, is found in cocoa. Methylxanthines are found in many other plants, including the kola nut originally used to make cola drinks.

Physiologically, caffeine is a central nervous system (CNS) stimulant. A dosage of 50–100 mg., the amount in one cup of coffee, will produce an apparent temporary increase in mental clarity and energy level while reducing drowsiness. For many users, it specifically improves muscular-coordinated work activity, such as typing. Through its CNS stimulation, caffeine increases brain activity, but it also stimulates the cardiovascular system, raising blood pressure and heart rate. It generally speeds up our body, increasing the basal metabolic rate (BMR), which can help burn more calories. Initially, caffeine may lower blood sugar, leading to increased hunger or craving for sweets. After the adrenal stimulation, the blood sugar rises again. Caffeine also increases the respiratory rate, and for people with tight airways, it opens the breathing passages, as do the other xanthine drugs. Caffeine is also a diuretic and a mild laxative, an effect that many coffee drinkers appreciate.

The amount needed to produce the wake-up and stimulation effect increases with regular use, as is typical of addictive drugs. Larger and more frequent doses are needed for the same effect, and symptoms can develop if we do not get our "fix." Eventually, we need the drug to function; without it, fatigue and drowsiness occur. So caffeine is a natural stimulant with both physical and psychological addiction potential and with withdrawal symptoms similar to the symptoms of its abuse.

A nutritional concern of most caffeine products is that they do not contain any of the nutrients (coffee and tea have a little manganese and copper) needed to support the increased activity that they cause. Also, the diuretic effect of caffeine leads to the urinary loss of many nutrients.

There are many possible symptoms and signs of caffeine intoxication and abuse. People who are already overstimulated, busy types (adrenal or fiery types) do not necessarily like the effects of caffeine. I have never been inclined to drink coffee because of both the taste and the effects, yet I understand that many people thoroughly enjoy the experience. The key to its use is moderation and avoiding addiction (even daily use can be considered as addiction). Allergy-type addiction is also fairly common, especially with coffee, but also with tea, chocolate, and cola. With allergy, withdrawal from the substance may lead to even worse symptoms.

Overall, addiction to caffeine is not as bad as addiction to most other drugs, but it is a problem for many. Completely stopping its use or tapering it off over time before stopping may produce several symptoms. Usually, the slower the tapering, the easier the withdrawal. After withdrawal and detox from caffeine, it is possible that it can still be used in moderation, but for many people, it can easily become a habit and addiction again. We cannot really know the severity of our addiction until we get off caffeine.

SIGNS AND SYMPTOMS OF CAFFEINE INTOXICATION OR ABUSE

nervousness	headache	increased heart rate
anxiety	upset stomach	irregular heartbeat
irritability	GI irritation	elevated blood pressure
agitation	heartburn	increased cholesterol
tremors	diarrhea	nutritional deficiencies
insomnia	fatigue	poor concentration
depression	dizziness	bed wetting

CAFFEINE WITHDRAWAL SYMPTOMS

headache	constipation	runny nose
craving	anxiety	nausea
irritability	nervousness	vomiting
insomnia	shakiness	cramps
fatigue	dizziness	ringing in the ears
depression	drowsiness	feeling hot and cold
apathy	inability to concentrate	tachycardia

The most common withdrawal symptom is a throbbing and/or pressure headache, usually located at the temples but occasionally at the back of the head or around the eyes. A vague muscular headache often follows. Of course, caffeine cures the symptom; but this is not the answer. Dietary guidelines and supplements may help with this and other withdrawal problems.

Let us now look at the wide range of uses of caffeine in the food and drug industries. Caffeine and caffeinelike xanthines are contained in coffee, many teas, cola, and chocolate. Of the teas, all "black" teas or common teas contain theophylline and theobromine, as do some "green" teas. Both contain less caffeine than coffee. These teas and coffee also contain tannic acid, which is a mild irritant to the gastrointestinal mucosa, and may further bind and reduce absorption of minerals, such as manganese, zinc, and copper. Most herbs do not contain caffeine, although maté and guarana are fairly high in caffeine. The kola nut and the cocoa bean also contain caffeine. All of these are natural products that have been used as stimulants throughout history; today, caffeine and its related stimulating xanthines are used in many artificial products, including soft drinks such as Coca-Cola, Pepsi Cola, Mountain Dew, Dr. Pepper, and Jolt, plus many chocolate bars. (Some of the soft drink companies are now making caffeine-free drinks.)

CAFFEINE-CONTAINING FOOD PRODUCTS

yerba maté	guarana root
kola nut	cocoa/chocolate
some soft drinks	tea
coffee	

Both extracted and synthesized caffeine may be added to other products. Many common pharmaceutical preparations contain caffeine for its stimulating effects to counteract sedating antihistamines or for its cerebral vasodilating effects to re–lieve vascular headaches. Cafergot is a prescription drug containing caffeine and is used for migraines; thus, caffeine can help reduce headaches or cause them, which is more common.

CAFFEINE DRUGS AVAILABLE OVER THE COUNTER

Stimulants—NoDoz, Vivarin, Refresh'n
Weight control—Dexatrim, Dietac
Pain Relief—Excedrin, Anacin, Vanquish, Empirin Compound
Menstrual pain relief—Midol, Premens, Aqua-Ban, Cope
Cold remedies—Dristan, Sinarest

Some people run their bodies on caffeine and not on their basic life force and the natural energy of their hormones, such as adrenal and thyroid. Caffeine, although it is not seriously addicting, is very habit forming. It is not particularly good for athletes or anyone seriously interested in their health. Although it may improve muscular work and short-term performance in both physical and mental athletes, it creates depletion by its diuretic nutrients, and foods can help balance this.

CAFFEINE LEVELS* IN COMMON SUBSTANCES**

Coffee and Other Drinks/6 oz. cup	Amount of Caffeine (mg.)	OTC Medicines	Amount of Caffeine (mg.)
Drip	120–150	NoDoz	100
Percolated	80–110	Vivarin	200
Instant	60–70	Dexatrim	200
Decaf	3–10	Dietac	200
Black tea	50–60	Cafergot	100
Green tea	30–40	Excedrin	65
Cocoa	10–30	Fiorinal	40
Chocolate milk	10–15	Anacin	30
Cocoa (dry, 1 oz.)	40–50	Vanquish	33
Chocolate (dry, 1 oz.)	5–10	Aqua-Ban	100
		Midol	32

Soft drinks, per 12 oz. serving	
Colas	30–65
Mountain Dew	50

*These caffeine levels and caffeine equivalents may depend on length of brewing time or amount of product used.

**Information gathered and integrated from at least six different sources.

Negative Effects of Caffeine

Most of the negative effects are not a concern with occasional caffeine use, such as a cup of coffee, tea, or cola a few times a week or even once daily. However, with regular use of over 100 mg. daily, many problems arise. A limit of one cup of coffee daily is suggested, along with a week off every few months just to assure us that we are not addicted and that we do not have appreciable symptoms from stopping or restarting. If we do, then we should stop totally.

The risks discussed in the following list vary with the level of caffeine intake. A total of over 500 mg. daily could be a relatively high intake. The total includes coffee, tea, soft drinks, and drugs (that is, five cups of coffee a day or a few cups of coffee and a few caffeinated aspirins, as examples). Between 250 and 500 mg. might be classified as moderate intake, while under 250 mg. would be low. With chronic use, the risks of problems rise, and even lower amounts become more of a concern.

For a long time, the popularity of caffeine has led people to resist the initial negative findings. Now the dangers are fairly clear, and it is hard to refute the evidence of the many difficulties generated by this addictive drug. Possible negative effects from caffeine use and abuse include the following:

- Common side effects of caffeine use include excess nervousness, irritability, insomnia, "restless legs," dizziness, and subsequent fatigue. Headaches can also be very common, as is "heartburn." Psychological symptoms of general anxiety or panic attacks may also occur. Hyperactivity and bed wetting may also develop in children who consume caffeine.

- An acid irritant to the gastrointestinal tract and liver, caffeine directly increases stomach hydrochloric acid production, so it is clearly bad for people with or prone to ulcers or gastritis. Regular coffee drinking thus also increases the likelihood of peptic ulcer disease. Decaffeinated coffee is also acidic, though it is less stimulating.

- Caffeine's diuretic effect causes loss of potassium, magnesium, zinc and other minerals, and B vitamins, especially thiamine B_1. Caffeine also washes out vitamin C. Therefore, all of these nutrients can be deficient unless they are obtained from foods in increased amounts or taken as supplements.

- Caffeine, and particularly coffee, reduces absorption of iron and calcium, especially when it is drunk around mealtime. These minerals are extremely important for women. Osteoporosis and anemia are thus more common with regular coffee use. Also in children and adolescents, caffeinated drinks interfere with these essential minerals needed for growth and health.

- Diarrhea can also occur with increased amounts of caffeine, which relaxes the smooth muscle in the colon. The laxative effect of caffeine can also create a dependency.

- A number of negative cardiovascular effects are caused by caffeine. First, it raises the blood pressure. Hypertension is a risk factor in atherosclerosis and heart disease. Caffeine increases cholesterol and triglyceride blood levels, also risk factors in cardiovascular disease. Heart rhythm disturbances, arrythmias, though usually of a mild type, occur with caffeine; these include a generally increased heart rate (tachycardia) and excitability of the heart nerve conduction system, leading to both palpitations and extra beats. Caffeine also increases norepinephrine secretion, which causes some vasoconstriction—that is, restricted blood flow. Although caffeine may have a mild direct vasodilating effect in the heart and body (vasoconstricting in the brain), the adrenal stimulation may override this. Research reports regarding caffeine's role in increasing the risk of heart attacks are mixed; however, it seems reasonable with the cardiovascular stimulation of caffeine to assume that drinking four to five cups of coffee per day does increase the incidence of myocardial infarctions. Overall, caffeine clearly increases risk of cardiovascular disease.

- Fibrocystic breast disease (FBD) may also be a consequence of caffeine use. Although results of various studies seem to be contradictory as to whether caffeine is a cause of FBD, it is clear that some women are more sensitive to caffeine use and that they experience an increase in size and number of cysts with increased use and a reduction of the disease when they stop using caffeine.

- Birth defects have been noted with higher levels of caffeine use during pregnancy. Spontaneous abortions are also more frequent with coffee drinking early in pregnancy. It is clear that caffeine crosses the placenta and affects the fetus, but whether it is the caffeine itself or other chemicals in coffee which have a mutagenic effect is not clear. It is wise to limit or completely avoid the use of caffeine during pregnancy. Caffeine also gets into breast milk, so it is also wise to limit its use during the nursing period to prevent having a jittery baby.

- The incidence of certain cancers is increased with caffeine use. Bladder cancer may result, probably also from a nicotine and caffeine combination along with the mild dehydration that occurs from the result of using these two drugs. Ovarian cancer is increased in women with an association of long-term coffee intake. Pancreatic cancer, which is very deadly, has also been in question as occurring more frequently with increased coffee use (more than three cups per day). Whether this is caused by the caffeine or by the chemicals used in coffee that concentrate in its oils is not clear. Recent research has cast some doubt on this relationship, however. Prostate enlargement and cancer may also be attributed to increased caffeine intake.

- Caffeine may also be correlated with kidney stones, possibly as a result of the diuretic and chemical effects. The fluoride mineral that is found in coffee and tea can also cause problems when consumed in excess. In addition, caffeine use may increase fevers, both by a mild direct effect and by counteracting the effect of aspirin.

- The adrenal exhaustion/stress/fatigue/hypoglycemia syndrome is tied to caffeine use as well. Caffeine has an overall effect of increasing blood sugar (especially when it is sweetened), as it stimulates the adrenals. Both stress and sugar use tend to pressure and weaken the adrenal function. Recovery from the resulting fatigue requires rest, stress reduction, and sugar avoidance, but caffeine can override this fatigue and restimulate the adrenals. This process can eventually lead to chronic fatigue, adrenal exhaustion, and subsequent inability to handle stress and sugar intake. Caffeine will then be of little help.

What to do—Detox

Anyone with regular caffeine intake should truly consider withdrawing from their habit until they can reach a state of occasional use and enjoyment. For caffeine detoxification, it is important to support ourselves nutritionally while we eliminate or reduce our intake. If we are clearly addicted to caffeine products or if we become pregnant, we should quit totally. Breaking the habit by tapering down or going "cold turkey" will be better handled with a good diet and adrenal support.

An alkaline diet is helpful during detoxification. Fruits can be used as snacks; vegetable salads, soups, greens, seaweed, corn, some whole grains, sprouts, soy products, and some nuts and seeds are the basis of this high-nutrient diet. A decrease in acid foods, such as meats, sugar (avoiding sugar may really help minimize caffeine withdrawal), and refined flours, and avoiding overuse of baked goods, even whole grain products, and nuts and seeds are good ideas. Drinking at least six to eight glasses of filtered water and sipping on some mineral waters can help replace the coffee habit. Often, some baking soda or, even better, potassium bicarbonate tablets, will help make us more alkaline and reduce withdrawal symptoms.

Vitamin C supplementation also helps during withdrawal and supports the adrenals. As an antistress program, several grams or more of vitamin C can be taken over the course of the day, preferably in a buffered form, along with certain minerals such as potassium, calcium, magnesium, and zinc, all of which often need to be supplemented. B complex vitamins with extra pantothenic acid (250 mg. four times daily) along with 500 mg. of vitamin C every two hours can be helpful in withdrawal.

With general coffee usage, we need to support the commonly depleted nutrients. These include thiamine (B_1), riboflavin (B_2), pyridoxine (B_6), vitamin C, potassium, magnesium, and probably zinc, iron, calcium, and the trace minerals. Sometimes additional amino acids are helpful in balancing our energy level during use or withdrawal from caffeine. Water intake and additional fiber, even on top of a high-fiber diet, will help support the bowel function, which can slow down during caffeine withdrawal.

For caffeine detoxification, it is definitely easier to detox over a week or two to avoid significant headaches and other symptoms, although some regular users can stop fairly easily without many problems. Drinking grain-coffee blends, diluted or smaller amounts of regular coffee, or decaffeinated coffee (only if it is water processed) is a good way to reduce caffeine intake. Some people can substitute tea, which has less caffeine, and taper off of that more easily.

If headaches occur during detoxification, some mild pain relievers can be used for a few days, but not much longer. Increased water intake, vitamin C and mineral support, an alkaline diet, and white willow bark herb tablets, which contain a natural salicylate, may also ease withdrawal.

As we move away from coffee and caffeine beverages, there are a number of herbal substitutes that can be both stimulating and refreshing. The roasted herbal roots, including barley, chicory, and dandelion, are most common. These grain "coffees," such as Rombouts, Postum, Pero, Cafix, and Wilson's Heritage, are becoming very popular among former coffee drinkers. Ginseng root tea is preferred by some. The Chinese herb ephedra is a stimulant like caffeine and can be used for transitions, though I do not recommend its regular intake as we still want our body's natural energizing functions to work. Ephedra is found in a number of "natural" stimulant formulas. Herbal teas made from lemon grass, peppermint, ginger root, red clover, and comfrey can also be very energizing.

HERBAL CAFFEINE SUBSTITUTES

Roasted barley	Rombouts	Ginseng root
Chicory root	Rosataroma	Ginger root
Dandelion root	Wilson's Heritage	Ephedra
Postum	Cafix	Comfrey leaf
Pero	Miso broth	Lemon grass
Pioneer	Duran	Red clover
	Peppermint	Comfrey leaf

Some authorities feel that if we are to drink a cup of coffee a day, we should do it in the mid to late afternoon, the most harmonious time. For the English, this is teatime. This best fits our body's natural cycle, as it does not interfere with the usually "up," high-adrenal morning hours, it mildly supports our relaxing time of the day while we may still have work to do, yet it is not too late interfere with sleep for most people. Those who are sensitive to caffeine's effects may not relax or sleep well after using it; they should consider avoiding it totally or using it only rarely.

The pleasures of coffee or tea drinking are related to our culture, taste preferences, and conditioning in terms of both social graces and work/life demands. All of these are developed, not inherent, and anything we learn, we can also unlearn or relearn. This is often what it takes to change our regular drinking of caffeinated beverages to more healthful practices regarding liquid refreshments and energy generation.

The ranges for certain nutrients in the table above represent amounts that vary from the lower support levels to the higher amounts to be used during detoxification. The amounts shown are daily totals, usually taken two or three times during the day.

New and Healthful Coffee Break

Take three days free of caffeine every two to three weeks—allow the body to rest and recover from the repeated stimulation. Instead, drink hot lemonade with mint tea and honey, or your favorite herbal beverage.

—Bethany ArgIsle

CAFFEINE SUPPORT AND DETOX NUTRIENT PROGRAM

Water	2½–3 qt.
Fiber	15–20 g.

Vitamin A	10,000 IUs	**Iodine**	150 mcg.
Beta-carotene	25,000 IUs	**Iron**	men—10–20 mg.
Vitamin D	400 IUs		women—20–30 mg.
Vitamin E	400–800 IUs	**Magnesium**	500–800 mg.
Vitamin K	300 mcg.	**Manganese**	5–10 mg.
Thiamine (B$_1$)	75–150 mg.	**Molybdenum**	300–500 mcg.
Riboflavin (B$_2$)	50–100 mg.	**Potassium**	300–600 mg.
Niacinamide (B$_3$)	50–100 mg.	**Silicon**	100 mg.
Niacin (B$_3$)	50–100 mg.	**Selenium**	200 mcg.
Pantothenic acid (B$_5$)	500–1,000 mg.	**Zinc**	45–75 mg.
Pyridoxine (B$_6$)	50–100 mg.		
Pyridoxal-5-phosphate	25–50 mg.	**Adrenal**	50–50 mg.
Cobalamin (B$_{12}$)	100–200 mcg.	**L-amino acids**	500–1,500 mg.
Folic acid	400–800 mcg.	**Potassium**	
Biotin	300 mcg.	**bicarbonate***	600–1,000 mg.
Vitamin C	2–6 g.		
Bioflavonoids	250–500 mg.		
Calcium	800–1,000 mg.		
Chromium	200–400 mcg.		
Copper	2–3 mg.		

*Can use Alka-Seltzer Effervescent Antacid, one tablet 2–3 times daily.

Alcohol Detoxification

Even though alcohol is in such general use worldwide, the regular consumption of alcoholic beverages is a serious health hazard and definitely a nutritional problem. Alcoholic beverages made by the fermentation of grains or fruits have been used for thousands of years. As with caffeine, occasional use or moderate social use is not a great cause for concern (other than for sensitive people or those who already have some disease of the liver, gastrointestinal tract, kidneys, brain, or nervous system), but alcohol abuse can lead to addiction, emotional problems, and a number of specific degenerative processes. Obesity, gastritis and ulcers, pancreatitis, hepatitis, cirrhosis, hypoglycemia and diabetes, gout, nerve and brain dysfunction, cancer, nutritional deficiencies, immune suppression, and injury and death from falls and auto accidents are some of the more common problems. Overall, alcohol is a toxic irritant for the human being.

Some people can handle as much as a drink or two a day, but that depends on their individual sensitivity. Certain drug-liberal medical authorities claim that two drinks daily may enhance our health and even increase our longevity by improving digestion, relaxation, and circulation, but I believe this is stretching it a bit, especially in light of the many chemicals used in the fermentation and bottling processes. These evaluations are done on people with average habits, and not health-conscious individuals who are trying to avoid intoxicants. For them, regular alcohol use can be very irritating.

Still, alcohol does have some positive physiological effects. It can stimulate the appetite and has a mild stress-relieving effect, though not as much as exercise. It is a vasodilator, so it improves the blood flow. Alcohol may also affect a mild increase in the HDL "good" cholesterol; however, it also raises the total fat levels, which is not so good. Small to moderate amounts (one to two drinks daily) may lessen the progression of atherosclerosis and heart disease. Some studies have shown a decrease in heart attacks in moderate drinkers over nondrinkers of the same age, possibly due to increased HDL cholesterol levels; and thus reduced atherosclerosis. Higher amounts of alcohol, however, increase blood pressure and heart disease risk. More research is needed to understand the real alcohol–heart disease relationship to see if drinking really helps without causing more problems, such as obesity, ulcers, liver disease, or cancer. I am sure that regular physical activity and nurturing personal relationships are much better health supporters and stress reducers to replace those couple of drinks daily, and will not have the side effects of alcohol.

There are over 100 million regular drinkers in the United States alone and an estimated 10 million alcoholics. More than half of our population (some estimates are that 80 percent of adults are social drinkers) use some alcohol, and more than three-fourths have tried it. Approximately one in ten drinkers have an alchohol problem. This is an even bigger concern in teenagers, who are not prepared to handle this depressant drug. More and more children are trying alcohol, and an estimated 15–20 percent of those 15–17 years old are regular drinkers.

Alcohol itself contains empty calories—seven calories per gram, almost double the calories in regular carbohydrates and protein (four calories per gram each). The average social drinker obtains about 5–10 percent of his or her calories from alcohol, while alcoholics may consume more than 50 percent of their calories as alcohol. This is a lot of calories and little nutrition, so deficiency diseases can be serious. In addition, the alcohol molecule is small and easy to absorb, so it gets assimilated before other foods and goes directly into the blood for that quick lift (or down). Most beer, wine, and especially the mixed drinks also rapidly affect the blood sugar. The liver is the only organ that really metabolizes alcohol, which can be converted into immediate energy or fat and is stored in the body or in the liver when there is excess consumption. Alcohol is not converted to glucose for use or to glycogen for storage, which is a significant nutritional limitation. When stored as fat in the liver, it is an irritant and can eventually lead to cirrhosis, or scarring of the liver tissue. Some alcohol, about 5 percent, is eliminated in the sweat, urine, and breath.

The opposite of caffeine, alcohol is a central nervous system depressant. It acts as a tranquilizer and mild anesthetic, for which it has been used for centuries. On the negative side, alcohol slows us down mentally and physically, as it hampers our reflexes and judgment. Many people believe it to be stimulating, but this is because it reduces inhibitions and, in small amounts, increases social interactions. It is a sedative that lowers our function and coordination. This is why there are so many alcohol-related accidents, occurring both while walking (or trying to walk) and while driving. Yet alcohol is part of much of our business life and social life. If it were used only for an occasional toast or celebration, we would be able to handle it much better; but when we feel emotionally depressed, we may want to celebrate all the time.

Alcohol is clearly an emotional suppressant, and because of this, it is cause for serious concern. Many people drink to cover up their feelings or to block pain. Alcoholism and alcohol abuse are clearly emotional diseases. It is possible that for some people this disease is genetic, perhaps involving an enzyme deficiency, but this has yet to be demonstrated. A deficiency or improper function of chromium, a trace mineral important to blood sugar metabolism, may influence alcoholism as well. Alcohol problems definitely seem to run in families. Children of alcoholics grow up feeling emotionally deprived, as the alcoholic parent is really not there for them. Adult Children of Alcoholics have formed many support groups nationwide to help them deal with their common problems.

Alcohol can also be an allergy-addiction problem. Certain grains, grapes, sugar, and yeast can all produce allergy reactions, including intestinal and cerebral symptoms. Corn, wheat, rye, and barley may all cause allergic reactions, and alcoholism may be an advanced food addiction, wherein the drinker obtains a quick absorption of the addictive food/drug. The allergy itself stimulates addiction, as withdrawal produces immediate psychological and physical symptoms. Alcohol products can also be a problem for people with a yeast overgrowth, as it feeds the yeasts and stimulates their growth.

There are some who claim that alcoholic beverages are nourishing. Wine contains vitamin C from grape (or rice) juice. Most wines have about 9–12 percent alcohol; in sherry and port wines, it may be higher, at 12–18 percent. Beers and ale have B vitamins and minerals from the cereal grains and yeast; usually, the brews range from 3–6 percent alcohol. The alcohol distillates or "spirits," including gin, vodka, rum, and whiskey, are made from grain products. They range from 35–50 percent alcohol—that is, 70–100 proof. In reality, none of these beverages is very nourishing when we compare the calorie levels with the actual nutrient contents.

CALORIE CONTENT OF ALCOHOLIC BEVERAGES

Amount to Provide 0.5 oz. of Alcohol	Type of Beverage	Calories
1 oz.	100 or 110 proof liquor	80
1½ oz.	80 proof liquor	90–110
5 oz.	8–10 percent wine (French, German)	100
4 oz.	12–14 percent wine (most American)	95
3 oz.	17–20 percent wine (sherry, port)	80
2½ oz.	18 percent dessert wine	120
8 oz.	6–7 percent dark beer (stout, porter)	150
12 oz.	4.5 percent regular beer	140
12 oz.	light beer	90
6 oz.	mixed drinks (various juices, sodas, sweeteners)	100–250

Risks of Alcohol

Alcohol overuse, abuse, and addiction generate a huge complex of problems, both internally, affecting most of our body systems and our mental and emotional functioning, and externally, in our personal lives and careers. Alcohol is a toxin that generates symptoms, deficiencies, and degenerative diseases. The excessive calorie intake from alcohol abuse also leads to obesity with its many problems. Alcohol use is particularly of concern in young people, as most are not really prepared for its effects. Nearly 90 percent of high school seniors have tried alcohol, according to some polls. Among college students, consumption is incredibly high. Let's face it, alcohol is still the most popular recreational drug. It is reasonably priced, compared to other drugs, and easy to obtain, apparently even for teenagers. Some even relate their first sexual experience to an alcoholic high, and this could set a precedent for life. Generally, our culture is very drug-oriented, and the peer pressure for drinking is fairly high in some circles.

Fermented alcoholic beverages have been available to the human species for an estimated 10,000 years. They have always been used as a symbol of celebration, and they have always been abused by some, more so now than at many other times in history. Of the many countries whose cultures center around alcohol consumption, many are Western, such as France, Italy, and the Scandinavian countries. Most Third World or native populations are less abusive unless alcohol is introduced to them by others—for example, among native Americans and Mexican-Americans, alcohol problems are now commonplace.

Alcohol abuse is commonly associated with denial of the problem, which, I believe, is inherent in this emotional disease. It is especially important for alcoholics to avoid other addictions, such as cigarette smoking and caffeine drinking, as these add even more risks to the health problems of alcohol. But since most alcohol abusers have a generally destructive lifestyle and poor attitude toward life and self, nicotine and caffeine are common companions. Red-meat diets with many fatty and refined foods often go along with drinking, and may also contribute to problems of excess and deficiency. Often, our whole life needs to be corrected to deal with alcohol abuse. Alcoholism is a disease that needs treatment.

The risks of alcohol are directly related to the amount of alcohol consumed and the time period over which it is used. Individual sensitivity and associated nutritional balance, supplements, allergy, and lifestyle factors also contribute to the specific problems that may result from alcohol. Empirically, high risk may be assumed to be posed by more than five drinks daily; moderate risk by three to five drinks daily; and low risk by one or two drinks daily. Social drinking of one or two drinks a week is considered light use.

Given the general liberal viewpoint regarding low-level alcohol consumption that prevails in common medical literature, I should clarify who should not drink. Clearly, people with diabetes, hypertension, or heart disease and pregnant or nursing mothers (and those planning pregnancy) should avoid alcohol completely. People with hypoglycemic problems, liver disorders, especially hepatitis, viral diseases, candidiasis, mental confusion, fatigue, or hypersensitive reactions to alcoholic beverages should also avoid it.

Major Risks of Alcohol

1. *Symptoms from drinking itself.* These include dizziness, talkativeness, slowed reflexes, slowed mental functions, loss of memory, poor judgment, emotional outbursts, incoordination, inability to walk, and loss of consciousness.

2. *Symptoms of hangover.* These include dryness of mouth, thirst, headache (throbbing temples are common), nausea, vomiting, stomach upset, fatigue, and dizziness. Alcohol dehydrates the cells, removes fluid from the blood, swells the cranial arteries, and irritates the gastrointestinal tract. Hangovers are more common with distilled, stronger alcohol drinks and less so with red wine, champagne, white wine, and beer. One theory is that the hangover is primarily an effect of the chemical congeners produced through the formation of fermentation by-products and the many chemicals used in growing the foods and manufacturing the beverages, although no chemicals (even food dyes) need be listed on a label.

3. *Symptoms of withdrawal.* These include alcohol craving, nausea, vomiting, gastrointestinal upset, abdominal cramps, anorexia, fatigue, headache, anxiety, irritability, dizziness, dry mouth, fevers, chills, depression, hyperactivity, insomnia, tremors, weakness, hallucinations, seizures, and delirium tremens (DTs). These symptoms, of course, vary according to the degree of alcohol abuse and individual sensitivities.

4. *Injuries, auto accidents, violent crimes, and jail.* It has become clear that alcohol abuse affects others through the actions of the abuser, causing innocent people to be injured and killed. Alcohol is responsible for more than 25,000 deaths a year from auto accidents, about half of all driver deaths and about one-third of pedestrian mortalities. About 20 percent of home accidental deaths are also attributed to alcohol, as are many falls and drownings. Other drugs may also be involved in these accidents and injuries, but alcohol is by far the most common culprit. The suppressant action of alcohol also reduces self-control, judgment, and usual moral sense. Drunk people act out their aggressions, often on their loved ones or strangers as well as themselves. Alcoholics have higher than average suicide rates. The weakened adrenal response from alcohol makes us less able to handle stress. With the growing awareness of the menacing qualities of alcohol, more stringent laws are being enacted to prosecute drunk drivers, and jail is usually good negative feedback for changing alcohol abuse. However, this alone may not correct or cure this common disease.

5. *Liver disease.* Alcohol irritates the liver, raising the liver enzyme levels and leading to hepatitis (liver inflammation). Remember, 95 percent of alcohol consumed must be metabolized in the liver; this process requires a lot of work and takes precedence over many other necessary functions. Fat metabolism is decreased, and fatty buildup can occur in the liver. Alcohol converts to fat, not to glucose or glycogen. Obesity also occurs with high alcohol use. With chronic

use, fat continues to be stored in and irritate the liver, which eventually swells, scars, and shrinks (the process of cirrhosis) until only a small percentage is functional. Usually more than half the liver must be destroyed before its work is significantly impaired. Advanced liver disease leads to all kinds of complications, including ascites, a fluid buildup in the abdomen. Still, since the liver is our most regenerative organ, stopping drinking will usually allow for recovery. Hemorrhoids and varicose veins are commonly a result of liver disease in alcoholics. Thiamine (B$_1$), and niacinamide (B$_3$) help the liver detoxify alcohol, so if body levels of these are low, the liver may be more sensitive to inflammation.

6. **Stomach disorders—gastritis and ulcers**. Alcohol irritates and injures the mucosal lining of the upper gastrointestinal tract, including the esophagus, stomach, and upper small intestine. It also increases hydrochloric acid production. This combination, along with poor nutritional protection, often leads to stomach inflammation—that is, gastritis—associated with abdominal pain and difficulty in eating. Both gastric and duodenal ulcers are found with increased frequency in alcoholics. A reduction in digestive enzymes needed to break down foods and alkalize the gastrointestinal tract causes irritating acid fluids to go further down the tube and affect the intestinal mucosa. This can lead to the "leaky gut syndrome," which allows larger, incompletely digested molecules to be absorbed and generates more food allergic reaction. The irritation of the esophagus can cause a painful esophagitis. Dilated (varicose) veins also can occur there because of liver circulation back up, and these can rupture, creating a medical emergency.

7. **Pancreatitis and gallstones**. Inflammation of the pancreas is a painful problem that is thought to be caused by alcohol irritation in certain individuals. There are likely other factors contributing to this problem. Gallbladder disease and gallstones are also probably caused by a number of factors, including alcohol irritation, poor fat utilization, and improper nutrient metabolism.

8. **Nervous system disorders**. Alcohol crosses the blood-brain barrier and directly affects the brain. It can actually destroy brain cells, leading to brain damage as well as behavior and psychological problems. Chronic use of alcohol, probably with associated B vitamin deficiencies, may lead to painful nerve inflammations called polyneuritis. Premature senility occurs with alcohol abuse, as does a chronic degenerative brain syndrome, termed encephalopathy.

9. **Cardiovascular disease**. Although it appears that a small amount of alcohol may raise HDL cholesterol and protect against atherosclerosis, the overall effect of alcohol abuse is deadly to the heart and blood vessels. The blood pressure is elevated, which increases cardiovascular risk. Lipid metabolism is affected, which increases triglyceride levels, which in turn raises blood cholesterol. With the familial hyperlipidemia disorders, this alcohol influence can be worse. Alcohol also reduces the essential fatty acid and protective prostaglandin levels; this further sensitizes the cardiovascular system. Heart function, heart muscle action,

and electrical conductivity in the heart are all decreased with alcohol. This can lead to heart disease, congestive heart failure, and cardiac arrythmias. Cardiomyopathy, or enlarged heart, with poor function has been associated with alcohol and some ingredients in the beverages, such as cobalt.

10. ***Carbohydrate metabolism***—hypoglycemia and diabetes. Since alcohol is a simple sugar that is rapidly absorbed and utilized, and affects the digestion as well as liver and pancreatic functions, it has a tendency to weaken glucose tolerance with chronic use. The incidence of both hypoglycemia and diabetes is higher with alcohol abuse. Blood sugar problems are generally more frequent with regular use of alcohol. The poor blood sugar utilization can affect the nerve and liver health as well.

11. ***Nutritional excesses***—obesity. An increase in alcohol calories that specifically turn into fat will lead to weight gain and more body fat unless it is balanced by exercise and a good diet. Many athletes drink excessively and can handle alcohol better than the less active person; when exercise is reduced, however, there is more concern. Also, with regular alcohol use, there is much more danger of nutrient deficiencies.

12. ***Nutritional deficiencies***. Alcohol can interfere with a number of functions related to the metabolism of nutrients. In addition to the poor intake of food nutrients common with alcohol abuse, alcohol impairs digestion and absorption of many nutrients from the small intestine. These include most B vitamins, such as B_1, B_6, B_{12}, choline and folic acid, as well as some minerals; and with liver impairment absorption of the fat-soluble vitamins A, D, E, and K is also reduced. Alcohol's diuretic effect can lead to the loss of nutrients and create dehydration as well. Alcohol also uses nutrients that it does not provide for its own metabolism, impairs the metabolism of many others, and reduces liver stores of even more. For example, vitamins B_1 and B_3 are needed by the liver to metabolize alcohol, and these are often in short supply. Folic acid's function in the bone marrow, where it helps make red blood cells, is diminished by alcohol. Thus, anemia may develop more easily with alcohol abuse, especially with low levels of vitamin B_{12} and reduced absorption and storage of iron. The low vitamin D availability and poor calcium absorption can lead to an increased risk of osteoporosis. The loss of many minerals, such as zinc and magnesium, increases even more with caffeine use. The lack of appetite caused by alcohol abuse also makes it harder to get needed nutrients. In the elderly, where nutritional status is often unstable and alcohol consumption a problem, nutritional deficits can be exacerbated. Alcoholism in all ages is commonly associated with malnutrition. Other nutrients commonly deficient with alcohol abuse include vitamins B_2, B_6, A, and C, essential fatty acids, and methionine.

13. ***Low sexuality and impotence***. Alcohol increases levels of the liver enzyme that breaks down testosterone, a hormone that stimulates sexuality. Alcohol's depres-

sant effect on the nervous system can also reduce a man's ability to perform, although it may reduce inhibitions and increase his desires. In teenage boys, the reduction of testosterone may delay sexual maturity. In later life, alcohol abuse is more commonly associated with impotence.

14. ***Cancer factor***. Alcohol is probably a cofactor in cancer development and is implicated in malignancy of the mouth, esophagus, pancreas, and breast. All of these cancers are even more likely to occur when alcohol abuse is combined with cigarette smoking. One theory is that cigarette smoke and alcohol together chemically create ethyl nitrite, which is a mutagen. Cancer rates are higher in heavy drinkers than in more moderate ones. Nutritional deficiencies likely play a role as well.

15. ***Birth defects***. Alcohol can be a definite problem for the fetus, a fact that seemed to be acknowledged thousands of years ago, but had been forgotten for awhile. Alcohol crosses the placenta and gets into the fetal circulation, where it cannot be handled metabolically because of undeveloped liver function, so it is more toxic. The fetal alcohol syndrome recently described is associated with under-sized babies with small facial features and mental deficits due to brain damage. To some authorities, limiting consumption to less than two drinks daily is enough to prevent this problem; to most others, there is no safe level—women simply should not drink while pregnant! Even one to two drinks a day in the first trimester can lead to retarded growth and mental development. Since alcohol has this influence on the fetus even during the first couple of months, a woman who is planning to become pregnant or even open to the possibility should avoid or at least limit (one drink only) alcohol intake. For the mother-to-be, who needs to be very well nourished to handle pregnancy, alcohol is an added stress, irritant, and nutritional drain. Alcohol also gets into the breast milk, and this may adversely affect nursing babies, although not as seriously as when in utero. Nursing mothers are also better off without the depleting effects of alcohol.

16. ***Immune suppression***. Alcohol clearly sedates the immune system by decreasing phagocytic activity, lymphocyte action, and mucous lining protection. Drinkers tend to have more infections and more severe problems than nondrinkers, especially with heavy use. Pneumonia is not at all uncommon in alcoholics.

17. ***Other health problems***. Alcohol use may precipitate gout attacks in those prone to this disease of uric acid metabolism, as alcohol reduces its elimination. Alcohol also worsens PMS (premenstrual syndrome) symptoms in many women with this problem. Vaginitis from *Candida albicans* and other infections are more common with alcohol abuse, as are headaches. Anemia may arise from nutritional deficiencies or bleeding disorders; swelling and redness of the nose and dilated blood vessels in the face are also signs of alcohol abuse.

18. ***Social problems***. Alcohol use lessens both our inhibitions and our self-control. With increased drinking, we may make other bad choices that are detrimental to

the interest of our health and the welfare of others. Alcohol abuse can be very devastating to the family unit, to a marriage, and to the health of children. The social life of the alcoholic can influence the rest of his or her life because of forming unwise associations, spending time in bars, or getting lost for days at a time.

19. **Economic disaster**. Alcohol abuse in the work force costs an estimated 20 billion a year in absenteeism and lost labor. The personal and medical costs are extreme because of the cost of alcoholic beverages and the medical care needed to treat the problems that alcohol causes.

Alcoholism

The alcoholic is someone who has lost control over the drug. Clearly, alcoholism is a major problem in the United States and the rest of the world. A genetic deficiency may make it a disease rather than just a lifestyle problem. This deficiency may cause an intense biological craving for alcohol or the products from which it is made. A problem with blood sugar metabolism may be at the root, and allergy-addictions may also be a factor. More research is needed to clarify the causal associations of this important problem.

There are many warning signs to suggest a problem with alcohol. I believe that anybody who drinks daily has a problem, though he or she may not be an alcoholic. If we can easily stop drinking for a week or two at a time (we begin with one day, of course), that is a good sign. This is also important to our personal perspective on alcohol. Remember, most alcoholics deny that there is any problem.

Other warning signs of alcoholism include drinking alone, skipping meals and drinking instead, drinking before social or business functions, drinking in the morning or late at night, missing work because of drinking, and periods of amnesia or blackouts. People who have any of these drinking problems or who believe that they might have an alcohol problem should definitely seek treatment. Even in the absence of these drinking characteristics, there are many reasons to stop drinking, especially for those with regular or moderate to heavy alcohol intake. Our wallet, automobile, our liver, brain, muscles, gastrointestinal tract, and our mind and memory are a few important reasons; our family, job, and self-image are others.

To deal with an alcohol problem, we first need to admit that we have a problem and get the support of our spouse or a friend. Clear the alcohol from home, work, car, or wherever, and then see a physician or therapist. A medical checkup and blood test may be in order. We may need pharmaceutical support to get off drink; tranquilizers such as Valium or Ativan are commonly used to get through the first few days of withdrawal.

There is a fairly good chance that we can get off alcohol if we are willing to try. With a multileveled approach and the current community and professional support, our chances are better than 50 percent. Our doctor may help us find out whether allergy is a factor in our alcohol abuse. If corn, wheat, barley, rye, or yeast generates positive tests, avoiding these foods may help relieve alcohol cravings.

Psychological counseling, family therapy, Alcoholics Anonymous (AA), or some religious/spiritual practice may also improve our motivation, self-image, and ability to create a new life. Regular AA meetings continue the positive support for many recovering alcholics. Avoiding negative influences, such as our old drinking buddies, parties, and exposure to alcohol, for a while will be helpful. Regular exercise, especially at the usual drinking time, and learning and practicing relaxation exercises are also very useful. Massage therapy can be wonderful, helping to clear body toxins and promoting relaxation and self-love. Acupuncture has also been shown to be beneficial for many recovering alcoholics, during withdrawal and afterward.

Alcohol detoxification may be very difficult, depending on the level of abuse, and it may take months or even years to completely clear its effects. Alcoholics can get fairly sick during withdrawal. Even with mild elimination, there may be increased tension, headaches, and irritability for a few days. For more severe withdrawal, tranquilizers may be needed. Medical care in a hospital setting is not uncommon for acute alcohol withdrawal, although this is usually necessary only for heavy drinkers, those who consume more than eight to ten drinks daily.

If the willpower is poor, a drug, such as Antabuse (disulfiram) can be used. This produces terrible nausea and vomiting when alcohol is drunk. Antabuse is usually tolerated fairly well for a while, but it can have side effects, such as affects on the cardiovascular system or psyche. Lithium therapy has recently been shown to reduce the urge to drink. For recovering alcoholics, many authorities believe that it is imperative to avoid all alcohol, for life, because the addictive potential never disappears. Nonalcoholic beverages may be all right, but even some dealcoholized drinks still contain small amounts of the drug.

Alcohol Detoxification

Diet and megavitamin therapy may be helpful during withdrawal, detoxification, and recovery from alcoholism. Alcoholics while drinking generally need more supplements than most other people. And during the detox time, they may need even more. This extra support will give a greater chance of recovery than just having psychotherapy. As I just mentioned, attending AA meetings may aid alcoholics greatly.

During the actual withdrawal period, which may last from a few days to a week, the diet can be focused on fluids and the alkaline foods. The appetite is usually not great, and liquids will help in clearing alcohol from the body. Water, diluted fruit and vegetable juices, warm broths and soups, and teas using herbs, such as chamomile, skullcap (a nervine), or valerian root all will serve the needs. Some other herbs that may be helpful during withdrawal are white willow bark to reduce pain and inflammation, ginseng, cayenne, and peppermint. Small amounts of light proteins, such as nonfatty poultry, fish, or even chicken soup, will provide more nourishment. Amino acid powder can also be supportive. Up to 2–3 grams of L-tryptophan can be taken for sleep. L-glutamine, another amino acid, has been shown to reduce cravings for alcohol and sugar, and is used in many detox clinics.

I have seen intravenous vitamins be very helpful during withdrawal. Extra vitamin C, B vitamins, and a few minerals, such as calcium, magnesium, and potassium, are the usual ones used, especially if supplements taken by mouth are not well tolerated. A vitamin C powder buffered with those same minerals, taken orally mixed in a liquid, such as water or juice, may be helpful. This particular formula is also useful during the detox period.

Alcohol detoxification continues for at least several weeks after the withdrawal period. During this recovery time, the body will eliminate alcohol, its by-products, and other toxins and begin breaking down some of the fat that may have been stored during alcohol abuse. General supportive and balanced nourishment with a low-fat, moderate protein, basic complex carbohydrate diet is recommended. Since alcoholics often have blood sugar problems, basic hypoglycemic principles should be followed. These include avoiding sugars and refined foods, soft drinks, candy, and so on; small amounts of fruits and fruit juices may be tolerated. Regular eating every few hours is recommended. Small meals and snacks of protein or complex carbohydrate, including whole grains, pasta, potatoes, squashes, legumes, and other vegetables, can be the basic diet. Proteins such as soy products, eggs, fish, or poultry can also be added, but the basic aim is to maintain an alkaline diet, so the primary focus initially during withdrawal should be on vegetables and fruit.

Water should be drunk throughout the day as well; chamomile or peppermint teas can also be used. All alcoholic beverages should, of course, be eliminated. Foods containing potentially damaging fats, including fried foods, chips, burgers, hot dogs, fast foods, and ice cream should also be avoided. These foods are all congesting and more acid-forming as well. Caffeine and cigarette smoking are best minimized. Many recovering alcoholics take in large amounts of coffee and smoke intensely, as can be clearly seen at AA meetings. This is not recommended at all. These habits suggest a need for stronger psychological support to become generally less addictive. Luckily though, in recent years there is a strong faction for nonsmoking AA meetings, and this is a big plus.

During detoxification from alcohol (usually from other substances, too), many other important nutrients besides diet can be added. Amino acids can be used, including L-tryptophan for sleep. Calcium and magnesium supplements taken at night may also aid sleep, as may valerian root capsules. L-glutamine is an amino acid that generates glutamic acid, and this can get directly into the brain and be used for fuel. Glutamine is naturally found in liver, meats, dairy foods, and cabbage. It can diminish the craving for alcohol and sugar (chromium may also help with sugar cravings). A dosage of 500–1,000 mg. three times daily between or before meals is suggested, as capsules or as L-glutamine powder, taken before or after meals and before bed.

A basic "multiple" along with antioxidant nutrients can be employed during detoxification from alcohol. Extra minerals, such as zinc, iron, calcium, and magnesium, can be taken to replace those lost during alcohol abuse. Higher levels of niacin, even up to several grams, along with 5–10 grams of vitamin C daily, have been used with some success in alcohol withdrawal and detox. A more modest level of C would be 500–1,000 mg. taken four to six times daily.

Other detoxifying nutrients include additional fiber, which helps to bind toxins in the bowel and improve elimination. Choline and inositol, about 500 mg. each three times daily, will improve fat digestion and utilization. Lemon water with a couple of teaspoons of olive oil and a quarter teaspoon or capsule of cayenne pepper will help detoxify the liver. Taking fiber along with oil decreases the oil absorption, but olive oil alone is thought to be nourishing to the liver and helpful in clearing chemical toxins. Cold-pressed olive oil is part of many natural liver therapies. Goldenseal root powder, one or two capsules twice daily, is also helpful for toning and clearing the liver. Parsley tea improves kidney elimination and cleansing of the blood. The amino acid L-cysteine is another helpful detoxicant for the liver, blood, and colon.

Other nutrients and herbs that are helpful during detoxification of alcohol include pancreatic digestive enzymes after meals and brewer's yeast, which, if tolerated, supplies many B vitamins and minerals. The essential fatty acids help to decrease the inflammatory prostaglandins. Gamma-linolenic acid from evening primrose or borage seed oil helps to reduce alcohol toxicity. White willow bark tablets can be used for pain, and valerian root, a natural and milder form of Valium, can be taken to decrease anxiety. Chamomile will help to calm the digestive tract, as will licorice root.

Nutritional Support for Drinkers

The basic support plan for an active drinker varies only a bit from that used during alcohol detox. A generally balanced, nutritious diet will help minimize some of the potential problems from alcohol. Regular nourishment is important, although even the best diet and supplement program will not fully protect us and our liver from the toxic effects of ethanol. When our liver has to deal with alcohol metabolism, it is helpful to avoid fried foods, rancid or hydrogenated fats, and other drugs, such as cocaine, all of which are hard on the liver. Thioctic acid as a supplement of 100–200 mg. daily may help protect the liver against some of the drug toxicity.

Alcohol abusers need more nutrients than most other people to protect them from malnutrition. Obviously, basic multiple and antioxidant formulas are important. Part or possibly most of the toxic effects of alcohol may be caused by production of free radicals, so higher than RDA levels of vitamins A, C, and E, beta-carotene, and the minerals selenium, zinc, manganese, and magnesium are suggested (see supplement table). The nutrients that are commonly deficient with alcohol use also need extra support. Thiamine and riboflavin, in dosages of 50 mg. twice daily, and niacin, in dosages of 50 mg. three times daily, help circulation and blood cleansing and can reduce the effects of hangovers. Folic acid is needed in amounts of 800–1,000 mcg. per day, more than twice the RDA; leafy greens and whole grains, both rich in this vitamin, should be added to the diet.

Water and other nonalcoholic liquids are needed to counteract the dehydrating effects of alcohol. Calcium is also supportive, as is extra zinc, 45–75 mg. daily, as its absorption is diminished and its elimination is increased with alcohol use. Zinc is commonly deficient in drinkers. This supplemental intake should be balanced out with 3 mg. of copper. The essential fatty acids and gamma-linolenic acid from evening primrose oil or borage seed oil support normal fat metabolism and protect against inflammation caused by free radicals and prostaglandins (PGEs). Alcohol decreases the levels of the anti-inflammatory PGE_1, and these oils will increase them. Gluta-thione helps prevent fat buildup in the liver by its enzyme activities, so the tripeptide glutathione (or L-cysteine, which forms glutathione) may be supplemented along with basic L-amino acids. Many alcohol users are not able to get enough glutamic acid to their brain; additional L-glutamine will help get it across the blood brain barrier.

Social drinkers can use a lighter program, but still, I believe, need protection. A good diet is, of course, recommended. B vitamins, including 50 mg. each of B_1, B_2, and B_3, 400 mcg. of folic acid, and 100 mcg. of B_{12}, 15–30 mg. of zinc, and 300–500 mg. of magnesium should all be taken before drinking, along with some food. Drinking should be limited to two drinks per day.

A number of things can be done to prevent getting too drunk or developing a hangover. Our blood level of alcohol is affected by how much and how fast we drink. If we drink fast on an empty stomach, absorption is immediate. Ideally, it is best to have some food in the stomach unless we limit consumption to one drink and want a quick "buzz" before dinner. Food definitely helps prevent us from getting sick. Drinking slowly is suggested. Women seem to be more quickly affected by alcohol than men and so get drunk more easily with less alcohol, even taking body weight into consideration. Foods to eat before drinking should be low-salt complex carbohydrates, such as bread, some crackers, or even vegetable sticks. Carbohydrates delay alcohol absorption. Fat-protein snacks, such as milk or cheese, will decrease alcohol absorption and thus help reduce drunkenness and hangovers. Some people drink a little olive oil before parties to coat their stomachs so that they can handle their drinking better. A few capsules of evening primrose oil will also help.

It does take a while for alcohol to clear from the blood after it gets in there. With heavy drinking, extra coffee and exercise, such as walking, do not really help, other than by making more active drunks; however, with mild intoxication they can increase alertness. Definitely avoid other psychoactive drugs with alcohol; these include tranquilizers, narcotics, sedatives, antihistamines, and marijuana, all of which may increase the alcohol effect.

Blood levels of alcohol have been studied to see varying effects of this drug. Legally this level can be determined through testing and used to clarify degrees of safety or drunkenness. Usually one or two drinks will keep most people in a safe range, but over that can create problems.

Hangovers are caused by the dehydrating effect of alcohol and some toxic effects of the chemical congeners that are created during fermentation or are added to the beverages before, during, or after processing. Allergies to some of the ingredients, such as corn, wheat, barley, or yeast, may intensify hangovers and withdrawal.

Alcohol Blood Level	*Status*
0.05 percent	"Cruising," feeling good, some positive effects
0.05–0.1	Beginning loss of balance, speech or emotions
0.08	Legally drunk
0.2	Passed out
0.3	Comatose, unresponsive

There are many old remedies for hangovers. The best is to prevent them by not overdrinking and taking supportive fluids and nutrients. Cream, coffee, oysters, chili peppers, and aspirin are common, occasionally helpful hangover remedies. Time is the best, along with rest and fluids. If alcohol intake has been excessive, drink two or three glasses of water before going to bed, along with vitamin C and a B complex vitamin which helps to clear alcohol from the blood. The vitamin C can be in the form of mineral ascorbates containing potassium, calcium, magnesium, and even zinc, or 15 mg. of zinc can be taken separately. Do this again upon awakening; it can really help. Further benefit may be obtained by taking evening primrose oil and flaxseed oil, which is a rich source of the essential fatty acids. A morning-after plan suggested by Dr. Stuart Berger includes 100 mg. of thiamine, 100 mg. of riboflavin, 50 mg. of B_6, 250 mcg. of B_{12}, 1,000 mg. of vitamin C, and 50 mg. of zinc.

Overall, we need to watch ourselves when drinking and especially not let alcohol use turn into abuse and addiction. We need to pay special attention to children and teenagers and offer them education regarding alcohol and drugs, but if we do not lead them by example, and they model themselves on our drug-, alcohol- and smoking-oriented society, how can we expect them to lead a drug-free life? Let us all live so as to provide an example of how we would like the world to be now.

ALCOHOL NUTRIENT PROGRAMS

	Support	*Withdrawal*	*Detox/Recovery*
Water	2 ½–3 qt.	3–4 qt.	3 qt.
Protein	60–80 g.	50–70 g.	75–100 g.
Fats	30–50 g.	30–50 g.	50–65 g.
Fiber	15–20 g.	10–15 g.	30–40 g.
Vitamin A	10,000 IUs	5,000 IUs	10,000 IUs
Beta-carotene	25,000 IUs	20,000 IUs	20,000 IUs
Vitamin D	200 IUs	400 IUs	400 IUs
Vitamin E	400–800 IUs	400 IUs	800 IUs
Vitamin K	300 mcg.	300 mcg.	500 mcg.
Thiamine (B_1)	100 mg.	50–100 mg.	150 mg.
Riboflavin (B_2)	100 mg.	50–100 mg.	150 mg.
Niacinamide (B_3)	50 mg.	50 mg.	50 mg.
Niacin (B_3)	50–150 mg.	100–1,000 mg.	200–2,000 mg.
Pantothenic acid (B_5)	250 mg.	1,000 mg.	500 mg.
Pyridoxine (B_6)	100 mg.	200 mg.	100 mg.
Pyridoxal-5-phosphate	50 mg.	100 mg.	50 mg.
Cobalamin (B_{12})	100 mcg.	200 mcg.	250 mcg.
Folic acid	800–1,000 mcg.	2,000 mcg.	800 mcg.
Biotin	300 mcg.	500 mcg.	500 mcg.
Choline	500 mg.	1,000 mg.	1,500 mg.
Inositol	500 mg.	1,000 mg.	1,500 mg.
Vitamin C	2–4 g.	5–25 g.	5–10 g.
Bioflavonoids	250 mg.	500 mg.	500 mg.

ALCOHOL NUTRIENT PROGRAMS (CONT.)

	Support	*Withdrawal*	*Detox/Recovery*
Calcium	850–1,000 mg.	1,000–1,500 mg.	1,000 mg.
Chromium	500 mcg.	500–1,000 mcg.	300 mcg.
Copper	3 mg.	3 mg.	3–4 mg.
Iodine	150 mcg.	150 mcg.	150 mcg.
Iron	20–30 mg.	10–18 mg.	20 mg.
Magnesium	500–800 mg.	800–1,000 mg.	600–800 mg.
Manganese	5 mg.	15 mg.	10 mg.
Molybdenum	300 mcg.	300 mcg.	300 mcg.
Potassium	300–500 mg.	500 mg.	300 mg.
Selenium	300 mcg.	150 mcg.	200 mcg.
Silicon	100 mg.	50 mg.	200 mg.
Vanadium	150 mcg.	150 mcg.	150 mcg.
Zinc	45–75 mg.	50–75 mg.	50–100 mg.
Flaxseed oil	1 teaspoon	2 teaspoons	2 teaspoons
Gamma-linolenic acid	3 capsules (40–60 mg./cap.)	3 capsules	6 capsules
L-amino acids	1,000–1,500 mg.	1,500–3,000 mg.	5,000–7,500 mg.
L-glutamine	500–1,000 mg.	1,500–3,000 mg.	1,000–2,000 mg.
L-tryptophan (if needed for sleep)	500–1,000 mg.	2,000–3,000 mg.	500–1,000 mg.
Thioctic acid	100 mg.	100 mg.	200 mg.
L-cysteine	250 mg.	250 mg.	250–500 mg.
Glutathione (if available)	250 mg.	500 mg.	250 mg.
Digestive enzymes	—	—	1–2 after meals
Goldenseal root	—	—	3 capsules
White willow bark (if needed)	1–2 tablets	4–6 tablets	2–4 tablets

Nicotine Detoxification

Cigarette smoking, the main way we take in nicotine, is the single greatest cause of preventable diseases (these are the progressive, serious diseases) and probably creates the most difficult addiction of the commonly used drugs. Smoking is a high-priced addictive pleasure (and sometimes displeasure) that is costly, not only in dollars but in lives as well.

In the United States alone, cigarette smoking causes a third to a half million deaths per year (over 1,000 per day) and is responsible for about 25 percent of the cancer deaths and 30–40 percent of the coronary heart disease. It also increases the incidence of atherosclerosis, strokes, and peripheral vascular disease. Diseases of the lungs—colds, flus, acute bronchitis, pneumonia, COPD (chronic obstructive pulmonary disease), which includes emphysema and chronic bronchitis, and lung cancer—are all much more common in smokers. Other infections or allergies are also prevalent, and rapid aging of the body and especially the skin results from the generally poor oxygenation of tissues and the other chemicals and physiological effects of regular cigarette smoking.

Smoking clearly decreases life expectancy for all age groups. One-pack-a-day smokers double their chances of death between the ages of 50 and 60, while two-packers triple theirs. And smoking also affects the life expectancy of nonsmokers close to them in heart and proximity. Of all the common drugs, nicotine intake from cigarette smoking clearly has the least benefits and the most negative consequences.

The estimated cost of smoking is somewhere between $50 and $100 billion a year. Some 650 billion cigarettes are sold yearly in the United States in this $18–25 billion megabusiness. Marlboros and Winstons top the list with nearly 50 percent of the market. The 650 billion count averages about 4,000 cigarettes per year per person over age 18. Recent estimates suggest that about 38 percent of the over-18 population in the United States smoke. Percentages of adult smokers are even much higher in most European countries and some parts of Asia. In addition to the cost of the cigarettes, there are many billions spent medically to treat the problems that afflict smokers and many more billions in lost work and productivity caused from diseases generated by smoking.

I am happy to say that now only 10 percent of doctors in the United States smoke; the percentage used to be much higher. The number of cigarette smokers, which for many years has increased steadily, is tapering off somewhat. Worldwide however, there is still about a 2–3 percent yearly rise in smokers. The dangers of nicotine and smoking are now so generally accepted and well documented that it would seem that more people would be stopping or not even starting. The fact that fewer doctors smoke (or admit that they smoke) is at least representative of these health dangers. People want doctors to do healthy things and to set healthy examples.

Since most nicotine intake is from smoking cigarettes, that is the focus of this section. Cigar and pipe smoking, chewing tobacco, and snuff also pose some health risks, but far less than cigarette smoking. The regularly inhaled smoke contains tars composed of literally thousands of chemicals, including those used in tobacco cultivation as well as in cigarette making. These agents add other health risks in addition to the nicotine, which directly acts on the cardiovascular and nervous systems. There are over 30 potentially carcinogenic chemicals contained in cigarette smoke.

Tobacco comes from a large-leafed nightshade, or Solanaceae, plant. It is one of a few plants that contain the psychoactive alkaloid, nicotine. Tobacco causes joint pain in some people; this seems correlated to the theory that arthritis is in part a result of an allergy to the nightshades, which also include potatoes, tomatoes, eggplant, and peppers.

Nicotine has been widely used throughout history, first in North America. Supposedly, Columbus and other visitors were interested in it and carried some tobacco and seeds back to Europe, where its use caught on rapidly and eventually spread to Africa and the Orient. Tobacco was outlawed by several countries during the early 1600s, but to no avail; then the governments eventually found ways to profit from its use. This seems fair, since it costs them in the long run with lost health and productivity of their people. The addictive nature of nicotine has been clear for hundreds of years, as people have found ways to smoke during poverty, famine, and war.

Sigmund Freud was fascinated with tobacco and obsessed with cigars (smoking more than 20 a day). He fought his addiction to nicotine (and apparently to cocaine) through much of his life, though he experienced mouth cancer, angina pain, and multiple surgeries. Freud's dance with death and his inability to get off tobacco probably generated his theory of Thanatos, our deep subconscious longing for death, manifested in part by our destructive habits.

Smoking is clearly a deadly pastime. Its addictive nature is revealed by the fact that many strong-minded and strong-willed people cannot stop smoking, even if they are otherwise health conscious or faced with death. And most smokers, over 80 percent, declare that they want to stop smoking, and plan to at some time. In my years working in hospitals, I saw the most bizarre smoking phenomena, such as lung cancer or emphysema patients smoking between ventilator treatments or patients who breathed through tubes in their necks after tracheostomies, actually putting cigarettes into the tubes to inhale. Our passion for puffing is persistent.

Nicotine is the addictive drug found in tobacco. Even though some people start smoking for the image or the ritual, they may easily become hooked. The "up" feeling that smoking produces is likely correlated with the increased blood pressure and heart rate, as well as the production of fatty acids, steroids and possibly other hormones or neurotransmitters. Nicotine mimics acetylcholine, which then improves alertness, memory, and learning capacity. Other neurotransmitter stimulation of norepinephrine and endorphins by nicotine may help balance moods and increase energy. The liver's increase in glycogen release gives a satisfying lift in the blood sugar.

The addiction to nicotine is probably stronger than addictions to most other drugs. The initial irritating effects progress to chronic irritations, yet these are covered by the physiological and, in many instances, the psychological need (although the latter is usually secondary). Heroin addicts and people addicted to other powerful drugs have commonly referred to nicotine as the hardest drug to kick. The American Psychiatric Association has described smoking as an "organic mental disorder." Their statistics suggest that around 50 percent of people cannot stop when they try to and that, of the people who do stop, about 75 percent of them begin again within one year.

Are There Benefits in Smoking?

There obviously must be a few, or so many people would not smoke, but it is very clear that the risks outweigh the pleasures by far. Many people find smoking relaxing, but this may be a result of calming the hyperactive withdrawal symptoms. People do experience mental stimulation and improvement of hand-to-eye coordination and work activities, probably as result of nicotine's vascular-neurological stimulation. The benefits that smokers experience were well described in Dr. Tom Ferguson's book, *The Smoker's Book of Health*, from his interviews with hundreds of smokers. They felt better able to deal with stress and to unwind and relax. Smoking helped control their moods, improve concentration and energy levels, especially with fatigue, and reduce withdrawal symptoms, obviously. Social comfort, work breaks, reduced pain and anxiety, increased pleasure, and less boredom were also correlates for some who smoked. Smoking also usually reduces the appetite and taste for food, so it may help people to reduce food intake, a positive step for the weight conscious. The average smoker weighs six to eight pounds less than the nonsmoker. In *Life Extension*, Sandy Shaw and Durk Pearson note that nicotine seems to reduce distraction by outside stimuli in people working in highly stimulating environments—that is, it desensitizes people. I see this as creating a smoke screen that protects us from relating to others and keeps us in our own world. It is clear that people who work in crowded, noisy, busy offices with other workers, computers, machines running, and lots of hustle and bustle tend to smoke more frequently than do workers in more private situations.

Yet, most employers now know there is a distinct disadvantage in hiring smokers. The smoke interferes with office morale, and it is more costly. Some estimates suggest that employing a smoker costs businesses nearly 5,000 yearly. This cost comes from increased absenteeism, death risk, incident of accidents, and property damage or cleaning bills from smoke, as well as less productivity. Dr. Ferguson points out that most people are aware of this and the health hazards of nicotine and cigarette smoke. They clearly want to quit, but have not found a way to get rid of withdrawal and craving. Finding ways to reduce stress and clear those conditioned responses to want to smoke takes a great deal of effort.

What Does Nicotine Do?

Nicotine, the active and addictive ingredient of tobacco, is a mild central nervous system stimulant and a stronger cardiovascular system stimulant. It constricts blood vessels, increasing the blood pressure and stimulating the heart, and raises the blood fat levels. In its liquid form, nicotine is a powerful poison—the injection of even one drop would be deadly. It is the nicotine, not the smoke, that causes people to continue to smoke cigarettes, but it is the cigarette smoke that causes many of the problems.

Cigarette smoke is a combination of lethal gases—carbon monoxide, hydrogen cyanide, and nitrogen and sulfur oxides—and tars, which contain an estimated 4,000 chemicals. Some of these chemical agents are introduced by current tobacco manufacturing processes. Although tobacco has been smoked for centuries, only recently has it moved from the naturally grown and dried process. It appears that in the last century the negative effects of smoking have skyrocketed. My belief, which is shared by many authorities, is that much of the added risk is produced by the chemical treatment and unnatural processing of tobacco. The little research that has been done on this (it is not sponsored by the industry) suggests that natural tobacco poses much less cancer risk, as well as cardiovascular disease risk, though this is predominately from the nicotine, which is not changed by processing.

Dangers in modern tobacco products include pesticides used during growth and chemicals added to the tobacco to make it burn better or taste different. Chemicals added to the leaves and papers to enhance burning are among the major causes of fire deaths in this country, as cigarettes continue to burn after they have been put down. The forced burning also makes people smoke more of each cigarette in order to complete it. Sugar curing and rapid flue drying are also associated with increased toxicity of cigarettes. Kerosene heat drying contaminates the tobacco with another toxic hydrocarbon. Using a natural tobacco, such as some imported from France or Germany and a few U.S.-made cigarettes (possibly Shermans and More), may reduce the smoking risk. If a cigarette does not go out when left alone, it has been chemically treated.

Other toxic contaminants in cigarettes include cadmium (which affects the kidneys, arteries, and blood pressure), lead, arsenic, cyanide, and nickel. Dioxin, the most toxic pesticide chemical known to date, has been found in cigarettes. Acetonitrile, another pesticide, is also found in tobacco. The nitrogen gases from cigarettes generate carcinogenic nitrosamines in the body tissues. The tars in smoke contain polynuclear aromatic hydrocarbons (PAH), carcinogenic materials that bind with cellular DNA to cause damage. Antioxidant therapy, particularly with vitamin C, is protective against both PAH and nitrosamines, and extra C also blocks the irritating effects of smoke. Smoking itself reduces vitamin C absorption; blood levels of ascorbic acid average about 30–40 percent lower in smokers than in nonsmokers.

Radioactive materials are also found in cigarette smoke; polonium is the most common. Some authorities believe that cigarettes are our greatest source of radiation.

965

A smoker of one and a half packs per day may be exposed to radiation equal to 300 chest x-rays a year. Radiation is a strong aging factor. Acetaldehyde, a chemical released during smoking, causes aging, especially of the skin, as it affects the cross-linking bonds that hold our tissues together.

CIGARETTE CHEMICALS*

Carbon monoxide	Hydrogen cyanide	Ozone
Vinyl chloride	Formaldehyde	Napthalenes
Acetaldehyde	Hydrazine	Arsenic
Formic acid	Cadmium	Nickel compounds
Lead	Nitric oxide	DDT
Pyrene	Methyl chloride	Hydrogen sulfide
Benzene	Acetronitrile	Nitrosamines
Acrylonitride	Phenols	Benzopyrene
Polynuclear aromatic	Ammonia	Hydrocarbons
Polonium-210	Radioactive compounds	Endrin
Acids	Dimethylnitrosamine	Alcohols
	Ethylmethylnitrosamine	

*as shown in *The Smoker's Book of Health*, by Tom Ferguson, M.D.

Cigarette smoking causes three primary degenerative-disease-producing effects: 1) irritation and inflammation; 2) free-radical generation; and 3) allergy-addiction. It is clear that cigarette smoke is a constant and chronic irritant to the body tissues, most specifically the oral cavity and respiratory tract. The polluting effect from cigarettes results less from nicotine than from the thousands of chemicals, including hundreds of poisons and carcinogens, contained in the smoke and tar. Supporting the nicotine addiction without the smoke (by using chewing tobacco, snuff, or nicotine gum) will reduce many of the undesirable respiratory effects of cigarettes. Cigarette smoke is a potent free-radical generator, also primarily a result of the many chemical irritants. And tobacco users exhibit the classic allergy-addiction picture. Studies testing smokers and nonsmokers in a variety of ways have shown that tobacco is a common allergen. Smoking causes irritation and many symptoms; stopping smoking causes cravings and withdrawal symptoms, so that smoking is needed for relief from the withdrawal. The ups and downs are associated with the chemical release of adrenal hormone and endorphins, such as that seen in allergies.

The main risk factor is the number of cigarettes smoked over time. "Pack years" is a common measurement in medical lingo. Someone who smoked one pack per day for

15 years and then two packs per day for 20 years would have 55 pack years, which is fairly high; even 20 pack years will increase the risk of many chronic problems, chiefly lung disease (bronchitis and emphysema), lung cancer, and heart disease. Smokers have twice the risk of death prior to age 65 than nonsmokers, and there is an average reduced longevity of 5–10 years for smokers, varying from lighter to heavier users. For shorter-term problems, such as bronchitis, smoking more than 25 cigarettes per day is associated with a high risk and smoking between 10 and 25 per day with a moderate one; smoking fewer than 10 cigarettes daily poses a low risk. The length and depth of inhalations also contribute to nicotine and tar intake.

There are also different levels of addiction. Least addicted are those who smoke only socially—at parties with friends—and usually only during certain parts of the day or week. They may smoke primarily for psychosocial or image reasons. Next are those who smoke in response to stress, mainly at work. They may stop and start. These first two smoking types are usually less addicted than heavier smokers, and it is easier for them to cut down or stop. The third type of smoker is the more serious, all-day-long smokers who have a fairly strong physical and psychological addiction; for these people, going more than an hour without nicotine causes the onset of withdrawal symptoms, such as irritability, anxiety, or headache. Often, the psychological influences lead to more frequent smoking of cigarettes than even the physical needs require. The extreme, "graduate" level smoker is the "chain smoker." He or she puffs nearly constantly, usually consuming three packs or more a day, and is strongly addicted. The latter two types often need medical and psychological support unless some special circumstance or divine intervention motivates them to stop immediately. Specialized stop-smoking programs are often needed, and even these are only sometimes helpful. Currently, about a third of adult men and women smoke in the United States. Between 10 and 20 percent of previous smokers have quit, leaving only 40–50 percent of adults who have not been regular smokers, and even most of them have at least tried cigarettes. But now by popular demand, from medical and social support, over 1 million smokers of the 50 million in the United States are stopping yearly, and they will immediately begin to lower their cancer and cardiovascular disease risks as well as reduce the negative effects on their lungs and other tissues.

Contrary to current marketing hype about low-tar, low-nicotine cigarettes, there are no safe cigarettes. Some of the newer "lights" may be even worse than regular cigarettes. Users inhale more deeply and smoke more in order to is satisfy their nicotine needs. Unless they have a low ratio of tar to nicotine, there are more risks posed by the increased chemical tars in the cigarettes. More carbon monoxide, hydrogen cyanide, and nitrogen gases are consumed with many of these low-nicotine cigarettes, and this can increase the oxygen deficit, heart disease, and lung damage associated with smoking. What smokers really need are high-nicotine, low-tar cigarettes, so that they need to smoke less to get their nicotine and have less exposure to the more carcinogenic, destructive tars. Even better will be ways to get nicotine to the blood without smoke. Nicotine gum works well, nicotine skin patches and nasal sprays are being researched, and soon there may be capsules or tablets to satisfy the craving. They will still be hazardous to our health but much less so than cigarettes, and will clearly get rid of pollution and secondary smoker risks.

What Are the Risks of Smoking?

Cigarette smoking probably has more harmful effects than any other commonly used drug, and affects more organs and tissues than most others. The total destructive nature of this one drug in the worldwide population is surpassed by no other, even though there are many drugs for which one dose is much worse than one cigarette. This is because it is so addictive and people use it so frequently for so long.

DISEASES ASSOCIATED WITH SMOKING

Atherosclerosis	Acute bronchitis	Allergies
Hypertension	Chronic bronchitis	Rhinitis
Heart disease	Emphysema	Sinusitis
Coronary artery disease	Lung cancer	Other infections
Peripheral vascular disease	Mouth cancer	Burns
Myocardial infarction	Tongue cancer	Peptic ulcers
Stroke	Laryngeal cancer	Varicose veins
Polycythemia	Esophageal cancer	Hiatal hernia
Low birth weight infants	Bladder cancer	Osteoporosis
Increased infant mortality	Kidney cancer	Periodontal disease
Alzheimer's disease	Pancreatic cancer	Senility
Vitamin/mineral deficiencies	Cervical cancer	Impotence

Cardiovascular disease (CVD) is one of the biggest concerns with tobacco use, both because of the direct effects of nicotine on the circulatory system (irritation and increased atherosclerosis) and the effects of other agents, such as carbon monoxide in inhaled smoke, which displaces oxygen. Carbon monoxide reduces the delivery of vital oxygen, our key life force, to all of our cells. Even low-tar cigarettes have high levels of carbon monoxide. Because of reduced oxygen delivery, our body makes more red blood cells (polycythemia), which can thicken the blood and further slow the circulation.

The CVD problem is primarily responsible for the decreased life expectancy associated with smoking, even more so than lung cancer, which usually results from 20–30 years of use. Circulatory effects start immediately and precipitate the development of

CVD, mainly by increasing blood fats and blood pressure. Remember, the three primary contributors to CVD are smoking, hypertension, and high cholesterol, and smoking itself increases the incidence of the other two. Nicotine particularly lowers the level of the protective HDL cholesterol while increasing the supposedly destructive LDL cholesterol. It decreases circulation, especially of the hands and feet, and increases peripheral vascular resistance, so that the heart has to work harder with every beat. These factors contribute to the commonly elevated blood pressure of smokers. Nicotine's effect on increasing platelet aggregation leads to more cases of cerebrovascular accidents (CVAs), or strokes, and myocardial infarctions (MIs), or heart attacks. Diabetics who smoke are at a very high cardiovascular risk, as nicotine increases blood fats and blood vessel effects and may increase insulin needs.

SYMPTOMS AND PROBLEMS ASSOCIATED WITH SMOKING

Heartburn	Surgical complications
Allergies	Nutritional deficiencies
Angina Pectoris	Stains on teeth and fingers
Hoarseness	Increased pregnancy risks
Cough	Increased caffeine use
Headaches	Increased alcohol use
Memory loss	More divorce
Anxiety	More job changes
Fatigue	More home changes
Lowered immunity	Fires, at home and outdoors
Low sexuality	Higher insurance rates
Cold hands and feet	Wasted money
Leg pains	

Smokers are three times as likely as nonsmokers to suffer heart attacks, and many of these are the artery-spasm type. Heart attack risks are even higher for smokers who have elevated blood pressure or increased cholesterol or who use drugs such as birth control pills. The pre-heart-attack propensity to angina pectoris is also much higher in smokers, and nicotine has been known to generate "tobacco angina"—that is, chest pain with smoking. Nicotine (and other agents in smoke) also increases the incidence of problems with the heartbeat—that is, arrhythmias.

High blood pressure and atherosclerosis are associated with an increased risk of strokes. Cerebral aneurysm (ballooning of the artery wall) occurs more commonly in smokers than in nonsmokers, and ruptured aneurysms are often fatal or at least lead to lifelong impairment. Hypertension can also be more serious in smokers; a rapid rise in blood pressure requires prompt control or it may also be fatal.

Peripheral vascular disease—that is, disease of the extremity arteries—is much more common in smokers. This may manifest as intermittent claudication (pain in the legs with walking), as the poor circulation caused by atherosclerosis and vasoconstriction reduces oxygen delivery to the muscles, leading to arterial insufficiency and pain much like that of angina pectoris. Buerger's disease is a specific arterial disease in smokers that may be caused by a hypersensitivity or allergy to tobacco. The inflammation and scarring of the arteries of the arms and legs caused by this disease in a small number of smokers are associated with pain and decreased function. Amputation may be needed if stopping smoking or drug therapy does not help. It would seem much easier and wiser to give up smoking than body parts, or life itself.

Although snuff and chewing tobacco are less toxic because they cause less air contamination, with chronic use the nicotine absorbed from them affects the circulatory system almost as seriously as smoking. There are currently over 10 million chewers addicted to nicotine, and even though they are not exposed to smoke, and thus, have reduced lung damage and lung cancers, tobacco chewers still have the negative cardiovascular effects of nicotine and a higher incidence of mouth, tongue, and throat cancers than smokers. The smoke from cigars and pipes is not usually inhaled, so less nicotine and tars are absorbed with their use, though local irritation is possible. If we want to do ourselves a favor, particularly for our heart and blood vessels, we obviously will not use tobacco at all.

For smokers, the lungs are the other key area of concern. Chronic inhalation of tobacco smoke leads to eventual destruction of the lung tissues through a process of irritation, inflammation, and scarring. Our respiratory tract includes the oral airway, the nose and sinuses, the larynx area, the large bronchial tubes, the smaller bronchioles, and the millions of tiny alveolar sacs at the depth of lung tissue where the massive surface area that contacts the blood stream allows the various inhaled substances to be absorbed. Primarily oxygen and carbon dioxide are exchanged there, but nicotine and other liquids and gases may be absorbed as well. Carbon monoxide, sulfur and nitrogen gases, hydrogen cyanide, and various metals and chemicals may also get into the body through the lungs. The respiratory tract can be used as a route for medication, mainly to affect lung function.

Smokers have a higher than average incidence of respiratory infections, including colds and flus, bronchitis, and sinusitis. By most estimates, smokers have at least twice as great an incidence as nonsmokers of these diseases, particularly acute bronchitis and bad flus. Cigarette smoke causes a decrease in the action of the cilia, and even temporary paralysis of these fine hairs on the mucous linings, which help protect the deeper tissues by pushing out microorganisms and other foreign materials. Smoke also decreases phagocyte activity by diminishing macrophage function. The thinning and drying of the mucus itself cause the bronchial tubes to become dry and irritated. This not only decreases defenses, but leads to much of the inflammation, hoarseness, and chronic cough associated with smoking.

Chronic bronchitis, one form of chronic obstructive pulmonary disease (COPD), results from long-term irritation, loss of mucus protection, and recurrent infection secondary to smoke, with a subsequent loss of function and lung capacity. This limitation in respiratory function occurs even in early smoking. When smoking is stopped, much of the function returns, unless there is lung tissue scarring, which is irreversible. Generally, smoking decreases lung capacity and endurance and often even the desire or ability to exercise. Emphysema, the other form of COPD, results from progressive alveolar scarring and loss of lung elasticity, and thus, the diminished ability to expand and contract—the basic breathing function. The irreversible damage that occurs from the chronic inhalation of tars and nicotine can cause respiratory crippling in later years, totally limiting activity and requiring regular breathing treatments. Exposure to other chemicals, usually industrial types, can also lead to lung scarring and emphysema, especially bad when combined with smoking.

Tobacco smoke is a carcinogen (many of the poisons in cigarette smoke are known carcinogens) and is the main contributor to our most deadly cancer, cancer of the lungs. This problem used to be almost exclusive to males, but now females have been smoking more, and their rates of lung cancer and death from this disease are rapidly catching up with those of the men. Equal rights to life and death! Recent studies show that the incidence of lung cancer is higher in people with low beta-carotene levels, so this is a protective nutrient. Further research will likely reveal that other nutrient deficiencies increase cancer rates, especially low levels of the other antioxidants. This has already been shown to be true for selenium.

Smokers are from five to ten times more likely to contract lung cancer than nonsmokers. These rates are even further increased with occupational exposure to agents such as asbestos, coal, textiles, and other chemicals. With regular alcohol use, smokers have greater than fifteen times the risk of lung cancer of nonsmokers.

Many other cancer rates are higher for smokers, particularly for alcohol-drinking smokers who are exposed to other carcinogenic chemicals. Smokers also have higher rates of cancer of the bladder, cervix, pancreas, esophagus, lips, mouth, and larynx. The risks are increased even further with a high-fat diet and probably with other habits that contribute to cancer, such as emotional stress, low-fiber diets, obesity, and so on. Smoking is the major cause of cancer of the mouth, tongue, and larynx, the latter being almost exclusive to smokers. Regular alcohol use along with smoking brings an increase in gastrointestinal tract cancers as well.

The incidence of cervical cancer has recently been shown to be increased in smokers, theoretically because chemicals from the smoke get into the blood and are released into the uterus and cervix. Deficiencies of nutrients such as vitamin A and folic acid may also be contributing factors in this cancer. Smoking is further implicated in bladder cancer as the bladder is a site where cigarette carcinogenic chemicals can be concentrated.

Cigarette smoking is clearly a common allergy-addiction. Symptoms of both irritation and allergy may appear when smoking is first begun and then decrease with continued smoking. Symptoms will increase with avoidance and increase further with full withdrawal before they diminish. This is classic for allergies as well as drug addictions. In addition to tobacco smoke being an allergen, many people with other allergies or with lowered immunity are very sensitive to smoke. Some people with allergies have even noticed that certain foods may stimulate the desire to smoke; the mechanism for this is unknown.

Cigarette smoking itself lowers general immunity, causing sedation of the protective phagocytic cells and cilia, as well as other effects. Cigarette smoke may be a powerful brain allergen, as nicotine goes rapidly to the brain. Many people, nearly 50 percent according to some reports, also notice decreased thinking ability with smoking (others notice improvement). And in the long run, the increase in atherosclerosis and subsequent decrease in blood circulation to the brain lead to further memory and thinking problems and early dementia. Recent research shows a four times increased risk of Alzheimer's disease in smokers over nonsmokers.

Cigarette smoking also increases the aging process through many effects, including chronic irritation, free-radical formation, atherosclerosis, lung inflammation, and the breathing of other toxic gases, such as carbon monoxide. The poor oxygen delivery to the skin and general dehydration of the tissues caused by smoking seem to cause an increase in deep wrinkles, or "smoker's face." This begins soon after age 30 in smokers. By age 40–50, the facial wrinkles of smokers are similar to those of nonsmokers 20 years older. I can often correctly guess that people are smokers just by knowing their age and looking at their skin, if I have not already smelled smoke on their clothes or breath. The wrinkling and aging effects may also result from nutritional depletions associated with smoking, such as deficiencies of vitamins C, B_1, and B_2, folic acid, zinc, and calcium. In addition to the carbon monoxide in smoke, acetaldehyde can also weaken the tissue cross-linking, causing more skin aging.

Worldwide reports suggest that smoking also affects sexuality and reproduction. In men, it has been shown to lower sperm counts and motility and thus sexual potency and reproductive ability. Smoking may also cause genetic mutation. There appears to be a slightly higher incidence of congenital malformations in the offspring of men who smoke.

In women who smoke, there are clearly more miscarriages and smaller babies. There are many increased risks for pregnant smokers as well as for their fetuses and infants. Besides resulting in babies with lower birth weight than those of nonsmoking women, which may result from a decrease in blood circulation and thus a lower oxygen and nutrient supply to the fetus throughout pregnancy, smoking increases the incidence of miscarriages, stillbirths, congenital malformations, and early infant deaths. Nicotine gets into breast milk and may decrease its production. I believe that early nicotine exposure may cause a greater likelihood of smoking addiction in later life. Smoking around newborns and infants increases their susceptibility to many diseases, particularly colds, bronchitis, and pneumonia. The increase in the number of teenage girls who smoke creates more problems in pregnancy than occur in adult smokers; in pregnant teenagers, poor development and lack of placental circulation and oxygen lead to more fetal and newborn deaths, more hospitalized newborns, and babies that are slow to learn.

Women in general have a higher incidence of many problems since more of them have started smoking. In addition to the worst, lung cancer, these include bronchitis and emphysema, hypertension and heart attacks, strokes, and hemorrhages. The use of birth control pills increases the risk of circulatory problems even further; for example, women who smoke and use the pill are 25 times more likely to suffer heart attacks than women who do neither.

HIGH-RISK SMOKERS

Pregnant women	Alcoholics or alcohol
Nursing mothers	abusers
Diabetics	Those with existing
Birth control pill users	smoker's diseases
Family history of heart disease	Those who work with
Hypertensives	toxic chemicals
Patients with high cholesterol	Those having surgery
Heavy smokers	Ulcer patients
Obese people	Type A personalities
Very thin people	

Other problems of smokers include an increased incidence of a variety of diseases and problems. Peptic ulcers are more frequent, especially in women who smoke (they used to have a low incidence). Hiatal hernias and heartburn pain are more common in smokers. Because of poor calcium utilization, smoking creates an increased risk of osteoporosis. Nutritional deficiencies due to decreased availability of vitamin A, thiamine, folic acid, and vitamin C increase risks of other illnesses, ranging from colds to cancers.

Another hazard of smoking is burns, which may be caused directly by cigarettes as well as by fires generated by them, as smoking is a major cause of fires and fire deaths. Smoking also eats away at the teeth and gums, creating disease, and stains the teeth, tongue, and fingers. It reduces appetite and taste for food, which definitely tends to interfere with good nutrition. Smoking often decreases the taste for sweets but increases the taste for more stimulating fatty or spicy foods. More caffeine and alcohol tend to be consumed by smokers than by nonsmokers.

Smokers also have more frequent job changes, as well as home and spouse changes. Problems with alcohol are associated with smoking, and many people who try to withdraw from alcohol and other drugs tend to smoke more. Smoking can weaken the memory, and with its destructive nature, it tends to lessen the desire and positive attitude toward life, which may be the reason why smokers experience more of these life changes.

What About Secondary Smoke?

The smoke from cigarettes that nonsmokers breathe has become a big issue in the last decade, a clear human rights issue. I will limit my comments here to saying that I feel that being exposed to secondary or "sidestream" smoke is a violation of my right to breathe clean air. To broaden this, pollution of Earth is a violation of the rights of us all and our future generations. We need to all do our best to minimize pollution and exposure to pollutants and to improve our methods of handling of wastes and industrial by-products.

Secondhand smoking occurs at work, at home, and in restaurants and shops (minimally outdoors). Sidestream smoke may be even more dangerous than mainstream smoke, since it is not filtered. Of the 16 or so poisons that arise from burning cigarettes, most are known carcinogens. Much of the ammonia, formaldehyde, acetaldehyde, formic acid, phenol, hydrogen sulfide, acetonitrile, and methyl chloride is filtered through the tobacco and cigarette filters and is more concentrated in the smoke that passive, involuntary smokers inhale. The blood level of carbon monoxide in secondhand smokers is more than 50 percent higher than that of those not exposed and often exceeds that of light firsthand smokers. And what about houseplants that surround smokers? It would be interesting to see research on the changes in growth and health and the chemical makeup of common plants; they may indeed do better than we humans.

The *22nd Annual Surgeon General's Report on Smoking and Health* focused on "sidestream" or secondary smoking. Since tobacco is used by more than 30 percent of Americans, it is a major concern. This report suggested that in excess of 70 percent more tars, two to three times the amount of nicotine and carbon monoxide, and seventy-three times more ammonia than found in mainstream smoke are present in sidestream smoke, which also contains lead, arsenic, cadmium, vinyl chloride (a strong liver carcinogen), benzene, oxides of nitrogen, and various radioactive substances. This information was cited in Dr. Rollin Odell, Jr.'s, article "Deadly Effects of Side Smoke," printed in the *San Francisco Chronicle* (January 10, 1987).

The conclusions drawn from a review of more than 2,000 studies regarding sidestream smoke is that it increases the incidence of most of the smoking diseases. Children of smokers have increased incidence of respiratory infections, ear infections, and lower lung function than children of nonsmokers. Sidestream smoke increases the risk of COPD (emphysema and chronic bronchitis), heart disease, and lung cancer. An estimated 3,000 cases of lung cancer a year are caused by secondhand smoking. Nonsmoking wives of smokers have been shown to have a life expectancy four years shorter than that of nonsmoking wives of nonsmokers. This may even be more pronounced for nonsmoking husbands of smoking wives. A chronic nonsmoker's "smoker's cough" or hoarseness may develop as well. Sidestream smoke probably increases the cancer risk of everyone involved. More common secondary smoker symptoms include eye and nasal irritation, worsened allergies, headache, and cough.

Clearly, smokers endanger not only their own health but the health and lives of others as well. The surgeon general should change the warning on the cigarette package to say "Smoking is hazardous to the health of yourself and those around you." It is wonderful for nonsmokers now that smoking is not allowed on airplanes and in many public places. Many cities have passed ordinances restricting smoking in various ways publicly. Truly, people should be protected from cigarette smoke indoors. I believe it should be against the law for parents (and others) to smoke in cars when children are with them or in any closed area where children are present. I have seen many cases, and heard about more, where children have had low grade allergies or infections when exposed to regular household smoke. However, we also need to be compassionate, understanding, and supportive toward anyone with destructive health habits. I have noticed more and more smokers being courteous to those around them. Dr. Odell puts forth the goal of a smoke-free society by the year 2000. A radiation oncologist himself, he finishes his article with the assumption that "the brown plague will soon be only a footnote to the history of our time, just as the black (bubonic) plague is to the time of the Middle Ages." However, until we can rid our world of the "brown plague," we must protect ourselves from secondhand smoke. A good air filter can be very effective in removing from the air many of the toxins generated by burning cigarettes. A basic multiple vitamin-mineral and antioxidant formula will help protect us internally. The daily program should include at least:

SMOKER'S SIMPLE NUTRIENT PLAN

Vitamin C	1,000–2,000 mg.
Beta-carotene	15,000–25,000 IUs
Vitamin A	5,000–10,000 IUs
Zinc	15–30 mg.
Selenium	200 mcg.
Vitamin E	400 IUs

Dietary Recommendations

No support program for smokers will be as effective as stopping and then working to regain the health lost by smoking. A wholesome diet and nutritional supplements although even the best program cannot offer immunity to cigarettes.

While the diet is, of course, important, I believe that for smokers taking supportive, protective nutrients is even more essential. Many smokers do have an adequate diet; I have seen smoking macrobiotics, smoking vegetarians, and smoking health enthusiasts. However, there is a tendency for poor dietary habits to accompany the destructive smoking habit. Many smokers tend to eat more meats, fatty and fried foods, and refined foods than nonsmokers. It is important for smokers to avoid other addictions. Sugar, coffee, alcohol, and meats should be minimized or avoided if possible.

A basic, wholesome diet helps to at least reduce some of the risks of smoking addiction, which may be influenced by nutritional deficiencies. This plan, especially with adequate fruits, vegetables, and whole grains, will help to provide some of the necessary, protective antioxidant nutrients, beta-carotene, vitamins A, C, and E, and selenium, all of which will help lower risks of cancer and other smoker's maladies. In addition, some raw seeds and nuts, legumes, sprouts, and other proteins should be consumed. Water is an essential nutrient to balance out the drying effect of smoking. A daily intake of two to three quarts is suggested, depending on how many high-water-content fruits and vegetables, salads, and soups are consumed. Caffeine beverages increase the need for water, as they are also dehydrating. Smoking usually generates a mild acid condition in the body, and an alkaline diet is helpful to balance this. A high-fiber diet also helps in detoxification, maintaining bowel function, and reducing the risks of smoking. The overall plan for smokers is to increase the wholesome foods—fruits, vegetables, and whole grains—and to lower the intake of fats, cured or pickled products, food additives, and alcohol.

An alkaline diet is even more important during the cigarette withdrawal and detoxification periods. The increased blood alkalinity that results from a diet high in fruits and vegetables, even mainly raw food consumption, helps reduce the craving for and interest in smoking. Studies have shown this to be true, and I have heard this regularly from the hundreds of patients I have seen in smoking cessation programs.

The alkaline diet is not necessarily a lifelong program, although, as I discussed elsewhere in this book, it is wise for our diet generally to be more alkaline than acid. During cigarette withdrawal, a vegetarian or raw food diet may be sufficient for the average person to help reduce nicotine craving. This can be used for three to six weeks to aid in the detoxification process. Fasting has also been employed by some smokers to help eliminate their habit. It does allow for rapid transitions, but it can also be somewhat intense. It might be reserved for the more durable and strong willed or the overweight or hypertensive smoker.

STOP SMOKING DIET

Increase Alkaline Foods		Reduce Acid Foods	
fruits	figs	meats	beef
vegetables	raisins	sugar	chicken
greens	carrots	wheat	eggs
lima beans	celery	bread	milk
millet	almonds	baked goods	cheese

The vegetarian diet is high in chlorophyllic (green) vegetables and sprouts, grains, fruits, and liquids, such as water, juices, soups, and herbal teas. The raw foods diet is similar, with more seeds and nuts. Eating whole, unsalted sunflower seeds (or carrot or celery sticks) can help replace that hand-to-mouth addiction that is common in smokers; however, we must be careful not to replace nicotine addiction with food addiction.

The diet for detoxification is also low in fat and high in fiber. It is important to keep the energy and bowels moving. The raw foods (and vegetarian) diet helps with both. This includes several salads of leafy greens daily, and some snacks of fruits, vegetables, nuts, or seeds. Some of the high-protein algae, such as spirulina and chlorella, also help during withdrawal and detox. Since cigarettes are such a rapid ager and a key cancer risk, the dietary suggestions in *Cancer Prevention* and *Anti-Aging* programs are useful here as well (see Chapter 16).

Supplements

Many supplements are useful for smokers or during withdrawal and detoxification. An acid urine increases the elimination of nicotine and thus increases the craving. So, while an alkaline diet may slow down the detoxification of nicotine, it also reduces the desire for smoking. To support the body alkalinization during smoking cessation, I recommend sodium or potassium bicarbonate tablets, one to be taken with cravings for a total of five or six daily, along with the fruit- and vegetable-based, high-fiber diet.

A general "multiple " with additional antioxidant nutrients are part of the smoker's program. The antioxidants help reduce the toxicity of smoke in primary and secondary smokers and also help lessen the free-radical irritation during the detox period. Vitamin E, 400–800 IUs daily, specifically helps stabilize the cell membranes and protects them and the tissue membranes from the free-radical and chemical irritations generated by cigarette smoke. Selenium, as sodium selenite or selenomethionine, at a level of 200–300 mcg., supports vitamin E and also reduces cancer potential, which is so much higher with chronic smoking. Selenium also lessens sensitivity to cadmium. Vitamin A reduces cancer risk and supports tissue health, and beta-carotene specifically protects against lung cancer in smokers. Smoking clearly depletes body vitamin C levels, probably by increasing antioxidant demands and reducing absorption. Therefore, smokers need regular vitamin C intake to help neutralize the toxins. Supplementing 500–2,000 mg. four or five times daily is recommended. (Note: Both vitamin C and niacin are mild acids, which may increase ulcer risk, as well as nicotine elimination and craving in smokers. If these nutrients are used in higher amounts, extra alkaline salts such as the bicarbonates or calcium-magnesium ascorbates, may be used.) Extra zinc, 30–60 mg. a day, like vitamin A, helps protect the tissue and mucous membrane health.

There are many other helpful nutrients needed during smoking and detox. First, we need to support the B vitamins that are more easily depleted in smokers, mainly thiamine (B_1), pyridoxine (B_6), and cobalamin (B_{12}). The B_{12} may also help to decrease the cellular damage caused by tars and nicotine. Niacin (B_3) helps in opening up the circulation that is constricted with nicotine. It also lowers cholesterol, which may reduce the risk of atherosclerosis. Pantothenic acid may reduce the aging of the skin and support the generally stressful lifestyle. Folic acid should be taken in higher amounts, such as 1–2 mg. daily. Coenzyme Q_{10} is also helpful in dosages of 30–60 mg. daily. Extra choline may support the brain and memory.

Besides zinc and selenium, other minerals also are important. Magnesium and molybdenum are needed in higher amounts than usual. Copper is needed at levels of 3–4 mg. daily, when used along with a higher zinc intake (60–100 mg.). Zinc also helps reduce cadmium absorption and toxicity. Vitamins C and E, selenium, and L-cysteine also help to reduce cadmium toxicity.

L-cysteine is very helpful to smokers and during detoxification. Along with thiamine and vitamin C, it protects the lungs from smoking damage and from acetaldehyde generated by smoke. It helps reduce smoker's cough. Glutathione, formed from L-cysteine, is part of the protective antioxidant enzyme system. Heavy smokers might use 250–500 mg. of glutathione, up to 1,500 mg. (500–750 mg. more usually) of L-cysteine, with 5–6 g. of vitamin C, 150 mg. thiamine, and the total B vitamins and amino acids to balance the specific ones used.

To prevent obesity, it is very important to be aware of eating properly when stopping smoking. Smoking reduces appetites and the taste for foods and probably increases metabolism as well as nervous energy. It is natural to want to eat more and enjoy food more when not smoking. Over half of ex-smokers will gain weight, and this is more common in the heavier (use) smokers. If weight gain is undesirable (many smokers are underweight), a weight-control diet should be instituted as smoking is stopped. Research has shown that smokers crave and eat less sweets than nonsmokers. This changes with smoking cessation (the taste buds come alive again), so new nonsmokers need to watch out for this. The alkaline, high-fiber, low-fat diet is helpful in maintaining weight. Another amino acid, L-phenylalanine, can help reduce the appetite if taken before meals in amounts of 250–500 mg. Because it has a mild tendency to raise blood pressure, this should monitored if the blood pressure is of concern. Often, however, the blood pressure drops somewhat with smoking cessation. More choline may improve fat utilization and maintain weight, as may the amino acid L-carnitine. Regular exercise, walking, and getting used to breathing deeply of the fresh air are also part of our new plan.

Smoking Cessation

There are many reasons to stop smoking. Health benefits are clearly number one. Lower risks of cancer, heart disease, and lung problems and better resistance to disease, by-products of smoking cessation. Our life expectancy is improved when we do not smoke. Also, we can save a lot of money in three ways: 1) no cost of cigarettes, which are costing more and more, 2) reduced health and life insurance premiums, and 3) lower medical expenses with improved health.

Stopping smoking may require a major change in our whole relationship to ourselves and our health. We will need to decide to love, support, and nurture ourselves in the best way possible. Often, changing our attitude first makes it easier for us to give up our health-denying habits, such as smoking. If we want to be optimally healthy, we just cannot smoke.

Even though I do not smoke, I know that it is a very difficult habit to break. In general, it is difficult for nonsmokers to really appreciate and understand the connection smoking has to the smoker's psyche and to his or her whole life. The level of addiction, which is based on the amount and number of years of smoking, will determine the ease of stopping smoking. If you light up first thing in the morning or if you smoke more than two packs a day, you probably have a serious addiction, and it may be harder to stop than for lighter smokers.

There are many different plans for stopping or decreasing smoking. The best way is just to decide and stop cold turkey, go through the withdrawal, and forget it. Then there is no back and forth, no doubt; the decision is made, and strength and willpower provide the success. The program here will help in this. The success rate for those who make the decision and just stop is much better than for those who use other methods. They do not need tapes, counselors, or group support; they only count on themselves. Those who depend on others to stop smoking have more relapses.

Smoking withdrawal, however, may not be easy. The first three days to a week can be very difficult; for some people, the struggle may last for as long as a couple of months. Usually, the first 12–24 hours are the peak of withdrawal, when symptoms may appear. Cigarette craving is almost always present. Headaches, anxiety, irritability, dizziness, and insomnia are fairly common. Other smoking withdrawal symptoms include muscle aches, sore mouth, inability to concentrate, drowsiness, heart palpitations, depression, and gastrointestinal upset, such as nausea, vomiting, cramps, diarrhea, or constipation. Over time, weight gain is not uncommon; this may result from an increased appetite and slower metabolism, probably both. Those fire sticks tend to push our metabolic pedals.

During withdrawal, I suggest taking vitamin C (as a mineral ascorbate to reduce acidity) in amounts of about 1 gram every one or two hours. This may help reduce nicotine cravings. Other nutrients and dietary plans discussed earlier may also be used. The maximum dosages listed in the table at the end of this section can be used for support during withdrawal.

If you just cannot give up nicotine, there are other ways to get rid of cigarettes. Nicorette, a nicotine gum, is a very useful tool. This supports the nicotine addiction without providing the harmful smoke chemicals. It reduces withdrawal symptoms, and research shows a better long-term quitting percentage with the nicotine gum than with other methods. It is, however, a temporary aid which can be obtained only with a doctor's prescription. It is not ideal, but it is better than smoking tobacco. Nicorette still produces the cardiovascular effects of nicotine but a minimum of the lung and cancer problems. It may cause some symptoms, such as nausea, lightheadedness, hiccups, and muscle tension or jaw aches from chewing. It does, however, immediately help one to stop smoking, as most of the craving is for the nicotine. The psychological, conditioned, and social addiction patterns of smoking itself must also be handled, and the former smoker should be off the gum within two or three months. Nicorette should be avoided by people with ulcers or cardiovascular disease and by pregnant women and should be kept away from children. There are also "smokeless" cigarettes (Favor brand) available which provide nicotine, and these can be used for withdrawal and transition as well.

If Nicorette gum does not work or you cannot otherwise stop smoking, there are many self-help suggestions for cutting down. Smoking fewer cigarettes daily is a common practice, but usually this reaches a limit of about ten per day to satisfy the nicotine habit. You might also try taking fewer puffs per cigarette and smoking just the first half of it, where the least tars and chemicals are concentrated. Filters and cigarette holders decrease the amount of toxic elements inhaled. There are also devices that place tiny holes in the filters to allow dilution of smoke with outside air. One of these is called Phaseout. Changing brands to lower-tar, higher-nicotine cigarettes will help reduce total smoking. Even using brands you do not like helps reduce. For anyone who smokes, I suggest avoiding chemically-treated cigarettes, and using natural, untreated tobacco and untreated paper. Roll-your-own types, some French, German, and other cigarettes, and a few untreated American brands would be an improvement over processed tobacco.

Before you start to stop smoking, write out a plan and schedule of dates and stages of nonsmoking, as well as the reasons to quit. Pick a time of less stress to do it, such as during vacation or just after sick leave from work or school. New Year's Day, your birthday, or national stop smoking days are good choices as well. Don't try to stop during stressful times at work or home, during transitions, or prior to holidays. Write your plan in a diary or journal and keep notes of your process, feelings, and so on. Get to know yourself better through this process. The withdrawal can have both negative and positive effects. Many smokers release a lot of energy and excitement as they quit, so use this to construct new habits and a new life if that is appropriate.

Successful quitters were often dissatisfied with smoking and felt negative effects as well as oppression from being addicted. When you quit, make a committment. Know your cigarette triggers and work to defuse them when you quit. Get rid of ashtrays, clean your teeth, and your home, such as your drapes, carpets and clothes, to get rid of tobacco smoke. Make your home and life a nonsmoking zone. And take special care of yourself with good foods, drinking water, taking baths or showers, and walking— and get a massage.

It is crucial for people who stop smoking to learn to handle stress. Be aware of the potential for relapse. Most people who start again do so when they meet increased stress, which may trigger a desire to smoke, and they do not have the coping skills to deal with this. Relaxation tapes, classes, and counseling may be necessary to find

SUGGESTIONS FOR SMOKING CESSATION

- Cut down on other addictive substances, such as caffeine, sugar, and alcohol, all of which can increase the desire to smoke.
- Get a partner, another smoker, to stop with you or, even better, get an ex-smoker to support you while you stop.
- Tell friends or family and ask for their support—that is, go public with your plan to stop. Also let them know you may wish to use them during your transition.
- Stay busy to prevent boredom and to keep your mind off smoking.
- Exercise regularly to decrease withdrawal, increase motivation, and increase relaxation.
- Create a reward or goal for being successful, such as betting with a friend (bet on yourself, of course), or save cigarette money for a new outfit or trip; this money you will collect only after a certain time of nonsmoking.
- Get plenty of rest.
- Drink fluids and use water for therapy by taking showers, baths, hot tubs, or going swimming.
- Change daily patterns to avoid stimulating old smoking conditioning. This may include staying away from bars and alcohol or coffee, avoiding friends who smoke, not receiving or making phone calls at specific locations in which you usually smoked, and getting up and doing something right after a meal.
- Learn relaxation and breathing techniques and do them.
- Practice visualizations.
- Keep a positive attitude toward health and life.
- Get positive health treatments, such as massage, teeth cleaning to remove cigarette stains, a yoga class, and so on.
- Find temporary oral substitutes to deal with psychological ties to smoking—be careful not to overeat or choke on any of the following nonedibles. Oral fixation substitutes could include munchies such as vegetable sticks (carrot, celery, zucchini), apples, nuts, popcorn, sunflower seeds (unsalted) in shells, sugarless hard candies or gum; or chewing or sucking on ice cubes, toothpicks, licorice sticks, or drinking straws.
- If cravings arise, find ways to deal with them. Examples could include short relaxation exercises, taking a break, a walk, a shower, drinking tea, or doing things with your hands, such as rubbing a stone or crystal, or bending a paperclip.

appropriate coping strategies so that they can continue being ex-smokers. Stress-reduction plans and exercises, both mental and physical, are helpful in preparing for individual future potential stress areas, be they work demands, relationships, or health pressures. These plans for exercise and stress management may even be best initiated before stopping smoking, as many smokers experience that the transition to not smoking is enough to deal with without having other new programs to apply. Also, beginning regular exercise and learning to relax may offer positive reinforcement to cut down or quit smoking. In fact, regular exercise offers many of the positive qualities that smokers get from nicotine, such as an "up" feeling, confidence, and a greater ability to relax and concentrate.

It is important to keep a positive attitude and make positive statements. Affirmations such as "I am not a smoker" or "stopping smoking is a great benefit to my health" can be written down and posted in specific areas as well as repeated regularly. Many ex-smokers use negative imagery to stay away from cigarettes. They may see the lung damage, heart disease, wrinkled skin, or limited activity whenever they feel the urge to smoke. If we visualize these negative images when we take a deep breath and hold it, the negative feedback we feel while oxygen is decreasing and carbon dioxide is rising will help us stay off cigarettes. Even more important is visualizing the positive benefits, such as the new ability to taste and smell, better digestion, and the improved respiratory and circulatory functions. Increasing the love we have for ourselves as nonsmokers and continuing to see ourselves as nonsmokers are also important.

STOP SMOKING BREW

Lemon grass	3 parts
Dandelion root	3 parts
Raspberry	2 parts
Red clover	2 parts
Alfalfa	2 parts
Peppermint	2 parts
Mullein leaf	2 parts
Valerian root	1 part
Catnip	1 part

Simmer dandelion and valerian in water for 10 minutes, then pour into a pot containing other herbs and steep for 15 minutes. Use about 1 teaspoon of root and 1 tablespoon of leaves and flowers per cup. Drink one cup several times daily or as needed for cravings.

Both negative and positive visualizations will help when we feel the craving or urge to smoke. Exercising, staying busy, and resting and relaxing are all important. Drinking water and taking some nutrients, mainly the B vitamins and vitamin C, may also reduce cravings. Herbs such as valerian or skullcap will help calm the nervous system and reduce cravings as well.

Many herbs have been used with benefit to smokers, both for smoking as substitutes for cigarettes and to help in withdrawal and detoxification. Smoking herbs have been used to replace cigarettes temporarily or to treat bronchopulmonary problems. Mullein leaf is probably the most commonly used. Coltsfoot, yerba santa, sarsaparilla, and rosemary have also been smoked. Garlic (taken orally, not smoked) is also helpful during the tobacco detox period. Lobelia leaf, called "Indian tobacco," has been employed as a substitute for cigarettes; it acts and tastes a bit like tobacco. In China, other herbs are smoked to treat asthma and other respiratory problems. Datura and jimson weed have been used, but these can be slightly toxic. Ginseng leaf and other herbal cigarettes have been available. Smoking mugwort or catnip may help in relaxation; damiana is thought to have aphrodisiac properties, while peppermint added to a blend will give a cool, menthol feeling and licorice, a sweet flavor. Licorice sticks have also been chewed during cigarette withdrawal to replace the oral habit and settle down the system. Chewing on calamus root may cause a tobacco smoker to become nauseated, acting kind of like a nicotine Antabuse.

There are many supportive therapies to help in stopping smoking. Acupuncture has had some success. Some counselors I know have very good results with clients. Hypnosis is helpful for others. Massage therapy aids the detoxification and provides basic health support. A program that combines diet, supplements, exercise, counseling, hypnosis, acupuncture, and massage works wonderfully, but it is time consuming and costly. And there still must be a desire to stop and the willpower to continue not smoking and surpass the cigarette urge—that is, the nicotine addiction. There are a number of good stop smoking programs available in most cities. Often the cost commitment and group support add the extra incentive to make it successful. I do suggest avoiding the rapid smoking plans that make you sicker to get well, as the excessive nicotine can be toxic.

Concern for Children

Many more young people are smoking. They are beginning earlier and smoking more. The images of being cooler or older or feeling authority and power are portrayed by the media on billboards, in magazines, and in movies. Television has improved in this regard, but the cigarette companies would buy advertising on kid's cartoon shows if we let them. They are in business to sell cigarettes, not health. We need to find ways to dissociate cigarettes from vitality, virility, and sexuality.

Children need to be educated early to make accurate associations with cigarettes, such as poor health, foul smells, and serious disease. Children need to know that cigarettes are very addicting, that they are a drug. Initially, smoking creates sickness—nausea, vomiting, dizziness, and so on. If it becomes a regular habit, these symptoms subside, and the smokers just cough and become addicted until more problems arise.

Parents must not smoke, especially around their children. The sight of adults that they respect smoking lays the groundwork for smoking later, to say nothing of the dangerous effects of secondary smoke. Smoke-free homes, limiting public smoking, and increasing positive lifestyle habits and attitudes are a beginning. In addition, we need laws to stop misleading advertising; showing older smokers hooked up to respirators is more truthful. We should make smokers pay for the tremendous cost of smoking by increasing the costs of cigarettes and the taxes on cigarettes. This may help defray the loss in national productivity and rise in medical costs in the future. And we must all work together, not in accusation and attack but in support and love, to help each other rise above the smoking pollution habit and create a smoke-free society for the twenty-first century.

The nutrient levels in the following table can be spread out in several portions throughout the day. Vitamin C can be used even more frequently. The dosages range from smoker's support to withdrawal, with the three to six weeks of detoxification requiring a mid-range amount.

Hostages

2 be bourne & trained
2 be bourne & tamed
2 be bourne & chained
Hostages, we're all hostages in one way or another
chaining our NRG to wide-scream TV
what might we do or be?
We're hostages of time, hostages in line
until we can conceive and believe we're free

—*Bethany ArgIsle*

NICOTINE NUTRIENT PROGRAM

Water	2½–3½ qt.
Fat	30–50 g.
Fiber	15–45 g.

Vitamin A	10,000–15,000 IUs	**Iodine**	150–250 mcg.
Beta-carotene	20,000–40,000 IUs	**Iron**	women—20–40 mg.
Vitamin D	200–400 IUs		men—10–20 mg.
Vitamin E	400–800 IUs	**Magnesium**	500–1,000 mg.
Vitamin K	100–300 mcg.	**Manganese**	5–10 mg.
Thiamine (B$_1$)	100–200 mg.	**Molybdenum**	300–600 mcg.
Riboflavin (B$_2$)	50–100 mg.	**Potassium**	200–500 mg.
Niacinamide (B$_3$)	50–100 mg.	**Selenium**	200–400 mcg.
Niacin (B$_3$)	100–1,000 mg.	**Silicon**	50–150 mg.
Pantothenic acid (B$_5$)	250–1,000 mg.	**Vanadium**	150–300 mcg.
Pyridoxine (B$_6$)	50–200 mg.	**Zinc**	30–75 mg.
Pyridoxal-5-phosphate	25–75 mg.		
Cobalamin (B$_{12}$)	200–1,000 mcg.	**Coenzyme Q$_{10}$**	20–60 mg.
Folic acid	800–2,000 mcg.	**L-amino acids**	1,000–2,000 mg.
Biotin	200–500 mcg.	**L-cysteine**	500–1,500 mg.
Choline	500–1,000 mg.	**Glutathione**	250–500 mg.
PABA	500–1,500 mg.	**(if available)**	
Vitamin C	3–12 g.	**Essential fatty acids**	4–6 capsules
Bioflavonoids	250–750 mg.	**or Flaxseed oil**	2–3 teaspoons
Calcium	850–1,250 mg.	*For withdrawal and detox:*	
Chromium	200–500 mcg.	**Garlic**	3–6 capsules
Copper	2–4 mg.	**Valerian root**	4–6 capsules
		Lobelia leaf	1–2 capsules
		Carrot sticks	10–20

Fasting

Fasting is the single greatest natural healing therapy. It is nature's ancient, universal "remedy" for many problems. Animals instinctively fast when ill. When I first discovered fasting, 15 years ago, I felt as if it had saved my life and transformed my illnesses into health. My stagnant energies began flowing, and I became more creative and vitally alive. I still find fasting both a useful personal tool and an important therapy for many medical and life problems.

Of course, most of the problems for which I recommend fasting as treatment are ones that result from overnutrition rather than malnutrition. Dietary abuse problems, more common in the Western world than in Third World countries, generate many of the chronic degenerative diseases that I have written so much about; these include atherosclerosis, hypertension and heart disease, allergies, diabetes, and cancer. I believe that fasting is therapeutic and, more importantly, preventive for many of these conditions and more.

As I use the term here, fasting is the avoidance of solid food and the intake of liquids only (true fasting would be the total avoidance of anything by mouth). The most stringent form of fasting is taking only water; more liberally, fasting includes the use of fresh juices made from fruits and vegetables as well as herbal teas. All of these limited diets generate varying degrees of detoxification—that is, elimination of toxins from the body. Individual experiences with fasting depend on the condition of the body (also mind and attitude). Detoxification might be intense and temporarily increase sickness or might be immediately helpful and uplifting.

Juice fasting is commonly used (rather than water alone) as a mild and effective cleansing plan; this is suggested by myself and other doctors and authors and by many of the European fasting clinics. Fresh juices are easily assimilated and require minimum digestion, while they supply many nutrients and stimulate our body to clear its wastes. Juice fasting is also safer than water fasting, because it supports the body nutritionally while cleansing and probably even produces a better detoxification and quicker recovery.

Fasting (cleansing, detoxification) is one part of the triology of nutrition; balancing and building (toning) are the others. I believe that fasting is the "missing link" in the Western diet. Most people overeat, eat too often, and eat a high-protein, high-fat, rich-food, building and congesting diet more consistently than they need. If we regularly eat a more balanced and well-combined diet, such as my Ideal Diet, we will have less need for fasting and toning plans, although both would still be required at certain intervals throughout the year.

In a sense, detoxification is an important corrective and rejuvenative process in our cycle of nutrition. It is a time when we allow our cells and organs to breathe out,

986

become current, and restore themselves. We do not necessarily need to fast to experience some cleansing, however. Minor shifts in the diet such as including more fluids, more raw foods, and fewer congesting foods will allow for better detoxification; for a carnivore, for example, a vegetarian or macrobiotic diet will be cleansing and purifying. The general process of detoxification is discussed thoroughly in the *General Detoxification* program; here we focus on fluid fasting—its history, therapeutic use, benefits, contraindications, and, of course, how to do it, along with other aspects of lifestyle that support fasting.

Fasting is a time-proven remedy. Its use goes back many thousands of years, really to the beginning of life forms. As a healing process and spiritual-religious process, it has continued to be more intelligently applied, we hope, in the last several thousand years.

Voluntary abstinence from food has been a tradition in most religions and is clearly a spiritual purification rite. Many religions, including Christianity, Judaism, and the Eastern religions, have encouraged fasting for a variety of reasons, such as penitence, preparation for ceremony, purification, mourning, sacrifice and union with God, and the enhancement of knowledge and powers. From Moses, Elijah, and Daniel to Christ, the Bible is filled with fasters, who employed it to assist their purification and communion with God. Fasts as long as 40 days were employed to cleanse people of sins and the "devil."

The Essenes, authors of the Dead Sea Scrolls, also advocated fasting to purify themselves and commune with God. This was one of their primary healing methods. *The Essene Gospel of Peace*, transcribed by Edmond Bordeaux Szekely from the third-century Aramaic manuscript, suggests that Satan, his evil spirits, and his plagues will be cast out of our being by fasting and prayer. The Essenes believed that disease came from Satan (they claimed that it took three days without food to starve Satan) and from sins upon our body—the temple, which must be purified for God to reside there. To bring God into our life more completely, we would fast on water and "go to the waters (stream, lake) and find a hollow reed, insert it in our rear ends and flush the evils from our bowels."

For many philosophers, scientists, and physicians, fasting was an essential part of life, health, and the healing process needed to recreate health where there was sickness. Socrates, Plato, Aristotle, Galen, Paracelsus, and Hippocrates all used and believed in fasting therapy. Most spiritual teachers also recommend fasting as a useful tool. In a booklet from the 1947 lecture entitled *Healing by God's Unlimited Power*, Paramahansa Yogananda suggested that fasting is a way to increase our natural resistance to disease, stating that "Fasting is a natural method of healing. When animals or savages are sick, they fast." He continued, "Most diseases can be cured by judicious fasting. Unless one has a weak heart, regular short fasts have been recommended by the yogis as an excellent health measure." Yogananda referred to an Armenian doctor, Grant Sarkisyan, who had treated many patients successfully with fasting therapy for such disorders as asthma, skin diseases, digestive problems, and early stages of atherosclerosis and hypertension.

Throughout the centuries, many doctors have treated a variety of patients and maladies with fasting, **acknowledging that ignorance (of how to live in accordance with nature) may be our greatest disease**. Knowledge, not necessarily from books, but our inherent and experienced knowing of how to live according to the natural laws and spiritual truth, leads to the sacred wisdom of life and subsequent good health. Knowing when and how long to fast is part of this knowledge. Through fasting, we can turn our energies inward, where we can use them for healing, clarity, and change.

Physicians with a spiritual orientation tend to be more inclined than others to employ fasting, both personally and medically. Many of my life transitions were acknowledged, stimulated, and supported through fasting; and when I felt blocked or needed creative juice in my writing, fasting would be very useful. In *Spiritual Nutrition and the Rainbow Diet*, Gabriel Cousens, M.D., a California physician and spiritual teacher, includes an excellent chapter on fasting in which he describes his concepts of fasting and his own 40-day fast. According to Dr. Cousens,

> . . . fasting in a larger context, means to abstain from that which is toxic to mind, body, and soul. A way to understand this is that fasting is the elimination of physical, emotional, and mental toxins from our organism, rather than simply cutting down on or stopping food intake. Fasting for spiritual purposes usually involves some degree of removal of oneself from worldly responsibilities. It can mean complete silence and social isolation during the fast which can be a great revival to those of us who have been putting our energy outward.

From a medical point of view, I believe that fasting is not utilized often enough. We go on vacations from work to relax, recharge, and to gain new perspectives on our life; why not take occasional breaks from food? Or, for that matter, we might consider fasts from phones, cars, computers, talking, or from whatever activity/consumption we feel is excessive. Most people cannot break out of the conditioned pattern of eating three meals daily. Eating is a habit, an addiction. Most of us do not need nearly the amounts (and types) of food we consume. I have discussed allergy-addiction in many sections of this book; in a sense, eating itself is an allergy-addiction. When we stop and let our stomach remain empty, our body goes into an elimination cycle, and most people, especially when toxicity exists, will experience some "withdrawal" symptoms, such as headaches, irritability, or fatigue (only pure hunger is a clear sign of need for food). When they eat again, their withdrawal symptoms subside, and they feel better. This situation is worse when it involves allergic people eating allergenic foods.

I believe that fasting is one of the best overall healing methods because it can be applied to so many conditions and people. Those who are acid, sympathetic, or yang types, who tend to develop congestive symptoms and diseases rather than those of deficiency, do better on fasting than do other types. Some acid conditions, including colds, flus, bronchitis, mucus congestion, and constipation, can lead to headaches, other intestinal problems, skin conditions, and many other ailments. Those who follow a basic, wholesome, and balanced diet such as outlined in this book have less need to fast or detoxify, although on occasion it is a good idea for anyone, provided that they are not undernourished. Most of us living in Western, industrialized nations are mixed types, with both overnutrition and undernutrition. We may take in excessive amounts of potentially toxic nutrients, such as fats and chemicals, and inadequate amounts of many essential vitamins and minerals. Juice fasting supplies some of these needed nutrients and allows the elimination of toxins. Excess mucus and clogging of the eliminative systems constitute the basic process of congestive diseases; deficiency problems result from poor nourishment or ineffecive digestion/assimilation.

In the *General Detoxification* program, a number of symptoms and diseases of toxicity that can be alleviated by detoxification are discussed. Juice fasting is mentioned as part of the treatment plans in many other sections as well. It can be used to detoxify from drugs or whenever we want to embark on a new plan or life transition, provided that there are no contraindications to fasting (discussed later in this section). Fasting is very versatile and generally fairly safe; however, when it is used in the treatment of medical conditions, proper supervision should be employed, including monitoring of physical changes and biochemistry values. Many doctors, clinics, acupuncturists, nutritionists, and chiropractors feel comfortable overseeing people during fasting.

CONDITIONS FOR WHICH FASTING MAY BE BENEFICIAL

colds	atherosclerosis
flus	coronary artery disease
bronchitis	angina pectoris
headaches	hypertension
constipation	diabetes
indigestion	fever
diarrhea	fatigue
food allergies	back pains
environmental allergies	mental illness
asthma	obesity
insomnia	cancer
skin conditions	epilepsy

The use of fasting to treat fevers is controversial. Eastern medicine thinks of fasting as increasing body fire, so that it might worsen fever. In actuality, when we consume liquids, we generate less heat, so this really helps to cool the body. With fever, we need more liquids than usual; with high temperatures and sweating, we need even more.

Some cases of fatigue will respond well to fasting, particularly when the fatigue results from congested organs and energy. With fatigue that results from chronic infection, nutritional deficiency, or serious disease, more nourishment is probably needed, rather than fasting.

Back pains that are due to muscular tightness and stress rather than from bone disease or osteoporosis are usually alleviated with a lighter diet or juice fasting. Many tight muscles and sore areas along the back may result from referred pain from colon or other organ congestion. In my experience, poor bowel function and constipation are fairly commonly associated with back pains.

Many patients with mental illness, from anxiety to schizophrenia, may be helped by fasting. The purpose of fasting in this case, however, is not to cure these problems but to help understand the relationship of foods, chemicals, or drugs to the mental difficulties. Allergies and hypersensitive environmental reactions are not at all uncommon in people with mental illness. Care must be exercised with the use of fasting in mental patients as the toxicity or lack of nourishment may worsen their problems. If, however, the patient is strong and congested, fasting may be indicated.

Obesity can be remedied by fasting. Obesity is the problem for which fasting is currently most often used (mainly protein drinks) in the traditional medical system, although it is not the best use of this healing technique. Fasting is not even a good treatment for those who are overweight; it is too temporary and may generate *feasting reactions* in people coming off the fast. Better would be a change of diet and a longer-term weight-release plan; something that will allow new dietary habits and food choices to replace the old ones. A short fast, perhaps of five to ten days, can be useful as a motivator and catalyst for making these necessary dietary changes and new commitments and to help release a pound or two daily.

Some very obese patients have been monitored by doctors while on water fasts done in hospitals for months at a time to shed weights of a hundred pounds or more. With other patients, the jaws have been wired shut so that they can take in only fluids drunk through straws. Newer fasting programs substitute a variety of protein-rich powders for meals. These are usually medically supervised programs for people who are at least 30–50 pounds overweight and make use of a prepackaged, low-calorie powder, such as Optifast or Medifast. This high-protein, low-calorie diet allows patients to burn more fat. These programs are not nearly as healthful as vital juice fasts, but they are nutritionally supportive over a longer time period and can be used on a outpatient basis fairly safely if people are monitored regularly. They provide all the needed vitamins, minerals, and amino acids to sustain life and help many obese people to lower their weight, blood fats, blood pressures, and blood sugars. However, as with any weight-loss program, if it does not motivate the participants to change their diets and habits, they then may stay in the "yo-yo" syndrome (weight going up and down and up), which may actually be more harmful than just remaining overweight.

A balanced, low-calorie diet with lots of exercise is still the best way to reduce and maintain a good weight and figure. Many obese people are also deficient in nutrients because they eat a highly refined, fatty, sweet diet. Often, these obese people are fatigued, and they need to be nourished first before they will do well on any fast.

Fasting to treat cancer is also a controversial topic. Many alternative clinics outside the United States use fasting in the treatment of cancers. Since cancer can be a devitalizing, debilitating disease, this may not be wise. Possibly with early cancer, and definitely as a cancer preventive to reduce toxicity, juice fasting may be helpful. Anyone with cancer needs adequate nourishment, and adding fresh juices to an already wholesome diet can help induce a mild detoxification and enhance vitality.

The Process and Benefits of Fasting

Although the process of fasting may generate various results, depending on the individual condition of the faster, there are clearly a number of common metabolic changes and experiences. First, fasting is a catalyst for change and an essential part of transformational medicine. It promotes relaxation and energization of the body, mind and emotions, and supports a greater spiritual awareness. Many fasters feel a letting go of past actions and experiences and develop a positive attitude toward the present. Having energy to get things done and clean up old areas, both personal and environmental, without the usual procrastination is also a common experience. Fasting clearly improves motivation and creative energy; it also enhances health and vitality and lets many of the body systems rest.

In other words, fasting is a multidimensional experience. Physiologically, refraining from eating minimizes the work done by the digestive organs, including the stomach, intestines, pancreas, gallbladder, and liver. Most important here is that our liver, our body's large production and metabolic factory, can spend more time during fasting cleaning up and creating its many new substances for our use. Breakdown of stored or circulating chemicals is the basic process of detoxification. The blood and lymph also have the opportunity to be cleaned of toxins as all the eliminative functions are enhanced with fasting. Each cell has the opportunity to catch up on its work; with fewer new demands, it can repair itself and dump its waste for the garbage pickup. Most fasters also experience a new vibrancy of their skin and clarity of mind and body.

Initially, the reduction of calories allows the liver to convert glycogen stores to glucose and energy. Body fat can be used for energy (ATP) but it cannot generate or reform glucose; although many cells can metabolize fatty acids for energy, the brain and central nervous system need direct glucose. Proteins can be broken down into amino acids; of these, alanine and serine can be used to produce glucose. With fasting, some protein breakdown occurs, less if calories are provided by juices. When there is no stored glycogen left, our body will convert protein to amino acids and to energy. Fatty acids can also be a fair source of energy, usually after being converted to ketones. With total fasting, ketosis occurs as an adaptation by the body to prevent protein loss by burning fats. Still, protein and fats can be used to provide energy for brain cell function. With juice fasting, there is less ketosis, and the simple carbohydrates in the juices are easily used for energy and cellular function. The high-protein diets and fasts do burn fat and generate ketosis and weight loss, but they also add more toxin buildup

991

in the body from the foods or powders used. Also, they do not rest and cleanse the digestive tract and other organs as well.

Fasting increases the process of elimination and the release of toxins from the colon, kidneys and bladder, lungs and sinuses, and skin. This process can generate discharge such as mucus from the gastrointestinal tract, respiratory tract, sinuses, or in the urine. This is helpful to clear out the problems that have arisen from overeating and a sedentary lifestyle. Much of aging and disease, I believe, results from "biochemical suffocation," where our cells do not get enough oxygen and nutrients or cannot adequately eliminate their wastes. Fasting helps us decrease this suffocation by allowing the cells to eliminate and clear the old products.

SOME BENEFITS OF FASTING

Purification	More energy
Rejuvenation	Better sleep
Revitalization	More relaxation
Rest for digestive organs	Better attitude
Clearer skin	More clarity, mentally
Antiaging effects	and emotionally
Improved senses—vision,	Inspiration
hearing, taste	Creativity
Reduction of allergies	New ideas
Weight loss	Clearer planning
Drug detoxification	Change of habits
Better resistance to disease	Diet changes
Spiritual awareness	Right use of will

This physiological rest and concentration on cleanup can also generate a number of toxicity symptoms. Hunger is usually present for two or three days and then departs, leaving many people with a surprising feeling of deep abdominal peace; yet, others may feel really hungry. It is good to ask ourselves, "What are we hungry for?" Fasting is an excellent time to work on our psychological connections to consumption.

As far as fasting symptoms, headache is is not at all uncommon during the first day or two. Fatigue or irritability may arise at times, as may dizziness or lightheadedness. Our sensitivity is usually increased. Common sounds like television, music, refrigerators may irritate us more now. The sense of smell is also exaggerated, both positively and negatively; I have had whole meals of smells while fasting. The tongues of most people will develop a thick white or yellow fur coating, which can be scraped or brushed off. Bad breath and displeasing tastes in the mouth or foul-smelling urine or stools may occur. Skin odor or skin eruptions such as small spots or painful boils, may also appear, depending on the state of toxicity. Digestive upset, mucusy stools, flatulence, or even nausea and vomiting may occur during fasting. Some people experience insomnia or bad dreams as their body releases poisons during the night. The mind may put up resistance, with doubt or lack of faith or a fear that the fasting is not right. (This can be influenced even more by listening to other people's fears.) Most of these symptoms, however, will occur early if they do appear and are usually transient. The general energy level is usually good during fastings, although there can be ups and downs. Every two or three days, as the body goes into a deeper level of dumping wastes, the energy may go down, and resistance and fears as well as symptoms may arise. Between these times, we usually feel cleaner, better, and more alive.

The natural therapy term for periods of cleansing and symptoms is "crisis," or "healing crisis." During these times, old symptoms or patterns from the past may arise, usually transiently, or new symptoms of detoxification may appear. This "crisis" is not predictable and is thus often accompanied with some question by the fasters as well as their practitioners—is this some new problem arising or is it part of the healing process? Usually only time will tell, yet if it is associated with the fasting and one or more of the common symptoms, it is likely a positive part of detoxification. We should use the maxim of healing, *Hering's Law of Cure*, to guide us—it states that healing happens from the inside out, the top down, from more important organs to less important ones, and from the most recent to the oldest symptoms. Most healing crises pass within a day or two, although some cleansers experience several days of "cold" symptoms or sinus congestion. If any symptom lasts longer than two or three days, it should be considered as a side effect or a new problem possibly unrelated to cleansing. If there is a problem that worsens or is severe and causes concern, such as fainting, heart arrythmias, or bleeding, the fast should be stopped and a doctor consulted.

A doctor or knowledgeable practitioner should supervise anyone for whom fasting is questionable—that is, anyone in poor health or without fasting experience. If the fast is extended for more than three to five days, regular monitoring, including physical examination and blood work should be done, probably about weekly. Fasting may reduce blood protein levels and will definitely lower blood fats. Uric acid levels may rise secondary to protein breakdown, while levels of some minerals, such as potassium, sodium, calcium, or magnesium, may drop. Iron levels are usually lower, and the red blood count may also drop during this time.

Nutritionally, fasting helps us appreciate the more subtle aspects of diet, since less food and simple flavors become more satisfying. My early fasts definitely reawakened my taste buds and allowed me to appreciate and desire more natural foods. Mentally, fasting improves clarity and attentiveness; emotionally, it may make us more sensitive and aware of feelings. I have seen on several occasions individuals making decisions based on new clarities brought out during fasts. Fasting clearly supports the transformational evolutionary process. For example, when we really "get" that our spouse is not going to change his or her habits of eating, watching TV, or being too busy to really relate to us—that the priority of the relationship is very low and the love is clearly not there—it may be time to make a change. With fasting, we can feel empowered to do things we only thought about before. Fasting can precipitate emotional cleansing as well. Attitude and general motivation are usually uplifted with cleansing. Spiritually, juice fasting offers a lesson in self-restraint and control of passions, which help us in many avenues of life.

Fasting is a simple process of self-cleansing. We do not need any special medicines to do it; our body knows how. Provided that we are basically well-nourished, systematic undereating and fasting are likely the most important contributors to health and longevity. Fasting is even more important to balance the autointoxication that results from common dietary and drug indiscretions.

I look at fasting as "taking a week off work" to handle the other aspects of life for which there is often little time. With fasting we can take time to nurture ourselves and rest. Fasting is also like turning off and cleaning a complex and valuable machine so that it will function better and longer. Resting the gastrointestinal tract, letting the cells and tissues repair themselves, and allowing the lymph, blood, and organs to clear out old, defective, or diseased cells and unneeded chemicals all lead to less degeneration and sickness. As healthy cell growth is stimulated, so is our level of vitality, immune function and disease resistance, and our potential for greater longevity.

Fasting Examples

J.R. did a 67-day fast on juices at age 20 when he joined a fasting and health-food-oriented community in 1975. He describes feeling great and very light. In fact, he lost a lot of weight. His only problems were skin sores that would not heal. These were of course, seen as a detox process. Medically, they could be attributed to protein/nutrient deficiency as well. This long fast on juice nutrients was a major transitional period for J.R. to change his diet to raw foods and strict vegetarianism. It also helped change his beliefs and motivation for life.

S.R. was very overweight and in a family relationship that was not supporting her growth. She clearly grasped for spiritual unfoldment. She was very strong, had loads of energy and various congestive symptoms—a prime candidate for fasting. After she began her fast, she decided to go 30 days on Master Cleanser with my support. She did wonderfully, lost 24 pounds, and wasn't through yet. For the next 30 days, she did my seven-food diet (apples, lemons, alfalfa sprouts, brown rice, carrots, almonds, and broccoli), picking seven primary foods to make up her diet, thus continuing her willpower and diet focus. After that, S.R. did another 30-day fast on Master Cleanser and other juices. She did well. During these months she moved from bookkeeping and typing into the healing arts. She left her husband and moved to the Midwest to take a job assisting a well-known physician in her healing research.

---

*There are many choices that will make up a relatively balanced diet.

B.D. and C.D.—This father (B.D., age 46) and son (C.D., age 15) attended a recent fasting group. B.D. was 50 pounds overweight (231, 5'9") and had high blood pressure. On exam B.D.'s cholesterol was 214. He had in the past followed a low-fat, Pritikin-like diet and felt better. He was really ready for a change and wanted to fast. He wanted me to see his son to evaluate whether he also could join the fasting group. C.D. was an overweight (181, 5'9") teenager on a typical teenage diet but inspired toward health.

B.D. did incredibly well on the Master Cleanser for 10 days, feeling fine and energetic and dropping his weight to 213. His new diet plan became more vegetarian, wholesome, and low fat, and included one- to two-day fasts weekly, plus a week-long fast every few months. A follow-up four months later found him well and busy in a new job. His weight had gotten to a low of 195 and he stabilized at about 202 with his diet. The positive value he received was that he realized that he could be in control of his diet. He was in much better shape and his self-esteem was much higher; of course he could see his feet and the earth again as his pant size dropped from 42" to 36".

C.D. dropped his weight from 182 to 171 with the fast and was an inspiration to the fasting group. His body and face changed dramatically. New activities and exercise were added to his regimen, and he now is a more serious bicyclist. C.D.'s diet also changed dramatically to enjoying salads and fruits, some grains, and fish and poultry. He got away from the sweets, sodas, salt snacks, and fried foods he was eating before. Now at 165, he feels great!

Hazards of Fasting

If fasting is overused, it may create depletion and weakness, lower resistance, and allow diseases to begin. Certain people are not good candidates for fasting or cleansing. Others may enjoy fasting so much that they overindulge in it and take it beyond the limits of normal elimination, resulting in protein and other nutritional deficits, reduced immunity, and loss of energy. While fasting allows the organs, tissues, and cells to rest, clean house, and handle excesses, the body needs the nourishment provided by food to function after it has used its stores.

Many people of the world are involuntary fasters, while those of the Western nations are more likely to be feasters. In Third World countries, many starvation deaths result from the disease of protein deficiency, termed kwashiorkor, and protein-calorie malnutrition, known as marasmus. What happens to these people is what happens with chronic fasting—loss of muscle mass, weight, and energy, and finally swelling and death.

Malnourished people should definitely not fast, nor should some overweight people who are undernourished. Others who should not fast include people with fatigue resulting from nutrient deficiency, those with chronic degenerative disease of the muscles or bones, or those who are underweight. Diseases associated with clogged or toxic organs respond better to fasting. Sluggish men or women who retain water or whose weight is concentrated in their hips and legs often do poorly with fasting. Those with low daytime energy and more vitality at night (more yin or alkaline types) may not enjoy fasting, either.

I do not suggest fasting for pregnant or lactating women. People who have weak hearts, such as those with congestive heart failure, or who have weakened immunity usually are not good candidates for fasting. Before or after surgery is not a good time to fast, as the body then needs its nourishment to handle the stress and healing demands of surgery. Although some of the nutritional therapies for cancer include fasting, I do not recommend fasting for cancer patients, especially those with advanced problems. Ulcer disease is not something for which I usually suggest fasting, either, although fasting may be beneficial for other conditions present in a patient whose ulcer is under control. Many clinics and fasting practitioners do believe in fasting for ulcers, however. In the first test case of the Master Cleanser (lemon juice, maple syrup, cayenne pepper, and water), Stanley Burroughs claims to have cured a patient with an intractable ulcer. Mr. Burroughs used the two main ingredients that all doctors suggested that this patient avoid, citrus and spice, which he figured were the only things left that might heal the ulcer. The fasting process itself probably is helpful for ulcers, since it reduces stomach acid and aids in tissue healing. And cayenne pepper, even though it is hot, has a healing effect on mucous membranes, and in herbal medicine, it is commonly recommended for ulcers. So, even though peptic ulcers are on the contraindication list, some ulcer people may do very well with fasting, especially with cabbage/vegetable juices.

CONTRAINDICATIONS FOR FASTING

Underweight	Pregnancy
Fatigue	Nursing
Alkaline type	Pre- and postsurgery
Low immunity	Mental illness
Weak heart	Cancer
Low blood pressure	Peptic ulcers
Cardiac arrythmias	Nutritional deficiencies
Cold weather	

As with any therapy that has some physiological effect and benefit, fasting also may have some hazards. The potential for the development of these problems is maximized with lengthy, noncaloric or water fasts and minimized with juice fasting of reasonable length, such as one to two weeks. Clearly, excessive weight loss and nutritional deficiencies may occur, again more marked with water fasts (juices provide calories and nutrients, although they do not provide complete nutrition). Weakness may occur, or muscle cramps may result from mineral deficits. Sodium, potassium, calcium, magnesium, and phosphorus losses occur initially but diminish after a week. Blood pressure drops, and this can lead to episodes of dizziness, especially when changing position from lying to sitting or sitting to standing. Uric acid levels may rise, which may result in acute gout attacks or a uric acid kidney stone, although this is rare. This problem is minimized with adequate fluid intake.

Some research reports have described hormone level changes with fasting. Initially, the level of thyroid hormone falls, but it rises again in association with protein-sparing ketosis. Female hormone levels fall, possibly as a result of protein malnutrition, and this can lead to loss of menstrual flow; that is, secondary amenorrhea. This cessation of the periods in women is also seen in longtime vegetarians, especially those who engage in extensive exercise programs.

Cardiac problems, such as abnormal rhythms (arrhythmias), can occur more easily with prolonged fasting and/or with subclinical preexisting problems. Extra beats, both ventricular and atrial, have been seen, and there have been deaths from serious ventricular arrhythmias, such as ventricular tachycardia, most often occurring during long water fasts. Similar problems have occurred recently in people using the nutrient-deficient protein powders that have been freely sold; many unhealthy weight reducers have been put at risk by using these powders over extended periods on unmonitored fasts. This risk is minimized with juice fasting (up to two weeks) or when basic minerals, mainly potassium, calcium, and magnesium, are supplemented during water fasts. Having our progress followed medically through physical exams, blood tests, and even electrocardiograms is a way to protect ourselves from the potential hazards of fasting.

Another side effect of fasting involves its transformative aspects and how they relate to personal life changes. Often we maintain certain relationships and attitudes toward other people or our careers by resisting inner guidance, feelings, and desires to do something new. Divorce, job changes, and moves are all more likely after fasts, because fasting often stimulates self-realization and change, enhances our potential, and leads us to focus on where we are going, rather than where we have been. During fasting transitions, many people question all aspects of their lives and make new plans for the future. They also have new sensitivity to and awareness of their job, mate, home, and so on. I warn fasters before they begin that these experiences may arise and their lives may change, especially when I sense that they are not really committed to or believe in what they are doing. Even though these insights and changes may be traumatic, my belief is that they are ultimately positive, as they support the evolutionary purpose of the human being. In this way, fasting helps us follow our true nature.

How to Fast

In the thousands of people I have observed during fasting and detox programs, the complications have been negligible, provided that proper procedures have been followed and attention paid to the ongoing body changes. Usually, people feel fine, even euphoric after a few days, although there may be ups and downs or various symptoms; yet, overall, in my experience, changes are positive.

997

The general plan for fasting works progressively, from a moderate approach for new fasters and unhealthy subjects to a stricter program for the more experienced. It is important to take the proper time with this potentially powerful process and not jump into a water fast from an average American carnivorous diet. Although many people do fine even if they make such extreme changes, it clearly maximizes the risks of fasting.

A sensible daily plan is one where fasting is mixed with eating. Each day can include a 12–14 hour period of fasting in the evening and during sleep before awakening and getting ready for the day. (Breakfast was given that name to denote the time where we break the fast of the night.) Many people eat very lightly or not at all in the early morning to extend their daily fast. This is more important if dinner or snacking tends to be extended into the later evening, though this is not ideal. On the other hand, if we eat a decent, not excessive, meal in the early evening and awaken hungry, a good breakfast can be consumed after water intake and some exercise.

In preparation for our first day of fasting, we may want to take a few days to eliminate some foods or habits from our diet. When many self-indulgent habits exist, longer preparations may be indicated. Eliminating alcohol, nicotine, caffeine, and sugar if possible is very helpful, although some people choose to wait until their actual fast days to clear these. Red meats and other animal foods, including milk products and eggs, could be avoided for a day or two before fasting. Intake of most nutritional supplements can also be curtailed the day before fasting; these are usually not recommended during a fast. Many people do well by preparing for their fasts with three or four days of consuming only fruit and vegetable foods. These nourish and slowly detoxify the body so that the actual fasting will be less intense.

The first one-day fast (actually 36 hours, including the nights—from 8 P.M. one night until 8 A.M. the following day) gives us a chance to see what a short fast can be like, to see that it is not so very difficult and does not cause any major distress. Most people will feel a little hungry at times and may experience a few mild symptoms (such as a headache or irritability) by the end of the day, usually around late afternoon or dinnertime, but this depends on the individual and the state of toxicity. In actuality, the first two days are the hardest for most people. Feeling great usually begins around day three, so longer juice fasts are really needed for the grand experience.

One of the problems with fasting is that it can be the most difficult for those who need it the most, such as the regular three-square-meals-plus-snacks consumers who eat whatever and whenever they want. Often such people must start with more subtle diet changes and prepare even more slowly for fasting. A transition plan that can be used before even going on the one-day fast is the one-meal-a-day plan. The one daily meal is usually eaten around 3 P.M. Water, juices, and teas and even some fresh fruit or vegetable snacks can be eaten at other times. The one wholesome meal is not excessive or rich. It can be a protein-vegetable meal, such as fish and salad or steamed vegetables, or a starch-vegetable meal, such as brown rice and mixed steamed greens, carrots, celery, and zucchini. People on this plan start to detox slowly, lose some weight, and after a few days feel pretty sound. The chance of any strong symptoms developing, as might occur with fasting, is minimal with this type of transition, and the actual fast, when begun, will be handled more easily, also.

The goal, then, is to move into a one-day fast and then a few two- and three-day fasts with one or two days between them when light foods and more raw fruits and vegetables are consumed, and also provide fluids, juices, soups, and a generally alkaline cleansing diet. This way, we can build up to a five- to ten-day fast. When the transition is made this slowly, even a water fast can be less intense and more profound for those wishing a powerful personal and spiritual experience. With a water fast, however, I strongly suggest medical monitoring and retreating from usual daily life.

A juice fast, which I usually recommend, can be longer and is much easier for most people. The fresh juices of raw fruits and vegetables are what most fasting clinics and practitioners recommend. They provide calories and nutrients on which to function and build new cells, and also provide the inherent enzymes contained in these vital foods. (Food enzyme theories, discussed throughout this century, have recently been described in books such as *Enzyme Nutrition* by Dr. Edward Howell.) Raw foods are considered the healing force in our diet because they contain active enzymes, which are broken down when foods are cooked. Many health enthusiasts consider a raw-food diet the most healing and most nutritious diet.

For the inexperienced faster, it is best to go slowly through the various steps and to avoid being excessive or impatient so that we learn about ourselves in the process. To do this, we need to make a plan and put it into effect, observing or "listening" to our body and even keeping notes in a journal. Get to really know yourself. Then, once we have fasted successfully, we could continue to do one-day fasts weekly or a three-day fast every month if we need them. This helps to reconnect us with a better diet and to remotivate us toward our goal of optimum health.

In a more adventurous mode, many people, even some who have never fasted, begin with a seven- to ten-day or even longer fast on fresh juices. I recommend this for most people who have any of the indications and none of the contraindications discussed in this program (also see *General Detoxification*). People planning these longer fasts, especially inexperienced fasters who have been eating a random diet, should spend a period about equal in length to the planned fast preparing for it. During this preparatory period we can follow some of the previous suggestions, such as eliminating sugar and refined foods, fatty foods, chemicals, and drugs from the diet and reducing consumption of meats and other acid-forming foods, and then moving into several days of consuming primarily fruits and vegetables and more fluids. This will lead into an easier and more energizing fast.

For any cleansing period, it is essential to plan times to meditate, exercise, get fresh air and sunshine, clear our intestines, get massages, take baths, clean our house, brush our skin, and more. Maybe you thought you were going to sit back and relax and have juice delivered to your room? With less shopping, food preparation, and eating time, we have more hours in the day to take care of ourselves in other ways. These supportive aspects of cleansing are discussed further below.

Timing of Fasts

The two key times for natural cleansing are the times of transition into spring and autumn. (This is discussed in other sections of this book, such as in Chapter 9 on *Diets* and the *General Detoxification* program earlier in this chapter, and emphasized in my first book, *Staying Healthy With the Seasons*.) In Chinese medicine, the transition time between the seasons is considered to be about ten days before and after the equinox or solstice. For spring, this period is about March 10 through April 1; for autumn, it is from about September 11 through October 2. In cooler climates, where spring weather begins later and autumn earlier, the fasting can be scheduled appropriately, as it is easier to do in warmer weather. With fasting, the body tends to cool down.

In the *General Detoxification* program, there is also a complete yearly cycle for cleansing with a variety of ideas and options. For spring, I usually suggest lemon and/or greens as the focus of the cleansing. Diluted lemon water, lemon and honey, or, my favorite, the Master Cleanser, could be used.

SPRING MASTER CLEANSER

2 Tablespoons fresh lemon or lime juice
1 Tablespoon pure maple syrup
1/10 teaspoon cayenne pepper
8 ounces spring water

Mix and drink 8–12 glasses a day. Eat or drink nothing else except water, laxative herb tea, and peppermint or chamomile tea.

Fresh fruit or vegetable juices diluted with an equal amount of water will also provide a good cleansing. Some vegetable choices are carrots, celery, beets, and lots of greens. Soup broths can also be used. Juices with blue-green algae, such as spirulina or chlorella, mixed in can provide more energy, as these are high-protein plants and easily assimilable.

Autumn is the second most important cleansing time, when we prepare for a new health program, focus on our career or school year, and let go of the fun and games of summer. At this time, a fast of at least three to five days can be done, using water or a variety of juices, including the Master Cleanser, apples and/or grapes (usually mixed with a little lemon and water to reduce sweetness), vegetable juices, and warm broths.

How do we know how long to fast? We may use a certain time plan, such as discussed above. Ideally, though, we should follow our own individual cycles and our body's needs. As we gain some fasting experience, we should become attuned to when we need to strengthen or lighten our diet and when we need to cleanse. Usually, if we are under stress or have been overindulging or develop some congestive symptoms, we want to lighten our diet to balance this. If more changes are needed, a more cleansing, raw-food diet or a fast can be begun.

A special light, purifying soup is offered by Bethany ArgIsle.

AUTUMN REJUVENATION RATION

3 cups spring water
1 Tablespoon ginger root, chopped
1–2 Tablespoons miso paste
1–2 stalks green onion, chopped
cilantro, to taste, chopped
1–2 pinches cayenne pepper
2 teaspoons olive oil
juice of ½ lemon

Boil water. Add ginger root. Simmer 10 minutes. Stir in miso paste to taste. Turn off fire. Then add green onion, some cilantro, cayenne, olive oil, lemon juice. Remove from burner and cover to steep for 10 minutes. May vary ingredient portions to satisfy flavors. Enjoy.

Breaking a Fast

When to stop fasting and make a transition back into eating also takes some inner attunement. Things to watch for include energy level, weight, detox symptoms, tongue coating, and degree of hunger. If our energy is up and then falls for more than a day or if our weight gets too low, these may be signs that we should come off the fast. If symptoms are intense or if any suddenly appear, it is possible that we need food. Generally, the tongue is a good indicator of our state of toxicity or cleansing and clarity. With fasting, the tongue usually becomes coated with a white, yellow, or gray film. This represents the body's cleansing, and it will usually clear when the detox cycle is complete. Tongue observation is not a foolproof indicator, however. Some people's tongues may coat very little, while others will remain coated. In this case, if we were to wait until it totally cleared, we may overextend our cleanse. If in doubt, it is better to make the transition back to foods and then cleanse again later. Hunger is another sign of readiness to move back into eating. Often during cleansing times, hunger is minimal. Occasionally, people are very hungry throughout a fast, but most lose interest in food from day three to day seven or ten and then experience real, deep-seated hunger again. This is a sign to eat (carefully!).

It is important to make a gradual transition into a regular diet, rather than just going out to dinner after a week-long fast. Breaking a fast must be planned and done slowly and carefully to prevent creating symptoms and sickness. It is suggested that we take several days, or half of our total cleansing time, to move back into our diet, which is hopefully a newly planned, more healthful diet. Our digestion has been at rest, so we need to go slowly and chew our foods very well. If we have fasted on water alone, we need to prepare our digestive tract with diluted juices, perhaps beginning with a few teaspoons of fresh orange juice in a glass of water and progressing to stronger mixtures throughout the day. Diluted grape or orange juice will stimulate the digestion. Arnold Ehret, a European fasting expert and proponent of the "mucusless" diet, suggests that fruits and fruit juices should not be used right after a meat eater's first fast because they may coagulate intestinal mucus and cause problems. More likely, a meat eater's colon bacteria are different than a vegetarian's; with fruit sugars, the active gram-positive anaerobic bacteria in the meat eater will produce more toxins. Initially, a transition from meats to more vegetable foods will then allow a smoother fast, mainly with vegetable juices and broths. They could also take extra acidophilus to begin to shift their colon ecology.

With juice fasting, it is easier to make the transition back into foods. A raw or cooked low-starch vegetable, such as spinach or other greens, can be used. A little sauerkraut, a fermented cabbage, helps to stimulate the digestive function. A laxative-type meal, such as grapes, cherries, or soaked or stewed prunes, can also be used to initiate eating, as it is important to keep the bowels moving. Some experts say that the bowels should move within an hour or two after the first meal. If not, take an enema. Some people may do a saltwater flush (drinking a quart of water with 2 teaspoons of sea salt dissolved in it) before their first day of food.

However you make the transition, go slowly, chew well, and do not overeat or mix too many foods at a meal. Simple vegetable meals, salads, or soups can be used to start. Fruit should be eaten alone. Soaked prunes or figs are helpful. Well-cooked brown rice or millet is handled well by most people by the second day. From there, progress slowly through grains and vegetables. Some nuts, seeds, or legumes can be added, and then richer protein foods if these are desired. Coming back into foods is a crucial time for learning individual responses or reactions to them. You may even wish to keep notes, following such areas as energy level, intestinal function, sleep patterns, and food desires. If you respond poorly to a food, avoid it for a while, perhaps a week, and then eat it alone to see how it feels.

Juice Specifics

Some juices work better for certain people or conditions. In general, diluted fresh juices of raw organic fruits and vegetables are best. Canned and frozen juices should be avoided. Some bottled juice may be used, but fresh squeezed is best, as long as it is used soon after squeezing.

Water and other liquids are what primarily cleanse our system, increasing waste elimination—rather like squeezing out a dirty sponge in clean water. Lemon tends to loosen and bring out mucus and is useful for liver cleansing. Diluted lemon juice, with or without a little honey, or the Master Cleanser can loosen mucus fast, so if this is used, we need to cleanse the bowels regularly to prevent getting sick. Most vegetable juices are a little milder than lemon juice.

Each juice has a certain nutritional composition and probably certain physiological actions, although these have not been studied extensively. We can think of fresh juices as natural vitamin pills with a very high assimilation percentage, and we do not need to do the work of digesting them.

In general, some juices are more caloric than others and might be used less if more weight loss is desired. The juices of apples, grapes, oranges, and carrots are good cleansing juices but might be minimized for weight loss. More grapefruit, lemon, cucumber, and greens, such as lettuce, spinach, or parsley, may be more helpful in this situation. Also, a variety of juices can be used in a fast with different ones squeezed daily.

FRUIT JUICES

Lemon—liver, gallbladder, allergies, asthma, cardiovascular disease (CVD), colds
Citrus—CVD, obesity, hemorrhoids, varicose veins
Apple—liver, intestines
Pear—gallbladder
Grape—colon, anemia
Papaya—stomach, indigestion, hemorrhoids, colitis
Pineapple—allergies, arthritis, inflammation, edema, hemorrhoids
Watermelon—kidneys, edema
Black cherry—colon, menstrual problems, gout

VEGETABLE JUICES

Greens—CVD, skin, eczema, digestive problems, obesity, breath
Spinach—anemia, eczema
Parsley—kidneys, edema, arthritis
Beet greens—gallbladder, liver, osteoporosis
Watercress—anemia, colds
Wheat grass—anemia, liver, intestines, breath
Cabbage—colitis, ulcers
Comfrey—intestines, hypertension, osteoporosis
Carrots—eyes, arthritis, osteoporosis
Beets—blood, liver, menstrual problems, arthritis
Celery—kidneys, diabetes, osteoporosis
Cucumber—edema, diabetes
Jerusalem artichokes—diabetes
Garlic—allergies, colds, hypertension, CVD, high fats, diabetes
Radish—liver, high fats, obesity
Potatoes—intestines, ulcer

These juices may be helpful for particular organs or illnesses, based on my experience as well as information contained in Paavo Airola's *How to Get Well*. To prepare juices, we obviously want to start with the freshest and most chemical-free fruits and vegetables possible. They should be cleaned or soaked and stored properly. If there is a question of toxicity, sprays, or parasites, a chlorine bleach bath can be used (see Chapter 11). If not organic, they should be peeled, especially if they are waxed. With root vegetables such as carrots or beets, the above-ground ends should be trimmed. Some people like to drop their vegetables into a pot of boiling water for a minute or so for cleansing as well.

The best juicers are the compressors, such as the Norwalk brand, but these are very expensive. The rotary-blade juicers, such as the Champion, are good at squeezing the juice with minimum molecular irritation. The centrifuge juicers are also fine, but they waste juice left in the pulp. Blenders are not really juicers; what they make is more like liquid salads. These are high in fiber. I once did a energizing week-long fast with two blender drinks a day, fruits in the morning and vegetables in the late afternoon, with teas and water in between.

Other Aspects of Healthy Fasting

- *Fresh air*—plenty is needed to support cleansing and oxygenation of the cells and tissues.
- *Sunshine*—also needed to revitalize our body; avoid excessive exposure.
- *Water*—bathing is very important to cleanse the skin at least twice daily. Steams and saunas are also good for giving warmth as well as supporting detoxification.
- *Skin brushing*—with a dry, soft brush prior to bathing; this will help clear toxins from the skin. This is a good year-round practice as well.
- *Exercise*—very important to support the cleansing process. It helps to relax the body, clear wastes, and prevent toxicity symptoms. Walking, bicycling, swimming, or other usual exercises can usually be done during a fast, although more dangerous or contact sports might be avoided.
- *No drugs*—none should be used during fasts except mandatory prescription drugs. Particularly, avoidance of alcohol, nicotine, and caffeine is wise.
- *Vitamin supplements*—these are not used during fasting; thus, no program of nutrients will follow at the end of this section. Some supplemental fiber, such as psyllium husks, can be part of a colon detox program. Special chlorophyll foods, such as green barley, chlorella, and spirulina, may also be vitality enhancers and purifiers during cleanses. Occasionally, some mineral support, especially potassium, calcium, and magnesium, or vitamin C will be suggested, usually in powdered or liquid forms (pills are not suggested) to help in preventing cramps, if there is a lot of physical activity, sweating, and fluid and mineral losses, or for an extended fast. Some people even use amino acid powders and other vitamin

powders with some benefit during cleanses. In general, most of these supplemental nutrients are best used with foods.

- *Colon cleansing*—an essential part of healthy fasting. Some form of bowel stimulation is recommended. Colonic irrigations with water are the most thorough. These can be done at the beginning, midpoint, and end of the fast. It is suggested that enemas be used at least every other day if these are the primary colon cleansing. Fasting clinics often suggest that enemas be used daily, even up to several times a day. With these, usually water alone is used to flush the colon of toxins. It may be helpful for an enema or laxative preparation to be used the day before the fast begins to lessen initial toxicity. Herbal laxatives are commonly taken orally during fasting, and many formulas are available, as capsules or for making teas. These include cascara sagrada, senna leaves, licorice root, buckthorn, rhubarb root, aloe vera, and the LB formula of Dr. Christopher. Laci LeBeau tea is also very effective. The saltwater flush, or internal bath, recommended by Stanley Burroughs to be used with the Master Cleanser, is useful for those who can tolerate it. A solution of 2 teaspoons of sea salt is dissolved in a quart of warm purified water (not distilled) and is drunk first thing in the morning on alternate days throughout the fast to flush the entire intestinal tract, an advantage of this cleansing formula. It does not, however, work well for everyone. For example, it is not recommended for salt-sensitive or water-retaining people, or for hypertensives. Whatever colon cleansing method is used, keep in mind that regular cleansing of the intestines and colon is a key component to healthy and stress-free fasting.

- *Work and be creative*—and make plans for your life. Staying busy is helpful in breaking our ties to food. We also need time for ourselves. Most fasters experience greater work energy and more creativity and, naturally, find lots to do.

- *Cleanup*—a motto during fasting. As we clean our body, we want to clean our room, desk, office, closet, and home—just like "spring cleaning." It clearly brings us into harmony with the cleansing process of nutrition. If we want to get ready for the new, we need to make space by clearing out the old.

- *Joining others* in fasting can generate strong bonds and provide an added spiritual lift. It opens up new supportive relationships and new levels of existing ones. It will also provide support if we feel down or want to quit. Most people feel better as their fast progresses—more vital, lighter, less blocked, more flexible, clearer, and more spiritually attuned. For many, it is nice to have someone with whom to share this. Call our clinic or another that offers this service.

- *Avoid the negative influence* of others who may not understand or support us. There are many fears and misconceptions about fasting, and they may affect us. We need to listen to our own inner guidance and not to others' limitations, but we also need to maintain awareness and insight into any problems should they arise. Being in contact with fasters will provide us with the positive support we need.

- ***The economy*** of fasting allows us to save time, money, and future health care costs. While we may be worried about not having enough, we may already have too much. Many of us are inspired to share more of ourselves when we are freed from food.
- ***Meditation and relaxation*** are also an important aspect of fasting to help attune us to deeper levels of ourselves and clear the stresses that we have carried with us.
- ***Spiritual practice and prayer*** will affirm our positive attitude toward ourselves and life in general. This supports our meditation and relaxation and provides us with the inner fuel to carry on our life with purpose and passion.

Conclusion

Fasting can easily become a way of life and an effective dietary practice. Over a period of time (different for each of us), through newly gained clarity, we can go from symptom cleansing to prevention fasting. Ideally, we should fast at specific times to treat symptoms and/or to enhance our vitality and spiritual practice. (See the cleansing schedule in the *General Detoxification* program.) Otherwise, we should support ourselves regularly with a balanced, wholesome diet. This diet may change somewhat through the year as we experience different needs, and occasional fasting or feasting may be valuable. We also must maintain good digestion and elimination.

Fasting is needed more frequently by those who have abused themselves with foods or other agents so readily available these days. We all need to return to the cycle of a daily fast of 12–14 hours overnight until our morning "break-fast," and then find our own natural pattern of food consumption. This usually means one main meal and two lighter ones. For low-weight, high-metabolism people, two larger or three moderately sized meals are probably needed. If we eat a heavier evening meal, we need only a light breakfast, and vice versa. Through awareness and experience, we can find our individual nutritional needs and listen to that inner nutritionist, our body.

Choosing healthful foods, chewing well, and maintaining good colon function minimize our need for fasting. However, if we do get out of balance, we can employ the oldest treatment known to us, the instinctive therapy for many illnesses, nature's doctor and knifeless surgeon, the great therapist and tool for preventing disease—**fasting!**

Immortality and Beyond

I have written this last program to be able to indulge in my idealistic philosophy of human potential and perfection. I hope and believe that many of these idealized concepts can be practically applied to our daily lives. It seems appropriate and synchronistic that I am beginning to write this program on Sunday, September 20, 1987, with these words in front of me:

I AM A SPIRITUAL BEING, AGELESS AND ETERNAL. The idea that the older one gets, the more one slows down may be a widely accepted belief, but I do not accept it. I am a spiritual being, expressing the ageless, eternal life of God. I do not look upon sickness as something that is synonymous with accrued age. I erase from my mind every thought and belief that would age or idle me either physically or mentally. (from the *Daily Word*, a spiritual publication of the Unity Church).

This section is not a discussion of death and dying per se, although that is an important topic, especially in this day of artificially prolonged life and unnatural, difficult death. The way in which I view death, which is also how it is described by those who have died and returned, is that our spirit and body separate, our body remaining on the earth and our spirit moving toward "Heaven" with complete awareness of the spiritual world from whence it came, full of timeless consciousness and life.

This discussion of immortality and optimum life obviously cannot be easily separated from religion and spirituality. This program is, in fact, about the spiritual awareness, or the "essence of things," existing in human life. It addresses many aspects of optimum lifestyle and consciousness.

What is immortality? It is usually defined as eternal life or exemption from death. In our Western culture, it seems to have more to do with fame, with one's actions in life being planted deeply in the memory of subsequent generations. Spiritual immortality arises from our ability to carry on life simply and to nourish ourselves, our family, and our world. Fame, however, may be more a matter of material immortality through monuments, books, and records. Movie and rock stars, writers, musicians, and political leaders seem to lead the lists of famous immortals. Although fame may catapult some people into mass immortality, we all are immortal insofar as our lives have touched others and are remembered through our family genealogies and our careers, as our work, children, and influences on others leave part of us with them. Our greatest sense of immortality may lie in our bonds with our children, grandchildren, and future generations. Many of these circumstances of notoriety, fame, or remembrance may last hundreds or even thousands of years; however, that does not make them truly eternal or immortal. "I dance for life, and death is something I am sure to live through," says Bethany ArgIsle, founder of The Moment Museum Corporation.

For most of us, immortality is the sense that "something," some essence of ourselves, lives on after our death. Many people believe that the spirit is eternal, that it never dies, while death of the body is inevitable; we accept death as natural, like birth. Native Americans believe in the awareness of the right time to die, which then opens the way for the new beings to populate Earth.

Many cultures also believe in the possibility of a future existence, when our spiritual being may again enter a physical form and carry on the evolution of consciousness. Some of us remember (experience "re–memories") previous lives that may influence us in our current life. Although science cannot easily prove or disprove this concept, this philosophy of reincarnation is prevalent in many religions and spiritual paths.

Our personal beliefs regarding death or eternal life may deeply affect our daily existence, attitudes, ideology, and activities. In regard to an "immortalist" philosophy, the question of whether we live forever in our physical body is not the issue here, but feeling as if we do allows us to live every day with a new attitude. We may be more relaxed, be less limited, overcome challenges more easily, feel more motivation and responsibility to our world, be more courageous and enthusiastic about learning new skills or trades (even in later years), forgive and let go of past experiences, and generally take life less seriously with a sense of being part of a greater universe.

Our ego seems attached to our physical form. Our spiritual nature or consciousness is what will live on eternally. Immortalists believe that awareness and consciousness, knowledge and wisdom, and harmonizing with the natural and universal laws, are all part of our eternal path. When we believe that life is a continuum of growth and evolution of our being, we become more responsible for our thoughts, actions, and health. We also believe in karmic patterns—that all of our actions create waves in the cosmic energy that affect the entire universe and ourselves again at some time. The "Golden Rule" is the essence here: "Do unto others as you would have them do unto you." In a sense, maybe even more appropriate for today is "do not do unto others as you would not have them do unto you."

Karma can also be seen as a balancing force in the universe. Even supposedly evil acts may be programmed through some karmic patterns. With ignorance and unconsciousness still part of the earth's energy vibration, we attract both light and dark experiences and cycles.

Being immortalist in concept and action enhances our responsibility for life—our planet, our children, our own bodies, and each other. We must serve life and do the best we can to care for our human body, supporting and allowing it to be a clean, clear temple of the living Spirit. We want to live at the peak of our potential and express our purpose. Most of us begin with health, vitality, full life potential, and a clean temple and then interfere with it by our lifestyle (and environment), which affects our thoughts and actions and subsequently our outcome and experience, or that of our children's, who must deal with our actions. When we are not in touch with or believe in a spiritual, "immortal" philosophy, we may then generate and perpetuate an acceptance of a more "deathist" philosophy where we treat our body with self-abusive habits, as if it matters very little, appearing as if we would just as soon destroy it and get out of here as fast as possible; this seems to correlate with a consciousness that also supports war or destructive relationships of any type—getting the most out of a situation rather than giving the most, or better yet, seeking balance and harmony.

Believing in death as an ominous presence and an end, as many people do, allows other feelings, such as fear, helplessness, apathy, limitation, and self-deception, to enter, as described in *Rebirthing: The Science of Enjoying All of Your Life*, by Jim Leonard and Phil Laut. We then have no choice in life and live as if it will be over sooner or later, so why try to be our best or create optimum health. The "death" that is hidden in each of our cells then affects our health, life, and consciousness. Accepting death (or illness or aging) is like accepting the concept that three meals a day is right or that consuming animal meats is necessary for health. That has been most people's experience and beliefs, yet if we do not allow other possibilities, we can never know for sure or may limit potential new experiences. Those with a deathist philosophy may actually develop an urge to die, become judgmental, and resist change. Many deathists struggle inwardly with life and its issues and challenges. Others live more through their children, whom they may see as life, than through their own capabilities, purpose, and potentials.

With this deathist philosophy, we can more easily accept destructive health- and life-destroying habits, eat dead foods, and take dangerous devitalizing drugs—because we are going to die anyway. In the Bible and other religious and spiritual writings, disease represents sin and the presence of Satan in the body. *The Essene Gospel of Peace*, as translated by Edmond Szekely, suggests that fasting can clear Satan (representing negative thinking, disease, and death) and sin from our body and shine new light on our life. After three days of fasting, Satan starves, and we start to feel more alive and positive (although we may meet our own shadow and darkness during those days). And then we can begin to live fully every day beyond fear of death or "the end." We realize that there is no end—life is eternal, consciousness is a forever-moving force of which we are its key vehicle. We are of it, and it is of us. Feeling more immortal than mortal can actually help us be even more involved with and grateful for life and enjoy it with greater abundance, grace, and success because we can look beyond the shortcomings and problems, handle stress, and be positive and motivated toward our future.

Much that I have written in this book is supportive of optimum life, vitality, and longevity. How we feed ourselves influences all of these by-products and also may provide the basis for our attitudes and activities in life. Remember, good foods, good thoughts, good actions—and in that order. And feeling good about ourself, loving ourself, will generate the desire for good foods.

Breathing provides our primary nutrition, oxygen, and is at the center of life experience, attitude, and feeling immortal, eternal, and connected to Spirit. Some breathing techniques may help us better deal with life and move away from degenerative and death activities. Rebirthing (or conscious breathing) is one such technique. It is said to help us open up to memories, both of this life and possibly of other lifetimes, to experience total recall. Some body therapies or certain therapists or healers may also help us release memory patterns stored in our body tissues. There may even be, as some advanced therapists suggest, specific acupuncture points connected to these energies.

Many teachers believe that unpleasant memories are what create disease. Past negative or painful experiences that still live inside us and generate emotions of anger, frustration, fear, isolation, and hate must be handled. Forgiveness and integration of the past is essential to living totally and healthfully in the present.

Remembering and processing these past experiences in a loving, supportive way helps us to heal aspects of our life that may have been painful and generated some "deathist" attitudes. Until we can become aware of previous experiences, we cannot really deal with them. As we release these patterns, the emotions that have been blocked can be integrated more easily and clearly. The process of moving from disease to healing requires bridging the subconscious-conscious separations through reacquiring self-knowledge. Re-memory that comes from breathing, therapy, and meditation allows us to listen and learn and helps us to gain access to our subconscious while conscious. Very deeply, we already know everything we need to know to heal and guide us through our life.

Although immortalists may do all they can to carry on life, support health, and bring about healing in and around them, paradoxically they may have little or no attachment to the physical form. So they care and they do not care—that is, they care about spiritual values more than about the body—and these values actually motivate deeper concern for the physical condition; the body is a vehicle to carry out their purpose and expression. Their beliefs may allow them to lay their life on the line and be capable of going all the way to serve their "divine mission," and this state of being usually follows a feeling of being tapped for a special purpose. Truly, we each have a special purpose, yet usually this becomes more significant when it goes beyond the self. The bigger Self is humanity and the spiritual realm, or God. St. Francis of Assisi attempted to bring unity to his followers and those around him. He wanted people to come together toward a greater vision, to stay connected, and build together—a church, a community, a spiritually bonded life. He found this difficult, as most were involved in their own "path" or reality. This message is likewise important today, in this "Aquarian Age"—where larger families might merge together for greater vision, grander feats, and greater service. Yet most of us are too busy to take the time to join with others to create new models for our future that might go beyond our "self" world.

Oftentimes, to reach this level of connection and commitment of immortalism, we must experience some ego death (even going through a near physical death experience), where our spiritual sense becomes dominant. The love emotion enters all aspects of our being and life. As our commandments begin "Love thy God with all thy heart" and "Love thy neighbor as thyself," it is clear that our spiritual guidance and others' well-being are top priorities in a devoted life. One practicing immortalist, Marilena Silbey, told me, "We create immortality every time we express love."

Yet to understand immortality, we must look at the duality of our universe. Even love has its opposite expressions, such as hate or aggression. Immortality in one sense is the opposite of death, although when we speak of the essence or oneness—the Tao or God that exists beyond duality—that itself is immortal or eternal. Immortality in a deeper sense offers us greater spiritual power, vitality, and wisdom, and the subsequent longevity enters as we support love, attract light, and approach and affirm unity within us and outside us. Death itself is a duality; it may represent an end, yet it may be a doorway to our future and other dimensions.

In the truest sense, even peace and war are dualities. On a personal level, most of us prefer peace and light and love, the positive aspects of life. Yet, in a universal dimension, the dark or negative side may dominate at times, expressing itself as violence and war, and even natural disasters. Darkness and light need each other to exist; this is the nature of duality.

The simple symbol of the Tai Chi, or universal unity, represented by the yin-yang circle, reveals a spot of light in the darkness and a spot of darkness in the light. Nothing exists exclusively as light or dark on the earth plane. At the extremes, they become their opposite. This dual nature of the world also is relevant in our individual search or struggle for healing and optimum health. Oftentimes, in seeking more light, we struggle with our shadow or dark side, which wants to exist also. Even the healthiest people have symptoms, illnesses, or personal struggles they must handle. Balance here is the key; integrating both sides is essential.

Our spiritual essence, however, can take us beyond this duality to discover the power and rhythm of the universe. Many people find this solace in meditation, religion, or chanting of spiritual words or songs. Part of our human challenge is to ascend beyond or above this earthly duality and associate with the spiritual level, and being a "carrier of the light" allows us to illuminate our individual and collective paths. As we go beyond our awareness of light and dark and the dealings with our personal doubts, fears and life struggles (the specific interactions of light and dark), as well as our ego and desires, we may then reach that point of nothingness and eternity together (a touch or feeling of the immortal essence). Yet, even as we might experience this advanced state for a moment, we must still live in and care for our body and life, integrating our divinity with our humanity.

Historically, the science of alchemy understood this interplay of duality and our earthly challenge to rise above a mundane existence. This polarity was represented by the light and dark, masculine and feminine, yang and yin, and sun and moon. The path toward unity takes us from the struggles and stresses we experienced toward greater peace and harmony in our lives. This unity, termed the "mystical marriage" of the inner male and female aspects, brought in the spiritual nature of life, great wisdom, power, and health. The "gold" or most brilliant prize was attained through the continued balance or our duality and the unification of our levels of body, mind, heart, and spirit.

In this day and age, politics deals with the basic issues of duality. To go beyond politics, we must deal with the basic nature of ego orientation, competition, and preconceived values. At some level, religion and politics represent duality, as the church and government have historically. On another dimension, religious or spiritual disciplines are what may help us rise above, in concept at least, this basic struggle we encounter in life. Experiencing love for God, self, parents, neighbors, nation, and world is the beginning of a new dimension of spiritual responsibility and immortalism. Doing what we need to do physically, psychologically, and emotionally to attain this level of love in life is essential to reaching our spiritual truths.

At times, our inner journey may help awaken unconsciousness and align us with our true eternal relationships. In a sense, ignorance is the darkness, disease, and demise of life. Ignorance here means unconsciousness, not the lack of school learning.

In the beautiful book of wisdom by Manly P. Hall, entitled *The Medicine of the Sun and Moon*, one paragraph states,

> Thus, to the Chinese, health is the natural or normal state of all living things. To become sick, (wo)man must destroy his (her) own health, and this can be done either objectively or collectively. Sickness is a symptom, a symbol of ignorance, neglect, or the disturbance of natural processes by intemperance. To the Chinese mind, therefore, moderation of action is considered the best defense against sickness. The individual who is uncertain should adjust his own life to natural patterns and try not to disturb universal processes. His concept of health should not be a victory over sickness, but rather a victory over his own shortcomings. The person who follows nature in all things is a healthy person.

Knowledge is essentially wisdom and knowing of truth from the spiritual-universal realm. As I said, listening within is a way to gain access to this "knowledge." Being attentive to nature's ways and to interactions with people can provide us with many insights into "natural law." There are also many things we can do to elevate our vibrations or consciousness and to live in an immortalist way. Let us now look at applying these aspects of lifestyle to enhance our daily existence.

Here's what we can do to feel greater power, spirituality, connectedness to heaven and earth, and health and vitality. This is the *Immortality* program, so to speak. To begin with, a harmony between our mind and heart that allows us to know and do what we believe and feel within will support our physical and psychological health. We must maintain balance and not lose our composure or become angry or upset over stresses. This is not necessarily easy in this day and age, but if we know how to center ourselves, it is possible much of the time.

If we can view immortality as optimizing each moment of life and maximizing our life span, we must portray an idealistic lifestyle with an avoidance of stress and strain (but not avoiding hard work) and a pursuit of natural living, being in "harmony with the universe." In a way, this involves a separation from much of modern technology, pollution, and city living, going back to more pioneering days yet with the health knowledge that we have acquired over the past century.

Although we probably cannot find any pollution-free environment, there are many relatively clean places still left on our planet where we can be nourished with good light, air, and water to vitalize our being. Our "utopian" environment will provide a home of natural elements, avoiding synthetic materials such as chemicals, plastics, and so on. Energy is generated by solar power, water power, or windmills, whichever would be most appropriate for our area. Electricity is available, yet our lifestyle is not focused around it, and there are no big power lines, which are now known to have negative effects on life. For example, minimum electricity and/or natural gas is needed for some refrigeration, lighting, cooking, or listening to music, while more affluent functions, such as television, microwaves, or other high-tech services, are avoided. This also reduces local radioactivity.

Our connection to the earth is essential. We work and nourish the earth and plant food, and the earth nourishes us with her bounty. Much of our food comes from our work or local farming. Besides working the earth and getting fresh air and exercise much of the day, we walk in nature often. We avoid driving in cars, especially on freeways and in traffic.

We are not totally isolated, though, and may live in supportive communities where commodities can be shared and where help is available in time of need. Human relationships and sharing feelings, love, and family seem necessary for most human beings. We are mainly a tribal species; living in isolation or having a feeling of isolation is correlated with more disease and more rapid demise.

We need to maintain a positive attitude toward life with a wonderful self-image. Avoiding worry and other supporting low-stress plans are helpful. The natural stresses arising from feeding ourselves, protecting our families, and dealing with nature's changes and turmoils are sufficient survival stresses for inner motivation and bodily function.

Embracing life and living it fully, letting our troubles wash clean with laughter and tears, hard work, and an inner attitude of faith, purpose, and immortality, exist in our essential core. Handling changes, making progress, and accepting and making transitions through our life stages are important.

Immortal ArgIsle-izm

Through birth is all life attained
through the breath of love—
that which is eternal is sustained.

Many people may struggle with aging and act as they were and not as they are. Immortality does not necessarily mean that our physical body does not age, though with healthy living, we can minimize that. It is our essential nature and spirit that are immortal. This guides our body, and immortality is enhanced as we follow our inner core (Soul) path and do what we are here to do.

Acknowledging changes at different ages is one of our many challenges. It is essential to accept and enhance change in age, function, forces, and vitality with the grace, joy, and dance of life, and really as blessings and guides in our life rather than the discords of our destruction.

"Flexibility is the key to immortality in body and mind," says the highly quoted, inspired Bethany ArgIsle. This flexibility in regard to changes of weather, relationships to others, and our own internal attitudes or beliefs is important to our continued positive evolution and to minimizing the stress incurred in daily life. Many of us may struggle with the common minor everyday experiences; this is not necessary or helpful, and it can be avoided with an open mind, faith in life, and a feeling of spiritual guidance surrounding our existence.

Often, we may be held back by the limits or viewpoints of our own mind or those of our family, friends, or chance opinions. This may be a great challenge or struggle to see clearly in these situations and progress beyond them. We often manifest these conflicts as a reflection of our own inner questioning. As in nature where there are stresses at the transition or shift points between seasons, so there are for us at our life changes. The evolutionary process of life is one of the threads that ties us all together.

Many people may measure themselves in comparison to the accomplishments or values of others or of the world at large. Essential to life is acknowledging our own unique true nature. Learning who we are and expressing this identity to others, feeling good about ourselves, is the process of growing. The challenges that are presented to us help us to fine tune our perceptions, beliefs, and identity. Yet those truths that are at our essential core will remain and shine forth as all the illusions about life are dissolved. From this core wisdom, a true knowledge may arise and be a strong guide in our life.

Acknowledging our true nature is helpful in creating our diet. From an immortalist viewpoint, "life and death is really not a moral issue," and this is true in regard to food. Carrots and apples have measurable life force, although different from a cow or chicken. We are really dealing with a vibrational matter and the effects of and needs for certain foods. At different times, we may want and need to eat animal foods; at other instances, we may be vegetarians. (Clearly though, being vegetarian is more ecological in terms of precious resources and worldwide nutrition.) Some people are more inclined to one diet for various reasons and stay with that for many years. However, as I have discussed throughout this text, there are many diets, and we may change regularly in terms of the foods we eat, as our seasonal diet and availability of foods are a basic component of what we will eat in our natural lifestyle.

In terms of our diet, why not the Ideal Diet for optimum health and vitality? Let me reemphasize its basic nutritional components that will apply to our immortality and longevity. First, we must eat simply and not excessively, avoiding too many foods at one meal. For optimum vitality, we would eat a high amount of raw foods and, possibly, an almost exclusively raw diet at certain periods and at warmer times of the years. If we want to support life, we eat more live or close-to-living foods. If we eat more overcooked or dead, low-vibration foods, we will potentiate our death sooner. At colder times, however, more heated foods and richer foods, even some of the animal proteins, may be desired and useful, much like a log in the "fireplace" to warm our home, our body. So the immortalist diet is seasonally based. No refined foods are used. It is primarily a vegetarian diet, with lots of complex carbohydrates and vegetables. Grains are used whole or fresh ground for the baking of breads, biscuits, or other goods.

As we garden outside, the kitchen becomes our indoor garden to nourish us within. Sprouting seeds and legumes will provide optimum foods—high-vibrational, vital, and high-quality foods from a nutritional standpoint. Sprouts are also helpful to the gastrointestinal tract in that they provide fiber, chlorophyll, and many vitamins, minerals, and proteins. Foods that may be sprouted include hard wheat, alfalfa seeds, sunflower seeds, radish seeds, chia seeds, buckwheat, mung beans, lentils, garbanzos, and aduki beans.

In the areas of the world where people commonly live to an age of over 100 years, the environment is much cleaner. People work the land and have clean air, water, and food. They exercise as they work and live, have less stress and take care of the elders who need a positive self-image and purpose (to feel connected and needed, not isolated) to want to continue living. The diet of these "peoples of longevity" tends to be lower in calories, fats, and protein than that of the Western world. They eat unprocessed fresh foods or, in the colder seasons, well-stored foods. And their activity levels are more connected to the natural daily and seasonal cycles. When we live attuned to Nature, we perpetuate and manifest in ourselves Her strength, vitality, endurance, and reverence for life.

Our diet should also support our spiritual practice. The first level of the golden rule applies to Mother Earth. If we nurture her soil and create beauty with growing foods, she will nourish us and our family. Light eating is important for our times of spiritual seeking. Periodic fasting, especially in the midst of good nutrition, also supports the spiritual connection and reverence for all life.

In our *Immortality* program, we are not supported by extra vitamin pills unless they can be helpful for specific medical conditions. We have cleared out many of the stresses and abuses for which we needed these extra insurance pills and are now supported by nutritionally vital foods and healthy digestion. We need to eat a variety of foods that will supply us with our specific nutrients. Instead of supplements, we can use more concentrated, high-nutrient foods, such as vegetable juices, nutritional yeast, bee pollen, ground nuts and seeds, various herbs, and sprouts. These can support us to stay healthy, so that we will not require more concentrated supplements or medicines.

Our day-to-day life is our basic exercise level. This immortalist-longevity plan does not find us working the world of business with the hustle and bustle of meetings and constant time pressure stress, but in the world of smaller communities and nature. Our gardening, building, and caretaking will help us in our physical conditioning. Other exercises and even aerobic activities will keep us even more fit. Dancing, hill walking, bicycling, cross-country skiing, and swimming are all good. Some community sports, such as soccer and volleyball, may inspire others. Exercise, however, should not be extreme or overdone, and heavy competition and intense contact sports are not necessary. If we can do these activities purely in the spirit of developing our personal performance or coordinating team or group functions rather than for winning, they may fit in with our immortalist-spiritual values—less competition, more cooperation.

A key to immortal vitality is the subtle Eastern exercises that promote flexibility and mind-body integration. These include yoga and tai chi. They unite stretching, coordination, balance, strength, mental discipline, and harmonious breathing. They can also be more replenishing and stimulating to the energy than many other activities, yet they are helpful in general stress reduction and tend to relax and loosen our muscles rather than tighten them. Both yoga and tai chi also help open up the internal energy circulation in our body, which is essential to good health.

Other aspects of lifestyle philosophy focus on inner attunement and evolution of our being. Learning to listen to our body and nature is essential here. Adapting to the changes around us and within us, with awareness of our inner life needs and food needs, is important. Our personal cycles fit within nature's, and although we eat a healthy, vital diet, we do have special fast times to uplift us and feast times to help us to slow down, nourish us, and rest more deeply. Our basic sleep cycle should be attuned to nature. We go early to bed so that we can arise with the light of day or just before to meditate and open to the light and spirit coming into our daily life. Writing and being creative, which are so important to life also, come out of this inner silence and depth.

Of course, the "antsy" personality may go through levels of resistance and readjustment in order to achieve this grace of quiet knowingness. In truth, the ego and will of the human being must submit to the powers of nature and the universe for the benefit of all. We learn from these larger forces. Our meditation or "receptive quietude" is the greatest power we have in attuning to the wisdom of the universe.

If we wish to understand our relationship to people or events around us or if we have questions about other areas of our life, "we need no books to teach us the answers, because if we are quiet, in our hearts we will know," as Manly Hall states in *The Medicine of the Sun and the Moon*. He continues,

> Only when we disobey the quiet reaction of our own inner lives do we get into trouble. If we merely follow the gratification of our emotions, we may be wrong; if we follow the inclinations of our intellects, we may be in error. But if we are very quiet in the presence of need, a light in us suddenly moves us to the solution of this need.

Some basic concepts for the natural laws of our life and body are described by Thurman Fleet in *Rays of the Dawn*; the following four laws are my adaptations.

The first law is proper nourishment, including eating a living-food diet, more alkaline than acid. Fleet categorizes our foods as cleansers, builders, and congestors. We want mostly the cleansing fruits and vegetables, some building proteins, and very few congestors—that is, refined or sweetened foods, excess starches, or too much of the building foods, such as cheese, meats, or even nuts, seeds, and beans. A vital, more raw-food diet is our suggestion.

The second law is proper movement. Exercise is the distribution process of our nourishment. It aids the assimilation, utilization, and elimination of foods. Moving every joint every day will maintain flexibility and function. We also want to be active enough to keep toned muscles and a toned heart.

The third law is proper rest and recuperation to balance out our activity. This includes sleep, rest, relaxation, and recreation, particularly important to help us de-stress. Having playful, enjoyable hobbies and laughing a lot are important to feeling good about ourselves and life; conversely, if we feel this way, it is easier to laugh and play.

The fourth law is proper cleanliness. This is both outer and inner. Cleaning our skin through regular bathing is important. Sweating helps cleanse our blood of impurities. And a wholesome, high-fiber diet will allow our bowels to keep our elimination current. Order and cleanliness in our surroundings both prevent disease and support creativity. Being clean and organized allows us to be current in our life and awareness.

We must view our actions in regard to both their immediate and their long-term effects. This is part of the immortalist philosophy. I believe that contrary or pollution of our beautiful planet. Economy has taken precedence over nature's dance. We may think only of what we can get to fulfill our immediate needs without being concerned about the polluting effects on the environment. We accept that what we need now is most important and, since we are not going to be here, let those who come later deal with the consequences of our actions and how they affect future generations. With the number of toxic chemicals and radiation in use today, one little mistake can be the only one we are ever allowed.

Many companies are oriented to acquiring profits by producing products such as chemicals and plastics and releasing their wastes, many of them toxic, into the environment—the local air, rivers, or lakes—or storing them underground, where they can leak and pollute soil and groundwater. Many of the products that are being made these days that use toxic materials in their creation are not really needed or are toxic themselves. Even though all of these new plastics in particular have become the mainstay of the technological age, we wonder whether this is indeed evolution. Many new and old products could be manufactured more efficiently and with less pollution with greater forethought and concern for continued environmental balance.

In a thousand years, people will look back on this last century as one of the most disastrous, from an immortalist viewpoint, in its long-range effects on the planet. Although some technological progress has been made, more conscious people are beginning to realize that the cost to the Earth and its inhabitants is greater than the short-term profits generated by the productivity, or the extra convenience of the products themselves. Unless we now use our technological skills to clean up our planet, we may be in even bigger trouble in the near future.

Pollution has affected the ozone layer in our stratosphere and the level of radiation in the air. This might give a new image of immortality from the deathist viewpoint—such as surviving while wearing special suits and eyeglasses to protect us from the sun and wearing masks to filter the air. Or, worse yet, we may need to live in underground cities. In a civilization where economy and greed take precedence over the dance of peaceful, evolutionary existence, death takes over. But we will not accept this. I believe solutions to these pollution problems are yet to be revealed; however, healing must begin in our time! (See Chapters 1 and 11 for discussions on cleaning our waters and life.) We want to care for our planet. We want to live with the sunshine, breathing clean air, having good water to drink, and being able to walk in nature, to talk to the trees and animals. **So let's wake up now!** Our health has to do with building the future and keeping the planet healthy. We want to keep alive and extend life by better health practices, medicine, and technology. We need to focus more on our appreciation of life, nature, and those other beings around us.

Releasing the past is essential to healthy living. Sickness lives in our memories, especially the painful or negatively charged ones we carry around. We need to live now in preparation for our future, creating with enthusiasm, vitality, and purpose. Utilizing and vitalizing our mind (especially our untapped areas) through meditation and all the aspects of a healthy lifestyle that I have mentioned here are ways to keep our hands on the pulse of life around us and to understand the universal laws. This helps us to become more conscious in our thoughts and words, allowing us to be more creative with our lives. Sensitivity and heartfelt experience give understanding and guide us to correct the aspects of civilization and humanity that may need renewal.

"We suffer to learn until we learn that we do not have to suffer to learn. Then we can recognize that we are choosing the intensity of our experiences. Remaining conscious through inner listening is the tool to learning without suffering. Loving and forgiving ourselves and others is the key to inner peace."

—Marilena Silbey

Macromedicine deals with the care of humanity; micromedicine deals with the care of the individual. We all need to incorporate both aspects of this knowledge into healing and our health care system. Caring for ourselves individually and as families can easily extend to populations and the earth itself. For long-term health, it is important to learn to care for our body in relationship to the world from a very early age. Much of the basic information in this book and much of my future life are dedicated to teaching young people. A collective work with my associate Bethany ArgIsle, to be entitled *The Earth Children's Universal Health Guide*, is currently in progress.

It is also essential to correct problems early and not let long-term negligence lead to chronic disease or emergencies. Most emergencies are a result of neglecting little issues and details of health or trying to remain unconscious and resist inner guidance and awareness. *In The Medicine of the Sun and Moon*, Manly P. Hall states:

> Health rests upon the simple concept that there is a universal harmony which can be found everywhere and in everything. Man, by his indiscretions, deprives himself of the natural benefits which heaven bestows. The individual who breaks the rules does not destroy rhythms of infinite life but inhibits the supply of vitality moving through his own body, thereby depriving himself of his proper share of this universal energy.

Learning preventive measures early is important, and treating current mild diseases effectively probably affects the likelihood of chronic illness and longevity. Stress both arises from and influences our physical health. When our physical health is poor, greater psychological and emotional stresses may occur as well. It is important to handle these early to avoid the vicious cycle of poor health, stress, lack of vitality, stress, poor health.

In terms of basic health care, nutritional and botanical medicine are the core healers and preventive measures. Homeopathy practice is a fascinating science with many supporters, and it seems to be a very useful natural therapeutic approach. Herbs and diet can help rebalance us and heal specific problems, especially when handled early. Foods and herbs are also aligned with seasonal medicine. The changes in weather affect the availability of certain foods and plants, and naturally they correlate with our cyclical needs. The spring cleansers and tonics are the many greens and roots. The summer rejuvenators are the fruits, vegetables, and flowers. In the autumn and winter, more roots and building foods are available, which provide more heat to feed our furnace and protect us from the changing climate. It all fits together perfectly as we let it.

Healing has to do with integrating the body, mind, and spirit and releasing the energy flows in the body. Pain is held in place by resistance generated by anger, frustration, or fear of the worst, be it disease or death. Increasing tensions lead to increasing tissue disease, which is then harder to heal. Problems can even go beyond healing potential, especially when surgery is done and organs are removed.

Pain and limitation lead to much disease. We need to handle this early. Acupuncture, both by needle and electrical stimulation, can help move energy/pain and reestablish homeostasis. Many body therapies can be an important mode of treatment, close in importance to foods and botanicals. Laying on of hands with love and openness can allow these body resistances and pains to be released. Massage, acupressure, chiropractic therapy, and many other modalities can all provide "natural" healing. Allowing the energy channels to open again will allow our life force to flow freely and create health and vitality. We need to have people around us who understand and are supportive of this process—that of living life!

1019

In our ideal life we want to associate ourselves with a philosopher-physician who can connect with the entire family and provide preventive and therapeutic care, knowledge of natural medicine, and guidance in harmonious living. If sickness requires stronger medicines or surgery, the doctor could provide these or recommend specialists in those fields. Knowing the limits of our own knowledge is essential to effective treatment, as is getting our ego out of the way and letting our intuition guide us in the best approach for healing. Doctors should know that they are servants of nature and God. We are here to support healing and create health, and ultimately we all must begin with ourselves.

We do this by turning to our spiritual essence and developing our communion with our inner guidance and God. An appreciation of the Heavenly Father, or Spirit, and the Heavenly Mother, or Earth, is inherent in this reverence for life. When we live within the natural laws of the universe, we approach immortality, and our spirit is enhanced. In an article called "Healing Ourselves and Healing Our Planet," Robert Muller suggests that our spiritual development allows us to be in greater harmony with

the planet,

the heavens,

the time cycles,

others and our family,

and our self.

Spiritual development arises from listening within and allows us to gain wisdom and elevate our consciousness. As immortalists, we believe that anything is possible. With Jesus' 40-day fast, he was allowed access to all planes of travel—horizontally through people, vertically between God and earth, inwardly through his depths, and interdimensionally through time and truth. Christ continues to be present as he lives on immortally in the hearts and minds of many of his followers, as do other saintly beings who have ascended from the bonds of Earth, such as Buddha, Lao-tse, Gandhi, and those who have become immortal in our hearts.

We, too, can live with this sense of immortality with our individual spiritual development. Understanding nature and the universe, we know that order and discipline are important to this spiritual path. Yet, with the pursuit and unfoldment of our individual path within the harmony of the universe, we can create both a healthy body and life and a healthy, vital, and eternal world. Healing our planet begins with each of us and our commitment to being the best and healthiest that we can be. Peace be in you.

Staying Healthy With Nutrition
Questionnaire

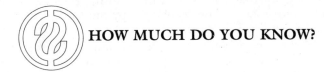 **HOW MUCH DO YOU KNOW?**

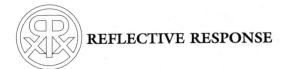 **REFLECTIVE RESPONSE**

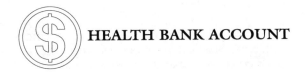 **HEALTH BANK ACCOUNT**

Conceived by Bethany ArgIsle. Compiled by Bethany ArgIsle, Sondra Barrett, Neil Murray, and Elson Haas

Dedicated to the inquisitive mind, compassionate heart, and passionate spirit that continue to make personal and planetary breakthroughs in health and peace.

Questionnaire

INSTRUCTIONS

There are three parts to this questionnaire. We have organized them so that they are easy for you to use and reuse. We suggest that you avoid writing in the book, and we have deliberately set margins to make it easier for you to photocopy the worksheets for *How Much Do You Know?* and the *Health Bank Account.*

We hope that you will answer this review before and after reading this book so that you can assess your new knowledge and see the changes as you adjust and align with any new lifestyle choices. You may also choose to review any section at different times of the year or on your own unique cycle.

Good Luck, and remember, Health is your Choice!

PART I: *HOW MUCH DO YOU KNOW?*

True-False

A quick review of what you know and how true or false your current information may be. Copy several worksheets and see how you and others do.

Multiple Choice

This is more in-depth and includes questions about general nutrition, specific nutrients, and environmental factors and concerns. Sharpen your pencils, copy the worksheets, and have friends, family members, or coworkers take this with you and see who knows what.

THE WORKSHEETS FOR ANSWERING TRUE-FALSE AND MULTIPLE CHOICE ARE TO BE FOUND AT THE END OF THE *HOW MUCH DO YOU KNOW?* SECTION.

THE CORRECT ANSWERS ARE LOCATED AT THE END OF THE ENTIRE QUESTION-NAIRE FOLLOWING THE HEALTH BANK ACCOUNT.

PART II: *REFLECTIVE RESPONSE*

This personalized portion of the questionnaire really has no single right answers—only what is right for you and how you view your life at the time you participate. This may help you see how you have gotten to be the you you are right now. Take a blank tablet, number the lines or spaces as you go, and then answer the questions or issues. Date this, tuck it away, and then check it in the future and see how you feel differently as your conditions are transformed through knowledge and application.

PART III: *HEALTH BANK ACCOUNT*

Now that you have warmed up your ability to answer in faith and truth to yourself, here's where the dividends and dollars are made obvious. Photocopy this portion for yourself and others, and then see what they and you are worth!

Please send any comments or answers to us in care of:

Celestial Arts, P.O. Box 7123, Berkeley, CA 94707.

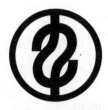

Questionnaire

Part I: How Much Do You Know?

True-False

1. Doctors and dentists must take nutritional medicine courses to become licensed.
2. Avoid all B vitamins when stressed or fatigued.
3. Vitamin A is thought to be a cancer deterrent.
4. Skin can take on an orange tint if too much beta-carotene is consumed.
5. Vitamin A is needed for night vision.
6. Sodium is concentrated inside the cells, while potassium is mainly on the outside.
7. Currently there are less than 7 million protein-deficient people in the world.
8. Water-soluble vitamins can be taken in large amounts and are relatively nontoxic.
9. Fat-soluble vitamins are stored in the body and can be toxic.
10. Calcium absorption is more efficient as we age.
11. Iron is the mineral in hemoglobin, the protein that transports oxygen throughout the body.
12. Riboflavin is needed on a daily basis as there are little or no reserves in the body.
13. Native Americans would soak their corn in ash water before or after grinding to release thiamine, which helped prevent pellegra.
14. Milk and poultry contain tryptophan.
15. The classic vitamin B_3 deficiency occurs mainly in rice-consuming cultures.
16. A niacin-deficient individual may have skin that is sensitive to light.
17. Pantothenic acid supports adrenal gland function and is called the "antistress" vitamin.
18. Without vitamin B_6, glycogen cannot be converted to sucrose.
19. Too much vitamin B_6 causes water retention, nausea, and vomiting.
20. Vegetarians and people on restricted diets need to be aware of adequate vitamin B_{12} intake.
21. Folic acid refers to "foliage" and is found in leafy green vegetables.
22. Folic acid deficiency anemia is also correctable with iron.

23. Lack of PABA production by the body's bacteria can result in gray or discolored hair.

24. Vitamin D is a water-soluble vitamin that is absorbed with fats and bile through the intestinal wall.

25. Age influences our need for vitamin D.

26. Vitamin E is found in both plant and animal foods.

27. Vitamin L (the Love vitamin) assists in the optimum use of all other vitamins.

28. Minerals are loaded with calories.

29. On its own the body manufactures enough of most minerals.

30. Due to soil depletion and loss of topsoil, our foods do not necessarily contain the minerals we need.

31. The acidity of the gastrointestinal tract influences its ability to absorb minerals.

32. There are no minerals in water unless they are artificially added.

33. Vitamin C is lost easily when cooking foods.

34. Soft water has too much sodium and is not good for those with high blood pressure or other cardiovascular concerns.

35. Most minerals are destroyed by heat.

36. Calcium functions in heart and muscle contraction.

37. The American diet readily supplies adequate calcium.

38. Diuretics stimulate magnesium loss.

39. High concentrations of sulfur are found in skin, hair, and nails.

40. Sulfur is found in fur and feathers.

41. Silicon is important in bone formation and gives strength to overall body tissues.

42. We could suck on car bumpers to get our daily dose of chromium.

43. Chromium in large dosages is potentially toxic to the body.

44. On the average, peoples of Africa have twice the levels of chromium than peoples of the United States.

45. One copper penny contains more copper than that measured in an average person's body.

46. Copper can be absorbed from cookware, utensils, and water pipes.

47. Geographic areas located near the ocean are more deficient in iodine.

48. Iron deficiency anemia is more common among women than men.

49. Vegetarians have trouble obtaining sufficient iron from the diet alone.

50. The expression "we're in the pink" refers to rosy cheeks, pink earlobes, and pink tongue, reflecting that there is adequate iron-oxygenated blood.

51. Minerals can interfere with the absorption of other minerals.

52. Taking lots of manganese can interfere with iron absorption.

53. Manganese levels in plants would be adequate even if grown in manganese-depleted soil.

54. Deficiency of essential trace minerals in the soil in a region of China influenced the incidence of esophageal carcinoma.

55. There is an association between low levels of selenium in the soil and an increased incidence of cancer.

56. Selenium is important in helping the body detoxify chemicals.

57. Low zinc levels may retard healing.

58. The amount of zinc we ingest depends on soil levels and food processing.

59. Alcohol intake, sweating, stress, and surgery all stimulate the production of zinc.

60. Zinc supports immune function by stimulating the production of T cells.

61. We eliminate nickel from the body when we sweat.

62. Newborn babies have greater levels of tin than adults because it helps them grow.

63. The trace mineral vanadium, found in petroleum, can become concentrated in the lungs.

64. Hair analysis is suggestive of body levels of aluminum.

65. Chelation therapy is used to treat heavy metal toxicity.

66. Aluminum is a common ingredient of antiperspirants.

67. Arsenic may be found in shellfish such as clams and oysters.

68. Lead is easy to detect because of its extremely bitter taste.

69. Sites at which old buildings are torn down may contain lots of lead.

70. Mercury fumes go directly into the lungs and bloodstream and can be found in breast milk.

71. The phrase "mad as a hatter" came from the manufacture of felt hats in which the lining contained mercury.

72. Mercury can be present in tattoo ink and house paints.

73. A pregnant woman or a woman contemplating pregnancy should avoid getting amalgam dental fillings.

74. The main effect of omega-3 fatty acids is to increase blood fat levels.

75. Wheat germ oil is more stable and less prone to rancidity than most other oils.

76. Taking individual amino acid supplements for prolonged periods may create other imbalances.

77. Carnitine deficiencies may occur on a vegetarian diet.

78. L-cysteine is an important vitamin antioxidant.

79. When taking antibiotics it may be dangerous to supplement with acidophilus.

80. Chlorella, spirulina and blue-green manna contain essential amino acids.

81. Fresh aloe vera juice can be used as a purgative and colon cleansing stimulant.

82. Garlic will elevate cholesterol.

83. Ginseng is safe for pregnant women.

84. Too much ginseng can cause increased blood pressure, diarrhea, insomnia, or skin eruptions.

85. Barley grass intake helps protect human cells from X-ray damage.

86. Insulin needs to be injected as it is easily destroyed through digestion.

87. Thyroid insufficiency can result from a lack of iodine or protein in the diet.

88. Groundwater contamination is currently irreversible.

89. The military is the largest polluting organization in the United States.

90. We can protect our personal water source from certain toxic substances by incorporating a home filtration system.

91. Once our drinking water supply has been tested, it is not necessary to check it again.

92. Most of the new chemicals being used now are harmless because it takes Earth and our bodies a long time to decompose them.

93. Most of the herbicides used during the early stages of plant growth are potentially carcinogenic.

94. One of the reasons we should avoid eating animal fats is that certain pesticide sprays used on animals become concentrated in their fat.

95. Bee pollen is a heart stimulant.

96. Honey is a natural antiseptic.

97. Even though lemons are acidic, they form alkaline residues in the body.

98. Even though fruit juices are low in calories, they are high in fiber.

99. Neither cherries nor apricots contain beta-carotene.

100. The U.S. government solved the earth-shaking riddle by deciding that tomatoes are a vegetable.

101. Pectin, which is found in apples, is a protein.

102. The most well-known source of laetrile is the pits of prunes.

103. Organic grapes may contain many chemicals used for their growth, shipping, and storage.

104. Olive oil contains saturated fats.

105. In Italy, when young virgins stomp on the olives, what they make is "virgin" olive oil.

106. The seeds of citrus fruits are high in bioflavonoids.

107. Citrus fruits are high in sodium.

108. A lemon juice cleanse is good for detoxifying the liver.

109. The British sailors were called "limeys" because they ate limes to prevent pellagra.

110. Melons have a diuretic quality.

111. If I live on a berry diet I won't get beriberi.

112. Peach fuzz should be saved as it is a good source of bioflavonoids in addition to being an excellent skin stimulant.

113. Papayas, mangoes, and other tropical fruits need a hot, dry climate to grow.

114. In Latin, the word for vegetable means to *enliven* or to *animate*.

115. A healthy diet contains more than 40 percent vegetables.

116. One quick way to make orange juice is to juggle the oranges.
117. Calcium is the central mineral of chlorophyll, just as iron is the center of hemoglobin.
118. Leafy greens are nutritious and high in calories.
119. Red cabbage is higher in vitamins A and C than green cabbage.
120. Leeks are a good diuretic and are very high in nutrients.
121. Root vegetables are most available in spring and summer.
122. Most root vegetables are high in protein.
123. Garlic can be used to kill some germs/microorganisms.
124. When you cut an onion your eyes tear because a sulfuric compound is released.
125. Radishes are one of the slowest growing plants in the garden.
126. Carrots are low in calories and high in the B vitamins.
127. When seeds or beans are sprouted, most of their nutrient levels increase, whereas their protein levels decrease.
128. Artichokes are actually flowers.
129. Pickles are grown on the same plant as cucumbers, but they are harvested at a different time of the year.
130. Eggplant is high in carbohydrates and low in fat.
131. Capsicum is also known as cayenne pepper and contains vitamins A and C.
132. Pumpkin seeds are high in zinc.
133. Only five varieties of mushrooms are edible.
134. Seaweeds are among the most vitamin-rich foods.
135. There are two types of edible seaweeds.
136. Animal foods have a much lower percentage of saturated fats than nuts.
137. Most nuts contain cholesterol.
138. Vegetable oils such as avocado, corn, and safflower contain linoleic acid.
139. Officially, peanuts are not nuts, they are beans.
140. Legumes are an important protein source for vegetarians.
141. Dried beans have a long shelf life if stored moist.
142. Beef cattle generate nearly 20 times the protein per acre as soybeans.
143. The kernel is the most nutrient-concentrated part of the grain.
144. Rice is the most commonly consumed grain on the planet.
145. Sprouted barley is the basis for malt syrup, which is used in beer and other foods.
146. Buckwheat is from the same plant family as wheat.
147. Popcorn is a complete protein because it contains all of the essential amino acids.
148. The main use for millet is bird seed.
149. A daily dose of oatmeal may help lower cholesterol.
150. The Chinese word for rice, "fan," is the same word for food.

151. Rye is the basis for whiskey.
152. Because of their high oil content, seeds and nuts should be kept dry or in the refrigerator to prevent rancidity.
153. Nuts are usually very low in oils and nutrients.
154. Nuts contain mostly unsaturated fats, which are better for us than saturated fats.
155. Coconut is a fruit rather than a nut.
156. Although sweet, coconut is also high in saturated fats.
157. Dairy products are required for our daily calcium intake.
158. Butter in small amounts may be safer than using spreadable margarines.
159. Dairy foods are high in natural fiber.
160. Sushi or any raw fish and/or shellfish can contain possible microbial or chemical contamination.
161. Approximately 500 mg. of the fat in two eggs is cholesterol.
162. Lean cuts of beef have very little effect on cholesterol levels.
163. The meats with the highest fat content are processed meats.
164. Meats are lowest in vitamin B_{12}.
165. Canned or bottled seasonings can be chemically treated or irradiated.
166. All the following foods may contain sugar: baby foods, catsup, chewing gum, salad dressing, bread.
167. Germs grow very well in honey.
168. The two most commonly consumed juices are orange and prune.
169. Headaches are the most frequent symptom of caffeine withdrawal.
170. Alcohol and caffeine are central nervous system stimulants.
171. A fortified food is one that was depleted during processing to which the missing vitamins and minerals are added.
172. An enriched food has vitamins and minerals added to it that were never there in the first place.
173. People who are milk sensitive have a maltose intolerance.
174. Currently foods are labeled when they have been irradiated.
175. Food irradiation improves flavor.
176. The name "Premarin" comes from the pregnant mare's urine from which that estrogen compound was originally extracted.
177. Agar is a natural food additive used to swell and gel.
178. Sodium alginate helps bind heavy metals within the intestinal tract and is derived from algae.
179. BHA and BHT are chemical antioxidants commonly used to protect foods.
180. Children can have hidden caffeine addictions from consuming chocolate bars and soft drinks.

181. Cyclamate is the most common artificial sweetener in the United States.

182. Caseinates come from soybeans.

183. Mono- and diglycerides are naturally occurring fats used as emulsifiers that are not easily metabolized in the body.

184. Lard may have preservatives such as BHT and other chemicals from the animal that are not listed on the package.

185. Many people react adversely to MSG, a common flavor enhancer in Asian cooking.

186. Meats cured with nitrate may form carcinogens in the body.

187. Sorbitol, commonly used in gum, is also the basis for Polysorbate 60 and 80.

188. Xylitol is a natural sweetener which affects blood sugar.

189. Yeast is a fungus that is grown on carbohydrates during fermentation.

190. Lacto-ovo-vegetarians avoid milk, eggs, and meat.

191. Vegans avoid fish, fowl, red meat, eggs, and milk.

192. Acetylsalicylic acid (aspirin) is made from coal tar or petroleum.

193. Silicates are salts of the earth that are used in food packaging to control moisture.

194. Baking soda can be used for cleaning toilets and teeth.

195. Many people can be sensitive to sulfite compounds used in dried fruit or wine.

196. Talc used to cover babies' bottoms can contain the dangerous contaminant asbestos.

197. Whole grains, legumes, and lots of vegetables should make up the main diet for the majority of Earth people.

198. Your diet should be more acid than alkaline.

199. Eating grapefruit makes the body more acidic.

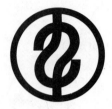

Part I: Worksheet—True-False

	True	False		True	False		True	False
1.	❑	❑	30.	❑	❑	59.	❑	❑
2.	❑	❑	31.	❑	❑	60.	❑	❑
3.	❑	❑	32.	❑	❑	61.	❑	❑
4.	❑	❑	33.	❑	❑	62.	❑	❑
5.	❑	❑	34.	❑	❑	63.	❑	❑
6.	❑	❑	35.	❑	❑	64.	❑	❑
7.	❑	❑	36.	❑	❑	65.	❑	❑
8.	❑	❑	37.	❑	❑	66.	❑	❑
9.	❑	❑	38.	❑	❑	67.	❑	❑
10.	❑	❑	39.	❑	❑	68.	❑	❑
11.	❑	❑	40.	❑	❑	69.	❑	❑
12.	❑	❑	41.	❑	❑	70.	❑	❑
13.	❑	❑	42.	❑	❑	71.	❑	❑
14.	❑	❑	43.	❑	❑	72.	❑	❑
15.	❑	❑	44.	❑	❑	73.	❑	❑
16.	❑	❑	45.	❑	❑	74.	❑	❑
17.	❑	❑	46.	❑	❑	75.	❑	❑
18.	❑	❑	47.	❑	❑	76.	❑	❑
19.	❑	❑	48.	❑	❑	77.	❑	❑
20.	❑	❑	49.	❑	❑	78.	❑	❑
21.	❑	❑	50.	❑	❑	79.	❑	❑
22.	❑	❑	51.	❑	❑	80.	❑	❑
23.	❑	❑	52.	❑	❑	81.	❑	❑
24.	❑	❑	53.	❑	❑	82.	❑	❑
25.	❑	❑	54.	❑	❑	83.	❑	❑
26.	❑	❑	55.	❑	❑	84.	❑	❑
27.	❑	❑	56.	❑	❑	85.	❑	❑
28.	❑	❑	57.	❑	❑	86.	❑	❑
29.	❑	❑	58.	❑	❑	87.	❑	❑

	True	False		True	False		True	False
88.	❏	❏	126.	❏	❏	164.	❏	❏
89.	❏	❏	127.	❏	❏	165.	❏	❏
90.	❏	❏	128.	❏	❏	166.	❏	❏
91.	❏	❏	129.	❏	❏	167.	❏	❏
92.	❏	❏	130.	❏	❏	168.	❏	❏
93.	❏	❏	131.	❏	❏	169.	❏	❏
94.	❏	❏	132.	❏	❏	170.	❏	❏
95.	❏	❏	133.	❏	❏	171.	❏	❏
96.	❏	❏	134.	❏	❏	172.	❏	❏
97.	❏	❏	135.	❏	❏	173.	❏	❏
98.	❏	❏	136.	❏	❏	174.	❏	❏
99.	❏	❏	137.	❏	❏	175.	❏	❏
100.	❏	❏	138.	❏	❏	176.	❏	❏
101.	❏	❏	139.	❏	❏	177.	❏	❏
102.	❏	❏	140.	❏	❏	178.	❏	❏
103.	❏	❏	141.	❏	❏	179.	❏	❏
104.	❏	❏	142.	❏	❏	180.	❏	❏
105.	❏	❏	143.	❏	❏	181.	❏	❏
106.	❏	❏	144.	❏	❏	182.	❏	❏
107.	❏	❏	145.	❏	❏	183.	❏	❏
108.	❏	❏	146.	❏	❏	184.	❏	❏
109.	❏	❏	147.	❏	❏	185.	❏	❏
110.	❏	❏	148.	❏	❏	186.	❏	❏
111.	❏	❏	149.	❏	❏	187.	❏	❏
112.	❏	❏	150.	❏	❏	188.	❏	❏
113.	❏	❏	151.	❏	❏	189.	❏	❏
114.	❏	❏	152.	❏	❏	190.	❏	❏
115.	❏	❏	153.	❏	❏	191.	❏	❏
116.	❏	❏	154.	❏	❏	192.	❏	❏
117.	❏	❏	155.	❏	❏	193.	❏	❏
118.	❏	❏	156.	❏	❏	194.	❏	❏
119.	❏	❏	157.	❏	❏	195.	❏	❏
120.	❏	❏	158.	❏	❏	196.	❏	❏
121.	❏	❏	159.	❏	❏	197.	❏	❏
122.	❏	❏	160.	❏	❏	198.	❏	❏
123.	❏	❏	161.	❏	❏	199.	❏	❏
124.	❏	❏	162.	❏	❏			
125.	❏	❏	163.	❏	❏			

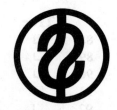

Questionnaire
Part I: How Much Do You Know?
Multiple Choice

1. Which four of the following elevate blood sugar?

a – epinephrine	d – insulin	g – eating food
b – exercise	e – glucagon	h – thyroid hormone
c – penicillin	f – calcium	i – chromium

2. Sugar match:

fructose	a – milk sugar
lactose	b – white refined sugar
sucrose	c – plant gum
mannose	d – malt sugar
maltose	e – monosaccharide

3. In which four of the following places will you find your mucous membranes?

a – eyes	c – bladder	e – GI tract	g – ears
b – sinus	d – blood vessels	f – muscles	h – armpits

4. Cholesterol has many *beneficial* uses in the body. Choose the correct answer.

a – bone metabolism	c – nerve excitement
b – precursor to sex hormones and bile acids	d – toenail growth

5. There are many differences between saturated and unsaturated fats. Match each property to one or both of these categories.

a – more stable	d – solid at room temperature
b – liquid at room temperature	e – becomes rancid more quickly
c – important in the synthesis of cholesterol	f – may be a factor in carcinogenesis

6. Trans-fatty acids are implicated in breast cancer. How are these formed? Choose one.

a – when ice cream is frozen	c – when olive oil is poured over spaghetti
b – when vegetable oils are hydrogenated	d – when butter is heated

7. Various dietary factors can increase (carcinogen) or decrease (cancer-preventive) the risk of cancer. Place each of the following in their correct column.

a – low-fat diet	d – peanut butter	g – smoked foods	j – vitamin C
b – cabbage	e – selenium	h – fried foods	k – fiber
c – nitrites	f – vitamin A	i – high-fat diet	

8. The most damaging effect of high fat intake is:

a – sagging skin   c – obesity   e – long eyelashes
b – fallen arches   d – diabetes   f – coronary artery disease

9. Match:

Chylomicron   a – made in intestines/liver to carry fats throughout the body
VLDL   b – circulates in blood, picks up unused cholesterol and takes it
                       to the liver for removal
LDL   c – made by liver to carry cholesterol to organs and cells and
                       most often is the highest component of cholesterol
HDL   d – made in the intestines to transport digested fats

10. Certain cultures have high-fat diets, but a low incidence of cardiovascular disease. Which one of the following fats/oils is the key to this?

a – polyunsaturated vegetable oils   c – corn oil
b – fish oils containing EPA   d – saturated animal fats

11. Which are three essential fatty acids we require for body function?

a – linoleic acid   c – stearic acid   e – linolenic acid
b – palmitic acid   d – oleic acid   f – arachidonic acid

12. Choose four special properties of olive oil.

a – mainly monosaturated fats   e – contains cholesterol
b – intestinal lubricant   f – liquid at room temperature
c – solid in the refrigerator   g – unstable during cooking
d – becomes rancid quickly

13. Vitamins are either fat soluble or water soluble. Which is which?

a – vitamin C   c – vitamin D   e – vitamin E
b – vitamin K   d – vitamin B_1 f – biotin

14. The first vitamins were officially discovered in 1912. Where were they first found?

a – in a milk mustache   c – in rice polishings
b – in bean dip   d – in a compost heap

15. Regular smoking may lead to dangerous free-radical formation. Antioxidants reduce free-radical formation. Choose the four antioxidant nutrients.

a – vitamin M   d – vitamin A/beta-carotene   g – manganese
b – vitamin D   e – vitamin E   h – magnesium
c – selenium   f – calcium   i – vitamin C

16. Choose five of the following foods that are good sources of vitamin A and/or beta-carotene.

a – carrots   d – broccoli   g – apricots
b – ice cream   e – toast   h – yams
c – cherries   f – tofu   i – sesame seeds

17. The richest, most concentrated source of most of the B vitamins is:

a – lamb   b – eggs   c – pizza   d – brewer's yeast

18. Choose the three factors that increase our need for vitamin C most significantly.
    a – smoking   c – run   e – have sex   g – are acutely stressed
    b – undergo surgery   d – drink alcohol   f – sunbathe   h – use a computer

19. Vitamin D performs which one of the following functions?
    a – regulates calcium metabolism and influences phosphorus utilization
    b – helps absorb the sun's rays and contributes to getting a suntan
    c – gives us athletic stamina by increasing breathing capacity
    d – increases the quantity of milk when a woman is lactating

20. Which vitamin contains the mineral cobalt?
    a – PABA   b – biotin   c – vitamin B_{12}

21. The best source of vitamin E is:
    a – pineapple juice   c – steak tartar   e – massage oil
    b – vegetable and seed oils   d – ginseng   f – cabbage

22. Vitamin B_{12} is found in which of these foods? Choose four.
    a – red meat   c – spinach   e – olive oil   g – yogurt
    b – liver   d – eggs   f – almonds   h – popcorn

23. Biotin is important in which one of the following functions?
    a – foot size at birth
    b – antiaging wrinkle cream
    c – metabolism of fat, protein, and carbohydrates
    d – whether or not we have moons on our fingernails

24. Eating too many raw eggs could contribute to a deficiency of which vitamin?
    a – vitamin A   b – folic acid   c – biotin   d – vitamin B_{12}

25. Two of the better PABA-containing foods are:
    a – Popsicles   c – tortillas   e – yeast   g – half-and-half
    b – molasses   d – mint julep   f – rice cakes   h – eggs

26. Which of the following is associated with a lack of vitamin C?
    a – shingles   b – scurvy   c – baldness   d – colic

27. Vitamin K is found in which of the following? Choose three.
    a – animal products   d – kelp
    b – fish liver oils   e – peanuts
    c – blackstrap molasses   f – alfalfa

28. Select the two richest sources of bioflavonoids (vitamin P).
    a – nuts and seeds   c – avocado pits   e – corn
    b – peach pits   d – white substance of citrus fruits   f – sprouts

29. The main function of bioflavonoids is:
    a – to regulate permeability by increasing the strength of the capillaries
    b – to increase muscle tone
    c – to increase long-term memory
    d – to help eliminate extra vitamin C

30. Which three of the following are essential trace minerals?

a – cobalt   c – sodium   e – calcium   g – arsenic   i – plutonium
b – iron   d – cadmium   f – lead   h – potassium   j – zinc

31. Choose the five macrominerals from the following list.

a – selenium   d – manganese   g – molybdenum   j – zinc
b – calcium   e – iron   h – sodium   k – lead
c – phosphorus   f – cadmium   i – magnesium   l – sulfur

32. The most abundant mineral in the human body is:

a – iron   c – lead   e – calcium
b – zinc   d – sodium   f – phosphorus

33. Which one of the nutrient groups below functions in all of the following roles: Nerve transmission, muscle contraction and acid-base balance?

a – vitamins   b – minerals   c – fats

34. Choose four factors that help in calcium absorption.

a – acid   c – grains   e – vitamin C   g – vitamin D   i – yogurt
b – iron   d – copper   f – beer   h – exercise   j – crying

35. For best calcium absorption which key vitamin is required?

a – vitamin C   b – vitamin D   c – vitamin E   d – vitamin B_6

36. Choose three factors that hinder calcium absorption.

a – acid   c – grains   e – vitamin C   g – vitamin D
b – cobalt   d – beer   f – yoga   h – iron

37. Foods high in oxalic acid can interfere with calcium absorption and contribute to kidney stones. Select five foods that are high in oxalic acid.

a – spinach   c – rhubarb   e – chard   g – chocolate
b – beet greens   d – tea   f – lemons   h – ox tails

38. The hardest substance in the body is:

a – bones   b – fingernails   c – hair   d – tooth enamel

39. The best time to take calcium is:

a – before meals   b – between meals   c – after meals   d – at bedtime

40. Magnesium is thought to be important in the prevention or treatment of which conditions? Choose four.

a – myocardial infarctions   c – kidney stones   e – PMS   g – muscle spasm
b – heartburn   d – pink eye   f – earaches

41. Choose the four best dietary sources of copper from the list.

a – whole wheat   d – chicken   g – liver   j – legumes
b – rutabagas   e – dried peas   h – oranges   k – nuts
c – oysters   f – lettuce   i – corn oil   l – safflower oil

42. What percentage of red blood cells is being recycled every day?

a – 1%   b – 10%   c – 25%

43. During times of blood loss, more iron is needed. If we donate a pint of blood, the 200 mg. of iron that it ideally contains will take how long to replenish?

    a – 24 hours   b – 7 days   c – 2–3 weeks   d – 3 months

44. Which three of the following foods are high in phosphorus?

    a – corn chips   c – animal meats   e – tap water   g – nuts
    b – eggs   d – bananas   f – alfalfa sprouts

45. Which is the most abundant mineral in the earth's crust?

    a – calcium   c – silicon   e – magnesium
    b – germanium   d – phosphorus

46. The best source of manganese is:

    a – skim milk   b – nuts   c – orange peel   d – potatoes

47. Molybdenum, important to the functioning of several enzymes, is found in which of the following foods? Choose four.

    a – oats   c – buckwheat   e – prunes   g – legumes
    b – yeast   d – lemons   f – liver   h – dark leafy greens

48. The nutrient most useful for selenium utilization is:

    a – vitamin E   b – vitamin C   c – magnesium   d – beta-carotene

49. Refining grain removes much of its zinc, found mainly in which part?

    a – the covering   b – the germ   c – the endosperm

50. Choose two of the following foods that are good dietary sources of zinc.

    a – garlic   c – pumpkin seeds   e – mustards   g – parsley
    b – egg yolk   d – pink foods   f – oranges   h – grape juice

51. Zinc helps maintain the levels of which vitamin?

    a – vitamin A   b – vitamin C   c – vitamin E

52. The lightest mineral used in medical treatment (psychological disorders) is:

    a – potassium   b – hydrogen   c – lithium   d – sodium

53. Which of the following is NOT a possible toxic effect of aluminum?

    a – muscle twitching   c – reduced absorption of selenium and phosphorus
    b – putrid sweat   d – Alzheimer's disease memory loss

54. It is believed that one mineral contaminated drinking and storage vessels and contributed to the downfall of the Roman Empire. Which one?

    a – arsenic   b – lead   c – tin   d – zinc

55. Which two of the following contain complete proteins, i.e., relatively equal amounts of all the essential amino acids?

    a – seaweed   c – nuts   e – milk
    b – eggplant   d – brown rice   f – turkey

56. In a vegetarian diet what are the most commonly deficient amino acids? Choose two.

    a – glycine   c – lysine   e – valine
    b – methionine   d – tyrosine   f – tryptophan

57. Match correctly:

Hormones   a – Have a dynamic effect on metabolism. Insulin is an example.

Antibodies   b – These protein catalysts stimulate biochemical reactions.

Enzymes   c – Formed in response to stimulus of something foreign,
usually a protein that enters the body.

58. The essential amino acid phenylalanine is the source for which hormone?

    a – thyroxine   b – epinephrine   c – insulin

59. Which essential amino acid has been used to promote sleep and treat premenstrual syndrome?

    a – threonine   b – tryptophan   c – methionine

60. Which three of these bacteria inhabiting the human colon are friendly/beneficial?

    a – Lactobacillus acidophilus   d – Lactobacillus bifidus

    b – Streptococcus faecium   e – Salmonella organisms

    c – Klebsiella pneumoniae   f – Pseudomonas aeroginosa

61. The inside of the aloe vera leaf is used for:

    a – burn relief   b – pain relief   c – an aphrodisiac   d – liver tonic

62. The bee provides us with many important products. Match the nutrient with its function or source.

Royal jelly   a – contains a natural antibiotic

Propolis   b – made in the salivary glands of worker bees

Bee pollen   c – collected off the legs of worker bees

63. Which two fruits contain helpful digestive enzymes?

    a – apple   b – pineapple   c – papaya   d – lemons

64. Dried fruit match:

Dates   a – George Burns eats these every day

Prunes   b – high in beta-carotene

Raisins   c – source of commercially made sugar

Apricots   d – rich source of iron made from grapes

65. Choose the four cruciferous vegetables from the list below.

    a – potatoes   d – cauliflower   g – red pepper   j – cabbage

    b – broccoli   e – carrots   h – rutabagas   k – eggplant

    c – bean sprouts   f – brussels sprouts   i – wheat berries

66. Spinach is high in two of the following minerals, which may be lacking in a vegetarian diet.

    a – calcium   b – magnesium   c – zinc   d – iron

67. Which four of the following are from the nightshade family of plants?

    a – cherry   c – tomato   e – pomegranate   g – potatoes

    b – artichoke   d – tobacco   f – raspberries   h – eggplant

68. Most seaweeds contain good levels of which three of the following?

    a – chromium   c – sodium   e – magnesium   g – pantothenic acid

    b – calcium   d – iodine   f – potassium   h – arachidonic acid

69. Which two of the following foods can be sprouted easily?

    a – clover seeds   b – spinach leaves   c – radish seeds   d – macadamia nuts

70. Which are the three top wheat-producing countries in the world?

    a – Ireland   c – Russia   e – Japan   g – United States
    b – Denmark   d – China   f – Mexico   h – Holland

71. Which four of the following grains contain gluten, an allergenic protein?

    a – millet   c – wheat   e – rice   g – oats   i – rye
    b – barley   d – lentils   f – corn   h – amaranth   j – polenta

72. Choose three nutrients that are commonly used to enrich foods.

    a – magnesium   c – vitamin B_{12} e – thiamine   g – selenium   i – folic acid
    b – riboflavin   d – pyridoxine   f – iron   h – vitamin C

73. Wheat is used to make which three of the following?

    a – couscous   c – pasta   e – bread   g – polenta
    b – beer   d – candles   f – tapioca   h – ice cream

74. Seeds are high in which four of the following nutrients?

    a – phosphorus   c – calcium   e – sodium   g – potassium
    b – vitamin E   d – vitamin D   f – vitamin A   h – vitamin C

75. Which nut is the highest in potassium and hence the most alkaline?

    a – cashews   b – almonds   c – peanuts

76. Our first nutritious sweet as babies should be:

    a – lactose   b – glucose   c – fructose

77. Which four of the following are most commonly associated with regular milk consumption?

    a – insomnia   c – excess mucus production   e – allergy   g – diarrhea
    b – diabetes   d – magnesium overload   f – cardiovascular problems   h – hair loss

78. Concerns over seafood consumption include which three of the following?

    a – heavy metal accumulation   c – high fat   e – incomplete protein   g – parasites
    b – excess omega-6 fatty acids   d – high sugar   f – ocean contamination

79. Shellfish can be high in which three of the following hard-to-obtain nutrients?

    a – vitamin C   c – calcium   e – selenium   g – vitamin E
    b – zinc   d – magnesium   f – sand   h – iron

80. Choose five foods that may commonly cause food poisoning.

    a – mayonnaise   c – brown rice   e – eggs   g – tofu   i – raw milk
    b – baked potatoes   d – cooked carrots   f – pesto pastas   h – crab   j – liverwurst

81. The average person in the United States consumes how many pounds of chicken each year?

    a – 10   b – 25   c – 50   d – 100

82. The fattiest part of the chicken is:

    a – thigh   b – breast   c – leg   d – skin

83. Eggs contain which four of the following?

a – complex carbohydrate   d – good-quality protein   g – fiber
b – cholesterol   e – ⅔ saturated fat   h – vitamin A
c – high in B vitamins   f – vitamin C   i – selenium

84. Most people in the world follow which type of diet?

a – carnivorous   c – vegetarian   e – omnivorous
b – macrobiotic   d – fast food   f – seafood

85. Vegetarians have a lower incidence of which four of the following?

a – heart disease   c – obesity   e – smoking   g – malnutrition
b – children   d – cancer   f – diabetes   h – dental cares

86. Vegetarians need to watch out for which four of the following deficiencies?

a – vitamin B_{12} c – iron   e – zinc   g – protein
b – vitamin A   d – manganese   f – potassium   h – linoleic acid

87. Which of the following compose the old basic four food groups?

a – cereal grains   c – fruits and vegetables   e – legumes   g – eggs
b – dairy   d – carbohydrates   f – meats   h – nuts

88. The "healthier" new basic fo ur food groups as discussed in this book are:

a – fruits   c – vegetables   e – pizza   g – grains and legumes
b – proteins   d – dairy   f – meats   h – microwave dinners

89. The four most common excesses of the Western diet are:

a – fat   c – iron   e – sugar   g – protein
b – calcium   d – fiber   f – chemicals   h – B vitamins

90. Which food is most commonly implicated in food allergies?

a – peanuts   b – cow's milk   c – seafood   d – cucumbers

91. What is the most common dietary deficiency in the United States?

a – iron   b – vitamin B_{12} c – fiber   d – zinc

92. How many calories does the average person have to burn to lose one pound?

a – 1,000   b – 2,500   c – 3,500   d – 5,000

93. What is the single most important preventable cause of disease in the United States?

a – alcoholism   b – fried foods   c – smoking   d – high cholesterol

94. Which has the most fat?

a – 1 cup of cottage cheese   b – 10 potato chips   c – 2 slices of bread

95. How many gallons of blood does the average adult heart pump each day?

a – 100   b – 600   c – 1,400   d – 4,800

96. Which three of the following are high-sodium foods?

a – whole wheat bread   c – cured meat   e – banana
b – pickles   d – pretzels   f – potatoes

97. Choose the four sodium-sensitive conditions.

a – PMS   c – hives   e – hypertension   g – asthma
b – pneumonia   d – edema   f – kidney disease   h – cancer

98. The amount of sugar that the average American adult consumes each year is:
   a – 10–20 pounds   b – 50–75 pounds   c – over 100 pounds

99. The amount of salt that the average American adult consumes each year is:
   a – 3–10 pounds   b – 15–20 pounds   c – 25–30 pounds

100. Which is closest to the amount of food additives consumed by the average American adult each year?
   a – less than 50 pounds   b – 50–100 pounds   c – more than 100 pounds

101. Which of the following foods are acid-forming and which are alkaline-forming in the body?
   a – grapefruit   c – cheese   e – cabbage   g – cauliflower   i – carrots
   b – wheat   d – cranberries   f – millet   h – peanuts   j – chicken

102. Choose three beneficial effects of food rotation.
   a – decrease food reactions   e – increase food reactions
   b – better variety   f – less defecation
   c – better digestion   g – less chance of nutritional deficiency
   d – better hearing and eyesight   h – more definitive defecation

103. According to food combining rules, pick the two correct statements.
   a – Do not eat more than one protein per meal.   c – Eat protein with vegetables.
   b – Eat protein with starches.   d – Eat fruit only after a meal.

104. Choose four of the main foods of the macrobiotic diet from the following.
   a – fish   c – whole grains   e – fruit   g – beans
   b – seaweed   d – cheese   f – vegetables   h – eggs

105. What is the most common commercial food additive in the United States?
   a – salt   b – BHA   c – sugar   d – BHT

106. Which of the following is closest to the number of additives currently used by our food industry?
   a – 50   b – 300   c – 1,200   d – 5,000

107. Contamination of our food supply comes from many sources: seed treatment, shipping, harvesting, packaging, handling. Approximately how many possible chemical contaminants are there?
   a – 1,000   b – 500   c – 12,000   d – 24,000

108. Of the following sources of pollutants in the United States, which group is the most dangerous?
   a – microorganisms   b – particulates   c – volatile chemicals

109. Which pesticide or chemical spray is used for which food?
   methyl bromide   a – bananas
   ethylene gas   b – grains/legumes
   sulfur dioxide   c – dried fruits

110. Each year in California alone, how many tons of pesticides are used?
   a – 2 million   b – 20 million   c – 200 million

111. Approximately how many food additives are approved for use?

      a – 60   b – 1,000   c – 3,000   d – 10,000

112. GRAS stands for:

      a – a controlled substance to smoke   b – a growing process for sprouts
      c – generally recognized as safe   d – great reaction after stimulation

113. Match each food additive to its correct category:

Flavoring	a – iron
Natural coloring agent	b – MSG
Preservative	c – annato
Alkali	d – diglycerides
Bleaching agent	e – ethylene gas
Moisture controller	f – calcium silicate
Activity controller	g – BHA
Emulsifier	h – baking soda
Texturizer	i – benzoyl peroxide
Nutritional additive	j – pectin

114. This book suggests avoiding which five of the following additives?

      a – calcium proprionate   d – saccharin   g – sodium benzoate
      b – sulfur dioxide   e – vanillin   h – potassium sorbate
      c – sodium nitrite   f – refined sugar   i – artificial colors FD & C

115. Which six of the following additives are probably safe?

      a – calcium proprionate   e – saccharin   h – artificial colors FD & C
      b – sulfur dioxide   f – sodium benzoate   i – Polysorbate 60
      c – sodium nitrite   g – sulfites   j – potassium sorbate
      d – glycerin   k – salt

116. The greatest number of food additives are:

      a – flavorings   b – colorings   c – texturizers   d – preservatives

---

THERE ARE A TOTAL OF 500 CORRECT ANSWERS
FOR *HOW MUCH DO YOU KNOW?*

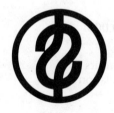

Part I: Worksheet—Multiple Choice

1. _____
2. Fructose _____   Lactose _____
   Sucrose _____   Mannose_____
   Maltose_____
3. _____
4. _____
5. Saturated _____
   Unsaturated _____
6. _____
7. Carcinogenic_____
   Cancer-preventive_____
8. _____
9. Chylomicrons __   VLDL __
   LDL _____   HDL ___
10. _____
11. _____
12. _____
13. Water _____   Fat _____
14. _____
15. _____
16. _____
17. _____
18. _____
19. _____
20. _____
21. _____
22. _____
23. _____
24. _____

25. _____
26. _____
27. _____
28. _____
29. _____
30. _____
31. _____
32. _____
33. _____
34. _____
35. _____
36. _____
37. _____
38. _____
39. _____
40. _____
41. _____
42. _____
43. _____
44. _____
45. _____
46. _____
47. _____
48. _____
49. _____
50. _____
51. _____
52. _____
53. _____

54. _____

55. _____

56. _____

57. Hormones ___ Enzymes ____
    Antibodies ___

58. _____

59. _____

60. _____

61. _____

62. Royal Jelly ___ Propolis ____
    Bee Pollen ___

63. _____

64. Dates _____ Prunes _____
    Raisins _____ Apricots _____

65. _____

66. _____

67. _____

68. _____

69. _____

70. _____

71. _____

72. _____

73. _____

74. _____

75. _____

76. _____

77. _____

78. _____

79. _____

80. _____

81. _____

82. _____

83. _____

84. _____

85. _____

86. _____

87. _____

88. _____

89. _____

90. _____

91. _____

92. _____

93. _____

94. _____

95. _____

96. _____

97. _____

98. _____

99. _____

100. _____

101. Acid _____
     Alkaline _____

102. _____

103. _____

104. _____

105. _____

106. _____

107. _____

108. _____

109. Methyl bromide _____
     Ethylene gas _____
     Sulfur dioxide _____

110. _____

111. _____

112. _____

113. Flavoring _____
     Natural coloring agent _____
     Preservative _____
     Alkali _____
     Bleaching agent _____
     Moisture controller_____
     Activity controller _____
     Emulsifier _____
     Texturizer _____
     Nutritional additive _____

114. _____

115. _____

116. _____

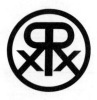

Part II: Reflective Response

See instructions on page 1022.

SELF: Health—Healing—Illness

1. How old do you want to live to be? Is this based on your family history? Is this based on a current health condition? Is this based on a fear of death or a fear of life? Is that based on the joy of life?

2. When was your last illness? How long did it last? How long until you came back into your preillness strength? What did you do to alleviate symptoms and/or hasten healing?

3. Do you currently have any disease? If so, what? Do you know whether or not nutritional changes might be able to influence your recovery or symptoms? If so, what are you doing to improve your health?

4. Who really cares about you? Who do you care about? Does your doctor really care about your health? Do you consider yourself educated? informed? a hypochondriac? Do you have enough money for your health? Do you spend more time for sickness than health?

5. In what shape is your immune system? Do you consider yourself immunosuppressed? If so, why? Are you satisfied with your communications to your immune system? If not, what are you willing to do to enhance it? When will you begin? How long before you expect results?

6. The last time you took antibiotics was for? The side effects you experienced were? Do you take antibiotics every time you experience the symptoms of a cold? Do you only take antibiotics for known bacterial infections?

7. What condition do you think your adrenal glands are in? Do you drink coffee or alcohol more than once a day? Is that too much? Are you on a diet low in vitamins and minerals? How often do you eat sweets? Do you currently have low blood sugar?

8. When did you or a family member have a wound? What type of wound, injury, post-surgery, etc. was it? How long did it take to heal? Was that what you expected? Did you use anything to accelerate the wound healing? If so, what—topical, internal, or mind? Have you had any surgery? If so, what? Did it help the problems it was meant to correct?

9. Have you or anyone in your family had cancer? How did it affect you?

10. The best diet to help prevent breast cancer is low in fats, high in complex carbohydrates and vegetables, and therefore, high in fiber. Rate your own daily intake:

% complex carbohydrates	% protein	grams of fiber
% simple carbohydrates	% fat	

11. Are you satisfied with your elimination habits? What can you do to improve them? What foods constipate you? What foods loosen you up? Do you know about colonic irrigation? Have you ever had one? Does the idea of one frighten you? Have you read *Staying Healthy with the Seasons*? Look up colonic irrigation there if you want to learn more about its benefits.

12. If you have any allergies what are they and what are your symptoms? How long have you had them? Are they seasonal? What medications do you use to combat the symptoms? What are the side effects from these drugs? What nutritional supplements have you used during an allergy attack or to prevent one?

13. Have you ever had *Herpes simplex* infections? If so, what seems to cause an outbreak or worsen the symptoms? How often does this occur? Have you ever found anything that helps eliminate the symptoms? If so, what?

14. When was your last immunization? What was it for? Was it injected? How did you feel before and after you got it? Did you experience any symptoms of the disease that the vaccine was protective against? Did you ever get symptoms of that illness again? Parents, what immunizations must your child get before attending school? Did your child have any reactions to this? Are you in favor of mandatory immunizations for school attendance?

15. Are you easily fatigued? Are you now, or have you ever been anemic? What were the symptoms that led to your diagnosis? Was there another reason for your fatigue? If so, is it treated with a supplement or food? Do you feel better when taking supplements? Are you seeing progress in your treatment? How could it be improved?

16. How is your thyroid? Have you ever had a weight problem? An energy deficiency? How would you rate your metabolism? Your overall energy level?

17. Do you know if your cholesterol level is high or low? Do you know your HDL and LDL levels? What about the levels of your family members? Do you feel that it is necessary for you to pay attention to your dietary fats?

18. Do you wear eyeglasses? For how many years? For what activities—driving, reading, constantly, other? Have you ever tried to improve your vision? How? Do you suffer from eye strain? How many hours per day/week do you use a computer, watch TV, read, rest your eyes in meditation or nature? Do you wear contact lenses? How do they feel? Do you use eyewash? If so, what are the ingredients? Do you wear sunglasses?

19. Do you cough up a lot of mucus? How often? Do you believe that the mucous membranes in your body are healthy and vital? Are you only aware of your body's mucus when you get a cough or a cold? How often is that?

20. Rate your skin: Dry or oily? Dry in some places, which areas? Do you have a skin condition? For how long? Has it been treated? What supplements have you tried to improve your skin condition? The best things for my skin seem to be?

21. Are you satisfied with your nail health? Do they grow rapidly? Are they strong or do they crack easily? Have you used false nails and/or acrylic nail polish? If so, do you know what your real nails are like?

22. Would you describe your hair as vital or lifeless? Have you ever tried any natural products or dietary supplements to improve the quality and appearance of your hair, and if so, what seemed to give you satisfactory results?

23. How often do you go to the dentist? When was your last visit? Do you experience fear or discomfort before you go? Are your visits to the dentist preventive or emergency? When was your last dental checkup? How was your dental health? How many teeth are your own? When was your last dental surgery? Did you know that zinc and vitamins A and C may help you recover more quickly? Do your gums bleed? If so, how often? How often do you use vitamin C and bioflavonoids to support the healing of your gums?

24. How many silver/mercury fillings do you have in your teeth? Can you taste any metal? Do you pick up radio stations or satellite communications on them? Do you feel any ill effects from these fillings?

25. What do you currently do to stimulate your circulation or body heat? Turn up the heater, get under the covers, put on extra clothes, eat more grains, go for a walk or exercise, have a drink, snuggle with someone, eat cayenne pepper?

26. Do you know your blood type? What is it? Do you know your family members' blood types? List them. Have you ever had a blood transfusion? Do you ever donate blood? If so, how often? Do you have any trouble with blood clotting or bruising?

SELF: Food—Diet

27. How much water do you drink daily? Other fluids? Does your body get rid of water easily? Do you sweat during physical exertion? How many times a day do you urinate? Do you have difficulty holding in your urine? Has urine ever been released when you coughed or laughed?

28. Do you drink fluoridated water? Do you believe that it helps prevent tooth decay? Do you believe that fluoride is toxic? Does your toothpaste contain fluoride? Does it contain sugar?

29. What are your current dietary strengths? What are your dietary weaknesses? During your life what different diets have you tried? Your current diet is?

30. Do you or does someone else prepare most of the foods you eat? What are your specialties? You learned cooking from classes, books, family, friends, videotapes, tasting other people's food and asking for recipes? Do you mostly use the microwave? Prepare only frozen foods? Start everything from scratch? Buy deli foods often? Only prepare food when someone else doesn't? Have you always had an interest in cooking? Cook only if someone else is around to feed? Feel it is important to develop your nurturing skills?

31. What are the most common methods you use for food preparation? Fry, bake, raw, microwave, broil, barbecue, wok? How often do you do each of these? Are you aware that some forms of cooking can destroy the vitamin content? Do you tend to under- or overcook your foods?

32. Your favorite flavor is: sweet, sour, hot, salty, bitter? Your favorite seasoning is? Your favorite food(s)? Is there a food you would never eat again—what is it?

33. Where do you eat your meals? Do you focus on it solely? Do you chew your food thoroughly? Do you sit quietly and nourish yourself? Do you usually eat on the run? In the car? In parking lots? Standing up? Do you need to be distracted while you eat— with music, TV, a book, a conversation? Do you indulge in TV dinners or other packaged meals? How often? Do you eat while you shop? At the movies, what do you usually consume?

34. With whom do you usually eat? Do you eat at the same times every day? Does the time vary considerably? What is the first thing you usually eat in the morning? Do you eat before you go to bed? If so, what? What's your favorite meal? Do you have a temper tantrum or bad mood if you don't eat or are hungry?

35. Do you think that your diet is as good as it's going to be? That it can be improved considerably? That you don't want to make any changes even though you are aware some could be made that would enhance your health? That your diet is really very good right now?

36. What are your food shopping habits? How often do you shop? Do you buy organically grown or chemically treated foods? Do you shop from a list? Does someone in your household do the shopping? Are they nutritionally aware? Does the same person who shops for food prepare it? Are these duties shared in your house? Fairly? How long do you keep leftovers in the refrigerator? What is the average time between preparation and storage? How long has the oldest food been in your refrigerator? What is it?

37. Do you buy your herbs and seasonings in bulk or already bottled? Which of the following seasonings do you use: sugar, artificial sweeteners, catsup, mustard, salt, pepper, garlic?

38. Is chocolate your biggest food craving? If not, what is? Do you use chocolate as: a seasoning, a food, drug, treat, sensual pleasure, never eat the stuff?

39. Your favorite restaurants are: fast food, Chinese, Italian, Indian, kosher, French, Mexican, Japanese, American, Middle East, Thai, deli, natural, other?

40. If you were in a situation in which you could only have seven foods, which ones would you choose for a healthy, balanced, and enjoyable diet?

41. Is your food sprayed with fungicides or pesticides, or is it pesticide-free? Do you know? Do you care only if you or a family member experiences some ill effects from these poisons?

42. What is your daily intake of dietary fats? Are you overweight? What is your ideal weight? Your most common fat intake is from? You currently consume fats in your diet in what ways? How often? Which vegetable oils do you use for: salad, sautéeing, wok cooking? What is your favorite vegetable oil?

43. Vegetables make up what percentage of your diet? Do you eat vegetables most frequently—steamed, raw, boiled, fried? The oldest vegetable in your vegetable bin is? It has been there—one week, several weeks, one month, you don't know?

44. Do you like vegetable juice and drink it—daily, regularly, never? Do you prefer it to fruit juices? Are your vegetable juices bottled or canned, fresh or frozen?

45. Your favorite leafy green is? The greens you eat most frequently are? The ones you like least are? How do you determine the freshness of green vegetables—by squeeze, look, taste, smell? The vegetable you eat most often is?

46. Do you currently use sprouts in your diet? The frequency with which you eat sprouts is? Do you sprout your own? Have you been successful in sprouting: wheatgrass, wheat berries, radish, wheat, aduki lentils, alfalfa, clover, garbanzo?

47. The fruit you eat most often is? Your favorite fruit is? Your favorite fruit combination is? Most fruit you eat is—raw, baked, sauced? Does fruit give you gas? You never eat fruit? Do you eat fruit alone or mixed with other foods? Are you aware of food combining and use fruit accordingly? The time of day you most frequently eat fruit is? You eat grapes in the following ways: wine, jam, raw, juice, fruit salad, other? Your favorite grape(s) are? How often do you eat berries? What are your favorite kind? Do you eat them fresh, only when in season, canned, frozen?

48. Your favorite fruit juice is? Do you drink it daily, more than once a day, weekly? Do you drink fruit juice that is frozen, canned, or fresh? Do you make it yourself? In your juice do you use the seeds and the pulp? Do you drink it at room temperature or cold? Do you only drink fruit juices if they are mixed with alcohol?

49. What's your main source of protein? How often do you eat it? How do you prepare it? What are your favorite protein foods? Did you know that more protein can be created from one acre of land by growing soybeans than by grazing cattle? Would this influence your protein choices?

50. You spend how much money on meat each month? How often do you eat meat? Is it raised on chemically treated land or feed? Do you seek out meat that is raised free of potentially toxic chemicals? If you eat little meat, do you take glandular products? The monthly frequency with which you use the following meat products: sausage, salami, bacon, ham, liver, steak, ground beef, turkey, beef, lamb, pork, veal, bologna? The meat you eat most frequently is—frozen, canned, fresh, dried, organic? Do you kill your own meat or pay others to do it for you? Do you experience prejudice against people who do not eat the same way you do?

51. When you eat meat, are your body and waste odors different? When you eat meat is your sexual desire up or down? Are you interested in the planetary effects of a meat-based diet? Have you read or are you aware of *Diet for a New America* by John Robbins, the book about the political and environmental effects of dairy and meat-based diet?

52. Most frequently do you eat nuts salted or unsalted? What's your favorite nut? Who's your favorite nut? When you eat nuts, are they canned, sugared, raw, roasted, or dry roasted?

53. How often do you use the following dairy foods on a weekly basis: whole milk, nonfat milk, yogurt, cheese, butter, ice cream? When you eat cheese, what's the most common form—melted, in sauce, in chunks, with bread? What is your favorite cheese?

54. Are you aware of the difference between free-range, untreated chickens and commercial chickens that usually contain chemicals, antibiotics, and hormones? Are you willing to spend more money to buy organic, chemical-free poultry? Do you prefer saving the money and are happy with commercially raised poultry? Can you taste the difference between the two? You eat chicken how many times per week, and it is usually prepared by: baking, deep-frying, stir-frying, boiling, other? Are you aware that fried chicken is high in fat? Do you avoid eating the skin of the chicken or other poultry? Being aware of the potential of Salmonella from raw chicken, do you bleach or disinfect your cutting board often?

55. Do you eat eggs: daily, weekly, rarely? Do you eat eggs in: breads, noodles, crepes, pancakes, omelettes, over-easy, ice cream, smoothies, egg nog?

56. Do you eat fish regularly? How often? How do you prepare it? What are your two favorite fish dishes? Do you take any fish oil supplements? If so, what type and how much?

57. Label detective work: Do you read food labels? Are you more interested in price or content? Why? Look in your cupboards, which of your foods contain BHA or BHT preservatives? Should you avoid either one of these? What are you going to do about eating additives in your food?

58. How often do you use cayenne pepper in your diet? How? Do you use cayenne to enhance your circulation or simply as a tasty spice? Do you ever take it in capsule form? Have you ever put it in your socks in the winter to keep your feet warm? Are you aware of the potential cancer-protective properties of fresh cayenne?

59. How much garlic do you use daily? Which forms do you use: pressed, raw, cooked, whole, salt, powder, deodorized tablets? Do you ever use it for medicinal purposes?

60. Do you use fresh ginger, and how? Do you use wheatgrass or barley juice for purification and rejuvenation?

61. Which of the following foods do you eat, and how many times weekly? Liver, whole grains, wheat germ, fish, poultry, eggs, soybeans, dried beans, peanuts, walnuts, bananas, prunes, potatoes, cauliflower, cabbage, avocado?

62. Do you eat according to the old basic four food groups? From which group do you eat the most: meat, dairy, cereals/grains, fruits/vegetables? If you could make a tasty one-bowl meal with your favorite foods, what would it contain?

63. Name the processed foods in your diet. What percentage of your foods are frozen or fresh? Name the natural foods in your diet. Name the imported foods you eat. Are they canned, fresh, bottled, frozen, or preserved? Do you mind if your food has been gassed, fumigated, or irradiated?

64. Are you salt-sensitive? Does your body bloat? Have you been instructed to alter your salt intake? Do you add salt to your food? Which foods do you regularly eat that are salty?

65. How many soft drinks do you have daily, weekly? Did you know that in one year, the average American drinks 39 gallons of soft drinks? What is your favorite beverage? What are its ingredients?

66. Which foods do you enjoy that you know are not good for you? Does eating these foods make you feel sated? Your favorite eating holidays are? How do you feel after these holidays? What do you do for a food hangover?

67. Which of these components of a healthy diet do you need to incorporate into your diet: natural, seasonal, fresh, nutritious, clean, tasty, rotating, moderate, food combining? Balanced in: macronutrients, micronutrients, food groups, flavors, acid/alkaline?

68. What are your personal dietary needs? Are you in charge of anyone else's diet? Whose? Do you consider yourself well informed about nutrition? How is your health and weight? What about your mate's? Other family members? Are you satisfied with your weight? When was your last diet? How long did you stay on it? Did you achieve your intended goal? When was your last cleansing fast? How long did you stay on it? What did you experience?

Supplements

69. Good sources of niacin and tryptophan are liver, organ meats, poultry, fish, and peanuts. How often are these in your diet? Daily, weekly, monthly? When taken, niacin or nicotinic acid can produce redness, warmth, and itching. Have you ever experienced a "niacin flush?"

70. Which of these excellent food sources of vitamin C do you take? Rose hips, acerola cherries, spruce needles, citrus fruits, sago palm?

71. Do you ever feel vitamin deficient? If so, is it seasonally specific? Do you get enough vitamin D from the sun? Do you spend more time indoors or outdoors? How many hours a day are you in the sun? During the summer? In the winter? Do you use a sunscreen when out of doors? Are you easily sunburned? If so, what do you do for protection or soothing? What activities do you enjoy in the sunshine? Do you live in a foggy or rainy area? Is there acid rain where you live? If you live where there's not much sunlight, where do you go for light? What kind of light do you spend the most time under: incandescent, fluorescent, full spectrum?

72. What vitamin/mineral supplements do you take? What form do you prefer: tablets, time-release capsules, powders, liquids, injection? When do you usually take them—with meals, in the morning, at bedtime? How does your body handle them? Can you taste them or feel them hours after taking? Are you aware of vitamin/mineral combining for optimal absorption? What combinations do you use? Do you vary what you take depending on season of the year or level of stress or illness? Do you know what the minimum recommended daily vitamin and mineral requirements are?

73. Take some time to evaluate what requirements are being met by the supplements you take now. List your current intake. List the other needed supplements.

74. Check the statements that best fit how you feel after taking supplements: I don't like taking pills. I feel better when I take them. I sleep better. I couldn't function without them. I only take them when I feel ill. I'm taking them on doctor's/nutritionist's instructions. I don't notice any effect.

75. How old are the supplements in your house? Are they stored in the dark, in sunlight, in the refrigerator? Why did you buy them? Have you stopped taking them? Why?

76. Have you experienced cracks at the corners of your mouth? This may be due to a folic acid or other B vitamin deficiency. How much do you get daily?

77. Have you used vitamin E (or vitamin A) oil topically for healing an injury or burn? Did you notice any difference in the healing process when you used it? Would you use it again?

78. Do you take regular amounts of vitamin C? When was your last cold? How long did it last? When you need extra strength or stamina what do you take/do/eat? Are you satisfied with the results? How often do you do this?

79. Which minerals do you take in supplements? Do you think that you are deficient in any minerals? If so, which ones and why? Your current calcium sources are?

80. The following are symptoms that may be related to magnesium deficiency. Have you experienced any of these: fatigue, irritability, muscle cramps, anorexia, insomnia, twitching?

81. Potassium with sodium regulates water and acid-base balance. How often do you sweat? Are you aware that alcohol, sweating, coffee, sugar, and diuretics deplete the body's potassium levels? This may affect blood pressure—what is yours?

82. Have you or a member of your family ever taken lithium therapeutically? If so, why? What effect did this have on daily functioning and health?

83. Do you know what organo-germanium is? Have you ever tried it? What kind of an effect did you experience?

SELF: Attitudes—Emotions

84. Are you an optimistic person? In what areas? Are you optimistic about your future? What have you specifically done daily to move towards a healthier future for yourself, your family, your community and the planet?

85. There are many types and sources of love, vitamin L. Where do you most readily get your dose? Spouse or partner, family, work, nature, alone, with others, the arts, serving others, religion or spiritual practices. Who do you nurture? How? Who nurtures you and how? Do you feel full or lacking?

86. Do you confuse love for possessiveness? Has anyone done this to you? Are any of these recurring issues in relationships: jealousy, control, irrational attachments, loving un-available or unattainable people, loving more than being loved? Are you usually the aggressor or the receptive one? Did you have a balanced emotional childhood? Have you been in any therapy to learn how to love and who is appropriate to share vitamin L with? How many hugs per day do you share? Do you hug and kiss when you meet an old friend or do you shake hands? Is physical contact important to you? Do you have a pet? If so, does this balance your need for affectionate contact with another life force? Do you get enough sensual support?

87. Have you ever had someone close to you die? How recently? What kind of personal ceremony did you do? What was the grieving process like for you? Did that open you to other grief or other losses? How do you work with loss and grief? Can you cry when you need to? What things make you cry?

88. Why did you purchase this book? Are you incorporating any of this book into your life?

SELF: Lifestyle

89. Have you ever smoked? If so, when and for how long? Do you still smoke? If so, how many packs a day? Do you take vitamin supplements to help counteract the harmful effects? Do any of your family members smoke? Every cigarette contains one microgram of the toxic mineral cadmium—30 percent goes into your lungs, 70 percent goes into the atmosphere around you that others breathe. Are you aware that secondhand smoke can be harmful to family and friends? Do you care? Do you or do they hack and cough?

Do your clothes and home smell like smoke? Have you ever tried to stop? What methods have you tried? Do you want to stop? What's preventing this? Have you chewed tobacco, smoked cigars, pipes?

90. When you exercise, run, or walk, is it by a freeway or busy road? Have you ever had chelation therapy to remove heavy metals from your blood? Some dietary supplements may be effective in removing toxic metals from the body. How much seaweed, kelp, sodium alginate do you eat and how often?

91. How frequently do you exercise? You currently work out or exercise how many times a week, month, year? Your favorite form of exercise is? Your most usual form of exercise is? Do you enjoy exercise? Have you eliminated any foods from your diet to optimize performance? Which ones? Do you drink adequate fluids after exercising?

92. How often do you have an alcoholic drink: daily, weekly, monthly, yearly? How do you feel before and after? Are there any alcoholics in your family? Do you consider yourself one? Do you consider yourself a social drinker? What is your favorite alcoholic beverage? Do you drink to reduce stress? What other things motivate you to drink alcohol? How does it affect your mood? Is the alcohol you drink chemically treated? Was your first sexual encounter surrounded with drug or alcohol use? Do your parents drink or abuse drugs? Does this bother you? Have you or they gone for support to stop? What has worked?

93. For stress reduction, have you ever tried: exercise, meditation, writing in a journal, walking? Do you have a regular stress reduction practice, and if so, what is it? How does stress manifest in your life? How often do you feel stressed—daily, weekly, monthly? What usually causes a stress reaction? Does it take a lot of stress before you notice your state? What is your usual first symptom of being "amped out"? How long after this warning does it take before you do something about it? Do you wait until you really need a "sick" day? Do you feel free enough to be able to take a "health" day when needed? How tuned in to your own system and rhythms are you?

94. Do you ever suffer from information overload? What do you do to rebalance? Is it hard to retrain your brain to refrain and/or retain? How do you focus on yourself?

95. How do you enjoy flowers? Will you count the ways? To smell, to grow, as decoration, to give bouquets to loved ones/for celebrations, for landscaping, to eat, give only to sick people, only on calendar occasions? Do you enjoy receiving flowers? Do you prefer live, still growing flowers over cut flowers?

96. Do you go to bed early or late in the evening? Do you work certain shifts and have to go to sleep on irregular schedules? Is it necessary for you to take sleeping pills or other aids to fall asleep easily? Do you sleep all the way through the night? How many times a week do you wake up in the middle of the night and have difficulty falling back to sleep? When you wake do you feel rested and ready to face the day? Do you remember your dreams? If so, do you record them? Do you often have nightmares? Do you fly in your dreams?

97. A class of chemicals called endorphins is released when we experience pleasure or pain. What do you do to create endorphins for pleasure in your life? Run, listen to music, eat, dance, have intimate contact, other sources of pleasure.

98. How often do you have sex? Do you feel tired afterwards? If so, how do you recover your energy? Do you enjoy for hours or only for minutes? Does your partner have similar desires and enjoy the same practices? Do you really enjoy sex with another person or do you have unfulfilled needs? Are you both satisfied with your sexperience?

99. Are you satisfied with your current method of "safe sex" or birth control? If so, which ones do you use? Do you abstain from sex rather than use a disliked method of protection? What other methods have you tried? If taking birth control pills, how many years have you been taking them? Do you supplement yourself for the vitamin depletions, such as vitamin B_6, they can cause? Have you ever had an accidental or unexpected pregnancy? How many times, and what did you do? Are you satisfied with your personal sexual lubrication? Do you use creams or gels? If so, which ones?

For Women:

100. If you have been pregnant, which dietary supplements did you take? Did you stop this program after the baby was born? Did you readjust it and if so, how? Do you have regular periods? Are they associated with cramps, breast tenderness, or other symptoms of PMS? What do you do nutritionally to lessen the PMS discomfort? For those of you taking birth control pills or if pregnant, copper levels rise dramatically. This has been associated with some forms of depression and hyperactivity. When did you last have your copper level measured? What was it?

101. If you are no longer menstruating, what age were you when you stopped? Did you have hot flashes or other symptoms during the transition time? Have you tried estrogen replacement therapy? What type? What was your response to this form of treatment? Are you still taking it? Did you have to try many types or dosages before finding something that worked for you? Would you recommend it to other women? Are you enjoying your post-menopausal years? Do you do something to honor your female self now that you are in the wisdom years beyond child rearing? If so, what? Are you using a calcium supplement and exercising regularly to help prevent osteoporosis? Did you take calcium while you had menstrual cycles? Do you feel that you have adequate vaginal lubrication, sexual libido, sensuality? Do you take vitamin E supplements, which are important in this time of life?

102. **Mothers,** did you breastfeed your children? **Men and women:** Were you breastfed or bottle-fed? How aware are you of your own breasts and those of your mate's? Are they a source of pleasure?

Men and women:

103. Does anyone you know have Alzheimer's disease? Aluminum toxicity may be a possible contributor. Do you use deodorant? What type—spray, stick, etc.? Does it contain aluminum? How much aluminum are you ingesting from food additives? Are you concerned about this? Which foods do you need to eliminate? Do you use aluminum cookware or foil? How often? Are you aware that storing acid foods such as orange juice or tomato sauce in aluminum containers may add aluminum to your food?

104. Which products did you buy because of seductive advertising? For personal hygiene, foods or nutrition aids, household care, lawn or garden, pets?

105. What ingredients are in your toiletries and cosmetics? Are you aware of what you put on your body? Do you care? Have you ever had any skin reactions to any of these?

106. Do you wash your hands before you eat? Do you wash your clothes regularly? Do you clean your house regularly?

107. Do you have health insurance that works and allows you to obtain health care you would not otherwise have? Can you use your insurance for massage therapy, acupuncture, preventive medicine, counseling, surgery, biofeedback, nutritional supplements, disease treatment, or disease prevention? Do you have a retirement fund?

108. Are the kind of images you watch/see for relaxation of violence, sexual, nature, people? The number of hours spent a day/week: watching TV, children watching TV, going to the movies? What are your favorite kinds of TV shows? What kind of movies do you enjoy the most? What do you never watch?

HOUSEHOLD

109. How many appliances are plugged into the walls in your home? How many appliances in your home are on right now? Could you live without electricity? Have you needed to in the last year due to natural disaster or power failure?

110. What are the pipes made of that supply your household water? Where does your water come from? Where does your used water go? Have you ever had your water tested? If so, for what and what were the results? Do you drink bottled water? Do you trust its quality? Why?

111. Parents, have you checked the toys that your children love to chew on? Are they safe? Have you checked whether contaminated water or poisonous fertilizers or sprays are used at your children's school or playground? Is it near a freeway or crowded roadway? What are the school's guidelines for safety?

112. How many products in your home or workplace are actively out-gassing? Can you smell or taste them? Do you ignore it waiting for it to go away? How is your home heated? Cooled? What do you know about the safety of products used for your heating? What about the safety of the fabrics in your household?

113. Are you aware of the potentially toxic chemicals you use in your house? Below is a list of the common products that need to be childproofed and person-proofed. What is your frequency of use of each: ammonia, drain cleaners, oven cleaner, furniture/floor polish, detergents, fabric softeners, spray starch, mothballs, spot removers, bleach, silver polish, glass cleaner, air freshener, disinfectants, mold cleaners, carpet/upholstery shampoo, dishwasher detergent, aerosol sprays, permanent ink markers, glues, typewriter correction fluid? What about your frequency of use per month of these personal items that may contain dangerous chemicals: toothpaste, mouthwash, antiperspirants, denture cleansers, talcum powder, perfume/after-shave, hair spray, hair dye, depilatory, dandruff shampoo, bubble bath, nail polish/remover, spermicides, douches? Which of these products can you find safe substitutes for?

114. Do you grow your own food or flowers? If so, do you use any chemicals in the soil, seed, water? What kind? Are you aware of natural pesticides and organic ways to enhance growing cycles? Do you use any sprays on your plants, inside or out? If so, which ones?

What type of soil is around your home? Do you use any pesticides inside your house and if so, which ones and what for? Do you have any symptoms of sensitivities to food spraying or pesticide exposure? What do you do about it? Are you sensitive to paint fumes or other chemicals?

Politics—Economics

115. Do you trust the government? The EPA and FDA? Who is your local Environmental Protection Agency representative? Do you know any other government official(s) who decide your future? If you do, what do you tell them?

116. What kind of education and/or activity would be best to teach people to clean up the environment? Do you feel that tax dollars, military, and prison time should pay for this, for planting trees, cleaning up the planet's waters? Do you think that the current concern about environmental dangers on our planet are real or just media hype? What are you most aggravated by in the field of health or ecology?

117. How much of the media that you see and read do you believe is true? Rate from 1–100 percent. How does this media affect you?

Earth—Environment

118. Check the statements that apply to your attitudes or sense about the correlations between people's actions around nature and disasters in the environment. Nuclear testing and earthquakes. Oil spills and beached baby whales. Cutting down the rain forests and drought. A meat-based diet and the destruction of the planet as well as personal health.

119. Are you aware of having ever been exposed to toxic minerals? If so, which one(s)? How did this occur? What have been the effects on your health and the environment of this exposure? How have you dealt with any symptoms you had? What were they? Are they still present? Did you take any medications and if so, what? Are you satisfied with the results or treatment? Did you report this incident? If so, how and to whom? What was the outcome?

120. Have you ever experienced an "environmental disease," and if so, what type? Have you ever sued anyone for environmental and/or toxic damage? How many times in your life have you been personally responsible for preventing a potentially harmful environmental situation? How did this make you feel about yourself and your planetary investment?

121. Through what means do you think you get the most chemical toxins: ingestants, inhalants, contactants, injectants? The source of these pollutants most often come from home, work, gym, outside, traveling, or other? Have you given up any activities due to this awareness or sensitivity, and if so, which ones?

122. How many items in your household do you REcycle? List them here. How do you REcycle them? How many items are you willing to PREcycle to prevent them getting into the environment? Be specific and list them here.

123. Make a list of the plastics you use every day. How much per week? What is the most common source of the plastic that you use—containers, packaging, dishes, etc? Do you REcycle them? If so, which ones and how? If not, why not?

124. Would you move near a nuclear dump site or power plant? What would you do if a chemical dump site was built near your home? Do you believe that the neighborhood in which you live has chemical/pollution problems?

125. Do you believe that we can reverse planetary pollution? How do you want to contribute to this?

126. Do you believe that your physician is educated about the effects of environmental toxins and pollutants? Do you think that he or she is aligned with drug or supplement companies? Is your physician or health practitioner environmentally aware? Do they REcycle? Does their office feel safe and is it free of strong chemicals? Do you seek help from those who are aligned with your own beliefs?

127. Do you believe that our natural resources are being adequately protected? Is it safe to entrust our lives and resources unconsciously to others? Are you aware of the many sources of pollution in your environment such as agriculture, industry, underground storage sites, mining? Which of these might affect your household, your neighborhood, your workplace?

128. Do you feel safe drinking your tap water? Is there water in your area that is safe for swimming or fishing? Do you know where your water comes from?

129. How often do you swim in the ocean? Do you feel differently about being in the ocean now that there have been oil spills, toxic waste, and nuclear waste added to our precious resource? Has this affected your relationship with the sea? Do you ignore what you cannot see? Do you feel helpless about what's happening to the ocean? Do you donate money to others who are trying to clean our planet's waters? Do you pick up trash when you go to the beach, even if it's not yours?

130. Do you live in an area of heavy smog? How do you react to it: ignore it, use eye drops, a lot of tissue? Do you spend more time indoors or outdoors? Are you sensitive to car fumes or smoke? Are there any indoor pollutants that bother you? If so, which ones? Where have you breathed the best air? Do you go there often? What are your environmental sensitivities?

131. Lead, a toxic metal contaminant, can be in paints, pottery glazes, and old buildings. Have you checked your ceramic containers to make sure that no lead was in the glaze? Do you or your children play in old building sites? Other sources of lead contaminants could be tin cans, pewter, insecticides. Do you use any lead-containing products? Does your vehicle use unleaded gasoline?

132. What changes are you willing to make now that will influence planetary survival? Suggestions for survival are addressed in Chapter 11 and are in the areas of Diet, Home, Work, Lifestyle, Political action, New activities.

133. What can you do generally to improve your life and the lives of those around you? Specifically? Nutritionally? Are you willing to find another way of dealing with your body, home, and agriculture instead of replacing germs with chemicals? How can you do this? Do you think we are living in a time of relative infinity on the planet Earth? Or is our time limited? What do you think/feel/sense about your/our future?

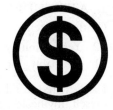

Part III: Health Bank Account

We have deposited $90,000 into your Health Bank Account (HBA); this is the value allotted to your Body-Mind-Heart-Spirit in the 1990s. That's $2.92 for your body minerals (up from $1.97, the worth of the mineral ash as scientifically valued in the 1980s), $14,198.99 for your mind (varies from person to person depending on how many brain cells they have left), $26,695.14 for your heart (or $60,000 if you've had heart bypass surgery), $49,099.95 for your soul-spirit (that's the most valuable), and $3 for the bank deposit service charge.

Have faith though. If you're taking good care of yourself—making conscious, alert and conscientious choices for your health and that of your family, local environment, and Earth as a whole—you may end up a "Health Millionaire." However, if you have poor health habits and believe you are a solitary planetary dweller and your actions are inconsequential, you may end up being "health bankrupt."

So, when you are ready, step up to the 24-hour truth teller window. Answer the following questions as honestly as you can, and see whether you make additional deposits to your Health Bank Account, or whether you must withdraw your savings to pay for the devaluation in longevity and your health. (And don't be too serious, that costs health dollars, too.) Relax and have a good time, it's your life!

This questionnaire/evaluation is divided into several sections that focus on various important lifestyle topics. Answer each question in the appropriate column, and tally your score at the end of each page. Then, you can multiply that amount by the HBA dollar factor, add or subtract it from your current balance, and enter your new total as indicated. See examples on pages 1059 and 1062.

Note: Based upon the way we have valued the various attitudes and lifestyle habits, and the relative importance placed upon mental, emotional, and spiritual levels as well as physical, it is possible that you could experience relatively good physical health, i.e., not be sick, and still not score very well. On the other hand, you could have cancer and still add dollars to your HBA based on your multidimensional approach to wellness.

Also note that certain habits, activities, or body states, such as smoking, alcohol use, or cholesterol and blood pressure levels, are listed multiple times throughout the various sections because we believe they have greater value upon your health and longevity and, thus, are worth more or less points and dollars for your Health Bank Account.

> REMEMBER, WE SUGGEST THAT YOU PHOTOCOPY
> THIS SECTION OF THE QUESTIONNAIRE SO
> THAT IT CAN BE USED MORE THAN ONCE.

I. ATTITUDES

(Rating System)

+2 Yes, definitely	+1 I think so	0 I'm not sure, maybe
−1 Probably not	−2 No, emphatically	

I am excited to fill out this lifestyle review and take an honest look at myself, my health, and my personal and planetary relationships—and become a Health Millionaire.	
I see illness as a positive process, helping me grow and change.	
I believe more in being well rather than getting well (i.e., health is an ongoing state of being/experience rather than something to attain).	
I have experienced greater health than illness in my life.	
I am reading this book to help me better understand my diet.	
I see the correlation between what I eat and how I feel.	
I believe the quality and the cleanliness (in regard to chemicals) of my food are important to my well-being.	
I am willing to pay a little more (10–20%) for cleaner or organic food.	
I believe "working" on myself and awareness of my actions are necessary to prevent illness.	
I first look within for answers to challenges or physical symptoms before I seek outer help.	
When I have demands on my time and energy from life's stresses, I am able to bypass frustration take positive action.	
I believe that harmony in relationships and personal peace influence planetary harmony and peace; on the other hand, personal frustration, anger, and, in general, lack of love, influence problematic relationships and planetary wars.	
I am satisfied by the actions I take daily and the way I feel.	
I am not in conflict with what I do and what I believe.	
Even though I am satisfied with my life as a whole, I know there is still more to do for a better future.	
I am satisfied with my overall diet and eating habits.	
I believe that if I have extreme frustrations or strong emotions about particular issues, a valuable method of dealing with these is talking with friends, family, or a therapist.	
I feel able both to hear another's opinions as well as express my own.	

Page Total	
× $3,000 =	
Beginning Balance	**$90,000**
New Balance	

(enter as Forward Balance next page)

I am able to adjust my attitudes when I feel it is appropriate.

I am willing to do what it takes to live a long, healthy, and productive life.

I really do care, and I can make a difference in the health and well-being of myself, others, and the planet.

After reading this section, my attitude/mood has improved.

Page Total	
× $3,000 =	
Forward Balance (from previous page)	
New Balance	
(enter as Forward Balance next page)	

EXAMPLE

I feel able both to hear another's opinions as well as express my own.	−1
I am able to adjust my attitudes when I feel it is appropriate.	+1
I am willing to do what it takes to live a long, healthy and productive life.	+2
I really do care, and I can make a difference in the health and well-being of myself, others and the planet.	+1
After reading this section, my attitude/mood has improved.	+1
Page Total	4 *
× $3,000 =	12,000 *
Sample Forward Balance	150,000
New Balance	162,000
(enter as Forward Balance next page)	

***NOTE: YOU CAN ALSO HAVE A MINUS SCORE.
SEE EXAMPLE ON PAGE 1062.**

II. GENERAL HABITS AND HYGIENE

Code—0 = never, d = day, wk = week, m = month, y = year, + = more than (e.g., +7/wk = more than seven times per week), minus sign (–) = less than (e.g., –1/wk = less than once per week)

Circle frequency in appropriate column. The scoring system is based on your experience of habits as they relate to current overall and long-range health.

	–3	–2	–1	00	+1	+2
Personal Hygiene						
Bathing/showering *weekly* } Circle one only *daily*	—	0–1/wk +4/d	2–3/wk 3–4/d	4–5/wk —	6–7/wk —	— 1–2/d
Brushing teeth	—	0–2/wk	3–4/wk	5–7/wk	+7/wk	2/d
Flossing	—	0	–1/wk	1–4/w	+4/wk	+1/d
Exercise to sweat (aerobic activity)	0 —	–1/m +10/wk	–1/wk +7/wk	1–2/wk —	3–4/wk —	+4/wk —
Take additional fluids and nutrients after sweating	—	0	–1/wk	1–2/wk	3–4/wk	+4/wk
Other active exercise (walking, sports)	0	–1/wk	1–2/wk	3–4/wk	5–6/wk	+6/wk
Regular stretching exercises	—	–2/m	–2/wk	2–3/wk	4–6/wk	+6/wk
Deep breathing/relaxation/ meditation	—	0	–1/wk	1–2/wk	3–4/wk	+4/wk
Sleep						
Falling asleep easily	—	–1/wk	1–2/wk	3–4/wk	5–6/wk	7/wk
Sleep through night	0	–1/wk	1–2/wk	3–4/wk	5–6/wk	7/wk
Dreaming activity	—	–1/wk	1–2/wk	3–4/wk	5–6/wk	7/wk
Dream recall	—	–1/wk	1–2/wk	3–4/wk	5–6/wk	7/wk
Sufficient sleep	0	–1/wk	1–2/wk	3–4/wk	5–6/wk	7/wk
Water Intake						
Glasses per day	—	–1/d	1–2/d	3–4/d	5–7/d	+7/d
Purified water—% of total	—	0	25	50	75	+95
Column Subtotals *						

Page Total

× \$3,000 =

Forward Balance (from previous page)

New Balance
(enter as Forward Balance next page)

** Remember to keep +
and – values when you
subtotal each column;
i.e., –3 and –3 = –6*

	−3	−2	−1	00	+1	+2
Driving						
Total hours per week	—	+15	+10	6–10	3–5	0–2
Wear seat belt (% of total)	0	1–20	21–40	41–75	+75	+95
Speeding in % of total time	—	+70	+50	+25	11–25	0–10
Moving violations in last 3 years	—	+5	3–5	2	1	0
Auto accidents in last 10 years	—	+5	3–5	2	1	0
Eating Habits						
Breakfast	—	0–2/m	−1/w	1–3/wk	4–6/wk	1/d
Meals, 3 moderate daily	—	0–2/m	−1/w	1–3/wk	4–6/wk	1/d
Snacking between meals	—	+2/d	+1/d	1/d	−1/d	−3/wk
Overeating	+2/d	+1/d	+3/wk	1–3/wk	−1/wk	−1/m
Eating within 2 hours of bed	—	1/d	4–6/wk	1–3/wk	−1/wk	−2/m
Eating rapidly	—	+2/d	+1/d	5–7/wk	2–4/wk	0–1/wk
Relaxing at meals	—	0–1/wk	2–4/w	5–7	+1/d	+2/d
Chewing thoroughly	—	0–1/wk	2–4/w	5–7	+1/d	+2/d
Fatigue after meals	—	+2/d	+1/d	2–7/wk	−2/wk	−1/m
Cleaning foods prior to eating	—	0–1/wk	−1/d	1/d	+1/d	+2/d
Eating organically grown foods	—	0–1/wk	−1/d	1/d	+1/d	+2/d
Restaurant meals	—	+1/d	+4/wk	1–4/wk	−1/wk	−2/m
Fasting on nutritious liquids (days per year)	—	0	1–3/y	+3/y	+7/y	+10/y
Substance Abuses						
Refined sugar* (1 tsp.)	—	+5/d	+1/d	1/d	−1/d	−1/wk
Other sugars (1tsp. honey, maple or corn syrup, fructose, etc.)	—	+6/d	+3/d	+1/d	1/d	0–1/d
Caffeine (1cup coffee, tea, soda)	—	+3/d	+1/d	1/d	−1/d	0–1/wk
Alcohol (1 drink)	+3/d	+2/d	1–2/d	−1/d	1–3/wk	0–1/m
Nicotine (1 pack)	+1/d	+3/wk	1–3/wk	−1/wk	−1/m	0
Secondary smoke (1 cigarette)	—	+9/d	1–9/d	−1/d	−1/wk	0
Column Subtotals						

Page Total

× $3,000 =

Forward Balance (from previous page)

New Balance
(enter as Forward Balance next page)

*Note: One average soda pop has over 5 teaspoons of sugar.

Code—0 = never, d = day, wk = week, m = month, y = year, + = more than (e.g., +7/wk = more than seven times per week), minus sign (−) = less than (e.g., −1/wk = less than once per week)

	−3	−2	−1	00	+1	+2
Marijuana (½ joint)	+3/d	+1/d	3–7/wk	−3/wk	−2/m	0
Narcotic drugs (e.g. codeine, Rx or street, 1 tablet or dose)	+3/d	2–3/d	1/d	−1/d	−1/m	0
Nonnarcotic drugs (1 dose)	—	+3/d	1–3/d	−1/d	−1/m	0
Television (hours/week)	—	+20	+10	8–10	4–7	0–3
Computer (hours/week)	—	+20	+10	8–10	4–7	0–3
Telephone (hours/week)	—	+20	+10	8–10	4–7	0–3
Column Subtotals						

Page Total
× $3,000 =
Forward Balance (from previous page)
New Balance
(enter as Forward Balance next page)

EXAMPLE

	−3	−2	−1	00	+1	+2
Narcotic drugs (e.g. codeine, Rx or street, 1 tablet or dose)	+3/d	2–3/d	1/d	−1/d	−1/m	(0)
Nonnarcotic drugs (1 dose)	—	+3/d	1–3/d	(−1/d)	−1/m	0
Television (hours/week)	—	(+20)	+10	8–10	4–7	0–3
Computer (hours/week)	—	(+20)	+10	8–10	4–7	0–3
Telephone (hours/week)	—	+20	(+10)	8–10	4–7	0–3
Column Subtotals		−4	−1	0		+2

Page Total | −3
× $3,000 = | −9,000
Sample Forward Balance | 229,000
New Balance | 220,000
(enter as Forward Balance next page)

Supplements

Answer yes or no under the appropriate column and then figure the total additions or subtractions. If a question or statement is inappropriate for you or you are indecisive over a simple yes or no, use 0 for that question.

	–2	–1	00	+1	+2
I use nutritional supplements regularly (at least 4 times a week) for preventive insurance.	no	—	—	—	yes
I use supplements regularly for optimal performance.	—	no	—	yes	—
I also observe myself and take special supplements when I sense I need them.	no	—	—	—	yes
When ill, I will take extra nutrients, such as:					
Vitamin C for colds or flus	—	no	—	yes	—
Zinc for sore throats	—	no	—	yes	—
B vitamins for stress	—	no	—	yes	—
Vitamin A for infections or skin problems	—	no	—	yes	—
I use herbs for healing or health support.	—	no	—	yes	—
When ill, I immediately turn to drugs, either prescription or over-the-counter.	yes	—	—	—	no
I am aware of supplement combinations and the best times to take specific nutrients.	—	no	—	yes	—
I am aware of safe intake levels for supplements I ingest.	—	no	—	yes	—
I take more than 20 tablets or capsules in the average day.	—	yes	—	no	—
I suggest supplements for others even though I may not know the person well.	—	yes	—	no	—

Emotional Interactions*

	–2	–1	00	+1	+2
My emotional life is connected to how I feel physically.	no	—	—	—	yes
I have people that I am close with to whom I can express my feelings.	no	—	—	—	yes
I have close friends or family.	—	no	—	yes	—
I have no one to talk to about my real feelings.	yes	—	—	—	no
I have regular affection in my life.	—	no	—	yes	—
Column Subtotals					

Page Total

× \$3,000 =

Forward Balance (from previous page)

New Balance

(enter as Forward Balance next page)

For interesting and R-rated questions about sexual/sensual activities and habits, see the Sextra Credit section at the end of the Health Bank Account.

1063

	−2	−1	00	+1	+2
I really love someone, and he or she also loves me.	—	no	—	yes	—
I express my feelings appropriately.	—	no	—	yes	—
I have deep frustrations or anger that influence how I feel and act.	—	yes	—	no	—
I can feel frustration, anger, or fear at times, then I deal with these and let them go.	—	no	—	yes	—
I am held back by my previous personal experiences.	yes	—	—	—	no
I have been able to understand, release, and forgive previous "negative" experiences.	no	—	—	—	yes
I respect my parents, and I had or do have good communication with them.	—	no	—	yes	—
I experience happiness or joy daily.	—	no	—	yes	—
I receive or give at least 3 hugs daily.	no	—	—	—	yes
I have intimate sensual or sexual experience that has meaning to me.	no	—	—	—	yes
Column Subtotals					

Page Total
× \$3,000 =
Forward Balance (from previous page)
New Balance
(enter as Forward Balance next page)

III. FAMILY HISTORY

	−2	−1	00	+1	+2
My family enjoys or enjoyed each other's company.	—	no	—	yes	—
Overall, treating each other with kindness was and is important in my family.	—	no	—	yes	—
I felt safe in the home in which I grew up.	no	—	—	—	yes
I was breastfed as an infant.	—	no	—	yes	—
In my family, we respect each other's opinions.	—	no	—	yes	—
I believe that overall I grew up with adequate to good self-esteem.	no	—	—	—	yes
My parent(s) were loving and nurturing to me.	—	no	—	—	yes
My parent(s) were good role models for me.	—	no	—	yes	—
My parent(s) were dissatisfied and lived beyond their means.	—	yes	—	no	—
There was much sibling rivalry in my family.	—	yes	—	no	—
My parent(s) or my sibling(s) were critical or negative with me.	—	yes	—	no	—
My parent(s) and sibling(s) allowed and even encouraged expression of feelings.	—	no	—	yes	—
My parent(s) read to me as a child.	—	no	—	yes	—
My parent(s) were "available" to me to discuss my feelings.	—	no	—	yes	—
I get (got) along with one parent much better than the other.	—	yes	—	no	—
I was open to the support and guidance that my parent(s) offered me.	—	no	—	yes	—
My parent(s) and family encouraged my growth and exploration.	—	no	—	yes	—
In my childhood, my family traveled together on outings or vacations at least twice yearly.	—	no	—	yes	—
One or both of my parents were "workaholics."	—	yes	—	no	—
Column Subtotals					

Page Total

× $3,000 =

Forward Balance (from previous page)

New Balance
(enter as Forward Balance next page)

1065

	−2	−1	00	+1	+2
My parents were divorced before I left home.	yes	—	—	no	—
My parents argued or fought often at home.	yes	—	—	no	—
Personal or family counseling improved our home life.	—	no	—	—	yes
I feel or felt like I should have been born into another family.	yes	—	—	no	—
My parents were very loving with each other at home.	—	no	—	—	yes
My parent(s) encouraged me to eat more than I needed.	—	yes	—	no	—
I believe my parent(s) fed me a good diet.	no	—	—	—	yes
My parent(s) rewarded me with sugar or other "treats."	—	yes	—	no	—
My family used guilt and blame in regard to me and my actions.	—	yes	—	no	—
In my upbringing, I was surrounded by the following activities:					
Alcohol abuse	yes	—	—	no	—
Smoking	yes	—	—	no	—
Verbal abuse	yes	—	—	no	—
Physical abuse	yes	—	—	no	—
Sexual abuse	yes	—	—	no	—
Drug abuse	yes	—	—	no	—
Money abuse	yes	—	—	no	—
Column Subtotals					

Page Total

× $3,000 =

Forward Balance (from previous page)

New Balance
(enter as Forward Balance next page)

Family Medical Factors

For the following diseases or problems, circle the appropriate number. Include your immediate family—parents, siblings, grandparents, and aunts or uncles.

	−3	−2	−1	00	+1	+2
Family longevity (succumbed to a disease before age 50)	+2	2	1	—	0	—
Parents (lived) over age 65	—	0	—	—	1	2
Grandparents lived over 65	—	0	1	2	3	4
Only count family members who had the following conditions prior to age 60:						
Heart disease	+2	2	1	—	0	—
High cholesterol	+2	2	1	—	0	—
Hypertension	+2	2	1	—	0	—
Cancer	+2	2	1	—	0	—
Diabetes	+2	2	1	—	0	—
Alcoholism/drug use	+2	2	1	—	0	—
Obesity	—	+2	1	—	0	—
Asthma	—	+2	1–2	0	—	—
Allergies or eczema	—	+2	1–2	0	—	—
Arthritis	—	+2	1–2	0	—	—
Ulcerative colitis	+2	2	1	0	—	—
Column Subtotals						

Page Total

× $3,000 =

Forward Balance (from previous page)

New Balance
(enter as Forward Balance next page)

IV. CURRENT HEALTH STATUS

	−3	−2	−1	00	+1	+2
Weight, by % from ideal.	+30	+20	+10	+5	1–5	0
(+ means over, − means under)	−20	−10	−5	—	—	—
I am satisfied with my energy level.	—	no	—	—	yes	—
I experience symptoms that interfere with my life activities and/or enjoyment.	—	+5/wk	+1/wk	1–4/m	−1/m	−2/y
Symptoms: # days per month						
Headaches	—	+10	+3	1–3	−1	−4/y
Allergies	—	+10	+3	1–3	−1	−4/y
Joint pains	—	+10	+3	1–3	−1	−4/y
Back pains	—	+10	+3	1–3	−1	−4/y
Fatigue	—	+10	+3	1–3	−1	−4/y
Chest pain	+5	+3	+1	1	−1/m	0
Shortness of breath	+10	+5	+1	1	−1/m	0
Abdominal pains	—	+5	+1	1	−1	0
Constipation/diarrhea	—	+10	+3	1–3	−1	−3/y
PMS (for men, irritability)	—	+5	+1	1	1–3/y	0
Colds or flus	—	+5	+2	+5/y	2–5/y	−2/y
I have a chronic condition that interferes with my life activities and enjoyment.	—	yes	—	—	no	—
Conditions:						
High blood pressure						
over 150/100	yes	—	—	no	—	—
over 140/90	—	yes	—	—	no	—
High cholesterol level						
over 250	yes	—	—	no	—	—
over 210	—	yes	—	—	no	—
Alcoholism	yes	—	—	no	—	—
Arthritis	—	yes	—	—	no	—
Asthma	—	yes	—	no	—	—
Heart disease	yes	—	—	—	no	—
Column Subtotals						

Page Total

× $3,000 =

Forward Balance (from previous page)

New Balance

(enter as Forward Balance next page)

	−3	−2	−1	00	+1	+2
Drug addiction	yes	—	—	—	no	—
Mental illness	—	yes	—	—	no	—
I am currently under treatment for some condition.	—	yes	—	—	no	—
I have an injury that inhibits my activity.	—	yes	—	—	no	—
I have had more than 3 injuries in the last year.	—	yes	—	—	no	—
Blood pressure level, systolic	+200 / —	+170 / 65–85	+150 / 86–95	126–150 / —	111–125 / —	96–110 / —
Blood pressure level, diastolic	+120 / —	+100 / −50	+90 / −60	81–90 / 60–64	71–80 / —	65–70 / —
Cholesterol level	+260 / —	+225 / 50–100	+200 / 101–129	181–199 / 131–139	165–180 / —	140–164 / —
HDL	0–30	31–35	36–40	41–45	46–55	+55
LDL	+180	+160	+140	+120	101–120	50–100
Cholesterol/HDL ratio	+10	+8	+6	4.6–6.0	3.1– 4.5	1–3
LDL/HDL ratio	+6	+5	+4	3.1–4	2.3–3.0	−2.3
Elimination/bowel function *weekly* ⎫ Circle one only *daily* ⎭	−1 / —	1–2 / +4	3–4 / +3	5 / +2	6 / —	— / 1–2
Constipation and/or diarrhea (% of time)	—	+50	+10	6–10	3–5	0–2
Stools normal in shape and color	—	—	no	—	yes	—
Cigarette smoking (cigs./day)	+40	+20	+5	1–5	−1	0
I have stopped smoking.	—	—	—	no	—	yes
Caffeine use (cups/day)	+4	+2	1–2	−1	−1/wk	−1/m
Decaffeinated coffee use (caffeine coffee users skip this question)	—	+3	+2	1–2	−1/wk	−1/m
Alcohol intake (drinks/day)	+3	+2	1–2	−1	−1/wk	−1/m
Column Subtotals						

Page Total ☐
× $3,000 = ☐
Forward Balance (from previous page) ☐
New Balance ☐
(enter as Forward Balance next page)

1069

	−2	−1	00	+1	+2
I am currently in a positive personal, intimate relationship.	—	no	—	yes	—
I have been divorced or had a significant relationship breakup.	yes	—	—	no	—
Marriage has been a positive experience for me.	no	—	—	—	yes
I have had other marriages or significant relationships that were not positive.	yes	—	—	no	—
Having children has been a positive experience for me.	—	no	—	—	yes
I have had or been involved in pregnancies which terminated in miscarriage or abortion.	yes	—	—	no	—
I have not had children and wished I had, or had them and wished I hadn't.	yes	—	—	no	—
I have overcome a disease by adapting new behavior.	—	—	no	—	yes
I have experienced needed weight reduction in the last year.	—	—	no	—	yes
I need to lose weight but have not been able to accomplish that.	—	yes	—	no	—
I have made some positive behavioral changes in the last year.	no	—	—	—	yes
I feel I maintain a good emotional balance.	—	no	—	yes	—
Column Subtotals					

Page Total

× $3,000 =

Forward Balance (from previous page)

New Balance
(enter as Forward Balance next page)

V. DIET

	−3	−2	−1	00	+1	+2
Meals per day	0	+4	1	4	2	3
I have snacks regularly, and I am overweight.	yes	—	—	no	—	—
I have a generally balanced diet.	—	no	—	—	—	yes
I prepare my own meals, % of total.	0	1–20	21–40	+40	+60	+80
I eat meals at a restaurant, % of total.	+80	+60	+30	16–30	6–15	0–5
I do food shopping for myself and/or my family.	—	no	—	—	yes	—
I am aware of the seasonal availability of foods and shop accordingly.	—	no	—	—	—	yes
I eat meals made from wholesome, natural foods (%).	0	1–25	26–50	+50	+70	+90
I use fresh, local produce when available.	—	no	—	—	—	yes
I eat completely vegetarian meals.	0	1–3/wk	4–6/wk	1/d	+1/d	+2/d
I take care to eat many fiber-containing foods, i.e., whole grains and vegetables.	—	no	—	—	—	yes
I eat meals containing animal products, i.e., meats, dairy, or eggs at least twice a day.	—	yes	—	—	no	—
I am careful not to overeat at or between meals.	—	no	—	—	—	yes
I rotate a variety of foods in my diet rather than consuming just a few.	—	no	—	—	—	yes
Column Subtotals						

Page Total

× $3,000 =

Forward Balance (from previous page)

New Balance
(enter as Forward Balance next page)

1071

	−3	−2	−1	00	+1	+2
I follow the principles of food combining.	—	no	—	—	—	yes
I follow the philosophy of undereating, yet I use wholesome foods.	—	no	—	—	—	yes
Food Choices						
Processed meats	+1/d	+2/wk	1–2/wk	−1/wk	−1/m	0
Fast foods	+1/d	+1/wk	+2/m	+1/m	−1/m	−3/y
Soda pops (w/sugar or chem.)	—	+1/d	+4/wk	1–4/wk	−1/wk	−1/m
Sugar-containing foods	—	+3/d	+1/d	4–7/wk	2–3/wk	−1/wk
Highly salted foods	—	+3/d	+1/d	4–7/wk	2–3/wk	−1/wk
Red meats	—	+3/wk	1–3/wk	1–3/m	−1/m	1–4/y
Fried foods	—	+7/wk	4–7/wk	1–3/wk	−1/wk	−1/m
Dairy products (whole milk)	—	+3/d	+2/d	+1/d	4–7/wk	−4/wk
Ice cream	+1/d	+4/wk	+1/wk	2–4/m	−2/m	−1/m
Baked goods, refined flour*	—	+7/wk	4–7/wk	2–3/wk	1/wk	−1/wk
Baked goods, whole grain*	—	+2/d	+1/d	5–7/wk	2–4/wk	−2/wk
Whole grains, cooked/sprouted	—	0–2/wk	−1/d	1/d	2/d	3/d
Vegetables, all (portions)	0	−1/d	1/d	+1/d	+2/d	+4/d
Vegetables, green (portions)	—	0–1/wk	2–3/wk	4–7/wk	+1/d	+3/d
Fruits, all (portions)	0	−3/wk	3–6/wk	1/d	2–3/d	+3/d
Sprouts	—	0–1/wk	2–3/wk	4–6/wk	1–2/d	+2/d
Raw nuts or seeds (handful) *weekly* } Circle one only	—	−1	−3	—	—	—
daily	—	+4	+2	−1	1	2
Food Preparations— Consumption of						
Fresh, whole foods (portions)	0	1–3/wk	4–6/wk	1–2/d	3–4/d	+4/d
Steamed or baked (portions)	—	−2/wk	3–6/wk	1/d	+1/d	+2/d
Frozen processed meals	—	+1/d	+4/wk	1–4/wk	−1/wk	−1/m
Column Subtotals						

Page Total ☐

× $3,000 = ☐

Forward Balance (from previous page) ☐

New Balance ☐
(enter as Forward Balance next page)

*Includes bread

	−3	−2	−1	00	+1	+2
Canned foods	—	+3/d	+2/d	1–2/d	−1/d	−1/wk
Processed foods	+2/d	+1/d	+4/wk	1–4/wk	−1/wk	0–1/m
Deep-fried foods	+2/d	+1/d	+4/wk	1–4/wk	−1/wk	0–1/m
Reheated foods	—	—	+1/d	+4/wk	1–4/wk	0–3/m
Microwaved foods	—	+2/d	+1/d	1/d	−2/wk	−2/m
Number of different foods/ meal, average	—	+12	+10	+8	6–8	1–5
Water intake, cups/day	0	1–2	3–4	5–6	+6	+8
Chemicals in foods	+3/d	+2/d	+1/d	5–7/wk	3–4/wk	0–2/wk
I take time to eat, and I chew my food well.	—	no	—	—	—	yes
I take time to relax during my meals.	—	no	—	—	—	yes
I eat the majority of my food before sundown.	—	—	no	—	—	yes
Column Subtotals						

Page Total ☐
× $3,000 = ☐
Forward Balance (from previous page) ☐
New Balance ☐
(enter as Forward Balance next page)

VI. HOME

	−2	−1	00	+1	+2
I feel comfortable and secure in my home and neighborhood.	no	—	—	—	yes
My neighborhood is dangerous or unclean.	—	yes	—	no	—
My neighborhood is either noisy or very close to a main road.	—	yes	—	no	—
I live in an area where exposure to agricultural chemicals or environmental pollution is likely.	yes	—	—	no	—
The industry around me pollutes the local air.	yes	—	—	no	—
My home is near electrical power lines.	yes	—	—	no	—
I sleep well in my home.	—	no	—	—	yes
I am interrupted by other people's sleep patterns.	—	yes	—	no	—
My sleep or rest is interrupted by home noises, such as the refrigerator hum or TV sounds.	—	yes	—	no	—
My home is filled with many electrical appliances.	—	yes	—	no	—
On any day, I use more than 10 electrical appliances, including 'fridge, TV, stove, clocks, computers, etc.	—	yes	—	no	—
I have forced air heating or cooling systems.	—	yes	—	no	—
Due to the climate in which I live, heating or cooling are needed in my home more than six months of the year.	—	yes	—	no	—
In my home, a microwave oven is used at least daily.	—	yes	—	no	—
For cooking, we use exclusively glass, ceramic, iron, or other safe materials.	—	no	—	yes	—
I avoid cooking food in aluminum or highly-treated cookware, such as Teflon.	—	no	—	yes	—
The structure and inner contents of my home may expose me to these toxic substances:					
Asbestos	yes	—	no	—	—
Synthetic fibers from rugs or furniture	—	yes	—	no	—
Paints, glues, and adhesives	yes	—	no	—	—
Radon	yes	—	no	—	—
Column Subtotals					

Page Total

× $3,000 =

Forward Balance (from previous page)

New Balance
(enter as Forward Balance next page)

	−2	−1	00	+1	+2
The majority of lighting in my home is from incandescent or full-spectrum bulbs.	—	no	—	—	yes
I totally avoid the use of aerosol sprays.	no	—	—	yes	—
I never use deodorant sprays and encourage others to avoid them.	—	no	—	yes	—
I would support legislation to make aerosol sprays illegal in public places.	—	no	—	yes	—
I am aware of the potential toxicity of synthetic cosmetics and attempt to use more natural ones that are also not tested on animals.	—	no	—	—	yes
I use chemical solvents for cleaning supplies.	yes	—	—	no	—
I/we maintain a clean home, especially the kitchen and bathroom(s).	no	—	—	—	yes
My home is cleaned thoroughly at least twice monthly.	—	no	—	yes	—
I, or my mate, specifically clean the kitchen counters regularly after meal preparation.	—	no	—	yes	—
I have a covered garbage container and empty it regularly.	—	no	—	yes	—
I separate my trash for recycling paper, glass, and cans.	no	—	—	—	yes
I have a compost pile for recycling organic waste.	—	no	—	—	yes
I am willing to go out of my way for safe disposal of potentially toxic products, such as motor oil, batteries, or chemicals.	no	—	—	—	yes
I store all prescription medicines and home chemicals out of the reach of children.	no	—	—	yes	—
I especially try to avoid pest spraying and the use of any toxic chemicals or paints in my children's rooms and my own bedroom.	no	—	—	yes	—
If I have pets, I check them out for parasites and worms at least yearly.	—	no	—	yes	—
I am careful to not let children play too close with my pet or near the litterbox.	—	no	—	yes	—

Column Subtotals

Page Total

× $3,000 =

Forward Balance (from previous page)

New Balance
(enter as Forward Balance next page)

VII. WORK (and Workout)

	−2	−1	00	+1	+2
The level of J-O-Y at my J-O-B (0–10)	0–2	3–4	5–6	+6	+8
I think positively about work in my time off.	—	no	—	yes	—
I look forward to going back to work on Monday.	—	no	—	—	yes
I am very bored at work and wish I could do something else.	—	yes	—	no	—
I am not really qualified for the work that I do, or I am overqualified.	—	yes	—	no	—
I have a fair amount of freedom or flexibility at my job.	—	no	—	—	yes
I experience some personal harassment at work.	—	yes	—	no	—
I work for myself and enjoy it.	—	no	—	—	yes
I have stress at work in these areas:					
Personality tensions that affect my work	—	yes	—	no	—
Wonderful cooperation among coworkers	—	no	—	yes	—
Time demands—more than I like giving	—	yes	—	no	—
Performance demands—more than I like	—	yes	—	no	—
Travel for work by airplane	+1/wk	+1/m	1/m	−1/m	−4/y
Car time for work—hours/day	+3	+2	+1	0.6–1	0–0.5
Commute time—avg. hours/day	+2	+1	0.5–1	−0.5	0–0.25
I use mass transit and can relax on my way to work (bus, train, ferry).	—	no	—	—	yes
I have two weeks or more vacation time and enjoy getting away.	no	—	—	—	yes
I have a car phone and use it often for work.	—	yes	—	no	—
I have significant electrical exposure at work.	yes	—	—	no	—
I use a fax machine and a computer at work.	—	yes	—	no	—
I work in a smoke-filled environment.	yes	—	—	no	—
There is some artificial temperature control (heating/cooling) at work at least 6 m/yr.	yes	—	—	no	—
Column Subtotals					

Page Total   [ ]

× $3,000 =   [ ]

Forward Balance (from previous page)   [ ]

New Balance   [ ]
(enter as Forward Balance next page)

	-2	-1	00	+1	+2
The air quality at work is very good.	—	no	—	yes	—
I work in an environment that provides natural light and fresh air.	—	no	—	—	yes
I work under fluorescent lights.	yes	—	—	no	—
The noise level at work is uncomfortable.	yes	—	—	no	—
My office is adjacent to a freeway or busy road.	—	yes	—	no	—
My office has a nice view and a natural setting in which I can walk on my breaks.	—	no	—	—	yes
I am exposed to smells (perfumes, chemicals) that affect me.	yes	—	—	no	—
Purified water is available to me at work.	—	no	—	yes	—
Good food is available to me at work or I bring my own nutritious meal.	—	no	—	—	yes
Toxin/chemical exposure:					
I personally use chemicals in my work.	yes	—	—	no	—
I use White Out or a similar product.	—	yes	—	no	—
I am exposed to chemicals used in my office by others.	yes	—	—	no	—
There is asbestos in the office structure.	yes	—	—	no	—
There are relatively new synthetic carpets or furniture in my office.	yes	—	—	no	—
Column Subtotals					

Page Total

× $3,000 =

Forward Balance (from previous page)

New Balance
(enter as Forward Balance next page)

VIII. EARTH—ENVIRONMENT

This section values your environmental awareness and activities in conserving resources and reducing wastes. It is important that we are all involved in these endeavors. Thank you.

	−2	−1	00	+1	+2
I am aware of and appreciate the need to maintain balance of Earth and its resources.	no	—	—	yes	—
I have been REcycling materials for 5 years.	—	no	—	—	yes
I have REcycling available in my area.	—	no	—	yes	—
I have curbside pickup for REcycled materials and I use it.	—	no	—	—	yes
I do not have curbside pickup, yet I still go out of my way to REcycle.	—	no	—	—	yes
I am aware of the concept of PREcycling—purchasing REcyclable products and minimally packaged products.	—	no	—	yes	—
I avoid purchasing products that are not REcyclable, i.e., plastics and chemical products.	—	no	—	—	yes
The following products I recycle at least monthly:					
Newspaper	—	no	—	—	yes
Other papers, junk mail	—	no	—	—	yes
Bottles	no	—	—	—	yes
Cans	no	—	—	—	yes
I try to conserve paper (and trees) by using it for scrap or using both sides.	—	no	—	—	yes
I have invested in tree replanting or donated to groups that replant or protect trees.	—	no	—	—	yes
I minimize my use of plastics and attempt to reuse what I have.	—	no	—	—	yes
If and when plastics become REcyclable, I will participate in this.	—	no	—	yes	—
I currently reuse the plastic bags that I get from the grocery or other stores.	—	no	—	—	yes
I minimize the use of chemicals that I know damage the environment.	—	no	—	—	yes
Column Subtotals					

Page Total

× $3,000 =

Forward Balance (from previous page)

New Balance
(enter as Forward Balance next page)

	−2	−1	00	+1	+2
If I change my own motor oil or use other hazardous environmental chemicals, I find safe ways to REcycle them—or I don't use them.	—	no	—	—	yes
I am aware of what my auto mechanic does with my old motor oil.	—	no	—	yes	—
I have a garden at home and grow food or flowers.	—	no	—	—	yes
I do not spray my garden, plants, or home with chemical pesticides.	no	—	—	—	yes
I would gladly participate in a community garden, or I already do.	—	no	—	—	yes
I have some composting area in my garden or yard in which to REcycle our food scraps.	—	no	—	—	yes
I regularly shop in a local farmer's market to purchase the freshest produce.	—	no	—	—	yes
I take my own bags to shop at the markets.	—	no	—	—	yes
I walk or hike in nature regularly.	no	—	—	—	yes
I also do other nonpolluting activities.	—	no	—	yes	—
I spend time observing or relating to the trees, plants, flowers, or animals.	no	—	—	—	yes
At home or work, I am aware of the need to conserve water.	—	no	—	yes	—
I do conserve water in as many areas as possible.	no	—	—	—	yes
I turn off the water while brushing my teeth, shaving, or in other activities when appropriate.	—	no	—	—	yes
I keep my auto maintained for optimum efficiency with regular checkups.	no	—	—	—	yes
The car I drive gets at least an average of 20 miles per gallon of gas.	no	—	—	—	yes
I maintain insurance on my auto.	—	no	—	yes	—
I have my car smog checked as regularly appropriate.	no	—	—	—	yes
Column Subtotals					

Page Total

× $3,000 =

Forward Balance (from previous page)

New Balance

(enter as Forward Balance next page)

1079

	−2	−1	00	+1	+2
If maintenance problems occur with my auto, such as an oil leak, I have it repaired immediately.	no	—	—	yes	—
I have some alternative to electricity, such as solar energy, at home.	—	no	—	—	yes
I invest more in environmental groups than in other areas of the economy.	—	no	—	—	yes
I have and will vote for issues that support the environment even if it costs me money.	no	—	—	—	yes
I do and will support politicians that support the environment.	no	—	—	—	yes
Column Subtotals					

Page Total

× \$3,000 =

Forward Balance (from previous page)

New Balance
(enter as Forward Balance next page)

IX. MISCELLANEOUS

Here are a few extra questions in the area of health, stress, and relaxation. If you are good to yourself, you'll be able to add some money to your Health Bank Account.

	−2	−1	00	+1	+2
My basic approach to illness is to take medicines when I have problems.	—	yes	—	no	—
When I become ill, my first approach is to stop, look, and listen to my life.	—	no	—	yes	—
I am willing to try natural approaches to medical problems first before drugs.	—	no	—	yes	—
I have tried nutritional, supplemental, herbal, or homeopathic approaches to medical concerns.	—	no	—	yes	—
I have massage or some other body therapy at least four times yearly.	—	no	—	yes	—
I trust my doctor/practitioner and believe I am in knowledgeable, competent hands.	no	—	—	—	yes
Overall, I enjoy my life and experience true pleasure in some important areas.	—	no	—	—	yes
I laugh at least daily.	—	no	—	—	yes
I take time away from work to play or have a good time.	—	no	—	—	yes
I have at least one healthy hobby that I enjoy.	no	—	—	yes	—
I take time to be in nature at least weekly and take several excursions yearly.	—	no	—	—	yes
I have learned and use some form of relaxation, stress reduction, or meditation regularly.	—	no	—	—	yes
I am able to express my feelings at both home and work.	—	no	—	yes	—
My feelings/emotions are something I value and will invest in keeping them harmonious.	—	no	—	—	yes

Column Subtotals

Page Total

× $3,000 =

Forward Balance (from previous page)

New Balance
(enter as Forward Balance next page)

X. SEXTRA CREDIT

For "*Sextraterrestrials*"—earthling-bound individuals involved in the personal interactive sexual experience for the art of sensuality, sport, and/or the instigation of the life-giving process of procreation.

If you are offended by sexual topics, skip this sextion and go to the end of this questionnaire, but subtract $25,000 from your total. Really, though, there are only about sexty questions in this sextion and you could easily make a couple hundred thou for your bank account.

Try it, you may have fun.

	−2	−1	00	+1	+2
I basically trust people.	no	—	—	—	yes
I enjoy my sexual life.	—	no	—	yes	—
I am a virgin, but I am interested in sex.	—	no	—	yes	—
I learned about sex in a healthy manner from my parents, school, or trusted other.	—	no	—	—	yes
I believe I have the appropriate frequency of sexual activity for me.	no	—	—	—	yes
I am divorced or separated and do not have a sexual partner currently.	yes	—	—	no	—
Other activities excite me as much as sex.	—	no	—	yes	—
My first sexual experience was drug or alcohol induced.	—	yes	—	no	—
I can only now have sex with some form of intoxication.	yes	—	—	no	—
I am only able to have sex under the covers or with the lights out.	—	yes	—	no	—
I have sexual problems and am afraid to become too close with others.	yes	—	—	no	—
I have had sexual problems and have done therapy to help me.	—	no	—	—	yes
I have been involved as one of the partners with an abortion.	—	yes	—	no	—
I am ashamed of my body.	—	yes	—	no	—
I have done things for which I am ashamed.	—	yes	—	no	—
Column Subtotals					

Page Total

× $2,000 =

Forward Balance (from previous page)

New Balance
(enter as Forward Balance next page)

	−2	−1	00	+1	+2
I sleep almost always alone.	yes	—	—	no	—
I have only one sexual partner.	—	no	—	—	yes
I have more than one sexual partner currently.	—	yes	—	no	—
I most often sleep with my pet.	—	yes	—	no	—
I actually sleep with my partner, kids, and pet.	—	no	—	—	yes
I practice safe sex to prevent getting infections.	no	—	—	—	yes
I know the sexual and health history of any sexual partner.	no	—	—	yes	—
I trust my partner(s) are well informed.	no	—	—	yes	—
I tell the truth to my sexual partners.	no	—	—	—	yes
I clean myself after most sexual experiences.	—	no	—	—	yes
I have had more than one sexually transmitted disease (STD).	—	yes	—	no	—
I currently have an STD which is being treated.	—	yes	—	no	—
I have a chronic, untreatable STD.	yes	—	—	no	—
If I am sexually active, I have regular medical exams and tests to make sure I am "clean."	—	no	—	—	yes
I do not engage in sexual practice because I choose to be celibate and enjoy the benefits of that.	—	no	—	—	yes
I am aware of spiritual sexual practices, such as tantric sex.	—	no	—	yes	—
I am aware of the Oriental philosophy of sexual practice.	—	no	—	yes	—
I have read books and practiced some of these sexual energy practices.	—	no	—	—	yes
I feel I have an appropriate level of sexual energy.	no	—	—	—	yes
I usually feel more invigorated and balanced after sexual experiences.	no	—	—	—	yes
I feel let down, irritable, or fatigued on the following day after sex.	yes	—	—	no	—
I have very special sexual fantasies.	—	no	—	yes	—
I would rather dream about them than do them.	—	yes	—	—	no
Some of my fantasies have become reality.	—	no	—	—	yes
Column Subtotals					

Page Total

× $2,000 =   2400

Forward Balance (from previous page)

New Balance

(enter as Forward Balance next page)

1083

	−2	−1	00	+1	+2
I have some beautiful sexual memories.	—	no	—	—	yes
I have wet dreams more than I have sex.	—	yes	—	no	—
I enjoy sexual activities outdoors in nature.	—	no	—	yes	—
Most often when I am having a sexual/personal experience, I am right there with it.	—	no	—	—	yes
I have certain foods that put me in the mood for sex.	—	no	—	yes	—
Watching things melt really turns me on.	—	no	—	yes	—
I know how to get my partner in the mood.	—	no	—	—	yes
I know how to communicate with my partner about our sexual life.	no	—	—	—	yes
I do not know what I want in sex.	—	yes	—	no	—
My desire for sex is similar to my partner's.	no	—	—	—	yes
My partner and I are both able to be thoroughly satisfied with our lovemaking.	no	—	—	—	yes
We really enjoy each other's company other than having sex.	no	—	—	—	yes
We have strong emotional bonds outside of sexual activity.	—	no	—	—	yes
We both enjoy a similar amount of foreplay.	—	no	—	—	yes
In most every sexual experience, my partner and I use multiple positions.	—	no	—	yes	—
I am willing to experiment with new positions.	—	no	—	yes	—
I hold and comfort my partner before and/or after our sexual experience.	no	—	—	—	yes
I am too passionate and need more than my partner.	yes	—	—	no	—
I am interested in sex primarily as a sport.	—	yes	—	no	—
I use sexual aids to enliven my sexual joys.	—	no	—	yes	—
The following items are in my home or that of my partner and are used at least on occasion.					
Lingerie	—	no	—	yes	—
Lace	—	no	—	yes	—
Feathers	—	no	—	yes	—

Column Subtotals

Page Total

× $2,000 =

Forward Balance (from previous page)

New Balance
(enter as Forward Balance next page)

1084

	−2	−1	00	+1	+2
Condoms	—	no	—	yes	—
Videotapes	—	no	—	yes	—
Vibrators	—	no	—	yes	—
Ice cubes	—	no	—	yes	—
Body paint	—	no	—	yes	—
Cameras	—	no	—	yes	—
Massage oils	—	no	—	yes	—
Ceiling mirrors	—	no	—	yes	—
Bubbles	—	no	—	yes	—
Hair dryer	—	no	—	yes	—
I feel that I have unhealthy sexual urges.	yes	—	—	no	—
I enjoy sex in water.	—	no	—	yes	—
I am aware of being turned on according to moon cycles.	—	no	—	yes	—
I enjoy whipped cream and honey.	—	no	—	yes	—
For me, music and sex enhance one another.	—	no	—	yes	—
Essensuality and toe sucking mean the same thing.	—	no	—	yes	—
I enjoy sex in moving vehicles (driver not included).	—	no	—	yes	—
Money turns me on.	—	no	—	yes	—
I have had intimate encounters with sextraterrestrials.	—	no	—	yes	—
I laugh and cry during sex.	—	no	—	yes	—
I love the aromas of sensuality.	—	no	—	yes	—
I enjoy being dominated.	—	no	—	yes	—
I enjoy dominating.	—	no	—	yes	—
I enjoy watching erotic film scenes.	—	no	—	yes	—
I have special clothing for sensual and sexual purposes.	—	no	—	yes	—
This special sextion has improved my HBA score, because I was nearly bankrupt before.	—	no	—	—	yes

Column Subtotals

Since there are so many Sextra Credit questions, each is valued at only $2,000.

Page Total

× $2,000 =

Forward Balance (from previous page)

Grand Total

Yes, you could come near to being a health two-millionaire with a near perfect score, yet we will be totally amazed if anyone is able to break the 1.8 million dollar mark.

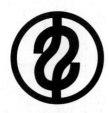

Part I: Answers—True-False

	True	False		True	False		True	False
1.	☐	☑	30.	☑	☐	59.	☐	☑
2.	☐	☑	31.	☑	☐	60.	☑	☐
3.	☑	☐	32.	☐	☑	61.	☑	☐
4.	☑	☐	33.	☑	☐	62.	☐	☑
5.	☑	☐	34.	☑	☐	63.	☑	☐
6.	☐	☑	35.	☐	☑	64.	☑	☐
7.	☐	☑	36.	☑	☐	65.	☑	☐
8.	☑	☐	37.	☐	☑	66.	☑	☐
9.	☑	☐	38.	☑	☐	67.	☑	☐
10.	☐	☑	39.	☑	☐	68.	☐	☑
11.	☑	☐	40.	☑	☐	69.	☑	☐
12.	☑	☐	41.	☑	☐	70.	☑	☐
13.	☐	☑	42.	☐	☑	71.	☑	☐
14.	☑	☐	43.	☑	☐	72.	☑	☐
15.	☐	☑	44.	☑	☐	73.	☑	☐
16.	☑	☐	45.	☑	☐	74.	☐	☑
17.	☑	☐	46.	☑	☐	75.	☑	☐
18.	☐	☑	47.	☐	☑	76.	☑	☐
19.	☐	☑	48.	☑	☐	77.	☑	☐
20.	☑	☐	49.	☑	☐	78.	☐	☑
21.	☑	☐	50.	☑	☐	79.	☐	☑
22.	☐	☑	51.	☑	☐	80.	☑	☐
23.	☑	☐	52.	☑	☐	81.	☑	☐
24.	☐	☑	53.	☐	☑	82.	☐	☑
25.	☑	☐	54.	☑	☐	83.	☐	☑
26.	☐	☑	55.	☑	☐	84.	☑	☐
27.	☑	☐	56.	☑	☐	85.	☑	☐
28.	☐	☑	57.	☑	☐	86.	☑	☐
29.	☐	☑	58.	☑	☐	87.	☑	☐

#	True	False		#	True	False		#	True	False
88.	☑	☐		126.	☐	☑		164.	☐	☑
89.	☑	☐		127.	☐	☑		165.	☑	☐
90.	☑	☐		128.	☑	☐		166.	☑	☐
91.	☐	☑		129.	☐	☑		167.	☐	☑
92.	☐	☑		130.	☑	☐		168.	☐	☑
93.	☑	☐		131.	☑	☐		169.	☑	☐
94.	☑	☐		132.	☑	☐		170.	☐	☑
95.	☐	☑		133.	☐	☑		171.	☐	☑
96.	☑	☐		134.	☐	☑		172.	☐	☑
97.	☑	☐		135.	☐	☑		173.	☐	☑
98.	☐	☑		136.	☐	☑		174.	☐	☑
99.	☐	☑		137.	☐	☑		175.	☐	☑
100.	☑	☐		138.	☑	☐		176.	☑	☐
101.	☐	☑		139.	☑	☐		177.	☑	☐
102.	☐	☑		140.	☑	☐		178.	☑	☐
103.	☐	☑		141.	☐	☑		179.	☑	☐
104.	☑	☐		142.	☐	☑		180.	☑	☐
105.	☐	☑		143.	☐	☑		181.	☐	☑
106.	☐	☑		144.	☐	☑		182.	☐	☑
107.	☐	☑		145.	☑	☐		183.	☐	☑
108.	☑	☐		146.	☐	☑		184.	☑	☐
109.	☐	☑		147.	☐	☑		185.	☑	☐
110.	☑	☐		148.	☑	☐		186.	☑	☐
111.	☐	☑		149.	☑	☐		187.	☑	☐
112.	☐	☑		150.	☑	☐		188.	☐	☑
113.	☐	☑		151.	☑	☐		189.	☑	☐
114.	☑	☐		152.	☑	☐		190.	☐	☑
115.	☑	☐		153.	☐	☑		191.	☑	☐
116.	☐	☑		154.	☑	☐		192.	☑	☐
117.	☐	☑		155.	☐	☑		193.	☑	☐
118.	☐	☑		156.	☑	☐		194.	☑	☐
119.	☑	☐		157.	☐	☑		195.	☑	☐
120.	☐	☑		158.	☑	☐		196.	☑	☐
121.	☐	☑		159.	☐	☑		197.	☑	☐
122.	☐	☑		160.	☑	☐		198.	☐	☑
123.	☑	☐		161.	☑	☐		199.	☐	☑
124.	☑	☐		162.	☑	☐				
125.	☐	☑		163.	☑	☐				

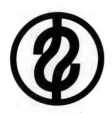

Part I: Answers—Multiple Choice

1. a, b, e, g
2. Fructose __e__   Lactose __a__
   Sucrose __b__   Mannose __c__
   Maltose __d__
3. a, b, c, e
4. b
5. Saturated a, c, d, f
   Unsaturated b, e, f
6. b
7. Carcinogenic c, d, g, h, i
   Cancer-preventive a, b, e, f, j, k
8. f
9. Chylomicrons d   VLDL a
   LDL c   HDL b
10. b
11. a, e, f
12. a, b, c, f
13. Water a, d, f   Fat b, c, e
14. c
15. c, d, e, i
16. a, c, d, g, h
17. d
18. a, b, g
19. a
20. c
21. b
22. a, b, d, g
23. c
24. c
25. e, h

26. b
27. b, d, f
28. d, f
29. a
30. a, b, j
31. b, c, h, i, l
32. e
33. b
34. a, e, g, h
35. b
36. c, d, h
37. a, b, c, e, g
38. d
39. d
40. a, c, e, g
41. c, e, j, k
42. b
43. c
44. b, c, g
45. c
46. b
47. b, c, f, g
48. a
49. a
50. b, c
51. a
52. c
53. b
54. b
55. e, f

56.   b, c

57. Hormones _a_   Enzymes _b_
    Antibodies _c_

58.   b

59.   b

60.   a, b, d

61.   a

62. Royal Jelly _b_   Propolis _a_
    Bee Pollen _c_

63.   b, c

64. Dates _c_   Prunes _a_
    Raisins _d_   Apricots _b_

65.   b, d, f, j

66.   a, d

67.   c, d, g, h

68.   b, c, d

69.   a, c

70.   c, d, g

71.   b, c, g, i

72.   b, e, f

73.   a, c, e

74.   a, b, c, g

75.   b

76.   a

77.   c, e, f, g

78.   a, f, g

79.   b, e, h

80.   a, e, h, i, j

81.   c

82.   d

83.   b, d, h, i

84.   e

85.   a, c, d, f

86.   a, c, e, g

87.   a, b, c, f

88.   a, b, c, g

89.   a, e, f, g

90.   b

91.   c

92.   c

93.   c

94.   a

95.   c

96.   b, c, d

97.   a, d, e, f

98.   c

99.   b

100.   c

101. Acid _b, c, d, h, j_
    Alkaline _a, e, f, g, i_

102.   a, b, g

103.   a, c

104.   b, c, f, g

105.   c

106.   c

107.   c

108.   c

109. Methyl bromide _b_
    Ethylene gas _a_
    Sulfur dioxide _c_

110.   b

111.   c

112.   c

113. Flavoring _b_
    Natural coloring agent _c_
    Preservative _g_
    Alkali _h_
    Bleaching agent _i_
    Moisture controller _f_
    Activity controller _e_
    Emulsifier _d_
    Texturizer _j_
    Nutritional additive _a_

114.   b, c, d, f, i

115.   a, d, f, i, j, k

116.   a

APPENDIX

Laboratories and Clinical Nutrition Tests

There are, of course, medical labs in most cities and within hospitals. Realize though, that there is current concern over the accuracy of many of these laboratories, and continuous, rigorous quality control is very important.

The following is a list of some of the clinical laboratories that provide the specialized tests I use in my practice; other labs that I do not use or use infrequently are also included because of particular nutritional interest. There are, of course, many other laboratories all over the United States that provide specialized testing. I have no financial interest in any of these labs, nor did any pay to be listed in this book; they are here to help spread the word about nutritional medicine.

LABS

Aeron Life Cycles
1933 Davis St., Suite 310
San Leandro, CA 94577
800-631-7900

Aeron specializes in the measurement of many bodily hormones through samples of saliva.

Antibody Assay Laboratories, Inc.
1715 E. Wilshire, #715
Santa Ana, CA 92705
800-522-2611

AAL performs a variety of immune, viral and biochemical tests, both basic and innovative, for practitioners who see complicated patients with chronic fatigue and chemical sensitivities.

Bay Area Laboratory Cooperative (BALCO)
1520 Gilbreth Rd.
Burlingame, CA 94010
800-777-7122

A popular California mineral lab that analyzes samples of blood, hair, urine, and water for levels of trace minerals and toxic minerals, and has been doing special assessments for athletes.

Chiralt Clinical Laboratories, Inc.
15644 Pomerado Rd., Suites F-S
Poway, CA 92064
800-354-2522

Chiralt Labs runs the special NutriProbe test, which measures mineral (elements) levels from cells in the mouth through a simple, painless collection procedure.

Diagnos-Techs, Inc.
6620 South 192nd Pl., Suite J-104
Kent, WA 98032
800-878-3787

Diagnos-Techs specializes in a wide variety of progressive medical and health testing, including the Adrenal Stress Index (ASI) saliva measurements of sequential cortisol levels, other salivary hormone (DHEA and female hormones) measurements, and many gastrointestinal tests.

Doctor's Data
170 W. Roosevelt Rd.
West Chicago, IL 60185
800-323-2784

A specialized lab for mineral levels, both essential (nutritional) and toxic minerals, which can be assessed in the blood (whole blood, plasma, or red blood cells), urine, and hair. Levels of minerals in water can also be measured if there is some concern over excessive quantities. Doctor's Data also performs a very specific amino acid profile. Mineral balances are very important for optimum body function and tissue health. Adequate levels in the body are also a result of a good diet and effective digestion and assimilation. Measuring at least blood and hair levels is part of the nutritional fine-tuning that I like to do for patients. Looking for deficiencies of such minerals as zinc, copper, magnesium, or manganese, as well as excessive levels of lead, mercury, or cadmium helps us to individualize the food and supplemental needs of each patient. (See samples of whole blood and hair mineral tests following this list.)

Great Smokies Diagnostic Laboratory
63 Zillicoa St.
Asheville, NC 28801
800-522-4762

Great Smokies does one of my favorite tests of recent years, the Comprehensive Digestive Stool Analysis (CDSA). This test evaluates the function and ecology of the digestive tract with more than 20 tests, including food components remaining in the stool, the biochemistry of the stool, and cultures for yeasts (fungi) and bacteria, followed up with antibiotic (for both natural and pharmaceutical antibiotics) sensitivity testing for any abnormal organisms. (See a sample test following this list.) Great Smokies also does state-of-the-art parasite testing, and many other general and specific tests for digestive integrity and other concerns.

Immunodiagnostic Lab (IDL)
P.O. Box 5755
San Leandro, CA 94577
800-888-1113

A specialized lab that I use for immunological evaluations through a T and B cell study, and for antibody levels to specific body tissues, such as thyroid or ovary, or to microorganisms, including Candida albicans, Herpes simplex viruses, or Epstein-Barr virus. I find these tests very helpful in the clinical evaluation of my patients.

Immuno Laboratories, Inc.
1620 W. Oakland Park Blvd.
Fort Lauderdale, FL 33311
800-231-9197

This lab's "food allergy" test measures antibody levels (IgG) of more than 100 foods. This test is helpful for the food-reactive or allergic patient or for those looking for health tuning because it will give all of the measurable reactions at one time. Elimination of these foods may then help relieve related symptoms. Food allergy testing is still a relatively controversial subject in medicine.

Immunosciences Lab, Inc.
8730 Wilshire Blvd., Suite 305
Beverly Hills, CA 90211
800-950-4686

This lab offers a variety of tests and panels for environmental and gastrointestinal problems.

Institute for Parasitic Diseases (IPD)
3530 W. Indian School Rd.
Phoenix, AZ 85018
602-955-4211

Dr. Amin and his lab are the best for finding parasitic infections.

Lab Corp
5601 Oberlin Dr.
San Diego, CA 92121
800-859-6046

A popular clinical laboratory with many national locations; this is the lab I currently use to evaluate blood counts, kidney and liver functions, blood sugar, protein levels, and cholesterol and other blood fat levels, including the cholesterol subfractions, HDL and LDL.

Medical Application Processing Services (MAPS)
1909 Studebaker Pl.
Gold River, CA 95670
916-638-0175

The nutritional analysis is a valuable, inexpensive test for people to see the levels of various nutrients in their diet, including the macronutrients, especially fats, and many micronutrients (see example following).

Meridian Valley Clinical Lab
515 Harrison St., Suite 9
Kent, WA 98032
800-234-6825

A specialized nutritional medicine laboratory with well-known practitioner, author, and educator Jonathon Wright, M.D. as consultant, this lab performs one of the few complete fatty acid profiles and a popular food allergy panel. They also run a wide range of other helpful tests.

Monroe Medical Research Laboratory
Route 17, P.O. Box I
Southfields, NY 10975
914-351-5134

A very specialized lab to support an exacting evaluation of essential nutrient status and function; they run tests for the biological activity of the B vitamins as well as many other vitamins and minerals.

Pantox Labs
4622 Santa Fe St.
San Diego, CA 92109
800-726-8696

Pantox offers a state-of-the-art blood profile of the major anti-oxidant nutrients, including CoQ10, Vitamins A, E and C.

Pacific Toxicology Laboratories
1545 Pontius Ave.
Los Angeles, CA 90025
800-23-TOXIC or 310-479-4911

This lab specializes in measuring blood, urine, and adipose tissue for toxic industrial chemicals, including organochlorine and organophosphate pesticides, chlorinated and aromatic solvents and their metabolites, PCBs and PBBs, and petroleum distillates.

Preventive Medical Center of Marin
25 Mitchell Blvd., Ste. 8
San Rafael, CA 94903
415-472-2343
Fax 415-472-7636

Many doctor's offices will do some specific tests, from blood counts to blood chemistries to X-rays. In my office, some of the tests we perform include urinalyses, electrocardiograms, all medical lab tests, mineral status, food allergies, and digestive analyses, utilizing many of the labs listed here.

Quest Diagnostics at Nichols Institute
33608 Ortega Hwy.
San Juan Capistrano, CA 92690
800-553-5445

A very reliable laboratory that many doctors and other labs refer to for specialized tests, such as for hormonal, immunological, and metabolic assessment.

Serammune Physicians Lab
14 Pidgeon Hill Dr., Suite 300
Sterling, VA 20165
800-553-5472

A lab directed by Russell M. Jaffe, M.D. that specializes in immune system reactions to pesticides, as well as measurement of food and chemical allergies through the new ELISA/ACT test.

SpectraCell Laboratories, Inc.
515 Post Oak Blvd., Suite 830
Houston, TX 77027
800-227-5227

SpectraCell Labs specializes in body nutrient measurements from blood samples.

Vitamin Diagnostics, Inc.
Route 35 and Industrial Rd.
Cliffwood Beach, NJ 07735
908-583-7773

A lab that runs a very specific vitamin profile. Many clinical labs test for certain common vitamin levels, such as vitamin B12 and folic acid; however, this lab runs most of the essential vitamins more economically because they specialize in this area.

These tests appear on the following pages:

1. Diet Analysis by MAPS
2. Comprehensive Digestive Stool Analysis (CDSA) by Great Smokies
3. Whole Blood Minerals by Doctor's Data
4. Hair Analysis Minerals by Doctor's Data

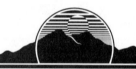

Comprehensive Digestive Stool Analysis

Great Smokies Diagnostic Laboratory℠

63 Zillicoa Street
Asheville, North Carolina 28801-1074

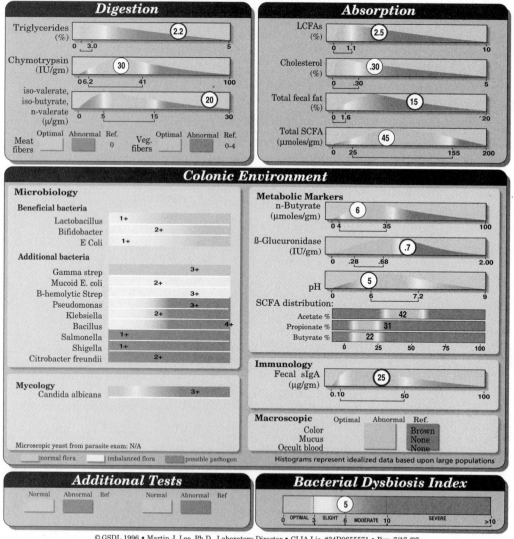

Digestion

Triglycerides (%)	2.2 — 0 3.0 ... 5
Chymotrypsin (IU/gm)	30 — 0 6.2 41 100
iso-valerate, iso-butyrate, n-valerate (µ/gm)	20 — 0 5 15 30

Meat fibers — Optimal / Abnormal / Ref. 0
Veg. fibers — Optimal / Abnormal / Ref. 0-4

Absorption

LCFAs (%)	2.5 — 0 1.1 ... 10
Cholesterol (%)	.30 — 0 .30 ... 5
Total fecal fat (%)	15 — 0 1.6 20
Total SCFA (µmoles/gm)	45 — 0 25 155 200

Colonic Environment

Microbiology

Beneficial bacteria
Lactobacillus	1+
Bifidobacter	2+
E Coli	1+

Additional bacteria
Gamma strep	3+
Mucoid E. coli	2+
B-hemolytic Strep	3+
Pseudomonas	3+
Klebsiella	2+
Bacillus	4+
Salmonella	1+
Shigella	1+
Citrobacter freundii	2+

Mycology
Candida albicans	3+

Microscopic yeast from parasite exam: N/A

normal flora | imbalanced flora | possible pathogen

Metabolic Markers
n-Butyrate (µmoles/gm)	6 — 0 4 35 100
ß-Glucuronidase (IU/gm)	.7 — 0 .28 .68 2.00
pH	5 — 0 6 7.2 9

SCFA distribution:
Acetate %	42
Propionate %	31
Butyrate %	22

0 25 50 75 100

Immunology
Fecal sIgA (µg/gm)	25 — 0.10 50 100

Macroscopic
	Optimal	Abnormal	Ref.
Color			Brown
Mucus			None
Occult blood			None

Histograms represent idealized data based upon large populations

Additional Tests

Normal Abnormal Ref | Normal Abnormal Ref

Bacterial Dysbiosis Index

5

0 — OPTIMAL 3 SLIGHT 6 MODERATE 10 SEVERE >10

© GSDL 1996 • Martin J. Lee, Ph.D., Laboratory Director • CLIA Lic. #34D0655571 • Rev. 7/17 /97

WHOLE BLOOD ELEMENTS

Doctor's Data Laboratories Inc.
c/o Doctor's Data Inc.
P.O. Box 111 170 W. Roosevelt Rd.
West Chicago, Illinois 60185-9986
CALL TOLL FREE (800) 323-2784
FAX (630) 231-9190

James T. Hicks, M.D., PhD, FCAP
Medical Director CLIA ID 14D0646470

Lab #:	97075-0002
Patient: Patient Name	Age: 43 Sex: F
Doctor: James T. Hicks, MD	Acct #: 15417
c/o: Darrell Hickok	
Collection Date: 3/14/97	Collection Time:
Date In: 3/16/97	Date Out: 3/17/97 R

ELEMENTS	PATIENT LEVEL	REFERENCE RANGE	2 Standard Deviations ←BELOW	1 Standard Deviation ←BELOW	M	1 Standard Deviation ABOVE→	2 Standard Deviations ABOVE→
Calcium	56.5 mcg/g	49- 69		★★★★★★			
Magnesium	30.6 mcg/g	28- 44	★★★★★★★★★★★★★★				
Sodium	78.2 mEq/L	66- 98		★★★★★★★			
Potassium	35.5 mEq/L	40- 60	<-★★★★★★★★★★★★★★★★★★★				
Phosphorus	347 mcg/g	300- 440		★★★★★★★			
Copper	.699 mcg/g	.61- 1.28		★★★★★★★★★★★★			
Zinc	5.47 mcg/g	4.2- 8.1		★★★★★★★★			
Manganese	.012 mcg/g	.003- .017				★★★★★★★★★★	
Iodine	.041 mcg/g	.018- .11				★★★★★	
Strontium	.02 mcg/g	.006- .031				★★★★★	
Sulfur	1140 mcg/g	920- 1710		★★★★★★★★★★★★★			

Potentially Toxic ELEMENTS	PATIENT LEVEL	EXPECTED RANGE	WITHIN 95% EXPECTED -->	> 95% OF EXPECTED-->	> 99% OF EXPECTED-->
Bismuth		dl- .005	level below detection limit of: .001		
Cadmium	.011 mcg/g	dl- .014	★★★★★★★★★★★		
Lead	.013 mcg/g	dl- .055	★★★		
Mercury	.002 mcg/g	dl- .013	★		
Nickel		dl- .019	level below detection limit of: .01		
Uranium		dl- .006	level below detection limit of: .001		

Comments:
k checked

Methodology:
ANALYZED BY ICP-MS
mcg/g = ppm
dl = detection limit

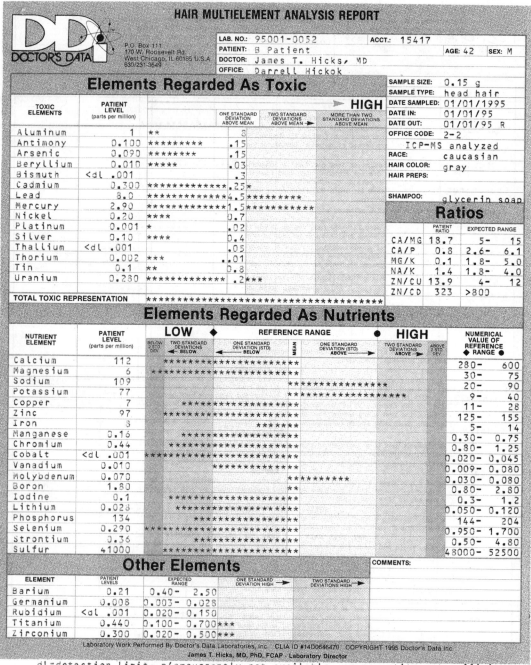

HAIR MULTIELEMENT ANALYSIS REPORT

P.O. Box 111
170 W. Roosevelt Rd.
West Chicago, IL 60185 U.S.A
630/231-3649

DOCTOR'S DATA

LAB. NO.: 95001-0052	ACCT.: 15417		
PATIENT: B Patient			
DOCTOR: James T. Hicks, MD		AGE: 42	SEX: M
OFFICE: Darrell Hickok			

Elements Regarded As Toxic

TOXIC ELEMENTS	PATIENT LEVEL (parts per million)		ONE STANDARD DEVIATION ABOVE MEAN	TWO STANDARD DEVIATIONS ABOVE MEAN ➤	MORE THAN TWO STANDARD DEVIATIONS ABOVE MEAN	HIGH ➤
Aluminum	1	**	8			
Antimony	0.100	********	.15			
Arsenic	0.090	********	.15			
Beryllium	0.010	*****	.03			
Bismuth	<dl .001		.3			
Cadmium	0.300	*************	.25*			
Lead	8.0	*************	4.5********			
Mercury	2.90	*************	1.5***********			
Nickel	0.20	****	0.7			
Platinum	0.001	*	.02			
Silver	0.10	****	0.4			
Thallium	<dl .001		.05			
Thorium	0.002	***	.01			
Tin	0.1	**	0.8			
Uranium	0.280	*************	.2***			
TOTAL TOXIC REPRESENTATION	***					

SAMPLE SIZE:	0.15 g
SAMPLE TYPE:	head hair
DATE SAMPLED:	01/01/1995
DATE IN:	01/01/95
DATE OUT:	01/01/95 R
OFFICE CODE:	2-2
	ICP-MS analyzed
RACE:	caucasian
HAIR COLOR:	gray
HAIR PREPS:	
SHAMPOO:	glycerin soap

Ratios

	PATIENT RATIO	EXPECTED RANGE	
CA/MG	18.7	5-	15
CA/P	0.8	2.6-	6.1
MG/K	0.1	1.8-	5.0
NA/K	1.4	1.8-	4.0
ZN/CU	13.9	4-	12
ZN/CD	323	>800	

Elements Regarded As Nutrients

NUTRIENT ELEMENT	PATIENT LEVEL (parts per million)	LOW ◆ BELOW 2 STD. DEV.	TWO STANDARD DEVIATIONS ◄ BELOW	ONE STANDARD DEVIATION (STD) BELOW	MEAN	ONE STANDARD DEVIATION (STD) ABOVE	TWO STANDARD DEVIATIONS ABOVE ►	HIGH ● ABOVE 2 STD. DEV.	NUMERICAL VALUE OF REFERENCE ◆ RANGE ●	
Calcium	112		********************						280-	600
Magnesium	6	**************************							30-	75
Sodium	109			*****************					20-	90
Potassium	77			********************					9-	40
Copper	7		*****************						11-	28
Zinc	97		*****************						125-	155
Iron	3			*******					5-	14
Manganese	0.16		*****************						0.30-	0.75
Chromium	0.44		*****************						0.80-	1.25
Cobalt	<dl .001	******************							0.020-	0.045
Vanadium	0.010		***************						0.009-	0.080
Molybdenum	0.070			**********					0.030-	0.080
Boron	1.80			**					0.80-	2.80
Iodine	0.1		*****************						0.3-	1.2
Lithium	0.028		****************						0.050-	0.120
Phosphorus	134		***************						144-	204
Selenium	0.290	*****************							0.950-	1.700
Strontium	0.36		****************						0.50-	4.80
Sulfur	41000		*****************						48000-	52500

Other Elements

ELEMENT	PATIENT LEVELS	EXPECTED RANGE		ONE STANDARD DEVIATION HIGH ➤	TWO STANDARD DEVIATIONS HIGH ➤
Barium	0.21	0.40-	2.50		
Germanium	0.008	0.003-	0.028		
Rubidium	<dl .001	0.020-	0.150		
Titanium	0.440	0.100-	0.700	***	
Zirconium	0.300	0.020-	0.500	***	

COMMENTS:

Laboratory Work Performed By Doctor's Data Laboratories, Inc. CLIA ID #14D0646470 COPYRIGHT 1995 Doctor's Data Inc.
James T. Hicks, MD, PhD, FCAP · Laboratory Director

dl=detection limit, n/a=currently not available, qns=quantity not sufficient

Nutritional Supplement Companies

This listing offers the most up-to-date addresses and phone numbers and a brief note about the product lines. If there is a toll-free number, I have given the national instead of the state one. Almost all of these companies are wholesale in nature and prefer first, written requests, and second, calls for information and catalogs. Obviously, they prefer interest from stores and practitioners rather than individual consumers, although most companies will answer important questions about their products. I know there are literally hundreds of companies nationwide, and I have included as many as I could access. Other companies that wish a review for later updates, please contact me. **To the consumer:** I suggest that you use your supplements wisely and be aware of the effects they may have on you; I am sure the companies would appreciate hearing from you about their products' effectiveness. NOTE: There is no financial involvement between me and any of these companies, other than I am a customer of some and am familiar with many of their products.

A. C. Grace Company
P.O. Box 570
Big Sandy, TX 75755
903-636-4368

Carries a high quality vitamin E product.

Advance Laboratories
120 Elm St.
Watertown, MA 02172
800-292-4343

Mainly carries Prostex and tea tree oil products.

Agape Health Products
P.O. Box 2277
Seal Beach, CA 90740
800-767-4776

The distributor of Perfect 7, one of the better intestinal fiber cleansers I know of.

Alacer Corporation
19631 Pauling
Foothill Ranch, CA 92610
800-854-0249

The makers of a popular electrolyte, powdered vitamin C, Emergen-C, and other fine products.

Allergy Research Group/Nutricology
400 Preda St.
San Leandro, CA 94577
800-545-9960

A company created and run by Dr. Stephen Levine, ARG sells many innovative and high-quality products for the clinical nutrition practice. I have several favorites; some are mentioned in this book.

American Health
4320 Veterans' Memorial Hwy.
Holbrook, NY 11741
800-445-7137

They have several lines of nutritional products, including El Molino Natural Foods and Radiance Vitamins. Their Super Papaya digestive enzymes are very popular.

Amni—Advanced Medical Nutrition, Inc.
2247 National Ave.
P.O. Box 5012
Hayward, CA 94540-5012
800-437-8888

Amni produces a variety of tableted multiples, the Basic Preventive series, and other specific products, such as Lipex dietary fiber.

Apex Energetics
(Futureplex Products)
1701 E. Edinger, Suite A4
Santa Ana, CA 92705
800-736-4381

Carries the Futureplex homeopathic and homeoenergetic products; also flower essences.

ApotheCure
13720 Midway Rd., Suite 109
Dallas, TX 75244
800-969-6601

A compounding pharmacy with a variety of supplements and difficult to find medicines.

Arizona Natural Products
8281 E. Evans Rd., Ste. 104
Scottsdale, AZ 85260
800-255-2823

Innovative products of garlic and desert plants, such as yucca, chaparral, and other herbals.

Atrium—Werum Enterprises, Inc.
1620 Sally Lane
Placerville, CA 95667
800-822-6193

A wide range of nutritional and herbal specialty products.

Bezweckin, Inc.
12535 SW 3rd St.
Beaverton, OR 97005
800-664-7800

Herbally based natural hormone products for women.

bio/chem Research (Nutrobiotic)
865 Parallel Dr.
Lakeport, CA 95453
800-225-4345

Producers of Citricidal, a grapefruit seed extract antimicrobial, and a variety of other products.

**Biologic Homeopathic
Industries (BHI)**
11600 Cochiti St. SE
Albuquerque, NM 87123
800-621-7644

The exclusive distributor of Heel homeopathics as well as the special formulas following the work of the eminent homeopathic physician H. H Reckeweg.

Biotec Foods
2639 S. King St. #206
Honolulu, HI 96826
800-331-5888

Special high-potency, enteric-coated antioxidant enzyme formulas, including superoxide dismutase and glutathione peroxidase.

Boericke & Tafel, Inc.
2381 Circadian Way
Santa Rosa, CA 95407
800-876-9505 (in CA)
800-272-2820 (outside CA)

"America's oldest and largest homeopathic pharmaceutical firm" with a full line of traditional and special homeopathics.

Bronson Pharmaceuticals
P.O. Box 46903
St. Louis, MO 63146
800-521-3322

A complete line of supplements for the entire family at a reasonable cost; popular items include their vitamin C crystals and Prenatal formula.

Cardiovascular Research/Ecological Formulas
106 "B" Shary Circle
Concord, CA 94518
800-888-4585

A very advanced nutritional medicine line with effective formulas for such areas as immune support, yeast problems, and allergies.

College Pharmacy
833 N. Tejon St.
Colorado Springs, CO 80903
800-888-9358

A compounding pharmacy with many natural hormone products and other innovative supplies.

Country Life Vitamins
180 Oser Ave.
Hauppauge, NY 11788
800-645-5768

A common natural food store line of supplements with multiple formulas and sports products.

DaVinci Laboratories/Food Science Corporation
20 New England Dr.
Essex Junction, VT 05453
800-325-1776

A complete line of nutritional supplements, including Gluconic DMG (N-N dimethylglycine), for health care practitioners.

deBuren Optimum International
35 Via Los Altos
Tiburon, CA 94920
415-383-1405 or 800-543-3831

Sharon deBuren, a nutrition-oriented nurse practitioner specializing in high-risk Ob/Gyn, has developed a top-quality, hypoallergenic multiple vitamin/mineral formula and a well-tolerated calcium-magnesium citrate that are very popular in my practice.

Doctor's Nutriceuticals
435 Croton Dam Rd.
Croton-on-Hudson, NY 10520
800-338-5200

A special line of nutrient formulas for specific health conditions available to practitioners.

Dolisos America, Inc.
3014 Rigel Ave.
Las Vegas, NV 89102
800-365-4767

A full-service homeopathic company that features a family kit with over 50 remedies.

Douglas Laboratories
P.O. Box 8583
Pittsburgh, PA 15220
800-245-4440

A full line of products that can carry your label or theirs, as well as customized products.

Dynapro International
P.O. Box 3002
Ogden, UT 84409
800-877-1413

A wide range of medical and nutritional products.

Eclectic Institute, Inc.
11231 S.E. Market St.
Portland, OR 97216
800-332-HERB

Many unique freeze-dried herbal products, extracts using organic alcohol, and therapeutic vitamin/mineral formulas.

Ecological Formulas
(see **Cardiovascular Research**)

Enzymatic Therapy
PO Box 22310
Green Bay, WI 54305
800-783-2286

A popular line of quality herbal and nutrient supplements available in many health food stores.

Flora, Inc.
805 E. Badger Rd.
Lynden, WA 98264
800-446-2110

Importers and distributors of the German made Floradix products, liquid herbal extracts of vitamins and minerals and a particularly well-tolerated and bioavailable iron formula.

Freeda
36 E. 41st St.
New York, NY 10017
800-777-3737

A wide range of very clean (no aluminum, coal tar dyes, or yeast in their products) nutritional formulas for all age groups with all completely vegetarian products.

Health Concerns
8001 Capwell Dr.
Oakland, CA 94621
800-233-9355

A speciality company for the field of Chinese herbology with individual and combination formulas.

Herbal Apothecary
2511 Nason Ave.
El Cerrito, CA 94530
415-456-1184

Some very special herbal extracts, mainly Chinese, created by pharmacist and herbalist, Tom Dunphy. Immu 8 and Immu Plus are their popular Chinese herbal extracts for the immune system.

Herb Pharm
P.O. Box 116
Williams, OR 97544
800-348-4372

A fine line of organically grown, custom Wild Crafted herbs and herbal extracts.

Herbs for Kids
151 Evergreen Dr., Suite D
Bozeman, MT 59715
800-735-0299

A product line of alcohol-free, good tasting herbal formulas for children.

Herbs of Light
PO Box 260456
Tampa, FL 33685
813-886-4114

A new company dedicated to conscious creation of a wide variety of herbal extracts.

J. R. Carlson Laboratories, Inc.
15 College
Arlington Heights, IL 60004
800-323-4141

A complete line of nutritional supple-ments specializing in high-quality vitamin E products.

Jarrow Formulas, Inc.
1824 S. Robertson
Los Angeles, CA 90035
800-726-0886

A popular company with a wide range of nutritional products popular in many health food stores.

Jones Medical, Inc.
1945 Craig Rd.
St. Louis, MO 63146
800-525-8466

Produces a clean porcine-based thyroid medicine, called Westhroid.

Karuna Corporation
42 Digital Dr., Ste. 7
Novato, CA 94949
800-826-7225

Karuna has some of my favorite powdered multiples, the Maxxum series, and a variety of effective nutrient and herbal products.

Key Company
1313 W. Essex
St. Louis, MO 63122
800-325-9592

Some basic, good quality yet inexpensive supplements and injectables for the nutritional practice.

King Bio Pharmaceuticals
1264 New Leicester Hwy.
Asheville, NC 28806
800-543-3245

A line of hypoallergenic formulas for special clinical needs.

Klaire Laboratories/Vital Life
1573 W. Seminole
San Marcos, CA 92069
800-533-7255 or 619-744-9680 (CA)

A very fine line of supplements, especially their colon flora products, Vital Plex and Vital Dophilus.

Klamath
PO Box 1626
Mt. Shasta, CA 96067
800-327-1956

A variety of quality products with the base of blue-green algae from Klamath lake.

Kroeger Herb Products
1122 Pearl St.
Boulder, CO 80302
303-443-0755

A line of special herbal products developed by Hanna Kroeger.

Legere Pharmaceuticals
7326 E. Evans Rd.
Scottsdale, AZ 85260
800-528-3144

A company that provides a variety of products to the practitioner, including oral and in-jectable drugs as well as vitamins and minerals.

Mayway Corporation
1338 Mandela Parkway
Oakland, CA 94607
510-208-3123

A wide collection of herbal products imported from China and the Orient.

Mega Foods
P.O. Box 325
Derry, NH 03038
800-848-2542

"Food Grown" and extracted supplements, which have become very popular in recent years.

Merit Pharmaceuticals
2611 San Fernando Rd.
Los Angeles, CA 90065
800-234-6825

Merit offers a wide variety of drugs and nutritional oral and injectable products for practitioners

Metagenics, Inc.
971 Calle Negocio
San Clemente, CA 92672
800-692-9400

Offering a wide range of innovative and top-quality products, this company follows the current research closely and provides special educational seminars for clinical nutrition-oriented practitioners.

Miracle Exclusives, Inc.
P.O. Box 8
Port Washington, NY 11560
800-645-6360

Importers and distributors for a variety of health appliances.

Natren
3105 Willow Lane
Westlake Village, CA 91361
800-992-3323 or 800-992-9393 (CA)

Promotes an improved "adhesion strain of acidophilus," Bio-Nate.

Nature's Answer
320 Oser Avenue
Hauppauge, NY 11788
800-439-2324

An extensve of quality liquid herbal extracts including Maitake mushroom.

Nature's Herbs
P.O. Box 336
Orem, UT 84059
800-HERBALS

A Twinlab company that provides top-quality herbal products that have certified potency and are certified organic.

Nature's Life
7180 Lampson Ave.
Garden Grove, CA 92841
800-854-6837

A wide line of quality supplements available in health food stores.

Nature's Plus
10 Daniel St.
Farmingdale, NY 11735
800-937-0500

A common line of natural food store nutritional supplements, including Source of Life multivitamins and Spirutein, a protein supplement/meal replacement.

Nature's Secret/Harmony Formulas
5485 Conestoga Ct.
Boulder, CO 80301
888-525-9696

A good selection of nutrient/herbal products for detoxification and health.

Nature's Way
10 Mountain Spring Pkwy.
Springville, UT 84663
800-9-NATURE

A complete line of nutritional and herbal supplements.

New Chapter Vitamins
(New Moon)
105 Main
Brattleboro, VT 05301
800-543-7279

A relatively new line of fine quality formulas for women and men.

NF Formulas, Inc.
805 S.E. Sherman
Portland, OR 97214
800-547-4891

Clinically useful naturopathic products including Echinacea–vitamin C tablets.

Nutricology

The health food store and public consumer line for the **Allergy Research Group** (see above) line of nutritional products.

Nutri-Dyn
222 N. Vincent Ave.
Covina, CA 91722
800-327-8355

A line of nutritional and glandular products with localized distributors throughout the country.

Nutrilite (Amway)
7575 E. Fulton St.
Ada, MI 49356-0001
800-253-6500

A multilevel distributor line of fine quality, food-extracted nutritional supplements.

Nutrition Resource
P.O. Box 238
Lakeport, CA 95453
800-624-9009 or 800-225-4345

Some very good quality, powdered supplement products, free of common allergens.

Nutritional Enzyme Support System (NESS)
100 NW Business Park Ln.
Riverside, MO 64150
800-637-7893

A professional line of high-quality vegetarian digestive enzymes, many of which focus on supporting the digestion of particular macronutrients or an area of healing.

Phyto-Pharmica
P.O. Box 1745
Green Bay, WI 54305
800-553-2370 or 800-376-7889

Nutritional, herbal, and glandular supplements are sold mainly to the naturopathic practitioner, but many of their quality products are also available to the public through Enzymatic Therapy, Inc.

Probiologic, Inc.
14714 N.E. 87th St.
Redmond, WA 98052
800-678-8218

A professional line of products that includes Liv 52, an Ayurvedic herbal preparation for the liver, and Capricin, a common intestinal antifungal made from caprylic acid.

Professional Botanicals
P.O. Box 9822
Ogden, UT 84409
800-824-8181

A very fine line of special herbal formulas for specific physiological effects and treatment of certain disease processes.

Professional Nutrition
811 Cliff Dr., Ste. C-1
Santa Barbara, CA 93109
800-336-9301

The company that markets Doctor-Dophilus, an excellent bio-culture mixture of beneficial intestinal flora.

Pure Body Institute
230 S. Olive St.
Ventura, CA 93001
800-952-7873

Producers and suppliers of a popular herbal detox product called Nature's Pure Body Program.

Rainbow Light Nutritional Systems
207 McPherson
Santa Cruz, CA 95060
800-635-1233

Food-grown nutrient supplements, the Living Source line, that are more "natural" than most products; even though they are relatively low-dosage, they are well absorbed.

Randal Nutritional Products
P.O. Box 7328
Santa Rosa, CA 95407
800-221-1697 or 707-528-1800

Have your own name on their special vitamin, mineral, or herbal products.

Richlife
222 N. Vincent Ave.
Covina, CA 91722
800-327-8355

A common line of natural food store supplements.

Schiff Products
180 Moonachie Ave.
Moonachie, NJ 07074
800-526-6251

Longtime mainstay of the nutritional market with a full line of products, available in many health food stores.

Scientific Consulting
466 Whitney St.
San Leandro, CA 94577
800-333-7414

Dr. Bela Balough provides many excellent powdered, readily usable nutritional metabolic products, including amino acid formulas, multiples, and injectables.

Solgar
410 Ocean Ave.
Lynbrook, NY 11563
800-645-2246

One of the longtime, quality companies of the industry, one that can be counted on for excellence in its many tableted formulas.

Source Cassette Learning Systems
Emmett Miller, M.D.
P.O. Box W
Stanford, CA 94309
800-528-2737

A great series; lifestyle, health, and healing tapes by the very creative and eloquent Dr. Miller.

Source Naturals/Threshold Enterprises
23 Janis Way
Scotts Valley, CA 95066
800-777-5677

A clean and effective vegetarian line of nutritional support and therapeutic supplements; the Wellness Formula is very popular.

Standard Homeopathic Company
P.O. Box 61067
Los Angeles, CA 90061
800-624-9659

A company that has provided top-quality homeopathics for decades, including the Hy-land's Homeopathic Combination Medicines.

Standard Process Laboratories
12209 Locksley Lane, Ste. 15
Auburn, CA 95603
800-662-9134 (in CA) or 916-888-1974 (outside CA)

An extensive, longtime line of special glandular supplements that are very popular with naturopathic practitioners. I think Zypan is an excellent nonvegetarian digestive formula.

Sunrider International
P.O. Box 2840
888-278-6743

A "multilevel" distribution company with high-quality and relatively expensive herbal products for balance and rejuvenation.

Superior Trading Company
837 Washington St.
San Francisco, CA 94108
415-982-8722

A variety of Oriental herbal products, such as ginseng, dong quai, and royal jelly.

Supernutrition/Nutritional Gold
2565 3rd St. #312
San Francisco, CA 94107
800-262-2116

I have used these advanced, potent products for more than a decade, especially for the active individual interested in high performance. My favorites are tableted vitamin C and the Energy (stress) Caps.

Systemic Formulas
P.O. Box 1516
Ogden, UT 84402
800-445-4647

A specific line of clinically applicable formulas designed by Master Herbalist, A. S. Wheelwright, and that are sold via a distributor network.

Thorne Research, Inc.
901 Triangle Dr.
Sandpoint, ID 83864
800-228-1966

Thorne manufactures an extensive practitioner line of nutritional, hypoallergenic products.

Twin Labs
2120 Smithtown Ave.
Ronkonkoma, NY 11779
800-645-5626

An extremely thorough line of primarily powdered, easily assimilable products for the entire family, from basic supplements to body-building formulas—"the leaders in sports nutrition."

Tyler Encapsulations
2204-8 NW Birdsdale
Gresham, OR 97030
800-869-9705

A wide variety of quality products specializing in digestive function and detoxification.

UAS Laboratories
5610 Rowland Rd., Suite 110
Minneapolis, MN 55343
800-422-DDS-1

The primary developer and distributor of the high-potency Lactobacillus acidophilus culture, DDS-1.

UltraVit Enterprises, Inc
116 W. Del Mar
Pasadena, CA 91105
800-758-4237

Specializes in their UltraPure products of bottled fermented juices and supplements ofr detoxification.

Vitaline Formulas
722 Jefferson Ave.
Ashland, OR 97520
800-648-4755

A good quality, yet relatively inexpensive line of products that I have used for years in my practice. I find that patients tolerate the Vitaline products very well.

Wakunaga of America
23501 Madero
Mission Viejo, CA 92691
800-421-2998 or 800-544-5800 (in CA)

Makers and distributors of Kyolic, an odorless garlic extract formula, and Kyogreen, a barley grass extract.

Wellness Health Pharmaceuticals
2800 S. 18th St.
Birmingham, AL 35209
800-227-2627

A distribution network for many fine nutritional and pharmaceutical products, including pure nystatin powder and some of the above-mentioned supplement lines, for the practitioner and consumer.

Werum Enterprises
(see **Atrium**)

Women's International Pharmacy
5708 Monona Dr.
Madison, WI 53716
800-279-5708

Women's is a compounding pharmacy specializing in natural hormone products.

Yerba Prima
P.O. Box 2569
Oakland, CA 94614
800-421-9972

A line of high-quality herbal products—"herbs to live by."

YSK American Corporation
4025 Spencer St., Ste. 103
Torrance, CA 90503
800-829-2828

Makers and distributors of the fabulous Sun Chlorella powder and tablets.

Zand Herbal Formulas
1722 14th St., Suite 230
Boulder, CO 80302
800-800-0405

A line of quality Western and Oriental herbal products including their popular echinacea-golden seal Insure formula and their throat lozenges.

○ BIBLIOGRAPHY

Aero, Rita, and Rick, Stephanie. *Vitamin Power: A User's Guide to Nutritional Supplements and Botanical Substances That Can Change Your Life*. New York: Harmony Books, 1987.

Airola, Paavo. *How to Get Well*. Phoenix, AZ: Health Plus, Publishers, 1974.

—— *The Airola Diet and Cookbook*. Phoenix, AZ: Health Plus, 1981.

Alabaster, Oliver. *The Power of Prevention: A Personal Plan to Reduce Your Cancer Risk by As Much As 70 Percent*. Washington, DC: Saville Books, Publishers, 1988.

American Institute for Cancer Research. *An Ounce of Prevention*. 4 vols. AICR Cookbook Series. Washington, DC: American Institute for Cancer Research, 1986.

ArgIsle, Bethany. *That Healing Feeling*. Forthcoming.

—— *Life Is a Fad*. San Rafael, CA: KeyWhole Publishing Co., 1992.

Badgley, Laurence. *Healing AIDS Naturally: Natural Therapies for the Immune System*. San Bruno, CA: Human Energy Press, 1987.

Ballentine, Rudolph. *Diet and Nutrition*. Honesdale, PA: Himalayan Publishers, 1978.

Becker, Robert O., and Selden, Gary. *The Body Electric: Electromagnetism and the Foundation of Life*. New York: William Morrow and Co., 1987.

Berger, Stuart M. *How to Be Your Own Nutritionist*. New York: Avon Books, 1988.

—— *Dr. Berger's Immune Power Diet*. New York: Signet Books, 1986.

Bianchini, Francisco; Corbetta, Francisco; and Pistoia, Marilena. *The Complete Book of Fruits and Vegetables*. New York: Crown Books, 1975. O.P.

Bland, Jeffrey. *Nutraerobics*. San Francisco: Harper & Row, 1985. O.P.

—— *Trace Elements in Human Health and Disease*. Redmond, WA: Eagle Print, 1979. O.P.

Bland, Jeffrey, ed. *A Year in Nutrition Medicine: 1986*. 2d ed. New Canaan, CT: Keats Publishing, 1986.

Braly, James, and Torbert, Laura. *Dr. Braly's Optimum Health Program: For Permanent Weight Loss and a Longer Healthier Life*. New York: Times Books, 1985. O.P.

Brody, Jane. *Jane Brody's Nutrition Book*. New York: Bantam Books, 1982.

Butler, Kurt, and Rayner, Lynn. *The Best Medicine: The Complete Health and Preventative Medicine Handbook*. San Francisco: Harper Religious Books, 1985.

Center for Science in the Public Interest. *Household Pollutant Guide*. New York: Anchor Books, 1978. O.P.

STAYING HEALTHY WITH NUTRITION

Chang, Jolan. *The Tao of Love and Sex: The Ancient Chinese Way to Ecstasy*. New York: E. P. Dutton, 1977.

Colbin, Annemarie. *Food and Healing*. New York: Ballantine Books, 1986.

Cousens, Gabriel. *Spiritual Nutrition and the Rainbow Diet*. San Rafael, CA: Cassandra Press, 1986.

Crook, William. *The Yeast Connection*. 3d ed. Jackson, TN: Professional Books/Future Health, 1989.

Dadd, Debra Lynn. *Nontoxic and Natural: How to Avoid Dangerous Everyday Products and Buy or Make Safe Ones*. Los Angeles: Jeremy P. Tarcher, 1984.

—— *Nontoxic Home: Protecting Yourself and Your Family from Everyday Toxics and Health Hazards*. Edited by Janice Gallagher. Los Angeles: Jeremy P. Tarcher, 1986.

Diagram Group Staff. *The Healthy Body: A Maintenance Manual*. New York: Plume Books, 1981.

Diamond, Harvey, and Diamond, Marilyn. *Fit for Life*. New York: Warner Books, 1987.

Eaton, S. Boyd; Shostak, Marjorie; and Konner, Melvin. *The Paleolithic Prescription: A Program of Diet and Exercise and a Design for Living*. New York: Harper and Row, 1989.

Ehret, Arnold. *Rational Fasting*. Beaumont, CA: Ehret Literature, 1971.

—— *Mucusless Diet and Healing System*. Beaumont, CA: Ehret Literature, 1972.

Erasmus, Udo. *Fats and Oils*. Burnaby, BC: Alive Books, 1986.

Ferguson, Tom. *Smoker's Book of Health: How to Keep Yourself Healthier and Reduce Your Smoking Risks*. New York: G. P. Putnam's Sons, 1987. O.P.

Fleet, Thurman. *Rays of the Dawn*. San Antonio, TX: Concept Therapy Institute, 1950.

Fox, Martin. *Healthy Water for a Longer Life: A Nutritionist Looks at Drinking Water*. Portsmouth, NH: Healthy Water Research, 1986.

Fuchs, Nan Kathryn. *The Nutrition Detective: Treating Your Health Problems Through the Food You Eat*. Los Angeles: Jeremy P. Tarcher, 1985.

Garrison, Robert H., Jr., and Somer, Elizabeth. *Nutrition Desk Reference*. New Canaan, CT: Keats Publishing, 1985.

Garvy, John W., Jr. *The Five Phases of Food: How to Begin*. 2d ed. Five Phase Energetics Series, no. 1. Newtonville, MA: Wellbeing Books, 1983.

Gerber, Richard. *Vibrational Medicine: New Choices for Healing Ourselves*. Santa Fe, NM: Bear and Co., 1988.

Gittleman, Ann Louise, and Desgrey, John M. *Beyond Pritikin*. New York: Bantam Books, 1989.

Gortner, Willis A., and Freydberg, Nicholas. *The Food Additives Book*. New York: Bantam Books, 1982.

Goulart, Frances Sheridan. *Nutritional Self-Defense: Protecting Yourself from Yourself*. Chelsea, MI: Scarborough House, 1990.

Graham, Judy. *Evening Primrose Oil: Its Remarkable Properties and Its Use in the Treatment of a Wide Range of Conditions*. Rochester, VT: Inner Traditions International, 1984.

Haas, Elson M. *Staying Healthy with the Seasons*. Berkeley, CA: Celestial Arts, 1981.

Haas, Robert. *Eat to Succeed*. New York: Onyx, 1987.

Hall, Manly P. *Medicine of the Sun and Moon*. Los Angeles: Philosophical Research Society, 1972.

Hamilton, Eva May Nunnelley, and Whitney, Eleanor Noss. *Nutrition: Concepts and Controversies*. 3d ed. St. Paul, MN: West Publishing Co., 1985.

Hatfield, Frederick C. *Ultimate Sports Nutrition: A Scientific Approach to Peak Athletic Performance*. Chicago: Contemporary Books, 1987.

Hendler, Sheldon Saul. *The Complete Guide to Anti-Aging Nutrients*. New York: Fireside Paperbacks, 1984.

Heinenman, John, et al. *Basic Natural Nutrition*. Provo, UT: Woodland Books, 1984.

Hoffman, David. *The Holistic Herbal*. Findhorn, Moray, Scotland: Findhorn Press, 1983.

Howell, Edward. *Enzyme Nutrition*. Garden City Park, NY: Avery Publishing Group, 1985.

—— *Food Enzymes for Health and Longevity*. Wilmot, WI: Lotus Light Publications, 1981.

Hunter, Beatrice Trum. *Consumer Beware!* New York: Touchstone Books, 1972. O.P.

Hurd, Frank J., and Hurd, Rosalie J. *Ten Talents Vegetarian Natural Foods Cookbook*, rev. ed. Chisholm, MN: Ten Talents, 1985.

Kalita, Dwight K., and Philpott, William H. *Victory Over Diabetes: A Bio-Ecologic Triumph*. New Canaan, CT: Keats Publishing, 1983.

Kerndt, Peter R., et al. "Fasting: The History, Pathophysiology and Complications." *Western Journal of Medicine* 137, no. 5 (November 1982): 379–399.

King, Jonathan. *Troubled Water: The Poisoning of America's Drinking Water*. Emmaus, PA: Rodale Press, 1985.

Kirschmann, John D., and Dunne, Lavon J. *Nutrition Almanac*. 2d ed. New York: McGraw-Hill Book Co., 1985.

Koch, Manfred. *Laugh with Health*. New York: Henry Holt, 1984. O.P.

Koop, C. Everett. *The Surgeon General's Report on Nutrition and Health—Summary and Recommendations.* Washington, DC: DHHS Publications, Department of Health and Human Services, 1988.

Kunin, Richard A. *Mega-Nutrition.* New York: McGraw-Hill Book Co., 1980.

Kushi, Michio. *The Cancer Prevention Diet.* New York: St. Martin's Press, 1985.

Lappé, Frances Moore. *Diet for a Small Planet.* New York: Ballantine Books, 1987.

Lark, Susan. *Premenstrual Syndrome Self-Help Book: A Woman's Guide to Feeling Good All Month.* Berkeley, CA: Celestial Arts, 1989.

Leonard, James, and Laut, Philip. *Rebirthing: The Science of Enjoying All of Your Life.* Cincinnati, OH: Vivation Publishing, 1983. O.P.

Lesser, Michael. *Nutrition and Vitamin Therapy.* New York: Grove-Weidenfeld, 1980. O.P.

Lettvin, Maggie. *Maggie's Food Strategy Book: Taking Charge of Your Diet for Lifelong Health and Vitality.* Boston: Houghton Mifflin, 1987.

Levine, Stephen A., and Kidd, Paris M. *Antioxidant Adaptation: Its Role in Free Radical Pathology.* San Leandro, CA: Allergy Research Group, 1985.

Locke, Steven E., and Hornig-Rohan, Mady. *Mind and Immunity: Behavioral Immunology.* Westport, CT: Praeger Publishers, 1983.

Makower, Joel. *Office Hazards: How Your Job Can Make You Sick.* Washington, DC: Tilden Press, 1981. O.P.

Manahan, William. *Eat for Health: Fast and Simple Ways of Eliminating Diseases without Medical Assistance.* Edited by Suzanne Lipsett. Tiburon, CA: H. J. Kramer, 1988.

McDougall, John A., and McDougall, Mary A. *The McDougall Plan.* Hampton, NJ: New Win Publishing, 1985.

McDougall, John A. *McDougall's Medicine: A Challenging Second Opinion.* Hampton, NJ: New Win Publishing, 1986.

McGee, Charles T. *How to Survive Modern Technology.* New Canaan, CT: Keats Publishing, 1981.

Mervyn, Leonard. *Thorsons' Complete Guide to Vitamins and Minerals.* New York: Thorsons Publishing Group, 1986.

Mindell, Earl. *Earl Mindell's New and Revised Vitamin Bible.* New York: Warner Books, 1989.

—— *Vitamin Bible for Your Kids.* New York: Warner Books, 1981. O.P.

Muller, Robert. "Healing Ourselves and Healing Our Planet." In *New Holistic Health Handbook: Living Well in a New Age,* edited by Shepherd Bliss. Lexington, MA: Stephen Greene Press, 1985.

Napoli, Maryann. *Health Facts: A Critical Evaluation of the Major Problems, Treatments and Alternatives Facing Medical Consumers.* New York: Overlook Press, 1984.

Ornish, Dean. *Stress, Diet, and Your Heart.* New York: Signet Books, 1984.

—— *Dr. Dean Ornish's Program for Reversing Heart Disease.* New York: Random House, 1990.

Passwater, Richard A., and Cranton, Elmer M. *Trace Elements, Hair Analysis and Nutrition: Fact and Myth.* New Canaan, CT: Keats Publishing, 1983.

Pauling, Linus. *How to Live Longer and Feel Better.* New York: Avon Books, 1987.

Pearson, Durk, and Shaw, Sandy. *Life Extension.* New York: Warner Books, 1987.

Pelletier, Kenneth R. *Mind As Healer Mind As Slayer.* New York: Delta Books, 1977.

Pennington, Jean A. T. *Food Values of Portions Commonly Used.* 15th ed. New York: Perennial Library, 1989.

Pfeiffer, Carl C. *Mental and Elemental Nutrients: A Physician's Guide to Nutrition and Health Care.* New Canaan, CT: Keats Publishing, 1976.

Pfeiffer, Carl C., and Braverman, Eric R. *The Healing Nutrients Within: Facts, Findings and New Research on Amino Acids.* New Canaan, CT: Keats Publishing, 1987.

Philpott, William H., and Kalita, Dwight K. *Brain Allergies.* New Canaan, CT: Keats Publishing, 1987.

Prevention Magazine Editors. *Understanding Vitamins and Minerals.* Prevention Total Health System Series. Emmaus, PA: Rodale Press, 1984.

Prevention Magazine Editors, and Nugent, Nancy. *Food and Nutrition.* Prevention Total Health System Series. Emmaus, PA: Rodale Press, 1984.

Price, Weston. *Nutrition and Physical Degeneration,* 9th ed. San Diego, CA: Price-Pottenger Nutrition Foundation, 1977.

Randolph, Theron G., and Moss, Ralph W. *An Alternative Approach to Allergies: The New Field of Clinical Ecology Unravels the Environmental Causes of Mental and Physical Ills,* rev. ed. New York: Perennial Library, 1990.

Reuben, David. *Everything You Always Wanted to Know about Nutrition.* New York: Avon Books, 1979.

Rinkel, Herbert J. *The Management of Clinical Allergy.* Cheyenne, WY: Russel I. Williams, M.D., 1983.

Robbins, John. *Diet for a New America: How Your Food Choices Affect Your Health, Happiness and the Future of Life on Earth.* Walpole, NH: Stillpoint Publishing, 1987.

Rodale, J. I., and Staff. *The Complete Book of Minerals for Health.* Emmaus, PA: Rodale Press, 1981. O.P.

Rodale Press Editors. *The Complete Book of Vitamins*. Emmaus, PA: Rodale Press, 1984. O.P.

Rohé, Fred. *The Complete Book of Natural Foods*. Boulder, CO: Shambhala Books, 1983.

Rose, Jeanne. *Herbs and Things: Jeanne Rose's Herbal*. New York: Grossett and Dunlap, 1972.

Rosenbaum, Michael, and Bosco, Dominick. *Super Fitness Beyond Vitamins*. New York: Signet Books, 1989.

Rosenfeld, Isadore. *Modern Prevention: The New Medicine*. New York: Bantam Books, 1987

Rossman, Martin L. *Healing Yourself: A Step-by-Step Program for Better Health Through Imagery*. New York: Pocket Books, 1989.

Saifer, Phyllis, and Zellerbach, Merla. *Detox*. Los Angeles: Jeremy P. Tarcher, 1984.

Samuels, Mike, and Bennett, Hal Zina. *Well Body, Well Earth: The Sierra Club Environmental Health Sourcebook*. San Francisco: Sierra Club Books, 1983.

Samuels, Mike, and Samuels, Nancy. *The Well Adult: Complete Guide to Protecting and Improving Your Health*. New York: Summit Books, 1988.

Saltman, Paul; Durin, Joel; and Mothner, Ira. *The California Nutrition Book: Food for the Nineties from University of California Faculty and American Health Magazine*. Boston: Little, Brown and Co., 1987.

Scala, James. *Making the Vitamin Connection*. New York: Harper & Row, 1985. O.P.

Schroeder, Henry A. *Trace Elements and Man*. Greenwich, CT: Devin-Adair, 1973.

—— *Trace Elements in Human Health and Disease*. Redmond, WA: Eagle Print, 1979. O.P.

Sehnert, Keith. *The Candidiasis Syndrome, Old Problem, New Mystery*. Minneapolis, MN: UAS Laboratories, 1986. O.P.

Serinus, Jason, ed. *Psychoimmunity and the Healing Process: A Holistic Approach to Immunity and AIDS*. Berkeley, CA: Celestial Arts, 1986.

Siegel, Bernie S. *Love, Medicine and Miracles: Lessons Learned about Self-Healing from a Surgeon's Experience with Exceptional Patients*. New York: Perennial Library, 1990.

—— *Peace, Love, and Healing: Bodymind Communication and the Path to Self-Healing: An Exploration*. New York: Perennial Library, 1990.

Szekely, Edmund Bordeaux. *The Essene Gospel of Peace*. Book 1. San Diego, CA: Academy Books, 1977.

Tierra, Michael. *Way of Herbs*. New York: Pocket Books, 1983.

Truss, C. Orian. *The Missing Diagnosis*. 3d ed. Birmingham, AL: Missing Diagnosis, 1986.

Weinberger, Stanley. *Healing Within: The Complete Colon Health Guide*. Larkspur, CA: Colon Health Center Publishing, 1988.

Weiner, Michael A. *People's Herbal: A Complete Family Guide for All Ages to Safe Home Remedies*. New York: Grossett and Dunlap, 1984.

Werbach, Melvyn, R. *Nutritional Influences on Illness: A Sourcebook of Clinical Research*. Tarzana, CA: Third Line Press, 1987.

—— *Third Line Medicine*. New York: Penguin Books, 1988.

Williams, Su Rodwell. *Basic Nutrition and Diet Therapy*. 8th ed. St. Louis, MO: Mosby Yearbook, 1988.

Winick, Myron. *Nutrition in Health and Disease*. Melbourne, FL: Robert E. Krieger Publishing, 1986.

Winter, Ruth. *A Consumer's Dictionary to Food Additives*. 3d ed. New York: Crown Publishers, 1987.

Yogananda, Paramahansa. *Healing by God's Unlimited Power*. Los Angeles, CA: Self Realization Fellowship, 1975.

INDEX

A

1113